Pathways

of the

PULP

Pathways

of the

PULP

edited by

Stephen Cohen, MA, DDS, FICD, FACD
Clinical Professor (Adjunct), Department of Endodontics
University of the Pacific School of Dentistry
San Francisco, California;
Diplomate, American Board of Endodontics

Richard C. Burns, DDS, FICD, FACD
Clinical Professor (Adjunct), Department of Endodontics
University of the Pacific School of Dentistry
San Francisco, California;
Diplomate, American Board of Endodontics

EIGHTH EDITION

with more than 2000 illustrations

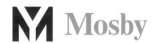 Mosby

A Harcourt Health Sciences Company

St. Louis   London   Philadelphia   Sydney   Toronto

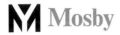

A Harcourt Health Sciences Company

Publishing Director: John Schrefer
Senior Acquisitions Editor: Penny Rudolph
Developmental Editor: Kimberly Frare
Project Manager: Linda McKinley
Production Editor: Rich Barber
Designer: Julia Ramirez
Illustrations provided by: NEW MENTOR GROUP
From their One-Visit Endodontic Treatment CD-ROM

EIGHTH EDITION

Printed in the United States of America

Mosby, Inc.
11830 Westline Industrial Drive
St. Louis, Missouri 64146

International Standard Book Number 0-323-01162-4

02 03 04 05 06 / 9 8 7 6 5 4 3 2 1

❖ Contributors

Robert E. Averbach, DDS, FICD, FACD
President's Teaching Scholar
Professor
Department of Endodontics
University of Colorado
School of Dentistry
Denver, Colorado
Diplomate, American Board of Endodontics

Edward J. Barrett, BSc, DDS, MSc
Assistant Professor
Department of Pediatric Dentistry
University of Toronto
Toronto, Ontario, Canada
Coordinator, Dental Trauma Research
Department of Pediatric Dentistry
The Hospital for Sick Children
Toronto, Ontario, Canada

J. Craig Baumgartner, DDS, MS, PhD
Professor, Chairman, and Director
Advanced Specialty Education
Program in Endodontics
Department of Endodontology
Oregon Health Sciences University
Portland, Oregon
Diplomate, American Board of Endodontics

David Clifford Brown, BDS, MDS, MSD
Associate Professor
Department of Endodontics
University of the Pacific
School of Dentistry
San Francisco, California
Private Practice of Endodontics
San Francisco, California
Diplomate, American Board of Endodontics

Richard C. Burns, DDS, FICD, FACD
Adjunct Clinical Professor
Department of Endodontics
University of the Pacific
School of Dentistry
San Francisco, California
Diplomate, American Board of Endodontics

Joseph H. Camp, DDS, MSD
Adjunct Associate Professor
Department of Endodontics
School of Dentistry
University of North Carolina
Chapel Hill, North Carolina
Private Practice of Endodontics
Charlotte, North Carolina

Peter F. Chase, DDS, MA
Associate Professor
Director-Orofacial Pain
Department of Medicine and Pathology
University of the Pacific
School of Dentistry
San Francisco, California
Vice President and Director of Craniofacial Research
The Chronic Pain Institute
San Francisco, California

Noah Chivian, DDS, FACD, FICD
Adjunct Associate Professor
Department of Endodontics
University of Pennsylvania
School of Dental Medicine
Philadelphia, Pennsylvania
Diplomate, American Board of Endodontics

A. Scott Cohen, DDS
Clinical Assistant Professor
Department of Endodontics
University of the Pacific
School of Dentistry
San Francisco, California
Private Practice of Endodontics
Concord, California
Diplomate, American Board of Endodontics

Stephen Cohen, MA, DDS, FICD, FACD
Adjunct Clinical Professor
Department of Endodontics
University of the Pacific
School of Dentistry
San Francisco, California
Diplomate, American Board of Endodontics

Lewis R. Eversole, MA, MSD, DDS
Professor
Department of Pathology and Medicine
University of Pacific
School of Dentistry
San Francisco, California
Oral and Maxillofacial Pathologist
Pathology Consultants of New Mexico
Roswell, New Mexico

Gerald N. Glickman, DDS, MS, MBA
Professor and Chairman
Director, Graduate Program in Endodontics
School of Dentistry
University of Washington
Seattle, Washington
Diplomate, American Board of Endodontics

James L. Gutmann, DDS
Professor and Director
Graduate Endodontics
Department of Restorative Sciences
Baylor College of Dentistry
Texas A & M University System
Health Sciences Center
Dallas, Texas
Diplomate, American Board of Endodontics

Kenneth M. Hargreaves, DDS, PhD
Professor and Chair
Department of Endodontics
University of Texas Health Science Center
San Antonio, Texas
Diplomate, American Board of Endodontics

Eric James Herbranson, DDS, MS
Adjunct Assistant Professor
Department of Endodontics
University of the Pacific
School of Dentistry
San Francisco, California

Jeffrey W. Hutter, DMD, MEd
Chair, Department of Endodontics
Director, Postdoctoral Program in Endodontics
Department of Endodontics
Goldman School of Dental Medicine
Boston University
Boston, Massachusetts
Diplomate, American Board of Endodontics

William T. Johnson, DDS, MS
Professor
Dows Institute for Dental Research
Department of Family Dentistry
University of Iowa
College of Dentistry
Iowa City, Iowa
Diplomate, American Board of Endodontics

Syngcuk Kim, DDS, PhD
Louis I. Grossman Professor and Chairman
Department of Endodontics
University of Pennsylvania
School of Dental Medicine
Philadelphia, Pennsylvania

Donald J. Kleier, DMD, FACD, FICD
Professor and Chairman of Endodontics
Department of Surgical Dentistry
University of Colorado
School of Dentistry
Denver, Colorado
Diplomate, American Board of Endodontics

Martin D. Levin, DMD
Consultant
Department of Pediatric Dentistry
Children's National Medical Center
Washington, DC
Diplomate, American Board of Endodontics

Frederick Liewehr, DDS, MS, FICD
Assistant Adjunct Professor
Department of Oral Biology and Maxillofacial Pathology
School of Graduate Studies
Assistant Clinical Professor
Department of Endodontics
School of Dentistry
Medical College of Georgia
Augusta, Georgia
Director
Endodontic Residency Program
Department of Endodontics
U.S. Army
Fort Gordon, Georgia
Diplomate, American Board of Endodontics

Stanley F. Malamed, DDS
Professor and Chair
Section of Anesthesia and Medicine
University of Southern California
School of Dentistry
Los Angeles, California

Kathy I. Mueller, DMD
Assistant Professor
Department of Fixed Prosthodontics
University of the Pacific
School of Dentistry
San Francisco, California
Diplomate, American Board of Prosthodontics

P. N. Ramachandran Nair, BVSc, DVM, PhD
Senior Scientist
Department of Oral Structural Biology
Centre of Dental Medicine
University of Zurich
Zurich, Switzerland
Adjunct Research Professor
Department of Endodontology
University of Connecticut Health Center
Farmington, Connecticut

Carl W. Newton, DDS, MSD
Professor of Endodontics
Department of Restorative Dentistry
Indiana University
School of Dentistry
Indianapolis, Indiana
Diplomate, American Board of Endodontics

Jacinthe M. Paquette, DDS
Associate Clinical Professor
Department of Restorative Dentistry
University of Southern California
School of Dentistry
Los Angeles, California
Executive Director
Newport Coast Oral Facial Institute
Newport Beach, California

Roberta Pileggi, DDS, MS
Assistant Professor
Director of Undergraduate Endodontics
Department of Stomatology/Endodontics
University of Texas
Houston Dental Branch
Houston, Texas

Franklin Pulver, DDS, MSc, FRCD, FICD, FACD
Adjunct Assistant Professor
Department of Pediatric Dentistry
Nova Southeastern University
College of Dental Medicine
Fort Lauderdale, Florida

Paul Rosenberg, BDS
Associate Dean of Graduate Programs
New York University
College of Dentistry
Professor and Chairman
Department of Endodontics
New York University
College of Dentistry
Program Director
Post Graduate Endodontics
Department of Endodontics
New York, New York
Diplomate, American Board of Endodontics

Clifford J. Ruddle, DDS, FACD, FICD
Assistant Professor
Department of Graduate Endodontics
Loma Linda University
Loma Linda, California
Adjunct Assistant Professor
Department of Endodontics
University of the Pacific
School of Dentistry
San Francisco, California
Consultant
Department of Graduate Endodontics
Long Beach Veterans Medical Center
Long Beach, California

Cherilyn G. Sheets, DDS
Clinical Professor
Department of Restorative Dentistry
University of Southern California
Los Angeles, California
Executive Director
Newport Coast Oral Facial Institute
Newport Beach, California
Private Practice
Newport Beach, California

Asgeir Sigurdsson, Cand. Odont., MS
Assistant Professor
Graduate Program Director
Department of Endodontics
School of Dentistry
University of North Carolina
Chapel Hill, North Carolina
Diplomate, American Board of Endodontics

Larz Spångberg, DDS, PhD
Professor and Head
Department of Endodontology
University of Connecticut
School of Dental Medicine
Farmington, Connecticut
Diplomate, American Board of Endodontics

Hideaki Suda, DDS, PhD
Professor
Department of Endodontics
Tokyo Medical and Dental University
Tokyo, Japan

Martin Trope, DMD, FICD, FACD
J.B. Freedland Professor and Chair
Department of Endodontics
School of Dentistry
University of North Carolina
Chapel Hill, North Carolina

Henry Trowbridge, DDS, PhD
Emeritus Professor of Pathology
University of Pennsylvania
School of Dental Medicine
Philadelphia, Pennsylvania
Attending Staff
I.B. Bender Division of Endodontics
The Albert Einstein Medical Center
Philadelphia, Pennsylvania

William F. Vann, Jr., DMD, PhD
Demeritt Distinguished Professor
Department of Pediatric Dentistry
School of Dentistry
University of North Carolina
Chapel Hill, North Carolina

Galen W. Wagnild, DDS
Associate Clinical Professor
Department of Restorative Dentistry
University of California–San Francisco
San Francisco, California
Diplomate, American Board of Endodontics

Richard E. Walton, DMD, MS
Professor
Department of Endodontics
University of Iowa
College of Dentistry
Iowa City, Iowa

Hom-Lay Wang, DDS, MSD
Director of Graduate Periodontics
Associate Professor
Department of Periodontics, Prevention and Geriatrics
The University of Michigan
School of Dentistry
Ann Arbor, Michigan

Lisa R. Wilcox, DDS, MS
Adjunct Associate Professor
Department of Endodontics
University of Iowa
Iowa City, Iowa
Diplomate, American Board of Endodontics

David E. Witherspoon, BDSc, MS
Assistant Professor
Department of Graduate Endodontics and Restorative Sciences
Baylor College of Dentistry
Texas A&M University System
Health Science Center
Dallas, Texas

Robert S. Wright, DDS, MSEd, MS
Private Practice of Prosthodontics
Newport Beach, California

Edwin J. Zinman, DDS, JD
Former Lecturer
Department of Stomatology
University of California, San Francisco
School of Dentistry
San Francisco, California

All textbooks of value are the result of the vision, commitment, and selfless efforts of many individuals. We dedicate this eighth edition to these extraordinary educators, researchers, and clinicians who have contributed to Pathways of the Pulp *over the last 25 years.*

Donald Arens, DDS, MSD, FICD, FACD
Robert E. Averbach, DDS, FICD, FACD
C. Richard Bennett, DDS, PhD
Scott K. Bentkover, DDS
Ronald Borer, DDS, FICD
Cecil E. Brown, Jr., MS, DDS
David Clifford Brown, BDS,MDS, MSD
L. Stephen Buchanan, DDS
Joseph H. Camp, DDS, MSD, FICD, FACD
Gary B. Carr, DDS
Noah Chivian, DDS, FICD, FACD
A.Scott Cohen, DDS
Charles C. Cunningham, DDS, FICD
Walter T. Cunningham, DDS, MS
Arthur W. Curley, JD
Quintilliano de Deus, DDS
Samuel O. Dorn, DDS, FACD
Thomas Dumsha, MS, DDS
Harold F. Eissmann, DDS, FACD
Lewis R. Eversole, MA, DDS, MSD
Ronald Feinman, DMD
Stuart B. Fountain, DDS, MSc, FICD, FACD
Alfred L. Frank, DDS, FICD, FACD
Jay W. Friedman, DDS, MPH
Shimon Friedman, DMD
Arnold H. Gartner, DDS
Dudley H. Glick, DDS, FICD, FACD
Gerald N. Glickman, DDS, MS, MBA
Alan H. Gluskin, DDS, FICD, FACD
Albert C. Goerig, DDS, MS, FICD, FACD
Fernando Goldberg, DDS
Ronald E. Goldstein, DDS
William W.Y. Goon, DDS, FICD, FACD
Daniel B. Green, DDS
Louis I. Grossman, DDS, Dr. Med, Dent, ScD
James L. Gutmann, DDS
Jerome R. Gutterman, DDS
Kenneth M. Hargreaves, DDS, PhD
Van B. Haywood, DMD
Eric James Herbranson, MS, DDS
Michael A. Heuer, DDS, MS, FICD, FACD
Harald O. Heymann, DDS, MEd

William T. Johnson, DDS, MS
James David Kettering, MS, PhD
Syngcuk Kim, DDS, PhD
Donald J. Kleier, DMD, FICD, FACD
Kenneth Knowles, DDS, MS
Anne-Li Knuut, DDS,
Alvin Arlen Krakow, DDS, FICD, FACD
Kaare Langeland, DDS, PhD
William S. Lieber, DMD
Stanley F. Malamed, DDS
F. James Marshall, DMD, MS, FICD, FACD
Howard Martin, DMD, FACD
Vincent B. Milas, DDS, FICD, FACD
Leo J. Miserendino, DDS, MS
Donald R. Morse, DDS, MA
Kathy I. Mueller, DMD
Thomas P. Mullaney DDS, MSD
Irving Naidorf, DDS, FACD
Elmer Joseph Neaverth, Jr., DDS
Carl W. Newton, DDS, MSD
Nguyen F. Nguyen DDS, FICD, FACD, FAAE
Edward M. Osetek, DDS, MA, FICD, FACD
Ryle A. Radke, Jr.. DDS, FACD, FACP
James B. Roane, MS, DDS, BS, FACP
Ilan Rotstein, CD
Clifford J. Ruddle, DDS, FICD, FACD
James T. Rule, MS, DDS
John Sapone, DDS, FICD, FACD, FAAE
Harvey Sarner, LLB
Herbert Schilder, DDS
Joseph Schulz, AB, DDS
Stephen Schwartz, DDS, MS, FADI
Alan G. Selbst, DMD, MS
Samuel Seltzer, DDS
Thomas P. Serene, DDS, MSD
Asgeir Sigurdsson, Cand Odont, MS
James H.S. Simon, DDS, FICD, FACD
Larz S.W. Spångberg, DDS, PhD
Adam Stabholz, DMD
Harold R. Stanley, DDS
H. Robert Steiman, MS, PhD, DDS, MSD, FICD
David Steiner, DDS, MSD

Aviad Tamse, DMD
Mahmoud Torabinejad, DMD,MSD, PhD
Calvin D. Torneck, DDS, MS
Martin Trope, DMD
Henry Trowbridge, DDS, PhD
Paul M. Vanek, DDS, MS, FICD, DABE
Robert M. Veatch, PhD
Galen W. Wagnild, DDS
Warren T. Wakai, DDS, MA, FICD, FACD
Richard E. Walton, MS, DMD

Leslie A. Werksman, DDS
John D. West, DDS, MSD
Lisa R. Wilcox, MS, DDS
David E. Witherspoon, BDSc, MS
Shannon Wong, DDS, MS
Fulton S. Yee, DDS
Robert Zelikow, DDS
Paul Eugene Ziegler, BA, DDS, FACD
Edwin J. Zinman, DDS, JD

❖ Preface

The editors find it especially challenging to prepare a completely current printed textbook in a digital world where scientific, medical, dental, and technological changes occur almost on a daily basis. Our purpose in this eighth edition of *Pathways of the Pulp* is to reframe the fundamental and universal concepts of endodontics—*accurate diagnosis, proper access, thorough cleaning and shaping, and meticulous obturation*—into an evidence-based, generously illustrated textbook that represents the highly evolved field of endodontics at the beginning of the twenty-first century.

It is our belief that a commitment to lifelong learning is the essential foundation for excellence in clinical practice, because the half-life of scientific knowledge now is less than 5 years! To reflect the many changes in our field since the last edition, every chapter has been completely rewritten or substantially revised. For the first time, computerized tomography, prepared by NASA research at Stanford University, will reveal three-dimensional views of human teeth and pulp spaces. An additional feature of this edition is a new section on facial space infections resulting from pulpal/periapical disease. A new chapter has been added to reflect the incorporation of computers and other technologies into the treatment room and their seamless integration into the administrative area.

We feel a deep sense of gratitude for the selfless devotion of our contributors; their willingness to share their knowledge stems from the original noble meaning of a doctor (i.e., a teacher). It is really our contributors who have collectively made this the seminal textbook on endodontics—it is for this reason that we dedicate this edition to them.

Finally, we would like to give special acknowledgment to Ms. Penny Rudolph as our editor and to Ms. Kimberly Frare for her expert development; they helped to segue the manuscripts and page proofs from daunting to delightful.

Stephen Cohen
Richard C. Burns

❖ Contents

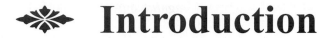

Introduction

A Historic Perspective
"I shall be telling this with a sigh
somewhere ages and ages hence;
Two roads diverged in a wood, and I—
I took the road less traveled by,
And that has made all the difference."
The Road Not Taken, 1916, Robert Frost

. . . And so it has been over the past century with the "pathways of the pulp." Ideas have arisen, challenges have emerged, materials have been developed, techniques have been devised, mistakes have been repeated, and personalities have been dominant. Yet within this time frame and within the confines of this "small and often-considered insignificant tissue," history has repeated itself, leading us to choose a variety of pathways—"less traveled by." As with the anatomy of the root canal system, the pathways have been winding and circular, deviating, or dead-ended—all with signposts along the way that have either highlighted advancement or regression, creativity or repetitiveness, biology or empiricism. As we move forward in this new millennium, it is not only important to revisit many of these divergent pathways but also to again heed the lessons of history and the past century—because they "have made all the difference" in the evolution of endodontology and endodontics.

At the turn of the twentieth century, the management of the pulp and periradicular tissues was bolstered by the discovery of x-rays and anesthetics, the refinement of the electric pulp tester, and the delineation of many of the principles of surgical endodontics that we use today. Additionally, asepsis and antisepsis were accepted as necessary aspects of endodontics as the pathway to focal infection began to be the road that characterized the predominant philosophy of managing infections of the pulp and their sequelae. In essence a new era had dawned, yet it was in conflict regarding the retention of the natural tooth. The pathway to the most probable pulpal diagnosis was enhanced significantly with the popularization of electric pulp testing and the availability of information from the dental radiograph. In the latter respect, Otto Walkhoff, who took the very first dental radiograph, and C. Edmund Kells, who used the radiographs for diagnosis and during root canal treatment, deserve our gratitude. Before this time, heat and cold were the only pulp tests used to determine whether the pulp was "dead or alive"—a painfully poor diagnostic choice that still lingers today. Moreover, all pathways of endodontic treatment could now be offered in a painless manner as the use of local anesthetic solutions emerged. Originally discovered in 1884 by Carl Koller, an ophthalmologist from Vienna who used a solution of cocaine as a topical anesthetic for eye surgery, its dental use received favorable reports by Guido Fischer and others in the dental literature. Glass and metal injection syringes used at the turn of the century gave way to the breech-loading syringe, developed by Harvey Cook in 1917. However, the dental professional was slow to adopt this instrument, favoring the pathway of cocaine pressure anesthesia to manage the inflamed and painful pulp.

Although the impact of asepsis and the tenets of antisepsis, as portrayed by William Hunter, brought to the dental profession the need for more careful and controlled root canal treatment, tooth retention was not favored. Identified as the source for a multitude of systemic maladies, infection of the pulp and periradicular tissues directed all health professionals to the pathway of extraction. In essence, Hunter had landed the "black-eye blow" to the dental profession that was to determine, for years, and in some respects even into this new century, the ultimate pathway of treatment for millions of patients. Fortunately, the scientific basis for microbiology, as delineated by W.D. Miller at the turn of the century (*Die mikroorganismen der mundhole*—The microorganisms of the human mouth), served as a basis for rationality for a number of dental clinicians and researchers, such as Edward Hatton, Edgar Coolidge, Charles Boedecker, J. Roy Blaney, W. Clyde Davis, William Skillen, Carl Grove, and others, who contributed so much toward a better understanding of the pathways of disease in the dental pulp and periradicular tissues. Not only was a better concept of the disease process detailed, but the means to prevent pulpal and periradicular injury was also provided. In some respects, however, this overwhelming focus on infection led to the excessive use of phenolic compounds to control complex microbial populations and unmanageable inflamed tissue, while at the same time creating irreversible damage to the same tissues . . . a pathway of therapy that still at times plagues contemporary endodontic treatment with no rationale for its choice.

The science of endodontics, "endodontology," owes a tremendous debt of gratitude to the pioneers of oral biology. During the 1920s, in particular in 1926 at the International Dental Congress in Philadelphia, the profile of American dentistry was one based heavily on the technical issues of restorative dentistry. However, the critical intersection of the biologic and technical was emerging, and a new pathway was beginning to develop—oral biology. Fostered by Bernhard Gottlieb from Vienna, who spent time in Chicago influencing local clinicians and researchers such as W. Skillen. E. Coolidge, and E. Hatton, the science of the oral biology had its roots. Subsequently, many of Gottlieb's assistants and colleagues, driven by the lure of science and the political upheaval in Europe, came to the United States and were the driving force in the emergent and exciting development of oral biology. These included Balint Orban and Rudolf Kronfeld, two of Gottlieb's closest assistants, along with Harry Sicher, Joseph Weinmann, and ultimately Gottlieb himself. To these gentlemen and many of their fledgling colleagues, such as Louis Grossman, Maury Massler, Edgar Coolidge, J. Henry Kaiser, Robert Kesel, Harry Johnston, W. Clyde Davis, and Ralph Sommer, who have influenced so many of the present day endodontists, we express our sincere thanks for the pathway to endodontology.

In the late nineteenth century there was a raging controversy over the performance of one-visit root canal treatment—a pathway revisited in the provision of present-day treatment. C. Edmund Kells, Jr. wrote, "putrescent pulp-canals can be successfully filled today at one sitting, just as was taught by Cassius M. Richmond over forty years ago, and being thus taught by him, I, for one, have followed the practice ever since." Additional authors, such as J. S. Dodge, C.T. Stockwell, G.O Rogers, M. S. Merchant, E. Noyes , L. Ottofy and A.W. Harlan were keen to point out or at least attempt to make claim to "who should be credited initially with this treatment modality," with each citing different criteria for choices or claiming different techniques to achieve success in one visit. This "heroic treatment," as L. Ottofy characterized it, was not only a radical step in thought concerning apical healing, but also supported the belief in the natural healing mechanism following root canal treatment. Possibly the most controversial position regarding immediate root canal filling was that taken by J. E. Cravens at the Ninth International Medical Congress in Washington, D.C. in 1887. He advocated the filling of all pulpless teeth without any previous use of medicinal agents, which "caused a storm of indignation among some of the best-known members of our profession." Ironically, since then there have been only a few well-designed published studies on the efficacy for one-visit treatment, this treatment protocol is still debatable based on evidenced-based information. However, as the new millennium commences, one-visit root canal treatment rages as the pathway to contemporary clinical endodontic success. Or, as put by one its strongest advocates, "The endodontic world is currently divided into those who do one-visit-endodontics; and those who do not. They end up with the same success rates, but those who do not do one-visit procedures make less per case, experience flare-ups, and unnecessarily subject their patients to another dreaded appointment for root canal therapy. What explains a clinician's reluctance to strike our for this promised land? . . . guilt, worry and fear." Sadly, this pathway of wisdom based solely on a monetary reward, comfort for the clinician, and empirical musings may have done more harm than good in the provision of predictable, evidenced-based patient care.

Significant changes in the way root canals were obturated in the 1930s fostered the development of new pathways to retreatment in the 1970s, 1980s, and 1990s. Silver cone root fillings, often attributed separately to Hugo Tribitsch and Elmer Jasper, were widely used in many areas of the world to fill root canals heretofore deemed impossible to obturate with gutta-percha. The silver cone fill was extolled for the management of small curved canals, which defied the use of gutta-percha, and its dense radiographic appearance. Only too often, however, the complex root canal system was not cleaned and shaped fully, leading to the ultimate demise of the silver cone fill. As reported by Sam Seltzer and others 40 years later, the corrosion products from silver cones in contact with apical or coronal leakage, bacteria, and retained tissue debris often led to the pathway of periradicular tissue destruction and failure of the root canal treatment.

During the first part of the last century, and well into the 1970s, periradicular surgery was the leading treatment of choice to manage teeth requiring revision of nonsurgical root canal therapy. The evolution of the surgical pathway to treatment must be credited to our European colleagues who detailed surgical flap designs and management of the resected root ends early in the twentieth century. Although these procedures were available to dental professional in the United States during the first half of that century, more often than not, the pathway of extraction was chosen because of the overwhelming influence of the focal infection/elective localization theories. In the latter half of the twentieth century, reason and rationale were brought to surgical endodontics with the extensive treatise on endodontic surgery by Jörgen Rud, Jens Andreasen, and J. E. Möller-Jensen. From their work, the biologic pathways of successful endodontic surgery were clarified and codified. Their exposé opened other pathways for both technological developments and treatment planning choices. In particular, their studies fostered the use of alternative root-end filling materials that favored tissue regeneration. More importantly, however, they established the major pathways for the failure of surgical endodontics. This latter achievement, by itself, led serendipitously to the enormous increase in the revision of nonsurgical endodontic treatment failures, because the leading cause identified for failure of surgical endodontic treatment was failure to clean, shape, and obturate the root canal system. Now, coupled with the use of the microscope that has provided the dental professional with a new visionary pathway for successful treatment in the new millennium, all phases of endodontic treatment can be managed with greater predictability.

In separate studies in the late 1800s, L. Friedel and J. Scheff attempted to determine the role of the periodontal ligament in tooth resorption, a process that was considered as a 'fait accompli' following tooth trauma. For years the specific pathway to tooth resorption could not be determined or prevented predictably, resulting in the loss of many teeth. The clarification of this destructive process and its prevention and treatment by Jens and Frances Andreasen, Lars Hammarström, Angela Pierce and others, subsequent to tooth trauma, have been a major boon to tooth retention and treatment planning—pathways founded in good science and clinical assessment "that have made all the difference."

Over the past century so many of the pathways to the treatment of the pulp and periradicular tissues have been determined and dictated by simple, single, empirical case reports or retrospective observations. For example, for more than 40 years authors and clinicians have cited a retrospective study in the 1950s that indicated that incomplete canal obturation, vis-à-vis apical leakage, was the major factor for failure of nonsurgical root canal treatment. Both historical and contemporary thought, however, supports the need for thorough cleaning and shaping of the canal system. As early as 1882, for example, Dr. R. H. Hofheinz set the stage for success with nonsurgical root canal treatment; "In attempting to assign the success or failure of operations upon diseased teeth to their proper causes, factors of the greatest importance are frequently left out of account, and the results ascribed to some agent that may have been entirely indifferent. One of these factors, which forms the very foundation of successful root-treatment, is the manner in which the mechanical cleansing of the canal is carried out."

Furthermore, in 1959 a single tooth case report appeared that indicated that a zinc carbonate precipitate from a zinc-containing root-end filling had caused failure of the surgical procedure. For the next two decades, the clinical edict was 'use only zinc-free amalgam' as a root-end filling material—a deviating pathway that lacked reason and rationale. Interestingly, this controversy provided the pathway for many postdoctoral students to fulfill their research expectations in their pursuit of specialization in the then newest recognized dental discipline. In another example, a single case report of multiple teeth in the 1970s that had been resected apically showed that the use of a heated instrument to burnish the gutta-percha was actually opening voids at the root apex. Therefore the edict in this clinical scenario was to burnish the apical gutta-percha with a cold instrument only, a technique that could not ensure the desired result. Even the use of super-EBA as a root-end filling was based on a single case report.

The pathway to success has been clear for decades, yet multiple meanderings on the part of a few have created dead-ended pathways pursued by the multitudes . . . "and that has made all the difference." Even contemporary thought and current clinician jargon has fostered the wrong idea for the determination of success and failure in endodontics. How often has it been said by the clinician upon viewing his or her handiwork on the radiograph, "look at those accessory canals and dense fill, the root canal is certainly sealed"—and *this* is accepted as the criteria for contemporary success?

Published reports by R. Ottolengui and E.S. Talbot in the late 1800s dealt with the crown-down approach to root canal treatment. The circular pathway to this technique has emerged 100 years later in the revival of this approach to treatment—but with new technologies and a new focus on the importance of cleaning and shaping. Needless to say, the pathway from carbon steel to stainless steel and ultimately to nickel titanium has been one of challenge, innovation, and apparent contemporary success—a far cry from the notched watch springs that were used by Edward Maynard in the early 1800s. One can only imagine what pathways would have been chosen if these types of advances in instrument design and metal would have been available early in the twentieth century.

For years, apical leakage studies were used to determine the quality and acceptability of the root canal obturation technique. Little effort went into determining the skill of the clinician in this pathway to success. It has only been in the last 25 years that the skill of the clinician was considered as the determining factor for achieving success. Needless to say, thousands of extracted teeth were subjected to gallons of dye, isotopes, bacterial inoculations, and even centrifugation to determine the extent of apical leakage. Ironically the pathway to success was at the other end of the canal—the coronal end, as a plethora of recent studies have identified that coronal leakage of bacteria and their by-products are the major causes of failure of endodontic treatment. So, for decades the dental profession was gleefully wandering down the wrong pathway for success—or were the lessons of history not heeded? As early as 1917 the impact of coronal leakage on the success of endodontic treatment was identified by B. E. Dahlgren. Apparently he had identified the pathway less traveled by, long before the virtues of Robert Frost's poetry were extolled.

The evolution of a focused body of endodontic literature and the vehicles for its dissemination loom as the major pathways that have influenced the development of endodontics and endodontology during the second half of the twentieth century. Initially the *Journal of Endodontia* appeared in the mid-to-late 1940s with only few editions making it to press. In the meantime, loosely formed endodontic societies resorted to occasional newletters to share news about endodontics—but a formal and focused voice for endodontics was unavailable. In the late 1940s a section on endodontics appeared in *Oral Surgery, Oral Medicine and Oral Pathology*. This section carried endodontics admirably into a contemporary position until the *Journal of Endodontics* was published in 1975. Before that, the only publication that focused strictly on endodontics was the *Journal of the British Endodontic Society*, first published in 1967 under the astute guidance of A.H.R. Rowe. In 1980 that journal became the *International Endodontic Journal* and has since provided the endodontic community with a global perspective or pathway to developments in all phases of endodontics. In 1975, the *Journal of Endodontics* was published under the editorial leadership of Worth Gregory. According to the then President of the American Association of Endodontists, Dr. Alfred L. Frank, it was "a tribute and living memorial to those pioneers in our field who have contributed tirelessly to achieve the recognition that their young discipline so richly deserved."

This journal has been the pathway to excellence in endodontics and endodontology for the past 25 years, and will, in conjunction with the *International Endodontic Journal*, and *Endodontics & Dental Traumatology*, provide continued leadership in the choice of pathways traveled as this specialty embraces the challenges of the new millennium. As other journals emerge as viable pathways for the dissemination of endodontic thought and treatment choices, they are encouraged to contribute to the overall global pathway to excellence.

Finally, you, the reader have arrived to the task at hand—and that is the new edition—the new *Pathways of the Pulp*—and the richness in fact, experience, knowledge, application, and integration that it contains for both generalist and specialist. The vast array of talent that has been assembled to provide the codification of endodontic thought that will guide us to the pathways of success for the twenty-first century is overwhelming. To the editors and the authors, a hearty congratulation is warranted. For it is with their guidance that the dental practitioner will be directed on pathways that are traveled on a continuous basis because they provide constant signposts and support areas that yield predictable success. Furthermore, this edition sets the stage for what is to come, as we forge ahead in this world of rapidly advancing technology and science—*a new pathway* that we must all embrace for the future of the specialty of endodontics and one that *must* be traveled. The future of endodontics as the premier dental specialty will require that all dental professionals, choosing to perform endodontic treatment, exercise judgment in their treatment planning choices and technique applications within evidenced-based parameters. In the future, evidence-based health care in endodontics will not be the road less traveled by . . . but rather the pathway to success for our patients...and that *will* make all the difference.

James L. Gutmann

Pathways
of the
PULP

PART ONE

The Art of Endodontics

Chapter 1

Diagnostic Procedures

Stephen Cohen, Frederick Liewehr

Chapter Outline

ART AND SCIENCE OF DIAGNOSIS

In the current computer-oriented world, some dentists want to reduce the diagnostic process to a spreadsheet. The human brain or ultimately electronic algorithms would then process the spreadsheet to arrive at a definitive diagnosis. Unfortunately, arriving at a correct diagnosis is not that simple. Although diagnostic testing of some common complaints may produce classic results, occasional testing will produce inconsistent or incomplete results that need to be carefully interpreted by the astute and curious clinician to resolve discrepancies. An accurate diagnosis can only result from the synthesis of scientific knowledge, clinical experience, intuition, and common sense. The process is thus both an art and a science.

The diagnostic process actually consists of four steps and is conducted in much the same manner as a detective might investigate a case in a mystery novel. The first step is to assemble all available facts. These "clues" are detected by considering the chief complaint, the medical and dental histories, and the history of the present condition. Additional information is gained from interviewing patients to determine what symptoms they may have experienced. A complete examination, including radiographic images, and laboratory tests, when necessary, will disclose objective physical signs.

In the next step, experienced investigators screen and interpret the assembled clues to discover which are germane to the case. They must decide whether the patient's symptoms are accurately reported and whether these and the objective signs and clinical test results represent significant departures from normal. Additionally, they must decide which findings require further follow-up.

Once the information has been gathered and interpreted, the investigator formulates a differential diagnosis, made up of all possible disease entities that are consistent with the signs, symptoms, and test results gathered. In the final step, the clinician carefully compares the patient's signs, symptoms, and test results to known disease entities in the differential diagnosis and selects the closest match. This becomes the operational or working diagnosis.

Most often, the operational diagnosis is the final diagnosis, which occurs when the signs and symptoms closely match a classic disease manifestation and leave little doubt as to the diagnosis. In some cases, the operational diagnosis is less certain and requires further procedures to confirm the diagnosis. Examples might be the construction of a bite splint for a suspected case of myofascial pain dysfunction syndrome; it might require intraligamentary anesthesia in the distal sulcus to confirm the source of radiating dental pain. In any case, the astute clinician always remains open to further input that could modify the diagnosis and potentially the treatment as the unfolding of information progresses.

The importance of making an accurate diagnosis cannot be overemphasized. There are times when the full range of diagnostic tests is applied and all experience and knowledge are drawn upon; yet, a satisfactory explanation for the patient's symptoms is not determined. In some complex cases, the etiology may be nonodontogenic. (Chapter 3 explores the diagnoses of these ostensibly odontogenic cases.)

Chief Complaint

Recording the history of the symptoms begins by making a note of what prompted the patient to consult a dentist in the first place. The form of the notation should be a few simple phrases *in the patient's own words* that describe the symptoms causing the discomfort. No diagnoses should be included, either by the dentist or by the patient. The reasons the patient's words are recorded are twofold. First, whatever prompted the patient to seek treatment is important and must be addressed first, even if something of greater interest to the dentist is discovered during the examination process. Second, the addition of diagnostic and historic information may cause the premature formulation of a diagnosis that could bias the examining dentist. If the clinician follows an unproductive lead, referral to the patient's original words can provide needed perspective to regain objectivity.

History of Present Illness

Completion of a preprinted dental history questionnaire, which inquires about the site, intensity, and nature of the pain (Fig. 1-1) affords patients the opportunity to record their observations in an organized and descriptive way. The report then provides the clinician with initial information about the patient's signs and symptoms, the duration and intensity of the pain, and the patient's experiences of what leads to relief or exacerbation of the symptoms. Additionally, the form should include questions about recent dental manipulations, past trauma to the area, any previous symptomatic episodes, and any prior treatment rendered by other practitioners. The dental history form thus provides a template for conversational discovery.

The development of the patient's history is an interview process during which the dentist attempts to evaluate the patient's symptoms accurately, completely, and objectively, avoiding the temptation to make a premature diagnosis. The history should be written as a clear, concise, chronologic narrative that details each of the patient's symptoms from its inception to the present. The patient is encouraged to omit nothing. Objectivity is supported with the use of questions phrased in such a way that the patient must provide information rather than simply answering "yes" or "no." The dentist might ask the patient, "Tell me about your problem," rather than "I understand you have been experiencing cold sensitivity in your upper front teeth for several weeks, is that correct?" Some patients will answer "yes" to be cooperative, some because they are suggestible, and others may answer "no" simply to be contrary. Open-ended, nonleading questions simply explore the patient's experience. Specific questions may then be asked about the nature of the symptoms experienced:

TELL US ABOUT YOUR SYMPTOMS

LAST NAME_____   FIRST NAME_____

1. *Are you experiencing any pain at this time? If not , please go to question 6.*   Yes ____ No ____
2. *If yes, can you locate the tooth that is causing the pain?*   Yes ____ No ____
3. *When did you first notice the symptoms?* _____
4. *Did your symptoms occur suddenly, or gradually?*_____

Please check the frequency and quality of the discomfort, and the number that most closely reflects the intensity of your pain:

LEVEL OF INTENSITY (On a scale of 1 to 10) 1= Mild 10=Severe	FREQUENCY	QUALITY
1__2__3__4__5__6__7__8__9__10__	___ Constant	___ Sharp
	___Intermittent	___ Dull
	___Momentary	___Throbbing
	___Occasional	

   Is there anything you can do to relieve the pain?   Yes ____ No ___
   *If yes, what?*_____
   Is there anything you can do to cause the pain to increase?   Yes ____ No____
   *If yes, what?*_____
   When eating or drinking, is your tooth sensitive to: Heat ____ Cold ____ Sweets ___
   Does your tooth hurt when you bite down, or chew?   Yes ___ No ___
   Does it hurt if you press the gum tissue around this tooth?   Yes ___ No ___
   Does a change in posture (lying down or bending over) cause your tooth to hurt? Yes ___ No ___

6. *Do you grind, or clench your teeth?*   Yes ___ No ___
7. *If yes, do you wear a night guard?*   Yes ___ No ___
8. *Has a restoration (filling or crown) been placed on this tooth recently?*   Yes ___ No ___
9. *Prior to this appointment, has root canal therapy been initiated on this tooth?*   Yes ___ No ___
10. *Is there anything else we should know about your teeth, gums or sinuses that would assist us in our diagnosis?*_____

Signed: Patient or Parent_____Date _____

Fig. 1-1 Dental history form that also allows the patient to record pain experience in an organized and descriptive manner.

- , Inception: "When did you first notice this pain? Have you ever noticed it before?"
- Frequency and course: "How often does this pain occur? Are the episodes becoming more or less frequent or about the same as when you first noticed the pain?"
- Intensity: "Is this pain mild, moderate, or severe?"
- Quality: "What is the nature of the pain? Sharp? Dull? Stabbing? Throbbing?"
- Location: "Could you point to the tooth that hurts or to the area that you feel is swollen?"
- Provoking factors: "Do heat, cold, biting, or chewing cause pain?"
- Duration: "When heat (or cold) causes the pain, is it momentary, or does it last longer?"
- Spontaneity: "Does the pain ever occur without provocation?"
- Attenuating factors: "Does anything relieve the pain—hot or cold liquids, sitting up or lying down?"

Careful, sensitive listening to the patient's responses to these queries allows the clinician to develop a narrative description of the patient's chief complaint and the history leading up to it. This dialog between doctor and patient is the first diagnostic step and serves two purposes. First, it allows the clinician to formulate a working diagnosis that is to be tested and further refined during the ensuing clinical examination. Secondly, it allows the patient to become acquainted with the doctor and to develop trust in the doctor's openness and receptivity—an important step in forming a good doctor-patient relationship. It is wise to remember the words of Sir William Osler (1849-1919), "Listen to your patient. He is trying to tell you what is wrong with him."

A question that sometimes arises is how thorough the development of the patient's history must be, particularly in cases where the diagnosis seems obvious. The answer is that clinicians can be thorough yet expedient, without failing to collect vital information if their focus remains on those questions that appear relevant to the obvious problem. If the patient points to a severely broken down molar as the offending tooth and cool air from the air-water syringe confirms that it is the source of the pain, there is little need for further testing. On the other hand, most diagnoses are not that simple, and "tunnel vision"—focusing on the suspected tooth while ignoring other teeth that may be the actual source of the problem—must be avoided to prevent misdiagnosis. Clinical experience and maintaining a proper degree of skepticism will produce the proper balance.

Pain

When the source of pain is discussed in this text, the origin of the pain—from where it comes—is the intended meaning. In most cases, the source of the pain is identical to the site of the pain-from where the patient thinks it comes. If a tooth acquires a carious lesion that extends into the pulp, a pulpitis and toothache ensue. This condition is called *primary pain*[41] and is relatively easy to conceptualize and diagnose.

The most common pain patients describe is a "toothache." The source of this pain arises either internally (i.e., pulpal pain) or externally (i.e., periodontal ligament) as discussed in the text that follows. Frequently, dental pain is the result of an inflamed or degenerating pulp. The *quality* of this pain may be described as *sharp* or *bright* if the Aδ fibers are functioning; sharp or bright pain is typical of acute tissue injury. In contrast, pain may be described as *dull, boring,* or *throbbing* if severe damage has occurred causing the C-fibers to respond (see Chapter 11 for a detailed discussion of pulpal neurophysiology). An attempt to replicate the symptoms by provocation (i.e., by isolating and washing the suggested tooth with cold [or very warm] water) is often productive. Since this pain arises in the pulpal tissue, the tooth will test vital to electric pulp testing and the pulpal diagnosis will generally be irreversible pulpitis.

The pain may also arise in the periodontal ligament. In this case, the tooth will be sensitive to percussion, chewing, and possibly palpation. The diagnosis may involve the pulp if the periodontitis is caused by an extension of pulpal disease; the cause may have a purely periodontic origin or be as simple as a new restoration in hyperocclusion. If the periodontal inflammation is a result of pulpal disease, the pulp

will be unresponsive to pulp testing. Thus pulpal vitality testing is the key to the diagnosis.

Another hint that the patient's pain may have a pulpal origin is the *intensity* of the pain. To gauge intensity, patients are asked to imagine a ruler with markings from 0 to 10. They are asked to consider 0 as having no pain and 10 as being the most painful response they can imagine. They are then asked to assign a number to their pain that corresponds to its place along this pain continuum. Pulpal pain produced by Aδ fibers can be excruciating and often approaches the upper limits of the scale. However, severe pain is rarely encountered in periodontal disorders. Mild-to-moderate pain can be found in either pulpal or periodontal pathosis, but acute pain is usually a reliable sign that the pain is of pulpal origin.[6]

The ability of the patient to locate the offending tooth accurately also depends on whether the inflammatory state is limited to the pulp tissue. Since the pulp contains no proprioceptive fibers, it may be difficult for the patient to localize the pain if the inflammation has not reached the periodontal ligament.[14,62] Once the inflammatory process extends beyond the apical foramen and affects the periodontal ligament, it will be easier for the patient to identify the source of the pain. In this instance, percussion and chewing tests can corroborate the patient's perception of the source of the pain.

Patients may report that lying down or bending over exacerbates their dental pain. They may also report that their toothache occurs shortly after they go to bed at night or that it wakes them up after they have fallen asleep. This type of pain occurs because the inflamed pulp has a lowered threshold for pain because of the action of the increased pressure on nerve endings from edema fluid confined within the inelastic walls of the tooth, as well as to sensitization of nerve endings by inflammatory mediators. When the patient lies down, the action of gravity no longer reduces the arterial pressure to the head as it does when the patient is standing. This, in turn, increases pressure on the inflamed, confined pulp.[14] The throbbing commonly experienced by these patients may be the result of the systolic pressure producing a suprathreshold stimulation, while the diastolic pressure drops below the threshold.

Far more baffling and difficult to diagnose than primary pain is *heterotopic* pain[41] in which the source and site of the pain are different. Cardiac-referred pain is a classic example of heterotopic pain. Often a patient suffering from an ischemic episode will feel pain that radiates down the left arm. Of more interest to the dentist, Natkin et al[38] stated that 18% of all cases of cardiac pain are localized solely to the teeth. The key point is that the true source of the pain must be identified to treat the underlying condition correctly. Little good is provided to the patient suffering from a cardiac episode by performing root canal therapy at the ectopic site of the pain.

Lack of an obvious reason for the pain, such as a carious or fractured tooth, should immediately cause concern. Diagnosis of suggested heterotopic pain is aided by the realization that pain will be increased when the source of pain is stimulated and decreased when it is anesthetized. In the case of a patient with suspected cardiac pain in the left mandible, attempting to reproduce the pain by palpation, percussion, and cold will fail to produce discomfort. Similarly, a mandibular block will fail to provide relief. In this case, investigative efforts must be directed elsewhere.

More commonly, pain will be referred from a diseased pulp to adjacent teeth or to those in the opposing quadrant.[14,60] Referred pain may be ipsilaterally referred to the periauricular area, down the neck, or up to the temple. In these cases, a posterior tooth is almost always the source of the pain. (Chapter 3 discusses ostensible toothache of nonodontogenic origin [e.g., neurologic, cardiac, vascular, mental, malignant, sinus diseases].)

Pain is a multifactorial experience that not only involves the perception of a noxious stimulus but also includes an emotional-affective reaction to it. Additionally, cognitive processes such as attention, beliefs, and learning can further modify the patient's pain experience.[52] The result can be a fearful patient whose perception of pain is out of proportion to the stimulus applied. In some cases, emotional disorders can manifest as dental pain. If no dental or other organic cause for the dental pain is found, the patient should be referred to a pain clinic or to a physician for medical consultation.

Vital Signs

An old maxim of medicine is: "Never treat a stranger." To evaluate patients accurately, all details of their physiologic condition must be known. When dentists know about their patients' health status and the medications they are taking, the diagnoses have better chances of being correct and the treatments better chances of being successful. Any treatment, whether a simple prescription for pain medication or a periapical surgery, is invasive to the patient's system and can produce unexpected results if the patient's system is not thoroughly known beforehand. Determination of the systemic blood pressure, as well as the patient's temperature, pulse, and respiration should ideally be routine procedures in any comprehensive dental examination. These measurements are discussed in detail in any standard medical textbook on physical diagnosis (see *Physical Diagnosis: Bedside Evaluation of Diagnosis and Function*[64]).

Medical History

One advantage of endodontic therapy is that it has few systemic contraindications and can be performed when other treatment alternatives may pose an unacceptable risk to the patient's health. Nonetheless, only a complete medical history can provide insight into systemic conditions that may produce or affect the patient's symptoms, enabling the clinician to determine whether a medical consultation or premedication is required before treatment is started. Completion of a preprinted comprehensive, yet succinct, medical history form (Fig. 1-2) is essential. Simply completing the form is not enough, however. The dentist must review the answers with the patient to elicit more information and to ensure that the information is properly understood and that questions are addressed. An additional safeguard is for the doctor to initial the form after its examination.

According to the 1997 standards of the American Heart Association, patients should be closely screened for specific cardiac conditions and specific dental treatments that are associated with a high risk of developing bacterial endocarditis. (These conditions and treatments are discussed more thoroughly in Chapter 5.) Additionally, immunocompromised patients also may require prophylaxis. Patients taking daily anticoagulant medications such as warfarin (Coumadin) may need a reduction in the dose or a suspension of the drug before the periodontal portion of the examination.

An aging population has resulted in an increasing number of patients with chronic disease processes for which they

---

TELL US ABOUT YOUR HEALTH

*LAST NAME*_____ *FIRST NAME*_____

How would you rate your health?   Please circle one.   *Excellent   Good   Fair   Poor*

*When did you have your last physical exam?*_____

If you are under the care of a physician, please give reason(s) for treatment.
_____

Physician's Name, Address and Telephone Number:

*Name*_____*Address*_____

*City*_____*State*_____*Zip*_____*Telephone*_____

Have you ever had any kind of surgery?   *Yes___ No___*

*If yes, what kind?*_____*Date*_____
_____*Date*_____

Have you ever had any trouble with prolonged bleeding after surgery?   *Yes___ No___*
Do you wear a pacemaker or any other kind of prosthetic device?   *Yes___ No___*
Are you taking any kind of medication, or drugs at this time?   *Yes___ No___*

If yes, please give name(s) of the medicine(s) and reason(s) for taking them:

*Name*_____*Reason*_____
_____   _____

Have you ever had an unusual reaction to an anesthetic or drug (like penicillin)? Yes___No___

*If yes, please explain:*_____

Please circle any past or present illness you have had:

Alcoholism	Blood Pressure	Epilepsy	Hepatitis	Kidney or Liver	Rheumatic Fever
Allergies	Cancer	Glaucoma	Herpes	Mental	Sinusitis
Anemia	Diabetes	Head/Neck Injuries	Immunodeficiency	Migraine	Ulcers
Asthma	Drug Dependency	Heart Disease	Infectious Diseases	Respiratory	Veneral Disease

Are you allergic to Latex or any other substances or materials?   *Yes___No___*

*If so, please explain*_____

If female, are you pregnant?   *Yes___No___*

*Is there any other information that should be known about your health?*_____
_____

*Signed: Patient or Parent*_____*Date:*_____

Fig. 1-2 Succinct, comprehensive medical history form designed to provide insight into systemic conditions that could produce or affect the patient's symptoms, mandate alterations in the modality of treatment, or change the treatment plan.

take medications. Additionally, many patients self-medicate with over-the-counter remedies that they may not realize are drugs about which the clinician needs to be informed. Finally, some use illicit drugs that can produce catastrophic interactions with common dental drugs such as local anesthetics. Before rendering endodontic therapy, the clinician must know *all* drugs the patient is taking to identify possible adverse drug interactions. Such cases may require consultation with the treating physician. The patient's record should include a summary of any conversations with other dentists and physicians and outline any treatment recommendations.

EXAMINATION AND TESTING

Extraoral Examination

The extraoral visual examination of patients should begin when they enter the operatory. Patients should be observed for any problems with gait or balance or unusual habits that may suggest underlying systemic disorders, drug or alcohol use, or psychologic states. While the clinician is conducting the verbal interview to establish the history of the present illness, the patient's facial features should be observed. As with all other portions of the examination, these observations should be recorded in a consistent, step-by-step manner to minimize the possibility of missing significant information because a portion of the examination is inadvertently omitted. This punctiliousness helps the clinician develop diagnostic discipline and good examination habits.

In observing the patient, the dentist should first look for facial asymmetry (Fig. 1-3, *A*) or distention that might indicate swelling of an odontogenic origin or be produced by a systemic condition. The patient's eyes should be observed for pupillary dilation or constriction, which may signal systemic disease, premedication, or fear. The patient's skin should be checked for the presence of any lesions, including lacerations, contusions, scars, and discolorations. If multiple lesions are noted, their distribution and relationship to the branches of the trigeminal nerve should be noted. Occasionally facial lesions (e.g., a sinus tract draining through the skin) can be traced to a tooth as the source (Fig. 1-3, *B*).

The head and neck examination continues with bimanual palpation of the muscles of mastication and temporomandibular joints. The clinician should again establish an organized, consistent sequence to ensure completeness of the examination. The muscles to be palpated are the masseter, temporalis, medial pterygoid, digastric, and mylohyoid. These muscles are observed for pain on palpation and for the presence of any trigger points. With the patient's mouth closed, the clinician places an index finger in each of the patient's external auditory meatuses and gently pulls anteriorly, watching for a painful response. The clinician then places a hand over each of the patient's temporomandibular joints and palpates, again looking for tender areas. The patient is asked to open the mouth. Any signs of tenderness are noted as the mouth is opened and the condyles translate forward beneath the clinician's fingers. While the mouth is in the open position, the clinician palpates in the depression behind the condyle to check for tenderness in the posterolateral aspect of the condyle and retrodiscal tissue.

Maximum opening should be noted and should correspond roughly to three finger widths in the adult. The clinician can assist the patient in opening by using the index finger and thumb of one hand in a scissorslike manner on the maxillary and mandibular incisors. This can help determine whether a limited range of motion is due to a nonreducing disk or to muscle guarding. Deviation or deflection during opening and closing typical of disk displacement should also be noted.[29]

Next, the neck musculature is examined for hypertrophy, atrophy, and tenderness. The entire neck should be palpated for nodes, with particular attention to the area in front of and behind the ears; at the base of the skull; superior, inferior, and posterior to the sternocleidomastoid muscle; and beneath the mandible. These nodes are assessed for size, mobility, and tenderness.

Intraoral Examination

After completing a thorough extraoral head and neck examination of the patient, the clinician should proceed with an oral examination. The necessary tools for a comprehensive oral examination include an explorer, two mouth mirrors, 2" x 2" gauze, cotton rolls, a saliva ejector, a headlamp, and good magnification (Fig. 1-3, *C*). Abnormalities are easily masked by saliva, so any tissue to be examined must be dried with an air syringe or gauze (Fig. 1-3, *D*). The clinician should search for signs of caries, toothbrush abrasion (Fig. 1-3, *E*), darkened teeth (Fig. 1-3, *F*), observable swelling (Fig. 1-3, *G*), fractured teeth (Fig. 1-3, *H*), and defective restorations. Additionally, the clinician should be alert for signs of attrition, cervical erosion, or developmental defects (e.g., external tubercles, lingual grooves) (Fig. 1-3, *I-K*). Any occlusal discrepancies should be noted.

As in the extraoral visual examination, a high index of suspicion will lead the clinician through a thorough, individualized oral examination. Any unusual alterations of the color, texture, consistency, or contour of the soft tissues should be noted. For example, the clinician should carefully look for lesions of odontogenic origin, such as sinus tracts (Fig. 1-3, *L*) or localized redness or swelling in the attachment apparatus. Generally, sinus tracts indicate underlying necrosis, producing periapical suppuration that has resorbed through the cancellous bone, the cortical plate, and the mucoperiosteum, and has finally reached the mucosal surface where it is draining. All sinus tracts should be traced with a gutta-percha cone (a number 35 is generally recommended) (Fig. 1-3, *M*) to locate the sources of the tracts, since they may not lie directly beneath the openings to the surface[60] (Fig. 1-3, *N-O*).

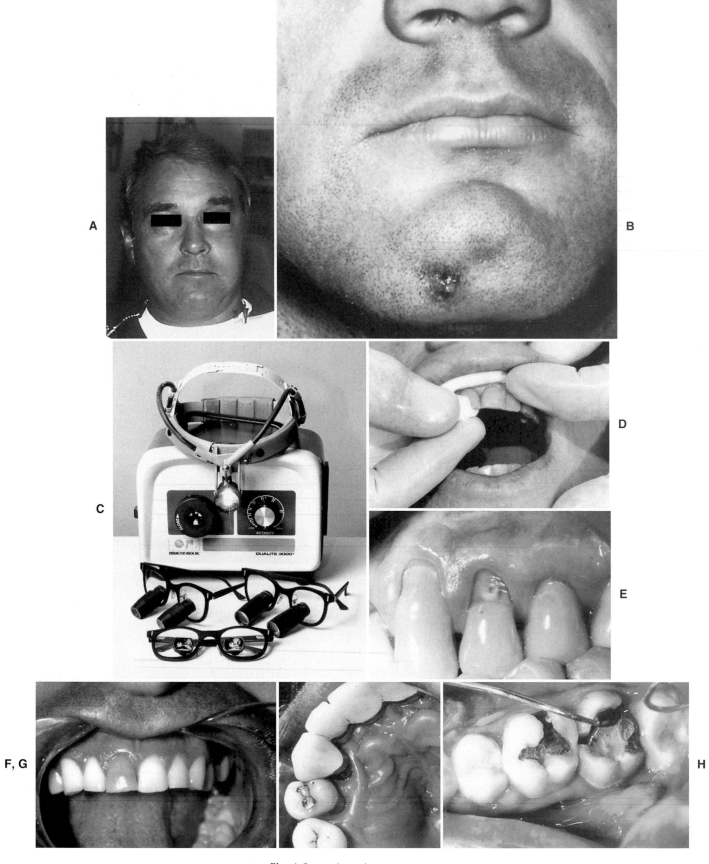

Fig. 1-3. For legend see opposite page.

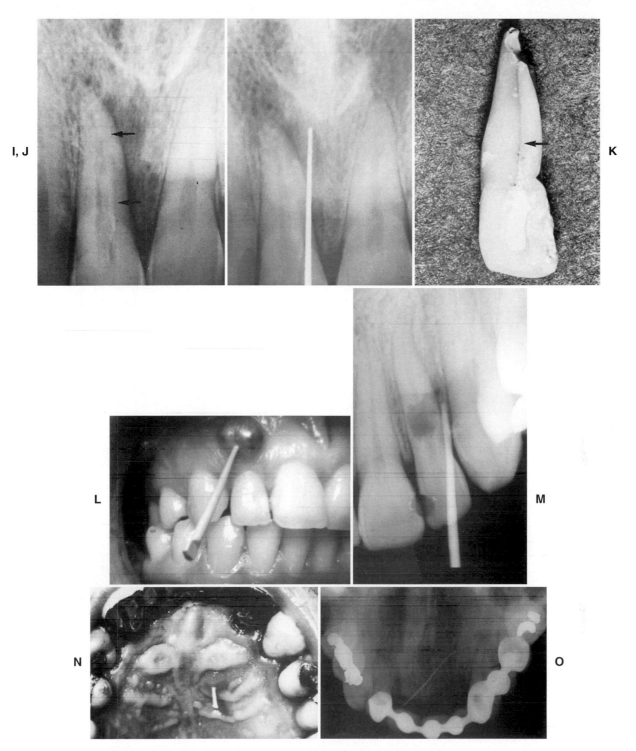

Fig. 1-3 **A**, During the gathering of the medical and dental histories, the patient's face should be examined for asymmetry and alertness. Patients who are suffering appreciate brevity, when possible. **B**, Occasionally an odontogenic infection can cause an extraoral lesion, such as this cutaneous fistula. **C**, Vision fiberoptic headlamps and magnifying telescopes provide improved illumination as well as magnification. **D**, A thorough clinical examination is facilitated by drying the tissues with gauze and cotton rolls. **E**, Common causes of pain from thermal stimuli, toothbrush abrasion, or Class V caries, are most likely to be detected during the visual examination. **F**, Tooth that discolored following a football injury. Because discolored teeth may remain healthy, vitality tests must be conducted before a diagnosis is made. **G**, In most cases intraoral swelling is found on the facial side. However, it may also occur on the lingual side or, as seen here, on the palate. **H**, Careful clinical examination may reveal crown fractures that may not be detected radiographically. **I**, Lingual developmental groove. Note that the canals of the central incisors are distinctly different. Arrows indicate the groove traced along the root. **J**, A silver cone placed in the lingual sulcular defect shows the extent of the associated periodontal breakdown. **K**, In this case the only treatment is extraction. In the future, fusing these grooves by laser surgery may allow the teeth to be retained. **L**, Whenever a sinus tract is found, it should be traced with a gutta-percha point. **M**, Radiograph taken with the gutta-percha cone in place. **N**, Palatal sinus tract traced with a gutta-percha cone. **O**, Occlusal jaw film revealed the remote source as the contralateral cuspid.

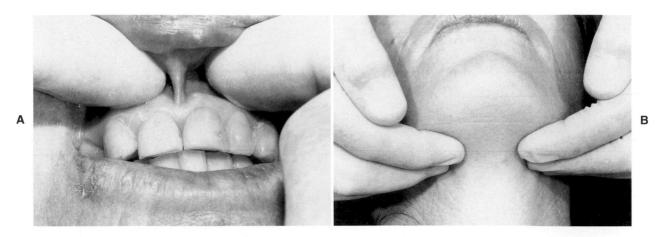

Fig. 1-4 **A**, Palpation test. The mucosa at the mucofacial fold should be gently pressed with the index finger to locate any spongy, fluctuant, or indurated areas or sites that elicit tenderness when palpated. If any tenderness is located, the degree of tenderness (+ = mild pain, ++ = moderate pain, +++ = severe pain) should be recorded. Palpating the same area contralaterally helps identify the normal range for each patient. **B**, Bimanual extraoral palpation to locate swollen submandibular or cervical lymph nodes. A swollen lymph node pressed against the ramus or between two fingers will also feel tender to the patient.

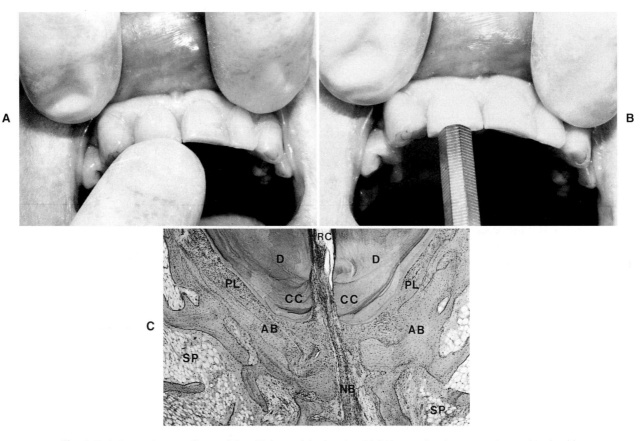

Fig. 1-5 **A**, Percussion test. If part of the chief complaint is pain with biting or chewing, percussion testing should begin with the index finger tapping the incisal or occlusal surface to avoid unnecessary pain. **B**, If no pain is elicited with digital percussion, a more definitive percussion test can be conducted with the handle of a mouth mirror. If a tooth is found to be tender to percussion, the degree of pain should be recorded as described in Fig. 1-4, *A*. **C**, A light, microscopic view of the healthy human periapex, showing the continuity of the pulp tissue and neurovascular bundle (*NB*) passing from the root canal (*RC*) to the periodontal ligament (*PL*). Magnification: ×46. (*C* from Nair PNR: Apical periodontitis: a dynamic encounter between root canal infection and host response, *Periodontology 2000* 13:122, 1997, Munksgaard International Publishers Ltd.)

Palpation   Palpation testing uses digital pressure to check for tenderness in the oral tissues overlying suspected teeth (Fig. 1-4, *A*). Sensitivity indicates that inflammation in the periodontal ligament surrounding the affected tooth has spread to the periosteum overlying the jawbone. In this manner, an incipient swelling may be detected before it is clinically evident by rolling the index finger over the mucosa and pressing it against the underlying bone. Additional information about fluctuation or induration of the soft tissues and changes in the underlying bony architecture can also be detected. Because of individual differences, bimanual palpation is most efficient, allowing the clinician to compare the patient's left and right sides for similarity or differences (Fig. 1-4, *B*).

Percussion   Tenderness noted upon percussing a tooth indicates some degree of inflammation in the periodontal ligament. This inflammation may be caused by occlusion, trauma, sinusitis, periodontal disease, or extension of pulpal disease into the periodontal ligament. Percussion is not a test of pulp vitality; thermal tests combined with electric pulp testing that evaluate pulpal nerve function are required to establish pulp vitality.

Before testing, the clinician should communicate the purpose of the test to the patient and explain how the patient should indicate any tenderness (e.g., raising a hand). Testing should begin with gentle tapping with the clinician's gloved fingernail, particularly if tenderness to biting is part of the chief complaint (Fig. 1-5, *A*). The clinician should randomly tap teeth in the suspected quadrant, beginning with one that is not suspected so the patient is aware of normal sensation. If the patient is unable to discern a difference in sensation with digital percussion, the blunt handle of a mouth mirror should be used (Fig. 1-5, *B*). Each tooth should be percussed on the facial, occlusal, and lingual sides. The technique is to gradually escalate the tapping pressure until it is just strong enough for the patient to discern a difference between a sound tooth and one with an inflamed periodontal ligament.

Patients' responses to percussion not only indicate that involvement of the periodontal ligament exists but also the extent to which it is inflamed. The degree of response will be directly proportional to the degree of inflammation. Histologically, there is no discernable division between the apical pulp tissue and the periodontal ligament (Fig. 1-5, *C*). Therefore when the pulp becomes inflamed, this inflammation will spread to the periodontal ligament. Additionally, endotoxin, cytotoxic materials, and bacteria emanating from the root apex may also produce a periapical inflammatory response. Conversely, where *chronic* periapical inflammation is present, percussion testing often yields a negative result.

Mobility   Tooth mobility provides an indication of the integrity of the attachment apparatus (i.e., whether inflammation of the periodontal ligament exists). As with percussion testing, pulp vitality testing is required to rule out or

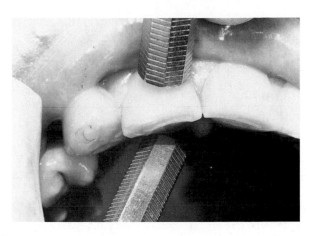

Fig. 1-6 Mobility test. With use of two mouth mirror handles, alternating lateral force should be applied in a facial-lingual direction. The degree of mobility detected should be recorded as Class 1 = barely perceptible movement, Class 2 = <1 mm movement, and Class 3 = >1 mm movement or depressibility.

support a diagnosis of pulpal involvement since periodontal inflammation can arise from multiple causes.

The clinician should use two mouth-mirror handles to apply alternating lateral forces in a facial-lingual direction to observe the degree of mobility of the tooth (Fig. 1-6). The degree of depressibility of the tooth within its alveolus should also be tested. The tooth should be pressed into its socket and any vertical movement should be noted.

All movement is subject to individual differences; consequently, the displacement of an individual tooth should be measured against that of the patient's other teeth. First-degree mobility is barely perceptible horizontal movement; second-degree mobility is no more than 1 mm of horizontal movement; third degree mobility is greater than 1 mm of horizontal movement and/or vertical depressability. However, a difference in mobility from the patient's other teeth should be noted to consider the movement significant.

The pressure exerted by the purulent exudate of an acute periradicular abscess may cause considerable tooth mobility,[5,25,60] but the mobility resolves quickly once drainage for the exudate is established. Root fracture, recent trauma, chronic bruxism, habits, and orthodontic tooth movement also cause tooth mobility.

Periodontal Examination   Although the mobility of a tooth increases when the integrity of the attachment is severely compromised, severe bone loss is often required before the damage is clinically detectable by tooth mobility alone. A far more sensitive test is to use a blunt, calibrated probe to explore the attachment level in the gingival sulcus around each tooth. All surfaces of the roots should be probed, along with any furcas. The findings should be recorded in the patient's clinical record (Fig. 1-7).

Periodontal probing should be carried out by "sounding,"—that is, "walking" the probe around the tooth while

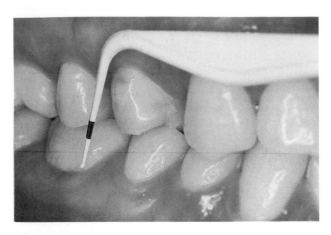

Fig. 1-7 Periodontal examination. A periodontal probe, such as this PSR instrument, should be used to check the integrity of the gingival sulcus. The findings of the periodontal examination should be recorded both in depths of the sulci and in tissue characteristics, such as contour, consistency, color, and bleeding.

pressing gently on the floor of the sulcus. Probing must be performed throughout the mouth, as with the periodontal screening and recording technique[30,44] to appreciate the patient's overall periodontal condition. Wide, gently sloping craters around multiple teeth characterize periodontal disease. Horizontal attachment loss on a suggested tooth in a patient with *generalized* pocketing is not as worrisome as *isolated* vertical bone loss, which is frequently indicative of a vertical root fracture. In some cases, a sinus tract can drain pus from the apex of a tooth with a necrotic pulp to the oral cavity through the periodontal ligament. This can also produce a narrow, deep pocket that will quickly close once endodontic therapy is completed.

Occasionally it is useful for diagnostic confirmation to place a gutta-percha cone or silver point in the sulcular defect and expose a radiographic film to confirm the depth and direction of the periodontal pocket. To distinguish a periodontal from an endodontic etiology, thermal and electric pulp testing must accompany periodontal probing.

Thermal Pulp Tests   One of the most common symptoms associated with the symptomatic inflamed pulp is pain elicited by thermal stimulation. Although some patients suffer pain when cold is applied to the tooth but are comfortable with warm substances and others require frequent applications of cold liquid to keep their pain bearable, there is no particular response to either heat or cold that is unique to a specific pulpal pathologic state.[56] The only conclusion the clinician may draw when a pulp responds abnormally to thermal stimulation, either in an exaggerated manner or not at all, is that it is not in a state of good health.

The rationale for innervation of any bodily structure is to provide a warning of damage that is occurring or impending. With this understanding, sharp, nonlingering pain with the application of thermal stimuli is normal and a vital part of

the patient's protective defense mechanism. The pain is proportionate to the stimulation; consequently, even teeth with intact enamel will react to extreme cold, such as ice or carbon dioxide snow. When teeth begin to react to stimuli that do not normally produce pain, such as tap water, the probability is that dentin has been exposed by caries, that the tooth structure is fractured, or that faulty restoration, abrasion, or attachment loss caused by periodontal disease exists. Additionally, an exaggerated response to thermal stimuli can indicate a lowered threshold to stimulus because of pulpal inflammation (e.g., immediately after placement of a restoration). In this case, the solution is not to "kill the messenger" by removing the pulpal tissue; rather, the solution is to address the cause of the dentin sensitivity by occluding the dentinal tubules by placing a temporary sedative restoration, such as intermediate restorative material (IRM). In the case of the new restoration, the clinician should simply wait to see whether the acute inflammation subsides in a short time.

When the chief complaint is pain to a thermal stimulus (usually cold), the clinician must distinguish between thermal testing to isolate the offending tooth by reproducing the patient's symptoms and attempting to determine whether a suspected tooth has a vital or nonvital pulp. In the former case, the patient is complaining of painful pulpal response to cold; therefore pulpal vitality is not at issue. A graduated method of applying the stimulus is required to avoid causing the patient unnecessary pain. Directed air, then water from the triple syringe, followed by isolating the tooth under a rubber dam and bathing it with cold water should elicit the patient's symptoms and quickly indicate the offending tooth. In contrast, when there is no complaint of cold sensitivity, the following methods for using cold to determine pulpal vitality are appropriate.

Cold Test   Various methods have been used to apply cold to the teeth for testing. The most commonly used methods are ice sticks, various compressed gasses, and carbon dioxide snow. Freezing water in the plastic covers from hypodermic needles can form sticks of ice (Fig. 1-8, *A*). When needed, one is removed from the freezer and held tightly in the clinician's hand for a few minutes. This melts the outside of the stick so that it can be removed from the plastic and held in a 2" x 2" gauze for use. The ice stick is applied immediately to the middle third of the facial surface of the crown of the tooth or on any exposed metal surface of crowns and kept in contact for 5 seconds or until the patient begins to feel pain.

Ethyl chloride is available as a compressed spray, commonly used in medicine as a skin refrigerant. Its use in pulp testing is no longer recommended because it has been found to be less effective than carbon dioxide snow or dichlorodifluoromethane, which is the refrigerant R-12 commercially packaged as a compressed spray (Endo-Ice).[4,18] The production of dichlorodifluoromethane, which has a boiling point of -21.6° F, was prohibited by the Clean Air Act in the United States on January 1, 1996, because of environmental con-

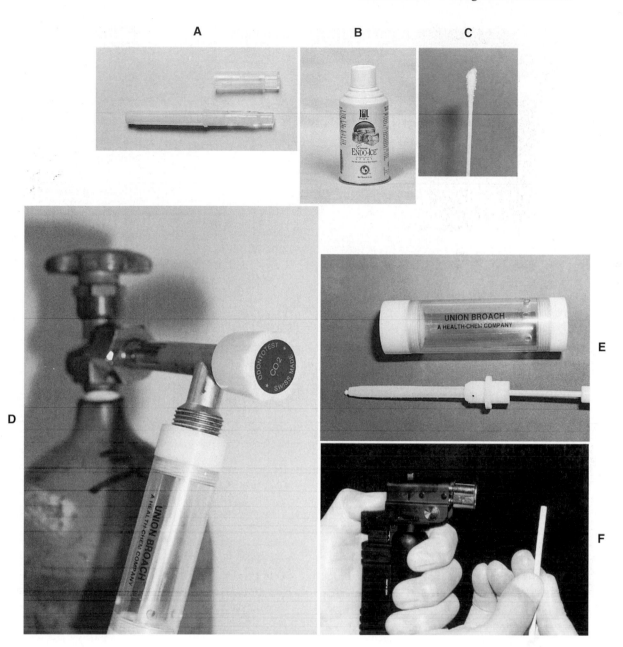

Fig. 1-8 **A**, A diagnostic ice stick for cold testing can be made by freezing water in a needle cover. **B**, Commercially available 1,1,1,2 tetrafluoroethane spray is convenient but not as accurate as an ice water bath. **C**, The material is sprayed liberally onto a cotton swab, which is then applied to the tooth for 5 to 10 seconds or until the patient feels pain. **D**, Preparing a carbon dioxide ice stick. **E**, Syringe used to form the CO_2 ice stick. **F**, A carbon dioxide dry-ice stick held in gauze and applied to the tooth.   *Continued*

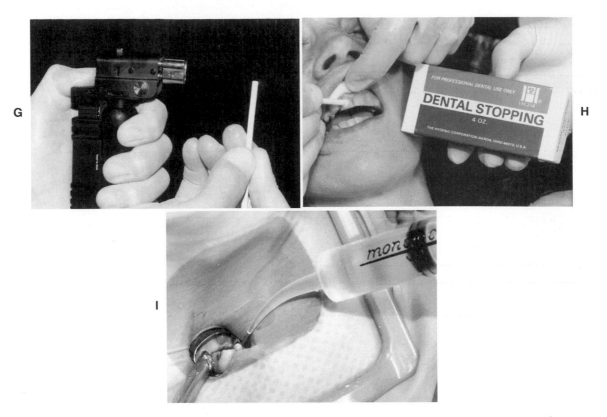

Fig. 1-8, cont'd **G**, Another technique for heat testing is to warm the temporary stopping until its surface begins to glisten. **H**, After the tooth is coated with petroleum jelly to prevent sticking, the warm gutta-percha is applied for 5 seconds or until the patient begins to feel pain. **I**, After the tooth has been isolated with a rubber dam, a plastic syringe is used to immerse the tooth in warm water. This method can also be used with ice water for cold testing. It is the most accurate testing method, because all surfaces of the tooth are exposed to the water.

cerns; it is mentioned nonetheless because several countries still permit its use. It has been replaced by the manufacturer with 1,1,1,2 Tetrafluoroethane, which is the nonchlorofluorocarbon refrigerant R-134a, available as Green Endo-Ice. No studies are yet available on the efficacy of this replacement compared with other testing methods. However, it also has a low boiling point (-15.1° F). The material is sprayed liberally onto a cotton pellet or swab, which is then applied immediately to the middle third of the facial surface of the crown of the tooth (Fig. 1-8, *B-C*). The pellet is kept in contact with the crown for 5 seconds or until the patient begins to feel pain.

Carbon dioxide snow formed into sticks (Fig. 1-8, *D*) is extremely cold (-77.7° C, -108° F). It is the most effective method of eliciting a response in vital teeth. No detrimental effects occurred in vital pulpal tissue, and no cracks or surface irregularities were produced in the enamel of tested teeth.[26,43,47] The carbon dioxide is released into a special syringe (Fig 1-8, *E*) in which it forms the "snow." It is compacted with a plunger, and the pellet is expressed onto a 2" × 2" gauze. It is applied immediately to the middle third of the facial surface of the crown of the tooth and kept in contact with the crown for 2 seconds or until the patient begins to

feel pain (Fig. 1-8, *F*). Although less convenient than the sprays, isolating the teeth individually with a rubber dam and bathing each tooth with ice water from a syringe for 5 seconds will elicit the *most accurate* patient response because it simultaneously cools all surfaces of the teeth.

Heat Test   As with cold testing, many methods for heat testing teeth have been suggested. Although all transfer heat to the tooth, the methods most commonly used are warm sticks of temporary stopping and the hot water bath. Warm sticks of temporary stopping are the most convenient for the clinician, but the hot water bath will yield the most accurate patient response.

Temporary stopping consists of gutta-percha in 3-inch sticks. To use this technique, the teeth to be tested are first protected with a light coating of petrolatum to prevent the warm temporary stopping from sticking to them. The stopping is warmed over a flame until it becomes soft and just begins to glisten (Grossman's method)[23] (Fig. 1-8, *G*), but not so that it slumps and becomes too limp to use. Application to the middle third of the facial surface of the crown usually results in a response in less than 2 seconds (Fig. 1-8, *H*). A 5-second application has been found to increase the temperature at the pulpodentinal junction less than 2° C; therefore it is unlikely that damage will occur to the pulp.[47]

Similar to the cold water bath, the hot water bath requires rubber dam isolation of the teeth to be tested individually (Fig. 1-8, *I*). The tooth is bathed in very warm water from a plastic syringe for 5 seconds or until the patient begins to feel pain. Since the patient's chief complaint is pain in response to heat, the temperature is gradually increased if no response is obtained, rather than producing unnecessary pain by beginning with excessively hot liquid.

Although the cold and hot water bath methods of thermal testing are time consuming, they are clearly superior in their accuracy compared to very warm temporary stopping or ice pencils. The use of water allows the entire crown to be immersed, not just one section of one surface of the tooth. Even when the tooth has been restored with a full crown (metal or porcelain), sufficient contact is made to allow cooling or warming of the pulp. In addition, the cold and hot water bath methods prevent damage to the tooth caused by excessive temperature change.

Responses to Thermal Tests

The sensory fibers of the pulp transmit only pain whether the pulp has been cooled or heated (see Chapter 11 on pulpal neurophysiology for further discussion). There are four possible responses to thermal stimulation:

1. No response
2. Mild-to-moderate degree of awareness of slight pain that subsides within 1 to 2 seconds after the stimulus has been removed
3. Strong, momentary painful response that subsides within 1 to 2 seconds after the stimulus has been removed
4. Moderate-to-strong painful response that lingers for several seconds or longer after the stimulus has been removed

If there is no response to thermal testing, a nonvital pulp is often the cause. However, no response to thermal testing can also indicate a false negative response because of excessive calcification, an immature apex, recent trauma, or patient premedication. A momentary mild-to-moderate response to thermal change is generally considered within normal limits. A somewhat exaggerated response that subsides quickly is characteristic of reversible pulpitis. A painful response that lingers for several minutes after the stimulus is removed is characteristic of irreversible pulpitis.

Electric Pulp Tests

The electric pulp tester (EPT) uses electric excitation to stimulate the Aδ sensory fibers within the pulp (Fig. 1-9, *A*). A positive response to electric pulp testing does not provide any information about the health or integrity of the pulp; it simply indicates that there are vital sensory fibers present within the pulp.[58] Often, irreversibly inflamed pulp is responsive to EPT because it still contains vital, functional nerve fibers that can produce a toothache. The EPT provides only a responsive or nonresponsive result that correlates, in many cases, with vital or nonvital pulpal

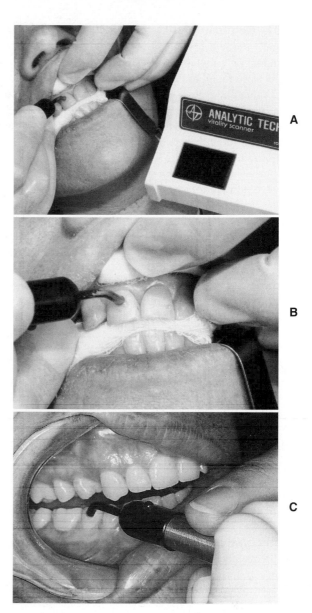

Fig. 1-9 A, Electric pulp testing. Before testing, the teeth must be isolated and dried, and a lip clip must be applied to the side of the mouth. **B,** After applying a conductor, such as toothpaste, between the electrode and the tooth, the rate of current increase is adjusted to a slow progression. **C,** A patient's finger placed on the probe acts as a "switch," preventing undue discomfort. Patients are instructed to release their hands from the probe as soon as they feel tingling or warmth in the tooth. Each tooth should be tested at least two or three times to ensure an accurate, reproducible response.

status. Therefore attempting to interpret the numerical values produced by the EPT is *not* recommended. The electric pulp test fails to provide any information about the vascular supply to the pulp, which is the true determinant of pulp vitality. As a result, teeth that temporarily or permanently lose their sensory function (e.g., teeth damaged by trauma, or teeth that have undergone orthognathic surgery), will be nonresponsive to EPT. However, they will have intact vasculature.[9]

EPT with the Analytic Technologies instrument is extremely reliable. Investigators failed to note any significant adaptation or habituation by patients to repeated testing. Results were found to be reproducible for consecutive trials on the same day and for trials on different days.[12] However, the accuracy of EPT has been questioned. Seltzer et al reported that 28% of teeth with necrotic pulps tested positive to EPT, and more than half of those with partially necrotic pulps were responsive.[56]

When a patient reports sensation in a tooth with a necrotic pulp, it is termed a *false positive response.* Circumstances that can cause false positive responses to electric pulp testing include patient anxiety, saliva conducting the stimulus to the gingiva, metallic restorations conducting the stimulus to the adjacent teeth, and liquefactive necrosis conducting the stimulus to the attachment apparatus.

A false negative response means that although the pulp is vital, the patient does not indicate that any sensation is felt in the tooth. This situation can be produced by premedication with drugs or alcohol, immature teeth, trauma, poor contact with the tooth, inadequate media, partial necrosis with vital pulp remaining in the apical portion of the root, and individual patients with atrophied pulps or high pain thresholds. Therefore it is essential that multiple tests be performed before a final diagnosis is made.[42]

EPT is an imperfect, though useful, way to determine the pulpal status of a tooth. In the case of a periapical radiolucency, EPT will help the clinician determine whether the pulp is vital. When used with thermal and periodontal testing, the EPT can help differentiate pulpal disease from periodontal disease or nonodontogenic causes.

EPT Technique   The teeth to be tested must be isolated and dried with 2" × 2" gauze, and the testing area must be kept dry with a saliva ejector to prevent false positive results caused by electrical conduction to the adjacent teeth (Fig. 1-9, *B*). If the tooth has a proximal metallic restoration, a rubber dam or celluloid strips should also be placed interproximally to prevent electrical conduction to the adjacent teeth.[37]

The clinician must prepare the patient by explaining the diagnostic value of the test and the procedure that will be followed. It is also important that the patient be informed about the sensations of heat or tingling felt during testing. Since the clinician will be wearing nonconductive latex gloves, the patient will have to place a finger on the handle of the testing device (Fig. 1-9, *C*) to serve as a "switch." The instrument will function only while the patient is touching the device, and any sensation will cease upon release; this reassures patients that they have control if any sensation occurs.

Many clinicians use the Analytic Technology Pulp Tester because the digital reading (indicating current flow) always starts at 0. In addition, a dial on the front of the unit easily controls the current flow rate. To use this device, the lip clip should be attached and the electrode of the pulp tester should be generously coated with a viscous conductor (e.g., toothpaste). The electrode should then be applied to the dry enamel of the tooth being tested on the middle third of the

facial surface of the crown. The current flow should be increased slowly to allow the patient time to respond before the attendant tingling sensation becomes painful. The electrode should not be applied to any restorations, because this could lead to a false reading. If a positive reading is not obtained, the electrode should be applied to several different locations on the lingual and facial surfaces of the tooth to ensure that the negative reading is not the result of electrode placement.

Each tooth should be tested at least two or three times, and an average result should be recorded. The patient's response may vary slightly with each test. However, a significant variation in response suggests a false reading. Enamel thickness influences response time: the thinner enamel of anterior teeth yields a faster response than does the thicker enamel of posterior teeth. In laboratory testing, EPTs did not interfere with pacemaker functioning, therefore they should be safe for use with patients with these devices. This may be because newer pulp testers contain improved shielding and filtering circuits.[35,59]

Laser Doppler Flowmetry   EPT uses electric current to stimulate the Aδ nociceptors in the pulp. When these fibers are intact, stimulation results in a painful sensation and the pulp is said to be vital. However, intact nerve functioning is not essential for pulp vitality. Teeth that have experienced recent trauma or are in a portion of the jaw that has undergone orthognathic surgery can lose sensibility while retaining an intact blood supply and vital pulp. Investigators[1] found that 21% of teeth in patients that tested nonresponsive to electrical stimulation after having undergone Le Fort I operations had intact blood supplies when tested with laser Doppler flowmetry. With EPT only, the pulps would have been considered necrotic, and endodontic therapy would have been needlessly undertaken.

To circumvent this limitation, other testing modalities have been suggested. Laser Doppler flowmetry uses a laser beam of known wavelength that is directed through the crown of the tooth to the blood vessels within the pulp. Moving red blood cells cause the frequency of the laser beam to be Doppler-shifted and some of the light to be back-scattered out of the tooth. This reflected light is detected by a photocell on the tooth surface, the output of which is proportional to the number and velocity of the blood cells.[15,19,50]

Laser Doppler flowmetry is complicated by the fact that the laser beam must interact with moving cells within the pulpal vasculature. To avoid artifactual responses, a custom-fabricated jig (i.e., mouth guard) is needed to hold the sensor motionless and maintain its contact with the tooth. The position on the crown of the tooth and the location of the pulp within the tooth cause variations in pulpal blood flow measurements.[46] Additionally, differences in sensor output and inadequate calibration by the manufacturer may mandate the use of multiple probes for accurate assessment,[34,49] and antihypertensive medications and nicotine may affect blood flow to the pulp, producing inaccurate results.[36] Finally, the equipment still is too expensive for the average dental office.

Current limitations aside, laser Doppler flowmetry promises an objective measurement of pulpal vitality and health. When equipment costs decrease and clinical application improves, this technology could be used for patients who cannot communicate effectively or whose responses may not be reliable (e.g., young children). Because this testing modality produces no noxious stimuli, apprehensive or distressed patients may accept it more readily than current methods.

Pulse Oximetry   Another optical diagnostic method currently under investigation is the adaption of pulse oximetry to the diagnosis of pulpal vitality. Pulse oximetry is a widely used technique for recording blood oxygen saturation levels during the administration of intravenous anesthesia. Increased acidity and metabolic rate produced by inflammation cause deoxygenation of hemoglobin and change the oxygen saturation of the blood. A pulse oximeter uses a probe con-

taining a diode that emits light in two wavelengths: (1) red light of approximately 660 nm and (2) infrared light of approximately 850 nm. This light is received by a photodetector diode, connected to a microprocessor. The device compares the ratio of the amplitudes of the transmitted infrared with red light. It uses this information, together with known absorption curves for oxygenated and deoxygenated hemoglobin, to determine the oxygen saturation levels.[21,40,54]

By monitoring changes in oxygen saturation, pulse oximetry may be able to detect pulpal inflammation or partial necrosis in teeth that are still vital. Several investigators[21,54] have successfully used modified finger probes or adapted the instrument to teeth to demonstrate the reliability of the system in the diagnosis of pulp vitality (Fig. 1-10, *A* and *B*). Other investigators indicate that the use of reflected light may be preferable to transmitted light[40] and that different or multiple wavelengths may be required to improve the sensitivity of the technique.[53]

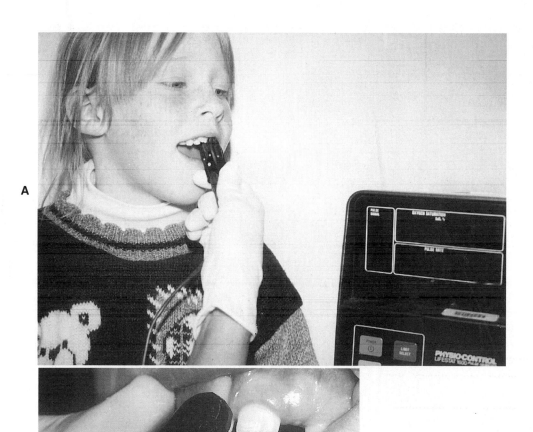

Fig. 1-10 **A**, Placement of a modified pulse oximetry ear probe on a partially erupted central incisor. **B**, The modified ear probe in place on the tooth. (**A** from Goho C: Pulse oximetry evaluation of vitality in primary and immature permanent teeth, *Pediatr Dent* 21:126, 1999. **B** courtesy Dr. C. Goho.)

Radiographic Examination

Although radiographs are arguably the single most useful diagnostic tool at the dentist's disposal, they are also the most misused. Too often the two-dimensional radiographic shadow is misinterpreted, which may cause a diagnostic error and thus improper treatment. Radiographs are only an *adjunct* to diagnosis: one more puzzle piece that helps form the entire picture. For this reason, diagnostic radiography should be used only after the history is recorded and the clinical examination is accomplished.[11]

Radiographs have several limitations. First, like a photograph, the radiograph provides a two-dimensional portrayal of three-dimensional reality. Although two-dimensional photos are flat, we can use optical clues to sense depth in the image. Optical clues are natural features that individuals have learned to recognize in their day-to-day lives. For example, *linear perspective*, which refers to the way objects appear to grow smaller as they recede into the distance, helps determine which objects in a photo are closer to the camera. Therefore if a photograph depicts two cars on a road and one car is smaller than the other, it is assumed that the smaller car is farther from the camera.

Similarly, optical features of radiographs must be learned, which is best accomplished by studying the anatomy of the jaws and teeth and relating these structures to their radiographic representations. In this way, for example, dentists become familiar with the fact that root canals often bifurcate and do not think that their radiographic appearance represents a calcification (Fig. 1-11, *A*).

Since clinicians make the radiographs themselves, they have a decided advantage over the casual observer of a photograph. To overcome the limitations of the film, they can create various views of the subject from multiple angles. Just as observers at sporting events or in theaters must move their

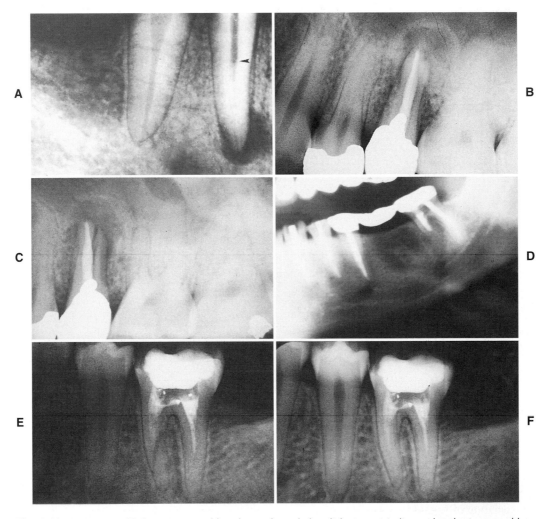

Fig. 1-11 **A**, Root canal bifurcation. A sudden change from dark to light (*arrow*) indicates that the root canal has branched into more than one canal. **B**, Tooth originally referred for retreatment. Note the "halo" (radiolucency) surrounding the tooth. **C**, A more distal angulation exposure reveals the vertical-root fracture. **D**, What appeared to be a periapical radiolucency on the mandibular second premolar is shown to be the mental foramen on the panoramic radiograph. **E**, Initially this molar appeared to exhibit a root fracture. However, careful scrutiny of the film revealed a fingernail bend. **F**, When a second radiograph was exposed, the "fracture" disappeared.

heads left and right to see around objects obstructing their vision, clinicians can make two films from the same vertical angulation, but with a 10- to 15-degree change in horizontal angulation of the tube head. In this way the buccolingual location of an object, such as a perforation, can be appreciated by noting the direction of movement of the object relative to the tube head (see Chapter 5). Canals that are superimposed can be separated and, in some cases, vertical fractures can be seen (Fig. 1-11, *B* and *C*). Lesions that appear to be attached to the root will move away from it when the angulation is changed. The tube head can also be shifted in a vertical manner. In this way, structures, such as the zygomatic arch that may be superimposed over root apices, can be moved. This approach enables the clinician to mentally construct a three-dimensional model of the anatomic reality that the radiograph is trying to convey.

The technique of exposing multiple radiographs is not limited to horizontally or vertically shifted periapical films. The clinician may need to use several types of films to get a complete picture of the tooth or teeth involved, as well as any surrounding structures. These films may include panographs, lateral jaw radiographs, occlusal radiographs or bitewing films. Because anatomic aberrations can be misinterpreted, a contralateral exposure of the same type of radiograph is helpful whenever there is a doubt as to the diagnosis. For example, a patient may have a suspicious radiolucent area overlying the periapex of a mandibular second molar. A contralateral exposure will reveal the same condition on the opposite side and identify the "lesion" as the mental foramen (Fig. 1-11, *D*). Finally, it should be remembered that when unusual or unexpected features appear on the radiograph, particularly those that appear to require treatment, another radiograph should always be taken to rule out artifactual aberrances (Fig. 1-11, *E* and *F*). (Chapters 2 and 5 offer an extended discussion of the particulars of dental radiology.)

The second limitation of the radiograph is that its interpretation is a learned skill and therefore subject to different assessments by various observers. Radiographic interpretation, like diagnosis itself, is part science and part art and intuition. As George Eliot, the English novelist said, "All meanings, we know, depend on the key of interpretation." Goldman et al[22] asked two endodontists, three second-year endodontic residents, and an associate professor of radiology to examine at a series of radiographs and determine whether there was an area of rarefaction. These six examiners agreed on less than 50% of the cases. When three of the original examiners viewed the same cases 6 to 8 months later, they agreed with their previous responses only 75% to 83% of the time. Finally, Gelfand and associates asked dentists at the 1981 American Association of Endodontists (AAE) meeting to view 10 of the radiographs from the previous studies and indicate if the cases were successful, failures, or questionable on the basis of the lesions. Within these cases, there were two identical radiographs. Not only did these dentists have greater than 50% agreement on less than half of the cases,

almost 22% of them marked different answers on the identical radiographs, despite viewing them only 2½ minutes apart![20]

As with any facet of diagnosis, certain radiographic phenomena are especially susceptible to multiple interpretations. These include the following:

Radiolucency at the Apex   At first glance the radiolucency at the apex may appear to be a periapical lesion. However, a positive response to thermal or EPT, an intact lamina dura, the absence of symptoms and probable cause, and the anatomic location of the mass clearly reveal that this is the mental foramen (Fig. 1-12, *A*).

Well-Circumscribed Radiolucency at or Near the Apex   Initially this well-circumscribed radiolucency at or near the apex may also appear to be a periapical lesion. However, the absence of symptoms, the history of apical surgery, and the intact lamina dura make it clear that the correct diagnosis is an apical scar (Fig. 1-12, *B*).

Ostensible periradicular lesion. The source of an ostensible periradicular lesion can be confirmed only through complete testing, including thermal and EPT. In this case the use of the radiograph alone for diagnosis could lead to treatment of the wrong tooth. Accurate differential diagnosis demands the careful consideration of anatomic landmarks in the region being examined (Fig. 1-12, *C-E*).

A third limitation of radiographs is that they cannot be used to determine the status of the health and integrity of the pulp. Only pulp testing, in concert with a comprehensive examination, can determine whether a pulp is vital. The discovery of deep caries, pulp caps, extensive restorations, pulpotomies, pulp stones, extensive canal calcification, resorption, radiolucencies at or near the apex, root fractures, a thickened periodontal ligament, or periodontal disease that has caused bone loss should heighten the suggestion of inflammatory or degenerative pulp changes.

Radiographic Interpretation

Accurate radiographic interpretation begins with properly exposed and processed radiographs. No clinician, no matter how astute, can be expected to interpret correctly a radiograph that exhibits improper density or contrast, lack of focus, or distortion. Only films of the highest quality should be accepted; any time or money saved by not re-taking questionable films would be forfeited by one misdiagnosis. Clinicians should strive to limit their patients' exposure to radiation and maximize their skills and the skills of staff members to achieve this end. However, because the benefits of radiographs outweigh the risks, diagnostic-quality radiographs should be obtained even at the expense of repeated images.

Once high-quality radiographs are obtained, the next step is to view them properly. Welander et al[63] studied the effect of various viewing conditions on the ability of observers to perceive radiographic details. They evaluated the perception

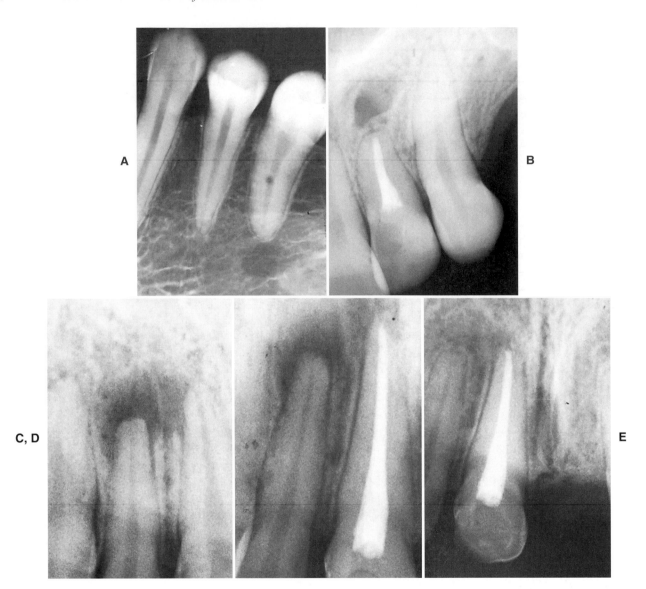

Fig. 1-12 **A,** Potential radiographic misinterpretation. Normal thermal and electric pulp tests, along with an intact lamina dura, indicate that this asymptomatic radiolucency is the mental foramen. **B,** With a history of prior apical surgery and an intact lamina dura, this asymptomatic radiolucency was identified as an apical scar. **C,** Vitality tests confirmed that the nonvital central incisor was the source of the radiolucency over the lateral incisor. **D,** Immediately after endodontic therapy. **E,** After 6 months, complete remineralization is visible. (Courtesy Dr. John Sapone.)

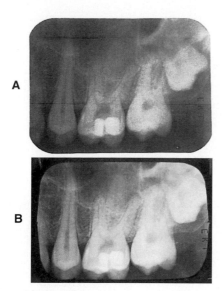

Fig. 1-13 **A**, Viewing an unmasked radiograph forces the eye to adapt to the bright view box, obscuring details on the film. **B**, Masking the film allows the eye to adjust to the radiograph itself.

of radiographic detail under various conditions and found extraneous light and improper masking reduced the perceived image contrast, because the observer's pupils constrict to adjust to the greater light from the viewbox (or room light) that surrounds the film. Thus the film is comparatively too dark for the eye to perceive the necessary detail (Fig. 1-13, *A* and *B*). On the other hand, viewing films in a room with subdued lighting on a viewbox with the periphery of the films masked resulted in perception as good as when an X-Produkter (a device that not only masks extraneous light but also magnifies the films) was used. Therefore it is critical to mount films in light-masking (opaque) frames, eliminate extraneous light from the viewbox, and dim room lights to achieve maximum diagnostic efficiency.

Just as with the clinical examination, properly lighted radiographs must be viewed in an orderly, consistent manner to avoid overlooking important features. The crown, the attachment apparatus, the root(s), the root canal system, and the periapical area must all be studied carefully. As long as they are all considered, the order in which these features are studied is not important.

Considering the variation in interpretation among different observers, investigators[28] evaluated 18 different radiographic features to determine which were most strongly correlated with the condition of the periapical area (i.e., which features most consistently allowed the observer to arrive at the correct pulpal diagnosis). They found that a diagnosis based on the continuity and shape of the lamina dura and the width and shape of the periodontal ligament space was the most accurate in identifying teeth with nonvital pulps.

In addition to inspecting the lamina dura and periodontal ligament space, the clinician should consider whether the bony architecture is within normal limits or whether there is evidence of demineralization. The clinician should also consider whether the root canal system is within normal limits, whether it appears to be resorbing or calcifying, and what anatomic landmarks could be expected in the area. A sound,

correct examination protocol includes a careful investigation of each of these considerations.

In addition to periapical films in the posterior region, it is helpful to prepare bite-wing films. Early caries, the depth of existing restorations, pulp caps, and pulpotomies or dens invaginitus can be identified in bite-wing films. Deep caries or extensive restorations increase the likelihood of pulpal involvement. A single root canal should appear as tapering from crown to apex; a sudden change in appearance of the canal from dark to light indicates that it has bifurcated or trifurcated (see Fig. 1-11, *A*).

The presence of "extra" roots or canals is more common than previously thought. For example, although molars are considered to have three roots and three root canals, studies of the maxillary molars suggest that approximately 95% of these teeth have four canals, and roughly 75% should be treatable clinically.[16,32,39] The clinician should always consider the possibility of "extra" canals (i.e., consider a molar to have four canals until proven otherwise). Three-rooted mandibular molars and maxillary premolars and two-rooted mandibular canines and incisors will be found with greater frequency as the clinician's understanding of anatomy, index of suspicion, and sophistication of diagnosis improve. The use of good illumination and magnification is also important in the identification process (Fig. 1-14, *A*).

A necrotic pulp will not cause radiographic changes until the enzymes produced by the inflammatory process have begun to demineralize the cortical plate.[7,45,55] For this reason, significant medullary bone destruction may occur before any radiographic signs begin to appear. Toxins and other irritants may exit through a lateral canal, causing periradicular (rather than periapical) demineralization. Conversely, a lateral canal in a tooth affected by periodontal disease can become a portal of entry for harmful toxins (Fig. 1-14, *B* and *C*).

Pulp stones and canal calcifications do not necessarily have pathologic origin; they can be the result of normal aging of the pulp.[58] Investigators[51] studying teeth from patients

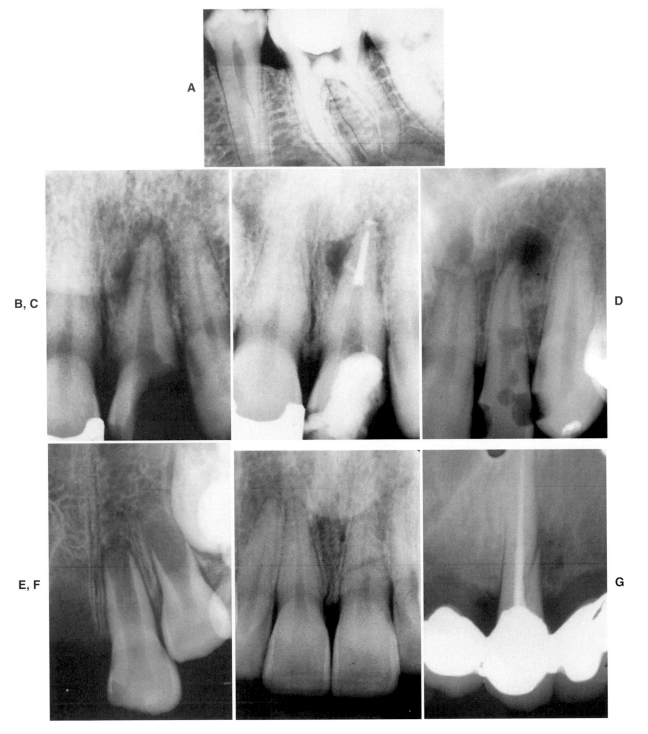

Fig. 1-14 **A**, Anticipation of "extra" root and canals. The astute clinician will not be surprised to find "extra" canals (premolar) or roots (molar). **B**, Periapical and periradicular demineralization. Bacteria or endotoxin or both irritants may cascade out of lateral canals and apical portals of exit, causing diffuse periradicular demineralization. **C**, When the portals of exit have been well sealed, remineralization will proceed uneventfully. In the presence of periodontal disease, these lateral canals could become infected and, ultimately, infect the pulp. **D**, Internal resorption, an insidious, asymptomatic, inflammatory process, will perforate the root unless endodontic therapy is initiated. **E**, Pulp vitality tests are unreliable when the apices are immature. **F**, Only horizontal root fractures are readily identifiable shortly after injury. **G**, Often oblique and vertical fractures are not identified until demineralization or root separation makes them evident.

with mild-to-severe periodontal disease found diffuse calcification and stones in 82% of pulps studied. These calcifications were not correlated with the severity of periodontal disease, did not produce higher EPT responses, and were not related to age. In traumatized teeth with pulp obliteration studied between 7 and 22 years posttrauma, 51% had a normal response to EPT. Another 40% did not respond but were clinically and radiographically normal. The investigators[48] calculated the average rate of pulp survival for 20 years at 84%. Consequently, in the absence of any additional signs or symptoms, the presence of pulp stones or canal calcification should not be interpreted as a pulpal disorder that requires endodontic therapy.

However, internal resorption (occasionally seen after trauma) *is* an indication for endodontic therapy (Fig. 1-14, *D*). The inflamed pulp recruits clastic cells, which asymptomatically resorb the radicular dentin, from the blood vascular system. In this case the pulp must be removed as soon as possible to eliminate these cells and avoid a pathologic perforation of the root. (Chapter 16 discusses this issue in depth.)

Periapical radiographs also allow the clinician to identify teeth with immature apices (Fig. 1-14, *E*). Recognizing the presence of immature apices allows the clinician to anticipate erroneous responses to thermal and electric pulp tests.

If the canal appears blurred when compared with the contralateral tooth on the radiograph and there is an irregular demineralized radiolucency surrounding the root, lingual developmental grooves would be suggested (see Fig. 1-3, *I-K*).

In a few cases, root fractures may cause pulp degeneration.[65] Only a horizontal root fracture will be identifiable in the early stage (Fig. 1-14, *F*) and then only if the fracture line is within ±15 degrees of the central radiographic beam.[13] In the case of a suggested horizontal fracture, two additional radiographs should be produced from angles ±30 degrees. Vertical and oblique root fractures will eventually cause demineralization and a resultant diffuse radiolucency adjacent to the fracture (Fig. 1-14, *G*). (Chapters 2 and 16 discuss these issues in detail.)

Special Tests

Crown Removal   Many times a patient will describe symptoms of irreversible pulpitis, but the suspected tooth is completely hidden from view clinically and radiographically by a prosthetic crown. Although thermal and EPT may be possible, if there are intact nerve fibers in the pulp, the results may be difficult to differentiate from normal. In this case it is often necessary to complete the examination by carefully removing the crown to inspect the tooth underneath. Many times, leakage from subgingival margins that were impossible to adequately explore clinically has resulted in a carious exposure of the pulp. Occasionally the result of this exposure is complete destruction of the crown of the tooth. Removal of the prosthetic crown not only confirms the

diagnosis, it also allows the clinician to assess the restorability of the tooth.

Selective Anesthesia Test   In special clinical situations, the use of intraligamentary anesthesia is an effective diagnostic tool. For example, an intraligamentary anesthesia test should be used when the clinician has determined, through prior testing, which tooth is the source of pain, although the patient reports severe, lingering, residual pain as a result of the thermal testing. Administration of 0.2 ml of local anesthetic into the distal sulcus will provide welcome relief for the patient (Fig. 1-15). Under these conditions, the use of intraligamentary anesthesia breaks the cycle of pain for the patient for several minutes and reconfirms, through the elimination of pain, what prior testing determined through the reproduction of pain.[61]

If the patient continues to have vague, diffuse, strong pain, and prior testing has been inconclusive, intraligamentary anesthesia may be used to help identify the source of pain. Administration of 0.2 ml of local anesthetic into the distal sulcus of the offending tooth will briefly stop the pain. However, investigators[60] who injected a radiopaque solution and colloidal carbon suspension into the periodontal ligament (PDL) of dogs and examined the distribution of the dye found carbon in the PDL, periapex, medullary bone, and pulp of injected teeth. They also found these substances in the same tissues of adjacent teeth, indicating that it does *not* provide selective, one-tooth anesthesia. Thus the clinician can not make a conclusive diagnosis between adjacent teeth on the basis of pain relief. Nevertheless, the use of anesthetic can help identify the probable source of pain and reliably rule out referred pain between arches.

If the patient's chief complaint concerns continuing pain and the pain is not relieved by the administration of intraligamentary anesthesia, the cause may be heterotopic pain. In this case the clinician must consider nonodontogenic causes. (Chapter 3 provides a comprehensive discussion of this kind of pain.)

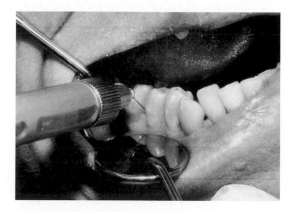

Fig. 1-15 Selective anesthesia test. Intraligamentary anesthesia, where 0.2 ml is injected into the distal sulcus, can be used to confirm the source of pain.

Test Cavity   Occasionally the clinician will encounter a tooth that exhibits mixed responses to pulp testing (e.g., it fails to respond to cold, but it does respond to EPT). Is this an example of a false positive response to EPT caused by gingival conduction? Although the pulp still responds to the EPT miniprobe placed subgingivally, is it so receded and sclerosed (or is the porcelain jacket crown sufficiently insulative) that the pulp is unable to respond to thermal testing?

The most accurate technique to discover whether a pulp is vital is to begin to make a preparation in a concealed area of the tooth without anesthetizing the patient, who has been adequately apprised of what to expect and how to respond if discomfort is felt. When the dentoenamel junction (DEJ) is passed, or as the pulp is approached, the patient should feel pain if the pulp is vital. Once a vital response is elicited, the cavity preparation should cease and the tooth should be restored. If no response is evoked, access preparation may continue and endodontic therapy completed. Although the damage can be repaired, this is not a reversible procedure. Therefore it should be reserved for cases when it is impossible to arrive at a pulpal diagnosis in another way.

Transillumination   Holding a fiberoptic illuminating device horizontally at the gingival sulcus in a dimly lit treatment room may reveal a vertical fracture line or it may make a suspected line more visible (Fig. 1-16, *A*). Normally the crown of an intact tooth will be illuminated uniformly by the fiberoptic light. If a fracture exists, the light will illuminate the side of the crown that it contacts. However, the portion of the crown on the opposite side of the fracture will remain dark. A specialized fiberoptic wand, an otoscope with a fiberoptic attachment, a bore light, or a fiberoptic handpiece may be used for this purpose (Fig. 1-16, *B*). Composite curing lights are not recommended, because they are excessively bright and, despite the fracture, may illuminate the entire crown. If the tooth contains a restoration, it may be necessary to remove it to expose the fracture line (Fig. 1-16, *C*). Although fiberoptic transillumination will also reveal discoloration caused by extravasation of blood after trauma or calcification of the pulp chamber, this discoloration is not reliably related to the health of the pulp. Therefore it should not be used to determine pulp vitality.[27,48]

Wedging and Staining   A wedging force exerted during mastication may result in pain for the patient while chewing. The most reliable technique for creating a wedging force is to ask the patient to bite on a Tooth Slooth that has been selectively placed on successive cusps until the offending cusp is located (Fig. 1-17, *A* and *B*). This technique helps the clinician identify both vertical crown root fractures and cuspal shear fractures (i.e., cracked tooth "syndrome") that may not involve the pulp.

The application of methylene blue or erythrosine dye to a cottonwood stick can be a helpful extension of the wedging technique, because it can highlight a subtle coronal fracture that might otherwise escape detection. The coronal surface of the tooth should be dried, and a cottonwood stick should be moistened with the dye and placed on the occlusal surface of the tooth. Then the patient should be instructed to bite firmly on the stick and to move the jaw from side to side (Fig. 1-17, *C*). Gauze dampened with 70% isopropyl alcohol should be used to wipe excess dye from the tooth surface. A close inspection of the tooth should reveal the elusive coronal fracture, darkened with dye. If a suspected fracture or crack is not evident under a restoration, dye can be incorporated into a mix of IRM and placed as a temporary restoration. By the next appointment, sufficient dye should have leached out of the restoration to stain the crack.

Cracked Tooth "Syndrome" and Vertical Fractures

One of the more baffling cases that the clinician will encounter is the patient who complains of sporadic, sharp

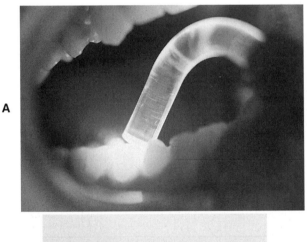

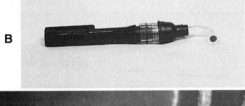

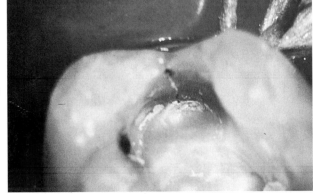

Fig. 1-16   **A,** A fiberoptic device will evenly illuminate the crown of a tooth where no fracture is present. **B,** A battery-powered bore light is ideal for transillumination. **C,** Removing the amalgam restoration revealed a fracture beneath. (**A** and **B** from Liewehr FR: An inexpensive device for transillumination, *J Endod* 2000 [in press].)

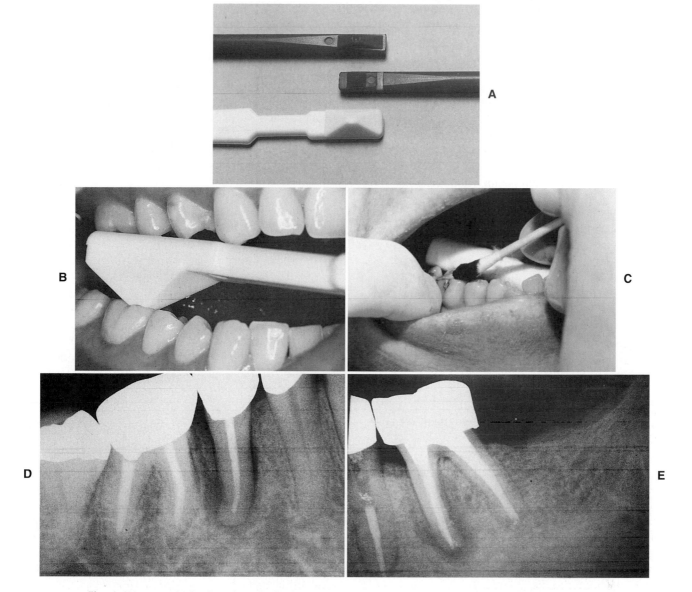

Fig. 1-17 **A,** Tooth Slooth and Tooth Slooth II are used to apply selective biting pressure to cusps and fossae. **B,** The patient is asked to bite on each cusp successively, until the pain is reproduced. **C,** After the occlusal surface is dried, methylene blue dye can be applied. The patient is directed to clench down on the cottonwood stick and move the jaw in a side-to-side motion. Gauze, moistened in isopropyl alcohol, should then be used to wipe away the excess dye. Vertical crown fractures will be stained by the dye. **D,** The "halo" surrounding the root of this mandibular second premolar strongly suggests a root fracture. **E,** A similar "halo" is seen around the mesial root of this mandibular molar.

pain while chewing, along with occasional pain from cold food or drink. Sometimes the patient may indicate that the pain occurs minutes after chewing or upon releasing from clenching. For example, the patient may recall an incident when a sudden jolt of pain was felt while the patient was chewing popcorn or ice or while accidentally biting into a bone or olive pit. Often the patient is unable to locate the source of the pain and can be otherwise asymptomatic. In this case the clinician must rely upon diagnostic testing to reproduce the patient's symptoms and to determine the source of the pain. Cameron[10] referred to this as the "cracked tooth syndrome," because the symptoms are the result of a

hairline, incomplete fracture of the tooth. When portions of the crown are spread apart by occlusal forces, the underlying dentin is momentarily exposed. As a result of hydrostatic movement of fluid within the dentinal tubules, the patient then experiences pain. Any tooth may be involved, but the mandibular molars are the most prone to fracture. Even though heavily restored teeth are subject to this syndrome, unrestored teeth are prone to fracture only half as often as those with large amalgams.[33]

The process may follow several different courses. In the event of a vertically oriented crack, continued use may widen the crack. If this occurs the tooth may develop the symptoms of an irreversible pulpitis or the pulp may become necrotic and asymptomatic. The fracture line may increase in width, and the fracture may progress apically to produce a vertical-root fracture.

If the crack extends in a more oblique direction and is sufficiently small or if it is hidden beneath a restoration, it may continue to produce the symptoms of a hypersensitive pulp and elude detection for years. Ultimately, it may proceed toward the pulp and produce the same results as the vertical crack, or the involved cusp may shear off, relieving the patient's symptoms.

Occasionally, clinical examination will reveal a crack that is often discolored and that extends over a marginal ridge. If this is the case, further investigation may be required. Often, however, an examination will reveal multiple craze lines on all teeth or it will reveal no craze lines at all. In the case of a severe fracture, a loose or fractured restoration may be discovered. The use of disclosing paper can highlight occlusal discrepancies that appear on balancing cusps. Often the existence of wear facets suggests which tooth may be fractured.

Generally, other clinical tests, such as percussion, palpation, mobility, and probing, will be within normal limits if the crack is confined to coronal tooth structure. The most useful test is to have the patient bite on successive cusps, using a Tooth Slooth, until the pain is reproduced (see Fig. 1-17, *A* and *B*). Staining can also help disclose subtle fractures. Often transillumination is effective in locating the affected portion of the crown. EPT will produce normal responses unless the pulp is involved. Cold testing may be productive, whereas heat testing may not be helpful. In most cases, radiographs will be unremarkable, because these fractures tend to run mesiodistally and are not in the plane of the x-ray beam. Therefore they will not be visible on the radiograph.

If the fracture extends beyond the crown onto the root, a periodontal defect may be observed in the form of a narrow, deep pocket adjacent to the fracture. By this time the pulp may have become necrotic, and sharp pain and cold sensitivity are not present. Only a dull ache on biting, caused by inflammation of the periodontal ligament fibers, may persist. In this case, percussion testing will be helpful, because of the involvement of the proprioceptive fibers within the PDL. Vertical fractures will often be recognized radiographically by their effect on the bony attachment apparatus that is seen as a diffuse radiolucency, or "halo," surrounding the root of the fractured tooth (Fig. 1-17, *D* and *E*). This can be differentiated from other periapical or periradicular radiolucencies by the fact that it surrounds the tooth uniformly, rather than being located at the portal of exit of the apical foramen or a lateral canal.

In addition to the progress of formerly incomplete fractures onto the root, sometimes vertical root fractures are caused by the incorrect use of a spreader or a plugger during the course of endodontic therapy. Gutta-percha is *not* compressible; spreading only serves to compact the accessory cones to eliminate voids. Increasing spreader pressure does not decrease leakage.[24] Typically a patient's dental history indicates that although the patient has undergone nonsurgical and, perhaps, surgical root canal therapy multiple times, the tooth in question remains symptomatic. Sometimes the patient may have undergone periodontal therapy that has failed to resolve a recurrent periodontal defect around one or two surfaces of a root, and no additional evidence of periodontal disease is evident. In these cases, reflecting a mucoperiosteal flap (with the aid of magnification and illumination, including the endodontic-operating microscope) may reveal the offending fracture.

CLINICAL CLASSIFICATION OF PULPAL AND PERIAPICAL DISEASE

In the 1960s a number of investigations revealed a lack of a correlation between clinical signs and symptoms and the actual histologic status of the pulp.[57] Since the histologic diagnosis of a pulp is impossible to determine without removing it and submitting it for histologic examination, a clinical classification system was developed. This system was based on the patient's symptoms and the results of clinical tests. It was developed to provide basic terms and phrases that clinicians could use to describe the extent of pulpal and periapical disease before selecting a method of treatment. A clinical classification of this sort is not meant to list every possible variation of inflammation, ulceration, proliferation, calcification, degeneration of the pulp, or attachment apparatus. Rather, its purposes are to suggest in the broadest possible interpretation whether the pulp is either healthy or unhealthy and to help the clinician determine whether it should be removed, based on clinical experience.

The terms listed in the following text outline the main clinical signs and symptoms of the degrees of inflammation or degeneration of the pulpal and periapical tissues. The clinical terms applied to periapical disease suggest the nature, duration, and type of exudation found in the disease processes.

Pulpal Disease

Within Normal Limits
A normal pulp is asymptomatic and produces a mild-to-moderate transient response to thermal and electrical stimuli. When the stimulus is removed, the response subsides almost immediately. The tooth and its attachment apparatus do not cause a painful response when percussed or palpated. Radiographs reveal a clearly delineated canal that tapers smoothly toward the apex. There is no evidence of root resorption, and the lamina dura is intact.

In the absence of other signs and symptoms indicating pathosis, teeth with canal calcifications are considered within normal limits. Aging; idiopathic patient characteristics; the physical stress of restorative procedures; periodontal disease or therapy; attrition; abrasion; or trauma may cause an otherwise healthy pulp to deposit excessive amounts of dentin throughout the canal system. Often canal calcification, like internal resorption, is detected through routine radiographic examination. Sometimes an anterior tooth will reveal coronal discoloration, suggesting chamber calcification. However, because it is rare for calcific metamorphosis to lead to necrosis,[48] monitoring these teeth for changes indicative of pathosis is all that is necessary.

Reversible Pulpitis   The pulp is inflamed to the extent that thermal stimuli—usually cold—cause a quick, sharp, hypersensitive response that subsides as soon as the stimulus is removed. Otherwise the pulp remains asymptomatic. Any irritant that can affect the pulp may cause reversible pulpitis, including early caries, periodontal scaling, root planing, microleakage, and unbased restorations.

Reversible pulpitis is *not* a disease; it is a symptom. If the irritant is removed and further insult is prevented by sealing the dentinal tubules communicating with the inflamed pulp, the pulp will revert to an asymptomatic, uninflamed state. Conversely, if the irritant remains, the symptoms may persist indefinitely or may become more widespread, leading to irreversible pulpitis. Reversible pulpitis can be distinguished from a symptomatic irreversible pulpitis in two ways:

1. Reversible pulpitis causes a momentary, painful response to thermal change that subsides as soon as the stimulus is removed. However, symptomatic irreversible pulpitis causes a painful response to thermal change that lingers after the stimulus is removed.
2. Reversible pulpitis does not involve a complaint of spontaneous (unprovoked) pain. Symptomatic irreversible pulpitis commonly includes a complaint of spontaneous pain. Therefore the key difference is that reversible pulpitis is *reactive*; it produces a response, albeit exaggerated, only when stimulated.

Irreversible Pulpitis   Irreversible pulpitis may be acute, subacute, or chronic; it may be partial or total, infected or sterile. Clinically, the acutely inflamed pulp is symptomatic, whereas, the chronically inflamed pulp is asymptomatic in most cases. The apical extent of irreversible pulpitis cannot be determined clinically until the periodontal ligament is affected by the cascade of inflammatory mediators and the tooth becomes sensitive to percussion.[3,58] Dynamic changes in the irreversibly inflamed pulp are continual; the pulp may move from quiescent chronicity to acute pain within hours.

Asymptomatic Irreversible Pulpitis   Although uncommon, asymptomatic irreversible pulpitis may be the conversion of symptomatic irreversible pulpitis to a quiescent state. Caries and trauma are the most common causes of this condition, which can be identified by information gathered from the patient's dental history and properly exposed radiographs.

Hyperplastic Pulpitis   A reddish, cauliflower-like growth of pulp tissue through and around a carious exposure is one

variation of asymptomatic irreversible pulpitis. The proliferative nature of this pulpal reaction, sometimes known as a "pulp polyp," is attributed to a low-grade, chronic irritation of the pulp and the generous vascularity characteristically found in young people.[58] Occasionally this condition may cause mild, transient pain during mastication.

Internal Resorption   Internal resorption is a painless condition resulting from the recruitment of blood-borne clastic cells, often stimulated by trauma, which produces dentin destruction. Often internal resorption is identified during routine radiographic examination (see Fig. 1-14, *D*). If undetected, internal resorption will eventually perforate the root. Before perforation of the crown, the resorption can be detected as a pink spot on the site. Only prompt endodontic therapy to eliminate these clastic cells will prevent tooth destruction. (Chapter 16 contains a further discussion of this issue.)

Symptomatic Irreversible Pulpitis   Symptomatic irreversible pulpitis is characterized by spontaneous (i.e., unprovoked), intermittent, or continuous paroxysms of pain. Sudden temperature changes (usually cold) elicit prolonged episodes of pain (i.e., pain that lingers after the thermal stimulus is removed). This pain may be relieved in some patients by the application of heat or cold. Occasionally, patients may report that a postural change (lying down or bending over) induces pain, resulting in fitful sleep. Even with the use of several pillows to stabilize themselves at a comfortable postural level, patients may continue to experience pain.

Generally, pain from symptomatic irreversible pulpitis is moderate to severe; it can be sharp or dull, localized or referred. In most cases, radiographs are not useful in diagnosing symptomatic irreversible pulpitis because the inflammation remains confined to the pulp. However, radiographs can be helpful in identifying offending teeth (i.e., teeth with deep caries, extensive restorations, pins, evidence of previous pulp capping, calcific metamorphosis).[2] In the advanced stage of symptomatic irreversible pulpitis, thickening of the apical portion of the periodontal ligament may become evident on the radiographs. (Chapter 2 offers a comprehensive discussion of referred pain from symptomatic irreversible pulpitis.)

Symptomatic irreversible pulpitis can be diagnosed through synthesis of the information provided in a thorough dental history, a complete visual examination, properly exposed radiographs, and carefully conducted thermal tests. If radiating or referred pain is involved, the application of 0.2 ml of intraligamentary anesthesia in the distal sulcus of the correctly identified tooth will immediately stop the pain. EPT is of little value in the diagnosis of symptomatic irreversible pulpitis, because the pulp, though inflamed, is still responsive to electrical stimulation.

The inflammatory process of symptomatic irreversible pulpitis may become so severe that it will lead to necrosis of the pulp. In the degenerative transition from pulpitis to necrosis, the usual symptoms of symptomatic irreversible pulpitis may subside as necrosis occurs.

Necrosis

Necrosis, the death of the pulp, actually refers to a histologic condition resulting from an untreated irreversible pulpitis, a traumatic injury, or any event that causes long-term interruption of the blood supply to the pulp. Pulp necrosis may be partial or total, and the remnants of the pulp may become liquefied or coagulated. Total necrosis is asymptomatic before it affects the periodontal ligament, because the pulpal nerves are nonfunctional. For this reason, there is no response to thermal or EPT. Some crown discoloration may accompany pulp necrosis in anterior teeth, but this diagnostic sign is not reliable.[27,48] Partial necrosis may be difficult to diagnose, because it can produce some of the symptoms associated with irreversible pulpitis. For example, a tooth with two or more root canals could have an inflamed pulp in one canal and a necrotic pulp in the other.

The bacterial toxins (and sometimes bacteria) that produced the necrosis in the pulp follow the pulp tissue through the apical foramen to the periodontal ligament, resulting in an inflammatory reaction in the periodontium (see Fig. 1-5, *C*). This inflammation will lead to thickening of the periodontal ligament and manifest itself as tenderness to percussion and chewing.[3,58] As these irritants cascade out of the root canal system, often periapical disease will occur.[5]

The difficulty with the use of the term "necrosis" is that pulp vitality testing has been limited to electrical and thermal stimulation of pulpal nerves. In the case of teeth that have been traumatized,[9] teeth in a segment of bone that has been surgically repositioned,[1] teeth with immature apices,[17,18,31] or teeth that have calcified with age,[8] nerve function can be diminished or cease altogether, while the pulp retains an intact vasculature. Thus reliance upon EPT and thermal pulp testing can result in the unnecessary removal of healthy, denervated pulps. Perhaps the use of more sophisticated testing techniques, such as laser Doppler flowmetry or pulse oximetry, will overcome this limitation and provide a clinical test that reliably indicates pulpal necrosis.

PERIAPICAL DISEASE

Acute Apical Periodontitis

Acute apical periodontitis is painful inflammation around the apex (periodontitis). This condition can be the result of an extension of pulpal inflammation into the periapical tissue, mechanical or chemical trauma by endodontic instruments or materials, or occlusal trauma caused by hyperocclusion or bruxism. Because acute apical periodontitis may occur around vital and nonvital teeth, *conducting EPT and thermal pulp tests is the only way to confirm the need for endodontic treatment.* As always, the need for endodontic treatment must be determined by pulpal status alone.

Although acute apical periodontitis is present, the apical periodontal ligament may appear within normal limits or appear only slightly widened on the pretreatment radiograph. However, the tooth may be slightly-to-extremely painful during percussion and chewing tests. If the tooth is vital, a simple occlusal adjustment will often relieve the pain. If the pulp is necrotic and the resulting acute apical periodontitis remains untreated, additional symptoms may appear as the disease advances to the next stage: acute periradicular abscess.

Acute Periradicular Abscess

An acute periradicular abscess consists of a painful purulent exudate (abscess) around the apex. This abscess is the result of the exacerbation of acute apical periodontitis from an infected, necrotic pulp. Although this disease can be very serious, the periodontal ligament may appear within normal limits or it may be only slightly thickened. This is because the rapid progress (acute in the temporal sense) of the infection has spread beyond the confines of the cortical plate before demineralization can be detected radiographically. Thus the periapical radiograph may only reveal a relatively normal or slightly thickened lamina dura.

The signs and symptoms of acute periradicular abscess include rapid onset of slight-to-severe swelling, moderate-to-severe pain, pain from percussion and palpation, and the possibility of a slight increase in tooth mobility. In more advanced cases, the patient is febrile. The extent and distribution of the swelling is determined by the location of the apex, the muscle attachments, and the thickness of the cortical plate.[5,25] The acute periradicular abscess can be differentially diagnosed from the lateral periodontal abscess and from the phoenix abscess in the following manner:

- In the case of a lateral periodontal abscess, EPT and thermal pulp tests confirm the vitality of the pulp, although symptoms of the lateral periodontal abscess may mimic those of the acute periradicular abscess. Additionally, with only rare exceptions a deep periodontal pocket is found associated with the lateral periodontal abscess.
- The symptoms of the phoenix abscess and the acute periradicular abscess are identical. (When a periapical radiolucency is evident, it is called a *phoenix abscess*.)

Chronic Apical Periodontitis

Generally, chronic apical periodontitis is an asymptomatic periapical lesion that is manifested radiographically. Bacteria and their endotoxins cascading out into the periapical region from a necrotic pulp cause an inflammatory reaction that produces extensive demineralization of cancellous and cortical bone. The resulting radiographically evident lesions may be large or small, diffuse or circumscribed. Occasionally there may be slight tenderness to percussion testing or palpation testing or to both testing methods. Often the patient will say that, although nonpainful, the tooth feels "different" or "hollow" when percussed. A sinus tract (incorrectly

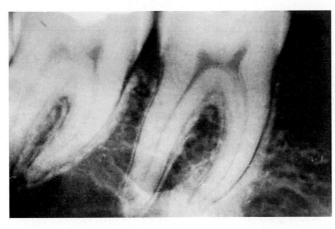

Fig. 1-18 Periapical osteosclerosis, possibly caused by a mild pulp irritant.

referred to as a "fistula" or "gum boil") represents frank suppuration and has been termed a chronic suppurative apical periodontitis or a chronic apical abscess. As pressure from pus is relieved by drainage through a sinus tract, the sinus tract may close temporarily. When the pressure from pus builds up again (along with slight tenderness to palpation), the sinus tract returns.

The general absence of symptoms, the presence of a periapical radiolucency, and the confirmation of pulp necrosis confirm the diagnosis of chronic apical periodontitis. A totally necrotic pulp provides a safe harbor for the primarily anaerobic microorganisms and their noxious allies: if there is no vascularity, there are no defense cells. For this reason only complete cleansing, shaping, and obturation of the root canal will eliminate the source of the periapical disease and create a microenvironment in which these periapical lesions can remineralize.

Phoenix Abscess

A phoenix abscess is always preceded by chronic apical periodontitis. The signs and symptoms of a phoenix abscess are identical to those of an acute periradicular abscess, but a radiograph will reveal a periapical radiolucency that indicates the existence of chronic disease. This condition can be produced if a chronic suppurative apical periodontitis worsens without a sinus tract to relieve the pressure; symptoms identical to those found with an acute periradicular abscess will appear. (Chapter 2 provides a full discussion of the causes of and the cures for this pathologic condition.)

Periapical Osteosclerosis

Periapical osteosclerosis is excessive bone mineralization around the apex of an asymptomatic, vital tooth (Fig. 1-18). This radiolucency may be caused by low-grade pulp irritation. Because this condition is asymptomatic and benign, it does not require endodontic therapy.

References

1. Aanderud-Larsen K, Brodin P, Aars H, Skjelbred P: Laser Doppler flowmetry in the assessment of tooth vitality after Le Fort I osteotomy, *J Craniomaxillofac Surg* 23:391, 1995.
2. Abou-Rass M: The stressed pulp condition: an endodontic-restorative diagnostic concept, *J Prosthet Dent* 48:264, 1982.
3. Andreasen JO: *Atlas of replantation and transplantation of teeth,* Philadelphia, 1992, WB Saunders.
4. Augsburger RA, Peters DD: In vitro effects of ice, skin refrigerant, and CO_2 snow on intrapulpal temperature, *J Endod* 7:110, 1981.
5. Baumgartner JC: Treatment of infections and associated lesions of endodontic origin, *J Endod* 17:418, 1991.
6. Bender IB, Seltzer S: The effect of periodontal disease on the pulp, *J Oral Surg* 33:458, 1972.
7. Bender IB, Seltzer S: Roentgenographic and direct observation of experimental lesions in bone (part 1), *J Am Dent Assoc* 62:152, 1961.
8. Bernick S: Effect of aging on the nerve supply to human teeth, *J Dent Res* 46:694, 1967.
9. Bhaskar SN, Rappaport HM: Dental vitality tests and pulp status, *J Am Dent Assoc* 86:409, 1973.
10. Cameron CE: Cracked tooth syndrome, *J Am Dent Assoc* 68:930, 1964.
11. Council on Dental Materials, Instruments, and Equipment: Recommendations in radiographic practices: an update, *J Am Dent Assn* 118:115, 1989.
12. Dal Santl FB, Throckmorton GS, Ellis E III: Reproducibility of data from a hand-held digital pulp tester used on teeth and oral soft tissue, *Oral Surg Oral Med Oral Pathol Oral Radiol Endod* 72:103, 1992.
13. Degering CI: Radiography of dental fractures, *J Oral Surg* 30:213, 1970.
14. Drinnan AL: Differential diagnosis of orofacial pain, *Dent Clin North Am* 31:627, 1987.
15. Ebihara A, Tokita Y, Izawa T, Suda H: Pulpal blood flow assessed by laser Doppler flowmetry in a tooth with a horizontal root fracture, *Oral Surg Oral Med Oral Pathol Oral Radiol Endod* 81:229, 1996.
16. Fogel HM, Peikoff MD, Christie WH: Canal configuration in the mesiobuccal root of the maxillary first molar: a clinical study, *J Endod* 20:135, 1994.
17. Fulling HJ, Andreasen JO: Influence of maturation status and tooth type of permanent teeth upon electrometric and thermal pulp testing procedures, *Scand J Dent Res* 84:286, 1976.
18. Fuss Z et al: S: Assessment of reliability of electrical and thermal pulp testing agents, *J Endod* 12:301, 1986.
19. Gazelius B, Olgart L, Edwall B, Edwall L: Non-invasive recording of blood flow in human dental pulp, *Endod Dent Traumatol* 2:219, 1986.
20. Gelfand M, Sunderman EJ, Goldman M: Reliability of radiographical interpretations, *J Endod* 9:71, 1983.
21. Goho C: Pulse oximetry evaluation of vitality in primary and immature permanent teeth, *Pediatr Dent* 21:125, 1999.
22. Goldman M, Pearson A, Darzenta N: Reliability of radiographic interpretations, *J Oral Surg* 32:287, 1974.
23. Grossman LI: *Endodontic practice,* ed 10, Philadelphia, 1981, Lea and Febiger.

24. Hatton JF, Ferrillo PJ, Wagner G, Stewart GP: The effect of condensation pressure on the apical seal, *J Endod* 14:305, 1988.

25. Hutter JW: Facial space infections of odontogenic origin, *J Endod* 17:422, 1991.

26. Ingram TA, Peters DD: Evaluation of the effects of carbon dioxide used as a pulpal test. I. In vivo effect on canine enamel and pulpal tissues, *J Endod* 9:296, 1983.

27. Jacobsen I, Kerekes K: Long-term prognosis of traumatized permanent anterior teeth showing calcifying processes in the pulp cavity, *Scand J Dent Res* 85:588, 1977.

28. Kaffe I, Gratt BM: Variations in the radiographic interpretation of the periapical dental region, *J Endod* 14:330, 1988.

29. Kaplan AS: History and examination of the orofacial pain patient, *Dent Clin North Am* 41:155, 1997.

30. Khocht A, Zohn H, Deasy M, Chang KM: Screening for periodontal disease: radiographs vs. PSR, *J Am Dent Assoc* 127: 749, 1996.

31. Klein H: Pulp response to electrical pulp stimulator in the developing permanent dentition, *J Dent Child* 45:199, 1978.

32. Kulild JC, Peters DD: Incidence and configuration of canal systems in the mesiobuccal root of the maxillary first and second molars, *J Endod* 16:311, 1990.

33. Maxwell EH, Braly BV, Eakle WS: Incompletely fractured teeth: a survey of endodontists, *Oral Surg Oral Med Oral Pathol* 61:113, 1986.

34. Mesaros SV, Trope M: Revascularization of traumatized teeth assessed by laser Doppler flowmetry: case report, *Endod Dent Traumatol* 13:24, 1997.

35. Miller CA, Leonelli FM, Latham E: Selective interference with pacemaker activity by electrical dental devices, *Oral Surg Oral Med Oral Pathol Oral Radiol Endod* 85:33, 1998.

36. Musselwhite JM, Klitzman B, Maixner W, Burkes EJ: Laser Doppler flowmetry: a clinical test of pulpal vitality, *Oral Surg Oral Med Oral Pathol Oral Radiol Endod* 84:411, 1997.

37. Myers J: Demonstration of a possible source of error with an electric pulp tester, *J Endod* 24:199, 1998.

38. Natkin E, Harrington GW, Mandel MA: Anginal pain referred to the teeth. Report of a case, *Oral Surg Oral Med Oral Pathol Oral Radiol Endod* 40:678, 1975.

39. Neaverth EJ, Kotler LM, Kaltenbach RF: Clinical investigation (In vitro) of endodontically treated maxillary first molars, *J Endod* 13:506, 1987.

40. Oikarinen K, Kopola H, Makiniemi M, Herrala E: Detection of pulse in oral mucosa and dental pulp by means of optical reflection method, *Endod Dent Traumatol* 12:54, 1996.

41. Okeson JP, Bell WE: *Bell's orofacial pains,* ed 5, St Louis, 1995, Mosby.

42. Peters DD, Baumgartner JC, Lorton L: Adult pulpal diagnosis. I. Evaluation of the positive and negative responses to cold and electrical pulp tests, *J Endod* 20:506, 1994.

43. Peters DD et al: Evaluation of the effects of carbon dioxide used as a pulpal test. I. In vitro effect on human enamel, *J Endod* 9:219, 1983.

44. Piazzini LF: Periodontal screening and recording (PSR) application in children and adolescent, *J Clin Pediatr Dent* 18:165, 1994.

45. Ramadan AE, Mitchell DF: A roentgenographic study of experimental bone destruction, *J Oral Surg* 15:934, 1962.

46. Ramsay DS, Artun J, Martinten SS: Reliability of pulpal blood-flow measurements utilizing laser Doppler flowmetry, *J Dent Res* 70:1427, 1991.

47. Rickoff B et al: Effects of thermal vitality tests on human dental pulp, *J Endod* 14:482, 1988.

48. Robertson A, Andreasen FM, Bergenholtz G, Andreasen JO, Noren JG: Incidence of pulp necrosis subsequent to pulp canal obliteration from trauma of permanent incisors, *J Endod* 22:557, 1996.

49. Roeykens H, Van Maele G, De Moor R, Martens L: Reliability of laser Doppler flowmetry in a 2-probe assessment of pulpal blood flow, *Oral Surg Oral Med Oral Pathol Oral Radiol Endod* 87:742, 1999.

50. Rowe AHR, Pitt-Ford TR: The assessment of pulp vitality, *Int Endod J* 23:77, 1990.

51. Rubach WE, Mitchell DF: Periodontal disease, age and pulp status, *J Oral Surg* 19:482, 1965.

52. Rugh JD: Psychological components of pain, *Dent Clin North Am* 31:579, 1987.

53. Schmitt JM, Webber RL, Walker EC: Optical determination of dental pulp vitality, *IEEE Trans Biomed Eng* 38:346, 1991.

54. Schnettler JM, Wallace JA: Pulse oximetry as a diagnostic tool of pulpal vitality, *J Endod* 17:488, 1991.

55. Schwartz SF, Foster JK: Roentgenographic interpretation of experimentally produced bony lesions (part 1), *J Oral Surg* 32:606, 1971.

56. Seltzer S, Bender IB, Ziontz M: The dynamics of pulp inflammation: correlations between diagnostic data and actual histologic findings in the pulp, *Oral Surg Oral Med Oral Pathol* 16:846, 1963.

57. Seltzer S: Classification of pulpal pathosis, *Oral Surg Oral Med Oral Pathol* 34:269, 1972.

58. Seltzer S: *Endodontology: biologic consideration in endodontic procedures,* ed 2, Philadelphia, 1988, Lea and Febiger.

59. Simon AB, Linde B, Bonnette GH, Schlentz RJ: The individual with a pacemaker in the dental environment, *J Am Dent Assn* 91:1224, 1975.

60. Smith GN, Walton RE: Periodontal ligament injection: distribution of injected solutions, *J Oral Surg* 55:232, 1983.

61. Colleagues for Excellence: Systematic endodontic diagnosis, endodontics, *Am Assoc Endod,* Winter 1996.

62. Walton RE, Torabinejad M: *Principles and practice of endodontics,* ed 3, Philadelphia, WB Saunders (in press).

63. Welander U, McDavid WD, Higgins NM, Morris CR: The effect of viewing conditions on the perceptibility of radiographic details, *Oral Surg Oral Med Oral Pathol Oral Radiol Endod* 56:651, 1983.

64. Willms JL, Schneiderman H, Algranati PS: *Physical diagnosis: bedside evaluation of diagnosis and function,* Baltimore, 1994, Williams and Wilkins.

65. Zachrisson BU, Jacobsen I: Long-term prognosis of 66 permanent anterior teeth with root fractures, *Scand J Dent Res* 83:345, 1975.

Chapter 2

Orofacial Dental Pain Emergencies: Endodontic Diagnoses and Management

A. Scott Cohen, David Clifford Brown

The duty of a Doctor:
   To cure sometimes
   To relieve often
   To care always
Above all, do no harm.

Chapter Outline

No area of dental practice has more potential to cause fear and discomfort for patients than the emergency visit for acute orofacial pain. Pain is the most common factor that motivates patients to seek dental treatment; therefore, the dentist is responsible for managing and diagnosing dental and other facial pain. This chapter describes the pathways leading to accurate and complete diagnosis, as well as the management of the endodontic emergency patient.

INCIDENCE OF PAIN

A large study was conducted to determine the reported incidence of orofacial pain[108]; it found that 21.8% of adults in the United States experienced orofacial pain symptoms within 6 months before the study. The most common pain was toothache, which was estimated to have occurred in 12.3% of the population. Because this survey was conducted on nonpatients within the entire population of the United States, it is clear that there are many people who avoid seeking treatment for the pain they are experiencing. The primary reason for avoiding dental treatment is fear.[39] Root canal treatment, in particular, is one of the most anxiety-producing procedures in dentistry.[49]

PAIN PATHWAYS

The Pain Phenomenon[173]

Current models of pain view it as a complex event. By its very nature, pain is no longer considered a single entity. Instead, it involves many overlapping components. "An unpleasant sensory and emotional experience associated with actual or potential tissue damage defines the physiologic and the psychologic components."[118]

Because of modulation and crossover in the central neural pathways, it may be difficult for patients to be objective when describing their pain. Modulation can intensify or suppress pain, giving it a multidimensional character. The pain process begins in the periphery, where specialized nerve fibers receive a painful stimulus. These nerve fibers transmit this information to the spinal cord and, ultimately, to the brain, where the information is interpreted and recognized as pain.

Detection of Pain

Odontogenic pain transmission is mediated primarily by peripheral sensory neurons of the trigeminal nerve. The peripheral terminals of these nerves innervate the dental pulp and other oral tissues, whereas the central terminals release neurotransmitters, such as substance P, which are involved in the initiation of pain. These trigeminal sensory afferent neurons, along with sympathetic branches of the superior cervical ganglion and blood vessels, enter through the apical foramen of a tooth. Together, these nerves and blood vessels form the neurovascular bundle.

There are myelinated and unmyelinated nerve fibers within the nerve bundles. The myelinated fibers, called A fibers, are grouped according to their diameter and conduction velocities. Predominantly, A fibers innervate the dentin.[6] The unmyelinated fibers, known as C fibers, innervate the body of the pulp and its blood vessels. Differences between the two sensory fibers enable the patient to discriminate and characterize the quality, intensity, and duration of the pain response.

The A and C fibers of the dental pulp are nociceptors; they perceive noxious stimuli. Some A-delta and C fibers function as nociceptive mechanoreceptors that warn of tissue damage, whereas others are polymodal, with a wide, dynamic range. Polymoydal receptors respond to mechanical, thermal, and chemical stimuli,[25] and they interact with the autonomic nervous system.

According to the specificity theory of pain, nociceptors are specialized neurons that are responsible for the detection of pain. Alternatively, the pattern theory proposes that pain results from stimulation of multiple classes of sensory neurons, not necessarily from the stimulation of nociceptors. The effect of this stimulation is to disinhibit, or unmask, ascending polymodal nociceptive channels.[34] According to this theory, noxious stimuli may not be necessary for the perception of pain. The pattern of the stimulus creates a pain sensation, rather than a pathologic entity. This mechanism may be one explanation for chronic pain, because innocuous stimuli can be perceived as painful.

A-Delta Nerve Fibers

Most of the myelinated nerve fibers of the pulp are A-delta fibers. They are referred to as nociceptive fibers because the threat of tissue damage is the most effective stimulus.[25] A-delta fibers are relatively large fibers, with fast-conduction velocities. They enter the root canal and divide into smaller branches, coursing coronally through the pulp. Once beneath the odontoblastic layer, the A-delta fibers lose their myelin sheath and anastomose into a network of nerves referred to as the plexus of Raschkow. This circumpulpal layer of nerves sends free nerve endings onto and through the odontoblastic cell layer, extending up to 200 μm into the dentinal tubules while also contacting the odontoblastic cell processes.[23] The intimate association of A-delta fibers with the odontoblastic cell layer and dentin is referred to as the pulpodentinal complex. Researchers have found that sensory innervation occurs only in dentinal tubules with viable odontoblasts, and that odontoblasts maintain their structural integrity only in innervated regions of a tooth.[25]

Disturbances of the pulpodentinal complex in a vital tooth initially affect the low-threshold A-delta fibers. Drilling, probing, drying with air, and application of hyperosmotic solutions to exposed dentin will cause pain. Movement of fluid in the dentinal tubules, known as the hydrodynamic theory of dentin sensitivity, stimulates the A-delta fibers.[20] The vital pulp responds immediately with symptoms of dentinal pain. Application of some hyperosmotic agents to dentin does not cause pain unless they are placed in a deep-cavity preparation. This finding supports an additional mechanism of dentin sensitivity, the direct ionic diffusion theory.[95]

Not all stimuli will reach the excitation threshold and generate a pain response. Irritants, such as incipient dental caries and mild periodontal disease, are seldom painful. However, they can be sufficiently irritating to stimulate the defensive formation of sclerotic or reparative dentin. The fact that a pulp can become necrotic in the complete absence of pain indicates that there are peripheral and central mechanisms that may control nociceptor sensitization and activation.

A-delta fiber pain must be provoked. Nociceptive signals, transmitted through fast-conducting myelinated pathways, are immediately perceived as a quick, sharp, momentary pain. The sensation dissipates quickly upon removal of the inciting stimulus, such as drinking cold liquids or probing exposed dentin. The clinical symptoms of A-delta fiber pain signify that the pulpodentinal complex is intact and capable of responding to an external disturbance.

A-Beta Nerve Fibers

A-beta nerve fibers are among the fastest conducting fibers of all intradental nerves. They may function as mechanoreceptors that trigger withdrawal reflexes so that potentially damaging forces may be avoided.[25] Intense cooling, serotonin, and hydrodynamic changes can also stimulate A-beta fibers. Although studies[91,131] suggest that they are capable of detecting prepain and pain, the role of A-beta fibers is not clearly understood. However, future research should clarify their purpose.

C Nerve Fibers

C fibers are small, unmyelinated nerves that innervate the pulp. They are high-threshold fibers, course centrally in the pulp stroma, and run subjacent to the A-delta fibers. Unlike A-delta fibers, C fibers are not directly involved with the pulpodentinal complex and are less easily provoked. The pain associated with C fibers is dull and poorly localized. In most cases, it occurs later, as a secondary pain. C fibers have a high threshold and can be activated by intense heating or cooling of the tooth crown or mechanical stimulation of the pulp. The receptive fields for these nerve fibers are exclusively in the pulp proper. Once activated, the pain initiated by C fibers can radiate to anywhere in the ipsilateral face and jaws.

C fiber pain is associated with tissue injury and is modulated by inflammatory mediators, vascular changes in blood volume and blood flow, and increases in tissue pressure. Stimulated C fibers are capable of releasing inflammatory modulating neuropeptides, such as calcitonin gene-related peptide (CGRP) and substance P. These neuropeptides enhance the inflammatory response by stimulating the release of histamine and arachidonic acid metabolites.[202]

When inflammation leads to pulp necrosis, a periradicular lesion may develop as an extension of the pulpal pathology. Even when a radiographic lesion is clearly visible, some nerve fibers may respond to vitality testing.[103,105] Both myelinated and unmyelinated nerves have been found in teeth with necrotic pulps and a periapical lesion.[104] For this reason, instrumentation of teeth with necrotic pulps may cause pain. Because C fibers are more resistant than A-delta fibers to compromised blood flow and hypoxic conditions, pain associated with a necrotic pulp is more likely to be caused by C fiber stimulation.

Processing[137]

Pain is perceived and recognized in the cortex because of incoming nociceptive (i.e., noxious stimulus) input. In most cases the input from the pulpal and periradicular tissues is transmitted through the maxillary or mandibular branches of the trigeminal nerve toward the central nervous system (CNS) for processing. The primary afferent neuron enters the brain stem at the level of the pons. The cell bodies of the trigeminal nerve are located in the Gasserian ganglion; the primary neuron synapses with a second-order neuron in the subnucleus caudalis region of the trigeminal spinal tract nucleus. The trigeminal spinal tract nucleus also receives input from the IX and X cranial nerves, as well as the upper cervical nerves. Once the second-order neuron receives the input, it is carried to the thalamus. The second-order neuron crosses the brain stem to the opposite side of the brain and ascends to the higher centers.

A-delta fibers from the pulp synapse in the lamina I area of the subnucleus caudalis, and C fibers synapse in the lamina II and III areas. A-delta neurons pass to the thalamus directly, by way of the neospinothalamic tract. The pathway ascends to the thalamus directly and is said to carry *fast pain*. The second-order C-fiber neuron carries impulses via the paleospinothalamic tract. This passes through the reticular formation, where the impulses are influenced by many modulating interneurons before they reach the thalamus. Because the impulses take longer to reach the thalamus, this type of pain is called *slow pain*. Fast pain tends to be sharp and easy to localize; slow pain tends to be dull and aching.

Once the nociceptive input reaches the higher centers of the brain, there are further interactions of neurons between the thalamus, cortex, and the limbic system. The CNS has the ability to control or modulate the pain-transmitting neurons. Several areas of the cortex and brain stem have been identified that can either enhance or reduce nociceptive input arriving by way of the transmitting neurons. When the impulses reach the sensory cortex, pain recognition occurs. The cortex may rely on memory for assistance in evaluating the sensation. It is at this point that previous experiences of toothache or suffering associated with past dental treatment begin to give meaning to the sensation.

The trigeminal system is not the only pathway responsible for transmission of painful sensations from the pulpal and periapical tissues. The seventh, ninth, and tenth cranial nerves and the first, second, and third cervical spinal nerves also innervate the oral region. It has been established that sympathetic afferent nerves, as well as some parasympathetic afferent nerves, mediate pain.[135] Sympathetic and parasympathetic fibers have been demonstrated in pulpal tissue. There are many afferent fibers in the trigeminal motor root, and motor nerves should be included among nociceptive pathways.

Perception

The final process involved in the subjective experience of pain is perception. When nociceptive input reaches the cortex, perception occurs. It is at this point that suffering may occur. Suffering refers to the manner in which the patient responds to pain. The different ways that individuals respond to pain is a common and dramatic clinical observation.[45] Patients may show very little evidence of clinical disease but seem to suffer intolerable, incapacitating pain. Others, with serious pathosis, may continue to function at a normal level and not feel ill or at risk.[153]

Factors, such as attention drawn to the pain, past dental experience, and expectation of treatment, determine to what extent the patient will suffer. Emotional factors, particularly anxiety, can decrease the pain threshold and heighten the patient's reaction to the pain.[214] Distraction has a particularly inhibitory effect on pain, as demonstrated by mental absorption and physical activities of different kinds. This may explain why toothache appears to worsen at night, when the patient is in bed and not preoccupied with daily events.

What individuals think about their pain involves the cognitive process. Cognition is implicated in virtually every aspect of the pain experience.[153] What patients understand about their pain is important in modulating how they react to it, and this understanding facilitates pain management. Patients who are told that a palatal swelling is from a pulpal disorder and not life threatening will react differently to the condition than uninformed patients. Prior experience with successful or unsuccessful treatment influences patient behavior. Reassurance that the dentist can treat and eliminate acute dental pain decreases anxiety. Personality and cultural factors are additional learned behaviors that can modify a patient's response to pain and, therefore, should be considered in pain management.

Pain behavior is the only communication the clinician receives regarding the pain experience, and it varies from patient to patient. It is important for the clinician to recognize that the information related to the dentist by the patient is not nociception, pain, or even suffering. The patient only relates pain behavior. Yet, it is through this communication that the clinician must gain insight into the patient's problem. For the clinician, managing patient pain disorders is not always an easy task.

Orofacial pain can generate unreasonable anxiety in a fearful patient. Speaking to the patient in a calm, knowledgeable manner, in words the patient can understand, significantly builds patient confidence. Providing information about typical procedures and sensations—sights, sounds, smells, vibrations, and other physical stimuli—is an invaluable management tool that removes much of the patient's uncertainty about the planned treatment.[81]

How patients perceive their control over pain is another important cognition. Often increased tolerance for potentially painful procedures can be seen when the dentist affords the patient a means to stop the procedure. Patients given control over what happens during procedures that may involve pain feel more comfortable and show a higher tolerance for these procedures.[33]

PHYSIOLOGY OF PULPAL PAIN [95,201]

Hyperalgesia and Allodynia[72]

Three characteristics define hyperalgesia: (1) spontaneous pain, (2) a decreased pain threshold (i.e., allodynia), and (3) an increased response to painful stimuli. The symptoms of hyperalgesia are frequently encountered in dental patients. Spontaneous pain usually indicates the presence of irreversible pulpitis or pulpal necrosis. The pulpal and periradicular tissues may have become sensitized during the inflammatory process, leading to a state of allodynia in which innocuous stimuli are perceived as painful.

Because of allodynia, spontaneous pain can arise from a reduced thermal threshold, causing pulpal nociceptors to be activated by the body temperature. Patients may describe sensitivity to heat and relief from cold, and they may sip a large cup of ice water to reduce discomfort. Some patients complain of a throbbing, pulsating pain, which is probably caused by a reduced threshold of mechanoreceptors that increases sensitivity to the point where the arterial pressure wave of the heartbeat stimulates perivascular nociceptors in the pulp.[72] Like pulpal nociceptors, periodontal mechanoreceptors acquire lower thresholds and increased firing frequencies. Therefore performing diagnostic tests, such as percussion and palpation, in the presence of allodynia can create painful responses. Similarly, performing pulp sensitivity tests can produce painful responses, because the pulpal nociceptors are sensitized.

These signs and symptoms indicate that the pulpal and/or periradicular tissues are in a state of hyperalgesia. A combination of neuroinflammatory mechanisms can induce hyperalgesia, some occurring at the site of inflammation and others occurring in the CNS.

Inflammatory Cycle

To set the stage for repair of inflamed tissues, activated pulpal defenses must be able to remove irritants hemodynamically and moderate the inflammatory process. Ideally, the inflammatory cycles of vascular stasis, capillary permeability, and chemotactic migration of leucocytes to injured tissues are synchronized with the removal of irritants and drainage of exudate from the area. With moderate to severe injury, an aberrant increase in capillary pressure can lead to excessive permeability and fluid accumulation. A progressive pressure front builds and begins to passively compress and collapse all local venules and lymphatic channels,[205] outpacing the capacity of the pulp to drain or shunt the exudate.[94,95] Blood flow to the area ceases, and the injured tissue undergoes necrosis. Leukocytes in the area degenerate and release intracellular lysosomal enzymes, forming a microabscess.

Inflammatory Mediators

Inflammatory mediators, such as histamine, bradykinin, prostaglandins, serotonin, substance P, CGRP, and leukotrienes, can cause pain directly by activating or sensitizing pulpal nociceptors.[95,190] They also cause pain indirectly by initiating a series of inflammatory events that result in increased vascular permeability, edema, and, ultimately, increased intrapulpal pressure.[202] Some mediators are short lived, but they are constantly replaced through the newly extravasated plasma.[71] The renewed presence of mediators sustains the inflammatory process beyond the initial traumatic event. Fluid leakage diminishes blood flow and results in vascular stasis. Platelets aggregated in the vessels release the neurochemical serotonin, which is leaked, along with plasma, into the interstitial tissues.[36] Serotonin and the other inflammatory mediators induce a state of hyperalgesia in the pulpal nociceptors.

The altered tissue conditions sensitize acute nociceptive activity and then activate an initially silent group of polymodal nociceptors. Nerve fibers that are activated by inflammation are termed silent, or sleeping, nociceptors.[25] Acute nociceptors respond as soon as a stimulus reaches threshold levels, whereas silent nociceptors are not activated until inflammation has been well established. Inflammatory mediators sensitize both types of nociceptors. When the dental pulp becomes inflamed, there is a significantly higher proportion of A-delta fibers responding to dentinal stimulation than in uninflamed pulps.[25] Additionally, the receptive fields (i.e., the size of the area where a stimulus activates a nerve fiber) become larger in inflamed pulps. This may be because of nerve sprouting or activation, or it may be because of sensitization of silent nociceptors.

When tissue becomes inflamed, the polymodal nociceptive fibers initiate and enhance this process by neurogenic inflammation. Substance P and calcitonin gene-related peptide (CGRP) can each contribute to the inflammatory process,[22] and research has shown that their vascular responses are potentiated with coadministration.[61] At the local level, neuropeptides stimulate the release of histamine, which refuels the vascular inflammatory cycle. The sustained inflammatory cycle is detrimental to pulpal recovery, terminating in necrosis of the tissues.

Central Mechanisms of Hyperalgesia and Allodynia

Sensitization of neurons can also occur within the CNS. Second-order neurons can be changed or sensitized when they receive a constant barrage of nociceptive input. Included in the list of receptors involved in this sensitization are the N-methyl-D aspartic acid (NMDA) receptors. Stimulation of these receptors by excitatory amino acids increases the sensitization of these neurons. Generally the changes are reversible, however, chronic sensitization may result in permanent changes to neuroprocessing. Permanent alterations may lead to chronic neuropathic pains. As central sensitization occurs, even normal input can be perceived as pain. Input carried by A-beta fibers, which do not mediate pain in most cases, can divert to nociceptive transmission. When this occurs, stimuli (e.g., a light touch to the tissues surrounding a symptomatic tooth) may be perceived as pain.

ODONTOGENIC PAIN

Odontogenic pain arises from the pulp and/or the periradicular tissues. These structures are functionally and embryologically distinct, and pain originating from each of them is perceived differently.

Pulpal Pain

There are two types of pulpal diagnoses: (1) those based on clinical findings and (2) those based on histologic findings. The aim of clinical diagnosis is to use relevant clinical information to establish which tooth is responsible for the symptoms, and to make an educated decision regarding the likely histologic condition of the dental pulp. *Clinical signs, symptoms and diagnostic tests do not, in many cases, correlate with the true histopathologic status of the pulp.*[169] One reason for this discrepancy is that pulpal and periapical inflammation is asymptomatic in many cases. When symptoms are present, the clinician can only speculate about the histopathologic condition of the pulp. Clinically, the pulp can be diagnosed as healthy; damaged but able to repair itself after removal of the irritant (reversible pulpitis) or damaged beyond repair (either irreversible pulpitis or necrosis). Histologically, pulpitis is described as acute, chronic, or hyperplastic.

Healthy Pulp   The healthy pulp is vital and free of inflammation. It is stimulated by cold and hot sensitivity testing, responding with mild pain that lasts for no more than 1 to 2 seconds after the stimulus is removed. Mainly, myelinated (A-delta) and unmyelinated (C fibers) afferent nerve fibers control the sensibility of the dental pulp. Operating under different pathophysiologic capabilities, both sensory nerve fibers conduct nociceptive input to the brain. Differences between the two sensory fibers enable the patient to discriminate and characterize the quality, intensity, and duration of the pain response.

Normally dentin is sensitive when exposed to irritants. The clinical symptoms of A-delta fiber pain serve to signify that the pulpodentinal complex is intact and capable of responding to an external disturbance. This is a *normal response of the vital pulp*. Many dentists have made the mistake of interpreting this symptom of dentinal pain as an indication of reversible pulpitis. However, they are not mutually exclusive. Thus dentinal sensitivity or pain should be distinguished from pulpal inflammation.

Dentin Hypersensitivity

The term dentin hypersensitivity has been used to describe a specific condition that is defined as pain arising from exposed dentin. Typically this pain is in response to thermal, chemical, tactile, or osmotic stimuli and is not caused by any other dental defect or pathology. The pain is consistent with an exaggerated response of the normal pulpodentinal complex, and it is severe and sharp on application of the stimulus to the exposed dentin. However, there is no lingering discomfort once the stimulus is removed.

Dentin hypersensitivity is probably a symptom complex, rather than a true disease; it results from stimulus transmission across exposed dentin. Although the precise mechanisms for dentin sensitivity are not known, the hydrodynamic mechanism, as postulated by Brännström,[18] is the theory that is most commonly cited.[200] In this mechanism sudden movements of fluid in the dentinal tubules are believed to deform mechanosensitive nerve fibers at the pulp-dentin interface. Consequently, the nerve endings fire, causing brief, localized, sharp pain.

Scanning electron microscopic studies show that hypersensitive dentin has more than seven times the number of surface tubules than insensitive dentin.[2] Although dentinal tubules of insensitive teeth are occluded, the apertures of the dentinal tubules in hypersensitive dentin are open, or widened.[139] Dye penetration studies indicate that the open tubules are patent to the pulp,[3] and as a result, bacteria or their toxic products can penetrate the dentin, causing inflammation.[16]

When symptoms are associated with exposed dentin, the diagnosis is dentin hypersensitivity. However, when there is a specific etiologic factor causing the sensitivity, such as caries, fractures, leaking restorations, or recent restorative treatment, teeth with vital pulps may exhibit symptoms that are identical to dentin hypersensitivity. When symptoms develop in these situations, a diagnosis of reversible pulpitis is appropriate. Thus a careful history, together with a clinical and radiographic examination, is necessary to conclude a definitive diagnosis of dentin hypersensitivity. The definitive diagnosis is more difficult when clinical causes of reversible pulpitis are present in combination with exposed dentin.

Reversible Pulpitis

An external irritant of significant magnitude or duration injures the pulp. Although a localized injury initiates tissue inflammation, the nature and extent of pulp injury and the dynamics of the inflammatory response will determine whether the process can be confined and the tissues repaired to restore pulpal homeostasis. Reversible pulpitis implies that from the clinical signs, symptoms, and diagnostic tests, the pulp is vital and inflamed but possesses the reparative capabilities to return to health on removal of the irritant. Emergency treatment of reversible pulpitis is discussed later in the chapter.

Differentiation between a normal pulp and a reversibly inflamed pulp can be difficult. For example, dental caries, microleakage of restorations, recession of the attachment apparatus, erosion of cervical tooth structure, as well as periodontal diseases and procedures can cause dentin hypersensitivity.[170] However, an assessment of pain intensity perceived at the time of stimulation, dental history, and a thorough dental examination allow the clinician to differentiate among the normal pulp, dentin hypersensitivity, and the reversibly inflamed pulp.

Pulpal pain is common after restorative treatment. Procedures, such as cavity and crown preparations, can make teeth feel especially sensitive. Damage to the pulp is caused by heat generation, pressure, dentin desiccation, toxic components of the restorative materials, and, especially, marginal leakage with bacterial colonization of the dentin-restoration interface. Often the histologic response to caries or a restoration is chronic inflammation. When a new operative procedure is performed on such teeth, the ensuing pain is, in most cases, related to an acute exacerbation of a previously existing, asymptomatic chronic pulpitis.

After insertion of amalgam restorations, teeth may be sensitive to thermal stimuli for several weeks. Initial contraction of the amalgam occurs after insertion, and it results in the formation of a 10 μm to 15 μm gap between the restoration and the dentin. Fluid in the gap may support the growth of bacteria, and dentin hypersensitivity and pain may result from the induced pulpitis. The application of cold stimuli may elicit pain, owing to contraction of the dentinal fluid in the gap. This rapid movement of fluid in the dentinal tubules stimulates nerve fibers in the pulp. This cold sensitivity often disappears after a few weeks, as amalgam corrosion products fill the gap[115] and plasma proteins and cell remnants from the pulp occlude the dentinal tubules. Reparative dentin formation occurs concurrently with the pulpal inflammatory response and tends to seal the dentinal tubules at the pulpal end.

Corrosion accelerates when an amalgam restoration encounters another object made of a different metal, such as a gold crown. The resulting galvanic currents run through the metals, as well as the dental pulp and the gingiva, leading to hypersensitivity and pain. As surface films are formed, the symptoms often abate in a relatively short time.

The use of composite resins can reduce, but not prevent, microleakage. Composite restorations may cause postoperative biting sensitivity after placement. In most cases, these symptoms may be caused by dentinal fluid movement in response to loading. Researchers have found that this fluid movement is greater than that which occurs in amalgam-filled teeth or unoperated controls.[79] The fluid supports the growth of microorganisms that may be left in the dentinal tubules, as well as that of any new microorganisms that penetrate the dentin through the dentin-restoration interface. The ensuing pulp inflammation results in hypersensitivity.

It has been demonstrated[24] that, after mild pulpal injury resulting from shallow cavity preparation, there is a rapid and extensive sprouting of new CGRP nerve fibers and substance P nerve fibers in the pulp. These newly developed fibers usually disappear within a few weeks. Postoperative pain immediately after cavity preparation might be caused by hydrodynamic stimulation of this increased density of neurons.

Irreversible Pulpitis   The pulp is enclosed in a rigid, mineralized environment and has a very limited ability to increase its volume during episodes of inflammation. In this low-compliance environment, an intense inflammatory response can lead to adverse increases in tissue pressure, outpacing the pulp's compensatory mechanisms to reduce it. The inflammatory process spreads circumferentially and incrementally through the pulp, perpetuating the destructive cycle.[205]

With provocation, an injured vital pulp with established local inflammation can emit symptoms of A-delta fiber pain. In the presence of inflammation, the response is exaggerated and out of character with the challenging stimulus, which is often thermal. Inflammatory mediators induce this type of hyperalgesia, and *one of the classic symptoms of irreversible pulpitis is lingering pain from thermal stimuli*. As the exaggerated A-delta fiber pain subsides, a dull, throbbing ache may persist. This second pain symptom signifies the inflammatory involvement of nociceptive C nerve fibers.

With increasing inflammation of pulp tissues, C fiber pain becomes the only pain feature. Pain that may begin as a short, lingering discomfort can escalate to an intensely prolonged episode or a constant, diffuse, throbbing pain. *Spontaneous (unprovoked) pain is another hallmark of irreversible pulpitis*. If the pulpal pain is prolonged and intense, central excitatory effects may produce pain referral to a distant site or to other teeth. When C fiber pain dominates A-delta fiber pain, pain is more diffuse and the dentist's ability to identify the offending tooth, through provocation, is reduced. Often clinicians have found[121] that pulps afflicted with irreversible pulpitis without periradicular pathosis are the most difficult to diagnose. If the periradicular proprioceptive nerve fibers are not inflamed, then the tooth will not be tender to percussion and the symptoms may be difficult to localize.

Occasionally the inflamed vasculature is responsive to cold, which vasoconstricts the dilated vessels and reduces tissue pressure. Momentary relief from the intense pain is provided; this explains why some patients bring a container of ice water to the emergency appointment. Relief provided by a cold stimulus is diagnostic and indicates that a vital irreversibly inflamed pulp is becoming increasingly necrotic. In the absence of endodontic intervention, the rapidly deteriorating condition will most likely progress to an acute periradicular abscess.[95]

C fiber pain is an ominous symptom that signifies that irreversible local-tissue damage has occurred. *Irreversible pulpitis is a clinical term that implies that the inflamed, vital pulp lacks the reparative ability to return to health*. The treatment indicated is either root canal treatment or tooth extraction.

Pulpal Necrosis   There are no true symptoms of pulpal necrosis, because the pulpal sensory nerves have been destroyed. (As described in Chapter 1, the pulp is nonvital.) However, pain may arise from the periradicular tissues that may be inflamed because of pulpal degeneration. Necrosis may be complete or partial, in which case various symptoms are present. This can be confusing, because of the presence of some remaining vital tissue in a portion of the root canal system. This condition is most common in multirooted teeth. In most cases there is no response to thermal or electric pulp sensitivity testing, however, a vital response is sometimes encountered. Radiographs may show no abnormalities, a widened periodontal ligament, or a periradicular radiolucency. Because of the potential for erroneous vitality responses, corroborating thermal tests and radiographs are necessary for a definitive diagnosis.

Periradicular Pain

Extension of pulpal disease into the surrounding periradicular tissues is the most common cause of periradicular pain. Proprioceptors of the periodontal ligament are capable of precise localization of pressure stimuli. Therefore pain of periradicular origin usually presents little diagnostic challenge, because the offending tooth is readily identified. Periradicular pain of endodontic origin may be associated with acute apical periodontitis or acute periradicular abscess.

Acute Apical Periodontitis   In most cases, acute apical periodontitis arises as a sequel to irreversible pulpitis, or it arises after endodontic treatment. The inflammatory process leading to irreversible pulpitis may extend into the periradicular tissues, resulting in a localized inflammation of the periodontal ligament. When the transition of pulpal inflammation to periradicular inflammation is rapid, the patients' pain experience is severe because of the simultaneous occurrence of irreversible pulpitis and acute apical periodontitis. The patient complains of symptoms consistent with irreversible pulpitis, and the tooth is extremely painful to touch, with a dull, constant, throbbing pain. Often the cause of acute apical periodontitis is obvious, and the symptoms are readily explained.

Radiographically a tooth with acute apical periodontitis may have deep, untreated caries, an extensive restoration, or a previous pulp cap. However, there may be no radiographic changes at the root apex or just a slight widening of the periodontal ligament. It must be understood that it is possible to have a periapical radiolucency associated with a tooth with irreversible pulpitis and simultaneous acute apical periodontitis.[105]

In most cases postoperative pain following endodontic treatment is caused by acute apical periodontitis. Root canal instrumentation, beyond the apex or extrusion of debris from the root canal into the periapical tissues, can produce an acute inflammatory reaction. In these situations the clinical differentiation between an acute apical periodontitis and a developing acute periradicular abscess is difficult.

Acute apical periodontitis may also occur because of traumatic occlusion, occlusal overloading, bruxism, orthodontic treatment, or a sinusitis. Other causes include a spreading inflammatory reaction incidental to nearby trauma or the healing of surgical wounds. Because there are many possible causes, it is imperative to perform vitality pulp testing to determine the cause of the problem and the best course of treatment.

Chronic apical periodontitis is asymptomatic; a periradicular radiolucency is the radiographic finding, and the pulp is necrotic. The patient may report a history of symptoms consistent with a previous irreversible pulpitis or acute periradicular abscess. Periodically the tooth may become sensitive to pressure and feel "different." Root canal treatment will usually result in resolution of chronic apical periodontitis. However, the chronic condition can "flare-up" as an acute periradicular abscess after initiation of root canal treatment (i.e., phoenix abscess). Because chronic apical periodontitis is not considered an emergency, it should be treated at a convenient time.

Acute Periradicular Abscess

Extension of pulpal disease into the surrounding periapical tissues may result in periapical infection. The acute periradicular abscess is an inflammatory reaction to pulpal infection and necrosis, characterized by rapid onset, spontaneous pain, tenderness of the tooth to pressure, pus formation, and eventual swelling of associated tissues.[7] The abscess may develop from a pulp that undergoes rapid degeneration from pulpitis to necrosis, with spread of infection into the periradicular tissues. Alternatively, it may arise as an exacerbation of a chronic apical periodontitis (i.e., phoenix abscess). Although the pulp is necrotic and not sensitive to thermal testing, the initial pain from an acute periradicular abscess can be intense. As bone resorption occurs, purulent drainage enters the surrounding tissue spaces and swelling occurs. However, as the intrabony pressure is reduced, the pain may subside slightly.

The location of any swelling is dependent on the orientation of the root apex and the relationship of the site of perforation of the cortical plate to muscle attachments on the maxilla or mandible.[99] Most commonly, drainage occurs to the buccal aspect of the tooth into the oral cavity, and drainage from the maxillary lateral incisor and maxillary molar teeth occurs to the palatal aspect. A complication is spread from maxillary and mandibular molars via the pterygoid venous plexus, causing a cavernous sinus thrombophlebitis and impairment of cerebral vascular drainage.[101] The most serious spread of infection from mandibular premolar or molar teeth is lingually, beneath mylohyoid muscle and into the

retropharyngeal space. Ludwig's angina is a bilateral retropharyngeal spread, from mandibular posterior teeth, that results in airway obstruction. An acute periradicular abscess associated with a mandibular premolar or molar may result in paraesthesia of the mental or inferior alveolar nerve. This is a result of the pressure from the abscess encroaching on the neurovascular tissues.[125]

Radiographically there may be no detectable lesion, a widened periodontal ligament, or an apical radiolucency (depending on the amount of bone destruction, the location of the root apex in the alveolar bone, and whether the abscess developed from chronic apical periodontitis or a pulp that has rapidly degenerated). On occasion there may be an acute periradicular abscess (with swelling) that shows no radiographic change. This is consistent with drainage into soft tissues through a fenestration in the cortical plate.

If the swelling associated with an acute periradicular abscess begins to drain through an intraoral or extraoral sinus tract, the painful symptoms will diminish as the pus discharges. Thus the acute periradicular abscess may subside into a suppurating chronic apical periodontitis.

Periodontal Abscess

The acute periodontal abscess is an inflammatory reaction originating in the periodontium. It is usually characterized by rapid onset, spontaneous pain, tenderness of the tooth to pressure, pus formation, and swelling. Frequently it is caused by foreign-body entrapment and associated with a tooth with a vital pulp.[7] The abscess develops from an infection of an existing periodontal pocket, or it develops as an apical extension of infection from a gingival pocket. The pain of a periodontal abscess is similar in nature to that of an acute periradicular abscess. However, it is often not as severe. A deep periodontal pocket is usually associated with the tooth, and localized swelling is often present.

The differentiation between an acute periradicular abscess and a periodontal abscess is established by confirming the status of the pulp. The pulp is always necrotic in the acute periradicular abscess and vital in the periodontal abscess. The differentiation between the two entities becomes more difficult if root canal treatment has been performed on the tooth previously. Researchers have found that the percentage of spirochetes in a periodontal abscess is greater than three times that seen in an endodontic abscess. They suggested a dark-field microscopic technique to detect these microbes and to aid differentiation of the two entities.[198] This technique is difficult, so careful clinical and radiographic examination must be used for diagnosis.

Referred Pain

Pain may be referred from teeth to other orofacial structures, or it may be referred from distant anatomic sites to teeth. Acute odontogenic pain often has a component that is felt in one or more adjacent teeth of the same arch, in teeth of the opposite arch, or in both locations. Clinically, it is rare for pain from pulpally involved teeth to be referred across the midline, except when the site of primary pain is located close to the midline. Referred odontogenic pain is most commonly associated with irreversible pulpitis, and it is frequently felt as a headache. The variable, spontaneous, unlocalized, and pulsatile qualities of the pain associated with irreversible pulpitis, together with its referral patterns, can imitate almost every pain disorder of the face and head.

NONODONTOGENIC PAIN

Toothaches can present a diagnostic problem for the clinician because pain felt in one tooth may be referred from another tooth or from other orofacial structures. To treat the "toothache" effectively, the clinician must first determine if the pain is truly odontogenic in origin. If it is not, the clinician is faced with the challenge of determining the true origin of the pain. It is up to the dentist to understand the mechanisms of pain, clinical characteristics of various categories of pain, the points of differentiation by which different types of pain are identified, the behavior characteristics of odontogenic pain, and the cardinal warning signs displayed by toothaches of nonodontogenic origin.

With a thorough knowledge of these painful conditions, the dentist is able to undertake the task of deliberate and selective elimination of nonessential pain characteristics. Through this process, the predominant pathognomonic pain patterns are identified, and a definitive diagnosis is achieved. Care must be taken that definitive dental treatment is not initiated until all doubt has been resolved as to the origin and cause of pain.

There are many conditions that mimic endodontic symptoms.[137] The most common nonodontogenic conditions that may be seen for urgent care will be reviewed briefly, with an emphasis on diagnosis. The discussion contrasts pain features that may imitate acute endodontic symptoms. However, there are distinct clinical features that will characterize the condition as nonodontogenic. (A thorough review of the causes and management of nonodontogenic pain entities is found in Chapter 3.)

Toothache of Neurovascular Origin

Toothache of neurovascular origin includes a group of pain disorders that have common mechanisms involving the trigeminal neurovascular system.[137] The most common type of pain is a migraine headache. Migraine pain can be referred to the teeth. However, because the toothache occurs in conjunction with one of the common forms of neurovascular headaches (e.g., migraine with aura, cluster headache, chronic paroxysmal hemicrania), diagnosis is rarely a problem. Importantly, the toothache subsides when the headache symptoms subside.

Some migraine variants are more of a diagnostic problem. For example, neurovascular variants, or migrainous neuralgias, can produce toothache without the traditional headache complaint. The pain of a neurovascular toothache is similar to that of irreversible pulpitis: spontaneous, variable, and throbbing. However, the neurovascular toothache is characterized by periods of remission and exacerbations over months or years, and there is a lack of reasonable dental cause for the pain.

Toothache of Neuropathic Origin

Pain from abnormal neural structures may present as a toothache. These pains may be either episodic or continuous. The clinician may begin to suspect one of the following conditions when, during the gathering of the dental history, the patient uses words not associated with odontogenic pathology (e.g., burning, electriclike, tingling).

Episodic Neuropathic Toothaches   A spontaneous, severe, sudden, sharp, lancinating, electrical shock pain that is felt in the tooth or radiates to a tooth characterizes episodic neuropathic toothache. The pain lasts for seconds to minutes, and then it disappears. It is consistent with trigeminal neuralgia (i.e., tic douloureux), which occurs between the fifth and eighth decade of life and causes distress for the patient.[42] Attacks of pain are confined to one side and involve one division of the nerve (although bilateral successive involvements have occurred).[145] The most prominent feature of episodic neuropathic toothache is the existence of trigger points. These areas are often located in the skin of the lips, cheeks, or gingiva. When touched, they provoke a painful response. Nevertheless, the possibility that these symptoms are being triggered by pulpal pathosis (instead of trigeminal neuralgia) must be ruled out.[145]

Attacks come in a series and can end abruptly. The period of remission is also free from the thermal and periapical sequelae seen with genuine endodontic pathosis. With each episode of pain, the patient learns to avoid the cutaneous or intraoral site that sets off the painful attack. Some patients are able to identify and describe vague prodromata of tingling just before an attack. Unfortunately, anesthetic blocking arrests the paroxysms of pain, which may lead to a mistaken diagnosis of odontogenic pain.[100] The cause of trigeminal neuralgia is still uncertain; the condition has been proposed to be viral in origin, secondary to stroke or cerebral tumor[52] or caused by dental trauma. A cause-and-effect relationship between advancing age and demyelination of the nerve may prove to be the most promising explanation.[159] Carbamazepine (Tegretol) is recommended as a first-line drug in the diagnosis and treatment of the condition, and it provides excellent initial results.[100]

Continuous Neuropathic Toothache   Some neuropathic toothaches produce a persistent, ongoing unremitting pain. These pains may be exacerbated by local provocation, such as percussion of the tooth or touching the surrounding gingiva, which adds confusion to the diagnosis. The neuropathic conditions that can produce continuous toothaches are neuritic pains (i.e., neuritis), deafferention pains, or sympathetically maintained pains.

Neuritic pains that arise in the maxillary and mandibular divisions of the trigeminal nerve can cause dental pains. Neuritic pains result from a spread of inflammation from surrounding structures to neural structures. The pain is often continuous, aching, and burning in nature.

Occasionally neuropathic pain may arise after dental treatment, such as a simple restoration, pulp extirpation, apicoectomy, or extraction. These conditions may appear as a *phantom toothache,* described by the term *atypical odontalgia.* This term is derived from the broad category of "atypical facial pain," which has served as a wastebasket diagnosis for any pain the clinician is unable to diagnose.

Atypical odontalgia Atypical odontalgia has been referred to as toothache with no obvious organic cause[148] and is characterized by prolonged periods of throbbing or burning pain in the teeth or alveolar process that occurs in the absence of any identifiable odontogenic cause. Usually the pain has been present for several months or longer, and repeated attempts at dental therapy have failed to resolve the pain. Commonly the patient has had multiple endodontic procedures, periapical surgical procedures, and even extractions, yet the pain persists in other teeth or the jaw.[102] Most commonly this condition affects middle-aged Caucasian women, and the maxillary canine and premolars are involved.

Although the pathophysiology of atypical odontalgia is not fully understood, it appears that the clinical characteristics best place it in the category of deafferention pains. Sympathetic activity may also contribute to the maintenance of the pain.

Phantom tooth pain is a syndrome of pain in the teeth and oral structures following pulp extirpation or extraction. In some rare cases, it may also follow an inferior alveolar block.[12,110,111]

Herpes Zoster (Shingles) A recurrence of herpes zoster infection involving the second and third division of the trigeminal nerve can manifest in a rare prodrome of symptomatic pulpitis.[189] The latent virus resides in the Gasserian ganglion following a primary chicken pox (i.e., varicella virus) infection. Like any trigeminal nerve involvement, pulp pain is unilaterally confined. Toothache pain can be localized in one or more teeth, and is described as sharp, throbbing, and intermittent. *The symptoms are believed to be genuine pulpal pain and not mimicked.*

During the prodrome, which can last for weeks, recognition of a recurrence of herpes zoster is nearly impossible. The symptoms are undeniably those of irreversible pulpitis, and the offending teeth are easy for the patient to identify. On examination, the dentist can be baffled to find the teeth intact, noncarious, and free of recent trauma.

The dilemma the dentist faces is whether to believe that the symptoms are genuine. A recent report suggests that varicella virus can lead to adverse pulpal responses; even

necrosis.[68] Other complications may include tooth exfoliation, internal resorption, and osteonecrosis. An early decision to intervene endodontically, during the prodrome of a suspected shingles infection, can relieve the intense pulpitis pain. However, the shingles infection may be followed to its clinical conclusion without intervention. Monitoring for development of pulpal or periapical pathosis is indicated[174] after a shingles infection.

Postherpetic neuralgia is a persistent pain syndrome resulting from infection with varicella-zoster virus, characterized as lancinating, burning, or itching. Areas affected by postherpetic neuralgia include the cranial-trigeminal nerve distributions of the face (the affected nerve pathways undergo degeneration and interruption, causing deafferention and subsequent nerve reorganization).

Toothache of Maxillary Sinus Origin

The apices of the maxillary canine to the molar teeth may be separated from the sinus by a thin osseous plate or by a thin membrane. Inflammation of the sinus lining mucosa can evoke facial pain that involves all of the related maxillary teeth. Maxillary sinusitis can produce a constant, dull, moderate aching pain in multiple teeth on the involved side.[42,161] Generally the teeth adjacent to the sinus have healthy pulps but behave identically to each other, because they are uniformly hypersensitive to percussion. Usually the teeth respond normally to pulp tests. Pain can increase with eating, involve the entire quadrant (up to the facial midline), or refer to the mandibular teeth on the same side.

The patient reports a fullness in the face, pain that increases with lying down or bending over, and tenderness of the skin overlying the sinus. In addition, the patient may describe pain that spreads to the scalp and toward the nose, often in association with a postnasal drip. Determining a history of a recent upper respiratory tract infection or nasal blockage and congestion help the clinician arrive at an early diagnosis. A Waters' radiographic view may show an air fluid level or thickened mucosa of the maxillary sinus.

In the differential diagnosis of maxillary sinusitis, the endoantral syndrome and barodontalgia barosinusitis originating from chronic pulpal pathosis or periapical pathosis, or both, must be considered to rule out a coexisting endodontically induced infection of the sinus lining.[165]

Toothache of Myofascial Origin

The muscles of mastication, particularly masseter, temporalis, and anterior digastric, can induce referred pain felt as toothache. Myofascial pain is nonpulsatile and may recur over several months or years, with periods of quiescence. It is common for a patient to complain of muscular pain after extensive dental treatment, during which the mouth has been open for extended periods. Pain usually increases with emotional stress or vigorous, extended use of the involved muscles.

Whenever a patient complains of a toothache and no clinical evidence exists of pulpal or periapical pathosis, palpation of the muscles of mastication should be attempted. Digital palpation of the trigger zones in the muscle will reproduce pain symptoms and confirm the diagnosis of pain of myofascial origin. This pain is not arrested by analgesic blocking of the painful teeth, but by locating the muscle that constitutes the site of primary pain and anesthetizing that source of nociceptive input.

Toothache of Cardiac Origin[42]

The presence of jaw pain related to angina pectoris and myocardial infarction highlights the importance of recording each patient's medical history, including relevant symptoms. Reports on the condition of cardiac induced jaw pain show approximately 10% of cases refer pain to the mandible.[159] Myocardial infarction is characterized by pain that is sudden, severe, and not induced by oral stimulation. In chronic angina and coronary (ischemic) artery disease, the pain may be less intense and associated with physical exertion and emotional excitement. In most cases, with the cessation of the inducing activity, pain originating from ischemia of the heart muscle dissipates.

Myocardial pain may manifest in the form of pain in the left arm, especially down the inner aspect, as well as pain in the neck, jaw, or teeth. Substernal chest discomfort may or may not be present. The attendant signs of shock, nausea, difficulty breathing, sweats, clammy skin, and pallor may accompany these symptoms.

With imminent myocardial infarct, pain symptoms are constant, and they spread to involve vast areas of the maxilla and mandible. Pain may travel down, into the neck, or it may travel up, into the temporal and zygomatic regions. During this time the patient becomes anxious and complains of pain that is increasingly unbearable.

A careful history is important in diagnosing the referred pain as myocardial in origin. Often the pain cannot be controlled with analgesics but is controlled with nitroglycerin. Radiographs and pulp tests of all the teeth in the painful area will appear ambiguous or normal. Sensitivity testing cannot reproduce the pain. Failure of analgesic blocking to arrest the pain promptly and completely confirms that the primary source of pain is not the tooth. If myocardial pain is suspected, the patient must be referred to the emergency room immediately.

Neoplastic Diseases

Neoplastic diseases are rare, but they can mimic symptoms of a toothache.[9,166] The nature of the pain can be severe, escalating with time and involving a developing paresthesia. The pain features are out of character with those seen with inflammatory pulpal disease, and they should prompt the dentist to seek immediate consultation with and referral to an oral surgeon or physician (Fig. 2-1).

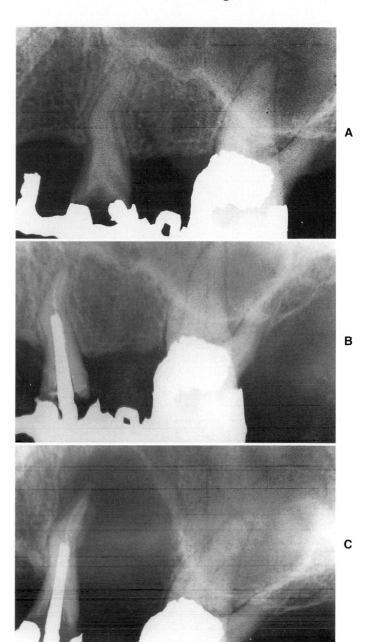

Fig. 2-1 **A**, Preoperative endodontic involvement of the left maxillary first premolar. **B**, Completion of the endodontic treatment. **C**, Reexamination at 6 months. Radiographic evidence of significant bone loss and apical resorption is seen, which is atypical of endodontic failure. Biopsy specimen revealed multiple myeloma, an malignancy of the lymphoreticular system. Discovery of systemic disease on the dental films was confirmed by head and chest films that demonstrated widespread involvement. The patient died 7 months later. (Courtesy Dr. Alan H. Gluskin.)

Toothache of Psychogenic Origin

On occasion a patient may report symptoms of toothache that do not fit any clinical orofacial pain entity. The symptoms may be the result of a somatoform pain disorder, a type of mental disorder in which a patient may complain of a physical condition that has no physical signs. When the pain complaint is confined to a tooth, the condition may be described as a psychogenic toothache. A dentist should suspect a psychogenic toothache only after eliminating other organic causes of toothache.

Munchausen's syndrome[42] is characterized by an elaborate description or creation of pain that is not real or is self-inflicted. The profile of these patients runs the gamut from the psychotic to the neurotic, the pathologic liar to the chemically dependent addict.

The psychotic or neurotic patient gives a history that is convincing for orofacial pain but that cannot be confirmed by clinical examination and testing. The patient may spend countless hours in a health science library "researching" the condition and may visit many dentists to determine the cause of pain. The pain is *real* to the patient, who insists on treatment.

The chemically abusive patient often gives detailed textbook descriptions of toothache. On examination, the dentist may actually find probable cause for the pain. The situation is self-induced or, at the insistence of the patient, "dentistogenic." The addicted patient shows up unannounced for "emergency visits" during the workday or before a holiday weekend. In some cases the patient may make an "emergency" call to the office on a holiday. This patient conveys convincing stories (e.g., "forgetting" or "losing" pain killers) and alleges dissatisfaction with other dentists. The patient then asks for sufficient medication to "tide them over" until the next workday. The addict may even allow the dentist to perform treatment, because it would be difficult to deny a prescription to someone when urgent care has been provided. The patient specifies what type of medication is being sought and often insists on a potent narcotic analgesic.

A summary of the signs and symptoms suggestive of nonodontogenic toothache are as follows[137]:

1. No local dental cause consistent with symptoms
2. Burning, nonpulsatile toothaches
3. Constant, nonvariable toothaches
4. Persistent toothaches over months or years
5. Multiple, spontaneous toothaches
6. Failure to eliminate the toothache after local anesthetic block of the suspected tooth
7. Failure to respond to reasonable dental therapy

DIAGNOSING OROFACIAL PAIN

To render care for any orofacial emergency patient, the dentist must make a prudent and thoughtful diagnosis regarding the cause and present state of the patient's disease. The clinician must collect relevant information regarding signs, symptoms, and history of the present complaint, together with results from the clinical examination and tests. A methodical and disciplined approach will help establish an accurate diagnosis.

The endodontic emergency is a pulpal and/or periradicular pathologic condition; it manifests itself through pain or swelling or both symptoms. An urgent endodontic emergency often interrupts the normal office routine and patient flow. In addition, after-hours accommodations may have to be made to care for the patient.

Before undertaking any definitive treatment for "toothache," two questions should be answered: (1) Does the pain emanate from a tooth? (2) If it does, which tooth is responsible for the pain? *The clinician is to be reminded that, even in a true endodontic emergency, it is most likely that only one tooth is responsible for an acute situation.* Clinically, it is quite rare that, on a biologic level, the set of circumstances that could produce the odontogenic emergency would occur in two teeth with the same intensity at the same time.

The clinician who reviews and prioritizes patient data in a deliberate and thorough manner for all emergencies can avoid the pitfalls of inaccurate diagnosis and inappropriate treatment.

Records

If the dentist is to provide a precise, structured appraisal of a patient's chief complaint, details of the comprehensive clinical and dental examination must be recorded. Forms allow the clinician to keep an efficient record and quantify diagnostic data (Figs. 2-2, 2-3, 2-4).

Triage of the Patient with Pain

Emergencies caused by orofacial pain demand immediate, professional attention. The urgency of the situation, however, should not preclude a thorough clinical evaluation of the patient. Orofacial pain can be the clinical manifestation of a variety of diseases involving the head and neck region. The cause must be reliably differentiated, odontogenic from nonodontogenic. Without a comprehensive knowledge of the pathophysiology of inflammatory pain of the pulp and periradicular tissues, this task is needlessly difficult.

Triage can expedite the differentiation process by systematically sorting through the signs and symptoms of the patient's pain. Each entity is characterized as having a dental or nondental pain feature; features that are shared and not exclusive to either source are also noted. With the signs and symptoms collected in this manner, triage is concluded by noting the preponderance of pain features in either the dental or nondental category. Thus a working differential diagnosis is methodically begun, and it directs the dentist to investigate further.

Triage of odontogenic symptoms should discriminate for sensory and proprioceptive sensations produced exclusively by inflammatory pulpal and periradicular diseases.

Identifying orofacial pain as endodontic pain becomes increasingly difficult as the focus shifts away from localized tooth pain to a wider area of the face. Numerous orofacial diseases can mimic endodontic pain and produce sensory misperception as a result of overlap between sensory fibers of the trigeminal nerve and adjacent cranial and cervical sen-

HAVE YOU EVER HAD ANY OF THE FOLLOWING? PLEASE CHECK EACH BOX.

	YES	NO		YES	NO		YES	NO		YES	NO
High blood pressure			Mitral valve prolapse			Tuberculosis			Diabetes		
Heart attack			Heart valve replacement			Hepatitis			Thyroid problems		
Stroke			Artificial joint			Jaundice			Epilepsy		
Arrhythmias			Asthma			Liver disorder			Nervous disorder		
Pacemaker			Seasonal allergies			Kidney disease			Blood transfusion		
Rheumatic fever			Sinus problems			Arthritis			AIDS/HIV-positive		
Heart murmur			Respiratory problems			Ulcers			Drug dependency		

If you answered YES to any of the above, list name of the medications and dosage below.

_____

_____

ARE YOU SENSITIVE OR ALLERGIC TO ANY OF THE FOLLOWING MEDICATIONS? PLEASE CHECK EACH BOX.

	YES	NO		YES	NO		YES	NO
Novocaine or xylocaine			Sulfa			Codeine		
Penicillin			Other Antibiotics			Latex products		
Erythromycin			Aspirin			Other medications		

List other medications: _____

What type of reation did you have? _____

1. Have you ever had surgery, x-ray treatment or chemotherapy for a tumor or growth? .... ❑ Yes ❑ No

2. Have you every had abnormal bleeding associated with previous extractions, surgery or trauma? .... ❑ Yes ❑ No

3. Do you have any disease, condition or problem not mentioned above? .... ❑ Yes ❑ No

4. Female Patients: Are you pregnant? ❑ Yes ❑ No   If Yes, what month? _____ Obstetrician _____

5. Have you ever taken Fen-Phen? .... ❑ Yes ❑ No

Other medical concerns:

_____

ARE YOU CURRENTLY TAKING ANY OF THE FOLLOWING? PLEASE CHECK EACH BOX.

	YES	NO		YES	NO		YES	NO
Antibiotics			Aspirin			Thyroid		
Medicine for high blood pressure			Anticoagulants (blood thinners)			Steroids		
Digitalis/other heart medications			Tranquilizers (Valium, Librium)			Birth control medications		
Nitroglycerine			Sedatives			Pain medications		
Antihistamines			Insulin/other diabetic drugs			Other medications		

6. Have you ever had endodontic (root canal) treatment before? .... ❑ Yes ❑ No

To the best of my knowledge, all the above answers are true and correct. I will Inform my dentist of changes in my health and/or medication.

Patient's signature _____ Date _____ Reviewed _____

Patient's signature _____ Date _____ Reviewed _____

Fig. 2-2 Chart of a medical systems review common to a comprehensive dental record.

DENTAL HISTORY:	CHIEF COMPLAINT	SYMPTOMATIC	ASYMPTOMATIC

SYMPTOMS	Location	Chronology	Quality	Affected By	Prior Tx	Initial:
		Inception	sharp intensity dull + ++ +++ Clinical Course: spontaneous pulsating provoked	hot palpation cold manipulation biting head position	Tx: restorative Yes No emergency Yes No RCT Yes No	TOOTH
localized diffuse	referred radiating	constant momentary intermittent lingering	steady reproducible enlarging occasional	chewing activity percussion time of day	Sx Pre-Tx: Yes No Sx Post-Tx: Yes No	R ——┼—— L

Fig. 2-3 Systematic format for charting the dental history.

CLINICAL FINDINGS

EXAMINATION	RADIOGRAPHIC		CLINICAL		DIAGNOSTIC TESTS						
Tooth	Attachment Apparatus		Tooth	Soft Tissues	Tooth #						
WNL caries restoration calcification resorption fracture perforation / deviation prior RCTx/RCF separated instrument canal obstruction post / build-up open apex	PDL normal PDL thickened alveolar bone, WNL diffuse lucency circumscribed lucency resorption apical lateral hypercementosis osteosclerosis perio:		WNL discoloration caries pulp exposure prior access attrition / abrasion fracture restoration amalgam composite inlay / onlay temporary crown abutment	WNL extra-oral swelling intra-oral swelling sinus tract lymphadenopathy TMJ perio: B M ———— D L	perio						
					mobility						
					percussion						
					palpation						
					cold						
					hot						
					EPT						
					transillum						
					cavity						
					bite / chewing						
					date:						

Fig. 2-4 Chart for clinical findings and diagnosis.

sory dermatomes. Convergence of signals in the medulla can cause sensory overload to occur. This, in turn, can cause a perceptual error by the cerebral cortex.

Triage of nonodontogenic symptoms should discriminate for pain patterns that are inconsistent with inflammatory pulpal and periradicular diseases. Nonodontogenic toothaches are often difficult to identify and can challenge the diagnostic ability of the clinician. The most important step toward proper management of toothache is to consider that the pain may not be of dental origin.

The process of diagnosis of the endodontic emergency, as set forth in this chapter, will concentrate on the acute emergency, or potentially complex orofacial pain emergency. The practitioner must collect the appropriate data (e.g., the set of signs, symptoms, test results) that will lead to a diagnosis.

When obtaining diagnostic data, the dentist must generate the following:

1. Subjective examination, including medical history, dental history, and chief complaint
2. Objective clinical examination
3. Diagnostic tests, including pulpal sensitivity testing and a radiographic examination

Medical History

The verbal, subjective examination of the patient must include a comprehensive evaluation of the patient's medical history. Although numerous authorities agree that there are almost no medical contraindications to endodontic therapy, it is important to understand how an individual's physical condition, medical history, and current medications might affect the treatment course or prognosis.

A medical history informs the clinician of any "high-risk patient" whose therapy may have to be modified (e.g., a cardiac patient who might tolerate only short appointments with limited procedural stress). The medical history would also identify patients who require antibiotic prophylaxis for congenital or rheumatic heart disease. The use of antibiotic prophylaxis to prevent infective endocarditis is justified in these patients. Antibiotic prophylaxis may be indicated in other patients at risk from a treatment-induced bacteremia, because of implanted prosthetic devices, hemodialysis, or impaired host defenses. Patients receiving chemotherapy or who have compromised immune systems may also require antibiotic prophylaxis.[109,140]

The medical history can identify patients for whom healing and repair of endodontic pathosis could be complicated or delayed, such as those who have uncontrolled diabetes or acquired immunodeficiency syndrome (AIDS). Having knowledge of specific critical blood values, as well as immune status and medications being used, is essential to any therapy provided to a patient with human immunodeficiency virus (HIV) or AIDS.[11] The patient whose ability to control bleeding has been altered by drugs or disease may be in grave danger unless the dentist identifies the problem and takes appropriate precautions before performing any dental treatment.

There are also aspects of a patient's medical background that might affect the chief complaint, the repair potential, or the radiographic appearance of disease. Sickle cell anemia, vitamin D–resistant rickets, and herpes zoster have been implicated in spontaneous pulpal degeneration.[168] Nutritional disease, stress, and corticosteroid therapy may also decrease the potential for pulpal healing and repair.[168]

The dentist should follow up by reviewing what the patient has written and seek additional detailed information that may not impress the patient as important. For example, some women are reluctant to discuss their use of birth control pills for contraception, yet a number of common antibiotics used to treat endodontic infections significantly decrease the efficacy of oral contraceptives.[32] Possible drug interactions between currently prescribed medications and those prescribed for the endodontic emergency must be understood by the dentist and noted in the patient's record.

To minimize the possibility of nondisclosure of important data by the patient, the diagnostician should ask supplemental questions in the following areas of concern:

1. Current medical condition

2. History of significant illness or serious injury
3. Emotional and psychologic history
4. Prior hospitalizations
5. Current medications, including over-the-counter remedies
6. Habits (e.g., alcohol, tobacco, drugs)
7. Any other noticeable signs or symptoms that may indicate an undiagnosed health problem

All significant medical data should be recorded in the patient's record (see Fig. 2-2). In the emergency setting, where there is evidence of worsening infection and the patient feels unwell, the dentist should measure and record the patient's vital signs (i.e., pulse rate, blood pressure, respiratory rate, and temperature). If any question exists regarding the patient's current medical status, the appropriate physician should be consulted.

Dental History

The dental history is unquestionably the most important aspect of the diagnostic workup and, if carefully done, will build rapport in the doctor-patient relationship. *It is important to listen carefully to the patient.* Specific information regarding the age of previous dental work, as well as symptoms before and after the work was done, should be sought from the patient. (The form in Fig. 2-3 may help the clinician and patient to focus on the chief complaint, the affecting factors, as well as the duration and intensity of any dental symptoms in an efficient way.)

Chief Complaint

The subjective questioning should attempt to provide a narrative from the patient that addresses the patient's chief complaint, expressed in the patient's own words, including the following:

1. Location—site or sites where symptoms are perceived
2. Onset of symptoms
3. Characteristics of the symptoms:
   Temporal pattern of the symptoms
   Quality—How the patient describes the complaint
   Intensity of pain symptoms
4. Affecting factors—Stimuli that aggravate, relieve, or alter the symptoms
5. Supplemental history—Pain diary for the difficult diagnosis

The diagnostician should listen carefully to the patient's choice of words, remembering that the patient's descriptions are being filtered through a myriad of complex psychosocial and emotional components. These components affect the way the patient describes the pain and how the pain is perceived. The questions listed in the right column ensure comprehensive and logical evaluation of the chief complaint.

Location of the Chief Complaint
The patient is asked to indicate the location of the chief complaint by using one finger to point to it directly. Pointing avoids verbal ambiguity, and the dentist can note if the pain is intraoral or extraoral, precise or vague, and localized or diffuse. If the symptoms radiate, or if the pain is referred, the direction and extent can also be demonstrated.

The diagnostician should be well aware of referred pain pathways, because referred pain is common with irreversible pulpitis when the disease has not yet produced signs or symptoms in the periradicular tissues. In posterior molars, pain can be referred to the opposing quadrant or to other teeth in the same quadrant. Maxillary molars often refer pain to the zygomatic, parietal, and occipital regions of the head, whereas mandibular molars frequently refer pain to the ear, angle of the jaw, or posterior regions of the neck. Corroborating tests and data are necessary to make a definitive diagnosis whenever referred pain is suspected.

Onset of Symptoms
The patient should relate when the symptoms of the chief complaint were initially perceived. Additional information that may be useful includes a history of recent dental procedures, previous treatment performed to remedy the condition, trauma, or past episodes of pain or swelling.

The vast majority of patients with toothache have a previous history of pain in the same location. A previous history of pain correlates well with the presence of pulpal pathosis.[169]

Characteristics of Pain

Temporal Characteristics of Pain
Beyond the onset of symptoms, it is important for the dentist to record details of symptoms. The following points should be emphasized:

1. Do the symptoms have a temporal pattern, or are they sporadic or occasional?
2. Is the onset or abatement of symptoms spontaneous or provoked? Is it sudden or gradual? If symptoms can be stimulated, are they immediate or delayed?
3. Have the symptoms persisted since they began, or have they been intermittent?
4. How long do symptoms last? Are they stated as "momentary" or "lingering?" If they are persistent, the duration should be estimated in seconds, minutes, hours, or longer intervals. If the symptoms can be induced, are they momentary, or do they linger?

Quality of Pain
The patient is asked to give a description of each symptom associated with the odontogenic emergency. This description is important for the differential diagnosis of the pain and for selection of objective clinical tests to reproduce symptoms.

Certain adjectives describe pain of bony origin (e.g., dull, gnawing, aching). Other adjectives (e.g., throbbing, pounding, pulsing) describe the vascular response to tissue inflammation. *Sharp, electric, recurrent,* or *stabbing* pain is usually caused by pathosis of nerve root complexes, sensory ganglia, or peripheral innervation, which is associated with irreversible pulpitis or trigeminal neuralgia. A single episode of sharp, persistent pain can result from acute injury to a muscle or ligament, as in temporomandibular joint dislocation or iatrogenic perforation into the periodontal attachment apparatus.

Pulpal and periapical pathosis produce sensations that are described as *aching, pulsing, throbbing, dull, radiating, stabbing,* or *jolting* pain. Though such descriptions support suspicion of an odontogenic cause, the diagnostician cannot ignore the fact that many of these adjectives can also describe nonodontogenic pathosis.

Intensity of Pain

The patient's perception of and reaction to an acute pain emergency, especially one that is odontogenic in origin, is widely variable. For an unremitting toothache, the treating clinician usually decides to render emergency treatment based on its intensity. The dentist, therefore, should try to quantify the intensity level of the pain symptoms reported by the patient. There are methods to accomplish this:

1. The patient should try to quantify the pain. Assigning to the pain a degree of 0 (i.e., no pain) to 10 (i.e., most severe or intolerable pain) helps the clinician to monitor the patient's perception of the pain throughout the course of treatment.

2. The patient should classify the pain as mild, moderate, or severe. This classification has implications for the question, *How does the pain affect the patient's lifestyle?* The pain can be classified as severe if it interrupts or significantly alters the patient's daily routine. Generally, pain that interferes with sleeping, working, or leisure activities is significant. If potent analgesics are required, the pain is also considered extreme.

Pain usually indicates tissue damage and, to some extent, reflects the extent of that damage. However, sometimes fear of dentists and dental procedures causes an exaggeration of perceived pain, resulting in an inconsistency between symptoms and pulpal pathosis. Some clinicians have not found any correlation between specific pain characteristics and histologic status of the pulp.[204] Whenever symptoms are clinically reproducible, the intensity of the pain should alert the dentist to which clinical and diagnostic tests are most appropriate. If the clinician can reproduce these tests, more painful symptoms will help locate the chief complaint and provide corroborative information. Although it "creates data," reproducing less intense symptoms may not help differentiate the involved tooth from those responses that are within normal limits.

Affecting Factors

The objective of the next part of the examination is to identify which factors provoke, intensify, alleviate, or otherwise affect the patient's symptoms. Before any corroborative testing is attempted (such as thermal or percussion tests), it is imperative to know the level of intensity of each affecting stimulus and the interval between stimulus and response. The patient who describes a toothache that manifests itself about halfway through drinking a cup of hot coffee should alert the diagnostician that the tooth is exhibiting a delayed onset response to heat. This has a significant bearing on how clinical testing should proceed. Unless adequate time between stimulus and response is allowed, coincidence may have the dentist stimulating a second tooth at the same time a previously stimulated tooth is manifesting a delayed response.

The prudent clinician will be cautious when using the percussion test. If the patient indicates that percussion may elicit an extreme response, it would be unwise to begin by percussing teeth (this could provoke so much discomfort for the patient that it clouds the diagnosis). Symptoms can be more meaningful if the investigator takes the time to hear and understand the circumstances in which they occur.

The stimuli generally associated with odontogenic symptoms are heat, cold, sweet, percussion, biting, manipulation, and palpation. A history of prolonged, painful responses to thermal changes suggests a problem of pulpal origin. Clinical tests using the thermal test that most closely *reproduces the patient's complaint* are indicated to locate the source and intensity of the response. If the patient's chief complaint is pain with cold, a cold stimulus is needed for testing; if the complaint is pain with hot drinks, a hot stimulus should be used.

Just as there are factors that provoke odontogenic pain, there are factors that can precipitate the onset of symptoms that may indicate a nonodontogenic cause:

1. Postural changes—Head or jaw pain accentuated by bending over, blowing the nose, or jarring the skeleton (e.g., by jogging) may imply involvement of the maxillary sinuses.

2. Time of day—Stiffness and pain in the jaws and masticatory muscles upon waking may indicate occlusal disharmony or temporomandibular joint dysfunction.[215] Odontogenic pain is often perceived to be worse at night or when lying down. This may be a result of increased blood flow to the head and inflamed pulpal tissue in the supine position. The pain may also seem worse at night, when the patient is not preoccupied by daily tasks.

Pain upon strenuous or vigorous activity may indicate pulpal or periapical inflammation. Pulpal or sinus involvement may also be revealed by changes in barometric pressure, which can occur during deep diving or flying at high altitudes. Another significant implication would be jaw pain associated with exertion, which may be a warning sign of coronary artery disease.

For most endodontic emergencies, there is a definite cause-and-effect relationship. However, there will always be cases that perplex and confound even the most astute diagnostician. Every dentist will be asked to diagnose and treat emergencies with symptoms that are vague and causes that are difficult to determine.

The patient who complains of poorly localized, disabling pain that is not reproducible at the time of the emergency visit is a difficult challenge. There may be a great deal of pain for the patient but very little evidence that provides definitive information for the doctor. If the patient is demanding that something be done, this can compound the stress of the emergency visit. Faced with a dissatisfied, insistent patient, there is a strong temptation to do "something," even before a definitive diagnosis can be made. *The dentist should avoid this situation at all costs* to prevent claims of misdiagnosis or negligence. Patients who are made aware of the dentist's concern for their problem and empathy for their suffering will be far more inclined to accept a cautious approach during the diagnostic process. The clinician must emphasize the scientific nature of the diagnosis and the real possibility that it may take more than one visit to identify the problem and treat it appropriately.

The dentist should inform the patient that it may be necessary to wait a while for vague symptoms to localize. This conservative approach is sometimes necessary when pathosis is confined to the pulp, which can refer pain to other teeth or nondental sites. It may be necessary to wait for the inflammatory reaction to involve the periradicular tissues before it can be localized. Generally, patients can be supported with analgesics until a definitive diagnosis can be made. Patients taking analgesics at the time of presentation also introduce a difficult diagnostic challenge, as the pain may be reduced or eliminated at the time of the dental examination.

Supplemental history—the pain diary. A daily diary can provide valuable information to aid in the difficult diagnosis. Patients' verbal reports are often vague, overdramatized, or contradictory. Frequency and severity of symptoms can vary with time, and the patient who feels stressed may not report critical information accurately. In these rare cases a pain diary provides an hour-by-hour or day-by-day narrative that can help the clinician determine if the pain is odontogenic or nonodontogenic. Information, such as the severity of pain (on a 1 to 10 scale), the duration of pain, the time of day pain occurs, and the cause or activity associated with the pain, should be recorded. These patterns of discomfort may provide concise information for the dentist; they may also help the patient to modify behavior toward the pain.

After providing descriptive information about their chief complaint, the patient should recount any significant incidents in the affected area (e.g., trauma, previous symptoms or treatments, complications). Certain descriptions of pain, such as trigger zones or headaches, as well as medical conditions, such as coronary artery disease or a history of neoplasm, are details that should be considered in a differential diagnosis when seeking the cause of pain.

After organizing, analyzing, and assimilating all of the relevant descriptions, facts, and data, the dentist should be ready to proceed with the clinical-examination phase of the diagnostic process.

Clinical Examination

Extraoral Examination   All patients must be examined for abnormal asymmetries, swellings, changes in skin color, draining sinus tracts, or signs of trauma (Fig. 2-5). The extraoral examination should include visual examination and digital palpation of the face, lips, and neck. Extraoral swellings may indicate serious spreading of intraoral disease processes. Painful or enlarged lymph nodes are of particular importance, because they indicate spread of infection and the possibility of malignant disease. The extent and manner of jaw opening can provide information regarding spread of infection and possible myofascial pain dysfunction.

Intraoral Examination   The extraoral examination is followed by a thorough intraoral examination, including a visual inspection of the hard and soft tissues of the oral cavity. To prevent missing any subtle lesions, soft tissues and teeth of the area to be examined should be made free of saliva. An intraoral examination of the oropharynx, cheeks, alveolar mucosa, gingiva, hard and soft palate, tongue, and floor of the mouth to identify possible areas of inflammation, abrasion, ulceration, neoplasm, or other abnormality is mandatory. A good light and magnification source will make this phase of the examination easier and more effective (see Chapter 5).

Dental Examination

The dental examination has two components:
1. Physical inspection
2. Diagnostic tests

Physical Inspection   The physical inspection should include observations of periodontal health, tissue color, and tissue texture. The clinician should also note any restorations, caries, tooth discoloration, erosion, fractures, swelling, and sinus tracts. A thorough periodontal assessment, with careful probing of the sulcus and attachment apparatus and notation of mobilities, is a standard and essential element of the physical inspection. A periodontal examination should identify any loss of attachment or pocketing associated with a patient's symptoms.

An essential aspect of diagnosis is to determine the periodontal health of a tooth in question. For example, a tooth that is causing pain may have a vertical root fracture or a periodontal lesion that warrants extraction of the tooth. These determinations cannot be made without a careful exploration of the sulcus around a tooth. Failure to measure periodontal pockets and furcation involvement may cause the dentist to misdiagnose the patient's problem.

Any signs of periodontal disease must be considered in the differential diagnosis. Pockets of periodontal origin tend to be broad, whereas pockets of endodontic origin tend to be narrow. For example, a sinus tract that exits through the sulcus or a vertical root fracture is associated with deep, narrow probings along one aspect of the root. Symptoms associated with periodontal disease may be a dull, aching pain, whereas pain of endodontic origin may be more sharp or throbbing. Because pain symptoms of periodontal or endodontic origin can overlap, the practitioner must be careful when assessing the periodontal and pulpal status of a tooth to determine the nature of the pain and prognosis of the tooth.

Diagnostic Tests   Diagnostic tests enable the practitioner to:
1. Define the pain by evoking reproducible symptoms that characterize the chief complaint
2. Compare normal responses to abnormal responses, which may be indicative of pathosis

The usefulness of diagnostic testing is determined by the clinician's correct and systematic application and interpretation of appropriate tests. Diagnostic tests include the pulpal sensitivity tests for hot and cold thermal testing, as well as electric pulp testing. Mechanical tests include tooth percussion and tissue palpation. Transillumination and magnification, test cavity preparation, and anesthetic tests are additional means of confirming a diagnosis. However, this discussion focuses on clinical considerations (relative to testing) that are necessary for identification and treatment of endodontic emergencies. (Chapter 1 provides a detailed discussion of diagnostic testing.)

When diagnostic testing is required to evaluate a patient's chief complaint, the success of the analysis depends on the following clinician characteristics:
1. An understanding of how to administer the appropriate tests
2. An awareness of the limitations of the various tests
3. A biologic knowledge of the inflammatory process and the pain phenomenon, as well as an understanding nonodontogenic entities that mimic pulpal and periapical pathosis

Investigators have explained why teeth with radiographically discernible periapical lesions retain pulpal innervation, even when pulpal necrosis is anticipated.[105] This fact can confound the interpretation of pulp vitality testing, and it may engender inaction on the part of the dentist when true pathosis is present. This should reinforce the clinician's requirement to provide a thorough evaluation and corroborative data before making a definitive diagnosis.

The dentist should include adequate controls for any set of applied test procedures. To establish the patient's normal range of response, several adjacent, opposing, and contralateral teeth should be tested before testing the tooth in question. The dentist should use care not to bias a patient's response by indicating whether a normal or suspect tooth is being tested.

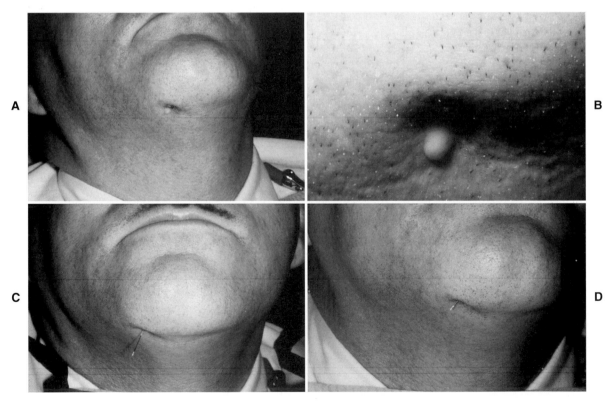

Fig. 2-5 **A,** Physical examination of the skin of a middle-age man who exhibits chronic drainage in the lower right chin area. The lesion was resistant to dermatologic therapy. **B,** Closer inspection of the area reveals active drainage. **C** and **D,** Presence of an extraoral sinus tract was confirmed by inserting a silver cone to the source, the mandibular first bicuspid. Confirmation was made by dental radiographs and pulp vitality testing.

Sensitivity Tests

This group of thermal and electric tests enables the dentist to determine the pulpal status of a tooth.

Thermal Tests   Endodontists have determined that misdiagnosis can result from misperception of symptoms, misinterpretation of data, or an incomplete diagnostic examination.[161] It has also been concluded that, in the difficult diagnosis of thermal sensitivity, it is imperative to accurately recreate the conditions that stimulate pain. Applying warm gutta-percha or a cold cotton pellet to a tooth surface may elicit symptoms. However, in many cases this method does not reproduce the patient's symptoms, because these tests only stimulate the tooth at a single point of contact.

Although the stimulus may be sufficient to produce a vital response, it is insufficient to reproduce the lingering response of an irreversible pulpitis. In such cases each tooth should be isolated with a rubber dam and bathed in hot water or ice water to reproduce the environment in which the pain is evoked. (See Chapter 1 for details.)

When the tooth is isolated using a rubber dam, all tooth surfaces are simultaneously stimulated (which is why this is the most reliable method for testing thermal sensitivity). This method is also very effective for evaluating teeth with full coverage restorations, whether porcelain or metal. Once the complaint is reproduced, the hot or cold fluid should be removed from the patient's tooth to provide relief. The dentist must use a methodical diagnostic technique to avoid producing conflicting and unreliable responses. The sensory response of teeth is refractory to repeated thermal stimulation. To avoid a misinterpretation of a response, the dentist should wait an appropriate time for tested teeth to respond and recover from any induced pain (Fig. 2-6).

Electric pulp testing   The clinician should be aware of the limitations of electric pulp testing. The electric pulp test should be regarded as an aid in detecting pulpal neural response, not a measure of pulpal health or pathosis. Basing

a diagnosis of necrosis solely on a nonresponsive electric pulp test ignores the possibility that the testing device has malfunctioned or the clinician has made an error in technique. In addition, secondary dentin, trauma, restorations, and dystrophic calcification may all contribute to negative responses on a normal tooth. Thermal and electric testing of the pulp depends on a subjective human response. Therefore the results must be interpreted carefully, and corroborating tests must be made. (Chapter 1 contains a discussion of the potential for erroneous results in electric pulp testing, including false positive and false negative results.[84])

Mechanical Tests

These tests allow the dentist to determine if the pulpal inflammatory process has extended into the periradicular region.

Percussion Tests   If the patient's chief complaint involves pain when biting or chewing, a combination of percussion and biting tests should be used to reproduce the symptoms. Selective percussion from various angles will help identify and isolate teeth with early inflammation in the periodontium. Care should be used when performing a percussion test, because some teeth may be extremely sensitive to touch. An asymptomatic tooth should be percussed before testing the suspect tooth so that the dentist is aware of the patient's typical response.

Sometimes percussion testing yields negative results, even when the patient complains of pain with chewing. Biting tests using a Tooth Slooth is one means of detecting dentinal fractures that may be hidden under restorations. A more subtle test is to have the patient bite down on and chew the end of a cottonwood stick. Because the teeth come much closer together in this test, it more closely replicates masticatory excursions. When the Tooth Slooth does not help in identifying the offending tooth (or cusp), the cottonwood stick test may be helpful. The diagnosis of a cracked tooth is

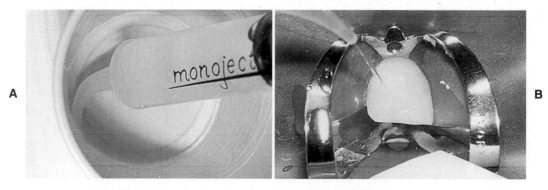

Fig. 2-6 **A**, Syringe for loading hot water to bathe the suspected tooth. **B**, Rubber dam isolation of a central incisor that is sensitive to heat. The patient should test the water with a finger to identify the affecting temperature.

most easily determined with biting tests, rather than percussion tests.

Palpation Tests

Palpation Tests   When the inflammatory mediators of an inflamed or necrotic pulp extend into the periradicular region, symptoms may manifest as sensitivity to tooth percussion and/or palpation of the mucosal tissues. Most frequently, percussion sensitivity precedes palpation sensitivity because, initially, the inflammatory process affects the immediate periradicular region. As the inflammation and infection penetrate through the cortical plate, palpation of the overlying mucosal tissue elicits pain. It may be possible to detect tenderness, fluctuation, induration, or crepitus before extensive swelling develops. It is important to check for buccal and lingual palpation sensitivity, because either may occur (depending on the affected roots and their position in the alveolar bone).

Supplemental Diagnostic Tests

Other tests are sometimes necessary to determine the diagnosis. Although magnification and transillumination, test cavities, and anesthetic tests are not routinely necessary, the benefits of these tests are discussed in the following sections.

Magnification and Transillumination

Magnification and Transillumination   The use of fiberoptic lighting and chair side magnification has become indispensable in the search for cracks, fractures, undetected canals, and obstructions in root canal therapy. Before searching for cracks and fractures, it may be necessary to remove all restorations from a tooth. The location and depth of a crack, along with the pulpal and periodontal status, establish the severity of the problem and the restorability of the tooth.

Test Cavity

Test Cavity   Under rare circumstances, when other tests have failed to determine the pulpal status of a tooth, a test cavity can be prepared. Without anesthetic, the tooth should be isolated under a rubber dam and a small bur should be used to enter the pulp chamber. A vital tooth will usually respond with pain or sensitivity once the dentin is reached. If the pulp is necrotic, the tooth is likely to be without symptoms as the pulp chamber is entered. At this time, anesthetic should be administered and root canal treatment should be continued.

Selective Anesthesia

Selective Anesthesia   Selective anesthesia involves the administration of local anesthetic to facilitate the identification of a tooth causing pain. This test is confined to a difficult diagnosis in which the results of earlier diagnostic tests are inconclusive. This should be the final test that is performed, because the tooth will be anesthetized and further sensitivity tests will not be possible during the visit. The purpose of this type of test is to anesthetize a single tooth and eliminate it as the source of pain. Delivering anesthetic to one tooth is best accomplished using an intraligamentary injection or the Stabident system. If anesthetizing one tooth alleviates all pain, then the source of pain has been determined. It is important to pulp test the suspected tooth *after* delivering the anesthetic to determine if it is profoundly numb. It also critical to pulp test the *adjacent teeth* to ensure that only one tooth has been affected by the anesthetic. It is often difficult to anesthetize one tooth without affecting adjacent teeth, so this test must be interpreted with caution. (Further discussion of this technique is found in Chapter 1.) Additional uses and interpretation of anesthetic tests are discussed later in the chapter.

Radiographic Examination

After collecting the details of the chief complaint from the patient's history, physical examination, and clinical examination, the doctor should obtain radiographic views that will contribute to the location and identification of the patient's problem. The interpretation of radiographs can be a source of enlightenment; it can also be a source of misinformation. Changes in the pulp chamber often constitute a record of past pulpal insults. Caries, secondary dentin under restorations, very large or narrow pulp chambers compared with adjacent teeth, deep bases, calcifications, and condensing osteitis can all indicate chronic inflammatory changes in the pulpal tissue. An optical magnifier (and proper illumination) will help the examiner discern these subtle and intricate details in the radiographic image. The patient's record should provide space to note radiographic changes (see Fig. 2-4).

Radiographs provide important information about the tooth and supporting structures. Proper selection of the appropriate type of radiographic views (see Chapter 5) is necessary to complete differential diagnosis. The attending dentist is cautioned to use discretion in accepting prior diagnostic radiographs from the patient or another dentist (regardless of how recently they were made), because they may not accurately reflect the present condition of the dentoalveolar structures. Investigations have shown that for a radiograph to exhibit a periapical radiolucency, the lesion must have expanded to the corticomedullary junction and a portion of the bone mineral must be lost.[15] This situation can occur in a short period of time in the presence of an aggressive infection.

New radiographs (taken when treatment is actually initiated) may corroborate a diagnosis or point to a different, unsuspected tooth. Furthermore, prior iatrogenic mishaps, such as ledge formation, perforation, or instrument separation, are critical for a newly treating dentist to uncover. The dentist who omits taking new radiographs assumes legal responsibility for earlier procedural errors, because there is no documentation that they occurred before the current treatment. (See Chapter 10 for a discussion of legal responsibilities.)

Good radiographic technique includes proper film placement, exposure, processing, and handling. These principles are the foundation for attaining a high-quality diagnostic radiograph, and they may provide the only legal defense in support of treatment outcomes. A thorough understanding of regional anatomic structures and their variations is critical to proper interpretation. In addition, a careful assessment of continuity in the periodontal ligament, lamina dura, and root canal anatomy will distinguish healthy structures from diseased ones.

Periapical Films

Periapical films need to show not only the apex of the tooth, but also a few millimeters of bone surrounding the root. If there is a lesion associated with the tooth, the film must show that lesion in its entirety. It is sometimes necessary to have more than one periapical film of a tooth, because different projections reveal different information about the size, shape, and symmetry of the roots. An untreated canal can often be detected in a properly angulated film. Periapical films are also valuable for examining the periradicular area of the root. However, they only provide limited information about the crown, crown/root ratio, the alveolar crest, and the presence of caries. The angulation of the exposure may distort or hide certain aspects of the tooth that are diagnostic. For this reason, bite-wing films are necessary for all posterior teeth.

Bite-Wing Films

Bite-wing films are excellent diagnostic aids. Unlike periapical films, bite-wings show the true dimensions of a tooth because there is minimal elongation or foreshortening of the image. There are many diagnostic elements that cannot be seen on periapical films, yet are clearly visible on bite-wing films. Recurrent caries, the depth of caries relative to the alveolar crest, the presence of open margins, and the size and depth of a post are best diagnosed with bite-wing radiographs (Fig. 2-7).

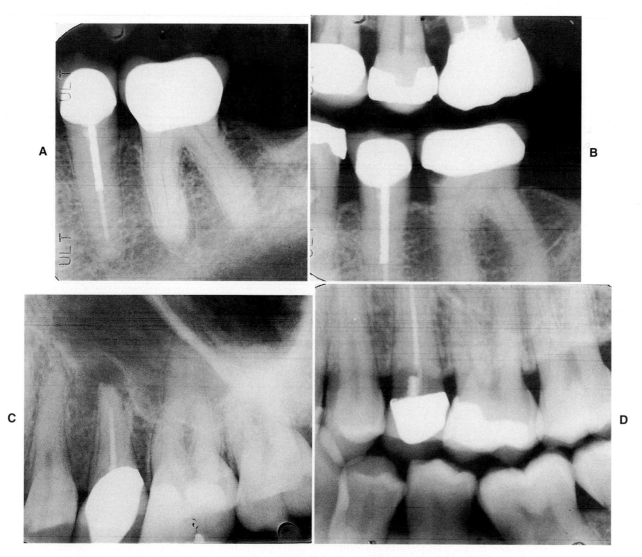

Fig. 2-7 **A**, A patient describes vague pain in the lower left quadrant. The periapical film shows no particular radiographic abnormalities. **B**, The bite-wing radiograph shows significant caries under the mesial margin of tooth #19. **C**, A patient has a buccal swelling associated with tooth #13. The periapical film shows a root canal filling that is short of the apex. Retreatment of this case appears uncomplicated. **D**, The bite-wing film shows extensive caries surrounding a post, none of which were visible on the periapical film. Retreatment of this case requires removal of the crown and post.

Supplemental Films

In addition to the periapical and bite-wing films, supplemental films may also be necessary. For example, a Panorex film is helpful if the maxillary sinus or mandibular canal need to be visualized. The use of supplemental films is especially important when evaluating a patient for apical surgery, because the proximity of the apex to certain anatomic structures may preclude surgery. Some lesions of the jaw may be so large that they cannot be seen clearly or completely on periapical films. Because the full extent of such lesions must be visible, Panorex films would be imperative. However, these films are not especially helpful for evaluating anterior teeth, because this is the area of greatest distortion.

When a cyst is suspected, occlusal films are particularly helpful to view the nasopalatine duct. Occlusal films are also very useful for evaluating the buccolingual location or the dimension of an object in the mandible. (For a further discussion of radiography, refer to Chapter 5.)

DETERMINING THE DIAGNOSIS

The final phase of the diagnostic sequence requires a systematic analysis of all pertinent data accumulated from the patient's history, as well as clinical, dental, and radiographic evaluations. The dentist must take a methodical approach to provide a diagnosis.

The first consideration when determining a diagnosis is whether the patient's chief complaint is reproducible. If the patient reports severe pain two days before the dental visit but diagnostic tests fail to reproduce that pain, the diagnosis is inconclusive. *Unless the symptoms can be duplicated, a diagnosis should not be made.* However, the dentist must remember that a patient who complains of past thermal sensitivity may have become insensitive to thermal testing because the pulp of the tooth in question has become necrotic.

Once a working diagnosis is established, the offending tooth should be anesthetized to confirm that it is the source of pain. When the offending tooth has been correctly identified, anesthetizing that tooth should eliminate all pain. If pain persists after administration of anesthetic, there are two possibilities for the continuing pain: (1) The tooth may not be anesthetized fully (a fully anesthetized tooth will be unresponsive to all aggravating factors, and the patient should feel asymptomatic). (2) The source of pain has not been correctly identified. A patient with referred pain may be certain that a particular tooth is the cause of pain, when the pain is coming from a different tooth or a nonodontogenic source.

When pain persists after administration of anesthetic, the diagnostic method used by the clinician needs to be reevaluated. Were all relevant pulp tests performed? If not, additional testing may lead to identification of the correct tooth. If doubt exists about the source of pain, it is appropriate to refer the patient to an endodontist for further evaluation.

Pulpal pain can be caused by caries, fractures, trauma, recent restorative treatment, and less obvious causes, such as developmental anomalies, orthodontic tooth movement, or viral agents.[68] When a correct diagnosis has been made, the cause of the pain must be clearly understood; *the diagnosis must be consistent with the etiology.*

Prognosis

Once the diagnosis has been established, it is critical to determine the prognosis of the tooth before beginning treatment. The important factors to consider are the periodontal, restorative, and endodontic prognosis. The overall prognosis may then be decided.

Periodontal Prognosis   Measuring the depth of the pockets and loss of attachment is the first step in assessing the periodontal status. Without proper intervention, deep periodontal pockets will enable putative periodontal pathogens to grow and sustain periodontal disease. Increasing loss of attachment will compromise the tooth and its long-term prognosis. If the pockets become so deep that they communicate with an endodontic lesion, the prognosis of this combined lesion is even worse. In posterior teeth, the furcation must also be checked for bone loss. If an explorer or probe can enter into the furcation, the long-term prognosis of the tooth may be questionable. When periodontal disease exists, the patient must be informed of this condition before beginning treatment. If severe periodontal disease exists, the patient may best be served by extraction of the diseased tooth.

Restorative Prognosis   The ability to place a good restoration on the tooth after root canal treatment (without invading the biologic width) should be the clinician's first consideration. If a restoration encroaches on the biologic width, periodontal crown lengthening may be necessary before beginning the restorative phase of treatment. The crown/root ratio of the tooth must be favorable, such that periodontal procedures will not compromise the tooth. (For a detailed discussion on restoring the endodontically treated tooth, see Chapter 22.)

When no esthetic, masticatory, or space-maintaining function can be attributed to the tooth in question, extraction may be a viable choice. Extraction may also be indicated if the tooth lacks adequate periodontal support, exhibits severe resorption, is unrestorable, or if the patient refuses endodontic treatment.

Endodontic Prognosis   The clinician's expertise and the technical difficulty of performing root canal treatment for a particular case are factors that determine the endodontic prognosis. Restricted access or the presence of calcified canals or curved roots increase the difficulty of treatment. Previously root-treated teeth with evidence of iatrogenic problems (e.g., a blocked canal, ledge, perforation) make root canal therapy challenging, even for the experienced clinician. In such cases the dentist may better serve the patient by referral to an endodontist.

Another factor affecting the clinician's ability to perform ideal endodontic treatment is patient management. Some patients may be so apprehensive that they create stress for the entire dental office. They may not permit treatment to be performed even though they desire it. These patients are best treated with oral or intravenous sedation to reduce anxiety. If the clinician is uncomfortable administering sedation, referral to a specialist is indicated.

Treatment Planning

Once a diagnosis has been made and the prognosis has been determined, a treatment plan is established. If the treatment required is within the skill and expertise of the dentist, then the patient can be treated right away. If uncertainty remains about the diagnosis or the required treatment is too challenging, the patient should be referred to an endodontist or other pain specialist for further evaluation and management.

MANAGEMENT OF THE DENTAL EMERGENCY PATIENT

In an acute pain emergency the physical problem and the emotional state of the patient should be considered. The dentist's reactions to the patient are important for both pain and patient management. The patient's needs, fears about the immediate problem, and defenses for coping with the situation, must be compassionately understood. This assessment and the clinician's ability to build rapport with the patient are key factors in proper interaction between the dentist and patient. This psychodynamic exchange involves five key aspects[58,81,153]:

1. The patient is to be treated responsibly. All symptoms and complaints are perceived as real. The patient must see that the dentist is giving all complaints and symptoms serious consideration. Concern and empathy must be shown for the individual.
2. A show of support for a patient's complaint is reflected through listening actively, expressing empathy, being nonjudgmental, and establishing and maintaining eye contact with the patient.[81] However, this support does not imply absolute agreement; the patient's symptoms and complaints must be evaluated thoroughly before a diagnosis is made.
3. A calm and confident professionalism should be displayed. This demeanor can be expressed verbally and nonverbally. Eye contact, supportive touching of the patient's shoulder, or body contact while moving the patient into the treatment chair is reassuring to the patient. Building rapport with patients requires sensitivity (providing care without positive statements or gestures is an obstacle to effective patient management).
4. A positive attitude to the patient's problem can make the individual aware that an efficient and effective treatment

or referral will be made. They must never feel that they will be abandoned.
5. Once a diagnosis is made and treatment determined, the patient should be informed about what to expect. Discussing the procedures and physical sensations that the patient will experience is useful; the patient's anxiety should be accepted as common and normal. Giving permission to be anxious can help to modulate the emotional responses of a patient in an emergency situation.[81,214]

Management of the orofacial pain emergency requires a comprehensive understanding of the patient's experience and feelings. The dentist who is perceptive, adaptable, and can actively participate in the dynamic interplay will avoid many potential hardships and failures in patient management.

The following treatment approaches pertain to permanent teeth with mature apices. (For a discussion of diagnosis and treatment of primary teeth, immature permanent teeth, and traumatic injuries, see Chapter 16.)

Anesthesia

Attaining profound anesthesia is paramount to rendering emergency treatment. This can be difficult, even for an experienced practitioner. Suppression of the nociceptive action potential is hampered by the numerous inflammatory pathways that are operating in the area. As the inflammatory process progresses, local tissue pH falls precipitously. The acidic environment prevents the anesthetic molecule from dissociating into ion form, and the cation is unable to migrate through the neural sheath. Further, the inflamed nerve fibers are morphologically and biochemically altered throughout their length by neuropeptides, such as CGRP and other neurochemicals. Therefore in a state of hyperalgesia, nerve block injections at sites distant from the inflamed tooth are rendered less effective.[129] (This issue is fully discussed in Chapter 20.)

To avoid this problem, the clinician must select alternate and supplementary sites for injecting anesthetic solution. Consideration must be given to the type and amount of anesthetic solution required for the conditions. There may be anatomic limitations, such as dense, bony plates, aberrant distribution of neural bundles, or accessory innervation, especially in the mandible. The clinician should be skilled in all of the anesthetic techniques that may be required (see Chapter 20).

The nerve block injection (of a nerve trunk central to an area or tooth) is the standard intraoral approach for achieving initial regional anesthesia. However, conventional local anesthetic techniques are sometimes unsuccessful in obtaining profound anesthesia for endodontic procedures. In difficult cases depositing a greater volume of anesthetic in the region increases the likelihood of achieving pain control. The periodontal ligament injection (i.e., intraligamentary injection)[30,208] and the intraosseous injection[43] are effective adjuncts to a conventional nerve block. If the pulp chamber is exposed and the pulp remains sensitive, the intrapulpal injection will anesthetize the remainder of the pulp tissue. Profound local anesthesia is essential. Only a complete lack of sensation will allow for effective therapy to ensue.

The "Hot Tooth"

Most dentists have seen a patient with a tooth that is difficult to anesthetize: the "hot tooth." Scientists have shown that there is a special class of sodium channels on C fibers, known as tetrodotoxin-resistant (TTXr).[67] Sodium channel expression shifts from TTX-sensitive to TTXr during neuroinflammatory reactions, and the TTXr sodium channels play a role in sensitizing C fibers and creating inflammatory hyperalgesia.

One of the clinically significant characteristics of these sodium channels is that they are relatively resistant to lidocaine.[160] Researchers found these channels to be five times more resistant to anesthetic than TTX-sensitive channels. After a mandibular block, a patient may describe profound anesthesia of the ipsilateral lip and tongue. However, entering the vital pulp chamber may initiate pain. This may be explained by the fact that the TTXr sodium channels have not been adequately blocked by the anesthetic. Additional anesthetic or supplemental injections are necessary to achieve profound anesthesia. Importantly, bupivicaine was found to be more potent than lidocaine in blocking TTXr channels[160] and may be the anesthetic of choice when treating the "hot tooth." Supplemental intraligamentary or intraosseous injections are most helpful to ensure profound local anesthesia.

EMERGENCY TREATMENT

Dentin Hypersensitivity

It is important to understand that symptoms consistent with reversible pulpitis may actually be dentin hypersensitivity devoid of pulpal inflammation. In such cases therapeutic dentinal-tubule occlusion is directed toward reduction or elimination of dentinal fluid movement. There has been limited success in treatment of exposed dentinal tubules and associated hypersensitivity caused by recession of attachment apparatus, abrasion of cervical tooth structure, or after periodontal treatment.

Reduction of the diameter of the dentinal tubules reduces the hydraulic conductance of dentin and, consequently, dentin hypersensitivity. Researchers[141] have discovered several physiological effects that reduce the diameter of dentin tubules. These include intratubular crystals from saliva and dentinal fluid, intratubular collagen plugs, the formation of irritation dentin, and leakage of large plasma proteins into tubules.

Dentinal hypersensitivity can be reduced by application of sodium fluoride,[141] fluorides and a thin layer of varnish,[19] potassium oxalate[5] and ferric oxalate,[41] as well as calcium

hydroxide,[69] cyanoacrylate,[89] and resin impregnation[217] to the exposed dentin. Other researchers[86,203] found that a high concentration of calcium phosphate solutions readily precipitate amorphous calcium phosphates on dentin discs. These salts obstruct the dentinal tubules and decrease dentin permeability by 85%. However, daily toothbrushing and the consumption of acidic beverages may remove the precipitates, thereby restoring hypersensitivity.

Dentin tubule occlusion is not the only way to reduce dentinal hypersensitivity. Hyperpolarization of the interdental nerves interferes with nerve transmission by raising the extracellular potassium ion concentration. Several studies have shown that dentifrices containing potassium nitrate are efficacious.[188] After applying potassium nitrate to deep cavities, investigators found that there was an initial burst of nerve firing, after which the nerves became insensitive to further stimulation.[130]

Laser irradiation has been reported to reduce dentinal permeability.[180,218] Various types of lasers, including Nd:YAG, carbon dioxide, and excimer, have been advocated. However, caution must be exercised in the use of lasers on dentin in vivo, because dentin heating may cause injury to the dental pulp.[163]

Reversible Pulpitis

Ideally pulp preservation measures should take priority in the management of reversible pulpitis. Removal of the cause of irritation should allow the pulpal inflammation to subside and symptoms to dissipate.

If caries is diagnosed, the tooth should be properly restored after thorough, atraumatic caries removal. If the clinician determines that reversible pulpitis has developed after operative procedures, the tooth should be allowed several weeks to recover before the need for endodontic intervention is considered. If symptoms do not resolve, or they progress to irreversible pulpitis, root canal treatment should be initiated. When examination of a recently placed restoration reveals marginal defects and probable microleakage, the restoration should be removed and replaced temporarily with a sedative dressing, such as zinc oxide eugenol. To assess the relative effectiveness of this treatment, the tooth must be allowed to recover before a judgment is made. If symptoms subside, a permanent restoration is placed. However, the patient must be informed that pulpal degeneration may occur in the future.

A recently placed restoration that is found to be in hyperocclusion should be adjusted to eliminate occlusal trauma as a source of discomfort. Hyperocclusion is not a cause of irreversible pulpitis.

In the management of reversible pulpitis, certain factors can alter subsequent treatment decisions. These factors include: evidence of previous "pulp stress," including significant fracture lines, large or deep areas of caries, extensive recurrent caries, or the *chronopathologic status* (i.e., age and current health) of the tooth in question. The defensive capabilities of the pulp diminish with successive treatment of the aging tooth, which adversely affects pulp vitality.[185] Chronopathologic factors include history of previous pulpal exposure and pulp capping procedures, history of trauma, periodontal disease, and history of extensive restorations (i.e., pins, buildups, crown).

The clinician must assess each factor on the basis of the adverse effect it may have had on pulpal health in the past, as well as any adverse affects it may have on pulpal health in the future. The dentist must then decide on the most appropriate treatment that will conserve the integrity of the pulpal tissue. At times, this may not be practical, and treatment may shift from pulp-preservation measures to elective removal of the pulp and sealing of the root canal system in anticipation of long-term restoration (especially if the restorative treatment plan for the tooth is extensive).

Cracked Tooth "Syndrome"

The cracked tooth "syndrome" consists of an incomplete fracture of a tooth with a vital pulp. The fracture involves the enamel and the dentin. In some cases it may also involve the dental pulp. Symptoms may vary; they include pain on chewing, varied patterns of referred pain, and sensitivity to thermal changes.[7] The most common symptom is sharp pain that occurs upon release of chewing pressure. Percussion of the teeth, careful probing with an explorer, and biting on a Tooth Slooth facilitates diagnosis. The Tooth Slooth is a small pyramid-shaped plastic bite block, with a small concavity at the apex of the pyramid to accommodate the tooth cusp. This small indentation is placed over the cusp, and the patient is asked to bite down. Force is directed to one cusp at a time, directing the desired force to the questionable cusp. Pain upon release of pressure is a strong indication of the presence of a cracked tooth. The use of a fiber-optic light to transilluminate a fracture line and staining the fracture with a dye, such as methylene blue, are valuable aids to detect a fracture. Most cracks run mesiodistally and are rarely detected radiographically when they are incomplete.

Molars of older individuals are the most frequently affected by cracked tooth "syndrome."[28] Most cases occur in teeth with class 1 restorations (39%) or that are unrestored (25%) but have an opposing plunger cusp occluding centrically against a marginal ridge. Mandibular molars are most commonly affected, followed by maxillary molars and maxillary premolars.[78]

Urgent care of the cracked tooth involves the immediate reduction of its occlusal contacts by selective grinding at the site of the crack or against the cusp or cusps of the occluding antagonist. Definitive treatment of a cracked tooth attempts to preserve pulpal vitality by requiring full occlusal coverage for cusp protection.[161] Cusp coverage may seem drastic, but a vertical crack that is left unprotected will migrate "pulpally" and apically. When the aging defect encroaches on the pulp, emerging endodontic symptoms, consistent with irreversible pulpitis, are indicative of the unavoidable need for root canal treatment. A long-standing defect can be apparent by heavy staining in a tooth that is asymptomatic. It is possible that slow pulp degeneration explains the absence of symptoms.

Endodontic treatment can alleviate irreversible pulpal symptoms in a vertically cracked tooth. Tooth retention, however, remains questionable. The apical extension and future migration of the defect down onto the root will decide the outcome.[161] If the fracture is not detected, pulpal degeneration and periradicular pathosis may be the initial indication that a complete vertical fracture is present.

When vertical root fractures occur, they are most commonly found in root-filled teeth. During obturation, the wedging effect of a spreader or plugger may cause a vertical fracture.[212] Structurally weakened root-treated teeth that have been restored with a short, wide, tapered post have the highest incidence of vertical fractures.[38] The chances of root fracture are increased if the coronal restoration fails to provide a ferrule affect on the remaining root structure.[87] Pain during mastication is the most common symptom. In severe cases, a root fracture may be visible radiographically; the presence of a lateral diffuse widening of the periodontal ligament is the characteristic radiographic appearance.[187] Periodontal probing may locate an isolated, narrow pocket adjacent to the fracture site. Frequently, a sinus tract is noted closer to the gingival margin than the apical area. If a fracture is suspected, a full thickness mucoperiosteal flap should be reflected. To corroborate the diagnosis, the root should then be stained and viewed under magnification.

The prognosis for a vertical root fracture extending apically from the alveolar crest is poor, and tooth extraction is often indicated.

Irreversible Pulpitis

Emergency management for painful, irreversible pulpitis involves initiating root canal treatment to alleviate the pain. Irreversible pulpitis can be predictably managed by complete removal of the pulp and total cleaning and shaping of the root canal system.

In multirooted teeth, a pulpotomy (i.e., the removal of the coronal pulp) or partial pulpectomy (i.e., the removal of the pulp from the widest canal) have been advocated for emergency treatment of irreversible pulpitis. However, because it is impossible to detect clinically the apical extent of the inflamed pulp and, therefore, provide predictable pain relief, it is important to perform a pulpectomy at the emergency visit.[59]

A file should not be introduced into any canal unless a pulpectomy is anticipated. Often inflamed vital pulp tissue that is lacerated with endodontic files will result in increased discomfort, because the pulp has become inflamed, shredded, and traumatized. Pain symptoms can persist or worsen if inflamed pulp remains in the root canals, because the inflammatory process will extend into the periradicular tissues. A popular idea that medicaments sealed in canals help control or prevent additional pain has not been fully substantiated. A dry cotton pellet is as effective in relieving pain as a pellet moistened with camphorated monochlorophenol (CMCP), Cresatin, eugenol, or saline.[77] *Complete removal of the pulp is the best treatment.*

There appears to be no contraindication to single-visit endodontic treatment for teeth diagnosed with irreversible pulpitis, providing there is no evidence of pretreatment apical periodontitis. Postoperative pain and the long-term prognosis after single-visit endodontics is similar to root canal treatment completed in multiple visits. Because temporary restorations eventually leak, obturation in one visit eliminates the possibility of interappointment bacterial contamination of the root canal system. However, time constraints at the emergency visit often make the single-visit treatment option difficult. If obturation is to be completed at a later date, medicating the canal with calcium hydroxide is indicated to reduce the chances of bacterial growth in the canal between appointments. Complete caries removal and an effective temporary coronal seal are mandatory to prevent contamination of the root canal system between appointments. Although it is usually unnecessary if the pulp has been removed, the occlusion should be reduced.[152]

Irreversible Pulpitis with Acute Apical Periodontitis

Complete pulp removal is particularly important in the emergency treatment of irreversible pulpitis with acute apical periodontitis. In this case pulpal inflammation has spread to the periradicular tissues, resulting in a combination of pulpal and periapical symptoms. Between visits, the canals should be medicated with calcium hydroxide to prevent bacterial regrowth.[31] Occlusal reduction has been reported to reduce postoperative pain in patients whose teeth initially exhibit pulpal vitality, percussion sensitivity, and preoperative pain.[152] Teeth with irreversible pulpitis should not be left open between visits because bacterial contamination of the cleansed canal will occur.

After root canal treatment, apical periodontitis can develop as a result of trauma to the periradicular tissues or from the inflammatory response to debris extruded beyond the confines of the root canal system. If all tissue has been removed from the root canal system, this is best managed with oral analgesic medications.

Apical periodontitis caused by traumatic occlusion often results in pain on biting, eating, or "when the teeth come together." Often a recent restoration has been placed with a high contact. Treatment includes occlusal adjustment to remove the premature contact.

Pulpal Necrosis with Acute Periradicular Abscess

No Swelling   The treatment of pulpal necrosis with periapical symptoms should involve thorough removal of necrotic pulp tissue from the root canal system. Complete cleaning and shaping of the root canals and placement of a calcium hydroxide dressing is the goal of emergency treatment. Some practitioners feel that if necrotic debris is not pushed beyond the apex, the patient will have less postoperative discomfort.[152] This is attempted by maintaining root canal instrumentation 2 mm to 3 mm short of the root apices. However, it is the opinion of the authors that complete instrumentation of the canal or canals is appropriate (at the emergency visit) to remove as much of the canal contents as possible. This includes introducing a small file (size 10 or 15) slightly beyond the apex to ensure patency of the canal. This is done to establish drainage from the periapical tissues. It is especially useful when the clinician has diagnosed pulpal necrosis with acute periradicular abscess, but where no drainage has been achieved by access into the root canals. Because of the possibility of iatrogenic damage (i.e., apical transportation), care must be taken to prevent aggressive extension with large files past the apical foramen.

Emergency treatment of previously root treated teeth that are symptomatic and have extensive restorations (including posts and cores, crowns and bridgework) can be difficult and time consuming. However, the goal remains the same: removing contaminants from the root canal system and establishing patency to achieve drainage. Gaining access to the periradicular tissues through the root canals may require removal of posts and failing root canal fillings, as well as negotiation of blocked or ledged canals. On occasion the canal may be obstructed with blocks or ledges that prevent canal negotiation. Failure to completely debride the canals and to achieve periapical drainage will likely result in continued painful symptoms. *Surgical trephination* may be of assistance in these cases.

Trephination is the surgical perforation of the alveolar cortical plate (over the root end of a tooth) to release accumulated tissue exudate that is causing pain.[7] This procedure may provide pain relief in patients with severe and recalcitrant periradicular pain. The technique involves making a small, vertical incision adjacent to the tooth in question. The mucosa is retracted with a tissue retractor, and a number six round bur is used to penetrate the cortical plate. An endodontic file has been suggested to bore a path through the cancellous bone toward the periradicular tissues or lesion, avoiding contact with the root structure or adjacent vital roots. This provides a pathway for drainage from the periradicular tissues.[70] Recently a rediscovered technique has been described that uses an engine-driven perforator to enter the medullary bone without the need for an incision.[29] When performed prophylactically along with root canal therapy, trephination has been shown to decrease postoperative pain in patients with chronic apical periodontitis.[144] However, a recent study failed to show a difference in postoperative pain when pulpectomy was performed with or without surgical trephination in patients with symptomatic apical periodontitis.[122] Indeed, the additional trauma of the surgical procedure may add to the pain process.

Research has indicated that there is little difference in postoperative pain in cases of pulpal necrosis obturated at the time of the emergency or obturated at a later date.[48] However, recent studies have questioned the long-term prognosis of such treatment. For example, a few investigators[178,199] have indicated that, in necrotic cases, single-visit treatment has a lower success rate when compared with single treatment in vital cases. They suggested that the reason for this discrepancy was the presence of bacteria that survive root canal instrumentation. However, a close examination of their methods and materials reveals this may have been due to an uncommonly high dilution of NaOCl to merely 0.5%. (For more information on this issue, see Chapter 8.) If bacteria are present in the root canal at the time of obturation, the long-term outcome of endodontic therapy is less predictable. For infected cases it is recommended that a calcium hydroxide dressing be placed in the root canal system between appointments to help eliminate remaining bacteria before obturation.[26,177]

With Swelling

Tissue swelling associated with an acute periradicular abscess may be seen at the initial emergency visit, as an interappointment flare-up, or as a postendodontic complication. Swellings may be localized or diffuse, fluctuant or firm. Localized swellings are confined within the oral cavity. A diffuse swelling or cellulitis is characterized by its spread through adjacent soft tissues, dissecting tissue spaces along fascial planes.

There are three ways to resolve swelling and infection:
1. Establish drainage through the root canal
2. Establish drainage by incising a fluctuant swelling
3. Antibiotic treatment

The cardinal rule for managing all of these infections is to *achieve* drainage.[73] When there is a localized swelling, it is the consensus among endodontists to clean and shape the root canal system with copious irrigation using = > 2.5% NaOCl. The drainage should be allowed to stop; then the root canals should be dried, medicated with calcium hydroxide, and closed.[59] Gentle finger pressure to the mucosa overlying the swelling and positive aspiration of the pulp chamber will aid drainage. On very rare occasions, if pus continues to drain through the canal and cannot be dried within a reasonable period of time, the tooth may be left open. If good drainage is achieved by access and instrumentation of the root canal system, then no incision and drainage procedure is needed (Figs. 2-8 and 2-9).

The systemic use of antibiotics in treating swellings caused by pulpal necrosis should be regarded as an aid to drainage.[59] The objective is to aid the elimination of pus from the tissue spaces. However, if bacteria remain within the root canal system, resolution of the acute condition is compromised.[59,116] Thorough removal of the diseased pulp, along with primarily anaerobic bacteria and their endotoxins, prevents these irritants from overwhelming the periradicular tissues. Generally the use of antibiotics alone (without concurrent attempts to establish drainage and clean the pulpal space) is not considered appropriate treatment.[73,83]

With localized swelling the clinician is dealing with an abscess that is confined within the oral cavity. The swelling

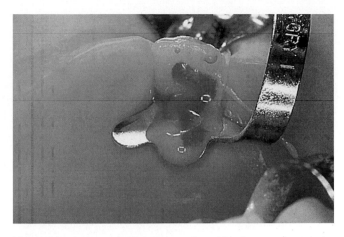

Fig. 2-8   Acute periradicular abscess relieved by drainage through the access opening. (Courtesy Dr. Eric Herbranson.)

does not have the same potential to spread as a diffuse swelling. Therefore it is treated less aggressively. A diffuse swelling indicates an advanced infection that is potentially dangerous for the patient (see Chapter 13 for a comprehensive discussion of how these infections must be managed). More aggressive treatment is necessary to minimize the possibility of the infection spreading. It is appropriate to use a systemic antibiotic for any diffuse swelling, whether or not drainage is obtained from the root canal or the soft tissue (Fig. 2-10).

Incision and drainage.   Management of a localized soft tissue swelling can be facilitated through incision and drainage of the area (Fig. 2-11). Fluctuance, the sensation (on palpation) that there is fluid movement under the tissue, indicates that pus is present. Profound anesthesia may prove more difficult in the infection site. Soft tissue infiltration of anesthetic around the periphery of the distended tissues may achieve a reasonable degree of anesthesia and permit tissue manipulation with minimum discomfort. Infiltration into the superficial mucosa overlying the swelling allows for anesthesia directly over the site of the infected tissues.

The following principles should be observed when employing incision and drainage therapy:
1. The clinician should make the incision at the site of greatest fluctuance.
2. The clinician should dissect gently, through the deeper tissues, and thoroughly explore all parts of the abscess cavity. This will allow compartmentalized areas of pus to be disrupted and evacuated. The dissection should then be extended to the roots of the teeth responsible for the pathosis.
3. To promote drainage, the wound should be kept clean with hot saltwater mouth rinses. (Intraoral heat application to infected tissues results in a dilation of small vessels, intensifying host defenses through increased vascular flow.[73,83])

Some clinicians recommend suturing an indwelling drain into the incision to maintain active drainage; others do

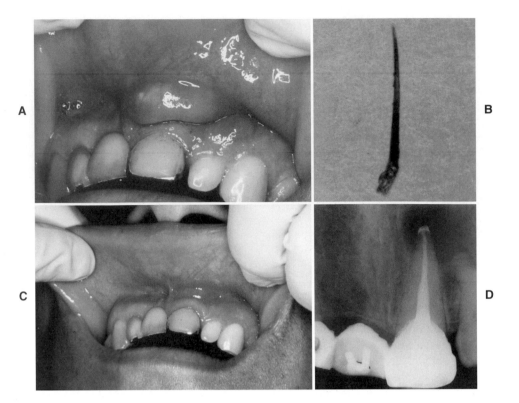

Fig. 2-9 **A**, large vestibular swelling associated with failing gutta-percha fill in tooth #9. Tooth #10 tested vital. **B**, After gutta-percha removal, the canal exhibited profuse drainage. Incision and drainage was accomplished. Black discoloration of the gutta-percha is likely pigmentation associated with bacterial growth. **C**, Near complete resolution of the swelling 1 week after cleansing and shaping of the canal. **D**, Postoperative radiograph.

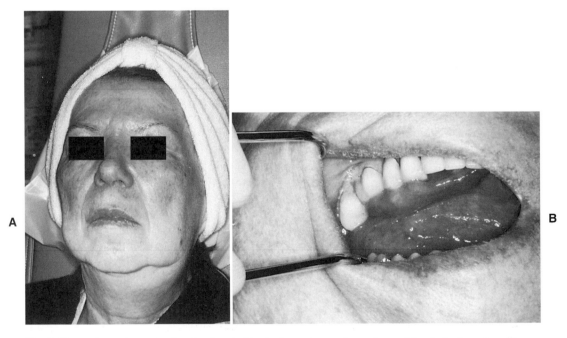

Fig. 2-10 **A**, This patient arrived at the dental office in the early morning and complained of pain and swelling on her left side. She said she had difficulty swallowing. **B**, An intraoral exam shows that the patient is so severely swollen that the floor of her mouth is elevated and protruding onto her front teeth. Her tongue is pushed up to the roof of her mouth, which makes it difficult for her to eat or swallow. Tooth #18 had a necrotic pulp, and the infection spread into her submandibular, submental, and masticator spaces. She was admitted to the hospital the same day, where she was placed on intravenous antibiotics. Her tooth was extracted, and she was released from the hospital 2 days later.

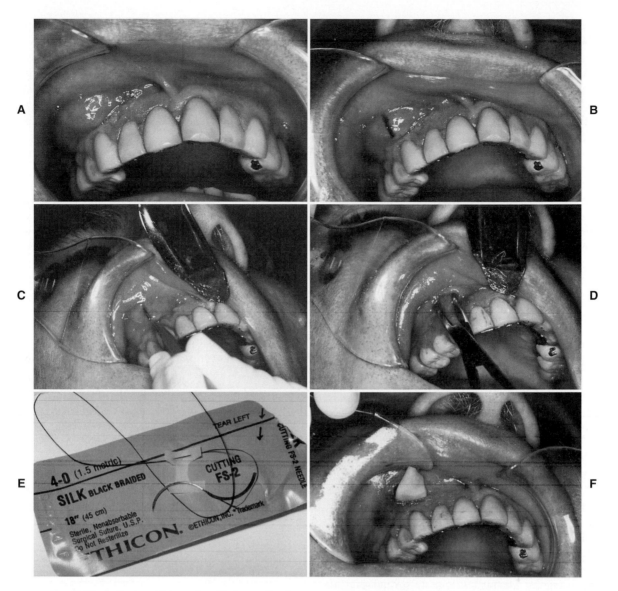

Fig. 2-11 **A,** Fluctuant intraoral vestibular swelling from a maxillary molar requires incision and drainage. **B,** Vertical placement of incision is marked for location. **C,** Incision is made through the swelling to the base of the alveolar bone. **D,** Surgical hemostat dissects and facilitates drainage. **E,** Suture placement through a rubber dam drain (optional). **F,** Indwelling drain may be removed in 24 to 48 hours. (Courtesy Dr. Alex McDonald.)

not place any drains into the incision site. In the region of the mental foramen, care must be taken to prevent damage to the underlying neurovascular bundle. A point of contention is whether to incise an indurated swelling or wait until the tissues become fluctuant. Early incision of an indurated swelling can reduce pain from increasing tissue distention, even if only hemorrhagic fluid is obtained. Medical therapy of the dentoalveolar abscess consists mainly of supportive care, hydration, soft diet, analgesics, and oral hygiene.

A diffuse swelling can turn into a medical emergency of potentially life threatening complications. For this reason, most endodontists[59] advise a more aggressive treatment approach. The tooth is opened, and the root canal is thoroughly instrumented and irrigated. If possible, apical patency should be achieved to encourage drainage from the periapical tissues. In the absence of drainage through the tooth, soft-tissue drainage must be established through incision of the diffusely swollen tissues. An indwelling drain may be sutured into the incision wound to promote tissue drainage. Individuals who show signs of toxicity, CNS changes, or airway compromise should be referred to an oral surgeon for immediate hospitalization, with aggressive medical and surgical intervention.[125]

Antibiotic therapy.   If drainage is achieved, antibiotic therapy is usually unnecessary for patients with localized swellings. Conversely, minor infections in immunocompromised patients should be treated with bactericidal drugs as soon as possible. Antibiotics are indicated for a diffuse swelling that drains inadequately, or in cases of pulpal necrosis, where it is impossible to gain access to the root canal terminus. Patients with spreading infections or systemic signs of illness (e.g., elevated temperature or malaise) also require antibiotics.[70]

Ideally the choice of antibiotic depends on the definitive laboratory results of culture and antibiotic sensitivity testing. Because most dentoalveolar infections and swellings occur in otherwise healthy patients, cultures are not routinely performed. If antibiotic choice is based on scientific data and clinical experience, empirical antibiotic selection is acceptable, both ethically and legally. Penicillin VK is effective against most aerobic and anaerobic oral bacteria, and it remains the drug of choice for many oral infections.[73,83,125] Amoxicillin, a derivative of penicillin, has a broader spectrum. However, there is an increased likelihood of inducing antibiotic resistance than with penicillin.[76] Metronidazole is a bactericidal synthetic antimicrobial that is effective against anaerobes. However, it is ineffective against facultative anaerobic bacteria. If penicillin is ineffective after 48 to 72 hours, the combination of penicillin and metronidazole is indicated (see Chapters 13 and 18).

Clindamycin is an appropriate antibiotic for patients who are allergic to penicillin.[116,192] It is beta lactamase resistant and is highly effective against orofacial infections. Erythromycin, which is commonly prescribed for patients with an allergy to penicillin, has been shown to be ineffective against most of the anaerobes associated with endodontic infections. Thus it is no longer recommended.

Proper drug dosage and selection of an antibiotic with a spectrum that covers the likely causative bacteria are important. To achieve a therapeutic concentration of the drug and to minimize the risk of developing resistant bacteria, antibiotic therapy should be short and aggressive. The patient should be instructed to adhere closely to the dosing schedule and to complete the entire course of antibiotics. A loading dose of 1000 mg of penicillin VK should be followed by 500 mg every 6 hours, for 7 days. The recommended oral dosage of metronidazole is a loading dose of 500 mg, with 250 mg every 6 hours, for 7 days. The usual adult dose of clindamycin begins with a loading dose of 300 mg, followed by 150 mg every 6 hours, for 7 days.

Laboratory diagnostic adjuncts. When an infection is severe or a patient is medically compromised, purulent samples should be collected and sent to a laboratory for culturing and isolation immediately. In these serious situations a clinical diagnosis of any infectious pathogens should be confirmed by laboratory methods (Fig. 2-12). However, some delay must be anticipated in awaiting a response from the laboratory, because culturing for anaerobic bacteria requires at least 1 to 2 weeks (see Chapter 13). Even when a culture is taken, antibiotic treatment should begin immediately. This is because oral infections progress rapidly, and the patient's condition may deteriorate while waiting for the laboratory results.

Specimens representative of the site of infection should be collected in an amount sufficient for both direct examination and culture. Specimens can be aspirated with a disposable syringe, recapped, and submitted *in toto*. This provides a safe method for collection of aerobic and anaerobic bacteria, and it allows for gram-staining procedures. Because anaerobic bacteria are always present in dentoalveolar infections,[4] specimens should be submitted in a transport medium that prevents desiccation and oxygen contamination. A variety of commercially prepackaged transport systems are suitable for this purpose. A maximum of 2 hours should be allowed to elapse between collection and microbiologic examination of the specimens.

It should be emphasized that the patient should contact the dentist at any time for additional instructions or an alternative course of action, should the situation worsen. Analgesics should be prescribed, and the patient should be monitored closely over the next several days until there is improvement.

Progressive deterioration of the patient's condition, as evidenced by increased swelling, a sustained high fever, mental confusion, and difficulty swallowing or breathing, is sufficient reason to hospitalize the patient for more specialized care and around-the-clock monitoring. The laboratory findings may guide the clinician or subsequent doctor in the proper choice of an antibiotic regimen.[73,83,125]

Pharmacologic Management

The pharmacologic management of the endodontic emergency patient consists of controlling pain and infection. As previously mentioned, patients who are prescribed antibiotics should be carefully instructed to follow the dosing

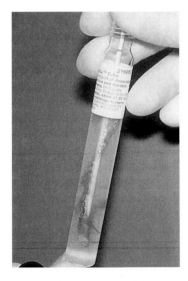

Fig. 2-12 Culture and antibiotic sensitivity testing of pathogenic microorganisms can be conducted with both aerobic and anaerobic techniques. Commercially available sample swabs and transport media are to be used as directed.

schedules and complete the entire course of medication. For pain, nonsteroidal antiinflammatory drugs (NSAIDs) are the drugs of choice because they inhibit portions of the inflammatory cascade, which acetaminophen cannot do. Therefore patients with moderate to severe pain benefit most from opioid analgesics in combination with NSAIDs. (For a complete discussion of pharmacology and specific regimens, please refer to Chapter 18.)

A summary of diagnosis and management of the endodontic emergency is given in Tables 2-1 and 2-2.

ENDODONTIC FLARE-UPS AND MIDTREATMENT URGENT CARE

Definition

Many researchers and clinicians who write about endodontic flare-ups define this expected treatment complication differently. Some have defined a flare-up as pain and/or swelling that requires an unscheduled patient visit and active intervention by the dentist.[209] The American Association of Endodontists defines a flare-up as an acute exacerbation of peri-

TABLE 2-1   CLINICAL EMERGENCY ENDODONTIC DIAGNOSIS

Signs and Symptoms	Pulpal Diagnosis	Periapical Diagnosis
Sharp pain from exposed dentin on application of thermal or osmotic stimuli or both. No relevant dental abnormality.	Normal (Dentin hypersensitivity)	Normal
Sharp pain on application of thermal or osmotic stimuli or both. Evidence of dental caries, fractured restoration, restorative treatment, cracked cusps.	Reversible pulpitis	Normal
Spontaneous, throbbing pain, sharp pain on application of thermal stimuli that persists following removal of stimulus.	Irreversible pulpitis	Normal
Spontaneous, throbbing pain, sharp pain on application of thermal stimuli that persists following removal of stimulus. Tenderness to bite or percussion or both. Radiographic widening of PDL likely.	Irreversible pulpitis	Acute apical periodontitis
Spontaneous, throbbing pain. No response to thermal stimuli. Tenderness to bite or percussion or both. Localized or diffuse swelling may be present. Radiographically may be inconclusive or lesion.	Necrosis	Acute periradicular abscess

TABLE 2-2   ENDODONTIC EMERGENCY TREATMENT

Diagnosis and Symptoms	Treatment	Postop Med
Irreversible pulpitis (asymptomatic)	Complete cleaning and shaping Obturate if time permits	NSAIDs Corticosteroids
Irreversible pulpitis (with acute apical periodontitis)	Complete cleaning and shaping * See below	NSAIDs (Narcotic) Corticosteroids
Pulpal necrosis (no swelling)	Complete cleaning and shaping Calcium hydroxide therapy	NSAIDs
Pulpal necrosis (localized swelling)	Complete cleaning and shaping Calcium hydroxide therapy Incision and drainage	NSAIDs
Pulpal necrosis (diffuse swelling)	Complete cleaning and shaping Calcium hydroxide therapy Incision and drainage	NSAIDs Antibiotics

* The extent of pulpal degeneration and periapical inflammation determine if a calcium hydroxide dressing should be placed at the initial appointment. Based on clinical and scientific principles, the practitioner must decide if the root canal treatment should be completed in one or more appointments.

radicular pathosis after the initiation or continuation of root canal treatment.[7] As the definition of flare-ups varies, so does the reported incidence of these exacerbations (1.4% to nearly 45%).[85,123,126,196,209] Because of the variability in the reported incidence of flare-ups, it is important to be cautious when comparing different studies to one another.

Causes

The causes of flare-ups are numerous and often multifactorial. The following discussion of urgent care for midtreatment exacerbations will focus on contributing factors, treatment modalities, and prevention.

Contributing Factors

Inadequate Debridement
Persistent pain or onset of acute pain often signals the presence of residual pulp tissue in inadequately instrumented or still-undetected canals. Inadequate debridement of a pulp that has degenerated or is degenerating allows bacteria and their toxins to remain in the root canal and act as a continuous irritant.[73] Overmedicating the tooth may also lead to acute onset of pain from medicaments that permeate into the periapical tissues. However, thorough debridement of the entire root canal system should eliminate the pain. Teeth with necrotic pulps (with or without associated periradicular lesions) are more prone to develop midtreatment flare-ups than are vital teeth. Complete elimination of the irritants from the root canal system is the treatment of choice; this usually results in the cessation of the inflammatory response. *Thorough debridement of the entire root canal space is a reasonable goal for initial management of all teeth.*

Debris Extrusion
Despite strict length control of instruments during root canal preparation, pulp tissue fragments, necrotic tissue, microorganisms, dentin filings, and canal irrigants are extruded beyond the apical foramen.[21,206] This may result in periapical inflammation and midtreatment or posttreatment pain. When flare-ups occur, pulpless teeth are the most problematic. Pulpless teeth with associated periradicular lesions are likely to be infected.[57,184] It is speculated that inadvertent extrusion of the infectious contents of the root canal predisposes the pulpless tooth to periapical exacerbation.[57,73]

Debris extrusion is a problem with all instrumentation techniques, however, some techniques cause less extrusion than others. Comparing the mean weights of apically extruded debris, researchers found that sonic instrumentation extruded the least debris. The cervical flaring technique and the ultrasonic technique followed closely.[51] Conventional hand instrumentation was shown to extrude the most debris; shaping the canal in the coronal aspect before apical preparation may reduce debris extrusion. Crown-down instrumentation techniques[154] and the balanced forces technique[117] have been shown to extrude significantly less debris

than step-back filing techniques (see Chapter 8). Both techniques rely upon early coronal flaring and a rotational manipulation of root canal instruments. A recent study reported that hand- or engine-driven instrumentation that uses rotation significantly reduces the amount of debris extruded apically, when compared with a push-pull (filing) technique.[146] Irrigation solutions may also be extruded during instrumentation. Forced irrigation of sodium hypochlorite beyond the apex of the tooth can cause violent tissue reactions and unbearable pain. In vital cases extruded irrigant has been found only in the space created by instrumentation. In necrotic cases the irrigant may go beyond instrumented areas.[158]

The presence of an apical dentinal plug may help prevent extrusion of debris beyond the apical foramen. The plug may reduce the potential for flare-ups, prevent overinstrumentation of the periapical tissues, and often prevent extrusion of the obturating material. However, because the plug could harbor infectious material, the long-term prognosis may be compromised.

Overinstrumentation
The correlation between endodontic overinstrumentation and postoperative pain has been demonstrated.[62] The incidence of moderate to severe pain is reported to be significantly higher if instrumentation occurs beyond the apical foramen. With care and attention, gross overinstrumentation is avoidable (see Chapter 8). Gross overinstrumentation may cause acute apical periodontitis, producing primarily inflammatory pain. If treatment is rendered using aseptic techniques, infection is not a factor in vital cases. However, a serosanguineous exudate (not pus) may be seen when a sterile paper point is placed into the apical extent of the canal or canals. In many symptomatic cases involving overinstrumentation, a profuse exudate will continue to be discharged, despite repeated and thorough reinstrumentation of the root canals. Placing a calcium hydroxide preparation (e.g., Ca[OH]$_2$ USP plus sterile water, Pulpdent, Hypo-Cal, VitApex [also contains iodoform]) against or slightly through the perforated foramen can control the problematic exudate. Once there is no discomfort in the tooth, treatment can be continued by removing the paste and maintaining instrumentation within the canal space.

Overfilling
The extrusion of sealer or gutta-percha or both into the periapical tissues of teeth with no periapical radiolucent areas is more likely to cause a higher incidence and degree of postobturation pain than similar teeth, filled flush or up to 1 mm short of their radiographic apices.[74,167,168] This, however, is not a universal finding, because some clinicians have found no correlation between the level of obturation, extrusion of sealer, and the intensity of postobturation pain.[194]

Even though overfilling with zinc-oxide eugenol sealers has been shown to cause chronic inflammation,[168] it may be that a small overfill of gutta-percha and/or sealer is not the primary cause of postobturation pain. Rather, some degree of overinstrumentation may have occurred before obturation, and gutta-percha protruding past the apex may be a sign of such an occurrence. Furthermore, it may not be possible to achieve a good apical seal in overinstrumented canals if the foramen has been transported. In these cases residual bacteria from the root canal are not sealed off, and percolation of apical tissue fluids into the root canal may provide the nourishment for these bacteria to grow. Symptoms may then ensue from bacterial proliferation inside the root canal system, which releases toxic substances periapically. Large overfills are a factor in postobturation pain. In addition, gross overfillings can cause nerve damage because of chemical toxicity of the extruded material and mechanical nerve damage caused by compressing or crushing forces of the foreign material.[132] Paraformaldehyde pastes are a classic example of neurotoxic substances that can cause irreversible nerve damage when released periapically. Surgical intervention is often required to remove such noxious irritants. A slight extrusion of gutta-percha is probably insignificant, affecting neither the long-term prognosis[106] nor the incidence of postoperative pain.[194]

One-Appointment Endodontics

Most patients experience little or no spontaneous pain after one-visit root canal therapy; only 2% may have severe pain.[55] In fact, the frequency of pain in single- or multi-visit root canal therapy does not differ.* Some studies have shown that single-appointment therapy produces postoperative pain less frequently than multi-visit treatments.[48,85,150] The reasons for the variability in studies are many, including the different criteria used to decide which cases can or should be treated in a single visit. The majority of endodontists have found that single-visit endodontics does not cause more flare-ups than multi-visit treatments.

Retreatment

Endodontists have found[85,192,197] that retreatment cases have a higher incidence of flare-ups. In these cases the host response to extruded filling materials and toxic solvents[213] may increase pain. Many retreatment cases have associated periapical pathoses, with symptoms that increase the likelihood of flare-ups.[192] Technically these cases are the most difficult and time consuming, with an increased chance for iatrogenic mishaps.

Microbiology and Immunology

Seven possible etiological factors for endodontic flare-ups have been described in the literature[171]:

1. The local adaptation syndrome—The introduction of a new irritant into inflamed tissue exacerbates a chronic problem.
2. Changes in periapical tissue pressure—Increased pressure causes pain because excessive exudate applies pressure to nerve endings; decreased pressure aspirates irri-

tants and microorganisms into the periapical space, exacerbating the inflammatory response.
3. The association between certain microorganisms and clinical signs and symptoms.
4. Chemical mediators of inflammation, such as prostaglandins, leukotrienes, Hageman factor, and the complement cascade.
5. Changes in cyclic nucleotides, such as cyclic AMP, affect biosynthetic and biodegradative pathways.
6. Immunologic responses—The production of antibodies plays a central role in the inflammatory response.
7. Psychologic factors—Fear and anxiety may exacerbate the patient's perception and tolerance of pain.

Periapical Lesion.   Some researchers have found apical radiolucencies to be correlated with an increased frequency of flare-ups.[85,126,196,209] The pulps of teeth with large periapical radiolucencies have more bacterial strains and are more infected.[104,126] These bacteria may cause an acute problem if inoculated periapically. Others found fewer problems when an apical lesion[114,123,127,192] or sinus tract is present, [85,192,209] because of the potential space for pressure release. In teeth with an intact periodontal ligament, the increased pressure that develops after an inflammatory response has nowhere to vent, so the area becomes more painful.

It is not clear what relationship periapical lesions have to the occurrence of exacerbations, because there is evidence supporting both sides of the controversy. It is also uncertain what significance pulpal status has on the incidence of flare-ups. Some investigators have found more flare-ups occurring in teeth with necrotic pulps[123,209] and others have not.[65,85,113]

Host factors   The intensity of preoperative pain and amount of patient apprehension are correlated to the degree of postoperative pain.[85,192,194,209] Patients with dental phobias are difficult to treat, because of their low psychophysiologic tolerance. Such patients may be best served by presedation, either oral or intravenous, to make their endodontic experience calmer. Other factors that have shown both positive and negative correlations with flare-ups include patients' age,* gender,* the presence of allergies,[191,209] and tooth position.* Race[127,209] and systemic disease[55,126,192] are not associated with increased flare-ups.

Treatment and Prevention of Flare-Ups

Studies have shown that postoperative pain will diminish to low levels within 72 hours.[65,74] This is a stressful time for the patient consumed by pain, as well as for the practitioner, whose job it is to help the patient. During this critical period, clinicians must know how to alleviate patients' pain quickly and effectively and prevent its recurrence.

---

*References 10,48,123,127,197,209

*References 10,48,55,65,85,123,126,127,192,209

Relaxing the Patient

The patient must feel relaxed and comfortable before treatment can begin and proceed smoothly and efficiently. Root canal treatment is one of the most anxiety-inducing dental procedures.[49] Researchers have shown that the amount of pain expected and experienced by dental patients is directly related to their anxiety.[96] Educating patients on the procedure to be performed will empower them with knowledge; it is often the misconception of the procedure that creates fear.

Some patients are so consumed with fear that they cannot be cooperative. These patients can make the dentist, assistants, and office personnel feel tense. General anesthesia and conscious intravenous sedation are excellent adjuncts for treating such patients. Unfortunately most dentists do not have the training to provide these services. A useful alternative is oral sedation with anxiolytic medication. Triazolam 0.25 mg (administered preoperatively) has been found to be a safe and effective medication.[47]

Compared with diazepam, it has a shorter half life and produces significantly more intraoperative amnesia, to the point where patients cannot recall local anesthetic administration. Other researchers have shown that traizolam has a greater anxiolytic effect when given sublingually, rather than orally. This is because of the increased bioavailability that occurs by avoiding the first-pass metabolism.[17] (For a complete discussion on management of pain and anxiety, refer to Chapter 20.)

Cleansing and Shaping

The single most effective method to reduce flare-ups is complete cleansing and shaping of the root canal system during the initial treatment visit. *The concepts of crown-down cleansing and shaping and confirming apical patency* (discussed in Chapter 8) *are two important factors in the strategic management of teeth that are likely to exhibit midtreatment flare-ups.*[66] As stated previously, symptomatic pulpless teeth and retreatment cases may be predisposed to interappointment exacerbations.[164,193] A crown-down shaping strategy is expeditious for removing the bulk of infected organic debris from the tooth with the least likelihood of midtreatment flare-up.

Calcium Hydroxide Therapy

Calcium hydroxide intracanal dressings are therapeutic in the prevention or treatment of flare-ups. Although the reasons for flare-ups are numerous, viable bacteria remaining within the root canal system is one of the most critical factors responsible for this problem.[26] Application of calcium hydroxide is intended to reduce bacterial colonies and their toxic by-products. It has been shown that the antimicrobial effects of calcium hydroxide are best achieved if the calcium hydroxide remains in the root canal system for at least 1 week[177] (Fig. 2-13). Removing the smear layer can facilitate the diffusion of calcium hydroxide through the dentinal tubules.[53] This step may be useful because bacterial lipopolysaccharides, which are involved in numerous inflammatory reactions,[156] can diffuse through dentin.[134] Furthermore, maintaining apical patency

may improve the therapeutic effects of calcium hydroxide. Researchers have found calcium ion diffusion to be greater through the apical foramen than through dentinal tubules.[149]

There are various methods by which calcium hydroxide can be placed in root canals. Using a Messing gun and vertical compaction, an injectable formulation of calcium hydroxide, a Lentulo spiral, a hand file, and paper points are all acceptable techniques.[175] A study comparing the use of a Lentulo spiral, the injection technique, and a hand file for placement of calcium hydroxide found that use of the Lentulo spiral most consistently delivered calcium hydroxide to working length with density, irrespective of the root canal curvature.[175] In contrast, the injection technique was limited by the root canal curvature and diameter, although others report that it may still be an effective delivery method.[181] Another delivery form for temporary dressing is calcium hydroxide gutta-percha points. However, studies have shown these to be inferior to the methods described previously.[27,44]

The possibility of calcium hydroxide reducing postoperative pain may depend on its ability to kill bacteria and neutralize their by-products. Studies have shown that calcium hydroxide hydrolyzes the lipid moiety of bacterial lipopolysaccharides, rendering it incapable of producing biologic effects, such as toxicity, pyrogenicity, macrophage activation, and complement activation.[156] Other investigators suggest that the antibacterial mechanism of calcium hydroxide may be related to its absorption of carbon dioxide, which would nutritionally starve capnophilic bacteria in the root canal system.[97] Additionally, calcium hydroxide may exert its effects by obliterating the root canal space, which minimizes the ingress of tissue exudate, a potential source of nourishment for remaining bacteria.[50,138,207]

Extrusion of calcium hydroxide into the periapical tissues may reduce inflammatory reactions by reducing the substrate adherence capacity of macrophages.[162] Researchers attribute the soft tissue dissolving potential and antibacterial effects of calcium hydroxide to its high pH.[8] The ability of calcium hydroxide to kill anaerobic bacteria may reduce the occurrence of flare-ups.[63] The exact therapeutic mechanisms of calcium hydroxide have not been clearly elucidated, but certain effects have been well studied. Because calcium hydroxide can dissolve necrotic tissue, the denaturing effect of calcium hydroxide on proteins allows sodium hypochlorite to dissolve remaining tissue more easily.[8,77] This tissue-dissolving effect works equally well in aerobic and anaerobic environments.[216] One of the only shortcomings of calcium hydroxide is its inability to effectively kill enterococcus species,[184] which are often associated with failed root canal treatment.[119,183,184]

Placement of calcium hydroxide between appointments is recommended for all teeth. Its therapeutic value is especially evident for symptomatic teeth, during long interappointment delays and when periapical infection is present.

Other Intracanal Medicaments

For root canals that require more than one visit to complete, there are sufficient

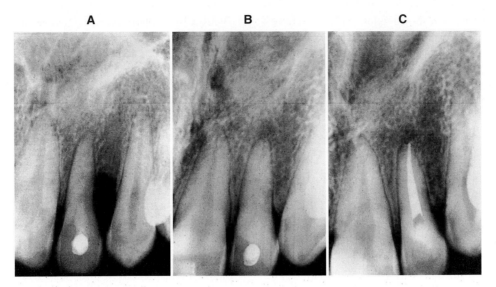

Fig. 2-13 **A**, Placement of calcium hydroxide one week after blunt trauma has devitalized the upper lateral incisor. After thorough cleaning and shaping, calcium hydroxide was placed to stimulate remineralization of the adjacent bone and to neutralize the acidic intracanal involvement. **B**, One week later. Remarkable remineralization of the alveolar matrix. **C**, Postobturation.

remaining bacteria within the system to grow and reinfect the root canal space between appointments.[14] Historically, placement of intracanal medicaments became a popular method of preventing bacterial regrowth. It may seem that eliminating bacteria would minimize any symptoms associated with reinfection, but numerous studies have found that the use of traditional intracanal medicaments has no effect on flare-ups.[74,191,196]

The decision to use an intracanal medicament should be guided by the antibacterial efficacy, toxicity, and specificity of the drug. For example, despite its superior antibacterial activity against anaerobes,[136] formocresol has been shown to cause periapical irritation and to be embryotoxic and teratogenic.[56] Cresatin and phenolic compounds, such as camphorated parachlorophenol, are bactericidal,[63,136,138] but also demonstrate toxicity to human cells.[179] Clindamycin-impregnated fibers have recently been suggested as an antimicrobial vehicle, however further research is needed to determine their safety and efficacy *in vivo*.[64] Chlorhexidine gluconate has been shown to have an antimicrobial efficacy that is comparable to sodium hypochlorite,[37,90,172] with a similar ability to penetrate dentinal tubules.[138] However, it is less toxic to periradicular tissues.[90] Iodine potassium iodide also has potent antibacterial effects, with minimal toxicity.[136,138,157]

Calcium hydroxide and chlorhexidine gluconate are the two primary medicaments to consider. Chlorhexidine is easy to deliver and can be dispensed through a syringe directly into root canals. Moreover, it has been shown to be as safe and effective as sodium hypochlorite[90,138,172]; its effect lasting as long as 72 hours.[211] Calcium hydroxide is a safe and effective intracanal medication that may be potentiated if it is mixed with chlorhexidine gluconate or iodine potassium iodide.[119]

Occlusal Reduction   Teeth with periapical inflammation may be extremely sensitive to occlusal forces. Occlusal reduction or selective adjustment of cusps is indicated as a palliative measure.[35,58,59,73] Researchers have found that the patients most likely to benefit from occlusal reductions are those whose teeth initially exhibit preoperative pain, pulp vitality, percussion sensitivity, the absence of a periradicular radiolucency, or a combination of these symptoms.[152] Temporary fillings that are overcontoured may cause intense periapical pain because of hyperocclusion, and they should be adjusted using articulating paper to ensure that the tooth does not hit prematurely.

Leaving Teeth Open   When a tooth is opened and purulence escapes, the exudate should stop after just a few minutes. Patients are instructed that their tooth will be allowed to drain for up to 20 minutes while the rubber dam is still in place. It is best to close all teeth immediately after treatment to prevent contamination by the oral cavity[13,59] and to prevent future problems, because *teeth left open are frequently involved in midtreatment flare-ups*.[171] On the rare occasion when exudate continues to well out of a tooth and prevent closure, the tooth may be left open to the oral environment if a cotton ball or similar barrier is used to prevent food impaction. These teeth can usually be closed the next day without incident, after additional cleaning and shaping.

Although some practitioners recommend routinely leaving teeth open between appointments, this is rarely indicated and not based on sound scientific research. Teeth left open to the oral environment show higher levels of secretory IgA than teeth that are not left open.[195] The significance of this finding is that epithelial growth factor, a polypeptide found in saliva, may stimulate the rests of Malassez found in periapical lesions to proliferate,[107,195] The result is that leaving canals open to the oral cavity may increase periapical cyst formation.[186] For this reason all teeth, with rare exception, should be closed aseptically under the rubber dam after treatment.

Incision and Drainage for Swelling

Treatment of an interappointment or postoperative swelling is similar to the treatment of a preoperative swelling: It involves establishing drainage and prescribing antibiotics, as indicated.[75,128] If the root canal has not been obturated or is inadequately obturated, reinstrumentation through the root canal should be attempted to achieve drainage. Surgical trephination may be necessary for teeth with an apical blockage. If the obturation appears adequate, drainage may be achieved through an incision and drainage procedure. Attempting periradicular surgery at the time of an acute infection is contraindicated because of difficulty in obtaining profound anesthesia.

Periapical Surgery

For most flare-ups, nonsurgical root canal therapy is the preferred treatment method because the root canal contents can be thoroughly cleaned in a noninvasive manner. In certain situations, however, periapical surgery may be the emergency treatment of choice. For example, nonsurgical treatment may be impractical because of restorative issues, failing retreatment, gross overfills, or necessary correction of procedural accidents. In some instances, surgical trephination can be used as a palliative measure. However, trephination is not generally recommended because of the additional trauma, invasiveness, and questionably beneficial result.[122]

Antibiotics and Analgesics

When it is necessary to give an antibiotic to control infection, phenoxymethyl penicillin (V-Cillin-K, Pen-VK) should be considered the drug of choice; metronidazole can be added to the regimen to enhance the killing of anaerobes. When there is an allergy to penicillin, clindamycin is recommended.

As previously mentioned, if drainage is achieved, antibiotic therapy is often unnecessary for localized swellings. One double-blind study found that emergency patients with pulp necrosis, periapical pain, and/or localized swelling did not recover faster when given concurrent penicillin than those given a placebo.[54] For most patients, NSAIDs are appropriate and sufficient to control pain.[88] When this is not the case, opioid analgesics may be used to supplement the NSAIDS.

Although drugs should never be prescribed to satisfy the patient's desire or addiction,[124] a reasonable request must be considered (not only for the pharmacologic effect but also for the psychologic value).

Antibiotic Prophylaxis

There is an ongoing controversy as to whether giving patients antibiotics prophylactically before root canal therapy will reduce the incidence of flare-ups in certain situations. In a double-blind, prospective study, administration of penicillin prophylactically was unrelated to reducing posttreatment signs and symptoms after root canal preparation.[210] A recent study[210] also supports the conclusion that antibiotic prophylaxis does not reduce the incidence of flare-ups.

However, there is also evidence to support the use of prophylactic antibiotics in preventing flare-ups.[126,193,194] For patients in moderate to severe pain, erythromycin base was the most effective medication for reducing the incidence of postoperative pain after instrumentation.[193]

Other researchers prefer penicillin because of its bactericidal action and efficacy.[126] In a series of studies, they reported their flare-up occurrence to decrease from about 20% to 2%.[126] Their rationale is that teeth showing pulpal necrosis with periapical lesions have anaerobic bacteria proliferating inside the root canal system. Penicillin given before root canal therapy is intended to treat an existing infection before it has the opportunity to spread. In addition, penicillin is given to inhibit the synergistic activity between certain microorganisms responsible for flare-ups, such as the gram-positive bacteria that provide vitamin K to porphyromonas species.

Prescribing patients antibiotics carries inherent risks of morbidity and mortality. Patients may suffer adverse side effects, such as nausea or diarrhea, or they may even develop an anaphylactic reaction. Other complications include sensitization to antibiotics, superinfections, and the development of microbial resistance. A dentist who prescribes an antibiotic of questionable benefit places a patient at risk and may be held accountable if the patient experiences a severe adverse reaction.[210]

The question then remains as to whether antibiotics should be given to patients with pulpal necrosis and periapical lesions. Although there is evidence to support either view, the most recent research supports the idea that antibiotics are generally unnecessary for prophylactic use. Careful cleaning and shaping of the root canal system and using crown-down techniques and copious irrigation should result in a low flare-up rate. This low rate, in conjunction with the knowledge of side-effects and risks associated with antibiotic use, should convince the clinician that the antibiotics are unnecessary for prophylactic use.

NSAIDs—Oral and Injectable

The use of pretreatment and posttreatment analgesics may significantly reduce the incidence of flare-ups,[191,193] especially for patients in moderate to severe pain. Because endodontic pain results from numerous inflammatory and immunologic pathways, most endodontists prefer NSAIDs to narcotics for interfering with this process and reducing pain symptoms.

Studies have evaluated ketorlac tromethamine (Toradol) when given as a local infiltration[143] or as an intramuscular injection.[36,143] Ketorlac is the first NSAID available for intramuscular injection. By blocking cyclooxygenase, ketorlac is a potent inhibitor of prostaglandin synthesis and may be equivalent or superior to morphine sulfate when delivered through the intramuscular route.[36,143] One research group found that nearly all patients in severe pain who were given ketorlac as an intramuscular injection experienced a pain reduction of 67% within 40 minutes, and that pain reduction increased to 99.5% after 90 minutes.[36] Others found that local infiltration of ketorlac produced a significant analgesic effect, especially in the mandible, when compared with the maxilla. From these results they concluded that the pharmacokinetics of ketorlac differ significantly from those of local anesthetics, and that ketorlac's ability to provide adjunctive pain relief was promising.

Two NSAIDs, diclofenac and ketoprofen, have been used as intracanal medicaments to control pain.[133] When injected into root canals, both medications were superior to a placebo in reducing pain subsequent to instrumentation of the canals. In one recent study, researchers injected ketorlac into root canals to deliver it periapically.[151] However, they found that the majority of the medication was expressed back out of the canal. In addition, ketorlac was found to be no more effective than oral ibuprofen in reducing postoperative pain, possibly due to the difficulty of delivering an adequate dose of the medication periapically. In oral form, however, ketorlac was found to be superior to an acetaminophen-codeine combination in reducing pain from acute apical periodontitis.[155]

Testing a novel combination of flurbiprofen (an NSAID) and tramadol (a centrally acting analgesic) by oral administration, researchers found that the combination of an NSAID and tramadol provides superior short-term pain relief when compared with either drug alone.[40] A good pain management strategy should include NSAIDs, because pretreatment with this group of analgesics has been shown to reduce postoperative pain significantly.[88] (For a complete pain management discussion, refer to Chapter 18.)

Corticosteroids—Oral and Injectable
Corticosteroids inhibit the enzyme phospholipase A_2, which is responsible for conversion of membrane phospholipids into arachidonic acid. Arachidonic acid is the precursor of various inflammatory mediators, including the prostaglandins, thromboxanes, prostacyclin, and leukotrienes. Thus corticosteroids reduce inflammation and pain by blocking the inflammatory cascade.

Researchers have shown that a local infiltration of dexamethasone produces a histologically significant antiinflammatory effect on the periapical tissues of overinstrumented teeth.[135] Studies of dentin and pulp confirm that dexamethasone reduces the immunoreactivity for calcitonin gene-related protein and substance P; it also reduces nerve-sprouting responses to dentin cavity injuries.[80,82] This inhibition of neural reactions to injury may contribute to the effect of steroids on clinical dental pain.

Oral methylprednisolone is effective in reducing postoperative symptoms when given prophylactically (with penicillin) to patients in moderate to severe pain.[193] Methylprednisolone also reduces the frequency and intensity of postobturation pain after single-visit treatment.[93] The Medrol Dosepak, which contains 21 tablets that the patient takes in decreasing amounts for 6 days, makes this medication easy to dispense.

Researchers evaluating postinstrumentation pain (at 8, 24, and 48 hours) in patients given either oral dexamethasone or placebo, found that those taking placebo experienced significantly more pain at all time periods.[65,98] Other studies evaluating the effect of intramuscular injections of corticosteroids on postoperative pain recorded similar results.[113,114]

Corticosteroids seem to have their greatest impact in the first 24 hours, postoperatively. For patients in severe pain, it may be beneficial to prescribe or administer some form of corticosteroid. Among the various methods of delivering corticosteroids, intracanal placement may be the least effective because of the difficulty of delivering sufficient quantities periapically.

There is no evidence of dexamethasone injections leading to an increase in infections, such as cellulitis, fever, or lymphadenopathy, regardless of the pulpal or periapical status of teeth to be treated.[113] For this reason, antibiotics may be given at the discretion of the practitioner, depending on the other treatment and health variables of the particular patient. *However, it is critical that the practitioner is confident that the recommendation to use corticosteroids is made for the pain of inflammation and injury, not for pain associated with infection and swelling.*

One-Appointment Endodontics
Endodontists and clinical researchers have found that obturation of root canals is associated with fewer flare-ups and a decrease in pain.[194,209] After obturation, the highest degree of pain occurs in the first 24 hours, and it diminishes substantially thereafter.[74,194] The popularity of single-visit treatment can be credited to favorable reports that found no difference in treatment complications or success rates when compared with teeth treated in multiple visits.[48,142,150,209] The preference of the single-visit approach, however, must be tempered with the understanding that careful case selection and the clinician's expertise factored heavily in achieving the reported outcomes.

Because bacteria are the source of pulpal and periapical infections, eliminating the bacteria will resolve associated symptoms. One author suggests "the root canal should ideally be completely cleaned at the initial treatment visit when the bacteria are particularly vulnerable to eradication by a disturbance in their sensitive ecology."[182] Between appointments, when the tooth is coronally sealed, "the anaerobiosis is restored and an influx of tissue fluid into the canal can support the regrowth of bacteria." If an intracanal dressing is not placed in the root canal, then resistant bacteria, which have survived the biomechanical treatment, may proliferate and resurrect infections that are difficult to treat.[26,182]

Placement of calcium hydroxide as an intracanal dressing has been shown to improve long-term healing in teeth with apical periodontitis by reducing the remaining bacteria in the root canal system.[92,199] Another group of investigators found that 40% of root canals that are treated in a single visit yield positive cultures before obturation.[178] They determined that the long-term success rate is 26% lower when bacteria are present at the time of obturation than it is when they are eliminated. Examination of their failures showed *Actinomyces* species in each case, whereas other clinicians have also found *Actinomyces* to be present in refractory lesions.[1,120,183] Placement of calcium hydroxide has been recommended to eradicate bacteria from infected canals before obturation,[177] which may be particularly effective because calcium hydroxide is capable of killing *actinomyces* species.[176]

Compared with single-visit treatment, these studies show an increased prognosis for a multivisit treatment sequence that includes placement of a calcium hydroxide dressing between appointments. Other research has shown that calcium hydroxide is difficult to completely remove from the canal walls before obturation,[112] and the presence of residual calcium hydroxide may adversely affect the quality of the apical seal. Based on clinical and scientific principles, the practitioner must decide if the root canal treatment is to be completed in one or more appointments.

HYPOCHLORITE ACCIDENT

Accidental injection of sodium hypochlorite into the periapical tissues is an experience that neither the patient nor practitioner will soon forget. The literature contains numerous case reports describing the morbidity associated with such occurrences.[14,46,60,147]

Definition

A hypochlorite accident refers to any event where sodium hypochlorite is expressed beyond the apex of a tooth and the patient immediately manifests some combination of the following symptoms:

1. Severe pain, even in areas that were previously anesthetized for dental treatment
2. Swelling
3. Profuse bleeding, both interstitially and through the tooth

Causes

Some of the reasons that a hypochlorite accident may occur include forceful injection of the irrigating solution; having an irrigating needle wedged into a root canal; and irrigating a tooth with a large apical foramen, apical resorption, or an immature apex. Most patients have several days of increasing

edema and ecchymosis, accompanied by tissue necrosis, possible paresthesia, and secondary infection (Fig. 2-14). Although most patients recover within 1 or 2 weeks, long-term paresthesia and scarring have been reported.[60,147] The volume, concentration, and temperature of the NaOCl expressed beyond the apical foramen, combined with the practitioner's timely response to the incident (see below), will determine the ultimate outcome.

Management

1. The clinician must recognize that a hypochlorite accident has occurred.
2. The immediate problem of pain and swelling should be attended to first. A regional block, with a long-acting anesthetic solution, should be administered. With the irrigant spreading rapidly over a wide region, pain management is difficult because symptoms from distant anatomic structures will continue to cause discomfort. This also explains the extreme pain felt during the incident, despite establishment of adequate local anesthesia before treatment. A reported incident describes flushing the palatal canal of a maxillary molar with sterile water to dilute the effects of the hypochlorite that was expressed into the sinus through the same route.[46]
3. The clinician should assure and calm the patient. The reaction, although alarmingly fast, is still a localized phenomenon and will resolve, with time. If available, nitrous oxide sedation can help the patient cope through the remainder of the emergency.
4. The tooth should be monitored during the next 30 minutes. A bloody exudate may discharge back into the canal; this bleeding is the body's reaction to the irrigant. To encourage further drainage from the periapical tissues, the fluid should be removed with high-volume evacuation. If drainage is persistent, the clinician should consider leaving the tooth open over the next 24 hours.
5. The clinician should consider antibiotic coverage. If the treated tooth is pulpless and cleaning and shaping procedures have not been completed, prescribing penicillin (500 mg, 5 times a day, over the next 7 days) may be helpful.
6. The clinician should consider an analgesic. Because of possible bleeding complications with aspirin and other NSAIDs, an acetaminophen-narcotic analgesic combination may be more appropriate. If swelling is extensive, the patient should be cautioned to expect bruising or pooling of blood as it subsides.
7. The clinician should consider prescribing a corticosteroid. Steroids will help minimize the ensuing inflammatory process.
8. The patient should be given home care instructions. For the first 6 hours the patient should use cold compresses; warm compresses thereafter.
9. The clinician should consider referring the patient. If the patient continues to be apprehensive, needs addi-

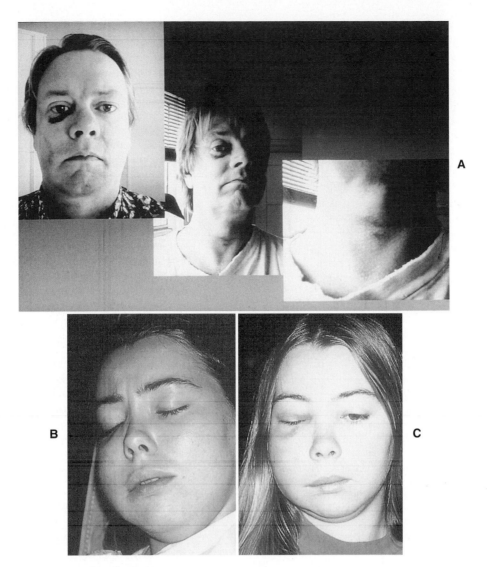

Fig. 2-14 A, Hypochlorite accident. The photograph on the far left shows the patient 24 hours after expression of 5.25% sodium hypochlorite through the distal buccal root of tooth #3. Note the intense ecchymosis around the right eye and slight swelling of the right cheek. The photograph in the center shows the progression of the swelling into the facial tissues 48 hours after the accident. The photograph on the far right shows the swelling extending into the neck after 72 hours. **B,** Immediately after mishap through a maxillary canine with 5.25% solution; the swelling had spread to involve the canine and infraorbital spaces. **C,** Swelling and ecchymosis are evident 24 hours later. (**B** and **C** Courtesy Dr. Ronald Borer.)

tional reassurance, or develops complications, referral to an oral surgeon or endodontist is recommended. Informing the specialist about the patient and the nature of the problem will ensure a smooth transition for the patient.

Prevention

A hypochlorite accident is completely avoidable. As an endodontic irrigant, hypochlorite solution is meant to flush debris from the root canal system. Part of the efficacy of hypochlorite depends on the volume of irrigation, as well as the depth of penetration of the irrigating needle. Even so, the solution must be delivered in a passive manner to avoid apical extrusion. As root canals are coronally flared during the cleansing and shaping process, the irrigating needle can penetrate deeper into the canal while still not binding against the walls.

The following measures are recommended to prevent a hypochlorite accident:

1. The irrigating needle should be bent at the center to confine the tip of the needle to higher levels in the root canal and to facilitate direct access to all teeth, regardless of angulation.
2. The needle should never be placed so deeply into the canal that it binds against the walls.

3. The needle should be oscillated in and out of the canal to ensure that the tip is free to express irrigant without resistance.
4. The irrigant should be expressed slowly and gently.
5. Irrigation should be stopped if the needle jams or if there is any detectable resistance on pressing against the plunger of the syringe.
6. The hub of the needle should be checked for a tight fit to prevent inadvertent separation and accidental exposure of the irrigant to the patient's eyes.

Although a hypochlorite accident requires immediate management, the definitive assessment and accurate identification of any dental emergency must follow the same process as outlined in this chapter.

The art and science of endodontic diagnosis and treatment have undergone a tremendous scientific and technologic evolution over the last half of the twentieth century. As a result the dental profession is prepared and able to remedy one of man's most painful and feared afflictions with compassion, knowledge, and skill.

References

1. Rass M, Bogen G: Microorganisms in closed periapical lesions, *Int Endodod J* 31:39, 1998.
2. Absi EG, Addy M, Adams D: Dentine hypersensitivity: a study of the patency of dentinal tubules in sensitive and non-sensitive cervical dentine, *J Clin Periodontol* 14:280, 1987.
3. Addy M: Etiology and clinical implications of dentin hypersensitivity, *Dent Clin North Am* 34:503, 1990.
4. Aderhold L, Konthe H, Frenkel G: The bacteriology of dentigerous pyogenic infections, *Oral Surg Oral Med Oral Pathol* 52:583, 1981.
5. Ahlquist M, Franzen O, Coffey J, Pashley D: Dental pain evoked by hydrostatic pressures applied to exposed dentin in man: a test of the hydrodynamic theory of dentin sensitivity, *J Endod* 20:130, 1994.
6. Ahlquist M, Franzen O: Pulpal ischemia in man: effects on detection threshold, A-delta neural response and sharp dentinal pain, *Endod Dent Traumatol* 15:6, 1999.
7. American Association of Endodontists: *Glossary: contemporary terminology for endodontics,* ed 6, Chicago, Ill., 1998, The Association.
8. Andersen M, Andreasen JO, Andreasen FM: In vitro solubility of human pulp tissue in calcium hydroxide and sodium hypochlorite, *Endod Dent Traumatol* 8:104, 1992.
9. Ardekian L et al: Burkitts lymphoma mimicking an acute dentoalveolar abscess, *J Endod* 22:697, 1996.
10. Balaban FS, Skidmore AE, Griffin JA: Acute exacerbations following initial treatment of necrotic pulps, *J Endod* 10:78, 1984.
11. Barr CE: Practical considerations in the treatment of the HIV-infected patient, *Dent Clin North Am* 38:403, 1994.
12. Battrum DE and Guttman JL: Phantom tooth pain: a diagnosis of exclusion, *Int Endod J* 29:190, 1996.
13. Baumgartner JC: Treatment of infections and associated lesions of endodontic origin, *J Endod* 17:418, 1991.
14. Becker GL, Cohen S, Borer R: The sequelae of accidentally injecting sodium hypochlorite beyond the root apex: report of a case, *Oral Surg Oral Med Oral Pathol* 38:633, 1974.
15. Bender IB: Factors influencing radiographic appearance of bony lesions, *J Endod* 8:161, 1982.
16. Bergenholtz G: Effects of bacterial products on inflammatory reactions in the dental pulp, *Scand J Dent Res* 85:122, 1977.
17. Berthold CW, Dionne RA, Corey SE: Comparison of sublingually and orally administered triazolam for premedication before oral surgery, *Oral Surg Oral Med Oral Pathol* 84:119, 1997.
18. Brännström M: The hydrodynamic theory of dentinal pain: sensation in preparations, caries, and the dentinal crack syndrome, *J Endod* 12:453, 1986.
19. Brännström M: The cause of postrestorative sensitivity and its prevention, *J Endod* 12: 475, 1986.
20. Brännström M: Etiology of dentin hypersensitivity, *Proc Finn Dent Soc* 88 (suppl 1): 7, 1992.
21. Brown DC, Moore BK, Brown CE Jr, Newton CW: An in vitro study of apical extrusion of sodium hypochlorite during endodontic canal preparation, *J Endod* 21:587, 1995.
22. Buck S et al: Pulpal exposure alters neuropeptide levels in inflamed dental pulp and trigeminal ganglia: evaluation of axonal transport, *J Endod* 16:718, 1999.
23. Byers MR: Dentinal sensory receptors, *Int Rev Neurobiol* 25:39, 1984.
24. Byers MR, Taylor PE, Khayat BG, Kimberly CL: Effects of injury and inflammation on pulpal and periapical nerves, *J Endod* 16:78, 1990.
25. Byers MR, Narhi MVO: Dentinal injury models: experimental tools for understanding neuroinflammatory interactions and polymodal nociceptor functions, *Crit Rev Oral Biol Med* 10:4, 1999.
26. Bystrom A, Sundqvist G: Bacteriologic evaluation of the efficacy of mechanical root canal instrumentation in endodontic therapy, *Scan J Dent Res* 89:321, 1981.
27. Calt S, Serper A, Ozxelik B, Dalat MD: PH changes and calcium ion diffusion from calcium hydroxide dressing materials through root dentin, *J Endod* 25:329, 1999.
28. Chan CP et al: Vertical root fracture in nonendodontically treated teeth: a clinical report of 64 cases in Chinese patients, *J Endod* 24:678, 1998.
29. Chestner SB, Selman AJ, Friedman J, Heyman RA: Apical fenestration: solution to recalcitrant pain in root canal therapy, *J Am Dent Assoc* 77:846, 1968.
30. Childers M et al: Anesthetic efficacy of the periodontal ligament injection after an inferior alveolar nerve block, *J Endod* 22:317, 1996.
31. Chong BS, Pitt-Ford TR: The role of intracanal medication in root canal therapy, *Int Endod J* 25:97, 1992.
32. Ciancio S: Oral contraceptives, antibiotics, and pregnancy, *Dent Manag* 5:54, 1989.
33. Corah NL: Effect of perceived control on stress reduction in pedodontic patients, *J Dent Res* 52:1261, 1973.
34. Craig AD, Reiman EM, Evans A, Bushnell MC: Functional imaging of an illusion of pain, *Nature* 384:258, 1996.
35. Creech TL, Walton RE, Kaltenbach R: Effect of occlusal relief of endodontic pain, *J Am Dent Assoc* 109:64, 1984.
36. Curtis P, Gartman LA, Green DB: Utilization of ketorlac tromethamine for control of severe odontogenic pain, *J Endod* 20:457, 1994.

37. D'Arcangelo C, Varvara G, De Fazio P: An evaluation of the action of different root canal irrigants on facultative aerobic-anaerobic, obligate anaerobic, and microaerophilic bacteria, *J Endod* 25:351, 1999.

38. Deutsh AS et al: Root fracture during insertion of prefabricated posts related to root size, *J Prosthet Dent* 53:786, 1985.

39. Dionne RA, Gordon SM, McCullagh LM, Phero JC: Assessing the need for anesthesia and sedation in the general population, *J Am Dent Assoc* 129:167, 1998.

40. Doroschak AM, Bowles WR, Hargreaves KM: Evaluation of the combination of flurbiprofen and tramadol for management of endodontic pain, *J Endod* 25:660, 1999.

41. Dragolich WE et al: An in vitro study of dentinal tubule occlusion by ferric oxalate, *J Periodontol* 64:1045, 1993.

42. Drinnan AL: Differential diagnosis of orofacial pain, *Dent Clin North Am* 31:627, 1987.

43. Dunbar D et al: Anesthetic efficacy of the intraosseous injection after an inferior alveolar nerve block, *J Endod* 22:481, 1996.

44. Economides N, Koulaouzidou EA, Beltes P, Kortsaris AH: In vitro release of hydroxyl ions from calcium hydroxide gutta-percha points, *J Endod* 25:481, 1999.

45. Ehlers I: Pain and new cultural diseases, *Endod Dent Traumatol* 15:193, 1999.

46. Ehrich DG, Brian JD Jr, Walker WA: Sodium hypochlorite accident: inadvertent injection into the maxillary sinus, *J Endod* 19:180, 1993.

47. Ehrich DG, Lundgren JP, Dionne RA, Nicoll BK, Hutter JW: Comparison of triazolam, diazepam, and placebo as outpatient oral premedication for endodontic patients, *J Endod* 23:181, 1997.

48. Eleazer PD, Eleazer KR: Flare-up rate in pulpally necrotic molars in one-visit versus two-visit endodontic treatment, *J Endod* 24:614, 1998.

49. Eli I, Bar-Tal Y, Fuss Z, Silberg A: Effect of intended treatment on anxiety and on reaction to electric pulp stimulation in dental patients, *J Endod* 23:694, 1997.

50. Estrela C, Pimenta FC, Ito IY, Bammann LL: Antimicrobial evaluation of calcium hydroxide in infected dentinal tubules, *J Endod* 25:416, 1999.

51. Fairbourn DR, McWalter GM, Montgomery S: The effect of four preparation techniques on the amount of apically extruded debris, *J Endod* 13:102, 1987.

52. Feinerman DM, Goldberg MH: Acoustic neuroma appearing as trigeminal neuralgia, *J Am Dent Assoc* 125:1122, 1994.

53. Foster KH, Kulild JC, Weller RN: Effect of smear layer removal on the diffusion of calcium hydroxide through radicular dentin, *J Endod* 19:136, 1993.

54. Fouad AF, Rivera EM, Walton RE: Penicillin as a supplement in resolving the localized acute apical abscess, *Oral Surg Oral Med Oral Pathol* 81:590, 1996.

55. Fox J et al: Incidence of pain following one-visit endodontic treatment, *Oral Surg Oral Med Oral Pathol* 30:123, 1970.

56. Friedberg BH, Gartner LP: Embryotoxicity and teratogenicity of formocresol on developing chick embryos, *J Endod* 16:434, 1990.

57. Fukushima H et al: Localization and identification of root canal bacteria in clinically asymptomatic periapical pathosis, *J Endod* 16:534, 1990.

58. Gatchel RJ: Managing anxiety and pain during dental treatment, *J Am Dent Assoc* 123:37, 1992.

59. Gatewood RS, Himel VT, Dorn SO: Treatment of the endodontic emergency: a decade later, *J Endod* 16:284, 1990.

60. Gatot A, Arbelle J, Leiberman A, Yanai-Inbar I: Effects of sodium hypochlorite on soft tissues after its inadvertent injection beyond the root apex, *J Endod* 17: 573, 1991.

61. Gazelius et al: Vasodilatory effects and coexistence of calcitonin gene-related peptide and substance P in sensory nerves of cat dental pulp, *Acta Physiol Scand* 130:33, 1987.

62. Georgopoulou M, Anastassiadis P, Sykaras S: Pain after chemicmechanical preparation, *Int Endod J* 19:309, 1986.

63. Georgopoulou M, Kontakiotis E, Nakou M: In vitro evaluation of the effectiveness of calcium hydroxide and para-monochlorophenol on anaerobic bacteria from the root canal, *Endod Dent Traumatol* 9:249, 1993.

64. Gilad JZ et al: Development of a clindamycin-impregnated fiber as an intracanal medication in endodontic therapy, *J Endod* 25:722, 1999.

65. Glassman G et al: A prospective randomized double-blind trial on efficacy of dexamethasone for endodontic inter-appointment pain in teeth with asymptomatic inflamed pulps, *Oral Surg Oral Med Oral Pathol* 67:96, 1989.

66. Goerig AC, Michelich RJ, Schulz HH: Instrumentation of root canals in molars using the step-down technique, *J Endod* 8:550, 1982.

67. Gold MS: Tetrodotoxin-resistant Na+ currents and inflammatory hyperalgesia, *Proc Natl Acad Sci USA* 96:7645, 1999.

68. Goon WWY, Jacobsen PL: Prodromal odontalgia and multiple devitalized teeth caused by a herpes zoster infection of the trigeminal nerve: report of case, *J Am Dent Assoc* 116: 500, 1988.

69. Green BL, Green ML, Mcfall WT: Calcium hydroxide and potassium nitrate as desensitizing agents for hypersensitive root surfaces, *J Periodontol* 48:667, 1977.

70. Guttman J, Harrison JW: *Surgical endodontics*, Boston, 1991, Blackwell Scientific Publications Inc.

71. Hargreaves KM, Troullos ES, Dionne RA: Pharmacologic rationale for the treatment of acute pain, *Dent Clin North Am* 31:675, 1987.

72. Hargreaves KM: Mechanisms of orofacial pain and hyperalgesia. Paper presented at the meeting of the American Association of Endodontists, Atlanta, April 1999.

73. Harrington GW, Natkin E: Midtreatment flare-ups, *Dent Clin North Am* 36:409, 1992.

74. Harrison JW, Baumgartner JC, Svec TA: Incidence of pain associated with clinical factors during and after root canal therapy. II. Postobturation pain, *J Endod* 9:434, 1983.

75. Harrison JW: The appropriate use of antibiotics in dentistry: endodontic indications, *Quintessence Int* 28:827, 1997.

76. Harrison JW, Svec TA: The beginning of the end of the antibiotic era? I. The problem: abuse of the "miracle drugs," *Quintessence Int* 29:151, 1998.

77. Hasselgren G, Olsson B, Cvek M: Effects of calcium hydroxide and sodium hypochlorite on the dissolution of necrotic porcine muscle tissue, *J Endod* 14:125, 1988.

78. Hiatt WH: Incomplete crown root fracture and pulpal—periodontal disease, *J Periodontol* 44:4, 1975.

79. Hirata T et al: Dentinal fluid movement associated with loading of restorations, *J Dent Res* 70:975, 1991.

80. Holland GR: Steroids reduce the periapical inflammatory and neural changes after pulpectomy, *J Endod* 22:455, 1996.

81. Holmes-Johnson E, Geboy M, Getka EJ: Behavior considerations, *Dent Clin North Am* 30:391, 1986.

82. Hong D, Byers MR, Oswald RJ: Dexamethasone treatment reduces sensory neuropeptides and nerve sprouting reactions in injured teeth, *Pain* 55:171, 1993.

83. Hutter JW: Facial space infections of odontogenic origin, *J Endod* 17:422, 1991.

84. Ikeda H, Suda H: subjective sensation and objective neural discharges recorded from clinically nonvital intact teeth, *J Endod* 24:552, 1998.

85. Imura N, Zuolo ML: Factors associated with endodontic flare-ups: a prospective study, *Int Endod J* 28:261, 1995.

86. Ishikawa K et al: Occlusion of dentinal tubules with calcium phosphate using acidic calcium phosphate solution followed by neutralization, *J Dent Res* 73:1197, 1994.

87. Isidor F, Brodum K, Raunholt G: The influence of post length and crown ferrule length on the resistance to cyclic loads of bovine teeth with prefabricated titanium posts, *Int J Oral Prosthodont* 12:78, 1999.

88. Jackson DL, Moore PA, Hargreaves KM: Postoperative non-steroidal antiinflammatory medication for the prevention of postoperative dental pain, *J Am Dent Assoc* 119:641, 1989.

89. Javid B, Barkhorder RA, Bhinda SV: Cyanacrylate—a new treatment for hypersensitive dentin and cementum, *J Am Dent Assoc* 114:486, 1987.

90. Jeansonne MJ, White RR: A comparison of 2.0% chlorhexidine gluconate and 5.25% sodium hypochlorite as antimicrobial endodontic irrigants, *J Endod* 20:276, 1994.

91. Jyvasjarvi E, Kniffki KD: Cold stimulation of teeth: a comparison between the responses of cat intradental A and C fibers and human sensations, *J Physiol* 391:193, 1987.

92. Katebzadeh N, Hupp J, Trope M: Histological repair after obturation of infected root canals in dogs, *J Endod* 25:364, 1999.

93. Kaufman E et al: Intraligamentary injection of slow-release methylprednisolone for the prevention of pain after endodontic treatment, *Oral Surg Oral Med Oral Pathol* 77:651, 1994.

94. Kim S: Microcirculation of the dental pulp in health and disease, *J Endod* 11:465, 1985.

95. Kim S: Neurovascular interactions in the dental pulp in health and inflammation, *J Endod* 16:48, 1990.

96. Klepac RK et al: Reports of pain after dental treatment, electrical tooth stimulation and cutaneous shock, *J Am Dent Assoc* 100:692, 1980.

97. Kontakiotis E, Nakou M, Georgopoulou M: In vitro study of the indirect action of calcium hydroxide on the anaerobic flora of the root canal system, *Int Endod J* 28:285, 1995.

98. Krasner P, Jackson E: Management of posttreatment endodontic pain with oral dexamethasone: a double-blind study, *Oral Surg Oral Med Oral Pathol* 62:187, 1986.

99. Laskin DM: Anatomic considerations in diagnosis and treatment of odontogenic infections, *J Am Dent Assoc* 69:38, 1964.

100. Law AS, Lily JP: Trigeminal neuralgia mimicking odontogenic pain, *Oral Surg Oral Med Oral Pathol* 80:96, 1995.

101. Li X, Tronstad L, Olsen I: Brain abscess caused by oral infection, *Endod Dent Traumatol* 15:95, 1999.

102. Lilly JP, Law AS: Atypical odontalgia misdiagnosed as odontogenic pain: a case report and discussion of treatment, *J Endod* 23:337, 1997.

103. Lin LM, Langeland K: Light and electron microscopic study of teeth with carious pulp exposures, *Oral Surg Oral Med Oral Pathol* 51:292, 1981.

104. Lin LM, Shovlin F, Skribner JE, Langeland K: Pulp biopsies from teeth associated with periapical radiolucency, *J Endod* 10:436, 1984.

105. Lin LM, Skribner J: Why teeth associated with periapical lesions can have a vital response, *Clin Prevent Dent* 12:3, 1990.

106. Lin LM, Skribner JE, Gaengler P: Factors associated with endodontic treatment failures, *J Endod* 18:625, 1992.

107. Lin LM et al: Detection of epidermal growth factor receptor in inflammatory periapical lesions, *Int Endod J* 29:179, 1996.

108. Lipton JA, Ship JA, Larach-Robinson D: Estimated prevalence and distribution of reported orofacial pain in the United States, *J Am Dent Assoc* 124:115, 1993.

109. Little JW: Prosthetic implants: risk of infection from transient dental bacteremias, *Compend Contin Educ Dent* 12:160, 1991.

110. Marbach JJ: Is phantom tooth pain a deafferentation (neuropathic) syndrome? Part II: psychosocial considerations, *Oral Surg Oral Med Oral Pathol* 75:225, 1993.

111. Marbach JJ: Orofacial phantom pain: theory and phenomenology, *J Am Dent Assoc* 127:221, 1996.

112. Margelos J, Eliades G, Verdelis C, Palaghias G: Interaction of calcium hydroxide with zinc oxide-eugenol type sealers: a potential clinical problem, *J Endod* 23:115, 1993.

113. Marshall JG, Walton RE: The effect of intramuscular injection of steroid on posttreatment endodontic pain, *J Endod* 10:584, 1984.

114. Marshall JG, Liesinger AW: Factors associated with endodontic posttreatment pain, *J Endod* 19:573, 1993.

115. Marshall SJ, Marshall GW: Dental amalgam: the materials, *Adv Dent Res*, 6:94, 1992.

116. Matusow RJ, Goodall LB: Anaerobic isolates in primary pulpal-alveolar cellulitis cases: endodontic resolutions and drug therapy considerations, *J Endod* 9:535, 1983.

117. McKendry DJ: Comparison of balanced forces, endosonic, and step-back filing instrumentation techniques: quantification of extruded apical debris, *J Endod* 16:24, 1990.

118. Merskey H et al: Pain terms: a list with definitions and notes on usage, recommended by the IASP subcommittee on taxonomy, *Pain* 6:249, 1979.

119. Molander A, Reit C, Dahlen G: The antimicrobial effect of calcium hydroxide in root canals pretreated with 5% iodine potassium iodide, *Endod Dent Traumatol* 15:205, 1999.

120. Molander A, Reit C, Dahlen G, Kvist T: Microbiological status of root filled teeth with apical periodontitis, *Int Endod J* 31:1, 1998.

121. Montgomery S, Ferguson CD: Endodontics-diagnosis, treatment planning, and prognostic considerations, *Dent Clin North Am* 533:548, 1986.

122. Moos H, Bramell JD, Roahen JO: A comparison of pulpectomy alone versus pulpectomy with trephination for relief of pain, *J Endod* 22:422, 1996.

123. Mor C, Rotstein I, Friedman S: Incidence of interappointment emergency associated with endodontic therapy, *J Endod* 18:509, 1992.

124. Morse DR: The use of analgesics and antibiotics in endodontics: current concepts, *Alpha Omegan* 83:26, 1990.

125. Morse DR: Infection related mental and inferior alveolar nerve paraesthesia: literature review and presentation of two cases, *J Endod* 23:457, 1997.

126. Morse DR et al: Infectious flare-ups and serious sequelae following endodontic treatment: a prospective randomized trial on efficacy of antibiotic prophylaxis in cases of asymptomatic pulpal-periapical lesions, *Oral Surg Oral Med Oral Pathol* 64: 96, 1987.

127. Mulhern JM, Patterson SS, Newton CW, Ringel AM: Incidence of postoperative pain after one-appointment endodontic treatment of asymptomatic pulpal necrosis in single-rooted teeth, *J Endod* 8:370, 1982.

128. Natkin E: Treatment of endodontic emergencies, *Dent Clin North Am* 18:243, 1974.

129. Najjar TA: Why can't you achieve adequate regional anesthesia in the presence of infection? *Oral Surg Oral Med Oral Pathol* 44:7, 1977.

130. Narhi MVO, Haegerstam G: Interdental nerve activity induced by reduced pressure applied to exposed dentin in the cat, *Acta Physiol Scand* 119:381, 1983.

131. Narhi MVO et al: Neurophsiological mechanisms of dentin hypersensitivity, *Proc Finn Dent Soc* 88 (suppl 1):15, 1992.

132. Neaverth EJ: Disabling complications following inadvertent overextension of a root canal filling material, *J Endod* 15:135, 1989.

133. Negm MM: Effect of intracanal use of nonsteroidal antiinflammatory agents on posttreatment endodontic pain, *Oral Surg Oral Med Oral Pathol* 77:507, 1974.

134. Nissan R et al: Ability of bacterial endotoxin to diffuse through human dentin, *J Endod* 21:62, 1995.

135. Nobuhara WK, Carnes DL, Gilles JA: Antiinflammatory effects of dexamethasone on periapical tissues following endodontic overinstrumentation, *J Endod* 19:501, 1993.

136. Ohara P, Torabinejad M, Kettering JD: Antibacterial effects of various endodontic medicaments on selected anaerobic bacteria, *J Endod* 19:498, 1993.

137. Okeson JP, Bell WE: *Bell's orofacial pains*, ed 5, Chicago, 1995, Quintessence Publishing Co.

138. Orstavik D, Haapasalo M: Disinfection by endodontic irrigants and dressings of experimentally infected dentinal tubules, *Endod Dent Traumatol* 6:142, 1990.

139. Oyama T, Matsumoto KA: Clinical and morphological study of cervical hypersensitivity, *J Endod* 17:500, 1991.

140. Pallasch TJ: Antibiotic prophylaxis: theory and reality, *Calif Dent Assoc J* 6:27, 1989.

141. Pashley DH: Dentin permeability, dentin sensitivity and treatment through tubule occlusion, *J Endod* 12:465, 1986.

142. Pekruhn RB: The incidence of failure following single-visit endodontic therapy, *J Endod* 12:68, 1986.

143. Penniston SG, Hargreaves KM: Evaluation of periapical injection of ketorlac for management of endodontic pain, *J Endod* 22:55, 1996.

144. Peters DD: Evaluation of prophylactic alveolar trephination to avoid pain, *J Endod* 6:518, 1980.

145. Pinsawasdi P, Seltzer S: The induction of trigeminal neuralgia-like symptoms by pulp-periapical pathosis, *J Endod* 12:73, 1986.

146. Reddy SA, Hicks ML: Apical extrusion of debris using two hand and two rotary instrumentation techniques, *J Endod* 24:180, 1998.

147. Reeh ES, Messer HH: Long-term paresthesia following inadvertent forcing of sodium hypochlorite through perforation in maxillary incisor, *Endod Dent Traumatol* 5:200, 1989.

148. Rees RS, Harris M: Atypical odontalgia, *Br J Oral Maxillofac Surg* 16:212, 1979.

149. Rehman K, Saunders WP, Foye RH, Sharkley W: Calcium ion diffusion from calcium hydroxide-containing materials in endodontically treated teeth: an in vitro study, *Int Endod J* 29:271, 1996.

150. Roane JB, Dryden JA, Grimes EW: Incidence of postoperative pain after single- and multiple-visit endodontic procedures, *Oral Surg Oral Med Oral Pathol* 55: 68, 1983.

151. Rogers MJ, Johnson BR, Remeikis NA, BeGole EA: Comparison of the effect of intracanal use of ketorlac tromethamine and dexamethasone with oral ibuprofen on post treatment endodontic pain, *J Endod* 25:381, 1999.

152. Rosenberg PA, Babick PJ, Schertzer L, Leung A: The effect of occlusal reduction on pain after endodontic instrumentation, *J Endod* 24:492, 1998.

153. Rugh JD: Psychological components of pain, *Dent Clin North Am* 31:579, 1987.

154. Ruiz-Hubbard EE, Guttman JL, Wagner, MJ: A quantitative assessment of canal debris forced periapically during root canal instrumentation using two different techniques, *J Endod* 13:554, 1987.

155. Sadeghein A, Shahidi N, Dehpour AR: A comparison of ketorlac tromethamine and acetaminophen codeine in the management of acute apical periodontitis, *J Endod* 25:257, 1999.

156. Safavi KE, Nichols FC: Alteration of biological properties of bacterial lipopolysaccharide by calcium hydroxide treatment, *J Endod* 20:127, 1994.

157. Safavi KE, Spangberg LSW, Langeland K: Root canal tubule disinfection, *J Endod* 16:207, 1990.

158. Salzgeber RM, Brilliant JD: An in vivo evaluation of the penetration of an irrigating solution in root canals, *J Endod* 3:394, 1977.

159. Sandler NA, Ziccardi V, Ochs M: Differential diagnosis of jaw pain in the elderly, *J Am Dent Assoc* 126:1263, 1995.

160. Scholz A et al: Complex blockade of TTX-resistant NA+ currents by lidocaine and bupivicaine reduce firing frequency in DRG neurons, *J Neurophysiol* 79:1746, 1998.

161. Schwartz S, Cohen S: The difficult differential diagnosis, *Dent Clin North Am* 36:279, 1992.

162. Segura JJ et al: Calcium hydroxide inhibits substrate adherence capacity of macrophages, *J Endod* 23:444, 1997.

163. Seka W et al: Light deposition in dentinal hard tissue and simulated thermal response, *J Dent Res* 74:1086, 1995.

164. Selbst AG: Understanding informed consent and its relationship to the incidence of adverse treatment events in conventional endodontic therapy, *J Endod* 16:387, 1990.

165. Selden HS: The endoantral syndrome, *J Endod* 3:462, 1977.

166. Selden HS, Manhoff PT, Hatges NA, Michel RC: Metastatic carcinoma to the mandible that mimicked pulpal/periodontal disease, *J Endod* 24:267, 1998.

167. Seltzer S: Long-term radiographic and histological observations of endodontically treated teeth, *J Endod* 25:818, 1999.

168. Seltzer S: *Endodontology: biologic considerations in endodontic procedures*, ed 2, Philadelphia, 1988, Lea and Febiger.

169. Seltzer S, Bender IB, Ziontz M: The dynamics of pulp inflammation: correlations between diagnostic data and actual histologic findings in the pulp, *Oral Surg Oral Med Oral Pathol* 16:846, 1963.

170. Seltzer S, Boston D: Hypersensitivity and pain induced by operative procedures and the cracked tooth syndrome, *General Dentistry* 45:148, 1997.

171. Seltzer S, Naidorf IJ: Flare-ups in endodontics. I. Etiological factors, *J Endod* 11:472, 1985.

172. Sen BH, Safavi KE, Spangberg LSW: Antifungal effects of sodium hypochlorite and chlorhexidine in root canals, *J Endod*, 25:235, 1999.

173. Sessle BJ: Neurophysiology of orofacial pain, *Dent Clin North Am* 31:595, 1987.

174. Sigurdsson A, Jacoway JR: Herpes zoster infection presenting as an acute pulpitis, *Oral Surg Oral Med Oral Pathol* 80:92, 1995.

175. Sigurdsson A, Stancill R, Madison S: Intracanal placement of Ca(OH)$_2$: a comparison of techniques, *J Endod* 18:367, 1992.

176. Siqueira JF Jr, De Uzeda M: Disinfection by calcium hydroxide pastes of dentinal tubules infected with two obligate and one facultative anaerobic bacteria, *J Endod* 22:674, 1996.

177. Sjogren U, Figdor D, Spangberg L, Sundqvist G: The antimicrobial effect of calcium hydroxide as a short-term intracanal dressing, *Int Endod J* 24:119, 1991.

178. Sjogren U, Figdor D, Persson S, Sundqvist G: Influence of infection at the time of root filling on the outcome of endodontic treatment of teeth with apical periodontitis, *Int Endod J* 30:297, 1997.

179. Soekanto A et al: Toxicity of camphorated phenol and camphorated parachlorophenol in dental pulp cell culture, *J Endod* 22:284, 1996.

180. Stabholz A et al: Efficacy of XeCl 308 nm excimer laser in reducing dye penetration through coronal dentinal tubules, *J Endod* 21:266, 1995.

181. Staehle HJ, Thoma C, Muller HP: Comparative in vitro investigation of different methods for temporary root canal filling with aqueous suspensions of calcium hydroxide, *Endod Dent Traumatol*, 13:106, 1997.

182. Sundqvist G: Ecology of the root canal flora, *J Endod* 18:427, 1992.

183. Sundqvist G et al: Microbiologic analysis of teeth with failed endodontic treatment and the outcome of conservative retreatment, *Oral Surg Oral Med Oral Pathol* 85:86, 1998.

184. Sundqvist G, Johansson E, Sjogren U: Prevalence of black-pigmented bacteroides species in root canal infections, *J Endod* 15:13, 1989.

185. Takahashi K: Changes in the pulp vasculature during inflammation, *J Endod* 16:92, 1990.

186. Takahashi K, Macdonald FD, Kinane DF: Detection of IgA subclasses and J chain mRNA bearing plasma cells in human dental periapical lesions by in situ hybridization, *J Endod* 23:513, 1997.

187. Tamse A, Fuss Z, Lustig J, Kaplavi J: An evaluation of endodontically treated vertically fractured teeth, *J Endod* 25:506, 1999.

188. Tarbet W, Silverman G, Fraterangelo PA, Kanapfa JA: Home treatment for dentinal hypersensitivity: a comparative study, *J Am Dent Assoc* 105:227, 1982.

189. Tidwell E et al: Herpes zoster of the trigeminal nerve third branch: a case report and review of the literature, *Int Endod J* 32:61, 1999.

190. Torabinejad M: Mediators of pulpal and periapical pathosis, *Calif Dent Assoc J* 14:21, 1986.

191. Torabinejad M: Management of endodontic emergencies: facts and fallacies, *J Endod* 18:417, 1992.

192. Torabinejad M et al: Factors associated with endodontic interappointment emergencies of teeth with necrotic pulps, *J Endod* 14:261, 1988.

193. Torabinejad M et al: Effectiveness of various medications on postoperative pain following complete instrumentation, *J Endod* 20:345, 1994.

194. Torabinejad M et al: Effectiveness of various medications on postoperative pain following root canal obturation, *J Endod* 20:427, 1994.

195. Torres JOC, Torabinejad M, Matiz RAR, Mantilla EG: Presence of secretory IgA in human periapical lesions, *J Endod*, 20:87, 1994.

196. Trope M: Relationship of intracanal medicaments to endodontic flare-ups, *Endod Dent Traumatol* 6:226, 1990.

197. Trope M: Flare-up rate of single-visit endodontics, *Int Endod J* 24:24, 1991.

198. Trope M, Tronstad L, Rosenberg E, Listgarten M: Darkfield microscopy as a diagnostic aid in differentiating exudates from endodontic and periodontal abscesses, *J Endod* 14:35, 1988.

199. Trope M, Delano EO, Orstavik D: Endodontic treatment of teeth with apical periodontitis: single vs. multivisit treatment, *J Endod* 25:345, 1999.

200. Trowbridge HO: Mechanism of pain induction in hypersensitive teeth: proceedings of symposium on hypersensitive dentin. In Rowe NH, editor: *Origin and management*, Ann Arbor, Mich, 1985, University of Michigan.

201. Trowbridge HO: Intradental sensory units: physiological and clinical aspects, *J Endod* 11:489, 1985.

202. Trowbridge HO, Emling RC: *Inflammation: a review of the process*, ed 5, Chicago, 1997, Quintessence Publishing Co.

203. Tung MS, Bowen HJ, Derkson GD, Pashley DH: Effects of calcium phosphate solutions on dentin permeability, *J Endod* 19:383, 1993.

204. Tyldesley WR, Mummford JM: Dental pain and the histological condition of the pulp, *Dent Pac Dent Rec* 20:333, 1970.

205. Van Hassel HJ: Physiology of the human dental pulp, *Oral Surg Oral Med Oral Pathol* 32:126, 1971.

206. Vande Visse JE, Brilliant JD: Effect of irrigation on the production of extruded material at the root apex during instrumentation, *J Endod* 1:243, 1974.

207. Waltimo TMT, Siren EK, Orstavik D, Haapasalo MPP: Susceptibility of oral candida species to calcium hydroxide in vitro, *Int Endod J* 32:94, 1999.

208. Walton RE: The periodontal ligament injection as a primary technique, *J Endod* 16:62, 1990.

209. Walton RE, Fouad A: Endodontic interappointment flare-ups: a prospective study of incidence and related factors, *J Endod* 18:172, 1992.

210. Walton RE, Chiappinelli J: Prophylactic penicillin: effect on posttreatment symptoms following root canal treatment of asymptomatic periapical pathosis, *J Endod* 19:466, 1993.

211. White RR, Hays GL, Janer LR: Residual antimicrobial activity after canal irrigation with chlorhexidine, *J Endod* 23: 229, 1997.

212. Wilcox LR, Roskelley C, Sutton C: The relationship of root canal enlargement to finger spreader induced vertical root fracture, *J Endod* 23:533, 1997.

213. Wolfson EM, Seltzer S: Reaction of cat connective tissue to some gutta-percha formulations, *J Endod* 1:395, 1975.

214. Wong M, Lytle WR: A comparison of anxiety levels associated with root canal treatment and oral surgery treatment, *J Endod* 17:461, 1991.

215. Wright EF, Gullickson DC: Identifying acute pulpalgia as a factor in TMD pain, *J Am Dent Assoc* 127:773, 1996.

216. Yang SF, Rivera EM, Baumgardner KR, Walton RE, Stanford C: Anaerobic tissue-dissolving abilities of calcium hydroxide and sodium hypochlorite, *J Endod* 21:613, 1995.

217. Yoshiyama M et al: Treatment of dentin hypersensitivity: effect of a light-curing resin liner on tubule occlusion, *Jpn J Conserv Dent* 34:76, 1991.

218. Zhang C et al: Effects of CO_2 laser in treatment of cervical dentinal hypersensitivity, *J Endod* 24:595, 1998.

Chapter 3

Nonodontogenic Orofacial Pain and Endodontics: Pain Disorders Involving the Jaws That Simulate Odontalgia

Lewis R. Eversole, Peter F. Chase

Chapter Outline

NATURE OF PAIN
PAIN DISORDERS THAT MIMIC ODONTALGIA
   Periodontalgia
   Neuralgias
   Vasogenic Craniofacial Pain
   Temporal Arteritis
   Otitis Media
   Sinogenic Pain
   Cardiogenic Jaw Pain
   Sialolithiasis
   Musculoskeletal Disorders
   Abnormal Joint Function (Internal Derangement)
   Myalgia
   Myofascial Pain
   Neoplasia
ATYPICAL PAIN DISORDERS THAT MIMIC ODONTALGIA
   Phantom Tooth Pain
   Neuralgia-Inducing Cavitational Osteonecrosis (NICO)
   Complex Regional Pain Syndrome
   Causalgia
CONCLUSION

Of all the symptoms that the dentist must confront, pain can be one of the most unpleasant. Sometimes pain is merely annoying and creates only a slight disruption in an individual's daily life; at other times it is excruciating, making it impossible for the individual to accomplish even minor tasks. Ridding the patient of pain is perhaps one of the most rewarding aspects of dental practice.

The ultimate purpose of the pain response is to inform the patient of anatomic, physiologic, or behavioral imbalances. These problems may range from mild to severe. A patient's oral and facial pain complaints may be based on a disorder in eight different areas: (1) periodontal tissues, (2) pulpal tissues, (3) tissues from adjacent sites (e.g., sinus, eye, ear, nose, throat, cervical spine, brain, heart), (4) neurologic system (e.g., peripheral, central), (5) psychologic systems, (6) vascular walls, (7) musculoskeletal tissues (i.e., temporomandibular, cervical), and (8) idiopathic processes (e.g., chronic atypical craniofacial pain).

It is the dentist's responsibility to diagnose and treat dental and periodontal disease and to recognize what is not pulpal or periodontal disease. In some cases the dentist may have the skills to expand treatment to include temporomandibular disorders; in other cases the dentist must make appropriate referrals.

Occasionally the pain-signaling system is triggered in the absence of noxious stimuli or may be exaggerated beyond the severity of the underlying pathologic process. In other conditions, pain may persist after the original cause has been eliminated. The pain experience can be likened to the immune response, because the immune system works to protect the host from foreign agents that have the potential to destroy tissue (e.g., pathogens). In some hosts, however, the immune response is triggered by harmless foreign particles. In the context of a hypersensitivity or allergic reaction, the host immune system is stimulated; the various cellular and biochemical components of this response often result in unpleasant symptoms, including pain.

Pain may be analogous to hypersensitivity in that symptoms may appear in the absence of a readily identifiable pathologic or detrimental process. Although some pain syndromes are associated with a low-grade inflammatory lesion, others seem not to be associated with an underlying disease process. Many of these pain syndromes are touted as psychogenic problems, but the precise cause and pathogenesis have yet to be deciphered. As more is learned about various neurotransmitter peptides, the mystery of chronic idiopathic pain, for which there is currently no explanation, will be solved.

NATURE OF PAIN

Normally the pain experience begins with the peripheral nervous system. Nerve fibers have a nucleus (i.e., the cell body) that is located either within the central nervous system or in ganglia located in the peripheral tissues. Emanating from the cell body are long processes referred to as *axis cylinders.* A single nerve is made up of hundreds of individual axis cylinders that are encased in a fibrous capsule known as the perineurium. Each axis cylinder is ensheathed by specialized Schwann cells. Thus the peripheral nerve can be envisioned as a bundle of electric cables, all with their own enveloping insulation.

Some axis cylinders, with their associated Schwann cells, have an additional insulating layer known as *myelin,* a specialized lipid synthesized by the Schwann cells. Those fibers capable of transmitting noxious stimuli (i.e., nociceptors) lack a myelin sheath. These nonmyelinated fibers are also referred to as *C fibers,* as opposed to certain A or B fibers that transmit nonpainful sensory stimuli. The nerve endings of nociceptor C fibers are found in the skin and mucosa and, of course, are prevalent throughout the jaws, teeth, and periodontal tissues. In the region of the jaws, the nociceptor fibers are components of the trigeminal nerve. All of these nociceptors in the trigeminal system have their cell bodies located in the Gasserian ganglion, and the afferent axis cylinders that feed into these cell bodies exit the ganglion and extend toward the central nervous system through the trigeminal trunk that enters the pons.

These fibers then progress from the pons into the upper aspects of the cervical region of the spinal cord. It is in this location where the axis cylinders terminate in a region referred to as the *caudate nucleus of V.* Nerves that are transmitting proprioceptive signals and light touch terminate higher in the spinal cord (mesencephalic nucleus). Fibers that terminate in the caudate nucleus are nociceptors that interdigitate with secondary neurons. These secondary neurons then pass (superiorly) into the brain itself. At this synapse in the caudate nucleus, neuropeptides are secreted that are capable of transmitting a noxious impulse from the C fiber across the synapse to the secondary nerve fiber. In addition, other fibers have been identified that modulate this neurotransmitter pathway. Interneurons also have fiber endings that contact the incoming nociceptor fibers and are capable of secreting yet other neurotransmitters capable of inhibiting propagation of noxious stimuli. Many of these inhibitory neurosecretory molecules fall into a special class of peptides known as *endorphins.*

Some time ago a theory was proposed to explain how noxious stimuli became consciously identifiable in the higher centers of the brain. This *gate theory of pain* is based on observation of a variety of interconnections in the region of the synapse. As noxious stimuli became more accentuated, the so-called gate would open and allow the impulses to be transmitted across the synapse. Indeed, neuroscience researchers have provided evidence that the gatekeeper is, in fact, represented by neurotransmitter molecules.

Once noxious stimuli, such as bacterial enzymes and toxins, as well as host mediators and cytokines, accumulate in an acutely inflamed dental pulp, stimulate nociceptor fibers, and the impulse is transmitted across the synapse in the caudate nucleus, the signal is further propagated through the secondary neuron to the midbrain. In this region the secondary fibers terminate in the vicinity of the thalamus. This section of the midbrain, the periaqueductal gray matter, is under significant neurosecretory molecular influences and is involved in a variety of emotions. Thus it is interesting to speculate how some pain syndromes may be modified by the patient's psychologic and emotional status. From this area of the brain, tertiary and quaternary neurons synapse and transmit the nerve impulse to the cerebral cortex. It is at this level that the patient actually becomes conscious of the pain symptom.

Nociceptor fibers are stimulated by a variety of physical and chemical stimuli. During an infection or in the face of trauma, the tissues release noxious chemicals, including both peptides and lipids. In acute inflammation the pH often drops below 5, and it is well documented that both acidic and alkaline solutions stimulate firing of nociceptor fibers. Excessive heat, such as that from an electrical burn or thermal injury, also stimulates nociceptor fibers. In the context of the inflammatory reaction, kinins and prostaglandins, small vasoactive molecules, also have strong nociceptor-stimulating effects. Acute compressive forces on nerve endings may also produce pain, and this compression may be the result of cellular infiltrates into tissues and edema formation. As a rule the patient is able to localize the specific region of pain where the tissue harbors the pathologic process that has engendered the pain sensation. As clinicians are well aware, severe and acute pain may not always be readily localized. The neuroanatomic basis for the inability to specifically localize severe pain is not well understood. Eventually, within several hours to several days, the pain becomes more precisely localized.

Pathologic processes, such as acute infections or acute trauma, often precipitate complaints of sharp, short-duration pain. Alternatively, low-grade or chronic inflammatory conditions are frequently expressed as dull pain of longer duration. In addition, *pain disorders that fail to show any organic basis commonly surface as aching, chronic pains of long duration.* Therefore pain symptoms must be precisely characterized before the clinician can arrive at a definitive diagnosis. However, the clinician is often confronted with varied, multiple complaints for which more than one diagnosis must be considered. This chapter will consider the facial pain disorders according to the type of pain symptoms that the patient describes, thus constructing differential diagnoses for specific types of complaints.

Pain may be classified as either typical (i.e., of expected character and duration) or atypical (i.e., of unexpected character and often more chronic duration). Typical, acute pains are of shorter duration, lasting seconds, minutes, hours, days, or even months, depending on the underlying problem. However, atypical, chronic pains are of longer duration and may last from months to years, and pain may be constant or intermittent. Some acute pains are singular in nature and nonrecurrent, whereas other complaints are characterized by multiple occurrences. With chronic pain, the pain experience frequently fluctuates, lasts beyond normal healing periods, and does not fit expected pain patterns. Some patients may complain of chronic pain that begins as a mere nuisance in the morning but builds to a more severe ache in the late afternoon.

Identification of precipitating, perpetuating, aggravating, or relieving factors is diagnostically important. Sometimes gravity influences the severity of the pain; simply by placing the head below the knees, the patient may experience an exacerbation of pain. Exposure of tooth surfaces to hot and cold is a well-recognized precipitating factor for pulpal pain. However, patients may relate exacerbation of pain to emotional stress, jaw clenching, turning the head from left to right, or they may note an increase in severity during mealtimes. Therefore it is important to explore any factors that could precipitate, perpetuate, aggravate or relieve symptoms and to evaluate these factors in the context of the differential diagnosis.

Although most pain localized to teeth or the jaw bones is odontogenic, anatomic considerations are also extremely important in the differential diagnosis of orofacial pains. From time to time the clinician may encounter nonodontogenic sources for tooth- and jaw-related pain symptoms.

The anatomic sites that must be evaluated in patients who complain of pain that does not appear to be of an odontogenic origin include the following:
- Periodontium (periodontalgia)
- Masticatory musculature (myalgia)
- Jaw joints (arthralgia)
- Salivary glands
- Sinus linings
- Middle ear (otalgia)
- Associated nerve or vascular structures

In the overall process of patient assessment, particularly when compiling physical findings, it is important to assess the function of cranial nerves. Clinicians are often concerned about the possibility that facial pain is a harbinger of malignancy. In reality, malignant tumors that cause facial pain symptoms are extremely rare. When they do occur, they often invade areas of the skull and cranial base, with resultant neural compression. Therefore motor deficits are common concomitant features. A brief evaluation of cranial nerve function takes only 1 minute and is easy to accomplish. Initially the patient is questioned about subjective complaints; questions are directed toward uncovering defects in

the special senses. The patient is asked about any changes or differences in the ability to see, smell, hear, or taste and about any numbness or paresthesia in the facial region.

Objective screening of cranial nerves is relatively simple. First, the three divisions of the trigeminal sensory pathways are evaluated by use of a cotton tip to test for light touch sensation of the forehead, the cheek, and the chin. This can also be done intraorally along the lateral border of the tongue and the palate and on the buccal mucosa. The sensory tract of nerve VII can be evaluated by stimulating the skin around the external auditory meatus. This is quickly followed by an assessment of pain sensation, which can be accomplished with a dental explorer. First, patients are allowed to feel a brief pinprick on their hands from the explorer (to show what sensation they should expect). Then the same areas of the face are stimulated with the sharp explorer point to the skin. The patient should feel all stimuli; if all sensory pathways are intact, the sensation should be the same in all sites.

Once sensory pathways have been evaluated, the objective examination turns to motor function. The cranial nerves that innervate the facial musculature are often grouped together. In this regard, those cranial nerves that innervate the extraocular muscles are evaluated together. Nerves III, IV, and VI can be evaluated by having the patient track a moving object with the eyes. The tracking involves vertical upward and downward movements of the object and side-to-side movements. The object is returned to the center of the patient's gaze and moved down and out, in both right and left directions. If the patient's eyes are able to follow the up, down, side-to-side, and down-and-out movements, nerves III, IV, and VI are intact.

The motor function of nerve VII is assessed by asking the patient to wrinkle the forehead, raise the eyebrows, close the eyes, pucker the lips, and smile. Hypoglossal function is evaluated by having the patient protrude the tongue and move it left and right. Finally, spinal accessory innervation is assessed by having the patient shrug the shoulders against the resistance of a hand placed on the top of the shoulder. Should a motor or sensory deficit such as paresthesia or hypoesthesia be encountered in a patient with facial pain, the clinician should suspect a serious organic disease.

PAIN DISORDERS THAT MIMIC ODONTALGIA

The alert practitioner is aware that pain problems mimicking dental problems can be separated into two major categories: (1) typical pain disorders, and (2) atypical pain disorders (Box 3-1). Typical pain disorders are those in which the pathogenesis is known; atypical pain disorders have no established etiopathogenesis. (Box 3-1 lists the major pain disorders included in the category of typical orofacial pain. For each of these disorders the clinical features, nature and duration of the pain, and precipitating factors should be considered.)

BOX 3-1   PAIN DISORDERS

Typical Pain Disorders
- Periodontalgia (inflammatory, infectious)
- Neuralgic (trigeminal neuralgia, postherpetic neuralgia, traumatic neuroma)
- Vascular (cluster headache, temporal arteritis, other)
- Otic (otitis media)
- Sinus (acute pyogenic sinusitis, chronic sinusitis)
- Heart (cardiogenic jaw pain)
- Salivary gland (sialolithiasis)
- Musculoskeletal (head; jaw and neck contusion, strain, and sprain; internal joint derangement; myofascial disorder; myalgia; other)
- Neoplastic (metastases of the jaws and skull base)

Atypical Pain Disorders
- Causalgia
- Reflex sympathetic dystrophy
- Atypical facial pain
- Phantom tooth pain
- Neuralgia inducing cavitational osteonecrosis

Typical orofacial pain complaints are usually of short duration, and they are consistent with similar pain problems that the patient has had in the past. Patients often describe these pains as sharp, stabbing, or lancinating. However, symptoms and clinical signs may vary, depending on the origins of the pain and the individual experiencing the pain. Once the usual and customary diagnostic approaches to rule out pain of pulpal or periodontal origin have been undertaken, other disease processes that cause pain must be considered. Pain syndromes that are episodic, paroxysmal, or of short duration usually represent neuralgias or vasodilatory pain syndromes. Sharp, acute pains that persist for many hours or days are more likely to represent a nociceptor response to organic disease, usually an acute infectious process. Some pain syndromes are diagnosed on the basis of exclusion, although most have unique signs and symptoms that direct the clinician to a definitive diagnosis (Table 3-1).

Periodontalgia

Periodontal pain complaints are often expressed as a localized deep pain and may involve periodontal tissues around one or more teeth. Soft tissue infection or inflammation or

---

TABLE 3-1   DIFFERENTIATING TYPICAL AND ATYPICAL OROFACIAL PAINS THAT MIMIC ODONTALGIA

Condition	Nature	Triggers	Duration
Odontalgia	Stabbing, throbbing, nonepisodic	Hot, cold, tooth percussion	Hours, days
Periodontalgia	Deep aching, throbbing, nonepisodic	Occlusion, percussion	Hours, days
Trigeminal neuralgia	Lancinating, electrical, episodic	1 mm to 2 mm locus on skin or mucosa, light touch triggers pain	Seconds
Postherpetic	Deep boring ache with burning neuralgia	Spontaneous after facial shingles	Weeks, years
Cluster headache	Severe ache, retroorbital component, episodic	REM sleep, alcohol	Minutes
Temporal arteritis	Throbbing, aching, erythema of skin	Spontaneous	Hours
Otitis media	Severe ache, throbbing, deep to ear nonepisodic, barometric pressure	Lowering head	Hours, days
Bacterial sinusitis	Severe ache, throbbing in multiple posterior maxillary teeth, nonepisodic	Lowering head, tooth percussion	Hours, days
Allergic sinusitis	Dull ache malar area, multiple posterior maxillary teeth, seasonal	Lowering head	Weeks, months
Cardiogenic	Short-lived ache in left posterior mandible, episodic	Exertion	Minutes
Sialolithiasis	Sharp, drawing, salivary swelling, episodic	Eating, induced salivation	Minutes
TMJ internal	Dull ache, sharp episodes, derangements	Opening, chewing	Weeks, years
Myalgia	Dull ache, degree varies	Stress, clenching	Weeks, years
Neoplastic	Variable, motor deficit, paresthesia facial pain	Spontaneous	Days, months
Atypical pain	Variable syndromes	Nonspecific	Seconds, years

both (e.g., swelling, redness, tissue sensitivity) is often associated with this disorder. Associated teeth are often sensitive to temperature and pressure and may feel elongated. Dental mobility may also be observed. Often examination will disclose localized bleeding and measurable pocket depth, and radiographs will reflect loss of supporting alveolar bone. When periodontal pain involves multiple teeth, including opposing teeth, occlusal trauma should be considered. This should include traumatic effects, dental malocclusion, and bruxing and clenching. In many instances, periodontalgia and odontalgia may coexist and involve multiple tissues.

Neuralgias

Trigeminal Neuralgia   Trigeminal neuralgia, or tic douloureux, is a facial pain disorder with specific clinical features.* The pain involves one or more of the trigeminal nerve divisions and, although the precise cause is unknown, empiric evidence suggests that the symptoms evolve as a consequence of vascular compression of the Gasserian ganglion. The precise neurophysiologic mechanism has not been uncovered, and other theories for this particular disorder include viral infection of either neurons or the Schwann cell sheath.

Two highly characteristic features of tic douloureux allow it to be differentiated from other facial pain syndromes. The character and duration of the symptoms are unique, and a specific anatomic trigger point can be identified. Although the pain may sometimes involve the ophthalmic division, it primarily involves either the maxillary or the mandibular division. In addition the pain is severe and lancinating, shooting into the bone and teeth. Frequently both patient and dentist are convinced that the source of the pain is pulpal; the electric-like quality of the pain is unique and is rarely encountered in odontogenic infections. Furthermore, the pain episode lasts only seconds at a time, although paroxysms may occur in rapid succession. A trigger zone exists somewhere on the facial skin or, occasionally, in the oral cavity. This trigger area may be only 2 mm wide. When it is touched with the finger or an instrument, the pain paroxysms are triggered. The patient is usually keenly aware of this small anatomic site and will do anything to avoid stimulating the spot.

Treatment modalities are varied and include medical intervention with specific drugs that alleviate the neuralgic pain and various surgical interventions. For the dentist the most salient advice is to establish a diagnosis and avoid any invasive dental procedures. Invariably patients with trigeminal neuralgia have undergone numerous endodontic procedures and extractions, but they continue to experience pain because pulpal and periodontal infectious processes have no role in this syndrome. Therefore despite the patient's insistence that the symptoms are tooth related, the diagnosis

should be established and the patient should be referred to a neurologist for definitive therapy.

Carbamazepine (Tegretol), the standard medical therapy for trigeminal neuralgia, is quite effective. Unfortunately this particular drug is a bone marrow suppressant and will eventually produce agranulocytosis. Because this side effect is dose dependent, many patients may be maintained on Tegretol without untoward effects. However, the dose must be restricted to a level where agranulocytosis does not occur, yet pain symptoms are alleviated. For patients who do not respond to medical treatment, a variety of surgical modalities have been advocated, including peripheral neurectomy, rhizotomy (i.e., severance of the nerve trunk at its exit from the ganglion), alcohol injections, glycerol injections, cryotherapy, radio frequency lesioning, and laser therapy. All of these therapies have met with some degree of success.

Two surgical procedures for the relief of trigeminal neuralgia are widely accepted by the neurosurgical community: (1) surgical decompression and (2) transcutaneous ganglionic neurolysis. Surgical decompression of the ganglion, which often results in prolonged reduction of pain symptoms, has shown that vascular compression on the ganglion may be a cause of pain. Transcutaneous ganglionic neurolysis has also been a successful surgical procedure for the relief of pain. This technique involves placing a probe into the ganglion to ablate the neurons by thermal means. Both of these procedures have 90% rate of success over a 5-year period. Again, it is stressed that dental extraction or endodontic therapy is contraindicated in trigeminal neuralgia.

Postherpetic Neuralgia   Primary infection with varicella zoster virus (VZV) causes chickenpox, a disease that affects over 95% of the population during early childhood.[6,13,29,55] In its secondary or recurrent form, the disease is referred to as *herpes zoster* or *shingles*. This disease represents a recrudescence of a latent virus located in sensory ganglia. In the head and neck area, it is the trigeminal ganglion that harbors latent virus. The factors that activate the virus and allow it to exit from the ganglion and enter the axis cylinder are unknown. Importantly, once the virus is liberated from the nerve endings, it enters epithelial cells and induces a rather characteristic vesicular eruption. Unlike herpes simplex, recrudescence of varicella zoster results in a vesicular eruption that outlines the entire distribution of the sensory pathways. Therefore the vesicles terminate at the midline and involve only one division of the trigeminal nerve. Occasionally more than one division may be involved, however, bilateral involvement is extremely rare.

The painful lesions of shingles cause a deep, boring ache, involving not only the superficial mucosal and cutaneous tissues but also the maxillary or mandibular bones. Before the onset of the vesicular eruption, it is common for the patient to experience prodromal pain, obscuring the diagnosis. These prodromal symptoms frequently simulate trigeminal neuralgia: they last only seconds and have an electric-like quality. However, once vesicles appear, the diagnosis is

---

*References 2,11,21,31,35,42,45,46,57,59,62,63

straightforward. If any doubts persist, samples of the vesicular fluid collected within the first 3 days can be cultured for virus or subjected to cytologic smear examination with immunoperoxidase staining to identify the specific viral capsid antigen.

Patients show clearing of vesicles in less than 5% of varicella zoster infections, and pain is likely to persist. In addition, postherpetic neuralgia may persist weeks, months, or years. The prodromal pain is acute and electric-like, and the pain associated with vesicular eruption is deep and boring. However, once the vesicles clear, the residual pain has a burning quality and is chronic. Occasionally deeper aching pains may be associated with this burning element, suggesting pain of odontogenic origin. Nevertheless, the classic sequence of events with an antecedent vesicular eruption is sufficient to make the diagnosis. The management of postherpetic neuralgia is problematic, and there is no way of knowing when the symptoms may resolve of their own accord. A variety of techniques have been used to manage the pain, including transcutaneous electrical nerve stimulation (TENS), antiseizure drugs, analgesics, and topical preparations. Prompt referral to a neurologist is recommended. Children are now vaccinated for VZV; shingles will become a disease of the past.

Vasogenic Craniofacial Pain

Cluster Headache   Cluster headache, also known as *Sluder's neuralgia* or *sphenopalatine ganglion neuralgia, is* an acute paroxysmal pain syndrome of no known cause.* The pathogenesis is hypothesized to be a consequence of vasodilatory phenomena that occur on an episodic basis. Presumably, nociceptor fibers that encircle vessels are stimulated during acute vasodilatation. If this is the case, cluster headache is a form of migraine.

Cluster headache is generally encountered among males in their thirties to fifties. Although precipitating factors are not always identifiable, many of these patients report onset of pain after consuming alcohol. There is a tendency for the patients who suffer from cluster headaches to have a unique facial appearance: they are often freckled and have a ruddy complexion. Onset and duration of the pain episodes are unique and easily diagnosed. In classic cluster headache the pain is located unilaterally in the maxilla, sinus, and retroorbital area.

Cluster headache is often mistaken for acute pulpitis or apical abscess of a posterior maxillary tooth. The pain frequently occurs just after the patient retires and is entering the early stages of rapid eye movement (REM) sleep. The onset is acute and severe with patients indicating that it feels like a hot poker has been jammed into the upper jaw and behind the eye. Typically, the pain continues to increase in severity and persists for 30 to 45 minutes. During this period the patient finds it difficult to remain seated and tends to pace the floor. In most cases the symptoms occur at approximately the same time, once each evening. However, some people suffer two such episodes a day. In the classic form of cluster headache the episodic symptoms persist only 6 to 8 weeks, then spontaneously disappear. The headache episodes cluster at a certain time of day and during a certain season; they seem to be more prevalent in spring. Hence the term *cluster headache.*

Another form of cluster headache is referred to as *chronic* cluster. These headaches are similar to the classic form in that they occur on an episodic basis and typically last 30 to 45 minutes. However, chronic cluster headaches affect the patient year round, rather than seasonally.

In the past, because vasodilatation is involved in their pathogenesis, cluster headaches were managed by prescribing ergotamine tartrate. This medication causes significant side effects, including nausea and vomiting, so it is prescribed as a suppository. Because ergot alkaloids induce vasoconstriction, they are contraindicated for patients with hypertension (many patients with cluster headache are also hypertensive). It was subsequently discovered that oxygen would lessen the headache attacks if administered at the onset of pain. Therefore administration of oxygen is often used as a diagnostic intervention.

The current therapy for cluster headache uses vasoactive drugs, particularly the calcium channel blockers. When prescribed on a regular basis, nifedipine (or one of its related compounds) prevents the pain paroxysms and is of benefit for both classic and chronic cluster headache. In addition, prednisone (in combination with lithium) has been shown to be effective in alleviating or preventing pain of cluster headache. Hyperbaric oxygen therapy has also been shown to have preventive effects. In addition, the vasoactive antimigraine drug sumatriptin succinate, a 5-hydroxytryptamine receptor agonist that is administered subcutaneously, is effective for treatment of cluster headache. However, oral administration of this drug is not particularly beneficial.

Temporal Arteritis

Also known as giant cell arteritis, temporal arteritis is a granulomatous inflammatory disease of the temporal artery wall in which the vessel wall is thickened and inflamed.[1,12] Temporal arteritis causes throbbing pain in the temple region. The disease usually appears in late life, and the temporal artery is often visibly thickened with erythema of the overlying facial skin. The sedimentation rate is elevated, and laboratory tests assist in confirming the diagnosis. Biopsy is also a means for diagnostic confirmation, because giant cells and granulomatous inflammation can be identified in the adventitia of the artery. Temporal arteritis can involve other carotid branches, including the facial artery, creating pain symptoms that may be experienced in the maxilla, mimicking toothache.

---

*References 10,14,17,30,40,41,43,50,58,61.

Otitis Media

Infection of the middle ear is common, particularly in children, and is caused by pyogenic microorganisms (e.g., streptococci).[18] It is well known that odontogenic infections of posterior teeth may refer pain back to the ear and temporomandibular joint (TMJ) areas. Similarly, middle ear infections may be confused with odontogenic pain because the symptoms radiate from the ear over the posterior aspects of the maxilla and mandible. It would be unlikely for middle ear infection to be exclusively expressed as jaw pain. The nature of the pain is acute; patients complain of a severe ache, and throbbing is a frequent accompaniment. Gravitational factors may also come into play; pain is often exacerbated as the patient lowers the head.

The pathogenesis is straightforward and is, in many ways, similar to that of acute pulp pain. In the dental pulp the noxious components of the inflammatory process and factors secreted by the pathogenic microorganisms accumulate in a confined space. In otitis media the infection occurs within the middle ear, which is confined laterally by the tympanic membrane and posteriorly by the oval window (laterally the eustachian tube serves as an outlet). In the process of acute inflammation, with accumulation of neutrophils, exudate, and associated mucosal edema, the eustachian tube lining mucosa swells and becomes occluded, thereby confining the noxious components of the infectious process to the middle ear chamber.

The definitive diagnosis is made by using an otoscope to examine the tympanic membrane, which is usually red and bulging. Treatment consists of antibiotic therapy, usually penicillin with P-lactase inhibitor or clindamycin; occasionally syringotomy is necessary. Once the diagnosis is established, referral to an otolaryngologist is recommended.

Sinogenic Pain

Acute Maxillary Sinusitis   Because the roots of the maxillary teeth extend to the sinus floor, it is axiomatic that acute infectious processes involving the sinus mucous membrane will simulate dental pain.[4,28] Most forms of sinusitis are allergic and are characterized by dull pain complaints in the malar region and maxillary alveolus.

When maxillary sinusitis is the consequence of an acute pyogenic bacterial infection, the symptoms are usually acute. The pain may be stabbing, with severe aching pressure and throbbing. Pain is frequently referred upward, under the orbit, and downward, over the maxillary posterior teeth. Importantly, pain is not referred to a single tooth but is perceived in all teeth in the quadrant. Percussion sensitivity of the molar teeth is a common finding, and when the head is placed below the knees, the pain is often exacerbated.

The aforementioned signs and symptoms are rather characteristic; however, other diagnostic approaches can be used to secure a definitive diagnosis. Transillumination is a diagnostic aid that is easy to perform. A fiberoptic light beam is placed against the palate; in a darkened room, a clear sinus will transilluminate. Antra that are filled with exudate are clouded and will not transilluminate. Radiographic imaging is also of considerable diagnostic utility. Although more advanced imaging, such as magnetic resonance imaging (MRI) and computed tomography (CT), may be used, a Waters' radiographic view of the sinus is usually sufficient.

Because maxillary root apices are separated from the antral floor by a few millimeters of bone, it is understandable that acute periapical infection could spread into the sinus. Therefore bacterial sinusitis can be a consequence of pulpal infection. It is essential to assess each maxillary tooth in patients with acute maxillary sinusitis, because treatment of the sinusitis without management of the dental source will only result in recurrence of symptoms.

Although acute bacterial sinusitis is generally readily responsive to antibiotic therapy, induced sinus drainage and lavage may occasionally be necessary when the ostia are closed because of edema. At the time of examination, culture and sensitivity tests should be performed to select the appropriate antibiotic (should preliminary therapy fail to resolve the infection). Referral to an otolaryngologist is recommended.

Allergic Sinusitis   As discussed in the differential diagnosis of acute facial pains, inflammatory disease of the antrum is more often chronic and allergic in nature.[4,28] Allergies tend to be seasonal, because most people with upperairway allergic reactions respond to various seeds and pollens. In northern climates the prevalence of sinusitis increases in spring and fall. However, in warmer climates, such as California and Florida, allergies may be encountered year round (some allergies may actually be more common during the winter months).

The contact of an allergen with the sinonasal mucous membranes results in an immediate-type hypersensitivity reaction that is mediated by an antigen that penetrates the respiratory epithelium, enters the submucosa, and is bound to an immunoglobulin E antibody. This antibody is complexed with mast cells and, on binding to the allergen, histamine is released. Vasoactive consequences evolve, with edema formation and transudation of fluids. Involvement of the sinus includes mucosal thickening and the presence of a fluid level within the maxillary sinus cavity. As the ostium becomes occluded, pain symptoms evolve. The pain is preceded by a feeling of pressure within the maxilla for a few hours or days, which evolves into a dull, chronic ache. Frequently the posterior maxillary teeth seem to "itch," and the patient feels compelled to clench. Percussion sensitivity is evident on all of the molar teeth, and frequently the premolars are percussion sensitive as well. This sensitivity is not acute; rather, it is experienced as a dull discomfort.

As with acute sinusitis, symptoms may be accentuated by having the patient place the head between the knees. The gravitational changes shift the fluid in the sinus and result in increased pain. Maxillary sinus pain is typically accentuated by changes in barometric pressure, therefore, traveling to high altitudes or flying may exacerbate the pain. Without treatment these symptoms persist throughout the period when allergens circulate in the air. The diagnosis is supplemented by antral transillumination, in which light will not illuminate an affected maxilla in a darkened room. Waters' sinus radiographs will disclose either soft tissue membrane thickening of the antral walls or an air fluid level will be discernable. Mucosal changes are also evident on MRI and CT scans.

Because chronic sinusitis is generally allergic in nature, the treatment differs from that of acute bacterial sinusitis. Decongestants and nasal sprays, along with antihistamines, are the treatments of choice. Identification of the allergen and desensitization may offer relief for some of patients, and referral to an otolaryngologist or an allergist should be considered.

Cardiogenic Jaw Pain[3,48]

Vascular occlusive disease is one of the most common afflictions. The accumulation of atherosclerotic plaque in coronary vessels (in association with vasospasm) will lead to angina pectoris. The most common manifestation of coronary vascular occlusion, particularly in its acute manifestation, is substernal pain with referred pain rotating over the left shoulder and down the arm. This pain is usually precipitated by exertion. Presumably the pain sensation is transmitted by nociceptor fibers that envelop the coronary vasculature and are stimulated by vasospasm. Because angina pectoris is a prelude to acute myocardial infarction, these symptoms are extremely significant and the appropriate diagnostic imaging studies are required to ascertain the degree of coronary occlusion. Such symptoms represent a life-threatening event. Occasionally angina pectoris is manifested as left shoulder and arm pain without a substernal component. Even less frequent is referral of pain up the neck into the left angle of the mandible. In these instances the referred pain may mimic odontalgia.

When a patient reports left posterior mandibular pain and there is no obvious odontogenic source of infection, referred cardiogenic pain should be considered. Importantly, the patient should be questioned about the onset of the symptoms. If they occur after exercise or other exertion, then coronary vascular disease should be considered.

Once suspected, specific diagnostic tests can be performed to assess the potential for coronary vascular occlusive disease. Specifically, electrocardiography or stress tests may be advisable. If these findings support a diagnosis of coronary ischemia, cardiac catheterization and angiography are indicated. Treatment consists of a variety of interventions, including restricted intake of lipids, administration of aspirin to prevent thrombosis, and surgical intervention by coronary angioplasty or bypass surgery should angiography show significant occlusive disease.

Sialolithiasis

Unlike kidney stones and gallstones, sialoliths are unrelated to increased levels of serum calcium or to dietary factors.[34,53] Although the pathogenesis is relatively well understood, the cause is unknown. Desquamated epithelial cells from the major salivary ducts may accumulate and form complexes with salivary mucin to form a nidus for calcification. The salivary stone evolves by sequential concretion of calcium phosphate salts, much like the growth rings of a tree. Once the stone reaches a critical size, the salivary duct becomes occluded and symptoms develop. Sialolithiasis is significantly more frequent in the submandibular duct; therefore pain associated with submandibular stones is more prone to mimic endodontic pain in the posterior aspect of the mandible. The occluded duct often leads to swelling of the submandibular area. Hence it may mimic lymphadenitis associated with an endodontic infection of a posterior mandibular tooth.

With close examination and questioning, the diagnosis is usually made quite easily because the pain has characteristic features. Although a chronic ache may extend into the mandible, the primary location is within the submandibular soft tissues. Typically, the pain is exacerbated by salivation (induced by a lemon drop or mealtimes). The floor of the mouth can be palpated using a milking motion; when the major duct is occluded, no saliva will flow from the duct orifice. The nature of the pain is also revealing in that the patient feels a stringent drawing in the area. When pain of this nature is encountered, salivary occlusion should be investigated before each tooth in the vicinity is evaluated. Typically, an occlusal radiograph will disclose the presence of a soft tissue calcification along the course of the duct in the floor of the mouth. It should be noted that panoramic radiographs may reveal an opacity in the mandible. In such instances the soft tissue calcification is simply superimposed (although it may mimic focal sclerosing osteomyelitis).

Although sialolithiasis of the parotid duct is quite rare, its pain can be mistaken for toothache. Again the symptoms are similar to those of submandibular sialolithiasis in that the pain is exacerbated during meals and with stimulation of salivation. The sialolith is generally demonstrable with a panoramic radiograph.

Treatment consists of physical attempts to remove the stone by manipulating it out the orifice. Larger stones cannot be removed in this fashion and will require a surgical cut down to the duct. Indeed, stones of large size and long duration usually culminate in ablation of the secretory component of the gland. In this case the nonfunctional gland becomes subject to retrograde bacterial infections, and sialoadenectomy, along with removal of the stone, is indicated.

Musculoskeletal Disorders

Musculoskeletal pain involving the jaw can be associated with trauma and dysfunction of the cervical, head, and jaw musculature.* The pain can be described as superficial or deep, as well as constant with variable intensity. Jaw function often exacerbates the pain complaints. Areas of pain complaints include the teeth, jaw joint (i.e., temporomandibular joint), cheek (i.e., masseter muscle), temple (i.e., temporalis muscle), sides of the neck (i.e., sternocleidomastoid muscle), and back of the head (i.e., suboccipital musculature). In most cases there is at least a partial myalgic or arthalgic basis to the overall pain complaints. Temporomandibular disorders (TMD) and disorders of the cervical spine are included in the musculoskeletal group. These problems tend to be relatively localized, but can involve other aspects of the musculoskeletal system. Musculoskeletal disorders may become more chronic in nature and more resistant to resolution the longer the patient experiences related pain.

Other organic joint diseases (e.g., rheumatoid, gouty, or psoriatic arthritis; arthritis-attending collagen diseases) may also involve the jaw and cervical joints and cause pain symptoms. All of these arthritides are quite rare in the TMJ region. Most pain symptoms referable to the musculoskeletal tissues of the jaws and neck are locally experienced. Nevertheless, some patients may relate the symptoms to their teeth.

Abnormal Joint Function (Internal Derangement)

Internal derangement of the TMJ is often associated with localized joint area pain complaints. Internal derangements of the TMJ include meniscus displacement, formation of intraarticular adhesions, and various forms of arthritis. A variety of etiologic factors have been implicated, but no single hypothesis has been universally accepted. It has been proposed that stress-related jaw clenching and bruxism may place stress on the meniscus and cause anterior displacement. Alternatively, traumatic events (e.g., motor vehicle accidents), yawning, and prolonged jaw opening have been suggested to cause compression or overextension of the ligaments, with secondary displacement of the meniscus. Once the meniscus has been anteriorly displaced, adhesions may form and the disk and retrodiscal tissues not designed for loading may degenerate, with adaptive osseous changes and a progression to degenerative joint disease. Although abnormal jaw posture may be a significant etiological factor, it is highly unlikely that occlusal discrepancies predispose (or even cause) these events.

The chief findings associated with internal derangement include limitation of jaw opening, deviation on opening, joint clicking or crepitus, and pain directly localized to the joint region in front of the tragus of the ear. The pain associated with internal derangement is generally a dull, boring ache, but it may be more acute when exacerbated by wide opening of the mandible or chewing. In some patients the chronic symptoms become progressively worse and the degree of pain increases. In such instances the pain symptoms may become more generalized. TMJ pain is often referred into the temple, cheek, and posterior dental areas of the maxilla or mandible. In such instances the patient may perceive a joint problem as a dental problem or as a temple area headache.

Myalgia

Myalgic pain disorders involving the masticatory musculature can be perceived as dental pain. These disorders appear to be the consequence of sustained muscle contraction usually associated with jaw clenching and bruxing, as well as muscle bracing and splinting. Muscle bracing and splinting (or muscle parafunction) can occur voluntarily or involuntarily as a protective response to injured tissue or structure. It can also occur as a response to other life stressors; facial myalgia is generally considered to be equivalent to tension headache. Myalgic pain is constant, variable in intensity, usually dull, aching, and it involves multiple muscle areas. In general most patients complain of symptoms over the mandible and temple. Palpitation of the masticatory muscles will often reveal the presence of localized tender areas. These tender areas should not be confused with the "trigger zone" of trigeminal neuralgia or referral patterns associated with myofascial disorders. Facial myalgia may exist as an isolated entity, or it may be associated with other pain disorders, such as cervicalgia, TMJ arthralgia, odontalgia, or periodontalgia. The pain symptoms can become quite variable and confusing to the examiner. In such instances, evaluations of jaw function, auscultation of the TMJ, masticatory muscle palpitation, and cervical evaluation, as well as endodontic and periodontal testing, should be performed. If an endodontic infection is uncovered, root canal therapy may relieve what appeared to be a myalgic pain problem. Treatment by a physical therapist (focused on the neck) may also relieve what appeared to be a jaw muscle pain problem.

Myofascial Pain

Myofascial disorders are characterized by continuous, dull pain of variable intensity, with localized tenderness in one or more muscles. Essential to the diagnosis of myofascial pain is discovery of localized hypersensitive areas (i.e., trigger points) with a positive jump sign response on palpation. Active trigger points (TrPs) are often associated with predictable pain referral patterns to adjacent or distant sites. Trigger points found in the superficial aspect of masseter muscles have consistent referral patterns to the maxillary and mandibular teeth; toothache is a common pain complaint. Other associated symptoms could include tinnitus, restricted jaw opening, deviation of jaw opening, jaw pain, and earache.

Temporalis muscle trigger points can refer pain to maxillary posterior and anterior teeth; headache and toothache are common associated complaints. Cervical muscle trigger points have also been shown to have referral pain patterns

---

*References 16,19,23,24,26,32,38,44,47,52,60

into the jaw and face area. Once trigger points have been located and a myofascial disorder diagnosis has been made, treatment can be instituted. The three most common techniques for eliminating trigger points and associated pain patterns include (1) physical therapy, (2) spray-and-stretch technique, and (3) trigger point injections.

When odontogenic sources have been ruled out and a diagnosis of internal derangement, myalgia, internal derangement with myalgia, or myofascial disorder is confirmed, appropriate therapy should be instituted. Psychologic and behavioral factors have been shown to play a role in TMJ and myofascial pain disorders, and a conservative approach to therapy is considered prudent. Treatment may include behavioral, psychologic, physical, dental, and medical therapies. Muscle relaxants, nonsteroidal antiinflammatories, physical therapy, stress management therapy, and occlusal splints are generally considered conservative procedures. Acupuncture has also shown some success in certain populations, but it is not universally effective.

Extensive tooth grinding (i.e., equilibration) aimed at curing the disorder should be avoided. When intractable pain persists after conservative therapy, surgery may be a consideration, including arthrocentesis, arthroscopic surgery, or open joint surgery. Even with surgical intervention, severe pain disorders often recur within months after the procedure, with continuing conservative management necessary. In selected cases, long-term splint therapy or stabilizing dental therapy may be necessary.

Neoplasia[9,22]

Although cancer involving the maxilla and mandible rarely manifests itself with pain, there is a published case report regarding prodromal facial pain from a glioblastoma.[8] Typically paresthesia or hypoesthesia is the complaint. Carcinoma arising in the maxillary sinus may proliferate and begin to erode the bony margins of the sinus walls. As the tumor extends into the floor of the orbit, encroachment on the infraorbital nerve induces paresthesia over the malar region and in the maxillary teeth. Similarly, a malignant tumor in the mandible, such as metastatic carcinoma from a distant site (e.g., lung, breast, colon), can invade the nerve. Therefore numbness is the ominous symptom of cancer in the jaws (although such tumors occasionally produce pain symptoms). In particular, multiple myeloma (e.g., malignant neoplasia of B lymphocytes) is notorious for causing intense bone pain. Therefore, in the jaws, such lesions could easily mimic toothache. However, myeloma rarely manifests itself only in the jaws because it is a disseminated disease. Therefore pain would also be experienced in other bones. The tumor induces "punched-out" radiolucencies that are poorly marginated. Such lesions should be investigated by obtaining a biopsy specimen.

A variety of cancer-associated pain syndromes of the face have been reported in the literature. These are rare conditions and are designated by a host of eponyms. In general they represent tumors that have metastasized to the base of the skull, where they encroach on exiting cranial nerves. Most such tumors will invade not only sensory nerves, they will also invade motor nerves. Therefore muscular weakness or paralysis in conjunction with pain are the usual accompaniments. When tumors affect the upper aspects of the nasopharynx and skull base, upper facial pain is experienced and the cranial nerves III, IV, and VI become involved, leading to ophthalmoplegia. Generally, tumors that arise around the exit of the trigeminal nerve affect the motor fibers of nerve V, and masticatory muscle weakness is identifiable. A combination of atypical facial pain with ocular, facial, or masticatory muscle paresis should alert the clinician that a malignant disease may be present. In this case more sophisticated imaging studies, such as MRI and CT scans, should be undertaken. If a tumor is present, it will be localized on such images, and referral to an oncologist is recommended.

ATYPICAL PAIN DISORDERS THAT MIMIC ODONTALGIA

Of all the facial pain syndromes, the group that most often simulates endodontic or odontogenic pain is "atypical facial pain."* Indeed, patients will insist the pain is of tooth origin and will often plead to have the offending tooth or teeth removed. When diagnosing jaw and endodontic pain, it is imperative that the clinician be well versed in the clinical features of this group of pain disorders because tooth extraction or endodontic therapy will fail to alleviate the symptoms.

Subsumed under the heading of atypical orofacial pain are a variety of disorders including phantom tooth pain, neuralgia-inducing cavitational osteonecrosis (NICO), causalgia, complex regional pain syndrome (CRPS), deafferentation pain, neuropathic pain, and sympathetically maintained pain. By definition, atypical facial pain represents a pain syndrome that does not conform to a specific organic disease and does not represent another well defined form of pain disorder. Although there is no identifiable cause, numerous experts consider the involvement of the autonomic nervous system.

Although the exact pathophysiology of atypical facial pain is unknown, it is possible that there could be different expressions of the same disorder identified with variable names (as noted previously). These types of atypical pains are chronic and aching; patients with atypical facial pain feel it deep within the bones and it is hard to localize. Indeed many patients with atypical facial pain will report that the symptoms seem to wander from site to site. In addition, many of these patients have pain complaints elsewhere in their bodies. The intensity of these atypical pains varies considerably from one patient to the next. Some complain of a

---

*References 5,7,8,15,20,25,27,33,36,37,39,49,51,54,56,64

constant nagging ache; others claim that the pain is excruciating at times. The cause of atypical pain has long been a mystery, and many clinicians have emphasized the probability that psychogenic factors play a major role.

A comprehensive evaluation should include psychologic and behavioral-dysfunction screening instruments that assess depressive, anxious, or hostile behaviors. Dental training establishes the belief that a physical condition is the basis of every disease or physical disorder, as well as any pain associated with that disease or disorder. However, it is possible that a psychologic disorder may be the primary causative factor of atypical pain. Therefore the astute clinician appreciates that no pain is without some influence from psychobehavioral factors, because these factors can contribute to (or be the cause of) a patient's orofacial pain. Additional diagnosis of hypochondriasis, somatoform pain disorder, malingering pain disorder, and conversion disorder may have to be considered in atypical facial pain problems. Psychologic or psychiatric consultation is appropriate.

Phantom Tooth Pain

The term *phantom tooth pain* is used to describe pain that persists in teeth or the area of a specific tooth after the pulp has been extirpated. Phantom tooth pain is estimated to occur in less than 3% of patients undergoing root canal therapy. It has been suggested that surgical extirpation of the pulp results in damage to nerve fibers at the apex of the teeth and should be considered a traumatic neuralgia. Another possible mechanism is formation of a small traumatic neuroma in the apical periodontium. Although psychologic factors have been suggested to be important in phantom tooth pain, there is not a great deal of evidence (on the basis of psychometric testing) that psychopathologic mechanisms are major factors. Because deafferentation in animals results in pain behavior, it has been suggested that phantom tooth pain is a form of deafferentation pain. However, although these postendodontic pain foci are subjected to surgical procedures, the pain often persists. The organic basis for phantom tooth pain remains an enigma.

Neuralgia-Inducing Cavitational Osteonecrosis (NICO)

Neuralgia-inducing cavitational osteonecrosis (NICO) is an atypical orofacial pain localized to edentulous foci, which can sometimes be alleviated with a subperiosteal injection of local anesthetic. In such instances it has been proposed that small residual inflammatory foci exist within the endosteum, and that focal necrosis occurs with neural damage. In selected cases surgical curettage has alleviated associated pain. Tissue curetted from these cavities often shows minor pathologic changes, such as fibrosis and mild inflammation. The validity of this theory of atypical facial pain arising in edentulous regions is not universally accepted and is considered somewhat controversial.

Complex Regional Pain Syndrome

Complex regional pain refers to pain complaints that have lasted longer than the normal healing period and have increased in complexity. Depending on the cause of the pain complaint, this diagnosis could be made in 4 to 6 weeks. However, some cases of complex regional pain take as long as 6 months to 1 year to diagnose. This phenomenon has been explained as an unusual pattern of pain with a higher level of central nervous system involvement. It has also been described as sympathetically maintained pain.

A variety of factors can contribute to the perpetuation of pain complaints, including a lack of healing, inappropriate therapy, missed diagnosis, increase in psychologic involvement, and secondary gain. Medical and psychosocial histories with references to depression, anxiety, addiction, dependence, low self-esteem, and hostility have been shown to characterize these patients. Unresolved litigation should also not be overlooked as a possible contributing factor. Five other characteristics leading to a diagnosis of chronic pain include (1) inconsistency of symptoms, with variable episodic or continuous pain complaints; (2) persistence of the pain despite therapy and passage of time; (3) pain complaints that appear disproportionate to stimulus; (4) pain complaints are not eliminated with routine anesthetic blocks; and (5) pain complaints that do not necessarily follow normal anatomic pathways or adhere to established referral patterns.

Causalgia

Causalgia pain can involve the jaws, head, and neck. When present, it may be confused with odontalgia. Causalgic pain is often associated with trauma, jaw fracture, or laceration, and it may evolve after surgery. It has been hypothesized that in causalgia, nociceptor fibers become retracked in association with autonomic fibers. The skin overlying the painful area often becomes erythematous during pain episodes. Patients have a tendency to rub and scratch the involved area, producing what are known as trophic foci; the skin can become encrusted and keratotic. The pain is characteristically paroxysmal and burning, and it may be both superficial and deep. When the predominant complaint is a deep component, it may be confused with toothache. To arrive at a definitive diagnosis of causalgia, historical trauma events and clinical features must be identified. Postherpetic neuralgia manifests similar features and should be considered in the differential diagnosis.

Whether atypical facial pains lie in edentulous areas, are poorly localized, or are centered in teeth, treatment should be approached cautiously. Many patients have submitted to numerous endodontic procedures and extractions for these pains; subsequent to the invasive procedures, the pain has persisted. Many dentists have undertaken such procedures at the insistence of the patient, who firmly believes there is an odontogenic source. When the symptoms are mild, the pain should be managed with analgesics and reassurance.

Many patients with atypical facial pain respond favorably to tricyclic antidepressants, particularly amitriptyline. This medication affects neurotransmitter substances and appears to have an analgesic property in addition to its antidepressant effects. In more severe cases, the therapy used for trigeminal neuralgia may be indicated. In particular, microvascular decompression and transcutaneous thermal neurolysis or radio frequency lesioning have been found to be effective in treating more severe atypical facial pain problems in some patients. Occasionally stellate and sphenopalatine ganglion blocks are employed successfully as therapeutic modalities.

CONCLUSION

A variety of pain disorders involving the jaws, head, face, and neck have the potential to simulate dental (i.e., odontogenic) pain. In evaluating pulpal and periapical pain, other disorders must be considered in the differential diagnosis. This is particularly true when the usual physical findings fail to implicate a particular tooth. Certain pain disorders have a higher morbidity than others with differential diagnosis, including entities from localized periodontal infections to invasive neoplasms to psychologic disorders. In addition, individual patients may suffer from more than one disorder. Therefore it is certainly possible for a patient who has one of these pain disorders also to harbor a dental or periodontal infection. For this reason, the importance of conducting a thorough history with a comprehensive physical examination to evaluate the dentition and other anatomic sites cannot be overemphasized.

References

1. Achkar AA, Lie JT, Gabriel SE, Hunder GG: Giant cell arteritis involving the facial artery, *J Rheumatol* 22:360, 1995.
2. Barker FG II et al: The long-term outcome of microvascular decompression for trigeminal neuropathy, *N Engl J Med* 334:1077, 1996.
3. Batchelder BJ, Krutchkoff DJ, Amara J: Mandibular pain as the initial and sole clinical manifestation of coronary insufficiency: report of case, *J Am Dent Assoc* 115:710, 1987.
4. Berg O, Lejdeborn L: Experience of a permanent ventilation and drainage system in the management of purulent maxillary sinusitis, *Ann Otol Rhinol Laryngol* 99:192, 1990.
5. Bouquot JE, Christian J: Long-term effects of jawbone curettage on the pain of facial neuralgia, *J Oral Maxillofac Surg* 53:387, 1995.
6. Bernstein JE et al: Topical capsaidcin: treatment of chronic postherpetic neuralgia, *J Am Acad Dermatol* 21:265, 1989.
7. Bouquot JE et al: Neuralgia-inducing cavitational osteonecrosis (NICO), *Oral Surg Oral Med Oral Pathol* 73:307, 1992.
8. Brooke RI: Atypical odontalgia, *Oral Surg Oral Med Oral Pathol* 49:196, 1980.
9. Cohen S et al: Oral prodromal signs of a central nervous system malignant neoplasm-glioblastoma multiform, *J Am Dent Assoc* 121:643, 1986.
10. Connors MJ: Cluster headache: a review, *J Am Osteopath Assoc* 95:533, 1995.
11. Dalessio DJ: Management of the cranial neuralgias and atypical facial pain. A review, *Clin J Pain* 5:55, 1989.
12. Das AK, Laskin DM: Temporal arteritis of the facial artery, *J Oral Surg* 24:226, 1966.
13. De Benedittis G, Besana F, Lorenzetti A: A new topical treatment for acute herpetic neuralgia and post-herpetic neuralgia: the aspirin/diethyl ether mixture. An open-label study plus a double-blind controlled clinical trial, *Pain* 48:383, 1992.
14. Dechant KL, Clissold SP: Sumatriptin. A review of its pharmacodynamic and pharmacokinetic properties, and therapeutic efficacy in the acute treatment of migraine and cluster headache, *Drugs* 43:776, 1992.
15. Donlon WC: Neuralgia-inducing cavitational osteonecrosis, *Oral Surg Oral Med Oral Pathol* 73:319, 1992.
16. Dworkin SF et al: Brief group cognitive-behavioral intervention for temporomandibular disorders, *Pain* 59:175, 1994.
17. Ekborn K et al: Cluster headache attacks treated for up to three months with subcutaneous sumatriptin (6 mg). Sumatriptin cluster headache long-term study group, *Cephalagia* 15:230, 1995.
18. Froorn J et al: Diagnosis and antibiotic treatment of acute otitis media: report from international primary care network, *BMJ* 300:582, 1990.
19. Gallagher RM et al: Myofascial face pain: seasonal variability in pain intensity and demoralization, *Pain* 61:113, 1995.
20. Graff-Radford SB, Solberg WK: Atypical odontalgia, *J Craniomandib Disord* 6:260, 1992.
21. Graff-Radford SB et al: Thermographic assessment of neuropathic facial pain, *J Orofac Pain* 9:138, 1995.
22. Greenberg HS: Metastasis to the base of the skull: clinical findings in 43 patients, *Neurology* 31:530, 1981.
23. Hapak L et al: Differentiation between musculoligamentous, dentoalveolar, and neurologically based craniofacial pain with a diagnostic questionnaire, *J Orofac Pain* 8:357, 1994.
24. Harness DM, Donlon WC, Eversole LR: Comparison of clinical characteristics in myogenic TMJ internal derangement and atypical facial pain patients, *Clin J Pain* 8:4, 1990.
25. Harness DM, Rome HP: Psychologic and behavioral aspects of chronic facial pain, *Otolaryngol Clin North Am* 22:1073, 1989.
26. Helms CA et al: Staging of internal derangements of the TMJ with magnetic resonance imaging: preliminary observations, *J Craniomandib Disord* 3:93, 1989.
27. Hoffman KD, Matthews MA: Comparison of sympathetic neurons in orofacial and upper extremity nerves: implications for causalgia, *J Oral Maxillofac Surg* 48:720, 1990.
28. Kennedy DW, Loury MC: Nasal and sinus pain: current diagnosis and treatment, *Semin Neural* 8:303, 1988.
29. Kishore-Kumar R et al: Desipramine? relieves postherpetic neuralgia, *Clin Pharmacol Ther* 47:305, 1990.
30. Kudrow L: Cluster headache. A review, *Clin J Pain* 6:29, 1989.
31. Lichtor T, Mullan JR: A 10-year follow-up review of percutaneous microcompression of the trigeminal ganglion, *J Neurosurg* 72:49, 1990.
32. Linde A, Isacsson G, Jonsson BG: Outcome of 6-week treatment with transcutaneous electric nerve stimulation compared

with splint on symptomatic temporomandibular joint disk displacement without reduction, *Acta Odontol Scand* 53:92, 1995.

33. Lipton JA, Ship JA, Larach-Robinson D: Estimated prevalence and distribution of reported orofacial pain in the United States, *J Am Dent Assoc* 124:115, 1993.

34. Lustmann J, Regev E, Melamed Y: Sialolithiasis. A survey on 245 patients and a review of the literature, *Int J Oral Maxillofac Surg* 19:135, 1990.

35. Main JH, Jordan RC, Barewal R: Facial neuralgias: a clinical review of 34 cases, *J Can Dent Assoc* 58:752, 1992.

36. Marbach JJ: Is phantom tooth pain a deafferentation (neuropathic) syndrome. I. Evidence derived from pathophysiology and treatment, *Oral Surg Oral Med Oral Pathol* 75:95, 1993.

37. Marbach JJ: Is phantom tooth pain a deafferentation (neuropathic) syndrome? II. Psychosocial considerations, *Oral Surg Oral Med Oral Pathol* 75:225, 1993.

38. Marbach JJ, Raphael KG, Dohrenwend BP: Do premenstrual pain and edema exhibit seasonal variability? *Psychosom Med* 57:536, 1995.

39. Marbach JJ et al: Incidence of phantom tooth pain: an atypical facial neuralgia, *Oral Surg Oral Med Oral Pathol* 53:190, 1982.

40. Mathew NT: Advances in cluster headache, *Neurol Clin* 8:867, 1990.

41. Mauskop A, Altura BT, Cracco RQ, Altura BM: Intravenous magnesium sulfate relieves cluster headaches in patients with low serum ionized magnesium levels, *Headache* 35:597, 1995.

42. McLaughlin MR et al: Microvascular decompression of cranial nerves: lessons learned after 4400 operations, *J Neurosurg* 90:1, 1999.

43. Medina JL, Diamond S, Fareed J: The nature of cluster headache, *Headache* 19:309, 1979.

44. Mock D: The differential diagnosis of temporomandibular disorders, *J Orofac Pain* 13:246, 1999.

45. Moller AR: The cranial nerve vascular compression syndrome. I. A review of treatment, *Acta Neurochir (Wien)* 113:18, 1991.

46. Moraci M et al: Trigeminal neuralgia treated by percutaneous thermocoagulation: comparative analysis of percutaneous thermocoagulation and other surgical procedures, *Acta Neurochir* 35:48, 1992.

47. Murakami K et al: Four-year follow-up study of temporomandibular joint arthroscopic surgery for advanced stage internal derangements, *J Oral Maxillofac Surg* 54:285, 1996.

48. Natkin E, Harrington GW, Mandel MA: Anginal pain referred to the teeth, *Oral Surg Oral Med Oral Pathol* 40:678, 1975.

49. Nicolodi M, Sicuteri F: Phantom tooth diagnosis and an anamnestic focus on headache, *N Y State Dent J* 59:35, 1993.

50. Pascual J, Peralta G, Sanchez U: Preventive effects of hyperbaric oxygen in cluster headache, *Headache* 35:260, 1995.

51. Okeson JP, Bell WE: *Bell's orofacial pains*, ed 5, Chicago, 1995, Quintessence Publishing.

52. Pertes R, Gross S: *Clinical management of temporomandibular disorders and orofacial pain*, ed 1, Chicago, 1995, Quintessence Publishing.

53. Pollack CV Jr, Severance HW Jr: Sialolithiasis: case studies and review, *J Emerg Med* 8:561, 1990.

54. Pollmann L: Determining factors of the phantom tooth, *N Y State Dent J* 59:42, 1993.

55. Robertson DR, George DP: Treatment of post-herpetic neuralgia in the elderly, *Br Med Bull* 48:113, 1990.

56. Schnurr RR, Brooke RI: Atypical odontalgia: update and comment on long-term follow-up, *Oral Surg Oral Med Oral Pathol* 73:445, 1992.

57. Sicuteri R et al: Idiopathic headache as a possible risk factor for phantom tooth pain, *Headache* 31:577, 1991.

58. Stovner LJ, Sjaastad O: Treatment of cluster headache and its variants, *Curr Opin Neurol* 8:243, 1995.

59. Taarhj P: Decompression of the posterior trigeminal root in trigeminal neuralgia: a 30-year follow-up review, *J Neurosurg* 57:14, 1982.

60. Truelove EL: The chemotherapeutic management of chronic and persistent orofacial pain, *Dent Clin North Am* 38:669, 1994.

61. Wilkinson M et al: Migraine and cluster headache—their management with sumatriptin: a critical review of the current clinical experience, *Cephalagia* 15:337, 1995.

62. Zakrewska JM: Medical management of trigeminal neuralgia, *Br Dent J* 168:399, 1990.

63. Ziccardi VB et al: Trigeminal neuralgia: review of etiologies and treatments, *Compendium* 14:1256, 1993.

64. Ziccardi VB et al: Peripheral trigeminal nerve surgery for patients with atypical facial pain, *J Craniomaxillofac Surg* 22:355, 1994.

Chapter 4

Case Selection and Treatment Planning

Paul Rosenberg

Chapter Outline

After the clinician has identified an endodontic problem, the process of case selection and treatment planning begins. The dentist must determine whether the patient's needs are best served by providing endodontic treatment and maintaining the tooth or advising extraction. If the patient elects to save the tooth, the next question to be asked is whether or not the patient should be referred to an endodontist. These decisions can be made only after a complete patient evaluation. Patient evaluation includes medical, psychosocial, and dental histories. Although most medical conditions do not contraindicate endodontic treatment, some can influence the course of treat-

ment. The following medical findings are offered as a sampling of selected situations and are not a thorough review of the subject. A number of excellent texts are available that review the subject of dental care for the medically compromised patient.[2,10,20,27]

Perhaps the most important advice for a practitioner is to be prepared to communicate with the medically compromised patient's physician. The dentist can review any proposed treatment with the physician and document any recommendations in the patient's record.

COMMON MEDICAL FINDINGS THAT MAY INFLUENCE ENDODONTIC TREATMENT PLANNING

Pregnancy

Although pregnancy is not a contraindication to endodontics, it does modify treatment planning. An extensive body of literature exists concerning the use of radiographs and drugs while treating pregnant patients.[7,12,16,23,24] The dentist should consult with the patient's physician to clarify individual treatment issues, especially when dental emergencies arise during the first trimester.

Unless emergency treatment is required, it is advisable to defer elective dental treatment during the first trimester because of the potential vulnerability of the fetus. The second trimester is the safest period during which to provide routine dental care. Treatment planning should be directed at eliminating potential problems that could arise later in pregnancy or during the immediate postpartum period.[10]

Cardiovascular Disease

Patients with some forms of cardiovascular disease are vulnerable to physical or emotional stress that may be encountered during dental treatment, including endodontics. Patients may be confused or ill informed concerning the specifics of their particular cardiovascular problem. In these situations, consultation with the patient's physician is mandatory before the initiation of endodontic treatment.

Patients who have had a myocardial infarction (i.e., "heart attack") within the past 6 months should not have elective dental care. This is because patients have increased susceptibility to repeat infarctions and other cardiovascular complications during the immediate postinfarction period. Such patients may be taking medications that could potentially interact with the vasoconstrictor in the local anesthetic. In addition, vasoconstrictors should not be administered to patients with unstable or progressive angina pectoris or to patients with high blood pressure. Vasoconstrictors may interact with some antihypertensive medications and should be prescribed only after consultation with the patient's physician. For example, vasoconstrictors should be used with caution in patients taking digitalis glycosides (e.g., Digoxin) because the combination of these drugs could precipitate arrhythmias.[10] Local anesthetic agents with minimal vasoconstrictors are usually adequate for nonsurgical endodontic procedures.

A patient who has a heart murmur as a result of a pathologic condition may be susceptible to an infection on or near the heart valves, which are caused by microorganisms entering the circulation. This infection is called *infective*, or *bacterial, endocarditis* and is potentially fatal. Patients who have a history of a murmur or mitral valve prolapse with regurgitation, rheumatic fever, or a congenital heart defect must be placed on antibiotic therapy prophylactically before endodontic therapy to minimize the risk of bacterial endocarditis.[10] Because the American Heart Association revises its recommended antibiotic prophylactic regimen from time to time for dental procedures, it is essential for the dentist to stay current concerning this important issue. A low-compliance rate exists among at-risk patients regarding their use of the suggested antibiotic coverage before dental procedures. Therefore the dentist must question patients concerning their compliance with the prescribed prophylactic antibiotic coverage before endodontic therapy. If there has not been compliance, the procedure must be delayed.

Patients with artificial heart valves are considered to be highly susceptible to bacterial endocarditis. Therefore consulting with this patient's physician regarding antibiotic premedication is essential. Some physicians elect to administer parenteral antibiotics in addition to or in place of the oral regimen.

The coronary artery bypass graft is a common form of cardiac surgery. Ideally, vasoconstrictors should be minimized during the first 3 months after surgery to avoid the possibility of precipitating arrhythmias. Ordinarily these patients do not require antibiotic prophylaxis after the first few months of recovery unless there are other complications.[10]

Cancer

Some cancers may metastasize to the jaws and mimic endodontic pathosis, whereas others can be primary lesions. A panoramic radiograph is useful in providing an overall view of all dental structures. When a dentist begins an endodontic procedure with a well-defined apical radiolucency, it is assumed to be because of a nonvital pulp that has been confirmed by pulp testing. If a local anesthetic is not administered, and if the patient experiences pain during access or canal instrumentation, it is advisable to reconsider the original diagnosis because the radiolucency may be a lesion of nonodontogenic origin. A definitive diagnosis of a periradicular osteitis can be made only after biopsy. When there is a discrepancy between the initial diagnosis and clinical findings, consultation with an endodontist is advisable. Patients undergoing chemotherapy and or radiation to the head and neck may have impaired healing responses. Treatment should be initiated only after the patient's physician has been consulted.

Human Immunodeficiency Virus and Acquired Immunodeficiency Syndrome

Although the problem of accidental instrument wounds is a concern in terms of potential transmission of human immunodeficiency virus (HIV) in the dental office, the actual occupational risk is very low. It should be noted that there is a much higher potential of developing hepatitis B or hepatitis C from a needlestick injury than there is of developing HIV. A major consideration for the management of patients with HIV or acquired immunodeficiency syndrome (AIDS) is the current CD4 lymphocyte count. It is also important to determine the presence of opportunistic infections and the medications that the patient may be taking. Patients who are HIV seropositive but are asymptomatic are usually candidates for endodontic treatment. Generally this is for patients with a CD4 count above 400.[10] Medical consultation is necessary before endodontic surgical procedures for HIV-infected patients.

Dialysis

Physicians should evaluate patients undergoing dialysis. Because hemodialysis tends to aggravate bleeding tendencies through physical destruction of platelets, it is important to review the patient's status with the responsible physician before endodontic procedures. Generally patients who have had a hemodialysis session are fatigued and could have bleeding tendencies. Therefore elective endodontic treatment should be postponed until the day after hemodialysis. The dentist should also be aware that hemodialysis removes certain drugs from the circulating blood, which can shorten the effect of prescribed medications. Some drugs used during endodontics are affected by dialysis. They include aspirin and acetaminophen, which may have to be avoided or have increased intervals between doses. Penicillin V requires increased doses, as do cephalexin and tetracycline. However, erythromycin requires no adjustment. It is advisable to consult with the patient's physician concerning specific drug requirements during endodontic treatment.[10]

Diabetes

Patients with diabetes, even those who are well controlled, require special consideration during endodontic treatment. The diabetic who is well controlled medically and free of serious complications, such as renal disease, hypertension, or coronary atherosclerotic disease, is a candidate for endodontic treatment. However, there are special considerations in the presence of acute infections. The noninsulin-controlled patient may require insulin, or the insulin dose of some insulin-dependent patients may have to be increased. When the pulp is nonvital bacteriologic, cultures should be taken from the infected area for antibiotic sensitivity testing to provide information in cases that do not respond to the initial antibiotic adjunct. Endodontic infections in the diabetic patient should be treated using the standard protocol, including chlorhexidine oral rinses before treatment, incision and drainage, pulpectomy, and antibiotics as indicated.[10]

Awareness of the patient's normal meal and insulin schedule is also important, along with an effort to reduce stress. The patient's physician should be consulted as needed. A treatment plan that includes periradicular surgery requires communication with the responsible physician to review the planned procedure and its systemic implications.

Prosthetic Implants

Increasing numbers of patients with prosthetic implants are being seen in dental offices, and some of them require endodontic treatment. An important issue concerns the need for antibiotic prophylaxis to prevent infection at the site of the prosthesis, secondary to transient bacteremias from endodontic therapy on nonvital teeth. Endodontic treatment has been shown to be an unlikely cause of bacteremia,[1,14] in contrast to extractions, periodontal surgery, scaling, and prophylaxis.

A major problem in determining the need for prophylactic administration of antibiotics to prevent infection at the site of prosthetic devices (e.g., heart valves, vascular grafts, pacemakers, cerebrospinal fluid shunts, prosthetic joints) is the underreporting of late infection of these devices. The most accurately reported infections are acute and occur while patients are still in the hospital. Each of these devices has its own implications, and varying amounts of evidence support the need for prophylaxis. It is advisable to consult with the patient's physician on a case-by-case basis to establish the need for prophylaxis.[10]

Behavioral and Psychiatric Disorders

Stress reduction is an important component in the treatment of patients with behavioral and psychiatric disorders. Sensitivity to the patient's needs must be a part of the entire dental team's approach. Significant drug interactions and side effects are associated with tricyclic antidepressants, monoamine oxidase inhibitors, and antianxiety drugs. Consulta-

tion with the patient's physician is essential before using sedatives, hypnotics, antihistamines, and opioids.

Psychosocial Evaluation

The initial visit, during which medical and dental histories are taken, provides an opportunity to begin to consider the patient's psychosocial status. Although some patients are quite anxious to maintain a tooth with a questionable prognosis, others lack the necessary sophistication to comprehend the potential risks and benefits. It is a mistake to lead patients beyond what they can appreciate, and patients should not be allowed to dictate treatment that has little chance of success. Part of the dentist's role is to educate the patient and present reasonable treatment plans.

DENTAL EVALUATION

The strategic value of the tooth with an endodontic problem must be considered at the outset of treatment planning. Although such decisions are often straightforward, they can also be intellectually challenging as the dentist considers multiple factors that will play a role in determining the ultimate success or failure of a case. Complicated cases should be referred because the input of dental specialists can be useful in evaluating the prognosis of the proposed treatment.

Periodontal Considerations

Extensive periodontal lesions frequently complicate the endodontic procedure being considered. Such lesions may necessitate consultation with an endodontist or periodontist or both to gather more information about the tooth's prognosis. Periodontal probing is an essential element in endodontic case selection. Multirooted teeth with periodontal complications offer a variety of multidisciplinary complexities and treatment possibilities. A tooth with a poor periodontal prognosis may have to be sacrificed, despite the probability of a favorable endodontic prognosis. In some situations it may not be clear if the primary problem is periodontal or endodontic. This fact can influence the treatment plan; the pathogenesis can be better understood after vitality testing, periodontal probing, radiographic assessment, and evaluating the dental history. The risk to the total treatment plan should be kept in mind when questionable procedures are considered. It is not prudent to build a chronic problem into a new, complex prosthesis (Figs. 4-1 and 4-2).

Surgical Considerations

Surgical evaluations are of particular value in the diagnosis of lesions that may be nonodontogenic. Biopsy is the only definitive means of making a diagnosis of such a lesion. In cases where retreatment is being considered and the prior

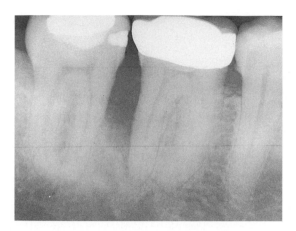

Fig. 4-1 Tooth no. 19 has a poor prognosis. Periodontal probing reached the apex of the distal root. Extraction is indicated and should be done as soon as possible to prevent further damage to the mesial bone associated with tooth no. 18. There are restorative questions concerning the ultimate treatment plan: Should the mesial root of tooth no. 19 be retained? Should tooth no. 20 be used as abutment? Should an implant be placed? (Courtesy Dr. Brian Licari.)

endodontic therapy was done well, biopsy is a valuable procedure to refine treatment planning after surgery.

Restorative Considerations

A satisfactory restoration may be jeopardized by a number of factors. Subosseous root caries (perhaps requiring crown lengthening), poor crown/root ratio, and extensive periodontal defects or misalignment of teeth may have a serious effect on the final restoration. Therefore it is wise to recognize these problems before endodontic treatment. For complicated cases, a restorative consultation with a prosthodontist may also be advisable for the dentist before initiating treatment. A restorative treatment plan should be in place before starting endodontic treatment in a nonemergency situation. Some teeth may be endodontically treatable but nonrestorable, or they may represent a potential restorative complication in a large prosthesis. Furthermore, reduced coronal tooth structure under a full-coverage restoration makes endodontic access more difficult because of reduced visibility and a lack of radiographic information about the anatomy of the chamber. Thus it is not unusual for restorations to be compromised during endodontic access (Fig. 4-3). Whenever reasonably possible, restorations should be removed before endodontic treatment.

Other Factors That May Influence Endodontic Case Selection

A variety of factors may complicate proposed endodontic therapy. Calcifications, dilacerations, and resorptive defects may compromise endodontic treatment of a tooth with potentially strategic value (Fig. 4-4). The inability to isolate a tooth is also a problem and may result in bacterial

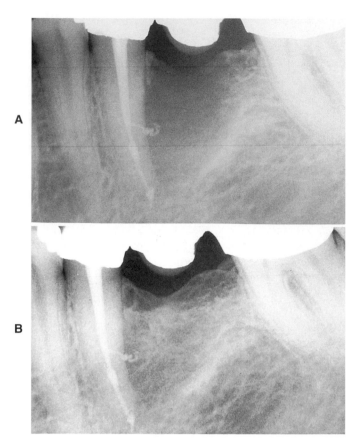

Fig. 4-2 **A** and **B**, The large, bony defect associated with tooth no. 29 healed after endodontic therapy. The tooth was nonvital and there was no excessive periodontal probing depth indicating pulpal disease.

penetration of the canal or canals. Extra roots and canals pose a particular anatomic challenge that radiographs do not always reveal (Fig. 4-5). Retreatment cases offer particular mechanical challenges (Fig. 4-6). Ledges, perforations, or posts may be present, all of which complicate treatment and alter the prognosis. The dentist should recognize these potential problems and have the ability to manage and factor them into the decision concerning the tooth's prognosis, including the possibility that the patient should be referred to a specialist. Rosenberg and Goodis suggest a method that permits a clinician to evaluate each patient to determine the level of anticipated difficulty and helps the generalist to identify which cases should be referred for specialty care.[19]

Some practitioners use a simple formula for determining which endodontic cases they treat and which they refer to a specialist. The number of roots may be the determining factor in a decision concerning referral, or the key factor may be the chronic or acute status of the case. If the generalist decides to treat the case, having specific goals at each visit helps to organize the treatment. For example, in an uncomplicated molar or premolar, some practitioners will set a specific goal for the first visit that includes access and thorough instrumentation, while deferring the obturation to a second

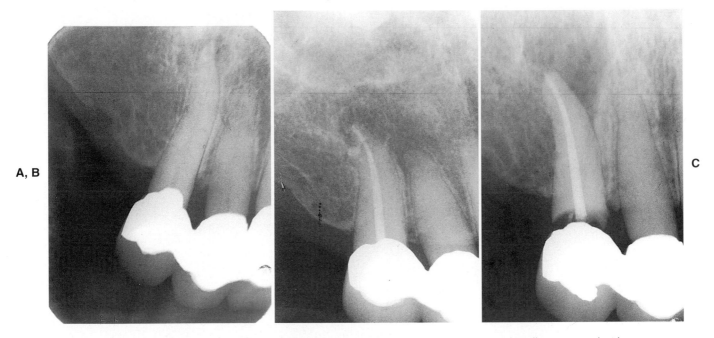

Fig. 4-3 **A-C,** Four years after endodontic therapy, the patient complained of pain and swelling associated with tooth no. 6. The initial impression was that apical surgery was indicated. However, further radiographs revealed the true cause of the endodontic failure. The initial endodontic access through the crown or caries may have damaged the coronal seal.

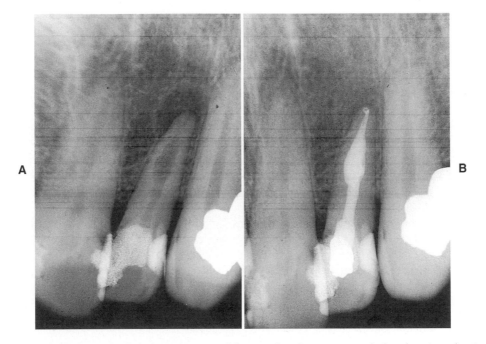

Fig. 4-4 **A** and **B**, Resorptive defects can be successfully treated. Early intervention, before there is perforation of the root, increases the chance of success. (Courtesy Dr. Leon Schertzer.)

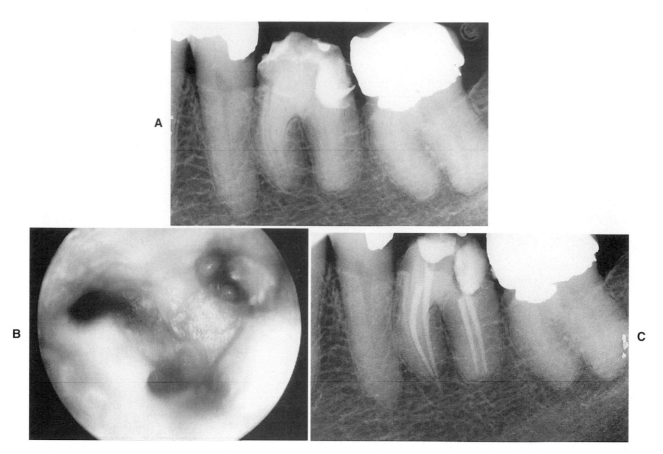

Fig. 4-5. Radiographs do not always demonstrate canal complexities. **A**, Initial radiograph. **B**, Highly magnified view of the pulp chamber. **C**, Completed endodontic treatment. (Courtesy Dr. Lee Adamo.)

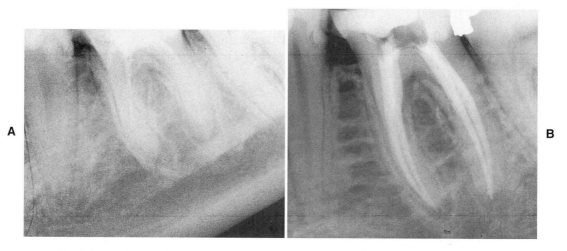

Fig. 4-6 **A** and **B**, Retreatment of tooth no. 30 was complicated by the presence of four canals.

visit. Uncomplicated single-rooted, vital teeth may be planned for a one-visit treatment; ample time should be allowed so that the procedure can be completed without stress. These recommendations have a biologic basis; it is not biologically sound to instrument incompletely and leave inflamed pulpal remnants in the canal because pulp remnants are likely to cause pain and be susceptible to infection. The practitioner would be well advised to begin canal instrumentation only if time permits for the extirpation of all pulp tissue. The most important variables in determining whether to refer a patient to a specialist are the skills of the practitioner and the complexity of the case.

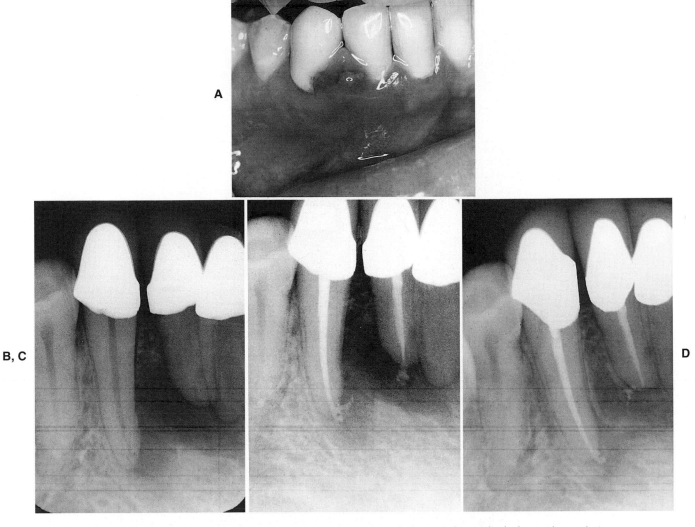

Fig. 4-7 The long-standing endodontic pathosis caused extensive destruction of periradicular bone. The overlaying gingival tissue became inflamed during an acute exacerbation of the chronic endodontic lesion. After 1 year, nonsurgical endodontic therapy resulted in healing. **A**, Edematous gingiva during acute exacerbation of the endodontic lesion. **B**, Periradicular demineralization. **C**, Completed endodontic therapy. **D**, Healing (remineralization).

Prognosis of Endodontic Treatment

It appears that the most important factor influencing the prognosis of endodontic treatment is the preoperative status of the tooth. Many studies have demonstrated that the success rate is significantly influenced by the existence of a pretreatment radiographic lesion.* Teeth with an apical radiolucency may have up to a 20% lower success rate than teeth without such lesions. In a classic study, Strindberg found that healing of periapical lesions could take up to 9 years after treatment.[28] More recently, Sjögren and associates noted that uncertainty exists concerning the influence of the size of the preoperative periapical lesion[26] and the effect of excess filling material on the outcome of endodontic treatment.[26] They

commented that the uncertainty might be because of insufficient duration of observation periods. Sjögren and associates evaluated 356 patients 8 to 10 years after endodontic treatment. Among factors analyzed, the preoperative status of the pulp and periapical tissue appear to be extremely important to the outcome of endodontic treatment. More than 96% of the teeth without preoperative periapical lesions were treated successfully, whereas only 86% of the cases with pulp necrosis and periapical lesions healed. Retreatment cases with periapical lesions had the least favorable results; only 62% of those cases were successful.[26] Other important endodontic and systemic variables exist. The patient's systemic resistance and the quality of instrumentation and obturation play a role in the ultimate outcome of endodontic treatment (Fig. 4-7).

---

*References 11,13,21,25,26,28

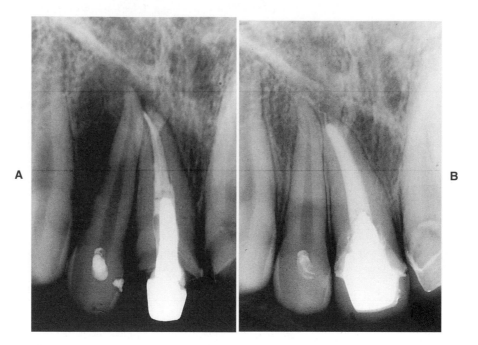

Fig. 4-8 **A** and **B**, Two years after endodontic therapy on tooth no. 8, the patient returned with pain and swelling. A dentist mistakenly began endodontic access on tooth no. 7, without confirming the apparent radiographic diagnosis with vitality testing. Tooth no. 7 was vital and tooth no. 8 was successfully retreated after removal of the post. (Courtesy Dr. Leon Schertzer.)

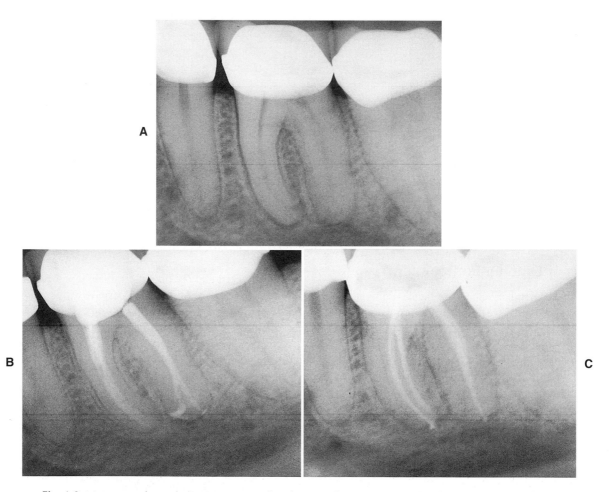

Fig. 4-9 Many years after endodontic treatment of tooth no. 30, the patient returned with a chief complaint of pain and an inability to chew on the tooth. Despite the radiographic appearance of excellent endodontic treatment, the tooth was retreated and the patient's pain disappeared. Note the unusual distal root anatomy, which was not apparent during the initial procedure. **A**, Initial radiograph. **B**, Completion of initial endodontic therapy. **C**, Retreatment.

DEVELOPING THE ENDODONTIC TREATMENT PLAN

The acute vital case is best managed with a biologically based approach. Performing a deep pulpotomy or establishing length control and instrumenting the canal system completely will reduce intrapulpal pressure. It has been shown that simply débriding the pulp chamber is a highly predictable method of providing pain relief.[8] Once a canal has been entered, the practitioner is committed to removing all tissue. Partial instrumentation (i.e., leaving tissue remnants) may leave the patient with more pain than at the outset of treatment. Where sensitivity to percussion is a problem, occlusal relief is a critical component of the emergency visit (see the section on occlusal reduction on p. 101). Teeth should be closed between visits.

The acute nonvital tooth may be extremely painful, because the pain comes from the periradicular tissue because of necrotic tissue and bacterial flora in the canal system. The goal in such cases is to decompress the periradicular tissues by thoroughly cleaning and shaping the canal(s). When indicated, incision and drainage may be performed in conjunction with canal instrumentation (see Chapter 2).

Retreatment Cases

Retreatment cases offer a particular set of challenges to the practitioner. Among the questions to be resolved are:
- Are prior radiographs available for review?
- Why did the case fail?
- Is there an obvious procedural problem that can be corrected?
- Is the canal system readily accessible for reentry?

- Are there additional factors (other than endodontic) that may have contributed to the failure?
- Is the tooth critical to the treatment plan?
- Does the patient understand the prognosis for the tooth and want to attempt retreatment?

A retreatment plan should be developed after the practitioner has determined the cause of failure and weighed other factors that may affect the prognosis (e.g., root fracture, defective restoration) (Figs. 4-8, 4-9, and 4-10). It is wise to avoid including a potentially chronic problem in a new treatment plan. Retreatment cases may require surgical endodontics in combination with nonsurgical retreatment. Referral to a specialist may be helpful when planning treatment for complex cases.

Immature teeth

Primary and immature permanent teeth may have pulpal pathosis caused by caries or trauma; preserving these young teeth is essential. Premature loss of an anterior tooth can lead to malocclusion, predispose the patient to tongue habits, impair aesthetics, and damage the self-esteem of the patient. (Chapter 23 contains a comprehensive discussion of these issues.)

Endodontic and Periodontic Considerations

The relationship between the pulpal and periodontal tissue complex begins during the embryonic stage of dental development. The richly vascularized dental papillae and the surrounding, future periodontal tissues have a shared circulation. This interrelationship provides the anatomic basis for potential pathosis. (Chapter 17 provides a comprehensive

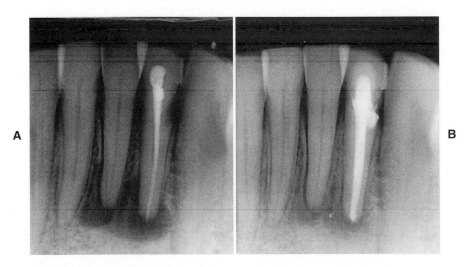

Fig. 4-10 **A** and **B**, Retreatment of tooth no. 26 resulted in healing of the periradicular lesion. The initial radiograph was misleading and implicated tooth no. 25 and tooth no. 26. Pulp testing indicated a vital pulp in tooth no. 25, so it was not treated. (Courtesy Dr. Leon Schertzer.)

discussion of the close relationship between the attachment apparatus and the pulp.)

Endodontic Surgery

Endodontic surgery may be performed at the outset or as a retreatment procedure. Before considering the actual treatment, the dentist should consider the most prudent measure to prevent recurrence of the problem. For example, if the cause of failure is a leaking coronal restoration, apical surgery will likely fail. As a primary treatment modality, apical surgery is usually performed when there is a completely calcified or blocked canal (e.g., a bonded post). As a retreatment procedure, apical surgery is performed as a secondary effort to salvage failed endodontic treatment. The primary reason for apical surgery is to improve the quality of the apical seal. In recent years there have been dramatic changes in the techniques and materials used for surgical resolution of complex cases.

Single Visit Versus Multivisit Treatment

There has been much debate concerning single visit versus multivisit endodontic treatment. Indications and contraindications exist for either choice. Recent studies have extended our understanding about postoperative pain associated with each approach; they have also extended our understanding of relative success rates.[6,9,15,17]

Indications   A vital case is often a candidate for single-visit treatment. The number of roots, time available, and dentist's skills are also factors to be considered. Some studies demonstrate that even with symptoms, a vital case may be treated in a single visit. Of course, anatomic or periodontal complications may modify such a treatment plan. Vital, asymptomatic teeth that cannot be well sealed between visits are ideal candidates for single-visit endodontics. For example, an anterior tooth fractured at the gingival margin is often treated in a single visit.

Contraindications   Some studies suggest a lower success rate in single-visit, nonvital cases with apical periodontitis than with the multivisit approach. It has been postulated that the intervisit use of an antimicrobial dressing is an essential factor in eradicating all infection from the root canal.[25,26,28] Retreatment cases are another group that would benefit from a multivisit approach.[29]

Research   A number of well-documented clinical research papers indicate that less postoperative pain results from a single-visit approach to treatment than the multivisit approach.[6,9,15,17] In dramatic support of this finding, Roane and his colleagues[17] reviewed the postoperative pain experience of 250 cases that were treated in a single-visit approach, compared with 109 cases using a multivisit methodology. In both study groups, they included even those patients with swelling and pain. Their results indicated that a higher frequency (2 to 1) of postoperative pain was associated with a multivisit treatment plan in both vital and nonvital cases, and they hypothesized that "immediate obturation prevents further communication to the apex via the canal." They went on to comment that obturation prevents reinfection of the canals as a result of leakage past the temporary filling.

More recently, in a prospective study, Imura and Zuolo assessed the incidence of flare-ups among patients who received endodontic treatment. Their results showed an incidence of 1.58% for flare-ups from 1012 endodontically treated teeth. Statistical analysis using the chi-square test ($P<0.05$) indicated that flare-ups were found to be positively correlated with multiple appointments, retreatment cases, periradicular pain before treatment, and the presence of radiolucent lesions.[9]

Although extensive literature and consensus exist concerning the issue of pain associated with the single-visit approach, the issue of long-term success is another matter. The determination of long-term success associated with a particular treatment modality remains a challenging research problem. Important issues include case selection, well-defined treatment procedures, and sufficient duration of recalls.

Recently, important information has become available concerning the question of success rates associated with single-visit and multivisit procedures.[25,26] Sjögren and associates investigated the influence of infection at the time of root filling on the outcome of endodontic treatment of teeth with apical periodontitis. Periapical healing was followed for 5 years. They found that, "Complete periapical healing occurred in 94% of cases that yielded a negative culture. Where the samples were positive before root filling, the success rate of treatment was just 68%—a statistically significant difference." They concluded that the objective of eliminating bacteria from the root canal system "cannot be reliably achieved in a one-visit treatment because it is not possible to eradicate all infection from the root canal without the support of an interappointment antimicrobial dressing."

Although a procedural question could be raised concerning the minimal 0.5% concentration of sodium hypochlorite used as an irrigant, it should be noted that this was a well-documented study. The use of sodium hypochlorite (as a canal irrigant) to destroy microbes and act as a tissue solvent is widely accepted by endodontists. Differences exist concerning the optimal concentration to recommend; the literature is mixed concerning what percentage to use.[3,4,5,30] Bystrom and Sundquist reported that they were in agreement with Cvek et al,[5] who "could not demonstrate any significant difference in antibacterial effect between 0.5% and 5% sodium hypochlorite solutions in a clinical study." Bystrom and Sundquist also reported that when 0.5% hypochlorite was used "no bacteria could be recovered from 12 of 15 root canals at the fifth appointment." Thus it would seem unwise to use 0.5% of sodium hypochlorite solution for single-visit endodontics because Bystrom and Sundquist found that five visits were necessary to eliminate bacteria in this study.

Trepagnier and associates reported that "dilution of 5% sodium hypochlorite with equal parts of water does not affect its solvent action appreciably, but a modified Dakins solution (0.5% NaOCl) has little solvent action."[30] They also noted that 5% sodium hypochlorite solution "used for five minutes was 65% more effective than Dakins solution (0.5%); the difference was significant (P=0.001)."[30] More recently, Sequeira and associates evaluated the antibacterial effect of endodontic irrigants against four black-pigmented gram-negative anaerobes and four facultative anaerobic bacteria by means of the agar diffusion test. Based on the averages of the diameters of the zones of bacterial growth inhibition, the antibacterial effects of the solutions were ranked from strongest to weakest as follows:

- 4% NaOCl
- 2.5% NaOCl
- 2% NaOCl
- 2% chlorhexidine
- 0.2% chlorhexidine
- EDTA and citric acid
- 0.5% sodium hypochlorite[22]

The preponderance of recent studies suggests that no less than 2.5% of sodium hypochlorite (or perhaps higher) is the best concentration for endodontic therapy. Further research findings concerning indications and contraindications for single-visit endodontics will be forthcoming.

Occlusal Reduction

In a recent clinical study by Rosenberg and associates at New York University College of Dentistry, 117 patients were examined for specific indicators that would signal the need for occlusal reduction.[18] Indicators mandating occlusal reduction were:

- Vital tooth
- History of pain
- Sensitivity to percussion
- Absence of periradicular osteitis

Cases with these findings had a very high probability of pain relief if the occlusion was relieved. When such cases did *not* have the occlusion relieved, there was a high probability of continued pain after instrumentation of the canal or canals.

When combined with long-duration local anesthesia and preoperative nonsteroidal inflammatory drugs (NSAIDs), occlusal reduction represents a particularly meaningful approach to the pain prevention strategy.

Scheduling Considerations

When vital cases are to be treated using a multivisit approach, it is wise to permit sufficient time between canal instrumentation and obturation. Generally 5 to 7 days provides sufficient recovery time for the periradicular tissues before obturation. It is frustrating for the clinician and patient to return for a proposed final visit only to find that transient, lingering apical periodontitis prevents obturation.

When a vital case is to be treated in a single visit, it is important that adequate time be scheduled. The clinician should be able to complete the planned procedure without stress. It is a good strategy to schedule patients who require mandibular block anesthesia to arrive 15 to 20 minutes before their treatment visit. This avoids the frustration of "losing treatment time" while the anesthetic agent becomes effective.

Nonvital case appointments should be scheduled more closely than vital-case appointments.

References

1. Bender IB, Naidorf IJ, Garvey GJ: Bacterial endocarditis: a consideration for physician and dentist, *J Am Dent Assoc* 109: 415, 1984.
2. Bricker SL, Langlais RP, Miller CS: *Oral diagnosis, oral medicine, and treatment planning*, ed 2, Philadelphia, 1994, Lea and Febiger.
3. Bystrom A, Sundqvist G: The antibacterial action of sodium hypochlorite and EDTA in 60 cases of endodontic therapy, *Int Endod J* 18:35, 1985.
4. Bystrom A, Sundqvist G: Bacteriologic evaluation of the effect of 0.5 % sodium hypochlorite in endodontic therapy, *Oral Surg Oral Med Oral Pathol* 55:307, 1983.
5. Cvek M, Nord CE, Hollander L: Antimicrobial effect of root canal débridement in teeth with immature roots. A clinical and microbiologic study, *Odontol Revy* 27:1, 1976.
6. Fava LRG: One appointment root canal treatment: incidence of postoperative pain using a modified double-flapped technique, *Int Endod J* 24:258, 1991.
7. Freeman JP, Brand JW: Radiation doses of commonly used dental radiographic surveys, *Oral Surg Oral Med Oral Pathol* 77:285, 1994.
8. Hasselgren G, Reit C: Emergency pulpotomy: pain relieving effect with and without the use of sedative dressings, *J Endod* 15:254, 1989.
9. Imura N, Zuolo ML: Factors associated with endodontic flare-ups: a prospective study, *Int Endod J*, 28:261, 1995.
10. Little JW, Falace DA, Miller CS, Rhodus NL: *Dental management of the medically compromised patient*, ed 5, St Louis, 1997, Mosby.
11. Matsumoto T et al: Factors affecting successful prognosis of root canal treatment, *J Endod* 13:239, 1987.
12. Mole RH: Radiation effects on prenatal development and their radiological significance, *Br J Radiol* 52:89, 1979.
13. Natkin E, Oswald RJ, Carnes LI: The relationship of lesion size to diagnosis, incidence and treatment of periapical cysts and granulomas, *Oral Surg Oral Med Oral Pathol* 57:82, 1984.
14. Pallasch TJ: Antibiotic prophylaxis: theory and reality, *J Calif Dent Assoc* 17:27, 1989.
15. Pekruhn BP: Single-visit endodontic therapy: a preliminary clinical study, *J Am Dent Assoc* 103:875, 1981.
16. Food and Drug Administration: Federal drug pregnancy categories for prescription drugs, FDA Bulletin 12:24, Washington DC, 1982, Government Printing Office.

Roane JB, Dryden JA, Grimes EW: Incidence of postoperative pain after single and multiple visit endodontic procedures, *Oral Surg Oral Med Oral Pathol* 55:68, 1983.

18. Rosenberg PA, Babick PJ, Schertzer L, Leung D: The effect of occlusal reduction on pain after endodontic instrumentation, *J Endod* 24:492, 1998.

19. Rosenberg RJ, Goodis HE: Endodontic case selection to treat or to refer, *J Am Dent Assoc* 123:57, 1992.

20. Scully C, Cawson RA: *Medical problems in dentistry,* ed 4, Boston, 1998, Reed Educational and Professional Publishing.

21. Seltzer S, Bender IB, Turkenkopf S: Factors affecting successful repair after root canal therapy, *J Am Dent Assoc* 67:651, 1962.

22. Sequeira JF, Batista MM, Fraga RC, de Uzeda M: Antibacterial effects of endodontic irrigants on black pigmented gram negative anaerobes and falcultative bacteria, *J Endod* 24:414, 1998.

23. Serman NJ, Singer S: Exposure of the pregnant patient to ionizing radiation, *Ann Dent* 53:13, 1994.

24. Shrout MK et al: Treating the pregnant dental patient: four basic rules addressed, *J Am Dent Assoc* 123:75, 1992.

25. Sjögren U, Figdor D, Persson S, Sundqvist G: Influence of infection at the time of root filing on the outcome of endodontic treatment of teeth with apical periodontitis, *Int Endod J* 30:297, 1997.

26. Sjögren U, Hagglund B, Sundquist G, Wing K: Factors affecting the long term results of endodontic treatment, *J Endod* 16:498, 1990.

27. Sonis S, Fang L ST, Fazio R: *Principles and practice of oral medicine,* ed 2, Philadelphia, 1995, WB Saunders.

28. Strindberg LZ: The dependence of the results of root canal therapy on certain factors. An analytic study based on radiographic and clinical follow up examinations, *Acta Odontol Scand* 14(suppl 21):1, 1956.

29. Sundquist G, Figdor D, Persson S, Sjögren U: Microbiologic analysis of teeth with failed endodontic treatment and the outcome of conservative retreatment, *Oral Surg Oral Med Oral Pathol* 85:86, 1998.

30. Trepagnier CM, Madden RM, Lazzari EP: Quantitative study of sodium hypochlorite as an in vitro endodontic irrigant, *J Endod* 3:194, 1977.

Chapter 5

 # Preparation for Treatment

Gerald N. Glickman, Roberta Pileggi

Chapter Outline

A number of treatment, clinician, and patient needs must be addressed before initiation of nonsurgical root canal treatment. These include proper infection control and occupational safety procedures for the entire health care team and treatment environment; appropriate communication with the patient, including case presentation and informed consent; premedication, if necessary, followed by effective administration of local anesthesia; a quality radiographic or digital-image survey; and thorough isolation of the treatment site.

PREPARATION OF THE OPERATORY

Infection Control

Because all dental personnel are at risk for exposure to a host of infectious organisms that may cause a number of infec-

tions (e.g., influenza; upper respiratory disease; tuberculosis; herpes; hepatitis B, C, D; acquired immunodeficiency syndrome [AIDS]), it is essential that effective infection control procedures be used to minimize the risk of cross-contamination in the work environment.[19-22,43,56] These infection control programs must not only protect patients and the dental team from contracting infections during dental procedures, they must also reduce the number of microorganisms in the immediate dental environment to the lowest level possible.

As the AIDS epidemic continues to expand, it has been established that the potential for occupational transmission of human immunodeficiency virus (HIV) and other fluid-borne pathogens can be minimized by enforcing infection control policies specifically designed to reduce exposure to blood and other infected body fluids.[12-14,43,56] Because HIV has been shown to be fragile and easily destroyed by heat or chemical disinfectants, the highly resistant nature of the hepatitis B virus, along with its high blood titers, makes it a good model for infection control practices to prevent transmission of a large number of other pathogens via blood or saliva. Because all infected patients are not readily identifiable through the routine medical history and many are asymptomatic, the American Dental Association (ADA) recommends that each patient be considered potentially infectious; this means that the same strict infection control policies or "universal precautions" apply to all patients.[20,56] In addition, the Occupational Safety and Health Administration (OSHA) of the U.S. Department of Labor, in conjunction with both the ADA and the Centers for Disease Control and Prevention (CDC), has issued detailed guidelines on hazard and safety control in the dental setting.[2,3,10-13,36,56] In 1992, laws specifically regulating exposure to blood-borne disease became effective through OSHA's Occupational Exposure to Bloodborne Pathogens Standard.[22] Primarily designed to protect any employee who could be "reasonably anticipated" to have contact with blood or any other potentially infectious materials, the standard encompasses a combination of engineering and work practice controls, as well as recommendations for the use of equipment and protective clothing, training, signs and labels, and hepatitis B vaccinations. It also authorizes OSHA to conduct inspections and impose financial penalties for failure to comply with specific regulations.[22]

In 1993 the ADA, CDC, and OSHA recommended or mandated that infection control guidelines include the following measures*:

1. The ADA and CDC recommend that all dentists and staff members who have patient contact be vaccinated against hepatitis B. The OSHA standard requires that employers make the hepatitis B vaccine available to occupationally exposed employees, at the employer's expense, within 10 working days of assignment to tasks that may result in exposure. An employee who refuses the vaccine must sign a declination form that uses specific language approved by OSHA. In addition, postexposure follow-up and evaluation must be made available to all employees who have had an exposure incident.

2. A thorough patient medical history, which includes specific questions about hepatitis, AIDS, current illnesses, unintentional weight loss, lymphadenopathy, and oral soft-tissue lesions, must be taken and updated at subsequent appointments.

3. Dental personnel must wear protective attire and use proper barrier techniques. The standard requires the employer to ensure that employees use personal protective equipment and that such protection is provided at no cost to the employee.

   a. Disposable latex or vinyl gloves must be worn when contact with body fluids or mucous membranes is anticipated or when touching potentially contaminated surfaces; they may not be washed for reuse. OSHA requires that gloves be replaced after each patient contact, when torn, or when punctured. If their integrity is not compromised, sturdy, unlined utility gloves for cleaning instruments and surfaces may be decontaminated for reuse. Polyethylene gloves may be worn over treatment gloves to prevent contamination of objects, such as drawers, light handles, or charts.

   b. Hands, wrists, and lower forearms must be washed with soap at the beginning of the day, before and after gloving, at the end of the day, and after removal of any personal protective equipment or clothing. An antimicrobial surgical hand scrub should be used for surgical procedures. The standard requires that any body area that has contact with a potentially infectious material, including saliva, must be washed immediately after contact. Sinks should have electronic, elbow, foot, or knee-action faucet controls for asepsis and ease of function. Employers must provide washing facilities (including an eyewash) that are readily accessible to employees.

   c. Masks and protective eyewear with solid side shields or chin-length face shields are required when splashes or sprays of potentially infectious materials are anticipated and during all instrument and environmental cleanup activities. When a facemask is

removed, it should be handled by the elastic or cloth strings, not by the mask itself. It is further suggested that the patient wear protective eyewear.

   d. Protective clothing, either reusable or disposable, must be worn when clothing or skin is likely to be exposed to body fluids, and it should be changed when visibly soiled or penetrated by fluids. OSHA's requirements for protective clothing (i.e., gowns, aprons, lab coats, clinic jackets) are difficult to interpret, because the "type and characteristics [thereof] will depend upon the task and degree of exposure anticipated." The ADA and CDC recommend long-sleeved uniforms. However, according to OSHA, long sleeves are required only if significant splashing of blood or body fluids to the arms or forearms is expected. Thus endodontic surgery would likely warrant long-sleeved garments. OSHA requires that the protective garments not be worn outside the work area. The standard prohibits employees from taking contaminated laundry home to be washed; it must be washed at the office or by an outside laundry service. Contaminated laundry must be placed in an impervious laundry bag that is colored red and labeled "BIOHAZARD." Although OSHA does not regulate nonprotective clothing (e.g., scrubs), such clothing should be handled like protective clothing once fluids have penetrated it.

   e. Patients' clothing should be protected from splatter and caustic materials, such as sodium hypochlorite, with waist-length plastic coverings overlaid with disposable patient bibs.

   f. High-volume evacuation greatly reduces the number of bacteria in dental aerosols and should be employed when using the high-speed handpiece, water spray, or ultrasonics.

   g. Use of the rubber dam as a protective barrier is mandatory for nonsurgical root canal treatment, and failure to use this barrier is considered to be below standard care.[14,15,25]

4. OSHA regulates only contaminated sharps. Contaminated *disposable* sharps (e.g., syringes, needles, scalpel blades) and contaminated *reusable* sharps (e.g., endodontic files) must be placed into separate, leakproof, closable, puncture-resistant containers. These containers should be colored red or labeled "BIOHAZARD," and they should be marked with the biohazard symbol. The standard states that before decontamination (i.e., sterilization), contaminated reusable sharps must not be stored or processed in a way that requires employees to use their hands to reach into the containers to retrieve the instruments. The OSHA ruling allows picking up sharp instruments by hand only after they are decontaminated.[19,36,43]

   a. The clinician should take the following steps when handling contaminated endodontic files: With tweezers, place used files in glass beaker containing a nonphenolic disinfectant and detergent holding solution.

*References 2,3,10-13,19,20,36,43,56

At the end of day, discard solution and rinse with tap water. Add ultrasonic cleaning solution, and place beaker in ultrasonic bath until thoroughly clean (i.e., 5 to 15 minutes). Discard ultrasonic solution, and rinse with tap water. Pour contents of beaker onto clean towel, and use tweezers to place clean files into metal box for sterilization. Files with any visible debris should be separately sterilized. Once sterilized, these files can be picked up by hand and débrided using 2 × 2 sponges. Once cleaned, files should be returned to metal box for sterilization. (As indicated in Chapter 8, all files should be regarded as disposable.)

b. Generally the standard prohibits bending or recapping of anesthesia needles. However, during endodontic treatment, reinjection of the same patient is often necessary, so recapping is essential. Recapping with a one-handed method and using a mechanical device are the only permissible techniques. Shearing or breaking of contaminated needles should never be permitted.

5. Countertops and operatory surfaces, such as light handles, radiograph unit heads, chair switches, and any other surface likely to become contaminated with potentially infectious materials, can be either covered or disinfected. Protective coverings (e.g., clear plastic wrap, special plastic sleeves, aluminum foil) can be used. These coverings should be changed between patients and when they become contaminated. OSHA mandates, however, that work surfaces be decontaminated or recovered or both at the end of each work shift and immediately after overt contamination. The coverings should be removed by gloved personnel, discarded, and then replaced with clean coverings after gloves are removed. Alternatively, countertops and operatory surfaces can be wiped with absorbent toweling to remove extraneous organic material and then sprayed with an environmental protection agency (EPA)-registered and ADA-accepted tuberculocidal disinfectant (e.g., 1:10 dilution of sodium hypochlorite, iodophore, synthetic phenol). With the advent of endodontic microscopy, appropriate barriers should be placed on the handles and controls of the microscope or the entire unit can be draped to prevent cross-contamination. If the system becomes contaminated, disinfection should be performed according to the microscope manufacturer's guidelines.

6. Contaminated radiographic film packets must be handled in a way that prevents cross-contamination. Contamination of the film (when it is removed from the packet) and subsequent contamination of the processing equipment can be prevented either by properly handling the film as it is removed from the contaminated packet or by preventing the contamination of the packet during use.[27] After exposure, "over-gloves" should be placed over contaminated gloves to prevent cross-contamination of processing equipment or darkroom surfaces.[35] For darkroom procedures, films should be carefully manipu-lated out of their holders and dropped onto a disinfected surface or into a clean cup without being touched. Once the film has been removed, gloves should be removed and discarded; the film can then be processed. All contaminated film envelopes must be accumulated (after film removal) in a strategically positioned impervious bag and disposed of properly. For daylight loaders, exposed film packets should be placed into a paper cup; gloves should be discarded and hands washed. Next, a new pair of gloves should be donned, and the paper cup with films and an empty cup should be placed into chamber. Using gloved hands, the chamber should be entered and packets should be carefully opened, allowing the film to drop onto a clean surface in the chamber. Empty film packets should then be placed into an empty cup, and gloves removed and discarded in the cup; films can then be processed.[36] Plastic envelopes, such as the ClinAsept Barriers (Eastman Kodak, Rochester, NY), have simplified the handling of contaminated, exposed films by protecting films from contact with saliva and blood during exposure. Once a film is exposed, the barrier envelope is easily opened and the film can be dropped into a paper cup or onto a clean area before processing. The barrier-protected film, however, should be wiped with an EPA-approved disinfectant as an added precaution against contamination during opening.[27]

7. In conjunction with the previously mentioned guidelines for infection control, a mouth rinse of 0.12% chlorhexidine gluconate, such as Peridex (Procter & Gamble, Cincinnati, OH), is recommended before treatment. This rinse will minimize the number of microbes in the mouth and, consequently, in any splatter or aerosols generated during treatment.[19,43,56]

8. After treatment, all instruments and burs must be cleaned and sterilized by sterilizers monitored with biologic indicators. Cassettes, packs, or trays should be rewrapped in original wrap and individually packaged instruments should be placed in a covered container. Air and water syringes must be flushed, cleaned, and sterilized. Antiretraction valves (i.e., one-way flow check valves) should be installed to prevent fluid aspiration and to reduce the risk of transfer of potentially infective material. Heavy-duty rubber gloves must be worn during clean up. The ADA and CDC recommend that all dental handpieces and "prophy" angles be heat sterilized between patients.[3,19,36,43] Before sterilization, all handpieces should be wiped with an EPA-registered disinfectant. In addition, high-speed hand pieces should be run for a minimum of 30 seconds to discharge water and air, with spray directed into a high-volume evacuation system. Dental unit water lines should be periodically flushed with water or a 1:10 dilution of 5.25% NaOCl to reduce biofilm formation. All regulated infectious waste must be immediately disposed of in containers that meet specific criteria. Disposal must be in accordance with applicable federal, state, and local regulations.

In 1987 the infection-control, decision-making process was transferred to the U.S. government through OSHA.[56] The ongoing goal of OSHA is to establish a routine and practical program of enforcing infection control standards (based on published CDC guidelines) to ensure the health and safety of all members of the dental health team. According to OSHA,[36,43,56] dentists must classify personnel and tasks in the dental practice according to levels of risk of exposure and must establish "standard operating procedures" to protect the patient and staff from infection transmission. OSHA requires the dentist to provide infection control training for all employees and to maintain records of such training; properly label all hazardous substances that employees are exposed to on the job; and have a written hazard communications program with manufacturers' Material Safety Data Sheets (MSDS) for all hazardous substances. With the enactment of OSHA's Bloodborne Pathogens Standard in 1991, employers must make exposure determinations and develop an exposure control plan. As mentioned previously, the rule encompasses a number of critical areas (e.g., universal precautions, engineering and work practice controls, employee training, specific record-keeping) designed to protect employees from exposure to blood-borne pathogens, particularly the HIV and the hepatitis B virus. Although the OSHA standard was written principally to protect employees, it does not encompass all of the infection control practices recommended by the ADA and CDC to protect dentists and patients.

In 1994 the CDC issued its position statement on the prevention of transmission of tuberculosis in dental settings. The statement suggested that elective dental treatments for patients suspected of having tuberculosis be deferred until it has been confirmed that they are free of the disease. The CDC also stated that emergency care for a patient with tuberculosis should only be provided in facilities with appropriate respirators, negative pressure treatment areas, and other respiratory engineering controls.[10] Compliance with OSHA regulations and with evolving infection control policies of the ADA and CDC will help provide a safer workplace for the entire dental-treatment team.[19,36,43,56]

PATIENT PREPARATION

Treatment Planning

Aside from emergencies that require immediate attention, endodontic treatment usually occurs early in the total treatment plan for the patient. Therefore any asymptomatic but irreversible pulpal and periradicular problems are managed before they become symptomatic and more difficult to handle. The most important rationale for the high priority of endodontics is to ensure that a sound, healthy foundation exists before further treatment is attempted. A stable root system within sound periradicular and periodontal tissues is paramount to the placement of any definitive restorations.

Regardless of the specifics of the case, it is the responsibility of the clinician to explain the nature of the treatment and inform the patient of any risks, the prognosis, and other pertinent facts. Because of bad publicity and hearsay, root canal treatment is reputed to be a horrifying experience. Consequently, some patients may be reluctant, anxious, or even fearful of undergoing root canal treatment. Thus it is imperative that the dentist educates the patient before treatment (i.e., "informing before performing")[15] to allay concerns and minimize misconceptions.

Good dentist and patient relationships are built on effective communication. There is sufficient evidence to suggest that dentists who establish warm, caring relationships with their patients through effective case presentation are perceived more favorably. These dentists also have a more positive impact on the patient's anxiety, knowledge, and compliance than those who maintain impersonal, noncommunicative relationships.[18] Most patients experience increased anxiety while in the dental chair. However, a simple but informative case presentation that answers all questions reduces patient anxiety and solidifies the patient's trust in the dentist.

Case Presentation

The ADA and the American Association of Endodontists (AAE) publish brochures (e.g., *Endodontics: Your Guide To Endodontic Treatment*[1]) to help patients understand root canal treatment. Valuable educational aids of this nature should be made available to the patient, either before or immediately after case presentation. This supportive information addresses the most frequently asked questions concerning endodontic treatment. These questions are reviewed in the following section. Accompanying each question is an example of an explanation that patients should be able to understand. In addition, the dentist will find it useful to have a set of illustrations or drawings to help explain the procedure. An excellent case presentation aid is the Endoboard (Fig. 5-1), a plastic-coated erasable drawing board that allows for visualization of various types of endodontic problems and treatment options. The American Association of Endodontists (AAE) also offers specialized case presentation forms with carbonless copies for record keeping and patient use.

What is Endodontic (Root Canal) Treatment?   Endodontics is the specialty in dentistry concerned with the prevention, diagnosis, and treatment of diseases or injuries to the dental pulp. The pulp, which some people call "the nerve," is the soft tissue inside the tooth that contains the nerves and blood vessels and is responsible for tooth development. Root canal treatment is a safe and effective means of saving teeth that otherwise would be lost.

What Causes the Pulp to Die or Become Diseased?   When a pulp is injured, diseased, and unable to repair itself, it becomes inflamed and eventually dies. The most frequent causes of pulp death are extensive decay, deep fillings, trauma (e.g., severe blow to a tooth), cracks in teeth, and

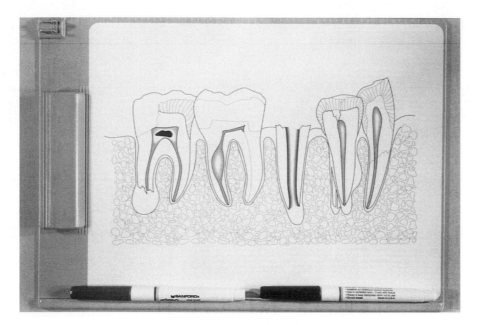

Fig. 5-1   The Endoboard is a handy erasable board for educating patients who need endodontic therapy. (Courtesy Kilgore International, Coldwater, Mich.)

periodontal or gum disease. When a pulp is exposed to bacteria from decay or saliva that has leaked into the pulp system, infection can occur inside the tooth and, if left untreated, can cause infection to build up at the tip of the root, forming an abscess. Eventually the bone supporting the tooth will be destroyed, and pain and swelling will often accompany the infection. Without endodontic treatment, the tooth will eventually have to be removed.

What Are the Symptoms of a Diseased Pulp?
Symptoms may range from momentary-to-prolonged, mild-to-severe pain on exposure to hot or cold or on chewing or biting. In some cases the condition may produce no symptoms at all. The patient should be informed that the radiographic examination may or may not demonstrate abnormal conditions of the tooth. The clinician should also make it clear that sometimes in the absence of pain there is radiographic evidence of pulpal or periradicular disease or both.

What Is the Success Rate of Root Canal Therapy?
Endodontics is one of the few procedures in dentistry that has a predictable prognosis if treatment is performed properly. Studies indicate that root canal treatment is usually 90% to 95% successful. Those in the failure group may still be amenable to retreatment or surgical treatment to save the tooth, though no treatment's success can be guaranteed. In addition, patients must understand that the prognosis may vary depending on the specifics of each case and that, without good oral hygiene and a sound restoration after endodontics, there may be an increased chance for failure. The need for periodic follow-up must be addressed to assess the long-term status of the tooth and periradicular tissues.

Will the Endodontically Treated Tooth Discolor After Treatment?
If the treatment is done correctly, discoloration seldom occurs. Bleaching with heat or chemicals can be used to treat discolored teeth. Some endodontically treated teeth appear discolored because they have been restored with tooth-colored fillings that have become stained or with amalgam restorations that leach silver ions. In these instances the fillings may be replaced, but often the placement of crowns or veneers is indicated.

What Are the Alternatives to Root Canal Treatment?
The only alternative is to extract the tooth, which often leads to shifting and crowding of surrounding teeth and subsequent loss of chewing efficiency. The patient should understand that often extraction is the easy way out and, depending on the case, may prove to be more costly for the patient in the long run. The patient always reserves the right to do nothing about the problem, provided the dentist has explained the associated risks of this decision.

Will the Tooth Need a Crown or Cap After the Treatment?
If there is no previously existing crown, the need for a crown or cap depends on the amount of sound tooth structure remaining after endodontic treatment. In addition, the need for a crown or cap depends on the type of tooth and the amount of chewing force to which the tooth will be subjected. Loss of tooth structure significantly weakens the tooth and renders it more susceptible to fracture; as a result, it may be necessary to protect what is left with a restoration, such as a crown. Significant loss of tooth structure with a concomitant loss of retentive areas for coronal buildups may necessitate the placement of a metallic, resin, or ceramic post

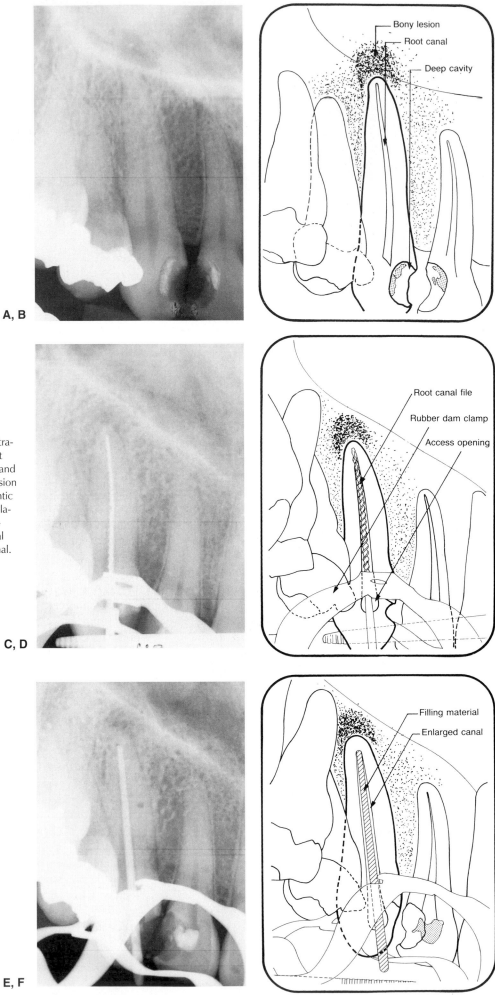

Fig. 5-2 Series of radiographs and illustrations demonstrating root canal treatment and restoration of a maxillary canine. **A** and **B**, Maxillary canine with periradicular lesion of endodontic origin. **C** and **D**, Endodontic file corresponding to length of canal; isolation with rubber dam throughout procedure. **E** and **F**, Endodontic filling material placed after cleaning and shaping of canal.

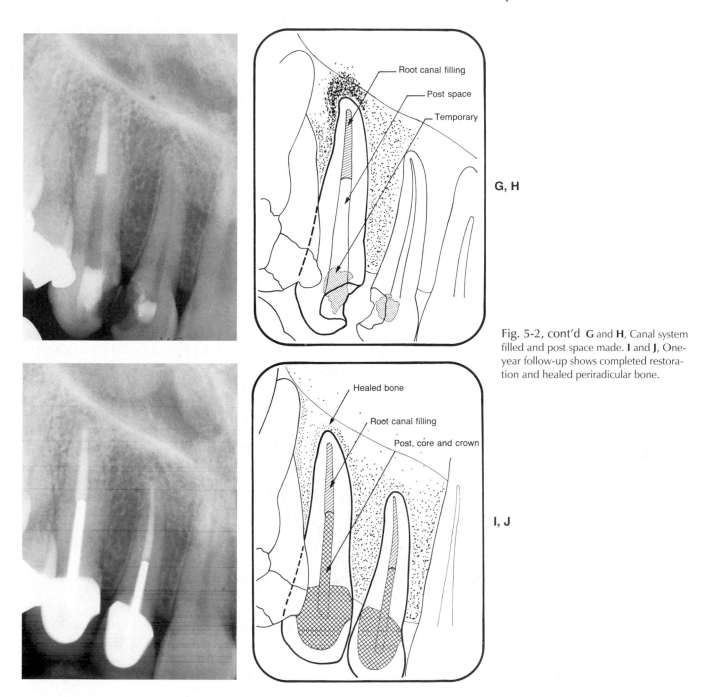

Fig. 5-2, cont'd **G** and **H**, Canal system filled and post space made. **I** and **J**, One-year follow-up shows completed restoration and healed periradicular bone.

in a canal to retain the buildup material (Fig. 5-2, *I, J*). (For further information on these issues, see Chapter 22.)

What Does Root Canal Treatment Involve?
Treatment may require one to three appointments, depending on the diagnosis, the number of roots, and the complexity of the case. During these appointments the clinician removes the injured or diseased pulp tissue. The root canals are cleaned, enlarged, and sealed to prevent recontamination of the root canal system. The following steps (see Fig. 5-2) describe the technical aspects of the treatment (illustrations, diagrams, radiographs, and digital images should be used as aids to the presentation):

1. Local anesthesia is usually administered.
2. The tooth is isolated with a rubber dam to prevent contamination from saliva and to protect the patient. This procedure is followed at each subsequent visit.
3. An opening is made through the top of the tooth to gain entrance to the root canal system.
4. The pulp tissue is painlessly removed with special instruments called *files*.
5. Periodic radiographs or digital images must be taken to ensure that these instruments correspond to the exact length of the root so that the entire tissue can be removed. Electronic apex locators can be used as adjuncts to help determine or verify lengths.

6. The root canal is cleaned, enlarged, and shaped so that it can be filled or sealed properly at the final appointment.
7. Sometimes medications are placed in the opening to prevent infection between appointments.
8. A temporary filling is placed in the crown opening between appointments.
9. At the final appointment the canal is sealed to safeguard it from further contamination.
10. Permanent restoration of the tooth is accomplished after completion of the root canal treatment.

Some additional points should be conveyed to the patient after treatment. The patient should not be given the impression that there will be no pain after the treatment.[54] In most cases, the mild discomfort the patient may experience is transitory and can usually be treated with an over-the-counter antiinflammatory or analgesic agent, such as aspirin or ibuprofen-containing compound. In fact, prophylactic administration of these drugs before the patient leaves the office will help reduce postoperative discomfort by achieving therapeutic blood levels of analgesic before the local anesthesia wears off (as discussed in Chapter 20). In certain cases simply handing the patient a written prescription for a stronger analgesic, "just in case," conveys a feeling of empathy and caring toward the patient and strengthens the doctor-patient relationship.

If the dentist wishes to refer the patient to an endodontist for treatment, skillful words of encouragement and explanation will convey the caring and concern behind this recommendation. Many patients already feel comfortable with their dentists and are fearful of "seeing someone new." In addition, they may not understand why a general dentist chooses not to do the root canal treatment. The referring dentist can help by carefully explaining the complex nature of the case and why it would be in the patient's best interests to visit the endodontist, who is specially trained to handle complex cases.[54]

Informed Consent

A great deal of controversy surrounds the legal aspects of informed consent. The current thinking in the courts is that for consent to be valid, it must be freely given; that all terms must be presented in language that the patient understands; and that the consent must be "informed."[15,16,46] For consent to be informed, the following conditions must be included in the presentation to the patient:

- The procedure and prognosis must be described. (This includes prognosis in the absence of treatment.)
- Alternatives to the recommended treatment must be presented, along with their respective prognoses.
- Foreseeable risks and material risks must be described.
- Patients must have the opportunity to have questions answered.[46]

It is probably in the best interests of the dentist and patient relationship to have the patient sign a valid informed consent form. With the continuous rise in dental litigation, it is important to realize that "no amount of documentation is too much and no amount of detail is too little."[46] (For further information on this subject, see Chapter 10.)

Radiation Safety

A critical portion of the endodontic case presentation and informed consent is educating the patient about the requirement for radiographs as part of the treatment. The dentist must communicate to the patient that the benefits of radiographs far outweigh the risks of receiving small doses of ionizing radiation, as long as techniques and necessary precautions are properly executed.[2] Although levels of radiation in endodontic radiography range from only 1/100 to 1/1000 of the levels needed to sustain injury,[42,52] it is still best to keep ionizing radiation to a minimum for the protection of both the patient and dental-delivery team.

Two simple analogies can be used to help the patient understand the small risk associated with dental radiographs. A patient would have to receive 25 complete full-mouth series (i.e., 450 exposures) within a very short time to significantly increase the risk of skin cancer.[42] One full-mouth survey (i.e., 20 ektaspeed [E]-speed films with rectangular collimation) has been found to deliver less than half of the amount of radiation of a single chest film and less than 1% the amount of a barium study of the intestines.[27] Nevertheless, the principles of ALARA—As Low As Reasonably Achievable—which are techniques used to reduce radiation exposure, should be followed as closely as possible to minimize the amount of radiation that both patient and treatment team receive. ALARA also implies the possibility that no matter how small the radiation dose, there still may be some deleterious effects.[27,42]

Principles of ALARA

In endodontic radiography, fast (i.e., sensitive) speed film, either ultraspeed (U) or E, should be selected.[42] Although E speed film allows for a reduction of approximately 50% of the radiation exposure required for D speed,[23] findings in observer preference studies have been mixed as it applies to the quality, clarity, and diagnostic capability of E film compared with D film. Processing of the E speed film is also more sensitive.[23,24,34] Specialized radiographic systems[27,45] (involving direct or indirect digital intraoral radiography) involve the digitization of ionizing radiation and use considerably smaller amounts of radiation to produce an image that is available immediately after exposure (see section on "Digitization of Ionizing Radiation" later in the chapter).

Meticulous radiographic technique helps reduce the number of retakes and obviates further exposure. Film-holding devices (discussed later in the chapter) along with correct film and tube head positioning are essential for maintaining film stability and producing radiographs of diagnostic quality.[27,42] A quality-assurance program for film processing should also be set up to ensure that films are properly processed.[27,42]

Dental units should be operated using at least 70 kVp. The lower the kilovoltage, the higher the patient's skin dose. Optimally, 90 kVp should be used. Units operating at 70 kVp or higher must have a filtration equivalent of 2.5 mm of aluminum to remove the extraneous low-energy x-rays before the patient absorbs them.[27,42]

Collimation also reduces exposure level. Collimation, essentially, is the restriction of the x-ray beam size by means of a lead diaphragm so that the beam does not exceed 2.75 inches (7 cm) at the patient's skin surface. Open-ended, circular, or rectangular lead-lined cylinders, known as *position-indicating devices* (PIDs), help direct the beam to the target (Fig. 5-3). However, the universal rectangular cylinder also collimates the x-ray beam by decreasing beam size even more, reducing the area of skin surface exposed to x-radiation, and reducing radiation burden by approximately 50% (Fig. 5-4). These PIDs, or cones, should be at least 12 to 16 inches long, because the shorter (i.e., 8-inch) cones that provide shorter source-to-film distances cause more divergence

of the beam and more exposure to the patient.[27,42] Pointed cones, illegal in some states, should not be used because of the increased amount of scatter radiation they produce.

The patient should be protected with a lead apron and a thyroid collar for each exposure (Fig. 5-5). When exposing films, the clinician should stand behind a barrier. Plaster, cinderblock, and at least 2.5 inches of drywall provide the necessary protection from the radiation produced by dental units. If there is no barrier the clinician should stand in an area of minimal scatter radiation: at least 6 feet away from the patient and in area that lies between 90 and 135 degrees to the beam.[27,42] All dental personnel who might be exposed to occupational x-radiation should wear film badges for recording exposure. If the concept of ALARA is strictly adhered to, no member of the dental team should receive doses close to the maximum permissible dose (MPD) (i.e., 50 mSv per year/whole body).[27]

For "declared" pregnant workers, the Nuclear Regulatory Commission limits the radiation dose to the fetus to 0.5 mSv during the gestation period. It is important to note that the MPD is specified as occupational exposure and should not be confused with exposure that patients receive as a result of radiographic procedures. Although no state-recommended maximum patient exposures exist, it is the responsibility of anyone who administers ionizing radiation to consult the respective state's bureau of radiation control to obtain information on current laws. Nonetheless, every effort should be made to keep the radiation dose to all individuals as low as possible and to avoid any unnecessary radiation exposure.

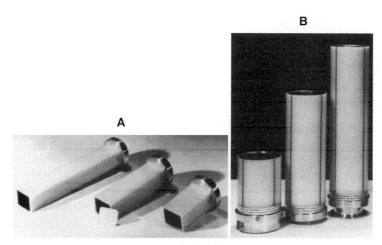

Fig. 5-3 Position-indicating devices: open-ended, lead-lined 8-inch, 12-inch, 16-inch. **A,** Rectangles. **B,** Cylinders. (Courtesy Margraf Dental Manufacturing, Jenkintown, Pa.)

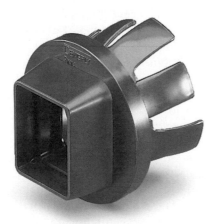

Fig. 5-4 Universal collimator snaps on aiming ring to extend the extra protection of a rectangular collimator to round, open-ended cones. (Courtesy Rinn Corporation, Elgin, IL.)

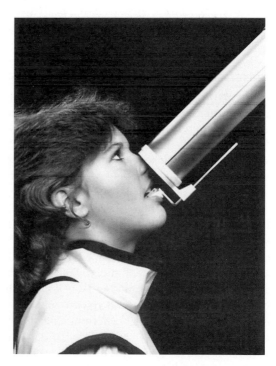

Fig. 5-5 Film-holding and aiming device (XCP instrument) with PID on a patient protected with a lead apron and thyroid collar. (Courtesy Rinn Corporation, Elgin, IL.)

Premedication with Antibiotics

Prophylactic coverage with antibiotics or antiinfectives is indicated for patients who are susceptible to systemic disease after bacteremia. Although it has been documented that the incidence of bacteremia associated with nonsurgical root canal treatment is essentially negligible as long as endodontic instruments are confined to the root system,[7,8] the American Heart Association (AHA) recommends prophylactic antibiotic coverage for patients who have prostheses, shunts, or certain diseases. The use of prophylactic antibiotics in these patients prevents blood-borne microorganisms from lodging on shunts and prostheses or from multiplying within a depressed system.[21,37,44,48]

With respect to premedication for dental patients with total joint replacements, there has been considerable controversy as to whether or not such patients require routine prophylaxis. In 1997 the ADA and AAOS (American Academy of Orthopedic Surgeons) drafted an advisory statement[4] on antimicrobial premedication for dental patients with total joint replacements. The joint organizations recognized that there was no agreed upon scientific evidence to support the contention that antibiotic prophylaxis is necessary to prevent metastatic infection in patients with total joint prosthesis. They also agreed that the analogy between late prosthetic joint infections with infective endocarditis was invalid, because the anatomy, blood supply, types of microorganisms involved, and mechanisms of infection are all different. The ADA and AAOS concluded that antibiotic prophylaxis is not indicated for dental patients with pins, plates, and screws, nor is it routinely indicated for most dental patients with total joint replacements.

However, because there is limited evidence that some dental procedures are high-risk procedures (e.g., extractions, intraligamentary local anesthesia, endodontic surgery, endodontic instrumentation "beyond the apex") and that some medically compromised patients with total joint replacements (e.g., insulin-dependent diabetes; inflammatory arthropathies, such as rheumatoid arthritis; immunosuppression; hemophilia; previous prosthetic joint infections) may be at higher risk for hematogenous infections, an antibiotic regimen should be considered. Prophylaxis should also be recommended during the first 2 years after joint replacement. The antibiotic regimen is cephalexin, cephradine, or amoxicillin (2 g PO, 1 hour before procedure). For those allergic to penicillin or cephalosporin, the recommended antibiotic is clindamycin (600 mg PO, 1 hour before procedure). It is recommended that patients who are not allergic to penicillin but who are unable to take oral medications should receive cefazolin (1 g) or ampicillin, (2 g) IM or IV, 1 hour before the dental procedure. For patients allergic to penicillin and unable to take oral medications, the recommendation is clindamycin (600 mg IM or IV, 1 hour before the dental procedure). Similar to the AHA guidelines, follow-up doses are no longer recommended. The advisory statement only represents recommended guidelines and is not intended as a standard of care, because it is impossible to make recommendations for all clinical situations in which late infection might occur in total joint prostheses. Practitioners must exercise their own clinical judgment in determining whether to premedicate a patient.

Patients with certain cardiac conditions are candidates for antibiotic coverage to prevent subacute bacterial endocarditis (SBE).[48] In 1997 the AHA revised its recommendations for the prevention of bacterial endocarditis that may be the result of an invasive procedure.[21] The major modifications include the recognition and emphasis that most cases of endocarditis are not the result of an invasive procedure; that predisposing cardiac conditions are stratified into high, moderate, and negligible risk categories based upon the potential outcome, should endocarditis develop; and modification of the drugs and dosages necessary for prophylaxis.

Based upon the new guidelines, prophylaxis is recommended for individuals in high-risk and moderate-risk categories. Individuals at high-risk are those who have prosthetic heart valves, previous history of endocarditis, complex cyanotic congenital heart disease, and surgically constructed systemic pulmonary shunts. Those conditions in the moderate-risk category include most other congenital cardiac malformations, rheumatic heart disease, hypertrophic cardiomyopathy, and mitral valve prolapse with valvular regurgitation or thickened leaflets or both. Conditions that are in the negligible-risk category (i.e., no greater risk than the general population) and for which prophylaxis is not recommended include previous coronary artery bypass graft surgery, mitral valve prolapse without valvular regurgitation, previous rheumatic fever without valvular dysfunction, and cardiac pacemakers (both intravascular and epicardial).

The AHA has developed a standard prophylactic antibiotic regimen for patients at risk and a set of alternative regimens for those unable to take oral medications, for those who are allergic to the standard antibiotics, and for those who are not candidates for the standard regimen.[21] The recommended standard prophylactic regimen for all dental, oral, and upper respiratory tract procedures is currently amoxicillin. This is because amoxicillin is better absorbed by the gastrointestinal tract and provides higher and more sustained serum levels than does penicillin.

The major modification in the new regimen is that the postoperative dose has been eliminated; the rationale for this is that amoxicillin has a sufficiently high plasma level for an adequate time to prevent endocarditis. Erythromycin has also been eliminated as a recommended drug in the penicillin-allergic patient because of the high incidence of gastrointestinal upset and the variability of the pharmokinetics of the various erythromycin preparations. The official AHA recommendations for prophylactic antibiotic regimens do not specify all clinical situations for which patients may be at risk. Thus it is the responsibility of the clinician to exercise his or her own judgment or consult with the patient's physician before giving treatment. (The current AHA guidelines for prophylactic antibiotic coverage are listed in Chapter 13.)

Antianxiety Regimens

Because patients have been often misinformed about root canal treatment, it is understandable that some may experience an increased anxiety about undergoing the procedure. Fortunately, however, the vast majority of patients are able to tolerate their anxiety, control their behavior, and allow treatment to proceed with few problems. Appropriate behavioral approaches can be used to manage most anxious dental patients. Retrospective studies[18] concerning dental anxiety have clearly demonstrated that explaining each procedure before beginning root canal treatment can effectively reduce a patient's anxiety. The clinician can also reduce patient anxiety by giving specific information during treatment, by advising the patient about possible minor discomfort, and by explaining how that discomfort can be controlled. Verbal support, reassurance, and personal warmth also help to ease patient anxiety during root canal treatment. Many of these measures can be taken during the case presentation.

Although the clinician's hope and desire may not cure a patient's fear of root canal treatment, each clinician should realize that all anxious patients are not alike; therefore, each patient should be managed individually. If behavioral solutions are not feasible or effective in a particular case, pharmacologic approaches to managing patient anxiety may be exercised. Selection of such pharmacotherapeutic techniques must involve a careful assessment of the relative risks and benefits of the alternative approaches. All pharmacologic treatment regimens include the need for good local anesthetic technique. For the management of mild to moderate anxiety states, these regimens range from nitrous oxide plus oxygen sedation to oral sedation to intravenous or conscious sedation. (For further information on these issues, see Chapter 20.)

Pain Control with Preoperative Administration of NSAIDs

During root canal cleaning and shaping, extrusion of small amounts of pulp tissue remnants and dentin filings is likely to occur. Often this extrusion results in additional inflammation and some postoperative discomfort. Prophylactic administration of a nonsteroidal antiinflammatory drugs (NSAIDs), such as 200 to 400 mg of ibuprofen, 30 to 60 minutes before the procedure, has been shown to reduce or prevent postoperative dental pain.[31] (See Chapter 18 for further information.)

Pain Control with Local Anesthesia

It is paramount to obtain a high level of pain control when performing root canal treatment; in no other specialty is this task as challenging or as demanding. The clinician must strive for a "painless" local anesthetic injection technique, with relatively rapid onset of analgesia (see Chapter 20).

PREPARATION OF RADIOGRAPHS

Radiographs are essential to all phases of endodontic therapy. They inform the diagnosis and the various treatment phases and help evaluate the success or failure of treatment. Because root canal treatment relies on accurate radiographs, it is necessary to master radiographic techniques to achieve films of maximum diagnostic quality. Such mastery minimizes retaking of films and avoids additional exposure of patients. Expertise in radiographic interpretation is essential for recognizing deviations from the norm and for understanding the limitations associated with endodontic radiography.

Functions, Requirements, and Limitations of the Radiograph in Endodontics

The primary radiograph used in endodontics is the periapical radiograph. In diagnosis this film is used to identify abnormal conditions in the pulp and periradicular tissues. It is also used to determine the number of roots and canals, location of canals, and root curvatures. Because the radiograph is a two-dimensional image (a major limitation), it is often advantageous to take additional radiographs at different horizontal or vertical angulations when treating multicanaled and multirooted teeth. Taking additional radiographs is also helpful when treating teeth with severe root curvature. These supplemental radiographs enhance visualization and evaluation of the three-dimensional structure of the tooth.

Technically, for endodontic purposes, a radiograph should depict the tooth in the center of the films. Consistent film placement in this manner will minimize interpretation errors, because the center of the films contains the least amount of distortion. In addition, at least 3 mm of bone must be visible beyond the apex of the tooth. Failure to capture this bony area may result in misdiagnosis, improper interpretation of the apical extent of a root, or incorrect determination of file lengths for canal cleaning and shaping. Finally, the image on the film must be as anatomically correct as possible. Image shape distortion caused by elongation or foreshortening may lead to interpretative errors during diagnosis and treatment.[26,27]

The bite-wing radiograph may be useful as a supplemental film. This film normally has less image distortion because of its parallel placement, and it provides critical information on the anatomic crown of the tooth. This information includes the anatomic extent of the pulp chamber, the existence of pulp stones or calcifications, recurrent decay, the depth of existing restorations, and any evidence of previous pulp therapy.[54] The bite-wing also indicates the relationship of remaining tooth structure relative to the crestal height of bone. Thus it can aid in determining the restorability of the tooth.

In addition to their diagnostic value, high-quality radiographs are mandatory during the treatment phase. Technique is even more critical, however, because working radiographs must be taken while the rubber dam system is in place. Visibility is reduced and the bows of the clamp often restrict precise film positioning. During treatment, periradicular radiographs are used to determine canal working lengths; the location of superimposed objects, canals, and anatomic landmarks (by altering cone angulations); biomechanical instrumentation; and master cone adaptation (see Fig. 5-2, *C* to *F*). After completion of the root canal procedure, a radiograph should be taken to determine the quality of the root canal filling or obturation. Recall radiographs taken at similar angulations enhance assessment of the success or failure of treatment (see Fig. 5-2, *I* and *J*).

The astute clinician can perceive that precise radiographic interpretation is undoubtedly one of the most valuable sources of information for endodontic diagnosis and treatment, but the radiograph is only an adjunctive tool and can be misleading. Information gleaned from proper inspection of the radiograph is not always absolute and must always be integrated with information gathered from a thorough medical and dental history, clinical examination, and various pulp-testing procedures (see Chapter 1).

Use of the radiograph depends on an understanding of its limitations *and* its advantages. The advantages are obvious: the radiograph allows a privileged look inside the jaw. The information it furnishes is essential and cannot be obtained from any other source, yet its value is not diminished by a critical appraisal of its limitations.

One of the major limitations of radiographs is their inability to detect bone destruction or pathosis when it is limited to the cancellous bone. Studies[50] have proven that radiolucencies usually do not appear unless there is external or internal erosion of the cortical plate. This factor must be considered in evaluating teeth that become symptomatic but show no radiographic changes. In most cases, root structure anatomically approaches cortical bone and, if the plate is especially thin, radiolucent lesions may be visible before there is significant destruction of the cortical plate. Nevertheless, inflammation and resorption affecting the cortical plates must still be sufficiently extensive before a lesion can be seen on a radiograph.

Principles of Endodontic Radiography

Film Placement and Cone Angulation   For endodontic purposes, the paralleling technique produces the most accurate periradicular radiograph. Also known as the *long-cone* or *right-angle* technique, it produces improved images. The film is placed parallel to the long axis of the teeth, and the central beam is directed at right angles to the film and aligned through the root apex (Fig. 5-6, *A* and *B*). To achieve

this parallel orientation it is often necessary to position the film away from the tooth, toward the middle of the oral cavity, especially when the rubber dam clamp is in position.[27] The long-cone (i.e., 16 to 20 inches) aiming device is used in the paralleling technique to increase the focal spot-to-object distance. This has the effect of directing only the most central and parallel rays of the beam to the film and teeth, reducing size distortion.[27,41,42] This technique permits a more accurate reproduction of the tooth's dimensions, thus enhancing a determination of the tooth's length and relationship to surrounding anatomic structures.[26] In addition, the paralleling technique reduces the possibility of superimposing the zygomatic processes over the apices of maxillary molars, which often occurs with more angulated films, such as those produced by means of the bisecting-angle technique (Fig. 5-6, *C* and *D*). If properly used, the paralleling technique will provide the clinician with films with the least distortion, minimal superimposition, and utmost clarity.

Variations in size and shape of the oral structures (e.g., shallow palatal vault, tori, or extremely long roots) or gagging by the patient can make true parallel placement of the film impossible. To compensate for difficult placement, the film can be positioned so that it diverges as much as 20 degrees from the long axis of the tooth, with minimal longitudinal distortion. With maxillary molars, any increase in vertical angulation increases the chances of superimposing the zygomatic process over the buccal roots. A vertical angle of not more than 15 degrees should usually project the zygomatic process superiorly and away from the molar roots. To help achieve this, a modified paralleling technique[17] that increases vertical angulation by 10 to 20 degrees can be used. Though this orientation introduces a small degree of foreshortening, it increases periradicular definition in this troublesome maxillary posterior region. The Dunvale Snapex System (Dunvale Corporation, Gilberts, IL), a film holder and aiming device originally designed for the bisecting angle technique, has been altered for the modified paralleling technique.[17] In conjunction with this technique, a distal angulated radiograph (i.e., a 10 to 20 degree horizontal shift of the cone from the distal, with the beam directed toward the mesial) tends to project buccal roots and the zygomatic process to the mesial, thus enhancing anatomic clarity.[17]

The bisecting angle technique is not preferred for endodontic radiography. However, when a modified paralleling technique cannot be used, there may be no choice because of difficult anatomic configurations or patient management problems.[17,27,41,42] The basis of this technique is to place the film directly against the teeth without deforming the film (see Fig. 5-6, *C* and *D*). The structure of the teeth, however, is such that with the film in this position there is an obvious angle between the plane of the film and the long axis of the teeth. This causes distortion, because the tooth is not parallel to the film. If the x-ray beam is directed at a right angle to the film, the image on the film will be shorter than the actual tooth (i.e., foreshortened). If the beam is directed perpendicularly to the long axis of the teeth, the image will be much longer than the

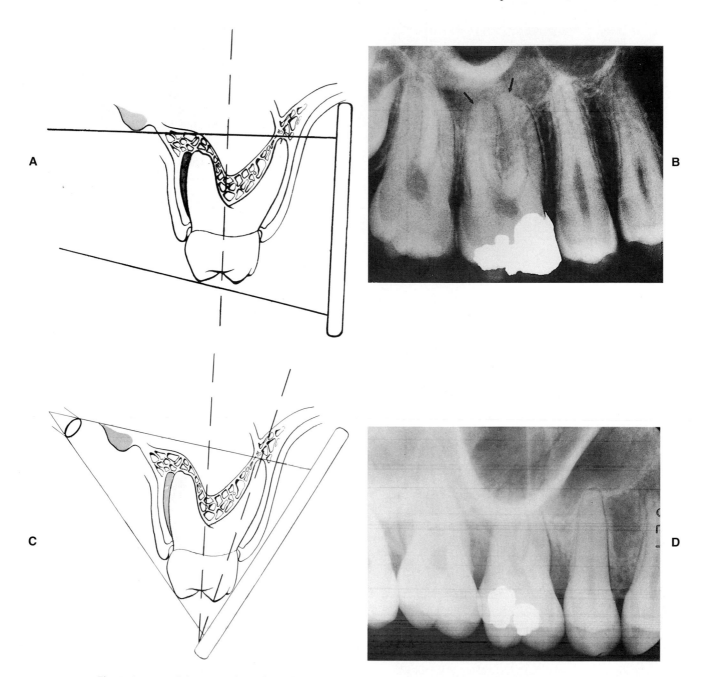

Fig. 5-6 **A**, Paralleling, or right-angle, technique. **B**, Projection of the zygomatic process above the buccal root apices with the right-angle technique, allowing visualization of the apices (*arrow*). **C**, Bisecting-angle technique. **D**, Superimposition of the zygomatic process over the buccal root apices of the maxillary first molar with the bisecting-angle technique.

tooth (i.e., elongated). Thus, by directing the central beam perpendicular to an imaginary line that bisects the angle between tooth and film, the length of the tooth's image on the film should be the same as the actual length of the tooth.

Although the projected length of the tooth is correct, the image will show distortion because the film and object are not parallel and the x-ray beam is not directed at right angles to both. This distortion increases along the image toward its apical extent. The technique produces additional error poten-

tial, because the clinician must imagine the line bisecting the angle (an angle that, in itself, is difficult to assess). In addition to producing more frequent superimposition of the zygomatic arch over apices of maxillary molars, the bisecting angle technique causes greater image distortion than the paralleling technique and makes it difficult for the operator to reproduce radiographs at similar angulations to assess healing after root canal treatment[27] (see Fig. 5-6, *C* and *D*).

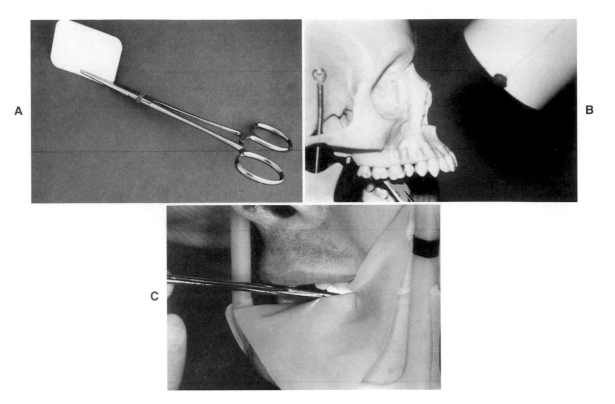

Fig. 5-7 **A**, Hemostat aids in film placement and in cone alignment. **B**, With the paralleling technique, the tube head is positioned at a 90-degree angle to the film. Note that the hemostat is resting on the mandibular anteriors so that the film is parallel with the long axis of the maxillary central incisors. **C**, Releasing a corner of the rubber dam aids in hemostat placement so that the film can be properly aligned. (*B,* Courtesy Dr. Eddy Tidwell. *C,* Courtesy Dr. Michelle Speier.)

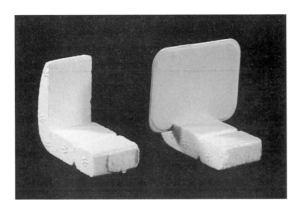

Fig. 5-8 The Greene Stabe disposable film holder.

Film Holders and Aiming Devices   Film holders and aiming devices are required for the paralleling technique because they reduce geometric distortion caused by misorientation of the film, central beam, and tooth.[17,27,41,42,54] They also minimize cone cutting, improve diagnostic quality, and allow similarly angulated radiographs to be taken during treatment and at recall. By eliminating the patient's finger from the x-ray field and thus the potential for displacing the film, these devices help to minimize retakes and make it easier for the patient and clinician to properly position the film.

A number of commercial devices are available that position the film parallel and at various distances from the teeth, but one of the most versatile film-holding devices is the hemostat (Fig. 5-7, *A*). The operator positions a hemostat-held film, and the handle is used to align the cone vertically and horizontally. The patient then holds the hemostat in the same position and the cone is positioned at a 90-degree angle to the film (Fig. 5-7, *B*). When taking working radiographs, a radiolucent, plastic, rubber dam frame, such as an Ostby or Young frame, should be used and not removed. To position the hemostat or other film-holding device, a corner of the rubber dam is released for visibility and to allow the subsequent placement of the device-held film (Fig. 5-7, *C*). Another film-holding device that is ideal for taking preoperative and postoperative films is the Greene Stabe disposable film holder (Rinn Corporation, Elgin, IL) (Fig. 5-8).

Besides the Dunvale Snapex System mentioned earlier, the major commercial film-holding and aiming devices include the XCP (extension cone paralleling) instruments, the EndoRay endodontic film holder, the Uni-Bite film holder, the Snap-A-Ray film holder, the Snap Ex System film holder with aiming device, and the Crawford Film Holder System (Figs. 5-9, 5-10, 5-11, and 5-12).

Fig. 5-9 XCP instruments hold the radiograph film packets and aid in cone alignment. Cone cutting is prevented, and consistent angulation can be achieved. (Courtesy Rinn Corporation, Elgin, IL.)

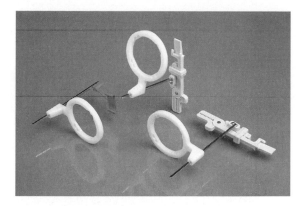

Fig. 5-11 Snap Ex System film-holder and aiming ring. The biting portion of the instrument is reduced to make it easier to place the instrument around the rubber dam. (Courtesy Rinn Corporation, Elgin, IL.)

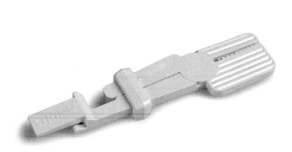

Fig. 5-10 Snap-A-Ray film-holding device. (Courtesy Rinn Corporation, Elgin, Ill.)

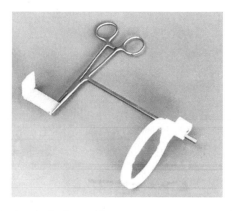

Fig. 5-12 Crawford Film Holder System. Components include Kelly hemostat with aiming rod (attached), aiming ring, and bite block. (Courtesy Dr. Frank Crawford, Indian Wells, CA.)

Variations in the use of the XCP system, for example, can prevent displacement of the rubber dam clamp and increase periradicular coverage during endodontic procedures. The film is placed off center in the bite block, and the cone is placed off center with respect to the aiming ring. This allows for placement of the bite block adjacent to the rubber dam clamp without altering the parallel relation of the cone to the film (Fig. 5-13). A customized hemostat (with rubber bite block attached) can also be made to assist film placement during the taking of working radiographs. Other specialized film holders, such as the EndoRay and the Crawford Film Holder System, have been designed to help the dentist secure parallel working films with the rubber dam clamp in place. Generally these holders all have an x-ray beam-guiding device (for proper beam to film relationship) and a modified bite block and film holder, for proper positioning over or around the rubber dam clamp (Figs. 5-14 and 5-15).

Exposure and Film Qualities The intricacies of proper kilovoltage, milliamperage, and time selection serve as examples of how the diagnostic quality of a film may be altered by changes in the film's density and contrast.[27,42] Density is the degree of darkening of the film, whereas contrast is the difference between densities. The amount of darkening depends on the quantity and quality of radiation delivered to the film, the subject thickness, and the developing or processing conditions. Milliamperage controls the electron flow from cathode to anode; the greater the electron flow per unit of time, the greater will be the quantity of radiation produced. Proper density is primarily a function of milliamperage and time. Kilovoltage also affects film density by controlling the quality and penetrability of the rays. Higher kilovoltage settings produce shorter wavelengths that are more penetrating than the longer wavelengths produced at lower settings.[27,42] The ability to control the penetrability of the rays by alterations in kilovoltage affects the amount of radiation reaching the film and the degree of darkening or density. Altering exposure time or milliamperage or both for each respective unit can control variations in density.[27,42]

Contrast is defined as the difference between shades of gray or the difference between densities. Most of the varia-

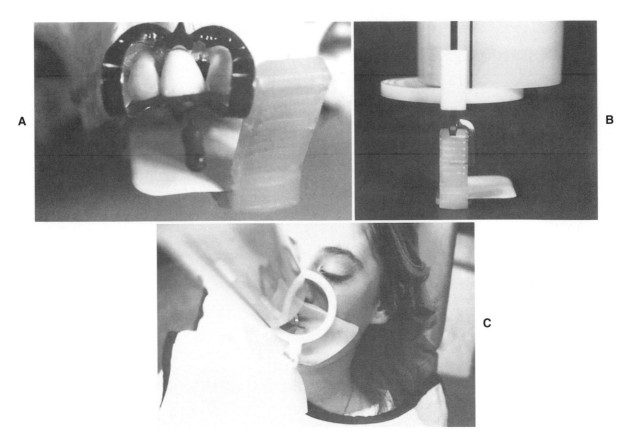

Fig. 5-13 **A**, Placement of a bite block on the tooth adjacent to the rubber dam clamp. **B**, Off-center placement of the film in the bite block. **C**, Alignment of the radiograph cone. (Courtesy Dr. Stephen F. Schwartz.)

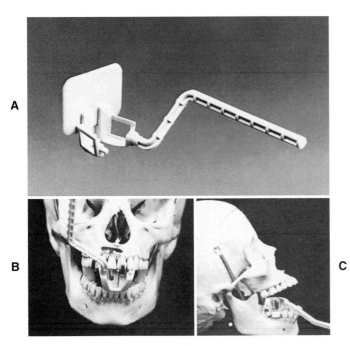

Fig. 5-14 **A**, EndoRay (posterior) film holder has a positioning arm to guide the cone to the center of the film. **B** and **C**, Anterior and posterior EndoRay film holders in place over the rubber dam clamp. Handle aids in determining cone position and angulation. (*A,* Courtesy Rinn Corporation, Elgin IL.)

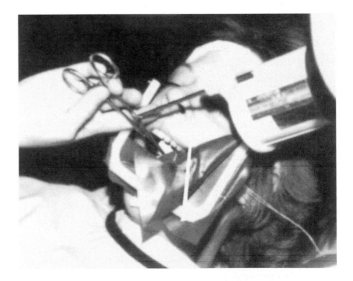

Fig. 5-15 Patient maintains position of film by holding handle of the hemostat of the Crawford Film Holder System. Note that the bite block is not used when rubber dam is in place.

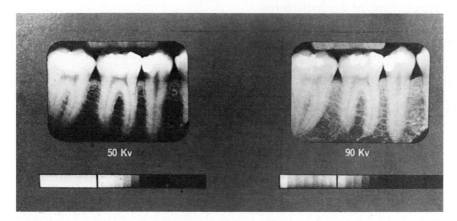

Fig. 5-16 Comparison of short-scale and long-scale contrast produced by altering the kilovoltage. Note the increased shades of gray in the film produced at 90 kVp. (Courtesy Rinn Corporation, Elgin, IL.)

tion observed in endodontic radiography is because of subject contrast, which depends on the thickness and density of the subject and the kilovoltage used. Thus kilovoltage is really the only exposure parameter under the clinician's control that directly affects subject contrast.[26,27,42] Exposure time and milliamperage only control the number of x-rays; therefore, they mainly influence the density of the film image. A radiographic film may exhibit a long scale, or low, contrast (i.e., more shades of gray or more useful densities); high-kilovoltage techniques (e.g., 90 kVp) produce this long scale of contrast as a result of the increased penetrating power of the rays. This results in images with many more shades of gray and less distinct differences (Fig. 5-16). Films exposed at low kilovoltage settings (e.g., 60 kVp) exhibit short-scale, or high, contrast, with sharp differences between a few shades of gray, black, and white.[27,42] Although they are perhaps more difficult to read, films exposed at higher kilovoltage settings (e.g., 90 kVp) make it possible to discriminate between images, often enhancing diagnostic quality; films exposed at a lower kilovoltage (e.g., 70 kVp) have better clarity and contrast between radiopaque and radiolucent structures, such as endodontic instruments near the root apex. Nevertheless, the optimal kilovoltage and exposure time should be individualized for each radiograph unit and exposure requirement.

Processing   Proper darkroom organization, film handling, and adherence to the time and temperature method of film processing play important roles in producing films of high quality.[42] For the sake of expediency in the production of working films in endodontics, rapid processing methods are used to produce relatively good films in less than 1 to 2 minutes (Fig. 5-17).[27,42] Although the contrast in using rapid-processing chemicals is lower than that achieved using conventional techniques, the radiographs have sufficient diagnostic quality to be used for treatment films and are obtained in less time and with less patient discomfort. Rapid-processing solutions are available commercially, but they

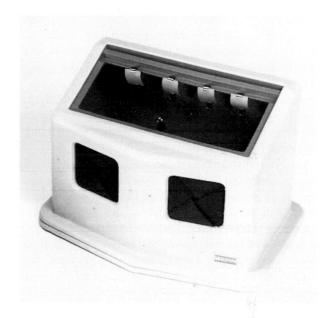

Fig. 5-17 Chair side darkroom allows rapid processing of endodontic working films. (Courtesy Rinn Corporation, Elgin, IL.)

tend to vary in shelf life, in tank life, and in the production of films of permanent quality.

To maintain the radiographic image for documentation, it is recommended that after an image has been evaluated it be returned to the fixer for 10 minutes more; then washed for 20 minutes and dried. An alternative is to reprocess the film by means of the conventional technique. Double film packets can also be used for working films: one can be processed rapidly and the other conventionally. Regardless of what method is used for working films, a controlled time and temperature method should be used for the diagnostic qualities desired in pretreatment, posttreatment, and recall radiographs. All radiographs taken during the course of endodontic treatment should be preserved as a part of the patient's permanent record.

Radiographic Interpretation in Endodontics

Examination and Differential Interpretation Radiographic interpretation is not strictly the identification of a problem and the establishment of a diagnosis. The dentist must read the film carefully, with an eye toward diagnosis and treatment. Frequently overlooked are the small areas of resorption, invaginated enamel, minute fracture lines, extra canals or roots, curved and calcified canals, and, in turn, the potential problems they may create during treatment (Fig. 5-18). If a thorough radiographic examination is conducted, problems during treatment, additional time, and extra expense can be avoided or, in the very least, anticipated. As mentioned earlier, additional exposures at various angulations may be necessary to gain a better insight into the three-dimensional structure of a tooth.

Many anatomic structures and osteolytic lesions can be mistaken for pulpoperiradicular lesions. Among the more commonly misinterpreted anatomic structures are the mental foramen (Fig. 5-19) and the incisive foramen. These radiolucencies can be differentiated from pathologic conditions by exposures at different angulations and by pulp-testing procedures. Radiolucencies not associated with the root apex will move or be projected away from the apex by varying the angulation. Radiolucent areas resulting from sparse trabeculation can also simulate radiolucent lesions. In such cases these areas must be differentiated from the lamina dura and periodontal ligament space.

A commonly misinterpreted osteolytic lesion is periapical cemental dysplasia or cementoma (Fig. 5-20). The use of pulp-testing procedures and follow-up radiographic examinations will prevent the mistake of diagnosing this as a pulpoperiradicular lesion. The development of this lesion can be followed radiographically from its early, more radiolucent stage through its mature or more radiopaque stage.

Other anatomic radiolucencies that must be differentiated from pulpoperiradicular lesions are maxillary sinus, nutrient canals, nasal fossa, and the lateral or submandibular fossa. Many systemic conditions can mimic or affect the radiographic appearance of the alveolar process. A discussion of these conditions is beyond the scope of this chapter, but the reader is encouraged to read further in any oral pathology textbook.

Lamina Dura: a Question of Integrity One of the key challenges in endodontic radiographic interpretation is understanding the integrity, or lack of integrity, of the lamina dura, especially in its relationship to the health of the pulp. Anatomically, the lamina dura[27] is a layer of compact bone (i.e., cribriform plate or alveolar bone proper) that lines the tooth socket. Noxious products emanating from the root canal system can effect a change in this structure that is visible radiographically. X-ray beams passing tangentially through the socket must pass through many times the width of the adjacent alveolus, and they are attenuated by this greater thickness of bone, producing the characteristic "white line." If, for example, the beam is directed more

obliquely so that it is not as attenuated, the lamina dura appears more diffuse, or it may not be discernible at all. Therefore the presence or absence and integrity of the lamina dura are determined largely by the shape and position of the root and, in turn, by its bony crypt, in relation to the x-ray beam. This explanation is consistent with the radiographic and clinical findings of teeth with normal pulps and no distinct lamina dura.[50]

Changes in the integrity of the periodontal ligament space, the lamina dura, and the surrounding periradicular bone certainly have diagnostic value, especially when recent radiographs are compared with previous ones. However, the significance of such changes must be tempered by a thorough understanding of the features that give rise to these images.

Buccal-Object Rule (cone shift) In endodontic therapy it is imperative that the clinician know the spatial or buccolingual relation of an object within the tooth or alveolus. The technique used to identify the spatial relation of an object is called the cone or *tube shift technique*. Other names for this procedure are the *buccal-object rule, Clark's rule*, and the *SLOB* (same lingual, opposite buccal) rule.[27,28,42,49] Proper application of the technique allows the dentist to locate additional canals or roots, to distinguish between objects that have been superimposed, and to distinguish between various types of resorption. It also helps the clinician to determine the buccal-lingual position of fractures and perforative defects, to locate foreign bodies, and to locate anatomic landmarks in relation to the root apex, such as the mandibular canal.[54]

The buccal-object rule relates to the manner in which the relative position of radiographic images of two separate objects changes when the projection angle at which the images were made is changed. The principle states that the object closest to the buccal surface appears to move in the direction opposite the movement of the cone or tube head, when compared with a second film. Objects closest to the lingual surface appear to move (on a film) in the same direction that the cone moved; thus "same lingual, opposite buccal" rule. Fig. 5-21 shows three simulated radiographs of a buccal object (circle) and a lingual object (triangle) exposed at different horizontal angles. The position of the objects on each radiograph is compared with the reference structure (i.e., the mesial root apex of the mandibular first molar). The first radiograph (see Fig. 5-21, *A* and *B*) shows superimposition of the two objects; in this case the tube head was positioned for a straight-on view. In the second radiograph (see Fig. 5-21, *C* and *D*), the tube head shifted mesially, and the beam was directed at the reference object from a more mesial angulation. In this case the lingual object (triangle) moved mesially with respect to the reference object, and the buccal object (circle) moved distally with respect to the reference object. In the third radiograph (see Fig. 5-21, *E* and *F*), the tube head shifted distally and the beam was directed at the reference object from a more distal angulation; here the triangle moved distally with respect to

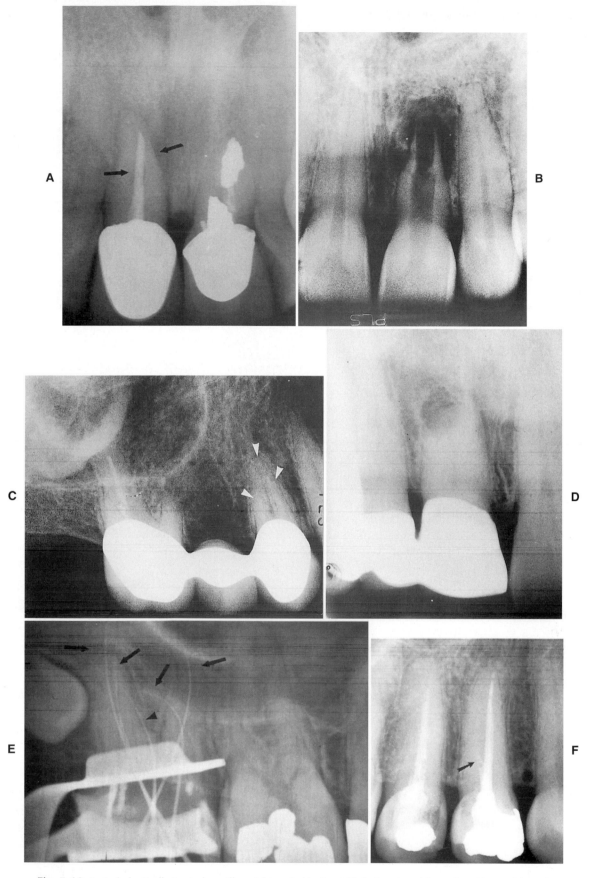

Fig. 5-18 **A,** Endodontically-treated maxillary right central incisor with both external (*arrow*) and internal (*arrow*) root resorption. **B,** Maxillary left central incisor with history of trauma and thin walls in the apical one third of the tooth. Once an apical barrier is formed, pressures exerted during obturation could cause fracture. **C,** Maxillary right first premolar with three separate roots (*arrows*). **D,** Maxillary right central with history of trauma. Apical resorption and calcification of the canal system complicate treatment. **E,** Working length radiograph of maxillary second molar demonstrates five separate roots (*arrows*): two mesiobuccal roots, two palatal roots, and one distobuccal root. **F,** Evidence of another canal in an endodontically treated maxillary first premolar. *Arrow* indicates root canal sealer in the unprepared canal.

continued

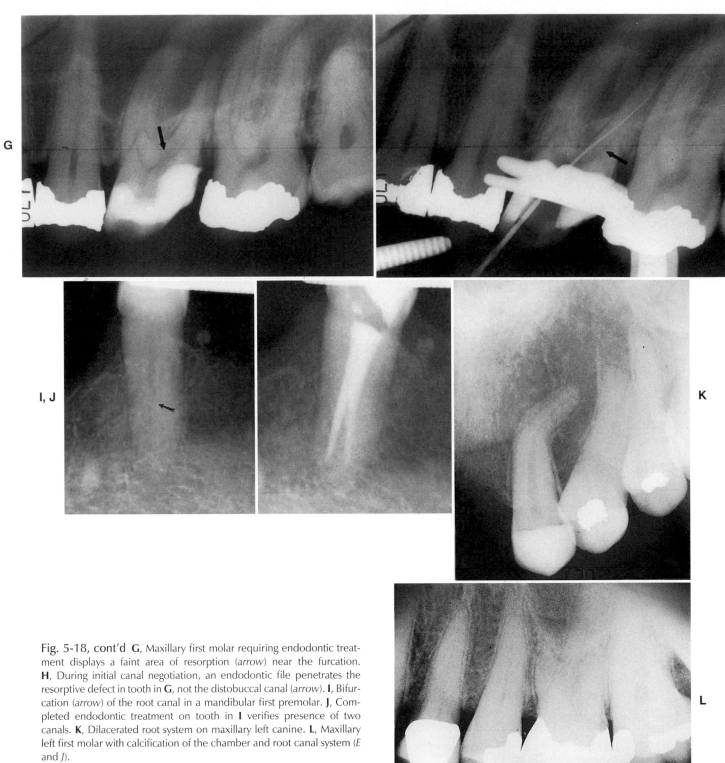

Fig. 5-18, cont'd **G**, Maxillary first molar requiring endodontic treatment displays a faint area of resorption (*arrow*) near the furcation. **H**, During initial canal negotiation, an endodontic file penetrates the resorptive defect in tooth in **G**, not the distobuccal canal (*arrow*). **I**, Bifurcation (*arrow*) of the root canal in a mandibular first premolar. **J**, Completed endodontic treatment on tooth in **I** verifies presence of two canals. **K**, Dilacerated root system on maxillary left canine. **L**, Maxillary left first molar with calcification of the chamber and root canal system (*E* and *J*).

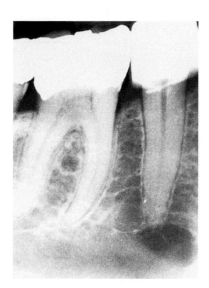

Fig. 5-19 A mandibular second premolar with an apparent periradicular radiolucency. Pulp-testing procedures indicated a normal response; the radiolucency is the mental foramen.

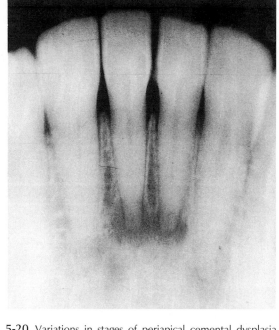

Fig. 5-20 Variations in stages of periapical cemental dysplasia (i.e., cementoma) on the four mandibular incisors. All teeth are vital.

the mesial root of the mandibular first molar, and the circle moved mesially. These radiographic relations confirm that the lingual object (triangle) moves in the same direction with respect to reference structures as the radiograph tube, and that the buccal object (circle) moves in the opposite direction of the radiograph tube. Thus, according to the rule, the object farthest (i.e., most buccal) from the film moves farthest on the film with respect to a change in horizontal angulation of the radiograph cone. In an endodontically treated mandibular molar with four canals (Fig. 5-22), a straight-on view results in superimposition of the root-filled canals on the radiograph. If the cone is angled from mesial to distal, the mesiolingual and distolingual canals will move mesially and the mesiobuccal and distobuccal canals will move distally on the radiograph, when compared with the straight-on view.

The examples cited previously involve application of the buccal-object rule, using changes in horizontal angulation. The clinician should be aware that this rule also applies to changes in vertical angulation (Fig. 5-23). To locate the position of the mandibular canal relative to mandibular molar root apices, radiographs must be taken at different vertical angulations. If the canal moves with or in the same direction as the cone head, the canal is lingual to the root apices; if the mandibular canal moves opposite the direction of the cone head, the canal is buccal to the root apices. The clinician should recognize the wide range of applicability of the buccal-object rule in determining the buccolingual relationship of structures not visible in a two-dimensional image.

Digitization of Ionizing Radiation The evolution of computer technology to radiography has allowed for nearly instantaneous image acquisition, image enhancement, storage, retrieval, and even transmission of images to remote sites in a digital format. The major advantages of using digital radiography in endodontics are that radiographic images are obtained immediately and radiation exposure is reduced from 50% to 90%, compared with conventional film-based radiography.[27,45] The primary disadvantages of digital imaging systems are their high initial cost and potential for reduction in image quality when compared with conventional radiography.

Digital imaging systems require an electronic sensor or detector, an analog-to-digital converter, a computer, and a monitor or printer for image display.[27] (See Chapter 26 for a further discussion of digital imaging systems and how they function.)

Digitization of ionizing radiation first became a reality in the late 1980s with the development of the original Radio-VisioGraphy (RGV) system by Dr. Francis Mouyen.[45] This system has evolved into the RVGui (Trex Trophy, Danbury CT). Other available systems include Dexis Digital X-Ray (Provision Dental Systems, Palo Alto, CA) and Computed Dental Radiography (CDR) (Schick Technologies, Long Island City, NY) (Fig. 5-24, *A* and *C*). The Food and Drug Administration has approved all of these systems.

Direct digital systems have three components: (1) the "radio" component, (2) the "visio" component, and (3) the "graphy" component. The "radio" component consists of a

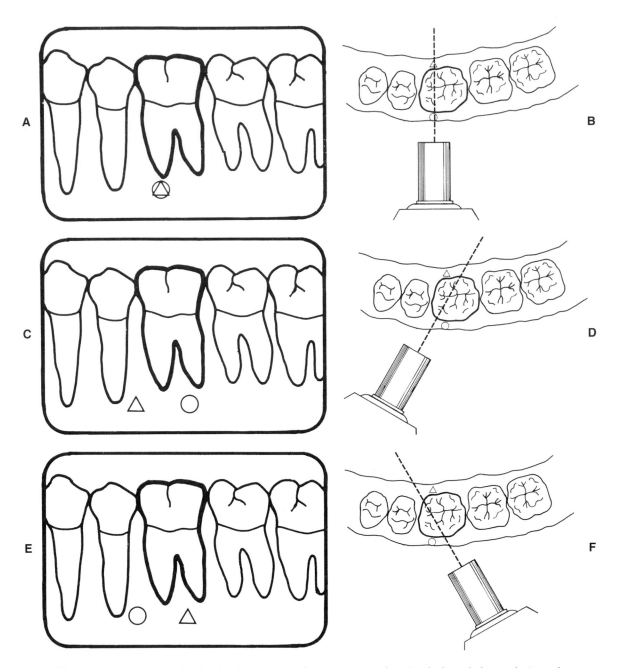

Fig. 5-21 Objects may be localized with respect to reference structures by using the buccal-object rule (i.e., tube-shift technique). **A** and **B**, A straight-on view will cause superimposition of the buccal object (*circle*) with the lingual object (*triangle*). **C** and **D**, Using the tube-shift technique, the lingual object (*triangle*) will appear more mesial with respect to the mesial root of the mandibular first molar, and the buccal object (*circle*) will appear more distal on a second view projected from the mesial. **E** and **F**, The object (*triangle*) on the lingual surface will appear more distal with respect to the mesial root of the mandibular first molar, and the object (*circle*) on the buccal surface will appear more mesial on a view projected from the distal aspect.

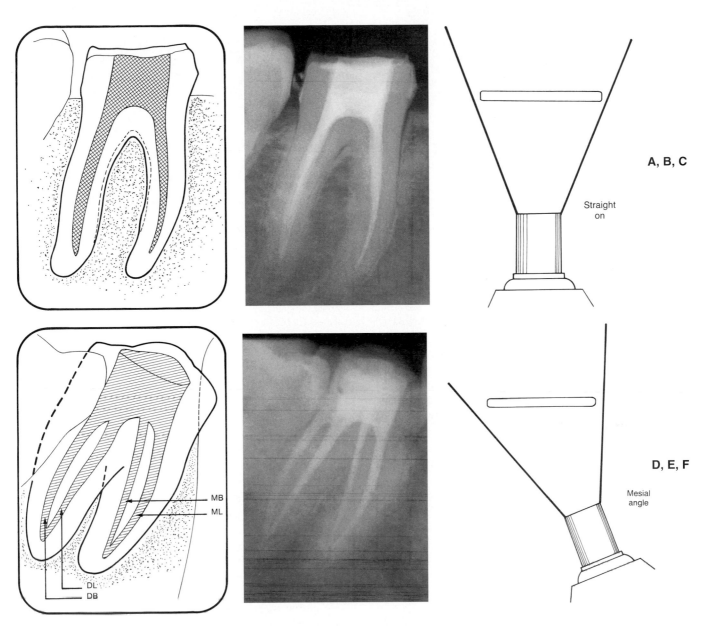

A, B, C

Straight on

D, E, F

Mesial angle

MB
ML

DL
DB

Fig. 5-22 Comparison of straight-on and mesial-angled views of an endodontically treated mandibular molar with four canals. **A**, **B**, and **C**, Straight-on view of the mandibular molar shows superimposition of the root canal fillings. **D**, **E**, and **F**, Mesial-to-distal angulation produces separation of the canals. The mesiolingual (*ML*) and distolingual (*DL*) root-filled canals move mesially (i.e., toward the cone), and the mesiobuccal (*MB*) and distobuccal (*DB*) root-filled canals move distally (i.e., away from the cone) on the radiograph.

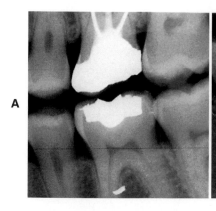
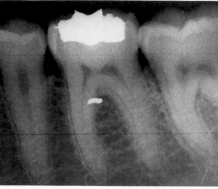
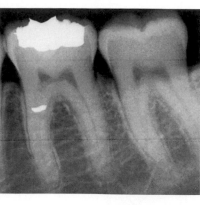

A

B, C

Fig. 5-23 Examples of the buccal-object rule using shifts in vertical and horizontal angulations. **A,** Bite-wing radiograph (straight-on view with minimal horizontal and vertical angulation) depicts amalgam particle superimposed over the mesial root of the mandibular first molar. To determine the buccal-lingual location of the object, the tube-shift technique (buccal-object rule) must be applied. **B,** The periapical radiograph was taken by shifting the vertical angulation of the cone (i.e., the x-ray beam was projected more steeply upward). Because the amalgam particle moved in the opposite direction to that of the cone (compared with the bite-wing radiograph), the amalgam particle lies on the buccal aspect of the tooth. **C,** The periapical radiograph was taken by shifting the horizontal angulation of the cone (the radiograph was taken from a distal angle). Compared with both **A** and **B,** each taken straight-on with minimal horizontal angulation, the amalgam particle moved opposite the direction of movement of the cone or tube head, confirming that the amalgam particle lies on the buccal aspect of the tooth.

high-resolution sensor with an active area that is similar in size to conventional film. However, there are slight variations in length, width, and thickness, depending on the respective system (Fig. 5-24, *B* and *D*). The sensor is protected from x-ray degradation by a fiber-optic shield, and it can be cold sterilized. Specially designed multiple types of sensor holders are available; for infection control, disposable plastic sheaths are used to cover the sensor when it is in use.

The second component of a direct digital system, the "visio" portion, consists of a video monitor and display-processing unit. As the image is transmitted to the processing unit, it is digitized and stored by the computer. The unit magnifies the image for immediate display on the video monitor; it also has the capability of producing colored images and can display multiple images simultaneously, including a full-mouth series on one screen. Because the image is digitized, further manipulation of the image is possible; this includes enhancement, contrast stretching, and reversing. A zoom feature is also available to enlarge a portion of the image up to full-screen size.

The third component of a direct digital system is the "graphy," a high-resolution video printer that provides a hard copy of the screen image, using the same video signal. In addition, a digital intraoral camera can be integrated with most systems. Indirect digital imaging or cordless systems, such as Digora (Soredex-Finndent, Conroe, TX) (Fig. 5-24, *E*) and DenOptix Digital Imaging System (Dentsply/Gendex, York, PA), involve the use of a reusable filmlike plate without wires (Fig. 5-24, *F*). The image to be scanned by a laser (to digitize it before viewing on the computer) is recorded on this plate. Although indirect digital imaging still

incorporates reduced radiation exposure and image manipulation, it usually takes slightly longer before the image can be viewed.

The advantages of both direct and indirect digital radiography seem numerous, but the primary ones include the elimination of standard radiograph film and processing chemicals, a significant reduction in exposure time (i.e., 80% to 90% reduction, when compared with D-speed film), and rapid image display. Virtually all systems can be linked with electronic record systems so that patient data can be stored, accessed, and transmitted easily. An exposure time in the range of hundredths of a second is all that is needed to generate an image.[27] One study showed that digital radiographic resolution was slightly lower than that produced with silver halide film emulsions, but the radiographic information may be increased with the electronic image treatment capabilities of the system.[45] These systems appear to be very promising for endodontics and for general dentistry.

Digital subtraction radiography[47] is a sensitive method for detecting changes in radiographic density over time. In endodontics, digital subtraction radiography may be especially useful for evaluating osseous healing after treatment and as an aid in diagnosis. By definition, subtraction radiography requires that two images have nearly identical image geometry; specialized positioning devices and bite registrations aid in matching the images. The subtracted image is a composite of the images, representing their variations in density. By subtracting all anatomic structures that have not changed between radiographic examinations, changes in diagnostic information become easier to interpret. If there is a change, it is displayed on the resultant image against a

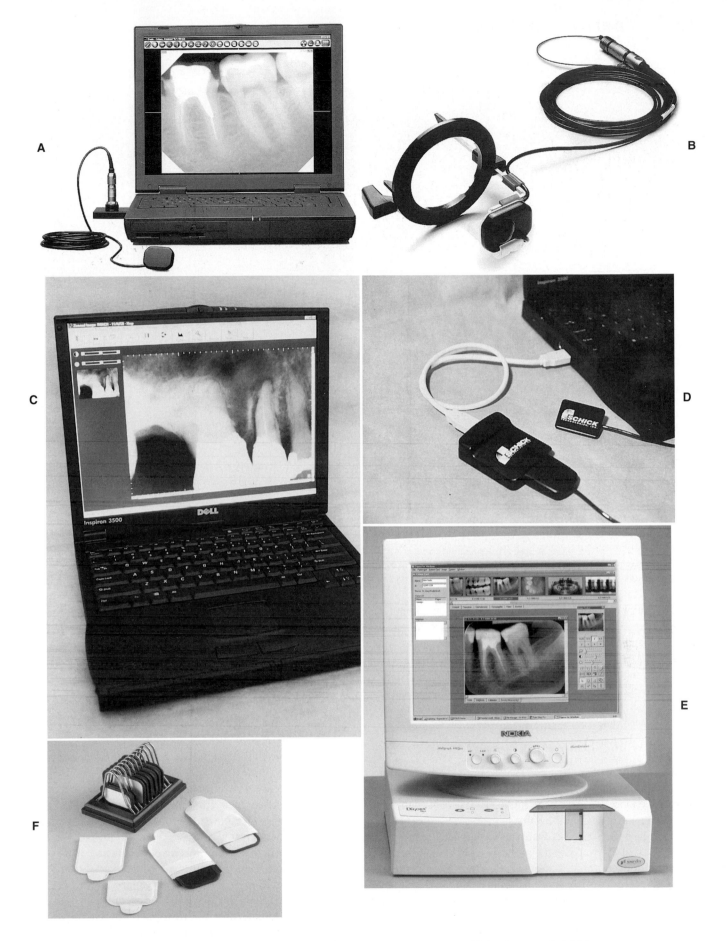

Fig. 5-24 Digital imaging systems. **A**, Dexis Digital X-Ray System. **B**, Positioner with Dexis sensor. **C,** CDR System. **D**, Schick intraoral sensor. **E**, Digora. **F**, Digora's reusable imaging plates are thin and flexible, like conventional film. (*A and B*, Courtesy Provision Dental Systems, Palo Alto, CA. *C and D*, Courtesy Schick Technologies, Inc., Long Island City, N.Y. *E and F,* Courtesy Soredex, Inc., Marietta, Ga.)

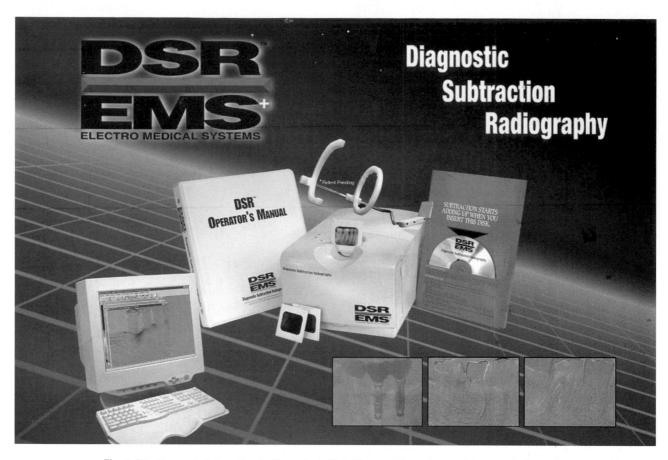

Fig. 5-25 Diagnostic Subtraction Radiography (DSR). (Courtesy Electro Medical Systems, Dallas, Tex.)

neutral, gray background. Recently, advances[47] in computer technology (Fig. 5-25) have incorporated built-in algorithms to correct for variations in exposure and projection geometry. These advances have also enabled colorization of density changes so that hard tissue gain is represented by one color and hard tissue loss is represented by another color.

Orascopy and Endoscopy

Orascopy[6] (Fig. 5-26, *A*), or endoscopy, is a new method for enhanced visualization in endodontics using a flexible, fiberoptic endoscope. These fiberoptic probes are available in two diameter sizes, 0.7 and 1.8 mm (Fig. 5-26, *B*); the probes provide a large depth of field and there is no need to refocus after the initial focus. Once the probe is applied, the operator views the conventional or surgical site from the magnified image displayed on the monitor. Endoscopic endodontics allow the clinician to have a nonfixed field of vision, and probes can be manipulated at various angles and distances from an object without loss of focus or image clarity. With orascopy, finite fracture lines (Fig. 5-26, *C*), accessory

canals, and apical tissues can be viewed. Evolving technology will likely enhance the precision and accuracy of the fiberoptic probes.

PREPARATION FOR ACCESS: TOOTH ISOLATION

Principles and Rationale

The use of the rubber dam is mandatory in root canal treatment.[14,16] Developed in the nineteenth century by S.C. Barnum, the rubber dam has evolved from a system that was designed to isolate teeth for placement of gold foil to one of sophistication for the ultimate protection of both patient and clinician.[54] The advantages[7,13,14,25,29] and absolute necessity of the rubber dam must always take precedence over convenience and expediency (a rationale often cited by clinicians who condemn its use). When properly placed the rubber dam facilitates treatment by isolating the tooth from obstacles (e.g., saliva, tongue) that can disrupt any procedure. Proper rubber dam placement can be done quickly and will enhance the entire procedure.

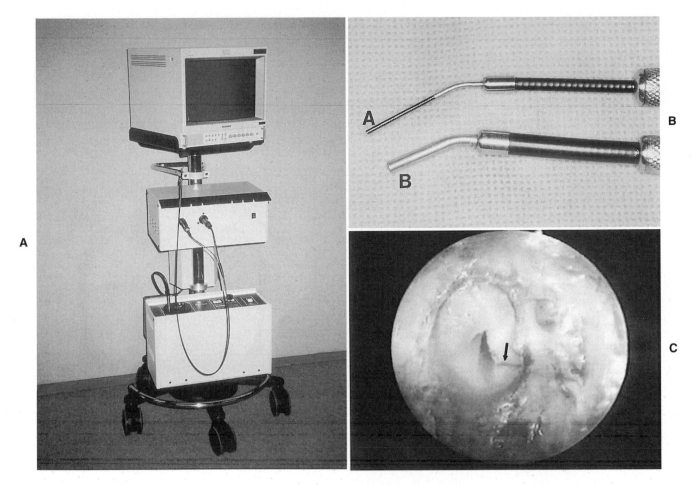

Fig. 5-26 **A**, Orascope. **B**, Flexible fiberoptic probes for orascopy (*A* is 0.7 mm in diameter, *B* is 1.8 mm in diameter). **C**, Endoscopic view of resected root showing fracture line (*arrow*). (*A*, Courtesy Sitca, Inc., Ann Arbor, MI. *C*, Courtesy Dr. Barnet B. Shulman.)

The rubber dam is used in endodontics because it ensures the following[5,14,25,32,54]:

1. Patient is protected from aspiration or from the swallowing of instruments, tooth debris, medicaments, and irrigating solutions.

2. Clinician is protected from litigation because of patient aspiration or swallowing of an endodontic file. *Routine placement of the rubber dam is considered the standard of care.*[15,16]

3. A surgically clean operating field is isolated from saliva, hemorrhage, and other tissue fluids. The dam reduces the risk of cross-contamination of the root canal system, and it provides an excellent barrier to the potential spread of infectious agents.[14,25] *It is a required component of any infection control program.**

4. Soft tissues are retracted and protected.

5. Visibility is improved. The rubber dam provides a dry field and reduces mirror fogging.

6. Efficiency is increased. The rubber dam minimizes patient conversation during treatment and the need for

frequent rinsing. It also relaxes the patient and saves time.

The dentist should be aware that in some situations, especially in teeth with crowns, access into the pulp system may be difficult without first orienting root structure to the adjacent teeth and periodontal tissues. Radiographically, the coronal pulp system is often obscured by the restoration and, as a result, the dentist may misdirect the bur during access. In these cases it may be necessary to locate the canal system before placing the dam. In doing so the dentist can visualize root topography, making it easier to orient the bur toward the long axis of the roots and prevent perforation. Once the root canal system is located, however, the rubber dam should be immediately placed.

Armamentarium

The mainstay of the rubber dam system is the dam itself. These autoclavable sheets of thin, flat latex come in various thicknesses (e.g., thin, medium, heavy, extraheavy, special heavy) and in two different sizes (5 × 5 inches and 6 × 6 inches). For endodontic purposes, the medium thickness is

---

*References 2,10-14,19,20,22,36,43,56

probably best because it tends to tear less easily, retracts soft tissues better than the thin type, and is easier to place than the heavier types. However, a thinner gauge may be desirable to decrease tension if retainer placement is questionable or if the retainer is resting on a band. The dam is also manufactured in a variety colors, ranging from light yellow to blue to green to gray. The darker-colored dams may afford better visual contrast, thus reducing eye strain. However, the lighter-colored dams, because of their translucency, have the advantage of naturally illuminating the operating field and allowing easier film placement underneath the dam. Depending upon individual preference and specific condi-

tions associated with a tooth, the dentist may find it necessary to vary the color and thickness of the rubber dam used. Glare and eyestrain can be reduced and contrast enhanced by routinely placing the dull side of the dam toward the operator.

For patients with latex allergies, a nonlatex rubber dam is available from Coltene/Whaledent (Fig. 5-27). This powder-

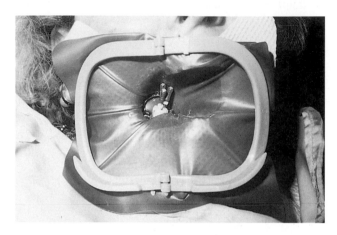

Fig. 5-29 Foldable plastic rubber dam frame (Plast-Frame) with hinge to allow for easy film-sensor placement. (Courtesy, Hager Worldwide, Odessa, FL.)

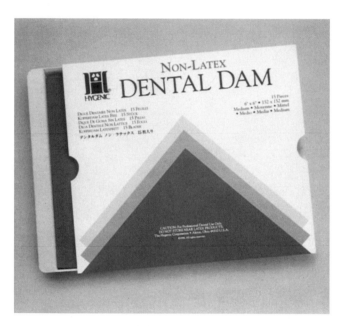

Fig. 5-27 Nonlatex, rubber dam is ideal for patients with known latex allergies. (Courtesy Coltene/Whaledent, Inc., Mahwah, N.J.)

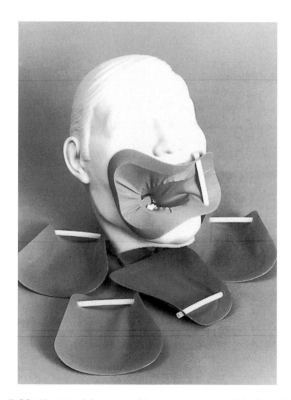

Fig. 5-30 The Handidam is a rubber dam system with built-in plastic frame. The disposable frame bends easily for film placement. (Courtesy Aseptico, Woodinville, WA.)

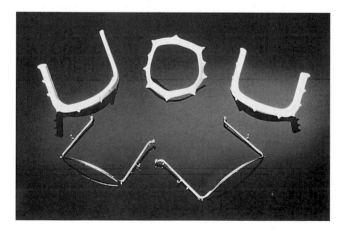

Fig. 5-28 Plastic radiolucent and metal rubber dam frames. *Top left, Young's frame. Top center, Nygaard-Ostby (N-O) frame.*

free, teal-colored, synthetic dam comes in one size (i.e., 6 × 6 inches) and in one thickness (i.e., medium gauge). It has a shelf life of 3 years but only one third the tensile strength of a latex dam. Other companies provide Nitrile rubber dams.

Another component of the rubber dam system is the rubber dam frame, which is designed to retract and stabilize the dam. Both metal and plastic frames are available, but plastic frames are recommended for endodontic procedures. They appear radiolucent, do not mask key areas on working films, and do not have to be removed before film placement. The Young's rubber dam frame (plastic type), the Star Visi frame, and the Nygaard-Ostby (N-O) frame are examples of radiolucent frames used in endodontics (Fig. 5-28). New to endodontics is a specially designed foldable plastic frame (Fig. 5-29), with a hinge to facilitate film or sensor placement without disengaging the entire frame. The disposable Handidam rubber dam system also provides a radiolucent plastic frame (Fig. 5-30). The Quickdam is another disposable single-isolation device with a flexible outer ring, eliminating the need for an additional frame (Fig. 5-31). Although metal frames (see Fig. 5-28) can be used, their radiopacity tends to block out the radiograph. If removed, this may result in destabilization of the dam and salivary contamination of the canal system, negating the "sterile" environment that was previously attained.

Rubber dam clamps or retainers anchor the dam to the tooth requiring treatment or, in cases of multiple-tooth isolation, to the most posterior tooth. They also aid in soft tissue retraction. These clamps are made of stainless steel, and each consists of a bow and two jaws. Regardless of the type of jaw configuration, the prongs of the jaws should engage at least four points on the tooth. This clamp-to-tooth relationship sta-

bilizes the retainer and prevents any rocking which, in itself, can be injurious to both hard and soft tissues.[33,40]

Clamps are available from a variety of manufacturers and are specifically designed for all classes of teeth with a variety of anatomic configurations. For most uncomplicated endodontic isolations, the dentist's basic armamentarium should consist of winged clamps, a butterfly type clamp for anterior teeth, a universal premolar clamp, a mandibular molar clamp, and a maxillary molar clamp (Fig. 5-32). The wings, which are extensions of the jaws, not only provide for additional soft tissue retraction but also facilitate placement of the rubber dam, frame, and retainer as a single unit (see the section on methods of rubber dam placement, which follows).

Other retainers are designed for specific clinical situations in which clamp placement may be difficult. For example, when minimal coronal tooth structure remains, a clamp with apically inclined jaws may be used to engage tooth structure at or below the level of the free gingival margin (Fig. 5-33). Retainers with serrated jaws, known as Tiger clamps, also may increase stabilization of broken-down teeth. Another type of retainer, the S-G (Silker-Glickman) clamp, should also be included in the dentist's armamentarium (Fig. 5-34). Its anterior extension allows for retraction of dam around a severely broken-down tooth, while the clamp itself is placed on a tooth proximal to the one being treated (Fig. 5-35).

The remaining components of the rubber dam system include the rubber dam punch and the rubber dam forceps. The punch has a series of holes on a rotating disc from which the dentist can select according to the size of tooth or teeth to be isolated. The forceps holds and carries the retainer during placement and removal.

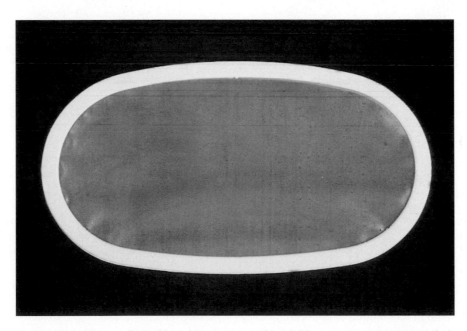

Fig. 5-31 The Quickdam is a disposable isolation system with a pliable outer ring. (Courtesy Ivoclar/Vivadent, Amherst, NY.)

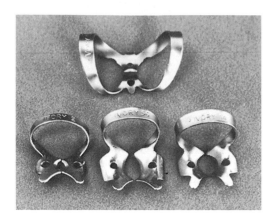

Fig. 5-32 Basic set of ivory-winged rubber dam clamps: *top*, no. 9 butterfly clamp for anterior teeth; *bottom* (from left), no. 2 premolar clamp, no. 56 mandibular molar clamp, and no. 14 maxillary molar clamp. (Courtesy Heraeus Kulzer, Inc., Dentist Products Division, South Bend, IN.)

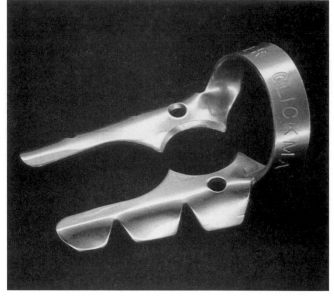

Fig. 5-34 The S-G clamp for isolation of severely broken-down teeth. (Courtesy The Smile Center, Deerwood, MN.)

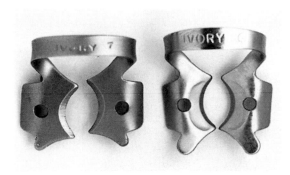

Fig. 5-33 Mandibular molar clamps. Clamp on right has jaws inclined apically to engage tooth with minimal tooth structure remaining. (Courtesy Heraeus Kulzer, Inc., Dentist Products Division, South Bend, IN.)

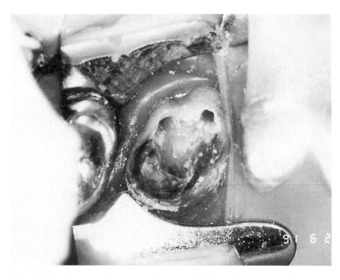

Fig. 5-35 The S-G clamp is placed on the maxillary second molar to isolate severely broken-down maxillary first molar.

Methods of Rubber Dam Placement

As mentioned earlier, an expedient method of dam placement is to position the bow of the clamp through the hole in the dam and place the rubber over the wings of the clamp (a winged clamp is required).[51] The forceps stretch the clamp to maintain the position of the clamp in the dam, and the dam is attached to the plastic frame, allowing for the placement of the dam, clamp, and frame in one motion (Fig. 5-36). Once the clamp is secured on the tooth, the dam is teased under the wings of the clamp with a plastic instrument.

Another method is to place the clamp, usually wingless, on the tooth and then stretch the dam over the clamped tooth (Fig. 5-37).[25,54] This method offers the advantage of enabling the clinician to see exactly where the jaws of the clamp engage the tooth, thus avoiding possible impingement on the gingival tissues. Gentle finger pressure on the buccal and lingual apron of the clamp before the dam is placed can be used to test how securely the clamp fits. Variations of this method include placing the clamp and dam first, followed by the frame, or placing the rubber dam first, followed by the clamp and then the frame.[54]

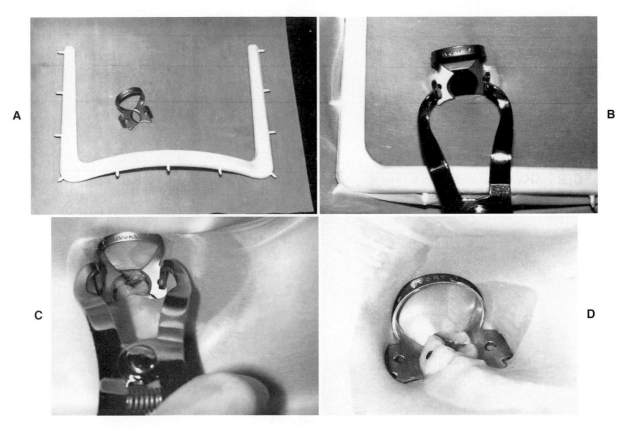

Fig. 5-36 **A**, Rubber dam, clamp, and frame. **B**, Clamp positioned in the dam with frame attached and held in position with rubber dam forceps. **C**, Dam, clamp, and frame carried to mouth as one unit and placed over the tooth. **D**, Clamp in place with four-point contact and rubber tucked under the wings.

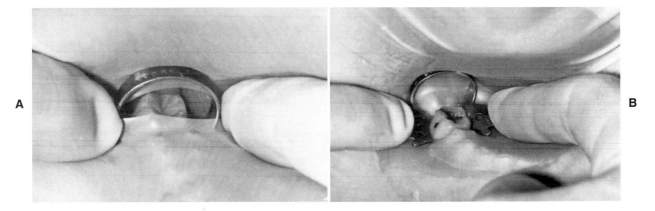

Fig. 5-37 **A**, After the clamp is placed, the dam is attached to the frame and gently stretched over the clamped tooth with the index finger of each hand. **B**, Clamp is tested for a secure fit with gentle finger pressure (alternately) on the buccal and lingual aspects of the clamp apron.

A third method, the split-dam technique, may be used to isolate anterior teeth without using a rubber dam clamp. Not only is this technique useful when there is insufficient crown structure, as in the case of horizontal fractures, but it also prevents the possibility of the jaws of the clamp chipping the margins of teeth restored with porcelain crowns or laminates. Studies[33,40] on the effects of retainers on porcelain-fused-to-metal restorations and tooth structure itself have demonstrated that there can be significant damage to cervical porcelain, as well as to dentin and cementum, even when the clamp is properly stabilized. Thus for teeth with porcelain restorations, ligation with dental floss is recommended as an alternate method to retract the dam and tissues, or the adjacent tooth can be clamped.

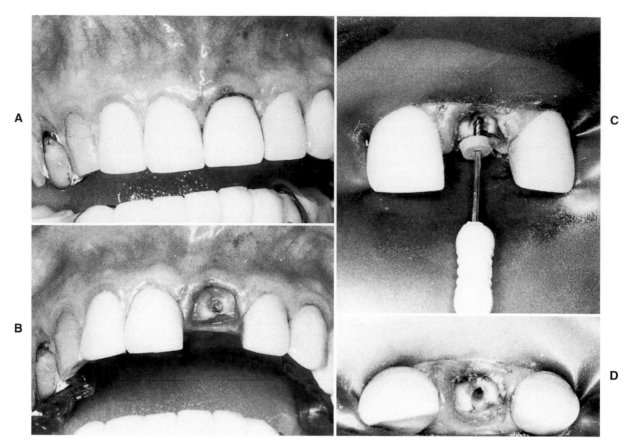

Fig. 5-38 Split-dam technique. **A,** Maxillary central incisor with a horizontal fracture at the cervical area. **B,** Appearance of the coronal fragment after removal. **C,** Cotton roll in place in the mucobuccal fold, and rubber dam stretched over the two adjacent teeth. **D,** Appearance after pulp extirpation.

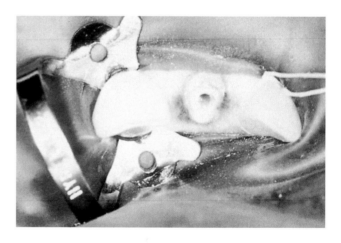

Fig. 5-39 Split-dam technique. Premolar clamp on maxillary central incisor along with ligation on the maxillary canine prevents dam slippage and aids in dam retraction during endodontic treatment on broken-down maxillary lateral incisor. (Courtesy Dr. James L. Gutmann.)

In the split-dam method, two overlapping holes are punched in the dam. A cotton roll is placed under the lip in the mucobuccal fold over the tooth to be treated. The rubber dam is stretched over the tooth to be treated and over one adjacent tooth on each side. The edge of the dam is carefully teased through the contacts on the distal sides of the two adjacent teeth. Dental floss helps carry the dam down around the gingiva. The tension produced by the stretched dam, aided by the rubber dam frame, secures the dam in place. The tight fit and the cotton roll help produce a relatively dry field (Fig. 5-38). If the dam has a tendency to slip, a premolar clamp may be used on a tooth distal to the three isolated teeth or even on an adjacent tooth (Fig. 5-39). The clamp is placed over the rubber dam, which then acts as a cushion against the jaws of the clamp.

Aids in Rubber Dam Placement

Punching and Positioning of Holes   The rubber dam may be divided into four equal quadrants, and the proper place for the hole is estimated according to which tooth is undergoing treatment. The more distal the tooth, the closer to the center of the dam the hole is placed. This method becomes easier as the clinician gains experience. The hole must be punched cleanly, without tags or tears. If the dam is torn, it may leak or permit continued tearing when stretched over the clamp and tooth.

Orientation of the Dam and Bunching   The rubber dam must be attached to the frame with enough tension to retract soft tissues and prevent bunching, without tearing the dam or displacing the clamp. The rubber dam should completely cover the patient's mouth without infringing on the patient's nose or eyes. To prevent bunching of the dam in the occlusal embrasure, only the edge of the interseptal portion of the dam is teased between the teeth. Dental floss is then used to carry the dam through the contacts. These contacts should always be tested with dental floss before the dam is placed. A plastic instrument is used to invert the edge of the dam around the tooth to provide a seal.

Problem-Solving in Tooth Isolation

Leakage   The best way to prevent seepage through the rubber dam is meticulous placement of the entire system. Proper selection and placement of the clamp, sharply punched, correctly positioned holes, use of a dam of adequate thickness, and inversion of the dam around the tooth all help reduce leakage through the dam and into the root canal system.[5,32,39,54] Nevertheless, clinical situations in which small tears, holes, or continuous minor leaks may occur. These often can be patched or blocked with Cavit, OraSeal Caulking, rubber base adhesive,[9] "liquid" rubber dam, or periodontal packing. If leakage continues, the dam should be replaced with a new one.

Because salivary secretions can seep through even a well-placed rubber dam, persons who salivate excessively may require premedication to reduce saliva flow to a manageable level. Failure to control salivation may result in salivary contamination of the canal system and pooling of saliva beneath the dam, as well as drooling and possible choking. Such occurrences can disrupt treatment and should be prevented. Excessive saliva flow can be reduced with an anticholinergic drug, such as atropine sulfate, propantheline bromide (Pro-Banthine), methantheline (Banthine), or glycopyrrolate (Robinul).[30] Therapeutic doses of atropine sulfate for adults range from 0.3 to 1 mg PO, 1 to 2 hours before the procedure. The synthetic anticholinergic drug propantheline bromide (Pro-Banthine) reportedly has fewer side effects than Banthine.[30] The usual adult dose of Pro-Banthine for an adult is 7.5 to 15 mg, taken orally 30 to 45 minutes before the appointment. Because they can cause undesirable autonomic effects, especially through various drug interactions, the anticholinergics should be used only in specific cases and only as a last resort.

Unusual Tooth Shapes or Positions that Cause Inadequate Clamp Placement   Some teeth do not conform to the variety of clamps available. These include partially erupted teeth, teeth prepared for crowns, and teeth fractured or broken down to the extent that their margins are subgingival. To handle these cases, rubber dam retainers may be customized by modifying the jaws to adapt to a particular tooth (Fig. 5-40).[55] In partially erupted teeth or cone-shaped teeth, such as those prepared for full coverage, one technique[53] is to place spots of self-curing resin on the cervical surface of the tooth. These resin beads act as a scaffold for the retainer during treatment. Another method[29] is to place small acid-etched composite lips on the teeth; these resin lips serve as artificial undercuts and remain on the teeth between appointments. When the root canal treatment is complete, the resin beads are easily removed. In multiple-treatment cases involving misshapen teeth, a customized acrylic retainer[51] can be used in conjunction with a dam to isolate the operating field.

Loss of Tooth Structure   If insufficient tooth structure prevents the placement of a clamp, the clinician must first determine whether the tooth is periodontally sound and restorable. Meticulous and thorough treatment planning often can prevent embarrassing situations for both the doctor and patient. One common example is the case in which the endodontic treatment is completed before restorability is determined; it is then discovered that the tooth cannot be restored.

Once a tooth is deemed restorable but the margin of sound tooth structure is subgingival, a number of methods should be considered. As mentioned earlier, less invasive methods,

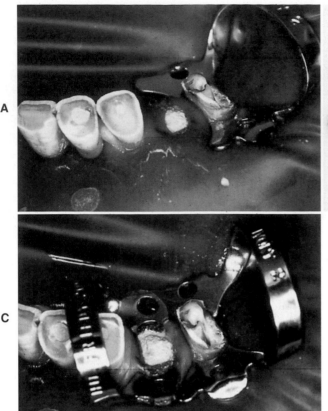

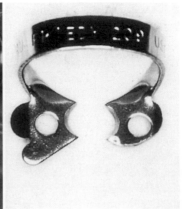

Fig. 5-40 **A**, Isolation rendered difficult by multiple, severely broken-down mandibular premolars. **B**, Modified premolar rubber dam clamp. **C**, Modified clamp in place on first premolar to accommodate wings of distal clamp. (Courtesy Dr. Robert Roda.)

such as using a clamp with prongs inclined apically or using an S-G clamp, should be attempted first (see Fig. 5-34). If neither of these techniques effectively isolates the tooth, the dentist may consider the clamping of the attached gingiva and alveolar process. In this situation it is imperative that profound soft tissue anesthesia exists before clamp placement. Although the procedure may cause some minor postoperative discomfort, the periodontal tissues recover quickly with minimal postoperative care.

Restorative Procedures   If none of the techniques mentioned above are desirable, a variety of restorative methods may be considered to build up the tooth so that a retainer can be placed properly.[38,39,54] A preformed copper band, a temporary crown, or an orthodontic band (Figs. 5-41 and 5-42) may be cemented over the remaining natural crown. This band or crown not only enables the clamp to be retained successfully, it also serve as a seal for the retention of intracanal medicaments and the temporary filling between appointments. These temporary bands or crowns have several disadvantages. One of their main problems is their inability to provide a superior seal. Another concern is that particles of these soft metals or cement can block canal systems during access opening and instrumentation. Third, these temporary crowns and bands, if they become displaced

or are not properly contoured, can cause periodontal inflammation.

Occasionally so little tooth structure remains that even band or crown placement is not possible. In these cases it becomes necessary to replace the missing tooth structure to facilitate placement of the rubber dam clamp and prevent leakage into the pulp cavity during the course of treatment.[38,39,54] Replacement of missing tooth structure can be accomplished by means of pin-retained amalgam buildups, composites, glass ionomer cements such as Ketac-Silver, Fuji II (Fig. 5-43), or Photac-Fil, or dentin-bonding systems such as Scotchbond 2, Tenure Bond, Gluma, Optibond, PermaQuik (Fig. 5-44), or C&B Metabond.[54] Although these newer dentin-bonding systems form a very strong immediate bond and are generally simple to use, any restorative method for building up a broken-down tooth is time consuming, can impede endodontic procedures, and may duplicate restorative treatment. Many restorations that have been hollowed out by access cavities are weakened and require redoing.

Canal Projection   The canal projection technique, using the Projector Endodontic Instrument Guidance System (CJM Engineering, Santa Barbara, CA), provides preendodontic reconstruction of debilitated coronal and radicular

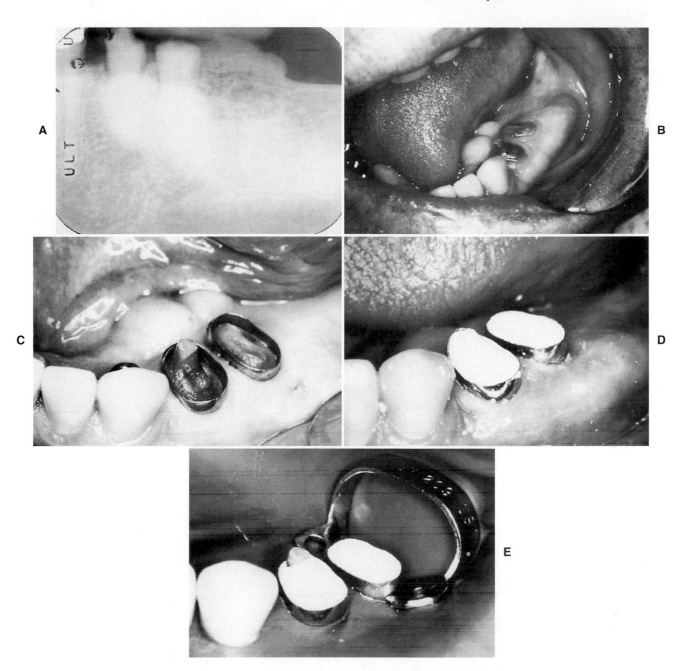

Fig. 5-41 **A**, Preoperative radiograph of mandibular premolar region depicts limited supracrestal tooth structure. **B**, Bony exostoses and minimal tooth structure make it a difficult case for tooth isolation. **C**, Fitted orthodontic bands on mandibular premolars. **D**, Orthodontic bands cemented in place with IRM (i.e., reinforced zinc oxide-eugenol cement). **E**, Effective isolation with rubber dam clamp placed on distal tooth. (Courtesy Dr. Robert Roda.)

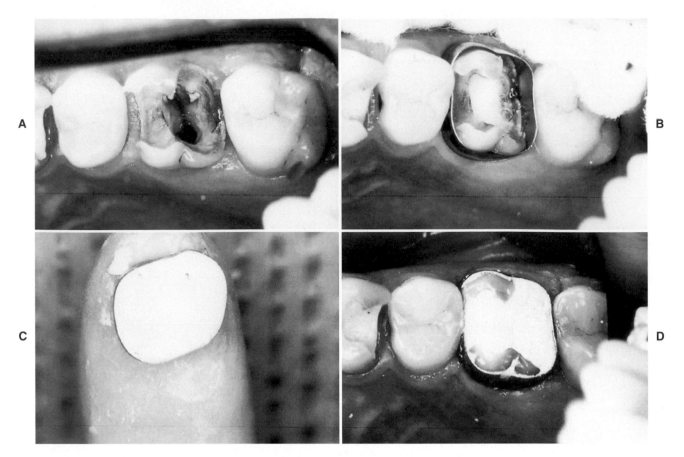

Fig. 5-42 **A**, Broken-down maxillary molar after removal of restoration, post, and caries. **B**, Fitted orthodontic band; cotton in access opening to protect orifices. **C**, IRM loaded into band before cementation. **D**, Completed temporary restoration before rubber dam placement. (Courtesy Dr. Robert Roda.)

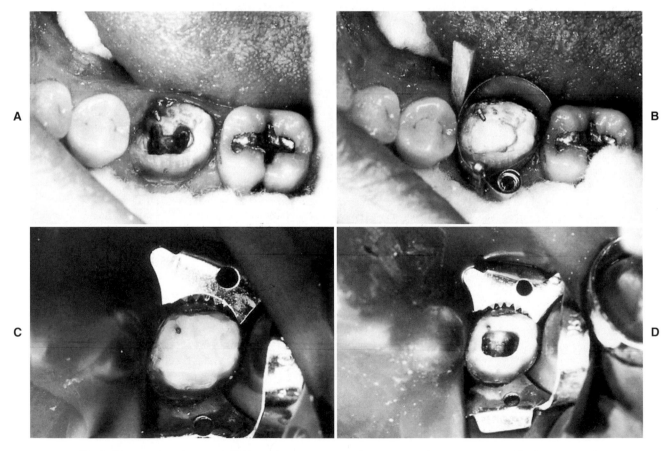

Fig. 5-43 **A**, Broken-down mandibular molar after crown and caries removal; preexisting pin will aid retention of restorative material. **B**, Isolation with wedged Automatrix. **C**, Completed temporary restoration using glass ionomer cement (Fuji II). **D**, Access through completed restoration after rubber dam placement. (Courtesy Dr. Robert Roda.)

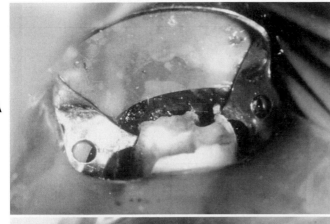

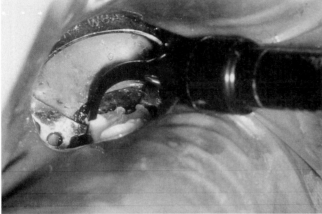

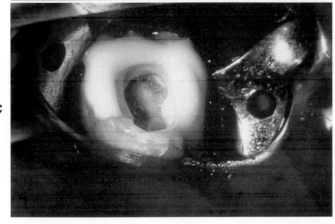

A

B

C

Fig. 5-44 **A,** Poor isolation due to a severely broken-down tooth. Jaws of the retainer are barely engaging the tooth. **B,** The dentin is etched and bonded using PermaQuik Primer and bonding resin. "Donut" shaped layers of Ultrablend, a light-activated glass ionomer, are added to the bonded resin and incrementally cured. **C,** "Donut" buildup can be accessed for endodontic treatment and can later serve as a matrix for a resin core once the endodontic treatment is completed. (Courtesy Ultradent Products, South Jordan, UT.)

tooth structure (Fig. 5-45, *A*) while preserving individualized access to the canals. The technique is as follows:

1. After gaining access, all orifices are dimpled to the depth of a no. 2, slow-speed, round bur.
2. An appropriate matrix system is applied, and all bondable surfaces are etched and primed with a moist-field primer.
3. Projectors (i.e., tapered plastic sleeves available in various diameters) are placed onto endodontic files, the files are inserted into the canals, and the Projectors are slid apically until they seat precisely into the dimples (Fig. 5-45, *B*).
4. Bonding agent is then applied to the primed surfaces and an autopolymerizing composite buildup material is injected from the chamber floor to the cavosurface of the access cavity.
5. After polymerization, the files are removed, leaving the Projector tops embedded in the resin.
6. A bull-nosed diamond is then used to contour the resin and flatten the occlusal surface, along with the embedded Projectors. Composite debris is prevented from collecting in the projected canals by leaving the Projectors embedded in the resin during this part of the procedure.
7. Engaging a no. 60 Hedstrom file in the walls of the lumen and withdrawing it removes the Projectors.
8. The external surfaces of the Projectors are treated with a releasing agent, enabling easy removal from all types of buildup material. Depending on how the Projectors are allowed to emerge from the chamber floor, the projected orifices will lie in various configurations on the occlusal surface. This procedure creates reliable endodontic reference points (Fig. 5-45, *C* and *D*)
9. After cleaning, shaping, and obturation, the projected portions of the canals are filled by injecting composite directly over gutta-percha from the level of the chamber floor to the cavosurface, creating a unique radiographic appearance (Fig. 5-45, *E* and *F*).

Periodontal Procedures   As a result of excessive crown destruction or incomplete eruption, the presence of gingival tissue may preclude the use of a clamp without severe gingival impingement. Various techniques of gingivectomy (Fig. 5-46) or electrosurgery have been suggested for cases in which the remaining tooth structure still lies above the crestal bone. With an inadequate zone of attached gingiva, osseous defects, or a poor anatomic form, an apically positioned flap with a reverse bevel incision is the technique of choice to "lengthen" the crown.[38,39]

Electrosurgery and the conventional gingivectomy are crown-lengthening procedures for teeth that have sufficient attached gingiva and no infrabony involvement.[38,39] The electrosurgery method offers the advantage of leaving a virtually bloodless site for immediate rubber dam placement. Electrosurgery units have become highly sophisticated and are capable of providing both cutting and coagulating currents that, when used properly, will not cause cellular coagulation. The

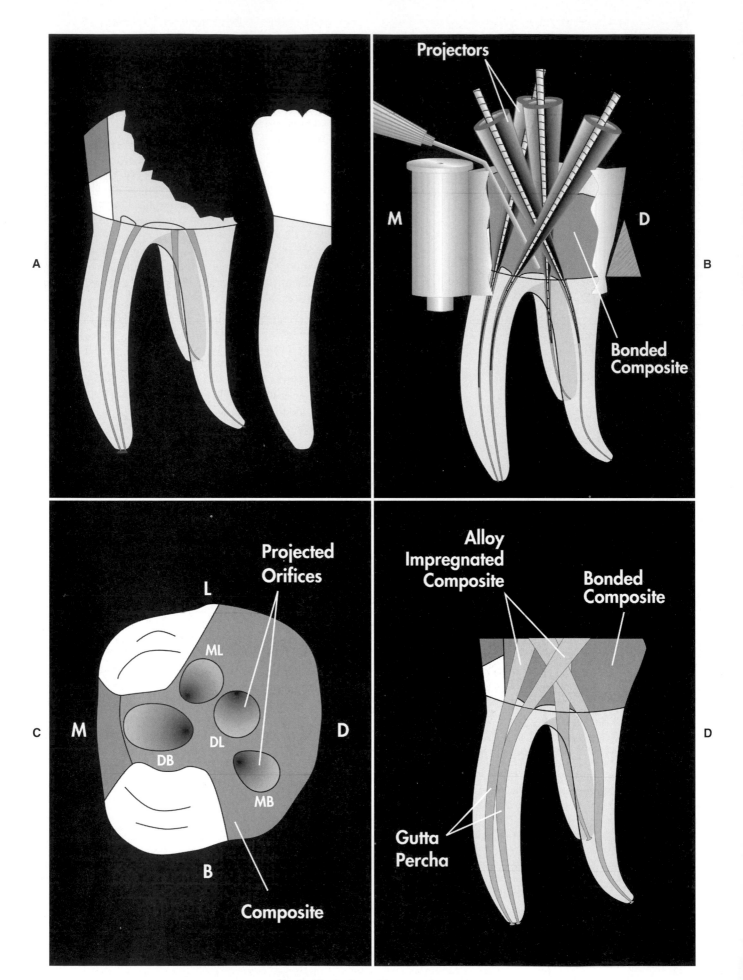

Fig. 5-45. For legend see opposite page.

wide variety of sizes and shapes of surgical electrodes enables the clinician to reach areas inaccessible to the scalpel. Furthermore, electrosurgery facilitates the removal of unwanted tissue in such a manner as to recreate normal gingival architecture. This feature, combined with controlled hemostasis, makes the instrument extremely useful in the preparation of some teeth for placement of the rubber dam clamp.

The main drawback of electrosurgery is the potential for damage to the adjacent tissues; if the electrode contacts bone, significant destruction of bone can occur. As a result this technique is not recommended when the distance between the crestal level of bone and the remaining tooth structure is minimal. Compared to electrosurgery, conventional gingivectomy presents the major problem of hemorrhage after the procedure; this forces delay of endodontic treatment until tissues have healed.

The apically positioned flap[38,39] is a crown-lengthening technique for teeth with inadequate attached gingiva, infrabony pockets, or remaining tooth structure below the level of crestal bone. With this technique as well, endodontic treatment should be delayed until sufficient healing has taken place.

Orthodontic Procedures   The most common indication for orthodontic extrusion is a fracture of the anterior tooth margin below the crestal bone.[38,39] The clinician should be aware that, because bone and soft tissue attachments follow the tooth during extrusion, crown-lengthening procedures after extrusion are often necessary to achieve the desired clinical crown length and restore the biologic and esthetic tissue relationships. Ultimately, the purpose of orthodontic extrusion is to erupt the tooth to provide 2 to 3 mm of root length above crestal bone level.

CONCLUSION

Success in endodontic therapy is predicated on a host of factors, many of which are controllable before the clinician ever initiates treatment. Proper and thorough preparation of both patient and tooth for endodontic treatment should lay the groundwork for a relatively trouble-free experience that will increase the chances for the ultimate success of the entire treatment.

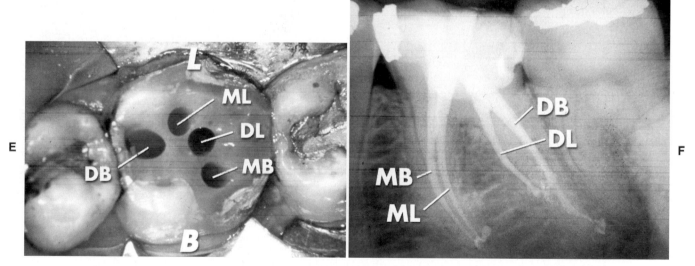

Fig. 5-45 A, Buccal view of severely broken-down mandibular molar with unusual second distal root following caries removal; isolation problems lead to severe leakage. **B,** Appropriate matrix system is applied, and all bondable surfaces are etched and primed. Files are selected that fit well into the body of each canal. **C,** Upon polymerization, the files are removed, leaving the Projectors embedded in the composite build-up. By projecting the canals, the risk of contamination has been eliminated. **D,** Cleaning, shaping, and obturation may now proceed as usual. **E,** Depending on how the operator elects to allow the Projectors to emerge from the chamber floor, the distribution of the projected canals on the reconstructed occlusal surface can have various configurations. In this example, the DB orifice is projected toward the mesial marginal ridge, the DL to the center of the occlusal surface, and the mesial canals towards the distal on either side of the projected DL orifice. **F,** According to the clinical circumstance, the bonded projection material may be removed following endodontic treatment in favor of an alternative build-up material, or it may remain as a block-out or build-up material in anticipation of a permanent coronal restoration. (Courtesy Dr. C. John Munce, CJM Engineering, Santa Barbara, CA.)

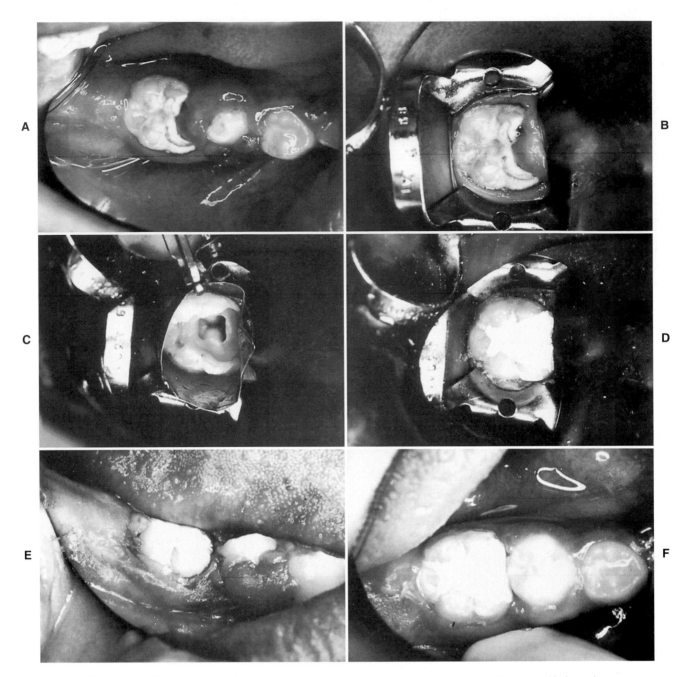

Fig. 5-46 **A**, Gingival hypertrophy on mandibular molar and erupting premolar of young patient; mandibular molar requires root canal treatment. **B**, Rubber dam clamp impinging on gingival tissues; tissue removed with scalpel. **C**, Automatrix placed immediately after tissue removal; bleeding was minimal. **D**, Placement of IRM temporary restoration after pulpectomy. **E**, Postoperative facial view immediately after gingivectomy; note homeostasis. **F**, Six-week postoperative occlusal view exhibits fully exposed mandibular molar and recently erupted premolar. (Courtesy Dr. Robert Roda.)

References

1. American Association of Endodontists: *Endodontics: your guide to endodontic treatment*, Chicago, 1996, The Association.
2. American Dental Association: *OSHA: What you must know*, Chicago, 1992, The Association.
3. American Dental Association: *Statement regarding dental handpieces*, Chicago, 1992, The Association.
4. American Dental Association and American Academy of Orthopaedic Surgeons: Advisory statement: antibiotic prophylaxis for dental patients with total joint replacements, *J Am Dent Assoc* 128:1004, 1997.
5. Antrim DD: Endodontics and the rubber dam: a review of techniques, *J Acad Gen Dent* 31:294, 1983.
6. Bahcall JK, DiFiore PM, Poulakidas TK: An endoscopic technique for endodontic surgery, *J Endod* 25:132, 1999.
7. Baumgartner JC, Heggers JP, Harrison JW: The incidence of bacteremias related to endodontic procedures. I. Nonsurgical endodontics, *J Endod* 2:135, 1976.
8. Bender IB, Seltzer S, Yermish, M: The incidence of bacteremia in patients with rheumatic heart disease, *J Oral Surg* 13:353, 1960.
9. Bramwell JD, Hicks ML: Solving isolation problems with rubber base adhesive, *J Endod* 12:363, 1986.
10. Centers for Disease Control: *Guidelines for preventing the transmission of mycobacterium tuberculosis in health care facilities*, Fed. Reg. 59:54242-54303, 1994, Washington DC.
11. Centers for Disease Control: Recommended infection control practices for dentistry, *MMWR Morb* 35:237, 1986.
12. Centers for Disease Control: Recommendations for prevention of HIV transmission in health care settings, *MMWR Morb* 36 (suppl 2S):1, 1987.
13. Centers for Disease Control: Recommendations for preventing transmission of human immunodeficiency virus and hepatitis B virus to patients during exposure-prone invasive procedures, *MMWR Morb* 40:1, 1991.
14. Cochran MA, Miller CH, Sheldrake MA: The efficacy of the rubber dam as a barrier to the spread of microorganisms during dental treatment, *J Am Dent Assoc* 119:141, 1989.
15. Cohen S: Endodontics and litigation: an American perspective, *Int Dent J* 39:13, 1989.
16. Cohen S, Schwartz SF: Endodontic complications and the law, *J Endod* 13:191, 1987.
17. Cohn SA: *Endodontic radiography: principles and clinical techniques*, Gilberts, IL, 1988, Dunvale Corp.
18. Corah NL, Gale EN, Illig SJ: Assessment of a dental anxiety scale, *J Am Dent Assoc* 97:816, 1978.
19. Cottone JA, Terezhalmy GT, Molinari JA: *Practical infection control in dentistry*, ed 2, Baltimore, 1996, Williams and Wilkins.
20. Council on Dental Materials, Instruments, and Equipment; Council on Dental Practice; and Council on Dental Therapeutics: Infection control recommendations for the dental office and the dental laboratory, *J Am Dent Assoc* 116:241, 1988.
21. Dajani AS et al: Prevention of bacterial endocarditis: recommendations by the American Heart Association, *J Am Med Assoc* 277:1794, 1997.
22. Department of Labor, Occupational Safety and Health Administration: *Occupational exposure to bloodborne pathogens, final rule*, Fed. Reg. 56(235):64004, Washington, DC, 1991.
23. Donnelly JC, Hartwell GR, Johnson WB: Clinical evaluation of Ektaspeed x-ray film for use in endodontics, *J Endod* 11:90, 1985.
24. Farman AG, Mendel RW, von Fraunhofer JA: Ultraspeed versus Ektaspeed x-ray film: endodontists' perceptions, *J Endod* 14:615, 1988.
25. Forrest W, Perez RS: The rubber dam as a surgical drape: protection against AIDS and hepatitis, *J Acad Gen Dent* 37:236, 1989.
26. Forsberg J: Radiographic reproduction of endodontic "working length" comparing the paralleling and bisecting-angle techniques, *J Oral Surg* 64:353, 1987.
27. White SC, Pharoah MJ: *Oral radiology: principles and interpretation*, ed 4, St Louis, 1999, Mosby.
28. Goerig AC, Neaverth EJ: A simplified look at the buccal object rule in endodontics, *J Endod* 13:570, 1987.
29. Greene RR, Sikora FA, House JE: Rubber dam application to crownless and cone-shaped teeth, *J Endod* 10:82, 1984.
30. Holroyd SV, Wynn RL, Requa-Clark B: *Clinical pharmacology in dental practice*, ed 4, St Louis, 1988, Mosby.
31. Jackson DJ, Moore PA, Hargreaves KM: Preoperative nonsteroidal anti-inflammatory medication for the prevention of postoperative dental pain, *J Am Dent Assoc* 119:641, 1989.
32. Janus CE: The rubber dam reviewed, *Compend Contin Educ Dent* 5:155, 1984.
33. Jeffrey IWM, Woolford MJ: An investigation of possible iatrogenic damage caused by metal rubber dam clamps, *Int Endod J* 22:85, 1989.
34. Kantor ML et al: Efficacy of dental radiographic practices: options for image receptors, examination selection, and patient selection, *J Am Dent Assoc* 119:259, 1989.
35. Kelly WH: Radiographic asepsis in endodontic practice, *J Acad Gen Dent* 37:302, 1989.
36. Kolstad RA: *Biohazard control in dentistry*, Dallas, TX, 1993, Baylor College of Dentistry Press.
37. Little JW, Falace DA, Miller CS, Rhodus NL: *Dental management of the medically compromised patient*, ed 5, St Louis, 1997, Mosby.
38. Lovdahl PE, Gutmann JL: Periodontal and restorative considerations prior to endodontic therapy, *J Acad Gen Dent* 28:38, 1980.
39. Lovdahl PE, Wade CK: Problems in tooth isolation and periodontal support for the endodontically compromised tooth. In Gutmann JL et al, editors: *Problem-solving in endodontics: prevention, identification, and management*, ed 3, St Louis, 1997, Mosby.
40. Madison S, Jordan RD, Krell KV: The effects of rubber dam retainers on porcelain-fused-to-metal restorations, *J Endod* 12:183, 1986.
41. Messing JJ, Stock CJR: *Color atlas of endodontics*, St Louis, 1988, Mosby.
42. Miles DA et al: *Radiographic imaging for dental auxiliaries*, ed 3, Philadelphia, 1999, WB Saunders Co.
43. Miller CH: Infection control, *Dent Clin North Am* 40:437, 1996.

44. Montgomery EH, Kroeger DC: Principles of anti-infective therapy, *Dent Clin North Am* 28:423, 1984.

45. Mouyen F et al: Presentation and physical evaluation of Radiovisiography, *J Oral Surg* 68:238, 1989.

46. Pollack BR, editor: *Handbook of dental jurisprudence and risk management*, Littleton, MA, 1987, PSG Publishing Co.

47. Reddy MS, Jeffcoat MK: Digital subtraction radiography, *Dent Clin North Am* 37:553, 1993.

48. Requa-Clark B, Holroyd SV: Antiinfective agents. In Holroyd SV, Wynn RL, Requa-Clark B, editors: *Clinical pharmacology in dental practice*, ed 4, St Louis, 1988, Mosby.

49. Richards AG: The buccal object rule, *Dent Radiogr Photogr* 53:37, 1980.

50. Schwartz SF, Foster JK: Roentgenographic interpretation of experimentally produced boney lesions. I. *J Oral Surg* 32:606, 1971.

51. Teplitsky PE: Custom acrylic retainer for endodontic isolation, *J Endod* 14:150, 1988.

52. Torabinejad M et al: Absorbed radiation by various tissues during simulated endodontic radiography, *J Endod* 15:249, 1989.

53. Wakabayashi H et al: A clinical technique for the retention of a rubber dam clamp, *J Endod* 12:422, 1986.

54. Walton RE, Torabinejad M: *Principles and practice of endodontics*, ed 3, Philadelphia, WB Saunders Co (in press).

55. Weisman M: A modification of the no. 3 rubber dam clamp, *J Endod* 9:30, 1983.

56. Wood PR: *Practical cross infection control in dentistry,* St Louis, 1992, Mosby.

Chapter 6

Armamentarium and Sterilization

Robert E. Averbach, Donald J. Kleier

Chapter Outline

ARMAMENTARIUM

Endodontic treatment has become an increasing part of comprehensive patient care in many general dental practices. A survey by the ADA indicated that recent graduates spend approximately 10% of their workweek providing endodontic treatment to patients.[1] A survey conducted by the Compendium of Continuing Education in Dentistry cited endodontics as one of the top areas of interest to its readership. The rapidly expanding market for new endodontic products and techniques has produced an extensive and, at times, bewildering array of approaches to root canal treatment. Although this chapter highlights many of these new trends, it is important for the clinician to maintain a sound scientific perspective based on biologic principles when considering new approaches. Critical thinking, based on independent long-term scientific studies, remains the bedrock of making sound choices. Aggressive commercial marketing of products or techniques should not replace evidence-based scientific validation and clinical experience.

Light and Magnification

The use of high-quality magnification in dentistry is becoming more common; users are convinced that magnification improves both the quality and speed of treatment.[7] Adding a headlight to the system of surgical telescopes significantly enhances both depth of field and magnified resolution, greatly increasing visual acuity. The headlight provides line-of-sight illumination, which is shadowless and avoids multiple adjustments to the traditional overhead dental operating light. The combination of light and magnification is especially useful in endodontics, because the clinician must search for small calcified root canals in hard-to-access areas following the completion of endodontic access.

Once they have tried working with additional light and magnification, it is not uncommon to hear clinicians remark, "How did I ever practice dentistry without these?" Although operating using magnification requires a brief learning period, most clinicians comment that returning to unaided vision is a distinct handicap. The most popular surgical telescopes provide magnification in the 2.0× to 3.5× range, with average working distances of 14 to 16 inches. Examples of some of the more popular light and magnification systems can be found in Figs. 6-1 and 6-2.

The use of the surgical operating microscope in endodontics is the next logical extension of the operating theory of enhanced light and magnification. Although initially introduced to aid a variety of endodontic surgical procedures, the operating microscope is being used more frequently for problematic, nonsurgical endodontic approaches (e.g., removal of posts, fracture diagnosis, endodontic retreatment). Surgical operating microscopes offer a wide range of magnification, usually from 4× to 25×. (See Chapter 19 for detailed information about surgical operating microscopes.) A recent addition to the field of visualization is a fiber-optic endoscope designed for intraoral use. The OraScope uses a fiber-

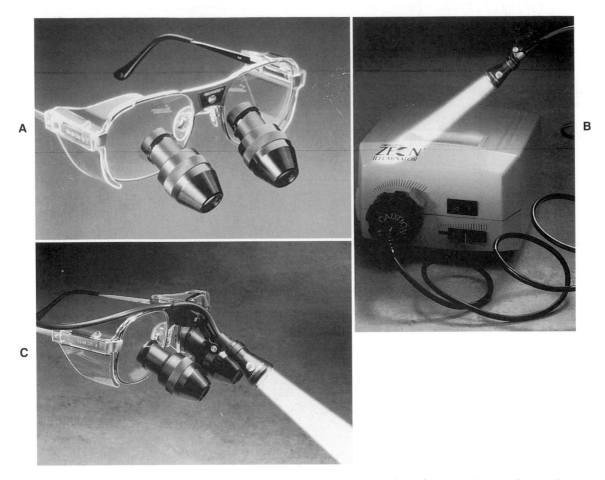

Fig. 6-1 **A**, Surgical telescopes. **B**, Headlight system. **C,** Headlight clipped to telescopes. (Courtesy Orascoptic Research Inc., Madison, Wis.)

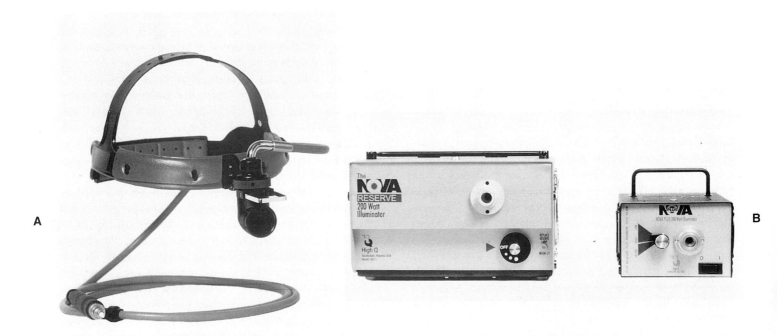

Fig. 6-2 **A**, Headband style headlight. **B**, Fiber-optic light source. (Courtesy High Q Systems, Scottsdale, Ariz.)

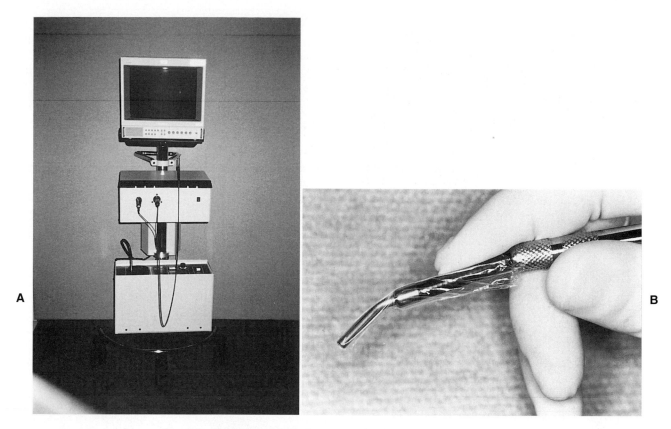

Fig. 6-3 **A**, Orascope unit. **B**, Orascope probe. (Courtesy Dr. James Bahcall.)

optic probe, xenon light source, and a medical-grade video monitor to provide a magnified image of the operating field (Fig. 6-3).

Radiographs

Obtaining a high-quality preoperative radiograph is essential before initiating endodontic treatment. As described in Chapter 5, the paralleling technique, using special film holders, produces radiographs with minimal image distortion. Tooth length measurements and diagnostic information from the radiograph tend to be more accurate when the paralleling technique is used.

The radiographs obtained during endodontic treatment pose a different set of challenges. These views include root length determination, verification of filling cone placement, and other procedures in which the rubber dam is in place. The rubber dam may make the positioning of working radiographs more difficult. A variety of film holders are available to overcome radiographic distortion problems (see Chapter 5, Figs. 5-14 and 5-15). All of these devices are specifically designed to aid in the placement of the film and tube head in proper relationship to the tooth undergoing endodontic treatment. Film holders help the clinician obtain accurate and distortion-free working films, with files or

filling points protruding from the tooth and the rubber dam in place.

The choice of film for endodontic radiographs has shifted from Ultraspeed to Ektaspeed (Eastman Kodak Company, Rochester, NY), because Ektaspeed is twice as fast and requires one-half the x-ray exposure of Ultraspeed film. Although it may be more grainy and demonstrate less contrast when compared with Ultraspeed film, careful attention to exposure and processing of Ektaspeed film produces an image of good diagnostic quality.[4] The use of a rapid, automated film processor is helpful in producing high-quality films. Daylight-loading, manual quick-processing boxes are also useful for working radiographs.

Digital radiography uses a conventional dental radiograph unit and a microprocessor. An intraoral radiation detector, more sensitive than conventional silver halide films, is used in place of radiographic film. The combination of the highly sensitive intraoral sensor (i.e., charged-coupled device) and the precision microprocessor results in a dramatic reduction in radiation. In addition, the displayed image may be altered with the computer, enhancing and enlarging details and converting negative images to positive images. Another type of system that uses a rechargeable storage phosphor plate instead of the charged-coupled device is also available. Both of these systems eliminate the need for conventional film and

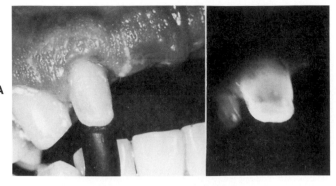

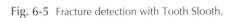

Fig. 6-4 Transillumination of pulpal "blush." **A**, Transillumination of lingual of full-crown preparation. **B**, Operatory lights out – demonstration of "blush."

darkroom chemistry, and they give the clinician the ability to store, retrieve, and transmit digital images via computer. Illustrations and a more complete explanation of these new high-tech digital radiography systems will be found in Chapter 26.

Diagnosis

The armamentarium for diagnosis has been detailed in Chapter 1. The technology of pulp testing continues to become more sophisticated and reliable. Examination techniques for disclosing tooth fractures with a fiberoptic light source have been shown in Chapter 1. This transillumination technique is also of value in determining the extent of a pulpal "blush"

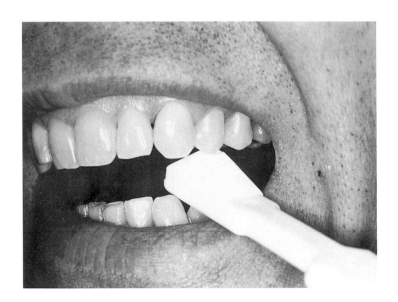

Fig. 6-5 Fracture detection with Tooth Slooth.

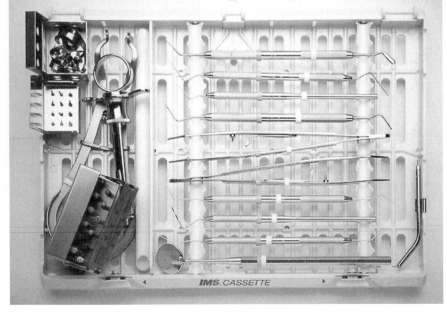

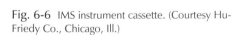

Fig. 6-6 IMS instrument cassette. (Courtesy Hu-Friedy Co., Chicago, Ill.)

after extensive tooth preparation. The operatory lights are dimmed and the transilluminator is placed on the lingual surface of the preparation (Fig. 6-4).

The technique of detecting a cracked tooth by wedging cusps with a cotton roll, cottonwood stick, or the equivalent has been described in Chapter 1. An additional wedging modality for the diagnosis of fractured teeth is the Tooth Sloth (Fig. 6-5). This plastic device is used as a selective wedge on or between the cusps as the patient bites. Sharp pain on *release* of biting pressure often indicates a cracked tooth.

Organization Systems

The trend toward using preset trays and cassettes in endodontics has simplified the organization, storage, and delivery of endodontic instruments. Although clinicians select different instruments and tray setups, certain basic principles are common to all systems. A standard cassette contains the most frequently used long-handled instruments, such as mouth mirror, endodontic explorer, long-spoon excavator, plastic instrument, and locking forceps. Items such as an irrigating syringe and needles, ruler, sterile paper points, burs, and rubber dam clamps often supplement standard cassettes. A sample cassette setup is shown in Fig. 6-6. A wide variety of file stands and file boxes are now available to provide organizational simplicity and sterility (Fig. 6-7). Whatever system is chosen, the emphasis is on keeping the setup easy for the staff to restock and sterilize, and convenient for the clinician, whether working alone or with a chair side assistant.

Rubber Dam

Rubber dam isolation is the standard of care in endodontics. However, a recent national survey revealed that only 59% of general dentists consistently use the rubber dam for endodontics, compared with more than 92% of practicing endodontists.[32] This important point needs to be reemphasized: Teeth undergoing endodontic treatment should always be isolated with a rubber dam unless the clinical situation makes tooth isolation physically impossible.

Rubber dam material for endodontic treatment is available in a variety of colors, thicknesses, scents, and materials. With the increased recognition of latex allergies, the traditional latex rubber dam has been supplemented by the availability of nonlatex dam material.[26] This nonlatex product is a synthetic elastomeric material that is 100% latex free and powder free (Fig. 6-8). Reportedly the tear resistance of this product is similar to latex, and it has a minimum 3-year shelf life.

When using a traditional latex rubber dam, many clinicians prefer the medium or lightweight dam material, citing its increased resilience and ease of application. Color is also a matter of personal preference. Dark-colored dam material provides sharp contrast between the tooth and dam; light-colored dam material permits visualization of the film holder's position when a radiograph during treatment is being exposed. Options include green dam material (scented with wintergreen) and royal blue, which yields good visual contrast plus "eye appeal." Regardless of which color or thickness is chosen, all dam material should be stored away from strong heat and light to prevent the latex from drying and becoming less flexible. Tearing of the dam upon applica-

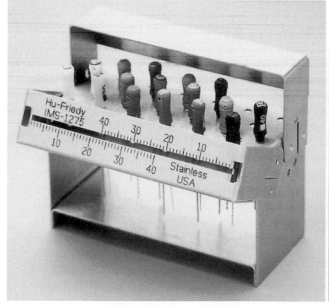
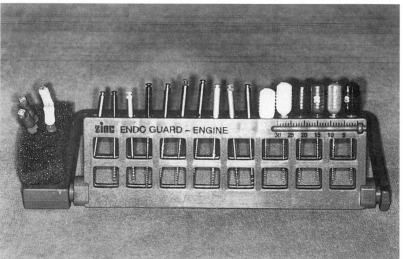

Fig. 6-7 A, File stand. **B,** File stand for rotary instruments. (*A* courtesy Hu-Friedy Co., Chicago, Ill. *B* courtesy Zirc Dental Products, Buffalo, N.Y.)

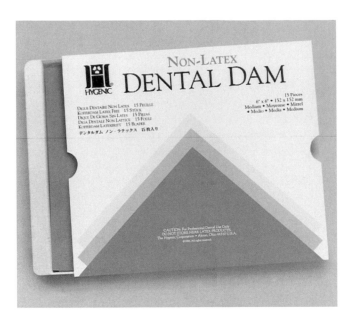

Fig. 6-8 Nonlatex dam. (Courtesy Hygenic Corp., Akron, Ohio.)

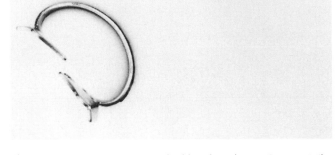

Fig. 6-9 Ivory "tiger-jaw" serrated rubber dam clamp. (Courtesy Miles Dental Products, South Bend, Ind.)

tion usually indicates the material is dried out and should be discarded. Refrigeration of dam material seems to extend its shelf life.

An almost endless array of rubber dam clamps is available to isolate special problem situations. The "tiger-jaw" clamps (Fig. 6-9) are especially useful for retaining the dam on broken-down posterior teeth. The winged style clamp is preferred, because it provides better tissue retraction and allows the use of the "unit" placement technique described in Chapter 5.

Any good-quality rubber dam punch will accomplish the goal of creating a clean hole for the tooth. Care must be taken to punch a hole without "nicks" in the rim to prevent accidental tearing and leakage. Small leaks can be conveniently patched using OraSeal, a flexible, puttylike product packaged in a plastic syringe (Fig. 6-10). A radiolucent, plastic rubber dam frame eliminates the need for removing the frame while exposing working radiographs.

Access Preparation through a Crown

Gaining access through a porcelain-fused-to-metal crown is more difficult than gaining access through natural tooth structure or other restorative materials. One approach is to use a small, round diamond with copious water spray to create the outline form in the porcelain. The metal substructure is then penetrated with either a tungsten-tipped or new carbide-end-cutting bur (Fig. 6-11). This two-stage technique reduces the possibility of porcelain fracture or chipping. (See Chapter 7 for more information on this technique.)

Uncovering receded or calcified root canal orifices is often a challenge. A useful adjunct for these types of problems is the use of low-speed Mueller burs. These burs have

an extralong, flexible shaft that allows visualization by the operator as the bur advances into the deeper portions of the access preparation. A clinical case illustrating their use can be found in Fig. 6-12.

Inadvertent perforation of the furcation is an unfortunate procedural accident that occasionally occurs during molar access preparation. Sealing of these perforations with mineral trioxide aggregate (MTA), known as *ProRoot*, has shown extraordinary healing results.[20, 29] One method of delivering and applying the mixed MTA is shown in Fig. 6-13.

Hand Instruments

A sample cassette for endodontics was shown in Fig. 6-6. The long, double-ended spoon excavator is specifically designed for endodontic therapy. It allows the clinician to remove coronal pulp tissue, caries, or cotton pellets that may be deep in the tooth's crown (Fig. 6-14). The double-ended endodontic explorer is used to locate and probe the orifice of the root canal as it joins the pulp chamber. Locking endodontic forceps facilitate the transfer of paper points and gutta-percha cones from assistant to dentist. Plastic filling instruments are designed to place and condense temporary restorations. A periodontal probe completes the basic setup.

Canal Preparation

Techniques for determining the "working length" of the root canal before instrumentation will be detailed in Chapter 8. Measuring blocks and special millimeter thumb rulers are useful for measuring endodontic files and gutta-percha cones (Fig. 6-15). The use of electronic apex locators as an adjunct to radiographic length determination is becoming more

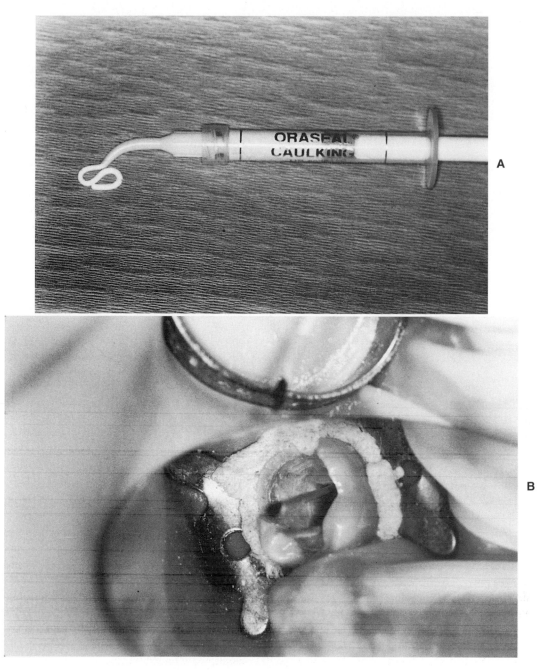

Fig 6-10 **A**, OraSeal caulking. **B**, OraSeal sealing rubber dam clamp.

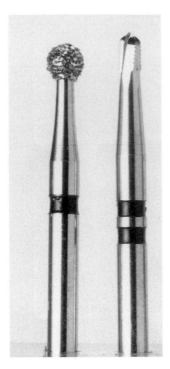

Fig. 6-11 Round diamond and carbide bur for porcelain-fused-to-metal crown access. (Courtesy Brasseler USA, Savannah, Ga.)

accepted (Fig. 6-16), and the accuracy of these devices is becoming more predictable.[11,24]

Cleaning, shaping, and sealing of the root canal, as described in Chapters 8 and 9, are primary components of clinical success. The barbed broach is used primarily for the gross removal of vital pulp tissue from large canals. The disposable broach is inserted into the canal and rotated to engage the tissue. Because these instruments are fragile and prone to breakage, they must be used with great care. The most commonly used hand instruments in canal preparation are endodontic files. Introduction of new file designs and metals has increased dramatically during the past few years. Triangular, square, and rhomboid blanks are usually used in the manufacturing of these hand instruments. Variations in metallurgy, taper, cutting-blade angle, degree of twist, flute spacing, and cutting or noncutting tip have complicated the clinician's choice of instruments. In addition, there is a growing body of evidence to suggest that flexible files of nickel-titanium, when compared with files of stainless steel, may produce more consistent root canal preparations.[12] A detailed description of these file variations can be found in Chapter 14.

The use of ultralow-speed, high-torque handpiece systems for canal preparation is accelerating with the proliferation of nickel-titanium, engine-driven files (Fig. 6-17). Two of the more popular rotary systems are illustrated in Fig. 6-18. Other contemporary nickel-titanium rotary instruments include the Light speed and Hero systems. Although all these rotary systems differ in file design, taper, and flute angle, they have certain common characteristics. For example, they all benefit from the unique ability that the blend of nickel-titanium has to follow canal curvature. In addition, all of these systems operate at a very low speed, have a high-torque handpiece system, and allow for full, 360-degree file rotation, as opposed to a reciprocal oscillatory movement. These systems should be used with a light touch (e.g., the same pressure as applied to writing with a sharp pencil) and minimal apical pressure to avoid instrument breakage. The emphasis is on preflaring of the upper portion of the root canal to allow more control in the preparation of the apical third. Clinical studies on these various systems demonstrate the ability of this new technology to provide smooth, clean canal walls, while maintaining natural anatomical curvatures.[14,27]

Conventional rotary instruments are used primarily as flaring devices for the coronal portion of the canal. The most commonly used is the Gates-Glidden drill, now available in a short version to facilitate use in posterior teeth (Fig. 6-19). The use of excessive force may either perforate the canal or fracture the instrument; the Gates-Glidden is designed to break high on the shaft if excessive resistance is encountered, allowing the clinician to remove the fragment easily. (See Chapter 7 for more information on the Gates-Glidden technique.)

Irrigation

Irrigation of the canal during instrumentation is described in Chapter 8. Systems for the delivery of irrigating solution into the root canal range from simple disposable syringes to complex devices capable of irrigating and aspirating simultaneously. The choice for the clinician is one of convenience and cost. The smaller syringe barrels (i.e., less than 10 ml) require frequent refilling during the instrumentation phase of therapy. Plastic syringes in the 10 to 20 ml range may offer the best combination of sufficient solution volume and ease of handling. "Back filling" of the syringe from a 500 ml laboratory plastic wash bottle filled with the irrigant of choice saves time and effort when compared with aspirating the solution into the barrel from a container (Fig. 6-20). The barrel tip should be a Luer-Lok design, rather than friction fit, to prevent accidental needle dislodgment during irrigation.

A side delivery design of an irrigating needle tip is shown in Fig. 6-21. This design helps prevent the accidental forcing of irrigating solution into the periapical tissues if the needle binds in the canal; it has been reported to provide superior apical third irrigation compared with other styles.[19]

Various sizes of paper points are available to dry the canal after irrigation. Paper points are used sequentially in the locking forceps until no moisture is evident on the paper point. To maintain asepsis, presterilized "cell" packaging is preferred over bulk packaging (Fig. 6-22).

If the root canal treatment cannot be completed in one visit, the use of calcium hydroxide as an intracanal medication has been advocated.[30,31] Different systems for applying intracanal calcium hydroxide are shown in Fig. 6-23.

Text continued on p. 161

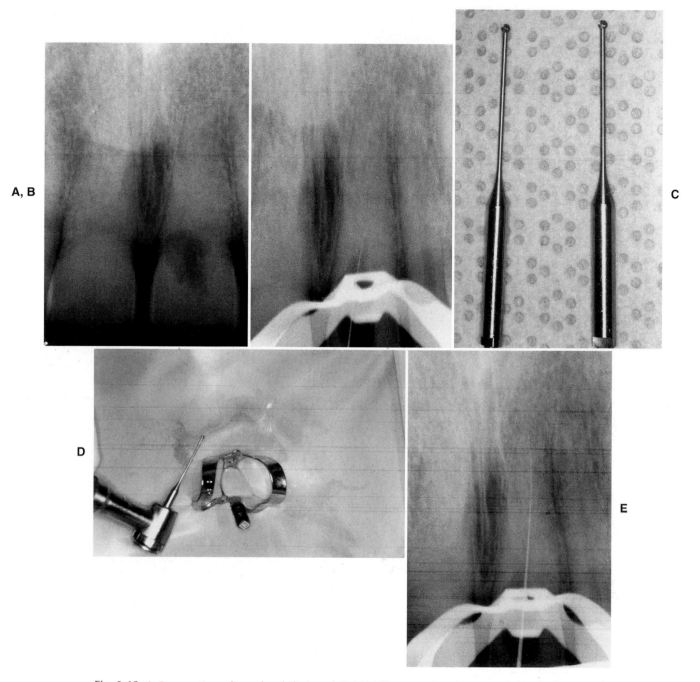

Fig. 6-12 **A**, Preoperative radiograph–calcified canal. **B**, Initial file penetration after access. **C**, Mueller burs. **D**, File penetration after use of Mueller bur. **E**, Working length radiograph.

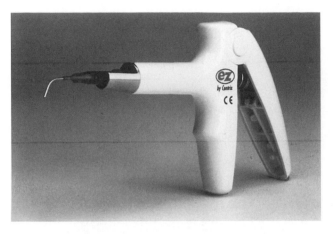

Fig. 6-13 Centrix syringe for application of MTA. (Courtesy Centrix Inc., Shelton, Conn. Application concept courtesy Dr. Jed Jultak.)

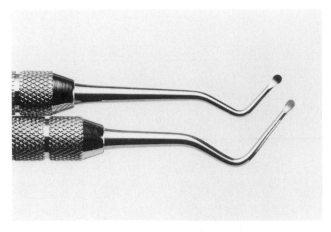

Fig. 6-14 Operative spoon excavator (*top*) and Endo Spoon excavator (*bottom*). (Courtesy Brasseler USA, Savannah, Ga.)

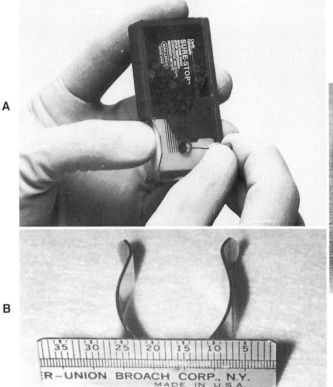

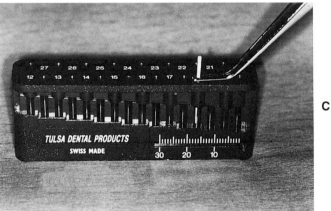

Fig. 6-15 **A**, Silicone stop dispenser. **B**, Millimeter thumb ruler. **C**, Measuring block. (*A* courtesy Caulk/Dentsply, Milford, Del.)

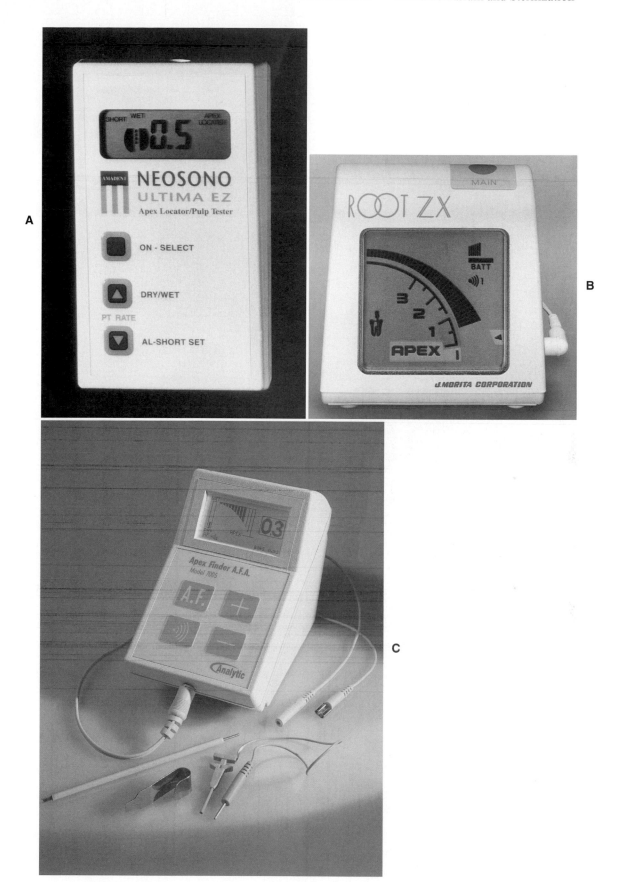

Fig. 6-16 Electronic apex locators. **A**, Neosono. **B**, Root ZX. **C**, Analytic apex finder. (*A* courtesy Amadent, Cherry Hill, N.J. *B* courtesy J. Morita USA, Tustin, Calif. *C* courtesy Analytic Endodontics, Orange, Calif.)

Fig. 6-17 Endodontic rotary handpieces. **A**, Endo-Mate 2. **B**, Quantec. **C**, Aseptico torque control. (*A*, Courtesy NSK America Corp., Schaumburg, Ill. *B*, Courtesy Analytic Endodontics, Orange, Calif. *C*, Courtesy Dentsply Tulsa Dental, Tulsa, Okla.)

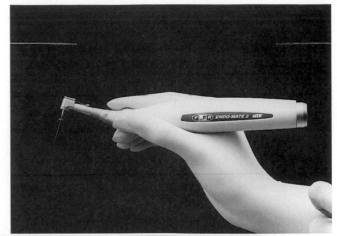

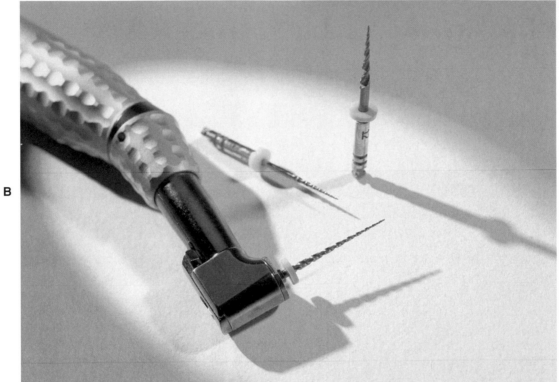

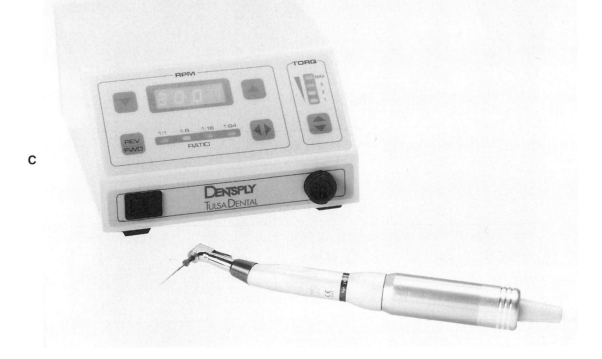

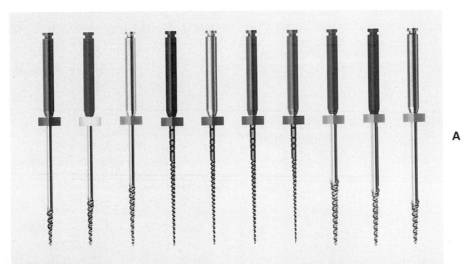

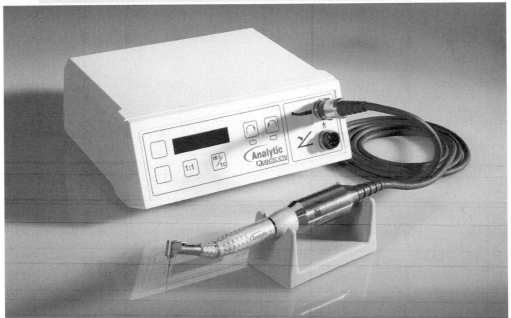

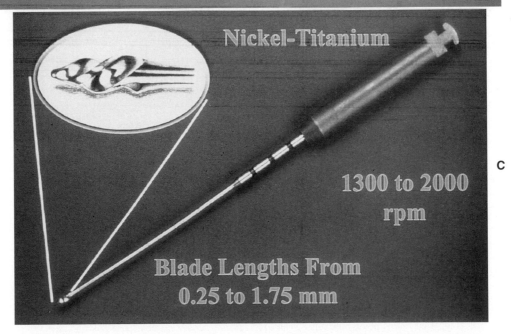

Fig. 6-18 **A**, ProFile GT rotary system. **B**, Quantec rotary system. **C**, Light-speed rotary system. (*A* courtesy Dentsply Tulsa Dental, Tulsa, Okla. *B* courtesy Analytic Endodontics, Orange, Calif.)

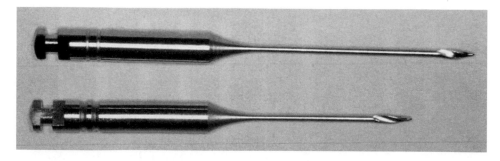

Fig. 6-19 Regular and short Gates-Glidden drills.

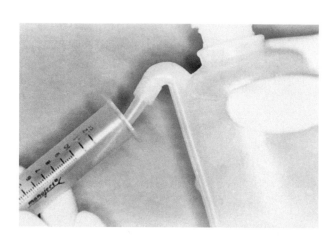

Fig. 6-20 Backfilling of irrigation syringe from wash bottle.

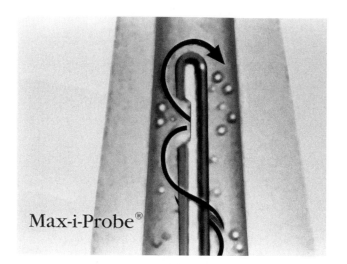

Fig. 6-21 Max-I-Probe irrigating needle. (Courtesy MPL Technologies, Franklin Park, Ill.)

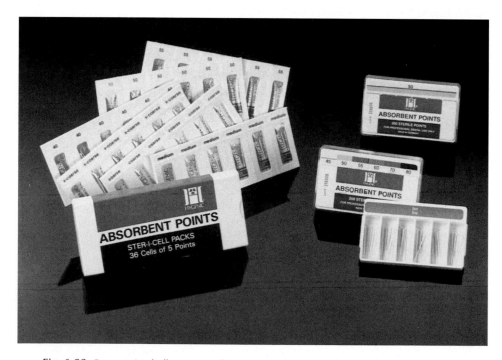

Fig. 6-22 Paper point–bulk versus "cell" packaging. (Courtesy Hygenic Corp., Akron, Ohio.)

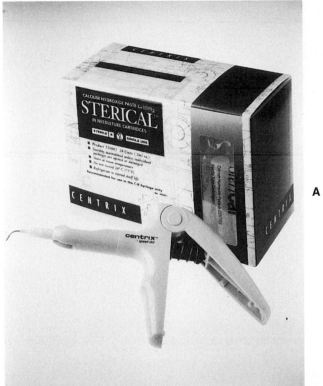

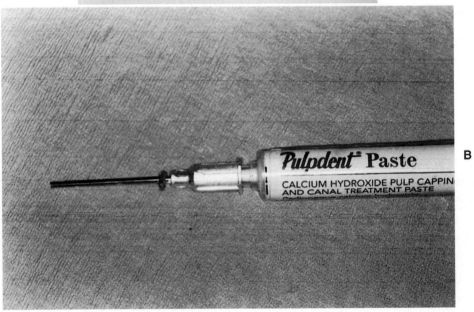

Fig. 6-23 **A**, Calciject calcium hydroxide system. **B**, Pulpdent calcium hydroxide paste.   *continued*

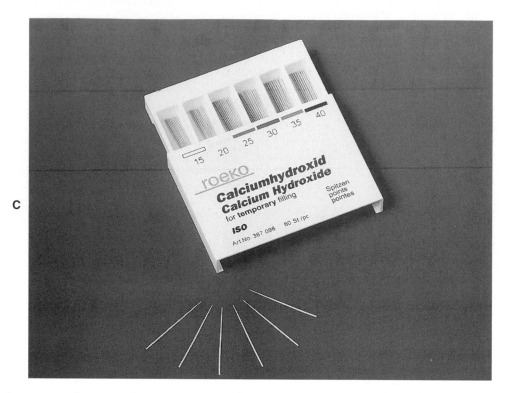

C

Fig. 6-23, cont'd   C, Cone-shaped calcium hydroxide intracanal medication, which activates upon contact with moisture. (*A* courtesy Centrix Inc., Shelton, Conn.)

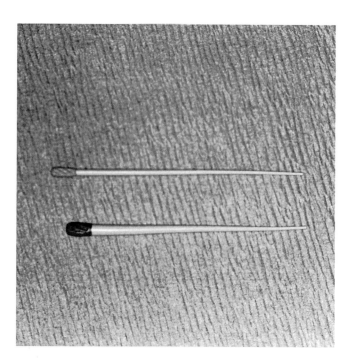

Fig. 6-24 Comparison of 0.02 taper gutta-percha cone (*top*) versus 0.04 taper gutta-percha cone (*bottom*). (Courtesy Charles B. Schwed Co. Inc., Kew Gardens, N.Y.)

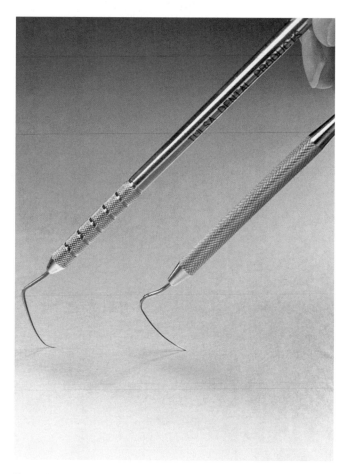

Fig. 6-25 Nickel-titanium spreader (*top*) versus stainless steel spreader (*bottom*) showing different tip flexibility. (Courtesy Tulsa Dental Products, Tulsa, Okla.)

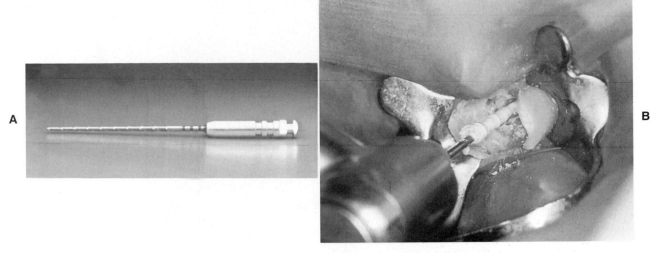

Fig. 6-26 **A**, GPX gutta-percha remover. **B**, Gutta-percha being removed by GPX. (*A* courtesy Brasseler USA, Savannah, Ga.)

Obturation

Most root canal filling methods employ root canal sealer as an integral part of the obturation technique. The most popular class of sealer cements used in endodontics is based on zinc oxide and eugenol formulations. These products require a glass slab and cement spatula for mixing to the desired consistency. Sealers containing calcium hydroxide are also available. Root canal obturation techniques are discussed in Chapter 9. Gutta-percha is the most commonly used canal filling material in contemporary endodontics. Gutta-percha is available as standardized cones that correspond to the International Standards Organization (ISO) tip size of root canal instruments, with a range of tapers from 0.02 to 0.06 (Fig. 6-24). Nonstandardized cones are even more tapered and are classified by size (from extrafine through extralarge).

Specialized hand instruments used in obturating the root canal with gutta-percha include spreaders and pluggers. Spreaders are available in a wide variety of lengths and tapers, and they are used primarily to compact gutta-percha filling material in the lateral compaction technique. Nickel-titanium spreaders offer increased flexibility, compared with spreaders made of stainless steel[18] (Fig. 6-25). Pluggers, also called *condensers*, are flat ended rather than pointed; they are used primarily to compact filling materials in a vertical fashion. A nickel and titanium rotary instrument for the removal of compacted gutta-percha is available (Fig. 6-26). This device breaks up and removes gutta-percha from the canal, facilitating retreatment procedures. The introduction of a system to remove posts from root canals has also been a welcome addition to the retreatment armamentarium (Fig. 6-27).

On the "high tech" front, devices for heating, delivering, and compacting gutta-percha in the prepared root canal are now available. A detailed description of these systems will be

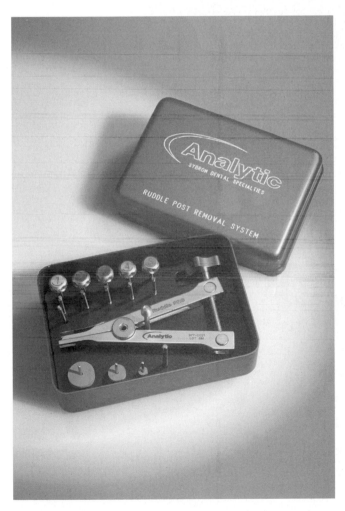

Fig. 6-27 Ruddle post remover. (Courtesy Analytic Endodontics, Orange, Calif.)

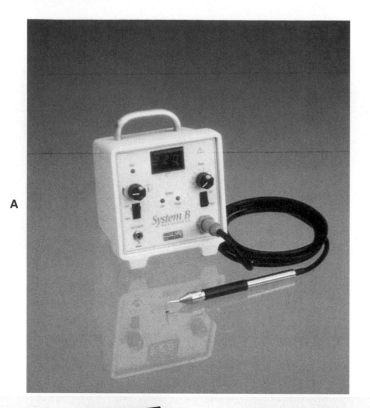

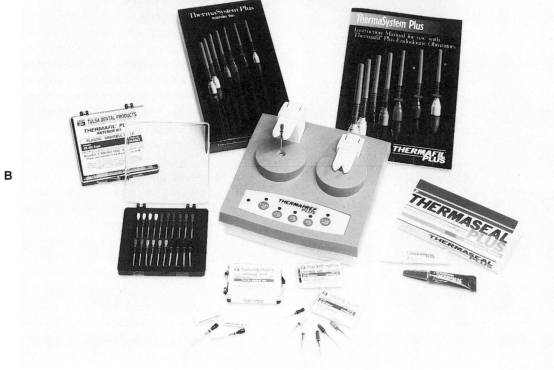

Fig. 6-28 **A**, System B. **B**, ThermaSystem Plus.

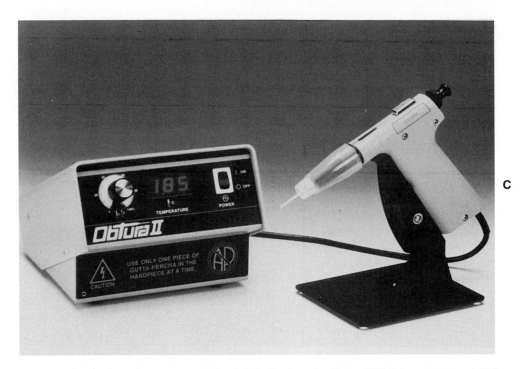

Fig. 6-28, cont'd   **C**, Obtura II. (*A* courtesy EIE/Analytic Technology, San Diego, Calif. *B* courtesy Dentsply Tulsa Dental, Tulsa, Okla. C courtesy Obtura Spartan, Fenton, Md.)

found in Chapter 9. Examples of these warm gutta-percha systems are shown in Fig. 6-28. Controversy abounds concerning the purported superiority of one system versus another.[16]

Temporary restorative materials used in endodontics must provide a high-quality seal of the access preparation to prevent microbial contamination of the root canal. Premixed products (e.g., Cavit) have become popular for temporary access cavity sealing. Cavit is a moisture-initiated, autopolymerized, premixed, calcium sulfate and polyvinyl chloride acetate.

STERILIZATION

Sweeping infection control changes have permanently altered the way dentists deliver patient care. Molanari recently catalogued the major advances that have affected dentistry.[22] Among these advances are the use of aseptic procedures, latex gloves, masks, protective eyewear, overgarments, scientific and safe handling of contaminated instruments, heat sterilization, chemical surface disinfectants, single-use disposables, and purpose-made disposable barriers. The sterilization portion of this chapter will examine these advances as they relate to the theory and practice of universal infection control precautions in the practice of dentistry and endodontics.

Vaccination

Dentists and dental health care workers who have direct patient contact are at risk of contacting or transmitting infectious diseases. Appropriate vaccinations for contagious diseases remain an important safety adjunct to infection control procedures. This is especially true for the hepatitis virus family. Dental health care workers should be immunized against hepatitis A and B.[9,13]

Barrier Techniques

The Occupational Safety and Health Administration (OSHA) requires that dentists follow infection control guidelines established by the Centers for Disease Control and Prevention (CDC).[10] These guidelines define the use of universal precautions to prevent cross-contamination while treating patients. The most effective method of preventing cross-contamination is the use of personal- and environmental-barrier techniques (Fig. 6-29). Hackney and Crawford showed a higher incidence of oral pathogens on dental operatory environmental surfaces, compared with similar surfaces in nondental settings. This occurred even when the best surface disinfection practices were used. Cleaning and disinfection are good practices, but they may not be the most effective or reliable method of infection control for busy dental offices. They recommended using single-use disposable plastic covers over surfaces to be touched during dental treatment.[15]

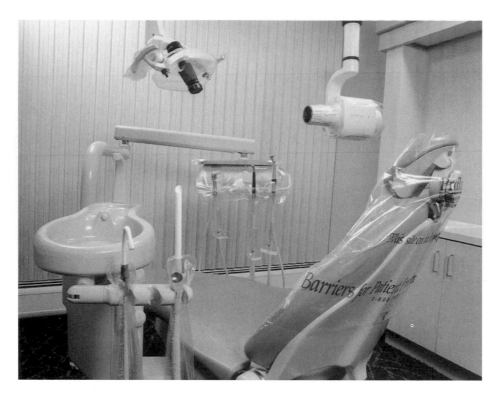

Fig. 6-29 Operatory plastic film barriers in place. (Courtesy Cottrell Ltd., Englewood, Calif.)

Definition of Terms

The clinician should be familiar with the following terms in relation to office infection control:

- Bacterial spore form (endospore)—A more complex structure than the vegetative cell from which it forms. Spores form in response to environmental conditions and are more highly resistant to sterilization methods than vegetative forms.
- Bacterial vegetative form—Active, multiplying microorganisms.
- Biofilm—The colonization and proliferation of microorganisms at a surface and solution interface. Especially problematic in the small-bore water lines of dental units. Bacteria, fungi, protozoa, and aquatic nematodes have been identified as inhabitants of water line biofilm.
- Biologic indicator—A preparation of microorganisms, usually bacterial spores, that serves as a challenge to the efficiency of a given sterilization process or cycle. Negative bacterial growth from a biologic indicator verifies sterilization.
- Cross-infection—Transmission of infectious material from one person to another.
- Disinfection—A less lethal process than sterilization. It eliminates virtually all pathogenic vegetative microorganisms, but it does not necessarily eliminate all microbial forms (spores). Usually this process is reserved for large environmental surfaces that cannot be sterilized (e.g., a dental chair). Disinfection lacks the margin of safety achieved by sterilization procedures. Disinfection is non-verifiable.
- Process indicator—Strip, tape, or tab applied to or packaged in a sterilizer load. Special inks or chemicals within the indicator change color when subjected to heat, steam, or chemical vapor and indicate that the indicator has been cycled through the sterilizer. Process indicators do *not* verify sterilization.
- Sterilization—The use of a physical or chemical procedure to destroy all microbial life, including highly resistant bacterial endospores. Sterilization is a verifiable procedure.
- Universal precautions—The same infection control procedures are used for all patients, regardless of medical or social history.

Instrument Preparation

The preoperative handling, cleaning, and packaging of contaminated instruments are frequently sources of injury and possible infection. Dental staff performing such procedures should wear reusable, heavy rubber work gloves similar to household cleaning gloves. Contaminated instruments that will not be cleaned immediately should be submersed in a holding solution so that blood, saliva, and tissue will not dry on the instrument surfaces. Ultrasonic cleaner detergent, iodophor solution, or an enzyme presoak is an effective holding solution.

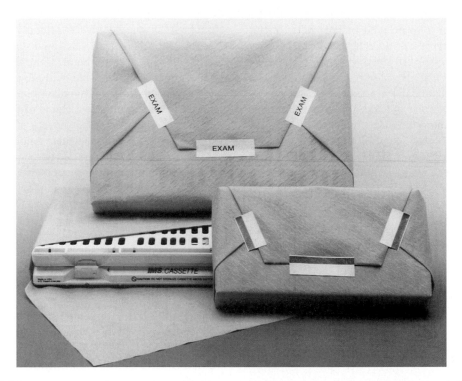

Fig. 6-30 Cassette wrapped in porous autoclave paper in preparation for sterilization. (Courtesy Hu-Friedy Co., Chicago, Ill.)

Use of an ultrasonic cleaner, which is many times more effective and safer than hand scrubbing, should be the choice for definitive instrument-cleaning sterilization. Instruments cleaned in an ultrasonic device should be suspended in a perforated basket. When an ultrasonic cleaner is on, nothing should come in contact with the tank's bottom, and its lid should be in place. The cleaner should be run for at least 5 minutes per load. Once the cycle is complete, the clean instruments must be thoroughly rinsed under a high volume of aerated water; placed on a clean, dry towel; rolled or patted; and air dried.[5] The ultrasonic solution becomes increasingly contaminated with each instrument load and should be discarded at least daily, and the tub of the ultrasonic machine should be disinfected. The contaminated instruments are now very clean, but they are not sterile. With cassette systems, the contaminated instruments are placed back in the cassette holder and circulated through an ultrasonic cleaner or thermal disinfector, resulting in minimal hand contact by staff during instrument preparation. Instruments packaged in a cassette may require additional time in an ultrasonic cleaner or thermal disinfector; the manufacturer's recommendations should be strictly followed. Continued precautions are necessary until the instruments have been sterilized.

Clean instruments or cassettes ready for sterilization should be packaged in materials designed for the specific sterilization process to be used (Fig. 6-30). The sterilizing agent must be able to penetrate the wrapping material and come into intimate contact with microorganisms. Contami-

nated endodontic hand files must be cleaned in an ultrasonic bath and autoclaved to completely eliminate microorganisms and measurable endotoxin.[28]

Methods of Sterilization

The most reliable agent for destroying microorganisms is heat. Methods for sterilization in endodontic practice include steam or chemical vapor under pressure, dry heat, and glutaraldehyde solutions.

Steam Under Pressure   The autoclave is the most common means of sterilization, except when penetration of steam is limited or heat and moisture damage is a problem. Moist heat kills microorganisms through protein coagulation, RNA and DNA breakdown, and release of intracellular constituents of low molecular weight.[3] The autoclave sterilizes in 15 to 40 minutes at 121° C (249.8° F), at a pressure of 15 psi. The time required for sterilization depends on the type of load placed in the autoclave and its permeability. Once the entire load has reached the desired temperature of 121° C, it will be rendered sterile in 15 minutes. An adequate margin of safety for load warm-up and steam penetration requires an autoclave time of at least 30 minutes. If there is any doubt as to the safety margin required, the clinician should always allow more time for load warm-up.

Existing chamber air is the most detrimental factor to efficient steam sterilization. Modern autoclaves use a gravity displacement method to evacuate this air, thus providing a fully saturated chamber with no cold or hot spots. Instruments and packages placed in an autoclave must be properly arranged so that the pressurized steam may circulate freely around and through the load. Because recirculation of water tends to concentrate contaminants in an autoclave, only fresh, deionized (i.e., distilled) water should be used for each cycle. Several manufacturers now provide countertop water distillers that simplify autoclave operation (Fig. 6-31). Caution must be exercised to never allow amalgam-containing teeth or instruments to be sterilized in an autoclave, because mercury vapor will be released during the heat of sterilization and could pose a health risk or contaminate the autoclave.[25] When instruments are heated in a steam autoclave, rust and corrosion can occur. Chemical corrosion inhibitors, which are commercially available, will protect sharp instruments.

Several rapid-speed autoclaves have been developed primarily for use in dentistry. Some of these devices may limit the chamber load size but have a sterilization cycle much shorter than the traditional steam autoclave (Fig. 6-32).

Advantages of rapid-speed autoclaves include:
1. Turnaround time for instruments is relatively quick.
2. Packages and internal areas of handpieces are penetrated.
3. Process will not destroy cotton or cloth products.
4. Sterilization is verifiable.

Disadvantages of rapid-speed autoclaves include:
1. Materials must be air dried at completion of the cycle.
2. Because certain metals may corrode or become dull, antirust pretreatment may be required. However, most stainless steels are resistant to autoclave damage.
3. Heat-sensitive materials or devices can be altered or destroyed with repeated sterilization cycles.

Unsaturated Chemical Vapor   This system, using a chambered device that is similar to an autoclave, is known as a Harvey Chemiclave or chemical vapor sterilizer (Fig. 6-33). The principle of chemiclave sterilization is that although some water is necessary to catalyze the destruction of all microorganisms in a relatively short period of time, water saturation is not necessary. Like autoclave sterilization, chemical vapor sterilization kills microorganisms by destroying vital protein systems. Unsaturated chemical vapor sterilization uses a solution containing specific amounts of various alcohols, acetone, ketone, and formaldehyde, and a water content well below the 15% level where rust and corrosion occurs. When the chemiclave is heated to 132° C (270° F) and pressurized to at least 20 psi, steriliza-

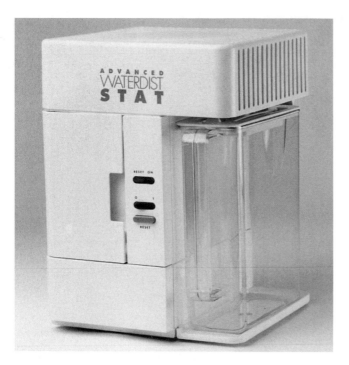

Fig. 6-31   Countertop water distiller. (Courtesy SciCan, Pittsburgh, Pa.)

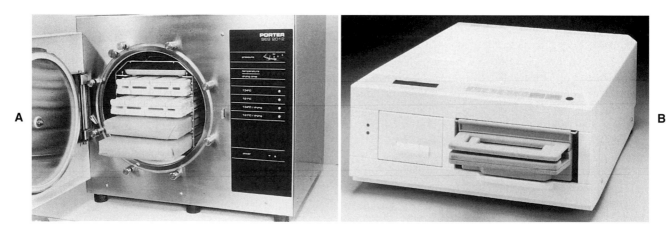

Fig. 6-32   Rapid-cycle autoclaves. **A**, Automatic, programmable autoclave. **B**, Statim cassette autoclave. (*A* courtesy Porter Instrument Co., Hatfield, Pa. *B* courtesy SciCan, Pittsburgh, Pa.)

tion occurs in 20 minutes. As in the autoclave, sterilization in the chemiclave requires careful arrangement of the load to be sterilized. The vapor must be allowed to circulate freely within the chemiclave and penetrate instrument-wrapping material. Chemiclave solution must not be recirculated; a fresh mixture of the solution should be used for each cycle.

Advantages of chemiclave sterilization include:
1. Process will not corrode metals.
2. Turnaround time for instruments is relatively quick.
3. Load comes out dry.
4. Sterilization is verifiable.

Disadvantages of chemiclave sterilization include:
1. Vapor odor may be offensive, requiring increased ventilation.
2. Special chemicals must be purchased and inventoried.
3. Process can destroy heat-sensitive materials.
4. Process may not penetrate the intricate internal workings of handpieces as well as steam.[21]

Dry Heat   There are complicating factors associated with sterilization by dry heat. The time and temperature factors may vary considerably according to heat diffusion, amount of heat available from the heating medium, amount of available moisture present, and heat loss through the heating container's walls. Dry heat kills microorganisms primarily through an oxidation process. Protein coagulation also takes place, depending on the water content of the protein and the temperature of sterilization. Dry-heat sterilization, like chemical vapor and autoclave sterilization, is verifiable. However, dry heat is very slow to penetrate instrument loads; it sterilizes at 160° C (320° F) in 30 minutes, but instrument loads may take 30 to 90 minutes to reach that temperature. A margin of safety requires instruments to be sterilized at 160° C for 2 hours. An internal means of determining and calibrating temperature is an essential component of any dry-heat sterilizer. If the sterilizer has multiple heating elements

on different surfaces, together with an internal fan to circulate air, heat transfer becomes much more efficient. It is important that loads be positioned within the dry-heat sterilizer so that they do not touch each other. Instrument cases must not be stacked one upon the other, and hot air must be allowed to circulate freely within the sterilizer.

High concentrations of mercury vapor can develop in a dry-heat sterilizer that has been used to sterilize amalgam instruments. Great care must be exercised to keep scrap amalgam out of any sterilizing device. Once contaminated with mercury or amalgam, a sterilizer will continue to produce mercury vapor for many cycles.

Small chamber, high-speed dry-heat sterilizers have been developed primarily for use in dentistry. Load limitations exist, but these devices are much faster than prolonged dry heat. This type of sterilizer has the advantages of prolonged dry heat (described previously), without many of the disadvantages of that sterilization method (Fig. 6-34).

Advantages of dry-heat sterilization include:
1. Process accommodates a large load capability.
2. Process offers complete corrosion protection.
3. Sterilization is verifiable.

Disadvantages of dry-heat sterilization include:
1. Process provides slow instrument turnaround because of poor heat exchange.
2. Sterilization cycles are not as exact as in moist-heat sterilization.
3. Dry-heat sterilizer must be calibrated and monitored.
4. If sterilizer temperature is too high, instruments may be damaged.

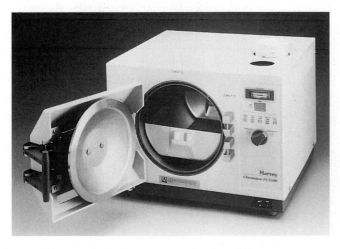

Fig. 6-33   Chemical vapor sterilizer. (Courtesy MDT Co., Gardena, Calif.)

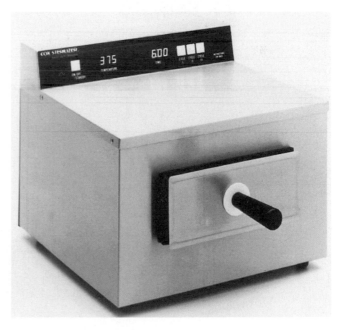

Fig. 6-34   Rapid heat transfer sterilizer. (Courtesy Cox Sterile Products Inc., Dallas, Tex.)

Handpiece Sterilization

Dental handpieces and related instruments should be sterilized between patients to help prevent cross-infection. Continued improvement in design has made repeated sterilization of dental handpieces possible. To reduce problems related to sterilization, such as loss of torque, turbine wear, and fiber-optic degradation, the manufacturer's instructions should be strictly followed. Christensen has recently outlined the problems associated with handpiece sterilization. He called for continued product development and the implementation of a sterilization system that does not require heat for handpiece sterlization.[8]

Dental Water Line Contamination

Dental handpieces, water syringes, and sonic and ultrasonic handpieces can be contaminated (before patient use but after sterilization) by biofilm-contaminated dental unit water lines. The usual source of this contamination is the commercial water supply entering the dental office. Biofilm is a complex, heterogenous microbial mass attached to surfaces bathed by fluids; it is formed by bacteria that attach themselves to surfaces, creating an intricate network of colonies. Because the flow rate in dental unit waterlines is very low, they provide an ideal environment for biofilm formation. The result of biofilm contamination is that the water emitted from handpieces, syringes, and ultrasonic devices may contain elevated concentrations of microorganisms. The ADA advises that each milliliter of unfiltered output water used in dental care contain less than 200 colony forming units (CFU) of biofilm.[2]

The U.S. Food and Drug Administration has approved several products for improving water used in providing dental care. These products fall into four groups:

1. Independent water systems (Fig. 6-35)
2. Chemical treatment protocols (whether intermittent or continuous)
3. Point-of-use filters
4. Sterile water delivery systems

Because some chemicals used in treating waterlines can be corrosive, it is important to follow manufacturers' instructions.

Glutaraldehyde Solutions

Whenever possible, reusable dental instruments should be heat sterilized by a method that can be biologically monitored. However, some dental and medical instruments are destroyed or damaged by the heat of sterilization. In these cases the use of aqueous glutaraldehyde preparations for high-level disinfection or sterilization can be used.

The biocidal activity of glutaraldehyde may be adversely affected by substandard preparation of "activated" glutaral-

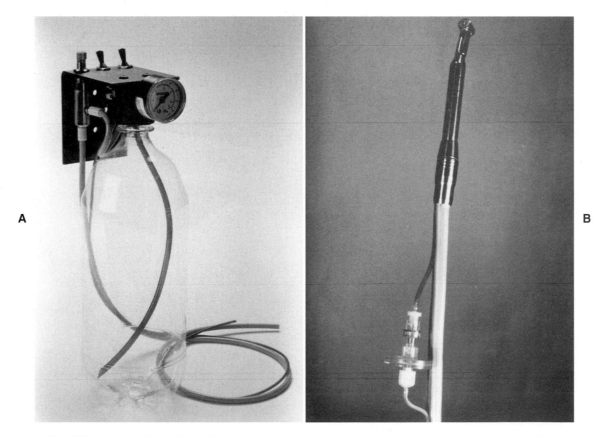

A   B

Fig. 6-35 **A,** Device for dealing with dental unit water line contamination. **B,** External solution container. (Courtesy EIE/Analytic Technology, San Diego, Calif.)

dehyde, contamination of the solution by protein debris, failure to change the solution at proper time intervals, water dilution of residual glutaraldehyde by washed instruments that have not been dried, and the slow but continuous polymerization of the glutaraldehyde molecule. Instruments contaminated with blood or saliva must remain submerged in glutaraldehyde long enough for spore forms to be killed. Sterilization may require 6 to 10 hours, depending on the product used.

Advantages of glutaraldehyde solution sterilization include:

1. Solution can sterilize heat-sensitive equipment.
2. Process is relatively noncorrosive and nontoxic.

Disadvantages of glutaraldehyde solution sterilization include:

1. Process requires long immersion time.
2. Solution has some odor, which may be objectionable, especially if the solution is heated.
3. Sterilization is nonverifiable.
4. Solution is irritating to mucous membranes (e.g., eyes).

Monitoring Sterilization

There are two methods commonly used to monitor in-office sterilization: (1) process indicators and (2) biologic indicators. Both types of indicators are necessary parts of infection control.

Process indicators are usually strips, tape, or paper products marked with special ink that changes color with exposure to heat, steam, or chemical vapor. The ink changes color when the items being processed have been subjected to sterilizing conditions. However, a process indicator usually does not monitor the length of time that such conditions were present. There are specific process indicators for different methods of sterilization. The process indicator's main role in infection control is to prevent accidental use of materials that have not been circulated through the sterilizer. A color change in a process indicator does not ensure proper function of the equipment or that sterilization has been achieved.

Biologic indicators are usually preparations of nonpathogenic bacterial spores that serve as a challenge to a specific method of sterilization. If a sterilization method destroys spore forms that are highly resistant to that method, then it is logical to assume that all other life forms, including viruses, have also been destroyed. The bacterial spores are usually attached to a paper strip within a biologically protected packet. The spore packet is placed between instrument packages or within an instrument package itself. After the sterilizer has cycled, the spore strip is cultured for a specific time. Lack of culture growth indicates sterility.

Every sterilizer load should contain at least one process indicator. A safer method is to attach a process indicator to each item sterilized. Each sterilizer should be checked periodically with a biologic indicator to ensure proper functioning of sterilizer equipment and proper loading technique. Records should be maintained, especially of the biologic

indicator results. Without periodic biologic monitoring, the clinician cannot be positive that sterilization failures are not occurring. An increasing number of universities and private companies provide mail-in biologic monitoring services (Fig. 6-36). Should sterilization failures occur, these monitoring services can offer consultation and recommendations.

Causes of sterilization failure include:

1. Improper instrument preparation
2. Improper packaging of instruments
3. Improper loading of the sterilizer chamber
4. Improper temperature in the sterilization chamber
5. Improper timing of the sterilization cycle
6. Equipment malfunction

Methods of Disinfection

Disinfection, which does not kill spore forms, should be reserved for the cleaning and decontamination of large sur-

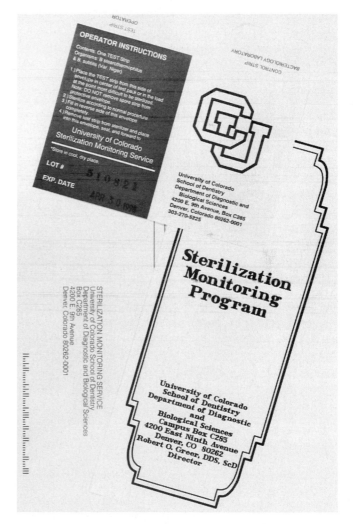

Fig. 6-36 Sterilization monitoring program: instructions, spore test strips, and microbiology report. (Courtesy University of Colorado School of Dentistry, Denver, Colo.)

faces, such as counter tops and dental chairs. Surface disinfectants approved by the Environmental Protection Agency (EPA) include iodophors, synthetic phenolics, and chlorine solutions. Surface disinfectants should have an EPA registration number and should be capable of killing *Mycobacterium tuberculosis* in 10 minutes.

Sodium hypochlorite, or household bleach, in a dilute solution (i.e., ¼ cup bleach to 1 gallon tap water) can be used to wipe down environmental surfaces. The surfaces to be disinfected should be kept moist for a minimum of 10 minutes (30 minutes is ideal). The free chlorine in solution is thought to inactivate sulfhydryl enzymes and nucleic acids and to denature proteins. Sodium hypochlorite is extremely biocidal against bacterial vegetative forms, viruses, and some spore forms. However, it is corrosive to metals and irritating to skin and eyes.

Iodophors are combinations of iodine and a solubilizing agent. The manufacturer's recommendations for dilution must be strictly followed to achieve the optimal amount of free iodine in the disinfecting solution. Iodophors have a built-in color indicator that changes when the free iodine molecules have been exhausted. This method of disinfecting offers an effective, practical approach without the problems associated with other disinfectants.

Sterilization of Gutta-Percha

The sterilization of gutta-percha cones is of importance in endodontic practice because this material may come in intimate contact with periapical tissue during obturation. Immersing gutta-percha cones in 5.25% sodium hypochlorite (i.e., full-strength household bleach) for 1 minute is very effective in killing vegetative microorganisms and spore forms. Gutta-percha can also be decontaminated by immersing cones for 1 minute in 1.0% NaOCl or for 5 minutes in 0.5% NaOCl.[6]

Effect of Repeated Sterilization on Instruments

The effect of repeated sterilization on the physical characteristics of endodontic files has been studied.[17,23] Repeated sterilization of stainless steel endodontic files, using any heat method described in this chapter, will not cause corrosion, weakness, or an increased rate of rotational failure.

References

1. American Dental Association: *Survey of dental practice,* Chicago, 1994, The Association.
2. American Dental Association Council on Scientific Affairs: Dental unit waterlines: approaching the year 2000, *J Am Dent Assoc* 130:1653, 1999.
3. Block S et al: *Disinfection, sterilization and preservation,* ed 4, Philadelphia, 1991, Lea & Febiger.
4. Brown R, Hadley J, Chambers D: An evaluation of Ektaspeed Plus film versus Ultraspeed film for endodontic working length determination, *J Endod* 24:54, 1998.
5. Burkhart N, Crawford J: Critical steps in instrument cleaning: removing debris after sonication, *J Am Dent Assoc* 128:456, 1997.
6. Cardoso C et al: Rapid decontamination of gutta-percha cones with sodium hypochlorite, *J Endod* 25:498-501, 1999.
7. Christensen G: Magnification, *Clinical Research Associates Newsletter,* 19:8, 1995.
8. Christensen G: The high-speed handpiece dilemma, *J Am Dent Assoc* 130:1494, 1999.
9. Cleveland J et al: Risk and prevention of hepatitis C virus infection, *J Am Dent Assoc* 130:641, 1999.
10. Department of Labor, Occupational Safety and Health Administration: *Occupational exposure to bloodborne pathogens, final rule,* Fed. Reg. 56(235):64004-64182, Washington, DC, 1991.
11. Dunlap C et al: An in vitro evaluation of an electronic apex locator that uses the ratio method in vital and necrotic canals, *J Endod* 24:48, 1998.
12. Gambill J, Alder M, del Rio C: Comparison of nickel-titanium and stainless steel hand-file, instrumentation using computed tomography, *J Endod* 22:369, 1996.
13. Gillcrist J: Hepatitis viruses A,B,C,D,E and G: implications for dental personnel, *J Am Dent Assoc* 130:509, 1999.
14. Glossen C et al: A comparison of root canal preparation using Ni-Ti Hand, Ni-Ti engine-driven, and K-Flex endodontic instruments, *J Endod* 21:146, 1995.
15. Hackney R et al: Using a biological indicator to detect potential sources of cross-contamination in the dental operatory, *J Am Dent Assoc* 129:1567, 1998.
16. Ingle J: A new paradigm for filling and sealing root canals, *Compendium* 16:306, 1995.
17. Iverson G et al: The effects of various sterilization methods on the torsional strength of endodontic files, *J Endod* 11:266, 1985.
18. Joyce A et al: Photoelastic comparison of stress induced by using stainless steel versus nickel-titanium spreaders in vitro, *J Endod* 24:714, 1998.
19. Kahn F, Rosenberg P, Gliksberg J: An in vitro evaluation of the irrigating characteristics of ultrasonic and subsonic handpieces and irrigating needles and probes, *J Endod* 21:277, 1995.
20. Koh E et al: Cellular response to mineral trioxide aggregate, *J Endod* 24:543, 1998.
21. Kolstad R: How well does the chemiclave sterilize handpieces? *J Am Dent Assoc* 129:985, 1998.
22. Molinari J: Dental infection control at the year 2000: accomplishment recognized, *J Am Dent Assoc* 130:1291, 1999.
23. Morrison S et al: The effects of steam sterilization and usage on cutting efficiency of endodontic instruments, *J Endod* 15:427, 1989.
24. Pagarino G, Pace R, Baccetti T: An SEM study of in vivo accuracy of the Root ZX electronic apex locator, *J Endod* 24:438, 1998.
25. Parsell D et al: Mercury release during autoclave sterilization of amalgam, *J Dent Educ* 60:453, 1996.
26. Safedi G et al: Latex hypersensitivity, *J Am Dent Assoc* 127:83, 1996.
27. Short J, Morgan L, Baumgartner J: A comparison of canal centering ability of four instrumentation techniques, *J Endod* 23:503, 1997.

28. Tittle K, Torabinejad M: Research abstract #50: Residual endotoxin on endodontic files after routine infection control procedures, *J Endod* 21:227, 1995.

29. Torabinejad M, Chivian N: Clinical applications of mineral trioxide aggregate, *J Endod* 25:197, 1999.

30. Trope M, Delano E, Orstavik D: Endodontic treatment of teeth with apical periodontitis: single vs. multivisit treatment, *J Endod* 25:345, 1999.

31. Wadachi R, Araki K, Suda H: Effect of calcium hydroxide on the dissolution of soft tissue on the root canal wall, *J Endod* 24:326, 1998.

32. Whitten B et al: Current trends in endodontic treatment: report of a national survey, *J Am Dent Assoc* 127:1333, 1996.

Chapter 7

 # Tooth Morphology and Cavity Preparation

Richard C. Burns, Eric James Herbranson

Chapter Outline

The hard tissue repository of the human dental pulp takes on many configurations that must be understood before treatment can begin. This chapter is designed to describe and illustrate tooth morphology and the rationale for the techniques that are critical to achieving unobstructed access to the pulp spaces. The information is divided into three sec-

tions: (1) the fundamentals of access design and preparation, (2) illustrative plates for internal and external visualization of real human teeth, and (3) the variables, problems, and resolution of access cavity difficulties.

COMPLEX ANATOMY

From the early work of Hess and Zurcher[18] to the most recent studies demonstrating anatomic complexities of the root canal system, it has long been established that the root with a graceful, tapering canal and a single apical foramen is the exception rather than the rule. Investigators have shown multiple foramina, fins, deltas, loops, furcation accessory canals, and more in most teeth. Kasahara et al[20] studied transparent specimens of 510 extracted maxillary central incisors for anatomic detail and found that 60% of the specimens showed accessory canals that were impossible to clean mechanically. Apical foramina located away from the apex were observed in 45% of the teeth. The student and the clinician must approach the tooth to be treated assuming that these "aberrations" occur so often as to be considered normal anatomy.

The first premolar in Fig, 7-1, *A*, is a good example of complex anatomy. The extra root is not obvious on a normal radiograph (Fig. 7-1, *B*). Fig. 7-2 shows the cross section of a similar tooth.[13] Instead of having two distinct canals, this tooth has a fine ribbon-shaped canal system. Both of these teeth present the clinician with a situation that is almost impossible to clean, shape, and seal thoroughly.

The teeth shown in Fig. 7-3 may be the longest on record. The maxillary cuspid measures 41 mm from incisal edge to apex; the central incisor is 30 mm long. These teeth, removed before placement of immediate dentures by Dr. Gary Wilkie of Korumburra, Victoria, Australia, belonged to a 31-year-old, 5-foot-2 inch tall European female.[3] The decision to remove the teeth was made jointly, by patient and dentist.[40]

It is humbling to be aware of the complexity of the spaces clinicians are expected to access, clean, and fill. However, dentists can take comfort in knowing that even under the dif-

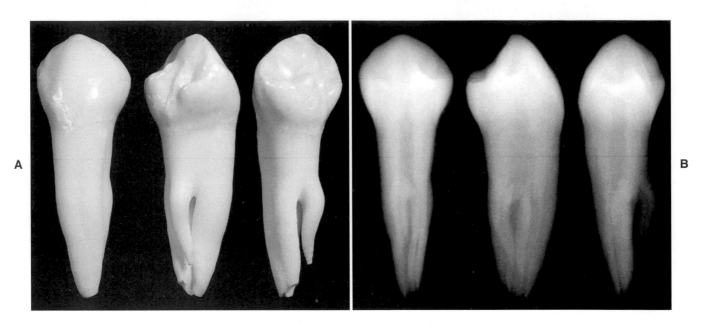

Fig. 7-1 **A,** An example of atypical and difficult morphology: this mandibular first premolar reveals three separate roots trifurcating at midroot. Small canals diverging from the main canal create a situation that is very difficult to instrument. **B,** Radiograph of three views.

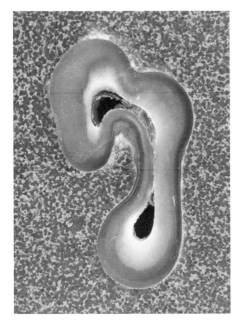

Fig. 7-2   Root section of a premolar similar to that shown in Fig. 7-1.

ficult circumstances of unusual morphology the current methods of root canal therapy result in an astonishingly high rate of success.

Ideal Access

A well-designed access preparation is essential for a quality endodontic result. A poorly executed access will make the procedure more difficult, compromising the final result and, consequently, the tooth's long-term survival.

The objective of an access preparation is to create a smooth, straight-line path to the canal system and, ultimately, the apex (see Figs. 7-11, 7-12, and 7-13). Correctly done this allows for complete irrigation and ease of shaping and, ultimately, quality obturation. Ideal access results in straight entry into the canal orifices, with the line angles forming a funnel that drops smoothly into the canal or canals. Projecting the canal centerline to the occlusal surface of the tooth produces the location of the line angles. Connecting the line angles creates the outline form. Modification of the outline form may be necessary to facilitate the location of canals and to create convenience form.

The clinician must find the balance between adequate access and removing too much dentin, which could compromise the final restoration. Intimate knowledge of tooth anatomy is mandatory to visualizing where the preparation should be made. Because dentin apposition during development takes place at essentially the same rate all around the circumference of the tooth, the external morphologic structure tends to predict the pulp chamber and canal locations. Shoji[29] showed that the height of contour of a root mimics the canal location. Taking advantage of all information available increases the chances that the visualization is correct. The cross section of a tooth at the cementoenamel junction almost always reveals the upper aspect of the pulp chamber; it is an important for the clinician to understand this part of the anatomy. A thorough investigation of the cervical outline, tooth angulation, and restorations is mandatory. Teeth with full coverage must be approached with caution because the axial alignment may have been changed (see Fig. 7-33, *A-C*).

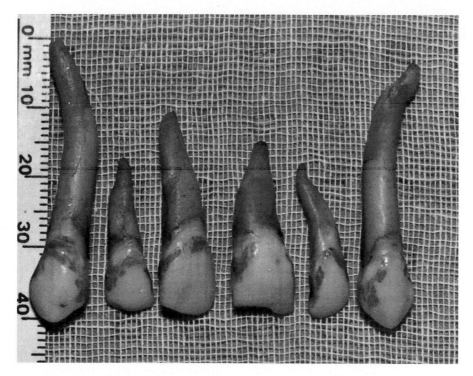

Fig. 7-3 The right maxillary cuspid measures 41 mm from the incisal edge to apex. Note the central incisor is 30 mm long. (From Booth JM: The Longest Tooth? *Aust Endod News* 13(3):17, 1988.)

Access Cavity Preparation in Maxillary Incisors and Cuspids

The maxillary central and lateral incisors have similar anatomy. They have a round root form and a shovel-shaped crown. A projection of the central axis exits incisally to the lingual. The ideal access preparation is an ovoid or rounded-triangle shape on the lingual surface of the tooth, with a slight curve lingually to avoid reducing the incisal edge. Post placement will require a straighter preparation that may involve the incisal edge (Fig. 7-4).

The maxillary cuspid is similar, but the tooth has a more ovoid root form. The access preparation follows this shape, with an ovoid preparation on the lingual surface.

Access Cavity Preparation in Mandibular Incisors and Cuspids

The mandibular incisors may be more problematic. They are significantly broader in the labiolingual dimension than they are mesiodistally. Because there is less tooth structure than the crown would imply, care must be taken to avoid lateral perforation. The cervical cross section varies from a long ovoid to a slightly hourglasslike shape. This cross section is not obvious on a normally angled radiograph, but it can be detected by changing the horizontal angle. Two canals are reported in approximately 41.4% of all mandibular anteriors.[2] Therefore the clinician must always suspect the existence of a second canal.

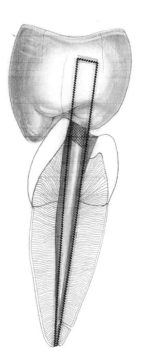

Fig. 7-4 Straight-line access to canals. In some circumstances, coronal tooth structure must be sacrificed to obtain direct access to pulp chambers. Most posterior endodontically treated teeth require full coronal coverage. Ultraconservative access preparation is usually contraindicated. The *hatched area* represents the removal of cuspal hard tissue necessary for ideal access.

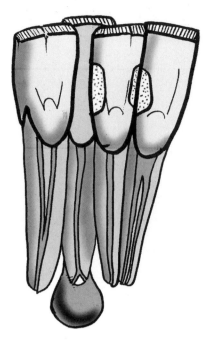

Fig. 7-5 Crowding makes lingual access impossible.

A projection of the central axis of the canal would exit at the incisal edge or even somewhat buccal to the incisal edge. The traditional access, for esthetic reasons, is from the lingual, but it becomes a compromise from the straight-line principle because it must be curved to avoid the incisal edge. In certain circumstances a buccal access may be more desirable for crowding (Fig. 7-5) or structural reasons, and it may involve less compromise of the straight-line principle[25] (Fig. 7-6). If the incisal edge is significantly worn, the access is positioned directly down the long axis of the tooth[9] (Fig. 7-7). The decision regarding which approach to use must be based on ease of access and conservation of as much tooth structure as possible. With modern restorative materials, the repair of a buccal access is esthetically acceptable. The mandibular cuspid has a more mesiodistal width, but otherwise the design principles are the same.

Access Cavity Preparation in Maxillary Premolars

The maxillary first and second premolars require similar access preparation design. Although the first premolar is usually two rooted and the second premolar single rooted, the preparation is ovoid and directed through the middle of the

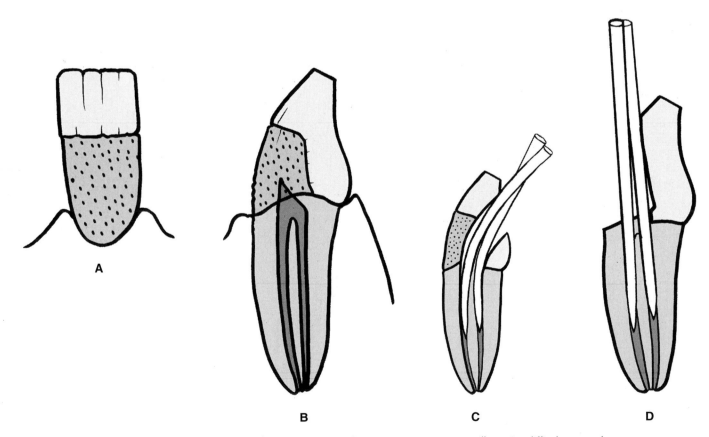

A   **B**   **C**   **D**

Fig. 7-6 **A,** Buccal view of restored incisor. **B,** Proximal view. **C,** Customary access illustrating difficult approach to chambers. **D,** After removal of old restoration. Note straight-line access.

occlusal surface. Teeth with divergent roots require a smaller buccolingual access preparation, and teeth with parallel canals require a more extended preparation. The width of the root at the cervical area is about two-thirds the width at the contacts, which gives the clinician a false sense of available tooth structure. There is mesial concavity common to the first premolar. Therefore a conservative canal preparation is needed to prevent strip perforation toward the mesial (Fig. 7-8).

Access Cavity Preparation in Mandibular Premolars

The mandibular premolars have a rounded cross section. Consequently, the primary canal tends to be located in the middle of the root. Although they usually have only one canal, the mandibular premolars can have significant aberrations in root form. A projection of the canal centerline will usually exit the tooth at the cusp tip (see Fig. 7-4). The ideal access is slightly ovoid, extends toward the buccal cusp tip from the central groove, and will involve the cusp ridge. The occlusal table of the mandibular premolar is rarely perpendicular to the long access of the root. A bur alignment that is perpendicular to the occlusal surface can lead to a perforation toward the buccal (Fig. 7-9).

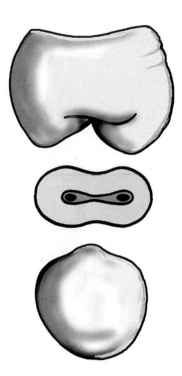

Fig. 7-8 Maxillary premolar showing narrow mesiodistal width and isthmus.

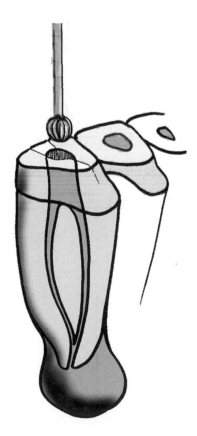

Fig. 7-7 Worn incisor simplifies straight-line access.

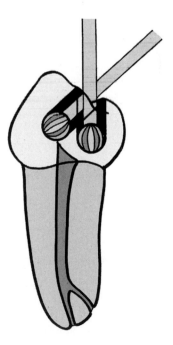

Fig. 7-9 Mandibular premolar showing potential misalignment of bur.

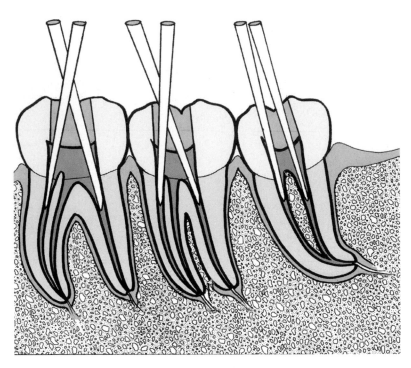

Fig. 7-10 Slight alteration in tooth alignment can create significant changes in the path of insertion of endodontic instruments.

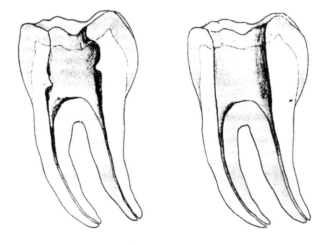

Fig. 7-11 Removal of natural internal protuberances (From Grossman LI: *Root canal therapy*, p. 201, Philadelphia, 1946, Lea & Febiger.)

Access Cavity Preparation in Maxillary Molars

The maxillary molar access preparation is traditionally described as having a triangular form that connects the line angle projections of the mesiobuccal, distobuccal, and lingual canals. The mesiobuccal root of the upper molar is the most complex root in the entire dentition. Various reports credit up to 90% of these roots as having either second canals

or major fins leading off the mesiobuccal canal.[15,23,28,32] These canals usually lie mesial to a line drawn between the mesiobuccal and lingual canals, lying under the mesial marginal ridge. The traditional outline form needs to be modified to a more trapezoidal shape, which must extend mesially to uncover this extra anatomy.

Access Cavity Preparation in Mandibular Molars

The mandibular molar access outline must be an extension of the canal projections to the occlusal surface. If the tooth has a single distal canal, the outline form will usually be triangular in shape (see Fig. 7-36, *B*). If there are two distal canals, the outline is more trapezoidal (see Fig. 7-36, *C*). It should be pointed out that the central groove of the occlusal surface is actually lingual to the central axis of the pulp chamber. The mesiobuccal canal openings of some molars actually lie under the mesiobuccal cusp tip. Slight changes in mesioangulation can change directions necessary for instrument placement (see Fig. 7-36, *A*).

Convenience Form of Molars

There are two important procedures for enhancing visualization and preparation of the radicular canal system after the clinician accesses the main chamber (see Fig. 7-12):

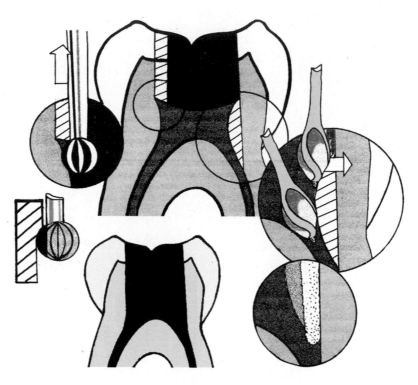

Fig. 7-12   Method for obtaining ideal convenience form.

1. Clearing the overhanging extension of the pulp horns (striped area in Fig. 7-12) is best accomplished using the "belly" of a round bur in a vertical direction.
2. The removal of the natural internal protuberance in the cervical region can be achieved using Gates-Glidden Drills and round-nosed, tapered, diamond instruments (Fig. 7-10). An early illustration appearing in Grossman's *Endodontic Practice*[16] reveals the historical importance of this procedure (Fig. 7-11).

To make file introduction easier, the maxillary molar mesiobuccal canal often requires the extension of convenience form. This convenience form may be enhanced with a Gates-Glidden drill or tapered diamonds used in a sweeping motion up the line angle of the access preparation (Fig. 7-12). Because the dentin may be thin toward the furcation, care must be taken to maintain a small diameter and to apply pressure away from the furca to prevent perforation.

ACCESS PREPARATION GUIDELINES

Most clinicians divide cleaning and shaping into access preparation, radicular shaping, and apical shaping. The clinician can use the following steps to create an excellent access preparation:
1. Because internal anatomy dictates the access shape, the first step in preparing an access is the visualization of the location of the pulp space (Fig. 7-13, *A*). Buccolingual angulations and coronal anatomy are judged visually. Cervical anatomy can be determined tactically, using an explorer under the sulcus to feel the cervical shape (see Fig 7-16, *D*). Palpation along the attached gingiva will help determine root location and direction (see Fig. 7-28). Diagnostic radiographs are then used to estimate pulp chamber position, degree of calcification of the pulp chamber, and the approximate canal length (see Fig. 7-13, *A*). The clinician uses information gained from these investigations to make a decision about the long-axis penetration of the initial bur. In difficult situations it is sometimes recommended that the initial access be prepared without a rubber dam in place.
2. Any restorative material impinging on straight-line access should be removed before the pulp chamber is accessed to prevent the lodging of debris in the canals (see Fig. 7-36, *E*) This is especially important in mandibular teeth. It is not necessary to remove all restorative material; only material that will be in the path of an ideal access. Caries is removed to prevent irrigating solutions from leaking past the rubber dam into the mouth and to prevent bacterial contamination of the canal system with saliva. Occasionally it is necessary to place an interim restoration, creating an efficient seal and facilitating rubber dam placement. A 1 mm to 2 mm occlusal adjustment of teeth may be done to establish a more accurate

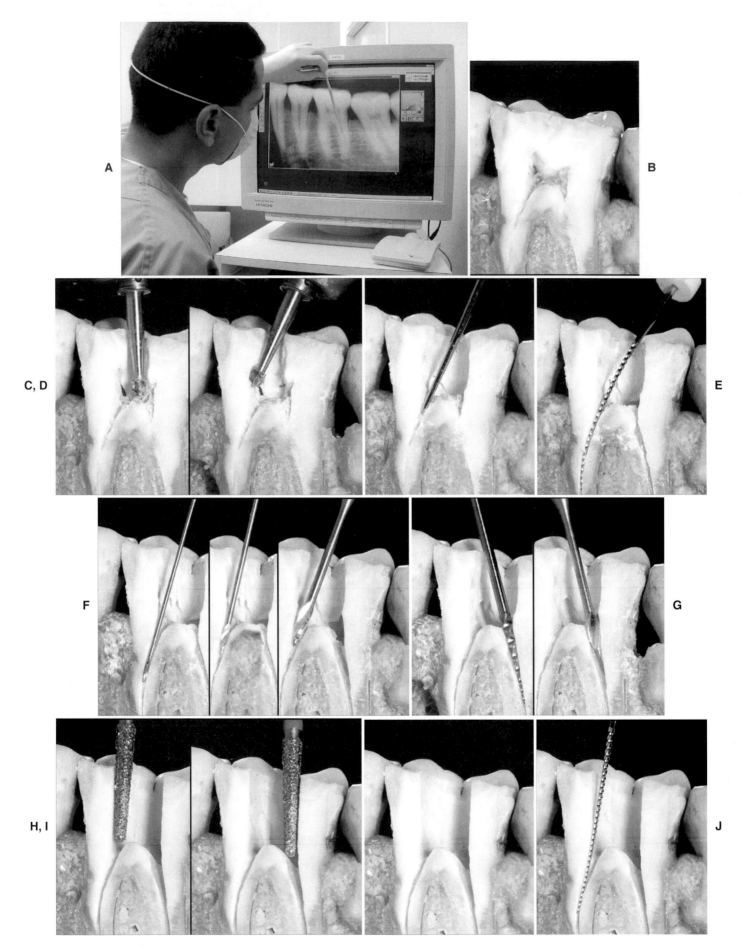

Fig. 7-13 **A-J,** Access preparation guidelines.

point for measuring canal length and to reduce postoperative pressure sensitivity.

3. The roof of the pulp chamber is best perforated with a round bur (see Fig. 7-13, *C*). A no. 2 bur should be used in anterior and premolar teeth, and a no. 4 bur should be used in molar teeth. For teeth with porcelain crowns, a water-cooled, round diamond instrument should be used until dentin is reached; this prevents fracture of the thin porcelain (see Fig. 7-15). The bur is best directed toward the largest part of the pulp chamber. In calcified, multi-rooted teeth, it is better to direct the access toward the largest canal. This will increase the likelihood of locating the canal and avoiding perforation.

4. Once the pulp chamber is located (with light upward pressure), the round bur is used to remove the roof of the pulp chamber from underneath; the "belly" of the bur should be used to cut on the out-stroke (see Fig. 7-13, *C* and Fig. 7-12). This should establish an initial outline form. The pulp chamber should be frequently flushed with a sodium hypochlorite solution to remove debris and bacteria.

5. A sharp DG 16 double-ended explorer is used to locate canal orifices and to determine their angle of departure from the main chamber (see Figs. 7-13, *D* and 7-14). In heavily calcified teeth the use of enhanced vision, transillumination, and the careful examination of internal dentin color aids in canal location (see Figs. 7-17 and 7-18). A fiber-optic light can be applied to the cervical aspect of the crown, which often reveals subtle landmarks that are otherwise invisible.

6. Once the canals are located, a no. 10 or no. 15 K type of file is introduced into the canal to determine patency (see Fig. 7-13, *E*). If the canal is large enough to place a no. 20 or no. 25 file, the clinician can progress to the next step. If the canal is narrow, the upper portion needs to be instrumented with K-type or Hedstrom files to provide space for the use of Gates-Glidden drills. Hedstrom files may be used with lateral pressure away from the furcation to move the canal laterally to avoid perforation. Tooth length may be determined at this point, but it can also be delayed until later. Care must be taken to keep the files within the canal system until the length is accurately determined. A lubrication agent, such as RC Prep, which is a water-based preparation that will not congeal vital pulp tissue, may be introduced. Congealed pulp tissue can potentially form a collagen plug at the apex that could block the apex from cleaning and shaping.[7]

7. The next step is to initiate the radicular access. There are two ways to accomplish this. The traditional and most popular method (as described in Chapter 8) is to use a Gates-Glidden drill in a step-back fashion (see Fig. 7-13, *F*). This technique involves forming a tapered shape by introducing the smallest Gates-Glidden drill to light resistance, followed by larger drills at progressively less depth. The clinician should introduce it into the canal until resistance is felt. It is important not to force the drill apically. The no. 1, no. 2, and no. 3 Gates-Glidden drills are used for the radicular step-back. The no. 4, no. 5, no. 6 Gates-Glidden drills are only used coronal to the canal orifice to create a funnel or flare shape to facilitate the ease of file introduction. This procedure will establish a convenience form that creates a more straight-line access into the canal. Convenience form is established by using the Gates-Glidden drill in a sweeping, upward motion, with lateral pressure away from the furcation. An alternative method is to use an 0.08 to 0.12 tapered, engine-driven nickel and titanium file to establish the upper canal shape; then to flare the orifice with a no. 5 or no. 6 Gates-Glidden drill (see Fig. 7-13, *G*).

8. Final outline form is established with a round-tip, tapered, diamond bur after the canals have been located and the initial opening has been completed (see Fig. 7-13, *H*). This important outline form (described in the *Ideal Access* section and illustrated in the plates provided in this chapter) is dictated by the internal anatomy and modified to improve visibility, establish convenience form, and conserve critical tooth structure (see Fig. 7-13, *I* and *J*).

USE OF PATHFINDER FOR LOCATING ORIFICES

After the pulp chamber is opened, the canal orifices are located with the endodontic pathfinder (Fig. 7-14). This instrument is to the endodontist what a probe is to the periodontist. Reaching, feeling, and often digging at the hard tissue, it is the extension of the clinician's fingers. Natural anatomy dictates the usual places for orifices, but restorations, dentinal protrusions, and dystrophic calcifications can

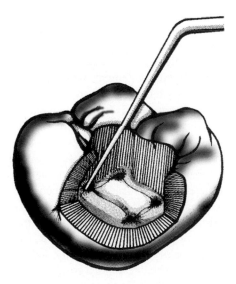

Fig. 7-14 The endodontic pathfinder is indispensable in endodontic treatment. It serves as an explorer to locate orifices, as an indicator of canal angulation, and as a chipping tool to remove calcification.

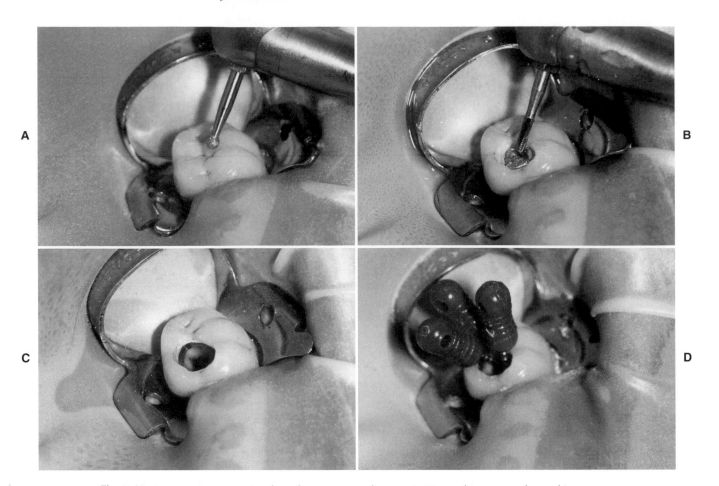

Fig. 7-15 Access cavity preparation through a ceramometal crown. **A,** Diamond-impregnated, round instrument. **B,** After access outline is made with the round diamond, an end-cutting or round-carbide bur cuts through the metal. **C,** Access cavity prepared, allowing direct approach to the canals. **D,** Test files placed without impingement on the access cavity walls.

alter the actual configuration the clinician encounters. While probing the chamber floor, the pathfinder often penetrates or dislodges calcific deposits blocking an orifice.

Positioning the instrument in the orifice enables the clinician to check the shaft for clearance of the orifice walls. Additionally, the pathfinder is used to determine the angle at which the canals depart the main chamber (see Figs. 7-10, 7-13, *D*, and 7-16).

The endodontic pathfinder is preferred over the rotating bur as the instrument for locating canal orifices (see Fig. 7-14). The double-ended design offers two angles of approach.

ACCESS THROUGH FULL-VENEER CROWNS

Properly made crowns are constructed with the occlusal relationship of the opposing tooth as a primary consideration. A cast crown may be made in any shape, diameter, height, or angle; this cast crown alteration can destroy the visual relationship to the true long axis (see Fig. 7-33, *A-C*). Careful

study of the preoperative radiograph identifies most of these situations.

Achieving access through crowns (Fig. 7-15) should be done with coolants, even when the rubber dam is used. Friction-generated heat can damage adjacent soft tissue, including the periodontal ligament; with an anesthetized or nonvital tooth, the patient is not aware of pain. Once penetration of the metal is accomplished, the clinician can change to a sharp, round bur and move toward the central pulp chamber. Metal filings and debris from the access cavity should be removed frequently, because small slivers can cause large obstructions in the fine canal system.

When sufficient access has been gained, the clinician should search margins and internal spaces for caries and leaks. The clinician should also search the pulpal floor for signs of fracture or perforation. Occasionally, caries can be removed through the occlusal access cavity, and the tooth can be properly restored. The interior of a crown can be a surprise package, containing everything from extensive caries to intact dentin (as seen in periodontally induced pulpal necrosis).

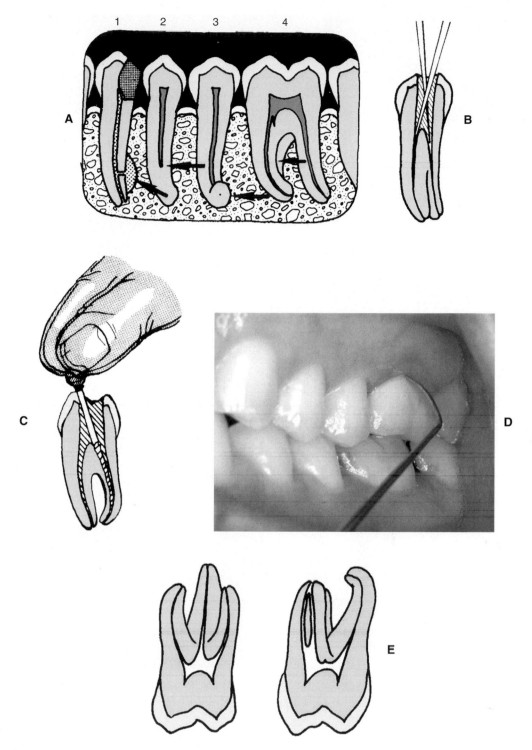

Fig. 7-16 **A,** A radiograph reveals many clues to anatomic "aberrations": (1) Lateral radiolucencies indicating the presence of lateral or accessory canals; (1 & 2) An abrupt ending of a large canal signifying a bifurcation; (3) A knob-like image indicating an apex that curves toward or away from the beam of the radiograph machine; (4) Multiple vertical lines shown in this curved mesial root indicate the possibility of a thin root, which may be hourglass shaped in cross section and susceptible to perforation. **B,** The endodontic pathfinder inserted into the orifice openings reveals the direction the canals take in leaving the main chamber. **C,** Digital perception with a hand instrument can identify curvatures, obstruction, root division, and additional canal orifices. **D,** Cervical anatomy can be tactilely identified with a pathfinder. **E,** Intimate knowledge of root formation can save the clinician difficulties with instrumentation. For example, root formation in what appears (radiographically) to be an average palatal root of a maxillary first permanent molar (1) is actually a root with a sharp, apical curvature toward the buccal aspect (2).

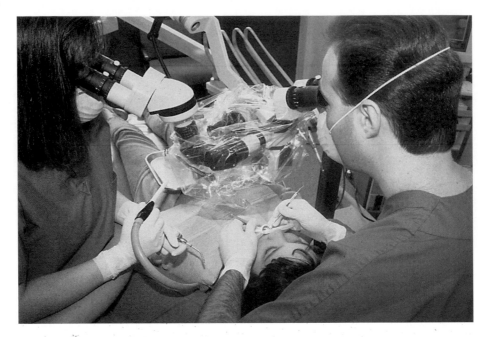

Fig. 7-17 The widespread adaptation of the operating microscope has provided exceptional advances in locating canal anatomy.

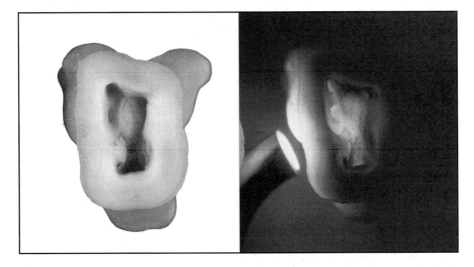

Fig. 7-18 As an adjunct to maximal visibility with magnification, the fiber-optic light can be applied to the cervical aspect of the crown. Transillumination often reveals landmarks otherwise invisible to the unaided eye.

INTRODUCTION TO PLATES

The anatomy represented in the following plates is taken from real human teeth, using recently developed three-dimensional (3-D) imaging technology. The teeth were scanned in a high-resolution, microcomputer-assisted tomographic scanner. This data was then manipulated with proprietary computer programs to produce the 3-D reconstructions and visualization. The following individuals made this project possible:

Tomograph scan: Courtesy Michael J. Flynn, PhD; Head, X-ray Imaging Research Lab; Henry Ford Health Science; Detroit, Michigan; Professor (Adjunct); Nuclear Engineering and Radiological Science; University of Michigan

3-D reconstructions and visualization: Courtesy Kevin Montgomery, PhD; Technical Director; Stanford-NASA National Biocomputation Center; Palo Alto, California

Facilitator: Dr. Paul Brown

Radiographs: Courtesy Dr. L. Stephen Buchanan and Dr. John Khademi

Anatomic variation illustrations: From the work of the late Quintiliano deDeus of Brazil*

Access cavity illustrations: Designed and formatted by Dr. Richard Burns and Dr. Eric Herbranson

---

*de Deus QD: *Endodontia,* ed 4, Rio de Janeiro, 1986, Medsi Editôra Médica e Cientifica, Ltda.

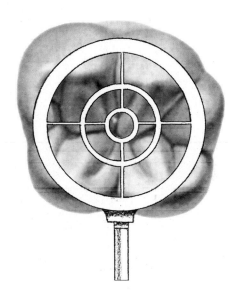

PLATE I
Maxillary Central Incisor

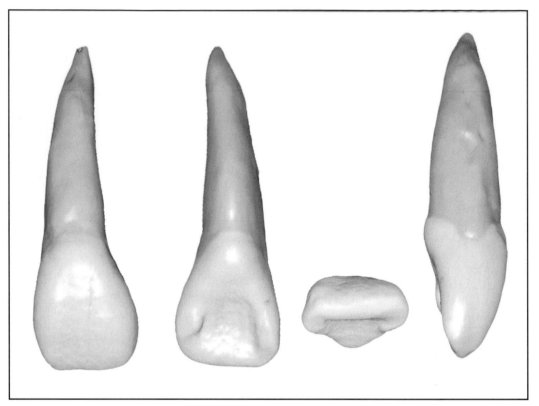

Average time of eruption: 7 to 8 years
Average age of calcification: 10 years
Average length: 22.5 mm

Somewhat rectangular from the labial aspect and shovel shaped from the proximal, the crown of the maxillary central incisor is more than adequate for endodontic access and is positioned ideally for direct-mirror viewing. This tooth is especially suitable for a first clinical experience, because more than one third of its canal is directly visible. Viewing of the canal proper may be enhanced with fiber-optic illumination.

The first entry point, with a round bur, is made just above the cingulum. The direction should be in the long axis of the root. A roughly triangular opening is made in anticipation of the final shape of the access cavity. Penetration of the shallow pulp chamber often occurs during initial entry. When the sensation of "dropping through the roof" of the pulp chamber is felt, the round bur is used to sweep out toward the incisal

edge. The clinician must be certain to completely expose the entire chamber. A long, round-nose, tapered, diamond bur may be used to extend and refine the access cavity.

Conical and rapidly tapering toward the apex, the root morphology is quit distinctive. Cross-sectionally, the radicular canal is slightly triangular at the cervical aspect, gradually becoming round as it approaches the apical foramen. Multiple canals are rare, but accessory and lateral canals are common. Kasahara et al[20] studied 510 maxillary central incisors to determine thickness and curvature of the root canal and locations of the canals. Data revealed that over 60% of the specimens showed accessory canals, and the apical foramen was located apart from the apex in 45% of the teeth.

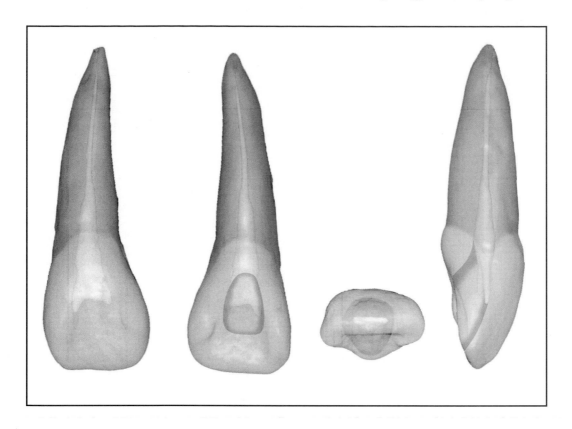

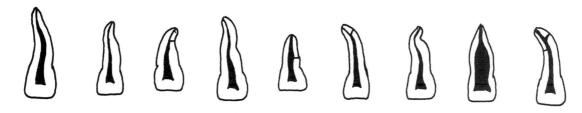

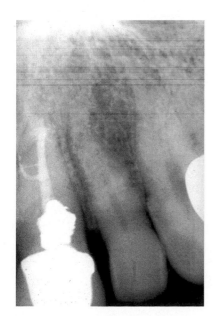

PLATE 7-I-1 Curved accessory canal with straight, lateral canal intersecting.

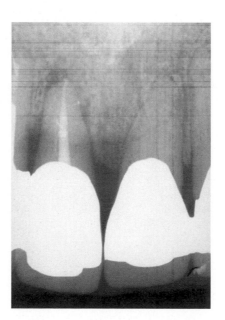

PLATE 7-I-2 Parallel accessory canal to main canal with simple lateral canal.

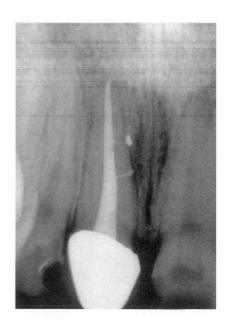

PLATE 7-I-3 Double lateral canals.

PLATE II
Maxillary Lateral Incisor

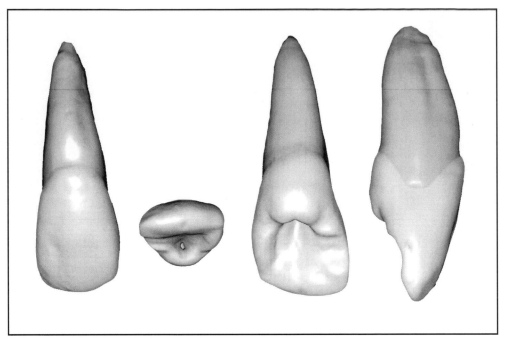

Average time of eruption: 8 to 9 years
Average age of calcification: 11 years
Average length: 22.0 mm

Tending toward an oval shape, the crown of the maxillary lateral incisor is nearly ideal for endodontic access. The initial entry, with a no. 2 or no. 4 round bur, is made just above the cingulum. The access cavity is ovoid. It is refined with either a round bur or a long, round-nose, tapered, diamond bur.

A number of rare morphologic oddities occur in the lateral incisor. Occasionally the crown is "pegged" and assumes the shape of a blunt-ended pencil. If the tooth is to be crowned after the endodontic procedure, the access preparation should extend down the middle of the crown; otherwise the access preparation is made on the lingual. Some lateral incisors have a deep cleft on the lingual, starting at the cingulum. On rare occasions this cleft extends apically into the root structure, creating an untreatable periodontal defect.

The radicular cross section of the pulp chamber varies from ovoid at the cervical foramen to round at the apical foramen. The root is slightly conical and tends toward a slight curvature, whereas the apex will often curve toward the distal.

Occasionally access may be complicated by a *dens in dente* (i.e., an invagination of part of the lingual surface of the tooth into the crown). A *dens in dente* most commonly occurs in the lateral incisor, having a frequency from 0.04% to 10%. These teeth are predisposed to decay because of the anatomic malformation, and the pulp may be involved before the root apex has completely developed.[19] Cases have been reported where pulps have remained vital.[33]

Goon et al[14] reported the first case of complex involvement of the entire facial aspect of a tooth root. An alveolar crest to apex facial root defect led to early pulpal necrosis and periapical rarefaction.[14]

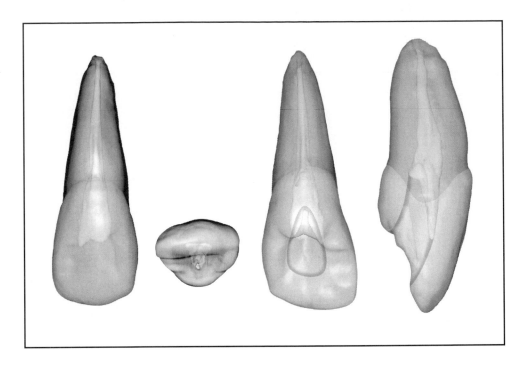

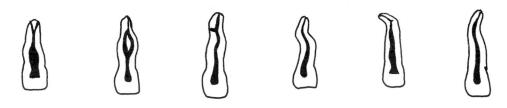

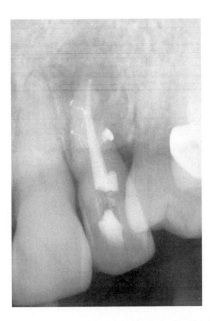

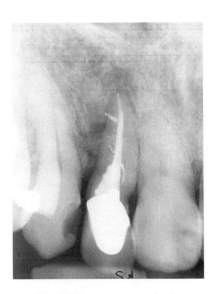

PLATE 7-II-1   Lateral incisor with a canal loop and multiple canals with associated lesions.

PLATE 7-II-2   Multiple portals of exit.

PLATE III
Maxillary Canine

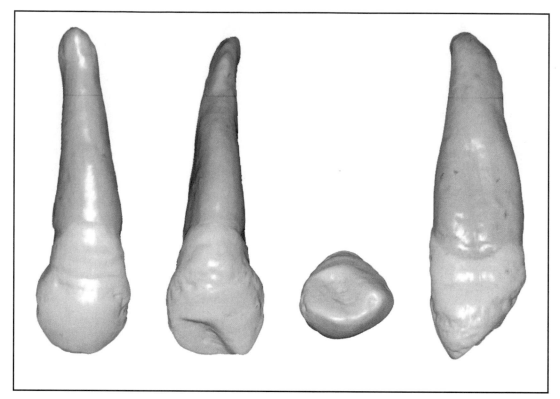

Average time of eruption: 10 to 12 years
Average age of calcification: 13 to 15 years
Average length: 26.5 mm

The longest tooth in the dental arch, the canine, has a formidable shape designed to withstand heavy occlusal stress. Its long, thickly enameled crown sustains heavy incisal wear and often displays deep cervical erosion from aging.

The access cavity corresponds to the lingual crown shape and is ovoid. To achieve straight-line access, the clinician must extend the cavity incisally. Care should be taken not to weaken the heavily functioning cusp excessively. Initial access is made slightly below midcrown on the lingual side using a no. 2 or no. 4 round bur, and it is refined with a long, tapered, round-tip diamond bur. If the pulp chamber is located apically, a long-shank bur may be necessary. The sweeping-out motion of this bur reveals an ovoid pulp chamber. The chamber remains ovoid as it continues apically through and below the cervical region. Attention must be paid to circumferential filing so that this ovoid chamber is thoroughly cleaned.

The radicular canal is reasonably straight and quite long; many canines require instruments that are longer than 25 mm. The apex often curves in the last 2 to 3 mm, and it can turn in any direction.

The thin buccal bone over the eminence often disintegrates, and fenestration is an occasional finding. Accurate length determination is critical. Another ramification of this fenestration is a slight, permanent apical pressure sensitivity that occasionally occurs after endodontic therapy. This sensitivity can best be corrected with apical surgery. The apical foramen is usually close to the anatomic apex but may be laterally positioned. In either case, the surgical access, if necessary, is relatively easy.

Canine morphology seldom varies, and lateral and accessory canals occur less frequently than in the maxillary incisors.

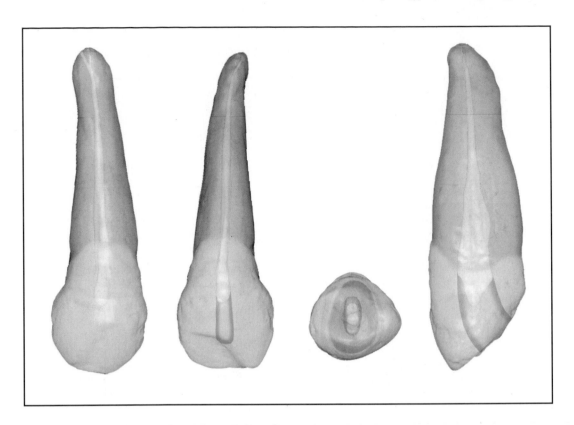

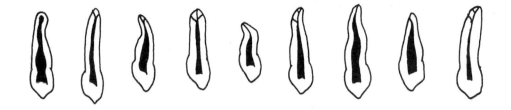

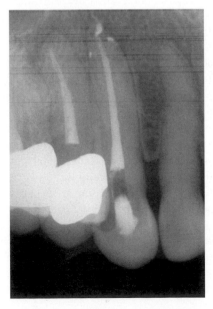

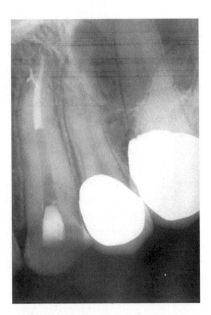

PLATE 7-III-1 Canine with multiple accessory foramina.

PLATE 7-III-2 Maxillary canine with lateral canal dividing into two additional canals.

PLATE IV
Maxillary First Premolar

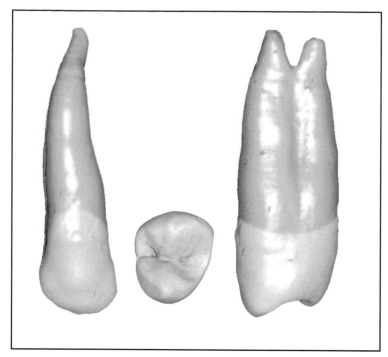

Average time of eruption: 10 to 11 years
Average age of calcification: 12 to 13 years
Average length: 20.6 mm

Most commonly two rooted, the maxillary first premolar is a transitional tooth between incisor and molar. The canal orifices lie below and slightly central to the cusp tips. The initial opening is made with a round bur into the central fossa and is ovoid in the buccolingual dimension. The preparation is refined with a round-nose, tapered, long diamond bur. When one canal orifice is located, the clinician should look for a developmental groove leading to other orifices.

Where posterior occlusion has been lost early in life, the premolars are exposed to excess occlusal loads and possibly torque loads from a removable appliance. These can induce heavy calcification of the pulp chamber and make locating canals difficult, if not impossible. Because the cervical width is narrower mesiodistally, the clinician must use caution to avoid perforation. Many of these teeth have a concavity on the mesial, which make the area below the pulp chamber laterally thin. This must be taken into account when locating canals, opening the orifice of the canals, and during post build up procedures. This is a less robust tooth than the crown size would indicate.

Radicular irregularities consist of fused roots with separate canals, fused roots with interconnections or "webbing," fused roots with a common apical foramen, and the unusual three-rooted tooth. In the last instance the buccal orifices are usually not clearly visible. Directional positioning of the endodontic pathfinder or a small file will identify the anatomy. Carns and Skidmore[7] reported that the incidence of maxillary first premolars with three roots, three canals, and three foramen was 6% of the cases studied.

The roots are considerably shorter and thinner than the cuspid. In two-rooted teeth the roots are most often the same length. The apical foramen is usually close to the anatomic apex, and the apical portion of the roots often tapers rapidly, ending in extremely narrow and curved root tips. The buccal root can fenestrate through the bone, leading to the same problems that occur with cuspids (i.e., inaccurate apex location, chronic post-operative sensitivity to palpation over the apex, increased risk of an irrigation accident).

This tooth is prone to mesiodistal root fractures and fractures at the base of the cusps, particularly the buccal cusp. If a fracture is suspected all the restorations should be removed and the coronal anatomy inspected with fiber-optic light and magnification. After endodontic therapy, full occlusal coverage is mandatory to ensure against cuspal and crown and root fracture.

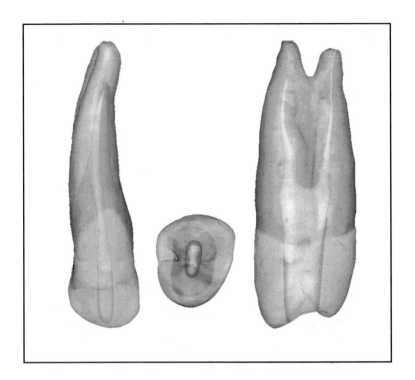

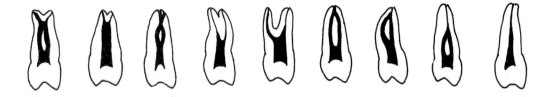

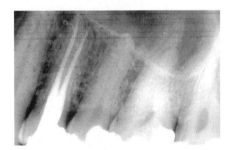

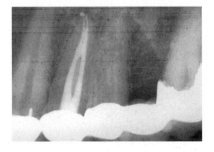

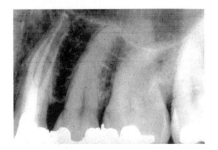

PLATE 7-IV-1 Lateral bony lesion associated with filled lateral canal.

PLATE 7-IV-2 Two canals fusing and redividing.

PLATE 7-IV-3 Three canals in a maxillary first premolar.

PLATE V
Maxillary Second Premolar

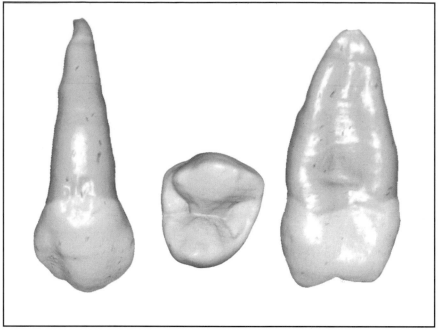

Average time of eruption: 10 to 12 years
Average age of calcification: 12 to 14 years
Average length: 21.5 mm

Similar to the first premolar in coronal morphology, the second premolar varies mainly in root form. Although the first premolar most often has two roots, the second premolar usually has one root. It may have two separate canals, two canals anastomosing to a single canal, or two canals with interconnections or "webbing." Accessory and lateral canals may be present, but they are present less often than in incisors. Vertucci et al[36] stated that 75% of maxillary second premolars had one canal at the apex, 24% had two foramina, and 1% had three foramina. Of the teeth studied 59.9% had accessory canals. These clinicians also reported that when two canals join into one, the lingual canal exhibits a straight-line access to the apex. They further pointed out that if the canal shows a sudden narrowing or even disappears, it means the canal has divided into two parts. These two parts can either remain separate or merge before reaching the apex.[36]

The root length of the maxillary second premolar is much like the first premolar and apical curvature is common, particularly with large sinus cavities. This proximity to the sinus can lead to a periapical abscess draining into the sinus and exposure of the sinus during apical surgery.

Like the maxillary first premolar, this tooth is prone to mesiodistal root fractures and fractures at the base of the cusps, usually the buccal cusp. If a fracture is suspected all the restorations in the tooth should be removed and the coronal anatomy inspected with fiber-optic light and magnification. After endodontic therapy full occlusal coverage is mandatory to ensure against cuspal and crown and root fracture.

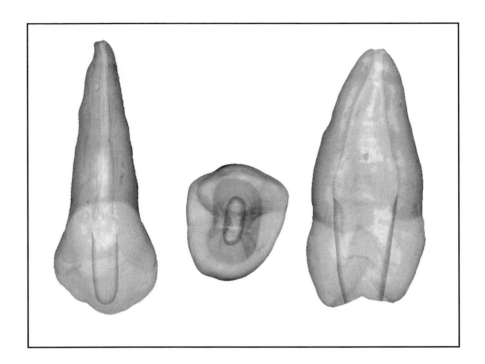

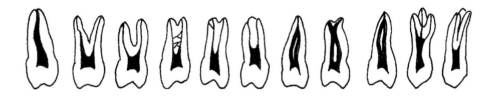

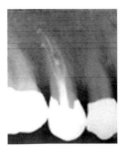

PLATE 7-V-1 An unusual three-canalled second premolar with a large lateral canal.

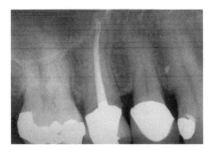

PLATE 7-V-2 Single canal dividing into two canals.

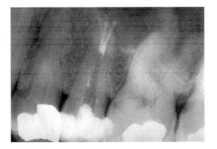

PLATE 7-V-3 Single canal splitting into three canals.

PLATE VII
Maxillary Second Molar

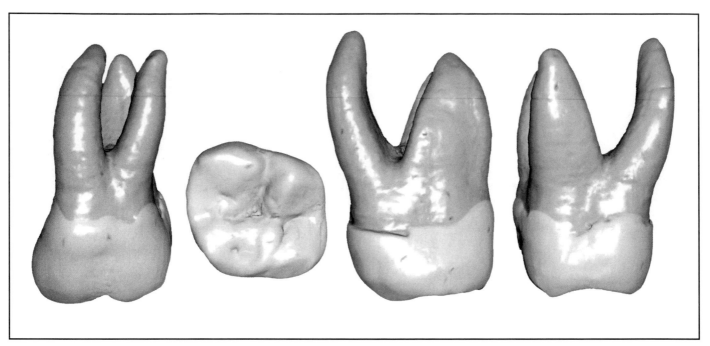

Average time of eruption: 11 to 13 years
Average age of calcification: 14 to 16 years
Average length: 20.0 mm

Coronally, the maxillary second molar closely resembles the maxillary first molar, although it is not as large. Access in both teeth can usually be prepared without disturbing the transverse ridge. The second molar is often easier to prepare because of the straight-line access to the orifice.

The distinguishing morphologic feature of the maxillary second molar is that its three roots are grouped closer together and are sometimes fused. They are usually shorter than the roots of the first molar and not as curved. The occurrence of four canals is less likely than in the first molar. The three orifices may form a flat triangle; sometimes almost a straight line. The floor of the chamber is markedly convex, giving a slightly funnel shape to the canal orifices. Occasionally the canals curve into the chamber at a more horizontal angle, making it necessary to remove a "lip" of dentin so that the canal can be entered more in a direct line with the canal axis. Teeth with fused roots occasionally have only two canals; rarely only one. Two-canalled teeth usually have a buccal and a lingual canal of equal length and diameter. These parallel root canals are frequently superimposed radiographically, but they can be imaged by exposing the radiograph from a distal angle. To enhance radiographic visibility, especially when there is interference with the malar process, a more perpendicular and distoangular radiograph may be exposed.

Initial access opening is with a round bur, which is ideally suited to uncover the pulp chamber followed by a round-nose, tapered, diamond bur to refine the outline form. The second molar is frequently tipped to the distal or buccal or both, which can complicate access, especially when the opening is limited or the mouth is small. A distally tipped tooth may require exaggerated convenience form to allow adequate access to the mesiobuccal canal. Buccal tipping can confuse the perception of long axis of the canals and lead to access errors. Fracture patterns are similar to that of the first molar.

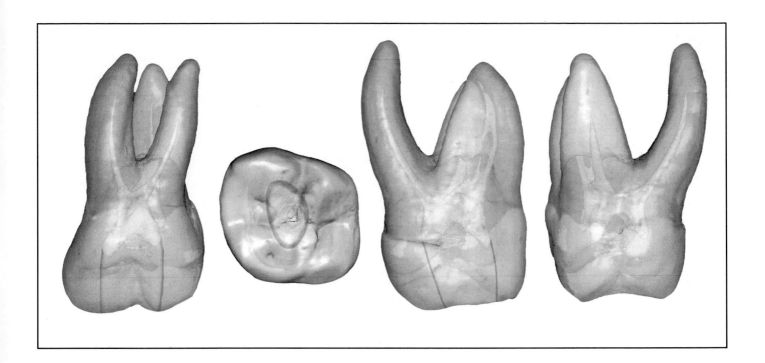

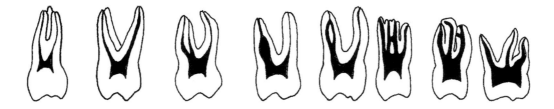

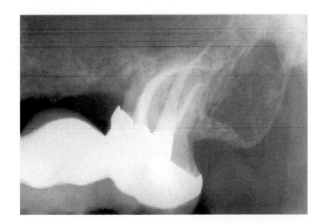

PLATE 7-VII-1 Severely curved mesiobuccal root, with right-angle curve in distobuccal root.

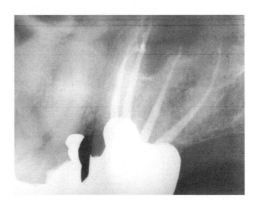

PLATE 7-VII-2 Four-rooted maxillary second molar.

PLATE VIII
Maxillary Third Molar

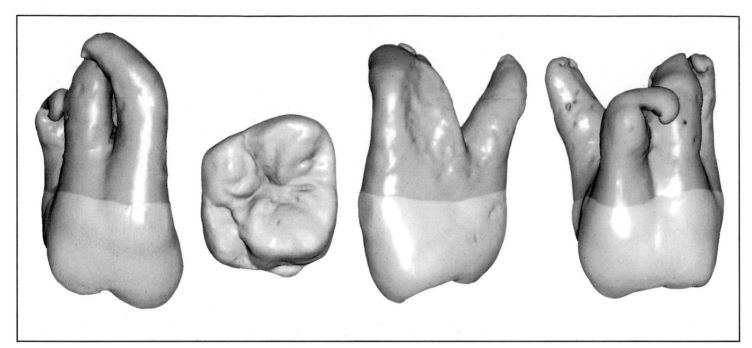

Average time of eruption: 17 to 22 years
Average age of calcification: 18 to 25 years
Average length: 17.0 mm

Loss of the maxillary first and second molar is often the reason for considering the third molar as a strategic abutment. Another indication for endodontic treatment and full coverage is a fully functioning mandibular third molar in an arch, with sufficient room for full eruption and oral hygiene.

Careful examination of root morphology is important before recommending treatment. The radicular anatomy of the third molar is completely unpredictable, and it may be advisable to explore the root canal morphology before promising success. However, many third molars have adequate root formation and, given reasonable accessibility, there is no reason why they cannot remain as functioning dentition after endodontic therapy.

There is significant variation in root anatomy. Some teeth have only one canal and some have two canals, but most teeth have three canals. Access preparation outline form is dictated by the internal anatomy. Many will be triangular; some will be nearly a straight line. There is the potential for significant tipping to the distal or buccal or both. This can create an even greater access problem than the second molar.

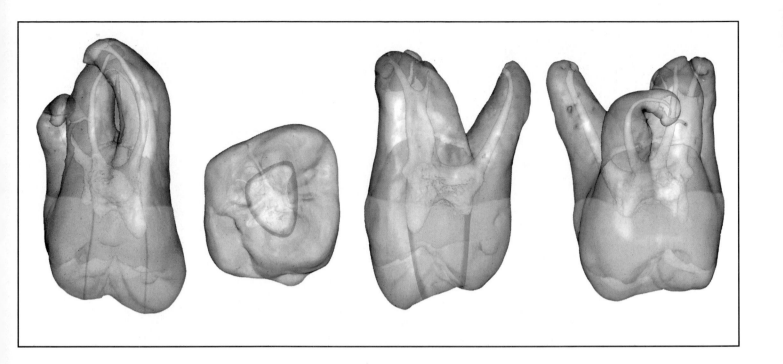

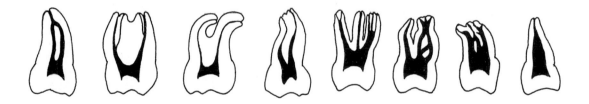

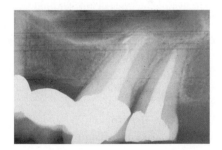

PLATE 7-VIII-1 Showing canals fusing into single canal. Note multiple accessories in second molar.

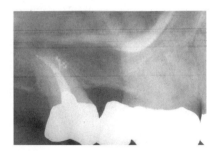

PLATE 7-VIII-2 Distal bridge abutment with major accessory canal.

PLATE IX
Mandibular Central and Lateral Incisors

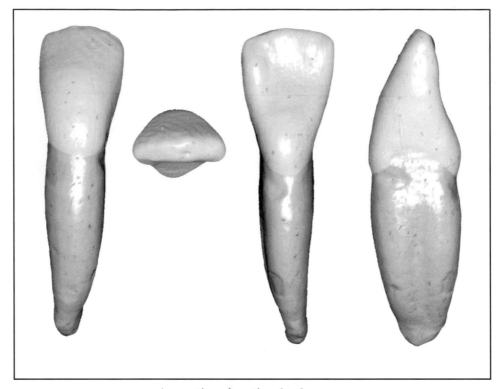

Average time of eruption: 6 to 8 years
Average age of calcification: 9 to 10 years
Average length: 20.7 mm

Narrow and flat in the buccolingual dimension, the mandibular incisors are the smallest human adult teeth. Visible radiographically from only two planes, they often appear more accessible then they really are and can be a treatment challenge. The narrow lingual crown offers a limited area for access. A no. 2 round bur is ideal for creating the access preparation. The access outline form is ovoid (see Fig. 7-4). The traditional access is from the lingual, but a labial approach may be more appropriate in some situations (see Fig. 7-6, *A-D*).

Frequently the mandibular incisors have two canals. One study[2] reported 41.4% of mandibular incisors had two separate canals; of these only 1.3% had separate foramina. The clinician should always search for a second canal. Radiographically, if an obvious canal suddenly disappears, the clinician should be suspicious of two canals. Endodontic

failure in mandibular incisors usually arises from uncleaned canals, most commonly toward the lingual portion of the pulp chamber. A labial access makes the lingual canal easier to find and clean. Two-rooted lower incisors are common (see Fig 7-7).

Although labial perforations are common, they may be avoided if the clinician remembers that it is nearly impossible to perforate in a lingual direction with a lingual access. A ribbon-shaped canal is normal and demands special attention in cleaning and shaping. The narrow mesiodistal root width (compared to the crown width) invites lateral perforation. Care must be taken to align the bur with the long axis of the tooth.

Apical curvatures and accessory canals are common in mandibular incisors.

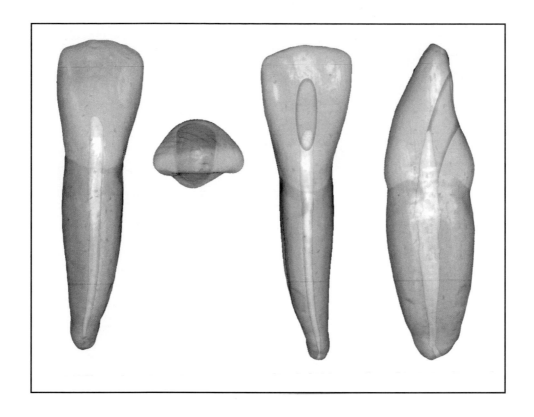

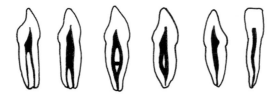

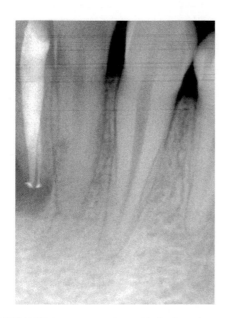

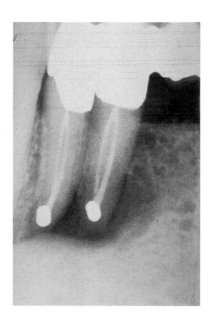

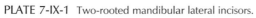

PLATE 7-IX-1 Two-rooted mandibular lateral incisors.

PLATE 7-IX-2 Mandibular lateral and central; both with two canals.

PLATE X
Mandibular Canine

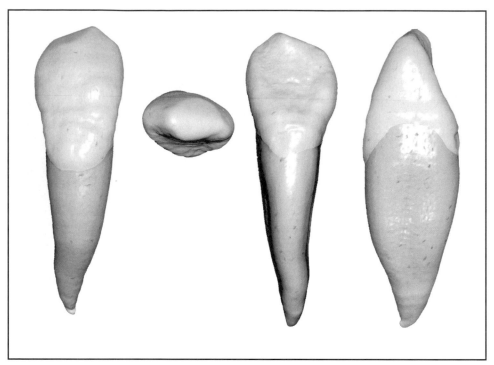

Average time of eruption: 9 to 10 years
Average age of calcification: 13 years
Average length: 25.6 mm

Sturdy and considerably wider mesiodistally than the incisors, the mandibular canines seldom display endodontic problems. Occasionally they have two canals and two roots.

The access cavity is ovoid and may extend incisally for access. The canal is somewhat ovoid at the cervical area, but it becomes rounder at the apex. Care must be taken to adequately débride the walls.

If there are two roots, one is always easier to instrument. The other must be opened and funneled in concert with the first canal to prevent packing of dentin debris and loss of access (see Fig. 7-30). Precurving of instruments at initial access enables the clinician to trace down the buccal or lingual root wall until the tip engages the orifice. When the difficult canal is located, every effort should be made to shape and funnel the opening to maintain continued access.

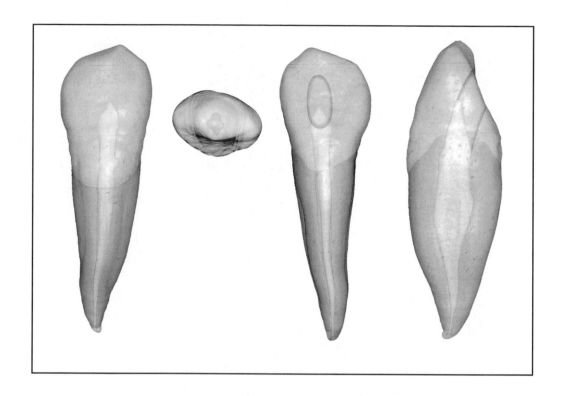

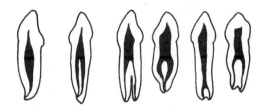

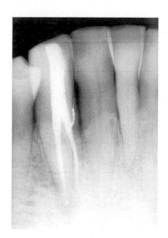

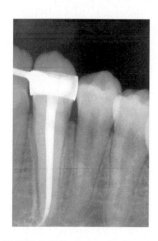

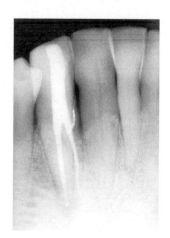

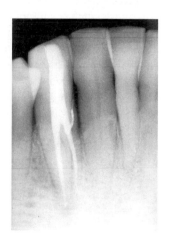

PLATE 7-X-1 Two-rooted mandibular canine.

PLATE 7-X-2 Sharp distal curvature at apex.

PLATE 7-X-3 Two lateral canals. The incisal canal is above the crest of bone; it was probably responsible for pocket depth.

PLATE 7 X-4 Twin-canalled mandibular canine, with significant lateral canals feeding a periodontal defect.

PLATE XI
Mandibular First Premolar

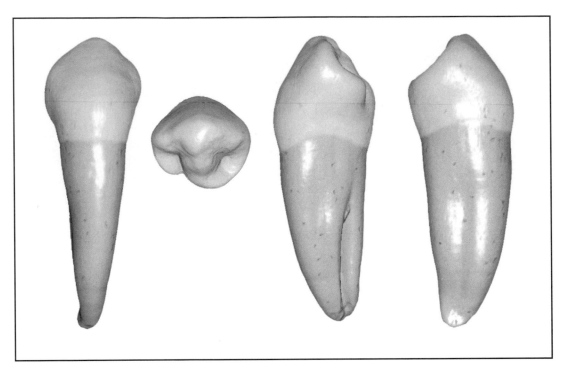

Average time of eruption: 10 to 12 years
Average age of calcification: 12 to 13 years
Average length: 21.6 mm

The mandibular first premolar can be very easy or very difficult to treat. The root anatomy can hide complexity that is not obvious on the radiograph.

The coronal anatomy consists of a well-developed buccal cusp and a small (or almost nonexistent) lingual cusp. The centerline of the root extends through the cusp tip; the access preparation starts at the central groove and extends toward the cusp tip, often involving the cusp ridge. This ovoid outline form is made with a no. 2 or no. 4 round bur, followed by a round-tip, long, tapered, diamond bur. Care must be taken to align the bur with the long axis of the root. Buccal perforation is a common untoward result (see Fig. 7-9). A cross section of the pulp chamber is almost round in single-canalled teeth and ovoid in two-canalled teeth. The centerline of the root extends through the cusp tip.

Zillich and Dowson[43] reported that "a second or third canal exists in at least 23% of first mandibular premolars." The canals may divide almost anywhere down the root. Because of the absence of direct access, cleaning, shaping, and filling of these teeth can be extremely difficult.

A study by Vertucci[35] revealed that the mandibular first premolar had one canal at the apex in 74% of the teeth studied, two canals at the apex in 25.5%, and three canals at the apex in the remaining 0.5% (see Fig 7-2). Baisden, Kulild, and Weller[1] reported the existence of C-shaped canals in 14% of the roots of mandibular first premolars that had one root canal and two apical foramina.

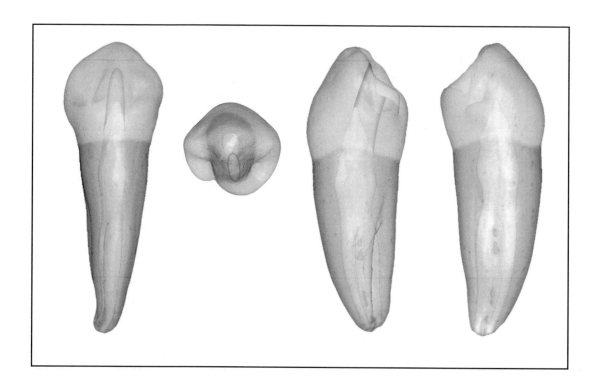

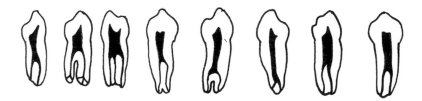

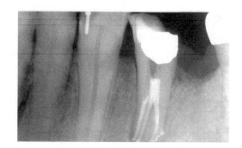

PLATE 7-XI-1 Three-rooted mandibular first premolar.

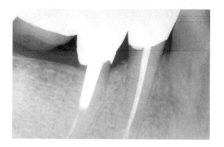

PLATE 7-XI-2 Single canal dividing at apex.

PLATE XII
Mandibular Second Premolar

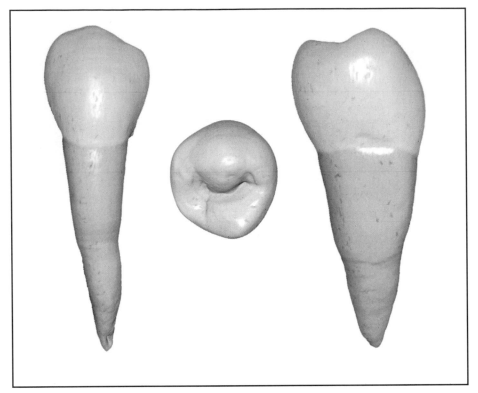

Average time of eruption: 11 to 12 years
Average age of calcification: 13 to 14 years
Average length: 22.3 mm

Very similar coronally to the first premolar, the mandibular second premolar presents less of a radicular problem. Its crown has a buccal cusp that is well developed and a lingual cusp that is better formed than the first premolar. Access is similar, with a slight ovoid outline form extending from the central groove toward the cusp tip and involving the cusp ridge.

Investigators[35] reported that only 12% of mandibular second premolars studied had a second or third canal. Vertucci, Seelig, and Gillis[36] showed that the second premolar had one canal at the apex in 97.5% of mandibular second molars and two canals in only 2.5% of the teeth studied. In 1991 Bram and Fleisher[4] reported a case of four distinct canals.

An important consideration that must not be overlooked with this tooth is the anatomic position of the mental foramen and the neurovascular structures that pass through it. The proximity of these nerves and blood vessels can result in temporary paresthesia from a fulminating inflammatory process when acute periapical abscess occurs with the mandibular second premolar. Exacerbations in this region seem to be more intense and resistant to nonsurgical therapy than other parts of the mouth.

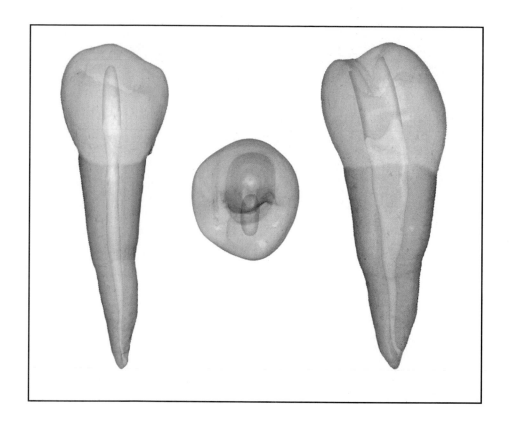

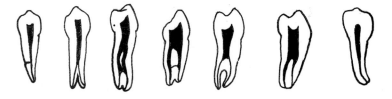

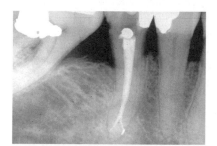

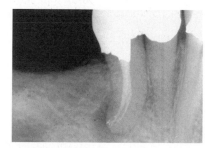

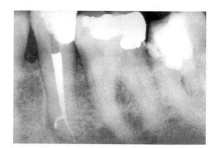

PLATE 7-XII-1 Single canal dividing at apex.

PLATE 7-XII-2 Single canal dividing and crossing over at apex.

PLATE 7-XII-3 Single canal with lateral accessory canal.

PLATE XIII
Mandibular First Molar

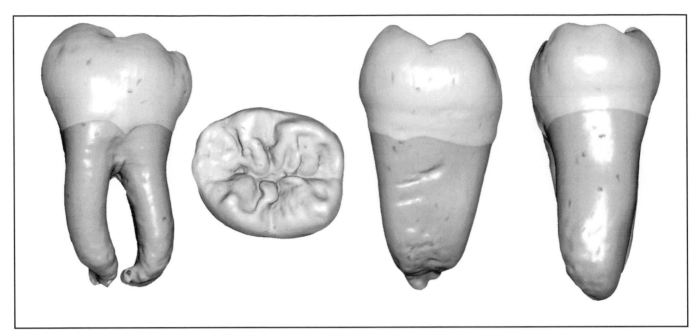

Average time of eruption: 6 years
Average age of calcification: 9 to 10 years
Average length: 21.0 mm

The earliest permanent posterior tooth to erupt, the mandibular first molar, seems to be the tooth most frequently in need of endodontic treatment. Although it usually has two roots, occasionally it has three, with two canals in the mesial and one or two in the distal root.

The distal root is readily accessible, and the clinician can frequently see directly into the orifice or orifices. The canals of the distal root are larger than those of the mesial root. A canal orifice that is wide buccolingually indicates the possibility of a second canal, or a ribbonlike canal with complex webbing that can complicate cleaning and shaping.

The mesial roots are usually curved, with the greatest curvature in the mesiobuccal canal. There can be significant curvature in the buccolingual plane that may not obvious on a radiograph. This can be detected with precurved instruments. The orifices are usually well separated within the main pulp chamber. The mesiobuccal orifice is commonly under the mesiobuccal cusp.

This tooth is often extensively restored. It is almost always under heavy occlusal stress, therefore the coronal pulp chambers are frequently calcified. The distal canals are easiest to locate; once located they can be used as landmarks to find the mesial canals. Access is started with a no. 4 round bur to locate the canals; then the outline form is defined with a long, round-nose, tapered, diamond instrument.

Because the mesial canal openings lie under the mesial cusps, they may be difficult to locate with conventional access-opening preparations. It may become necessary to remove the cusp or restoration to locate the orifice. As part of the access preparation, the unsupported cusps of posterior teeth should be reduced.[39] The mandibular first molar, like all

posterior teeth, should always receive full occlusal coverage after endodontic therapy (see Chapter 22). Therefore a wider access cavity to locate landmarks and orifices is better than overlooking one or more canals for the sake of a conservative preparation.

Skidmore and Bjorndal[30] stated that approximately one third of mandibular first molars studied had four root canals. When a tooth contained two canals, "they either remained two distinct canals with separate apical foramina, united and formed a common apical foramen, or communicated with each other partially or completely by transverse anastomoses. . . . If the traditional triangular outline were changed to a more rectangular one, it would permit better visualization and exploration of a possible fourth canal in the distal root."

On rare occasions a smaller and shorter third root is present. It is found on the distolingual aspect and may posses a sharp apical hook toward the buccal that is not obvious on the radiograph. Orifice locations of the two distally located canals may be found in extreme buccal and lingual position.

Multiple accessory foramina are located in the furcation areas of mandibular molars.[21] These foramina are usually impossible to clean and shape directly and are rarely seen, except occasionally on a postoperative radiograph if they have been filled with root canal sealer or warmed gutta-percha. Because sodium hypochlorite solutions have the property of dissolving protein degeneration products, the furcation area of the pulp chamber should be thoroughly exposed (calcific adhesions removed and so on) to allow the solutions to reach the tiny openings.

Fractures occasionally occur on proximal marginal ridges and extend down the root or under the lingual cusps.

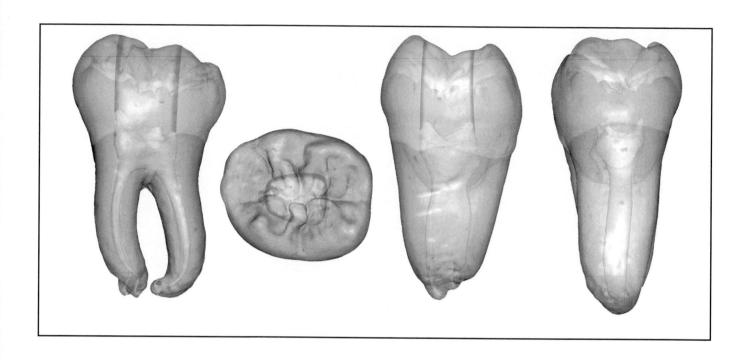

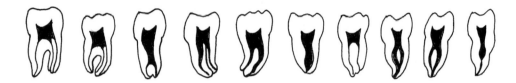

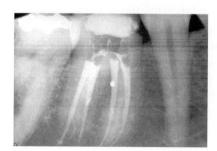

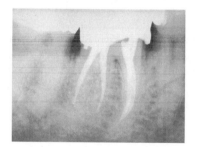

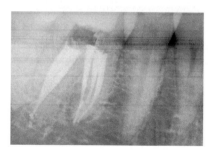

PLATE 7-XIII-1 Mandibular first molar with four roots.

PLATE 7-XIII-2 Mandibular first molar with four roots, with wide division of the distal roots.

PLATE 7-XIII-3 Mandibular first molar with three mesial canals.

PLATE XIV
Mandibular Second Molar

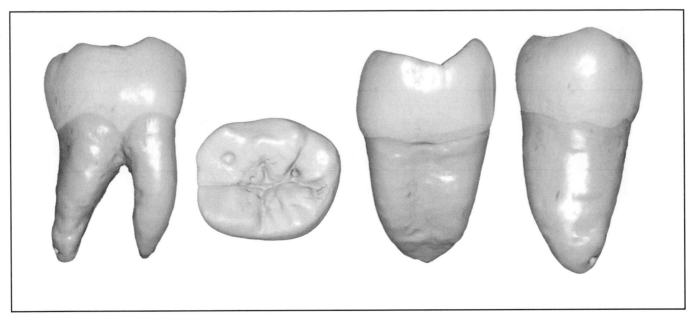

Average time of eruption: 11 to 13 years
Average age of calcification: 14 to 15 years
Average length: 19.8 mm

Somewhat smaller coronally than the mandibular first molar and tending toward more symmetry, the mandibular second molar is identified by the proximity of its roots. The roots often sweep distally in a gradual curve, with the apices close together. The degree of canal curvature and configuration was studied in the mesial roots of 100 randomly selected mandibular first and second molars; 100% of the specimens demonstrated curvature in both lingual and mesiodistal views.[11] In separate studies, Weine[38] reported that 4% and 7.6% of mandibular second molars had a C-shaped canal configuration. They also reported that 4% had two roots with two canals, a majority had two roots and three canals, and that two distal canals were less common than in the mandibular first molar.

Access is made in the mesial aspect of the crown, with the opening extending only slightly distal to the central groove.

A no. 4 round bur is used for the initial penetration and to locate the canals. The outline form is created with a round-tip, long, tapered, diamond instrument.

The mandibular second molar is the most susceptible to fracture because of its close position to the insertion of the muscle of mastication and the subsequent high occlusal loads. Fractures are usually on the distal marginal ridge or under the lingual cusps. After the access preparation is accomplished, the clinician should carefully examine the pulp chamber for evidence of fracture. The use of enhanced vision in the form of telescopes or a surgical operating microscope along with transillumination light will increase the possibility of finding fractures.

Because of the heavy occlusal loads and risk of fracture, full coverage restorations are mandatory after endodontic therapy.

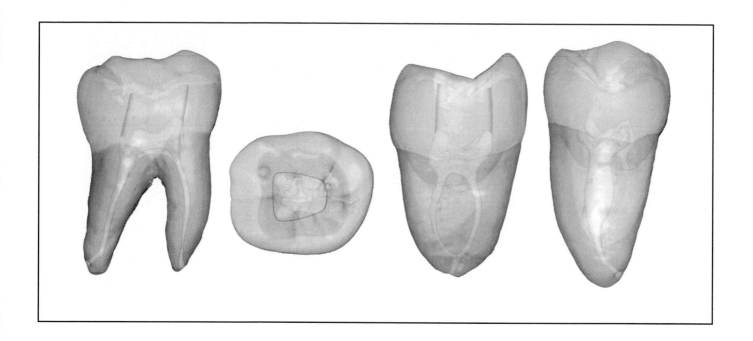

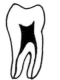

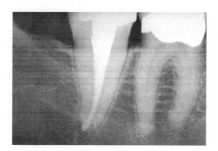

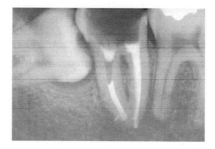

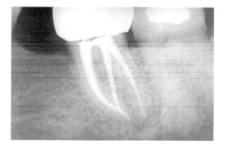

PLATE 7-XIV-1 Mandibular second molar with anastamosis of all canals into one.

PLATE 7-XIV-2 Accessory canal at distal root apex.

PLATE 7-XIV-3 Fusion of mesial canals at the apex.

PLATE XV
Mandibular Third Molar

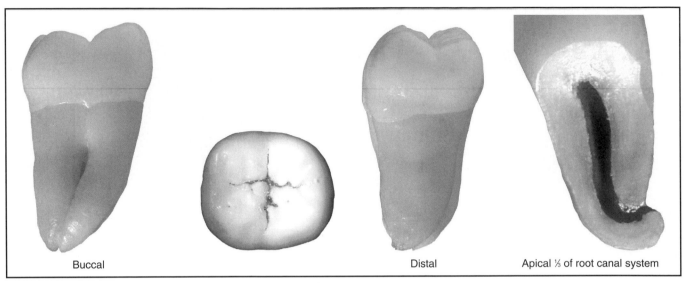

Buccal   Distal   Apical ⅓ of root canal system

Average time of eruption: 17 to 21 years
Average age of calcification: 18 to 25 years
Average length: 18.5 mm

Anatomically unpredictable, the mandibular third molar must be evaluated on the basis of its root formation. Fused, short, severely curved, or malformed roots often support well-formed crowns. Most teeth can be successfully treated endodontically, regardless of anatomic irregularities, but root surface volume in contact with bone is what determines long-term prognosis. A judgment should be made as to the benefit derived from treatment of a third molar balanced against its prognosis. In many cases the benefit is so marginal that extraction is the best choice.

The clinician may find a single canal that is wide at the neck and tapers to a single foramen. Access is gained through the mesial aspect of the crown. Distally angulated roots often permit less extension of the access cavity. If the tooth is in function, full cuspal coverage is indicated after endodontic therapy.

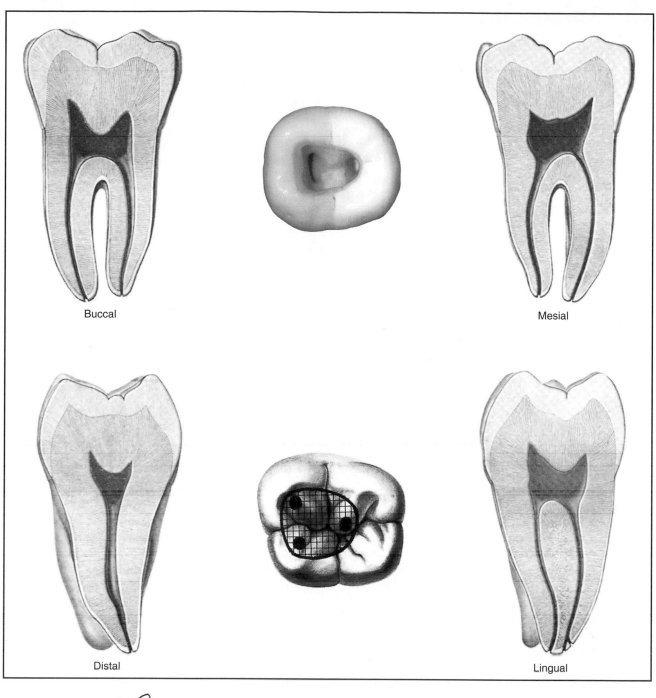

Buccal

Mesial

Distal

Lingual

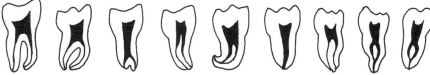

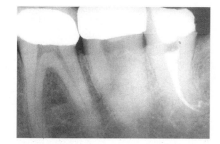

PLATE 7-XV-1 Third molar with accessory foramina at apex.

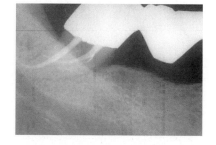

PLATE 7-XV-2 Complex curved root anatomy.

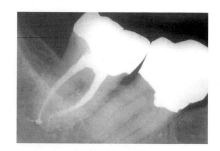

PLATE 7-XV-3 Complex apical anatomy.

PLATE XVI
The C-Shaped Mandibular Molar

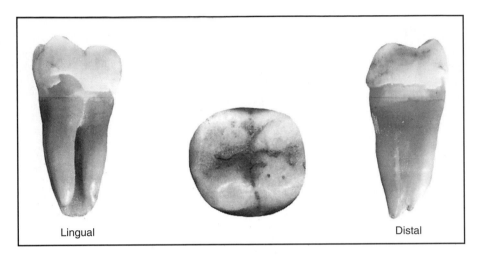

Lingual   Distal

The C-shaped molar is so named for the cross-sectional morphology of the root and root canal. Instead of having several discrete orifices, the pulp chamber of the C-shaped molar is a single ribbon-shaped orifice with a 180-degree arc (or more), starting at the mesiolingual line angle and sweeping around the buccal to end at the distal aspect of the pulp chamber.[10]

Below the orifice level, the root structure of a C-shaped molar can harbor a wide range of anatomic variations. These can be classified into two basic groups: (1) those with a single, ribbonlike, C-shaped canal from orifice to apex and (2) those with three or more distinct canals below the usual C-shape orifice.

Fortunately C-shaped molars with a single swath of canal are the exception rather than the rule. Melton, Krall, and Fuller[26] found that the C-shaped canals can vary in number and shape along the length of the root, with the result that débridement, obturation, and restoration in this group may be unusually difficult (see Plates 7-XVI-6 and 7-XVI-7). More common is the second type of C-shaped canal, with its discrete canals having an unusual form. The mesiolingual canal

is separate and distinct from the apex, although it may be significantly shorter than the mesiobuccal and distal canals (see Plate 7-XVI-4). These canals are easily overinstrumented in C-shaped molars with a single apex (see Plate 7-XVI-5).

In these molars the mesiobuccal canal swings back and merges with the distal canal, and these exit onto the root surface through a single foramen. A few of these molars with C-shaped-shaped orifices have mesiobuccal and distal canals that do not merge but have separate portals of exit.

Although the C-shaped-shaped molar creates a considerable technical challenge, the increased visibility afforded with the use of surgical operating microscopes has made treatment more successful.

There is significant ethnic variation in the incidence of C-shaped-shaped molars. This anatomy is much more common in Asians than in Caucasians. Investigations in Japan[22] and China[41] showed a 31.5% incidence of C-shaped-shaped canals, and Haddad, Nehma, and Ounsi[17] found a 19.1% rate in Lebanese subjects.

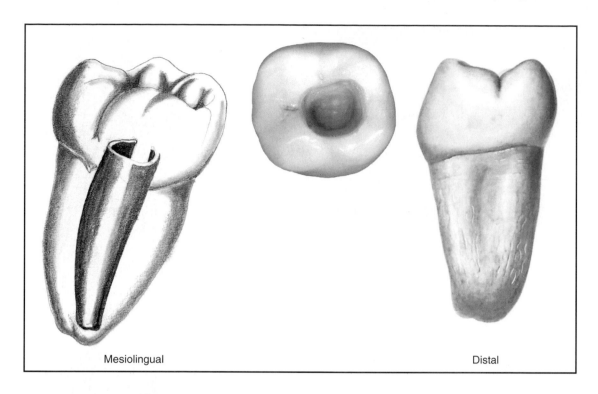

Mesiolingual   Distal

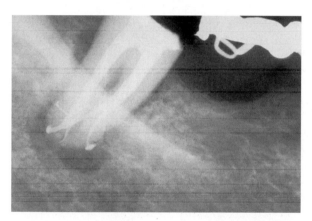

PLATE 7-XVI-1 Mandibular second molar with multiple foramina.

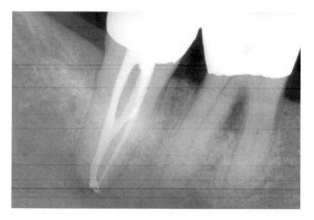

PLATE 7-XVI-2 Mandibular second molar with interconnecting canal anatomy.

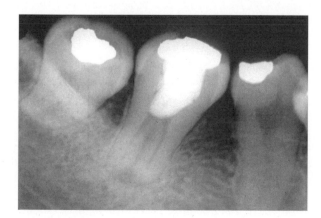

PLATE 7-XVI-3 Preoperative of mandibular first molar with C-shaped canal.

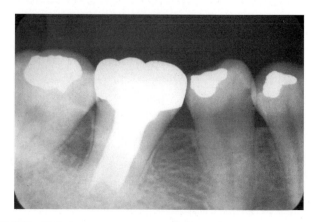

PLATE 7-XVI-4 Completed endodontic showing obturation of the ribbonlike canal spaces.

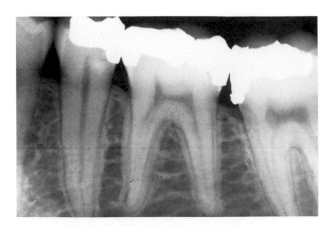

Fig. 7-19 Radiograph of actual case (taken in 1976) at the time of first symptoms. The tooth was not treated endodontically because tests showed it to be vital. Caries was removed from under the mesial amalgam; calcium hydroxide was placed over cavity proximal to pulp space.

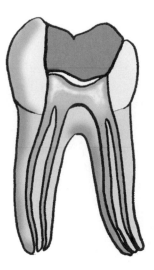

Fig. 7-21 Mandibular first molar with class I amalgam restoration and average pulp chambers.

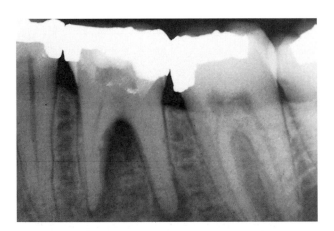

Fig. 7-20 Radiograph of tooth in Fig. 7-19 (taken in 1989) reveals severe calcification of the pulp chambers and periapical and furcal radiolucencies.

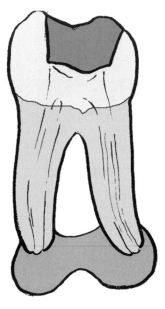

Fig. 7-22 Mandibular first molar with a class I amalgam, calcified canals, and periapical radiolucency. The assumption is that a pulpal exposure has occurred, causing calcification and ultimately, necrosis of the pulp tissue.

METHODS OF LOCATING CALCIFIED CANALS

Preoperative radiographs (Fig. 7-20) often appear to reveal total or nearly total calcification of the main pulp chamber and radicular canal spaces. Unfortunately the spaces have adequate room to allow passage of millions of microorganisms. Chronic inflammatory processes (e.g., caries, medications, occlusal trauma, aging) often cause the narrowing of these pulpal pathways.

Despite severe coronal calcification, the clinician must assume that all canals exist and must be cleaned, shaped, and filled to the canal terminus. Canals become less calcified as they approach the root apex. There are many methods of locating these spaces (Figs. 7-21 through 7-30). It is recommended that the illustrated sequences be followed to achieve the most successful result.

In the event of inability to locate a canal orifice, the prudent clinician will stop excavating dentin or tooth structure will be weakened. Serious errors can occur when overzealous or inappropriate attempts are made to locate canals (Figs. 7-33, 7-34, and 7-37). Root wall or furcal perforations can occur even with the most careful search for canals. Immediate attention must be given to repair communication with the ligament space and surrounding bone (Fig. 7-38). Retrograde procedures become conservative when compared with perforations or root fractures. There is no rapid technique for dealing with calcified cases. Painstaking removal of small amounts of dentin has proven to be the safest approach.

Text continued on p. 226

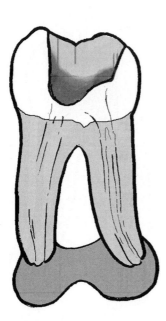

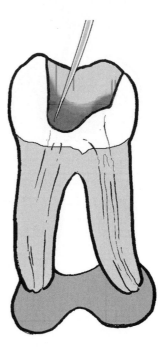

Fig 7-23 Illustration showing excavation of amalgam and base material. The cavity preparation should be extended toward the assumed location of the pulp chamber. At this phase of treatment the clinician must attempt to provide maximum visibility of the roof of the main chamber. All caries, cements, and discolored dentin should be removed.

Fig. 7-25 The endodontic explorer, DG 16 (Hu-Friedy Co., Chicago, Ill.), is used to explore the region of the pulpal floor. The endodontic explorer is as important to the clinician doing endodontic therapy as the periodontal probe is to the dentist performing a periodontal examination. It is both an examining instrument and a chipping tool, often used to "flake away" calcified dentin. Reparative dentin is slightly softer than normal dentin. A slight "tug-back" in the area of the canal orifice often signals the presence of a canal.

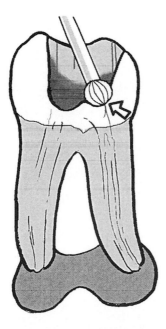

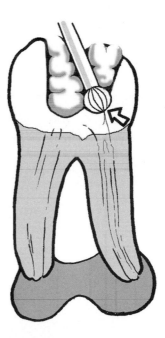

Fig 7-24 Using a long-shanked no. 4 or no. 6 round bur, the clinician explores the assumed location of the main pulp chamber.

Fig. 7-26 If access does not occur at this point in the search, the clinician should begin to feel concern about the loss of important tooth structure, which could lead to vertical root fracture. The bur may be removed from the handpiece and placed in the excavation site. Packing cotton pellets around the shaft maintains the position and angulation of the bur. The radiograph exposed at right angles through the tooth reveals the depth and the angulation of the search.

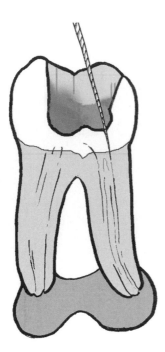

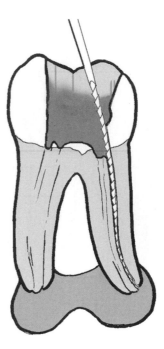

Fig. 7-27 At the first indication of a space, the smallest instrument (i.e., a no. .06 or no. .08 file) should be introduced. Gentle passive movement, both apical and rotational, often produces some penetration. A slight pull, signaling resistance, is usually an indication that the clinician has located the canal. It is suggested that the access to the canal orifice be widened using Gates-Glidden drills until the clinician can identify the orifice.

Fig. 7-28 A larger instrument is shown passing two curvatures to the apex by locating one canal in a multicanaled tooth. It is usually possible to locate the second, third, or fourth canal once the first one has been located.

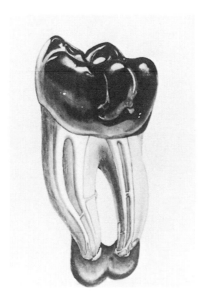

Fig. 7-29 Final canal obturation and restoration, revealing anatomic complexities. This drawing appeared on the cover of the fifth edition of *Pathways of the Pulp*. (Simulations of prepared and filled canals courtesy Dr. Clifford Ruddle, Santa Barbara, Calif.)

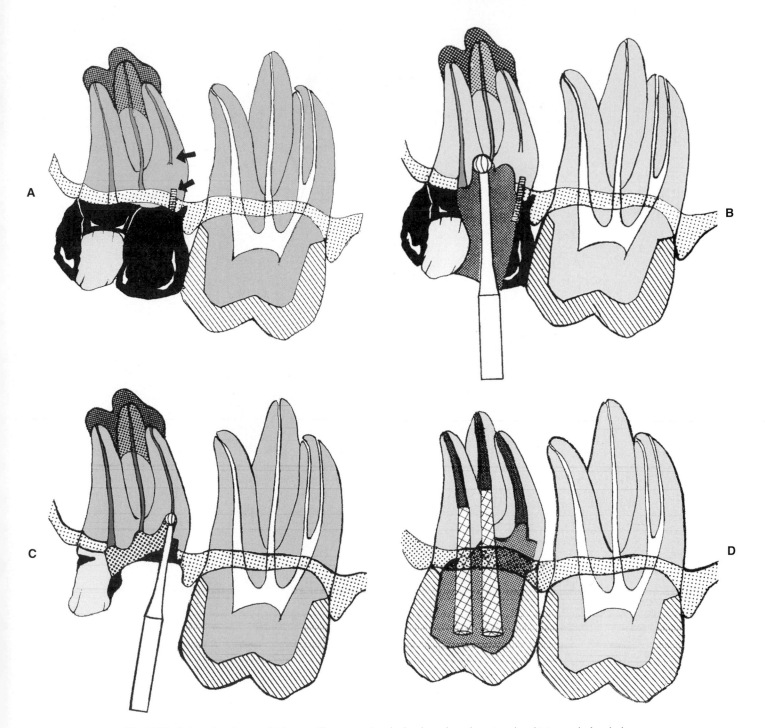

Fig. 7-30 **A,** In a situation in which a maxillary second molar has been heavily restored and is in need of endodontics, the clinician may elect to attempt access to the canals. The restoration itself provides three clues: (1) a reinforcing pin is visible (*arrow*), (2) at least two thirds of the coronal portion is restorative material, and (3) the mesiobuccal canal appears calcified (*arrow*). These factors alone suggest complete excavation. **B,** On occasion, however, a patient requests a clinician to attempt an unexcavated search for the canals, which might result in a furcal perforation, thereby compromising the prognosis. In this case the patient should be engaged in the decision to continue treatment, which most certainly involves removal the existing restoration. **C,** A safer and more conservative approach is to remove the amalgam, the pin, and any old cements. **D,** Careful excavation, using enhanced vision, results in access to the pulp chambers and gives the clinician the opportunity to perform routine endodontic therapy, followed by internal reinforcement and full coverage.

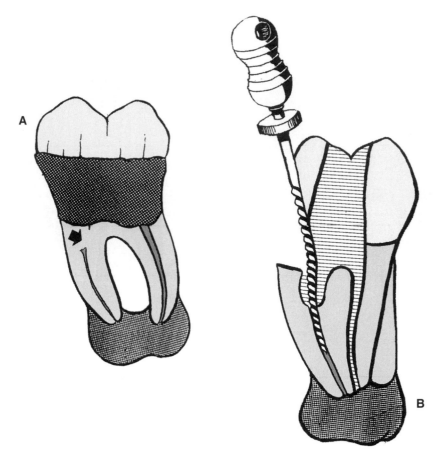

Fig. 7-31 **A,** Extensive class V restoration necessitated by root caries and periodontal disease leading to canal calcification (*arrow*). **B,** Gaining access to the canals occluded by calcification may require removing the facial restoration to obtain access from the buccal surface.

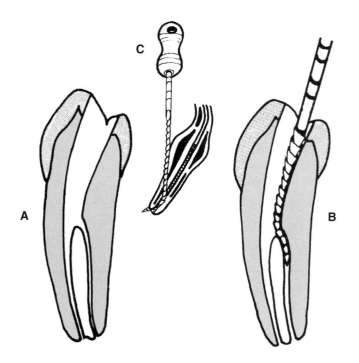

Fig. 7-32 **A,** Mandibular first premolar with division of the root canal system in the radicular portion of the tooth. **B,** The endodontic file is prebent to facilitate access. **C,** Sliding the precurved instrument down the root wall until the tip engages the point of bifurcation.

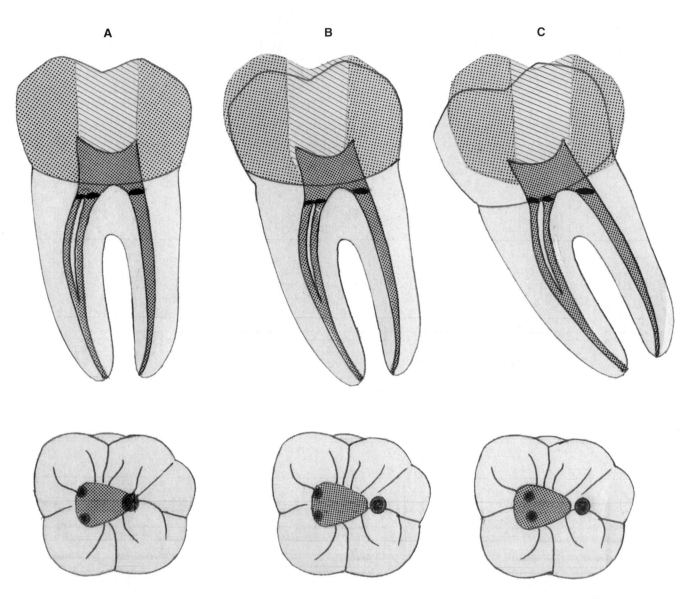

Fig. 7-33 Orifice positions in inclined molars. Inclined posterior teeth occur frequently after tooth loss. Often full-veneer crowns are placed with biting surfaces prepared to engage the opposing tooth. The appearance of the occlusal surface can be misleading to the clinician. Even an 11-degree incline can move subcervical orifices dramatically. Careful excavation is required, especially with teeth with 18-degree angulations or more. Severely tipped molars have a high incidence of root perforations. **A,** Conservative access made in full-veneer crown of a mandibular molar in a normal vertical position. **B,** Same access in an occlusal surface made to occlude with maxillary molar in a tooth with an 11-degree angle. **C,** A crown made on an 18-degree angle.

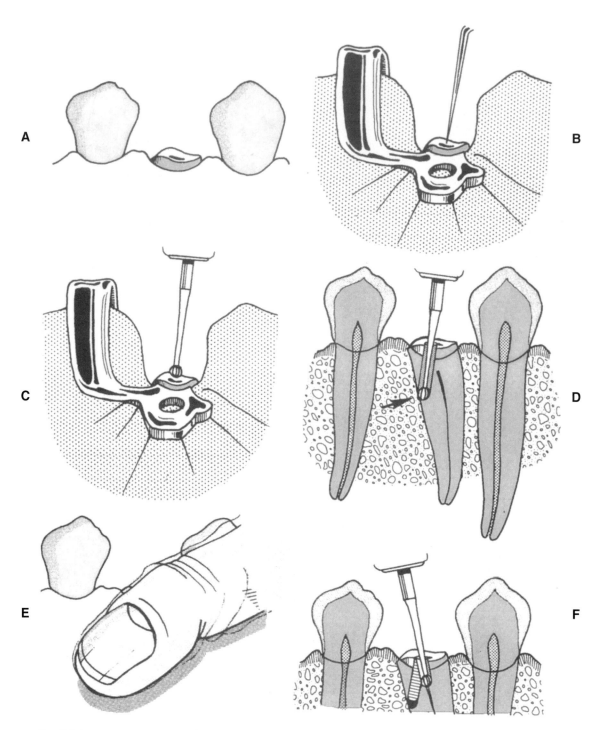

Fig. 7-34 Errors in access cavity when the anatomic crown is missing. **A,** Mandibular first premolar with the crown missing. **B,** An endodontic explorer fails to penetrate the calcified pulp chamber. **C,** Long-shanked, round bur directed in the assumed long axis of the root. **D,** Perforation of the root wall (*arrow*) because of the clinician's failure to consider root angulation. **E,** Palpation of the buccal root anatomy to determine root angulation. **F,** Correct bur angulation after repair of the perforation with MTA.[34]

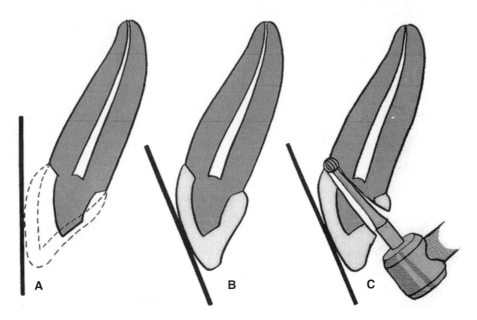

Fig. 7-35 Errors created by crown modification. Avoidable perforations occur when clinicians rely on the cast crown (**B**) and not on the long axis of the root. A modification of the labial tooth surface for esthetic reasons (**A**), (which belies the pulp location) results in a perforation (**C**). Careful exploration keeping root form in mind and using enhanced vision, results in ideal access preparation.

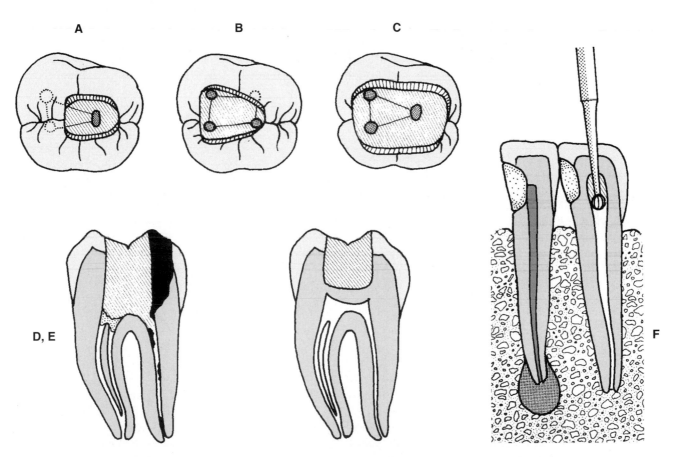

Fig. 7-36 Common errors in access preparation. **A,** Poor access placement and inadequate extension, leaving orifices unexposed. **B,** Better extension, not including the fourth canal orifice. **C,** Overextension, which weakens coronal tooth structure and compromises the final restoration. **D,** Failure to reach the main pulp chamber is a serious error, unless the space is heavily calcified. Bite-wing radiographs are excellent aids in determining vertical depth. **E,** Allowing debris to fall into the orifices creates an iatrogenic failure. Amalgam filings and dentin debris can block access and result in endodontic failure. **F,** The most embarrassing error with the most damaging medical and legal potential is entering the wrong tooth because of incorrect rubber dam isolation. When teeth appear identical, the clinician should begin the access cavity *before* placement of the rubber to avoid this problem.

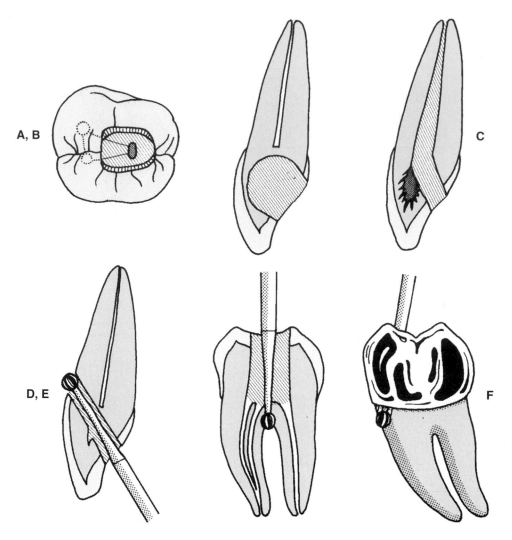

Fig. 7-37 Difficulties created by poor access preparation. **A,** Inadequate opening, which compromises instrumentation, invites coronal discoloration and prevents optimal obturation. **B,** Overzealous tooth removal, resulting in weakening and mutilation of coronal tooth structure, leads to coronal fracture. **C,** Labial perforation (lingual perforation with intact crowns, is all but impossible in incisors). **D,** Surgical repair is possible, but permanent disfiguration and periodontal destruction will result. **E,** Furcal perforation of any size, which is difficult to repair, causes periodontal destruction and weakens tooth structure, thus inviting fracture. **F,** Misinterpretation of angulation (particularly common with full crowns) and subsequent root perforation. Even when repaired correctly, the result becomes a permanent periodontal problem because it occurs in a difficult maintenance area.

ACHIEVING ACCESS THROUGH COMPLEX RESTORATIONS

Most teeth in need of endodontics have (or have had) major caries. Extensive coronal tooth loss requires many types of restoration. Subgingival caries requires complex restorative procedures, which often result in the recession of coronal and radicular canals. Therefore achieving access in these teeth requires major excavation of filling materials, caries, and calcified tooth structure. Coronal access most often is made through multiple layers of materials placed over long periods of time. Straight-line access can be difficult (Fig. 7-32), particularly in teeth with calcified canals (see Fig. 7-21) or malpositioned teeth (see Fig. 7-7, *C*). Inclined teeth that have been crowned can create difficult access situations

if the dentist uses only the anatomy of the cast crown as a guide. The orifices to the canals can be hidden (Fig. 7-36).

Ideal access can only be achieved by total removal of all restorative materials. In the case of gold crowns and porcelain-fused-to-metal crowns, financial constraints may influence the choice for gaining access. Under these circumstances the clinician is well advised to inform the patient of all the potential risks (e.g., perforation and fracture). If the patient accepts these risks, the clinician should make one careful attempt at access through the existing restoration, with the understanding that if the access opening is unsatisfactory, the restoration will have to be completely removed and a new restoration prepared after endodontic treatment (see Fig. 7-30, *A-D*).

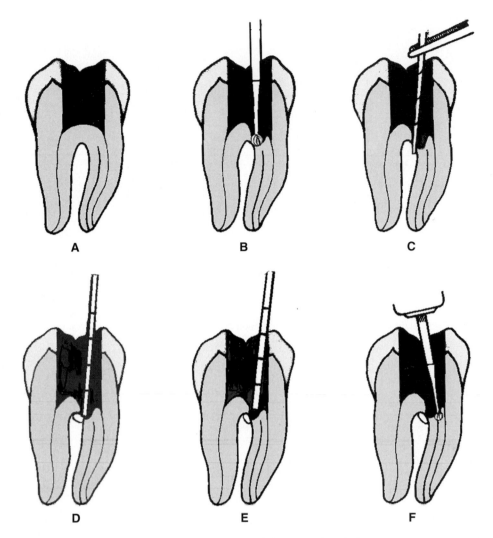

Fig. 7-38 Perforation repair. **A,** Access achieved in two canals but not in the calcified third canal. **B,** Minute furcal perforation during search for the elusive canal. **C,** Using absorbent points for hemorrhage control. **D,** Introducing Collacote to provide a base for repair material. **E,** Introducing MTA.[34] **F,** Attempt to locate missed canal on a subsequent appointment. Magnified vision, including the endodontic microscope, is recommended.

PERIODONTAL AND ENDODONTIC SITUATIONS

Complications of aging make locating canal orifices difficult. The problems of bone loss, chronic inflammation of the periodontal ligament, mobility, and leakage into the root canal system are a combined periodontal and endodontic situation. The gradual closure of the internal spaces may be observed as the attachment apparatus demineralizes away from the root surfaces. The height of the pulp space now moves apically, making occlusal access difficult. Perforations of root walls and furcations are real risks as the clinician reaches deeper with long-shanked burs. One means of locating the position of the bur tip and proper angle of approach is to stop,

remove the bur from the handpiece, replace it in the cavity, pack the cavity around the bur with cotton to stabilize it (see Fig. 7-26), and expose a periapical film.

Periodontal patients may have caries on exposed root surfaces and, thus require extensive class V restorations. These restorations and the calcification often accompanying them can make gaining occlusal access to some canals impossible. In unusual cases it may become necessary to remove the restorative material and then locate, clean, and shape the canals from the buccal aspect (Fig. 7-31).

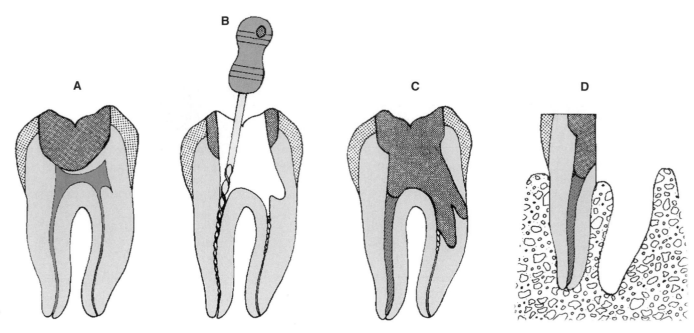

Fig. 7-39 Hemisection as an alternative when mutilation occurs during access preparation. **A,** Calcification after advanced caries and the application of calcium hydroxide can result in serious difficulties in making access. **B,** (1) An instrument has fractured in the mesial canal; (2) a second mesial canal seems totally calcified; and (3) the third canal in the distal root is patent. **C,** Searching for canals and instrument fragments can result in mutilation of tooth structure. **D,** Obturation of one root and placement of amalgam in access areas restores the intracanal spaces in preparation for routine hemisection. Reinforcement with a dowel and core may be performed before final restoration.

References

1. Baisden MD, Kulild JC, Weller RN: Root canal configuration of the mandibular first premolar, *J Endod* 18:505, 1992.
2. Benjamin KA, Dowson J: Incidence of two root canals in human mandibular incisor teeth, *J Oral Surg* 38:122, 1974.
3. Booth JM: The longest tooth? *Aust Endod News* 13:17, 1988.
4. Bram SM, Fleisher R: Endodontic therapy in a mandibular second bicuspid with four canals, *J Endod* 17:513, 1991.
5. Brand RW, Isselhard DE: *Anatomy of orofacial structures*, ed 5, St Louis, 1994, Mosby.
6. Buchanan LS: Management of the curved root canal: predictably treating the most common endodontic complexity, *J Calif Dent Assoc* 17:40,1989.
7. Carns EJ, Skidmore AE: Configuration and deviation of root canals of maxillary first premolars, *J Oral Surg* 36:880, 1973.
8. Carr GB: Surgical endodontics. In Cohen S, Burns RC, editors: *Pathways of the pulp*, ed 6, St Louis, 1994, Mosby.
9. Clements RE, Gilboe DB: Labial endodontic access opening for mandibular incisors: Endodontic and restorative considerations, *J Can Dent Assoc* 57:587, 1991.
10. Cooke HG, Cox FL: C-shaped canal configurations in mandibular molars, *J Am Dent Assoc* 99:836, 1979.
11. Cunninghham CJ, Senia ES: A three-dimensional study of canal curvature in the mesial roots of mandibular molars, *J Endod* 18:294, 1992.
12. Fogel HM, Peikoff MD, Christie WH: Canal configuration in the mesiobuccal root of the maxillary first molar: a clinical study, *J Endod* 20:135, 1994.
13. Gher ME, Vernino AR: Root anatomy: a local factor in inflammatory periodontal disease, *Int J Periodontics Restorative Dent* 1:53, 1981.
14. Goon WW et al: Complex facial radicular groove in a maxillary lateral incisor, *J Endod* 17:244, 1991.
15. Green D: Double canals in single roots, *J Oral Surg* 35:689, 1973.
16. Grossman LI: *Endodontic practice*, ed 10, Philadelphia, 1981, Lea & Febiger.
17. Haddad GY, Nehma WB, Ounsi HF: Diagnosis, classification, and frequency of C-shaped canals in mandibular second molars in the Lebanese population, *J Endod* 25:268, 1999.
18. Hess W, Zurcher E: *The anatomy of the root canals of the teeth of the permanent and deciduous dentitions*, New York, 1925, William Wood & Co.
19. Hovland EJ, Block RM: Nonrecognition and subsequent endodontic treatment of dents invaginatus, *J Endod* 3:360, 1977.
20. Kasahara E et al: Root canal systems of the maxillary central incisor, *J Endod* 16(4): 158, 1990.
21. Koenigs JF, Brillant JD, Foreman DW Jr: Preliminary scanning electron microscope investigation of accessory foramina in the furcation areas of human molar teeth, *J Oral Surg* 38: 773, 1974.
22. Kotoku K: Morphological studies on the roots of the Japanese mandibular second molars, *Shikwa Gakuho* 85:43, 1985
23. Kulild JC, Peters DD: Incidence and configuration of canal systems in the mesiobuccal root of maxillary first and second molars, *J Endod* 16:311, 1990.

24. Loushine RJ, Jurak JJ, Jeffalone DM: A two-rooted mandibular incisor, *J Endod* 19:250, 1991.

25. Mauger MJ et al: Ideal endodontic access in mandibular incisors, *J Endod* 25:206, 1999.

26. Melton DC, Krall KV, Fuller MW: Anatomical and histological features of C-shaped canals in mandibular second molars, *J Endod*, 17:8, Aug 1991.

27. Meyers VWE: Die anatomie der Wurzelkanale, dargestellt and mikroskopischen, Rekonstruktionsmodellen, *Dtsch Azhnarztl Z* 25:1064, 1970.

28. Pineda F: Roentgenographic investigations of the mesiobuccal root of the maxillary first molar, *J Oral Surg* 36:253, 1973.

29. Shoji Y: What is new or unchanged in shaping the pulp cavity? Proceedings of the fifty-sixth annual meeting of the American Association of Endodontists, Atlanta, April 1999.

30. Skidmore AE, Bjorndal AM: Root canal morphology of the human mandibular first molar, *J Oral Surg* 32:778, 1971.

31. Slowey RR: Radiographic aids in the detection of extra root canals, *J Oral Surg* 37:762, 1974.

32. Stropko JJ: Canal morphology of maxillary molars: clinical observations of canal configurations, *J Endod* 25:446, 1999.

33. Szajkis S, Kaufman A: Root invagination: a conservative approach in endodontics, *J Endod* 11:576, 1993.

34. Torabinejad M: Sealing ability of a mineral trioxide aggregate for repair of lateral root perforations, *J Endod* 11:541, 1993.

35. Vertucci FJ: Root canal morphology of mandibular premolars, *J Am Dent Assoc* 97:47, 1978.

36. Vertucci FJ, Seelig A, Gillis R: Root canal morphology of the human maxillary second premolar, *J Oral Surg* 38:456, 1974.

37. Weine FS et al: Canal configuration in the mesiobuccal root of the maxillary first molar and its endodontic significance, *J Oral Surg* 28:419, 1969.

38. Weine FS: The C-shaped mandibular second molar: Incidence and other considerations, *J Endod* 24:372, 1998.

39. Weine FS, Pasiewicz RA, Rice RT: Canal configuration in the maxillary second molar using a clinically oriented in vitro method, *J Endod* 14: 207, 1988.

40. Wilkie G: Personal communication, 1993.

41. Yang ZP, Yang SF, Lin YL: C-shaped canals in mandibular second molars in Chinese population, *Endod Dent Traumatol* 4:160, 1988.

42. Zeisz RC, Nuckolls J: *Dental Anatomy*, St Louis, 1949, Mosby.

43. Zillich R, Dowson J: Root canal morphology of the mandibular first and second premolars, *J Oral Surg* 36:738, 1973.

Chapter 8

 # Cleaning and Shaping the Root Canal System*

Clifford J. Ruddle

Chapter Outline

There are enormous differences in opinion regarding the best methods for preparing root canal systems for obturation. A review of the literature reveals virtually no agreement on a variety of fundamental clinical issues. There are ongoing controversies regarding the size of an access cavity, as well as the strength, temperature, and type of irrigants and their potential to clean. Debate continues regarding working length and patency files, the sequence of canal preparation, and the ideal percentage taper that ensures a root canal system can be three-dimensionally cleaned, shaped, and obturated. With such divergent opinions, the clinician can experience confusion when trying to identify, assimilate, and integrate the best and most relevant new technologies and instruments.

Findings from the dental literature must be balanced by clinical experience and long-term follow-up. A random review of countless endodontically treated cases begins to

reveal the factors that influence success; successful cases leave clues that can potentially guide clinical actions. However, the plethora of endodontic failures provides irrefutable evidence that our unresolved controversies perpetuate clinical breakdowns and decrease success rates. Ethical clinicians are continually trying to discover the most efficacious techniques supported by independent studies.

This chapter focuses on concepts, strategies, and practice-building techniques that will potentially produce superior results in cleaning and shaping a canal system in preparation for obturation. The mature clinician is continuously challenged to simultaneously hold conflicting views until the truth is determined. In the final analysis, objective scientific research will guide clinical endeavors. However, it is by clinical actions that success is measured.

RATIONALE FOR TREATMENT

Pulpal Breakdown and Disease Flow

Pulpal injury frequently leads to irreversible inflammatory conditions that proceed from ischemia to infarction to necrosis and, ultimately, periradicular extension of the disease process. This phenomenon originates in a space exhibiting infinite anatomical configurations and intricacies along its length (Fig. 8-1). Root canal systems commonly contain branches that communicate with the attachment apparatus furcally and laterally; these branches often terminate apically into multiple portals of exit (Fig. 8-2).[60] Consequently, any opening from the root canal system to the periodontal ligament space should be thought of as a portal of exit (POE) through which potential organic breakdown products may pass.[117,145] How clinicians manage the anatomy when performing endodontic treatment will ultimately influence the destiny of a tooth. When root canal preparation techniques are directed toward three-dimensional cleaning and disinfection, there is enormous potential for endodontic success (Fig. 8-3). Although spectacular change is occurring in technologies, instruments, and materials, the only thing that has not changed is the anatomy of roots and root canal systems.

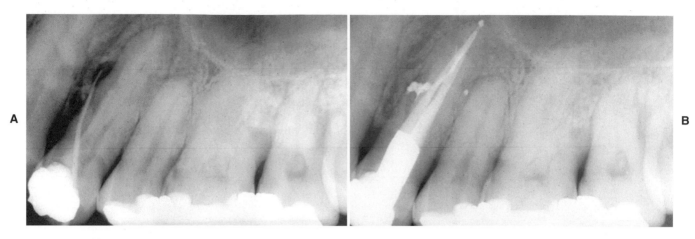

Fig. 8-1 **A,** Preoperative film of a maxillary first premolar. A trimmed gutta-percha cone traces a sinus tract and points to a lesion of endodontic origin. **B,** Five-year recall film demonstrates excellent remineralization; this emphasizes the importance of three-dimensional cleaning, shaping, and obturation.

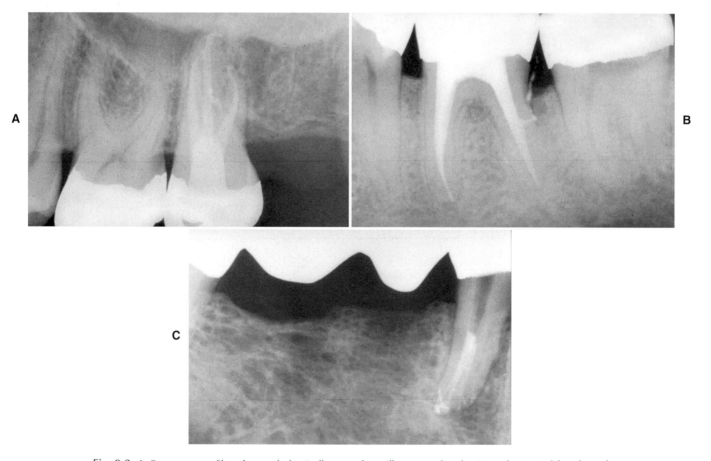

Fig. 8-2 **A,** Posttreatment film of an endodontically treated maxillary second molar. Note the treated furcal canal and the apical recurvature of the DB system. **B,** Postoperative film of an endodontically treated mandibular first molar. Note the lateral canals and the periodontal importance of treating root canal systems. **C,** Posttreatment film of an endodontically treated anterior bridge abutment. Two systems bifurcate at midroot and further divide apically.

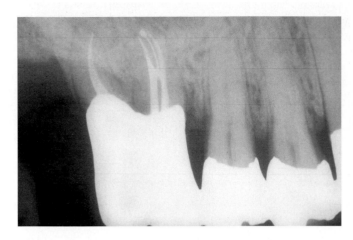

Fig. 8-3 Ten-year recall film of a maxillary first molar with a history of palatal root resection. Note a third system originates in the anastomosis between the MB^I and MB^{II} canals and has its own separate apical POE.

Improvement in the diagnosis and treatment of lesions of endodontic origin (LEOs) occurs with the recognition of the interrelationships between pulpal disease flow and the egress of irritants along these pathways of the pulp (Fig. 8-4).[116] In general, pulpal degeneration and disease flow move in a coronal to apical direction. It is fundamental to associate radiographic LEOs as arising secondary to pulpal breakdown and as forming adjacent to the portals of exit. Except in rare instances, LEOs will routinely heal after the extraction of pulpally involved teeth because the extraction removes the tooth and 100% of the contents of the root canal system. Discounting severely pathologically involved teeth and teeth with vertical fractures, endodontic treatment can approach 100% success if the contents of the root canal system are completely removed, because they are the source of irritation to the attachment apparatus (Fig. 8-5).[35,118]

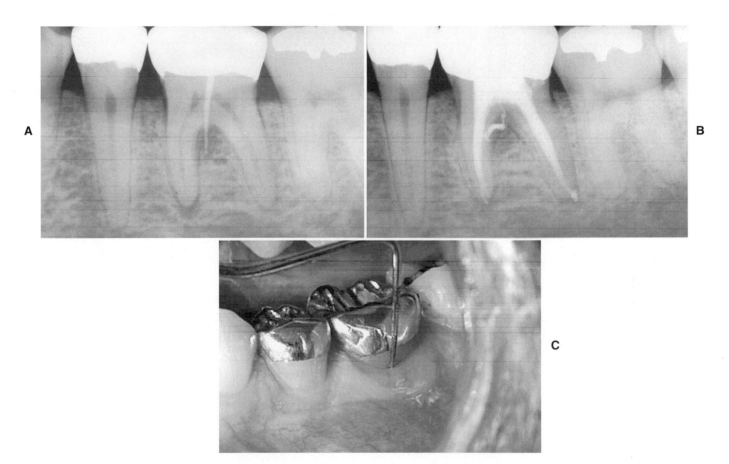

Fig. 8-4 **A,** Preoperative film of a mandibular first molar. A gutta-percha point traces through the sulcus to a furcal lesion of endodontic origin. **B,** Posttreatment radiograph reveals a treated furcal canal and emphasizes the endodontic-periodontic interrelationship. **C,** Periodontal reattachment is confirmed on the 30-day posttreatment examination.

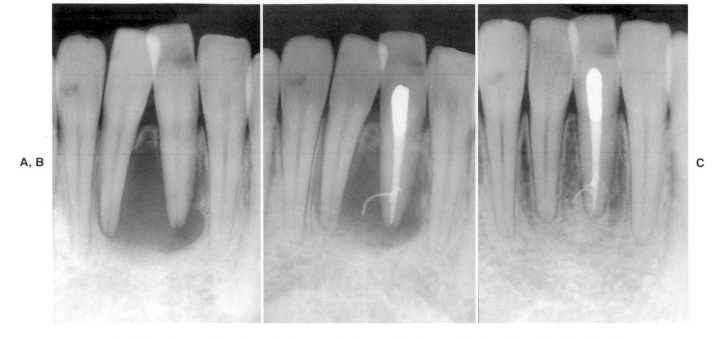

Fig. 8-5 **A,** Preoperative radiograph of the mandibular central incisors reveals a large lesion of endodontic origin encompassing divergent roots. **B,** Posttreatment film demonstrates several portals of exit including a thread of gutta-percha exiting toward the midline. **C,** Twenty-year recall film demonstrates root realignment, bone-fill; it also shows that surplus material after three-dimensional filling is well tolerated.

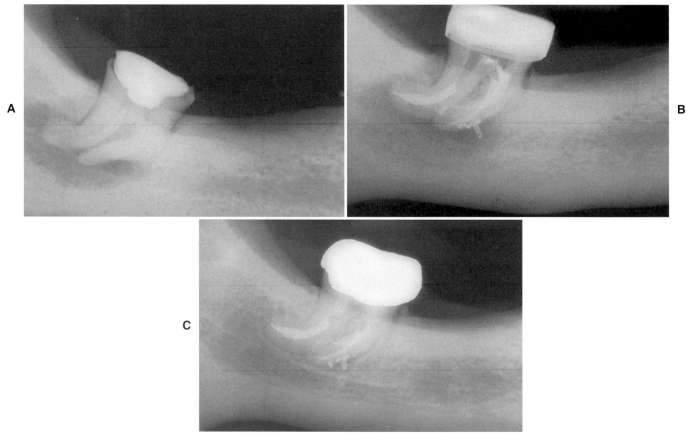

Fig. 8-6 **A,** Preoperative film of a coronally broken-down and endodontically involved mandibular third molar. Note the root curvatures and a diffuse apical lesion. **B,** Posttreatment radiograph demonstrates the build up and banding efforts, this illustrates the completed endodontic treatment of a complicated root system. **C,** Seven-year recall reveals excellent osseous repair.

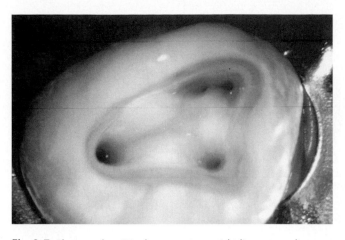

Fig. 3-7 Photograph at 15× demonstrates straight-line access, divergent axial walls, and that the orifices are just within this outline form.

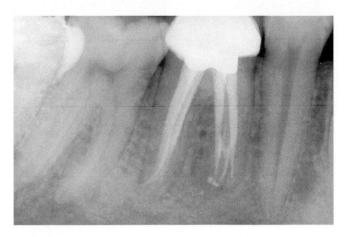

Fig. 8-8 Posttreatment film of a mandibular first molar. Note the mesial anastomosis and the multiple apical portals of exit associated with each root.

Clinical Objectives

There is an old expression: "Start with the end in mind." Certainly, endodontic performance is enhanced when clinicians view preoperative radiographs, envision an ideal result, and then use this mental image to guide each procedural step.[95] Before initiating treatment, the clinician must think, visualize, and plan so that all clinical actions are directed toward fulfilling the vision of producing optimal cleaning and shaping results.

Pretreatment   Before endodontic treatment, pulpally involved teeth must be evaluated to ensure they are restorable. At times it is advantageous to band and build up a tooth to facilitate subsequent endodontic procedures (Fig. 8-6). Seriously broken-down teeth should be evaluated for periodontal crown lengthening procedures so that the restorative dentist can achieve the ferrule effect and maintain a healthy biologic width.[76,91,129] When necessary, crown lengthening improves all phases of ensuing interdisciplinary treatment. Endodontically, crown lengthening addresses isolation issues, creates pulp chambers that retain irrigants, and facilitates interappointment temporary restorations.

Access for Success   Access preparations (fully described in Chapter 7) are essential elements to successful endodontics.[77] Preparing a well-designed endodontic access cavity is a critical first step in a series of procedures that leads to the three-dimensional obturation of the root canal system. Access cavities should be designed so the pulpal roof, including all overlying dentin, is removed. The size of the access cavity is dictated by the position of the orifice or orifices. The axial walls are extended laterally so that any orifices are just within the outline form (Fig. 8-7). The internal walls are flared and smoothed to provide straight-line access into the orifice and the root canal system. Additionally, access preparations are expanded to eliminate any coronal interference during subsequent instrumentation. Access objectives are confirmed when all the orifices can be visualized without moving the mouth mirror. Ideally, endodontic access cavities should parallel the principle of restorative dentistry, where the axial walls of a "finished" preparation taper and provide draw for a wax pattern. Cleaning and shaping potentials are dramatically improved when instruments are conveniently passed through the occlusal opening, effortlessly slid down smooth axial walls, and easily inserted into the orifice.

Shaping Facilitates Cleaning   There is consensus regarding the fundamental importance of packing the root canal system in three dimensions (Fig. 8-8). The breakthrough is to understand that unshaped canals cannot be cleaned.[43] Shaping *facilitates* "cleaning" by removing restrictive dentin, which allows an effective volume of irrigant to work deeper and more quickly to potentially circulate into all aspects of the root canal system.[80] Shaping also facilitates cleaning by serving to eliminate the pulp, bacteria, and their endotoxins (Fig. 8-9).[117] Shaping is the development of a "logical" cavity preparation that is specific for the anatomy of each root.[98] *It is important to appreciate that files produce shape, but it is essential to understand that irrigants clean a root canal system.*

Shaping Facilitates Obturation   Every clinician could compact the gutta-percha in root canals in three dimensions if they were shaped well.[13] The desired shape produces a three-dimensionally cleaned root canal system that any dentist can effectively pack (Fig. 8-10).[6,118] Shaping serves to remove all contents from the root canal space and creates the smooth, tapered opening to the terminus for three-dimensional obturation. Shaping *facilitates* three-dimensional obturation by removing restrictive dentin. This allows instruments to work deeply, unrestricted by dentinal walls, thus allowing ther-

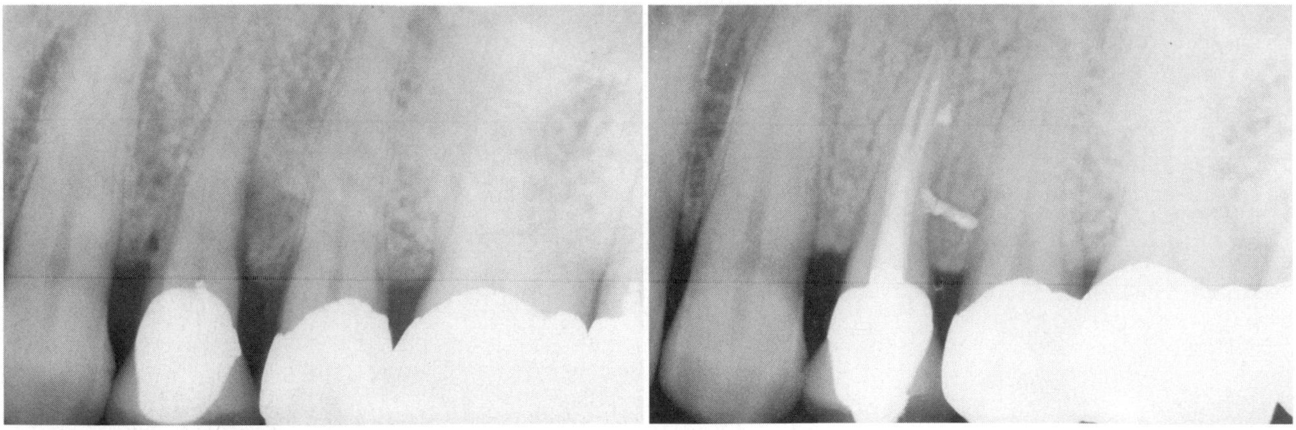

Fig. 8-9 **A,** Preoperative film of an endodontically involved maxillary first premolar. Note the distocrestal lesion threatening the sulcus. **B,** Ten-year posttreatment radiograph reveals excellent remineralization; this illustrates the importance of thoroughly treating root canal systems three-dimensionally.

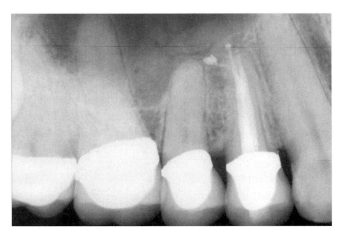

Fig. 8-10 Posttreatment radiograph of a maxillary first premolar emphasizes that shaped root canal systems promote 3-D cleaning and obturation.

mosoftened gutta-percha and sealer to be moved into all aspects of the prepared root canal system (Fig. 8-11).[110]

Traditionally, *cleaning and shaping* procedures were performed concomitantly and occurred over longer intervals of time. With the advent of nickel and titanium (NiTi) rotary-shaping instruments, many canals can be shaped in just a few minutes, although they may not be cleaned. The expression *shaping and cleaning* is intended to emphasize that canals are generally shaped first and then cleaned if irrigation protocols are followed. In summary, the shape is critical, not only for effective cleaning but also for three-dimensional obturation.[79] It is axiomatic that well-shaped canals produce well-packed canals (Fig. 8-12).[117,118] Consistently producing *the shape* is one of the strategic cornerstones in the foundation of endodontic success.

Restoration and Recall   Fundamental to endodontic success is a tooth with a protective restoration that is well-designed, marginally sealed, and esthetically pleasing.[72] An endodontically treated tooth with a restorative margin that is open inevitably invites microleakage and failure, and it necessitates retreatment or even extraction (see Chapter 25).[7] Many currently used bonding materials are hydrophilic and expand volumetrically when exposed to moisture, resulting in leakage.[5] As such, restorative dentists and endodontists must communicate and assign responsibility for definitively sealing off the pulp chamber and closing the access cavity. A timely restoration (see Chapter 22) is essential to prevent microleakage into the canal system.[130]

Recall examinations should be conducted periodically until healing is noted, then scheduled appropriately over the life of the patient to evaluate the endodontic and restorative status (see Figs. 8-1, 8-3, 8-5, 8-6, and 8-9).

Evidence-Based Success

The *biologic* objectives of cleaning and shaping procedures are to remove all the pulp tissue, bacteria, and their endotoxins from the root canal system. The *mechanical* objectives are intended to fulfill the biologic objectives and are additionally directed toward producing sufficient canal shape to achieve the hydraulics required for three-dimensional obturation.

Ongoing debate surrounds the question, "Can a root canal system be totally cleaned?" Some dentists vociferously debate the necessity of eliminating all the tissue from the root canal system. Other colleagues are uncertain if the root canal space can be completely cleaned; a few mistakenly think it is impossible. Many dentists correctly believe they can clean into all aspects of the canal anatomy.[146] Clearly, mechanical endodontic instruments alone cannot accom-

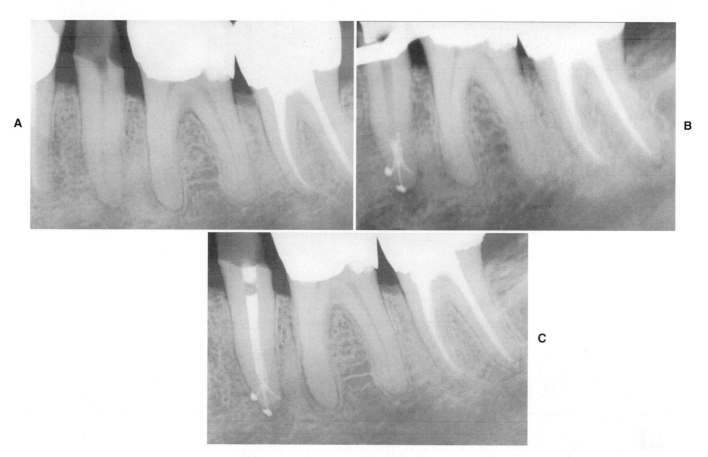

Fig. 8-11 **A,** Preoperative film of a mandibular second premolar that had been opened for drainage. **B,** Working film demonstrates that shaping facilitates cleaning, moving warm gutta-percha, and corking the root canal system. **C,** Posttreatment film reveals "the pack" and provisionalized tooth.

plish the biologic objectives when the typical configurations of any given root canal system are considered (Fig. 8-13).

Today, informed clinicians agree that "files shape and irrigants clean." How do dentists clinically know when the root canal system is cleaned? The answer is when there is sufficient shape to fit at least a nonstandardized "fine-medium" or "medium" master cone.[6,87,147] Canals prepared to accommodate these tapered master cones hold an effective volume of irrigant that, with sufficient time, can penetrate and clean the root canal system (Fig. 8-14).[80]

For the practicing clinician radiographically visualizing a three-dimensionally obturated root canal systems indicates efforts were directed toward fulfilling the biologic objectives of endodontic treatment and improving long-term success. Although the excitement of a well-packed case is deserved, scientific evidence should support dentists' enthusiasm. Moving gutta-percha or sealer or both into seemingly all aspects of the anatomy does not necessarily indicate that the canal system has been thoroughly cleaned and disinfected.

In dentistry a radiopaque contrast solution has been used experimentally to visualize root canal system anatomy and residual dentinal wall thickness; it has also been used to verify the shape of a canal preparation (Fig. 8-15).[80,114] Inter-

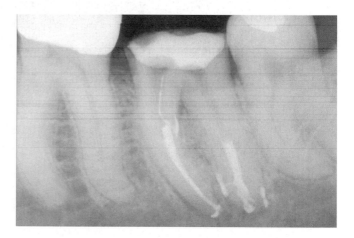

Fig. 8-12 Posttreatment film of a mandibular second molar demonstrates that well-shaped canals produce well-packed canals. Note the furcal canal.

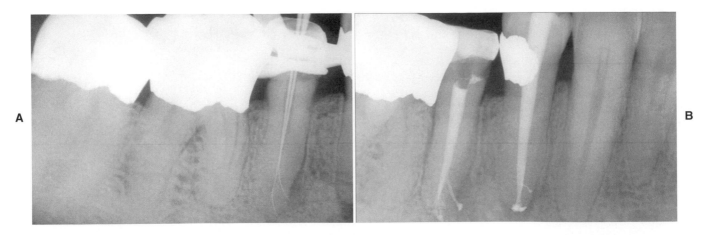

Fig. 8-13 **A,** Working film shows two files in a mandibular second premolar and confirms that a single canal coronally divides apically. **B,** Posttreatment film demonstrates that well-shaped canals can be obturated three-dimensionally.

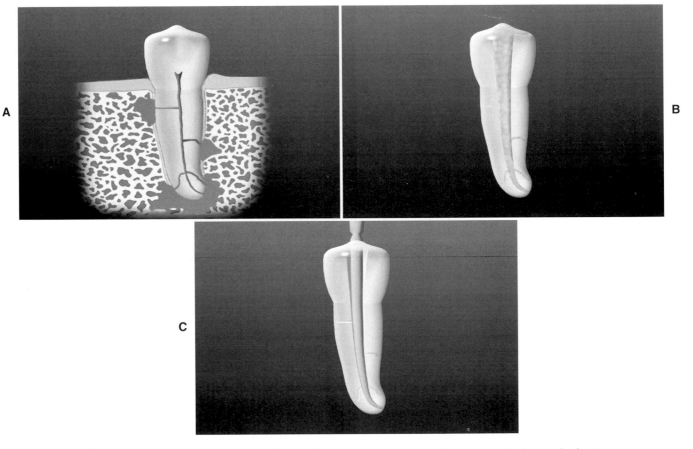

Fig. 8-14 **A,** Pulpal breakdown, disease flow, and lesions of endodontic origin form adjacent to the portals of exit. **B,** Shaped canals allow irrigants to penetrate and clean into all aspects of the root canal system. **C,** Shaped canals facilitate cleaning and fitting fully tapered gutta-percha master cones.

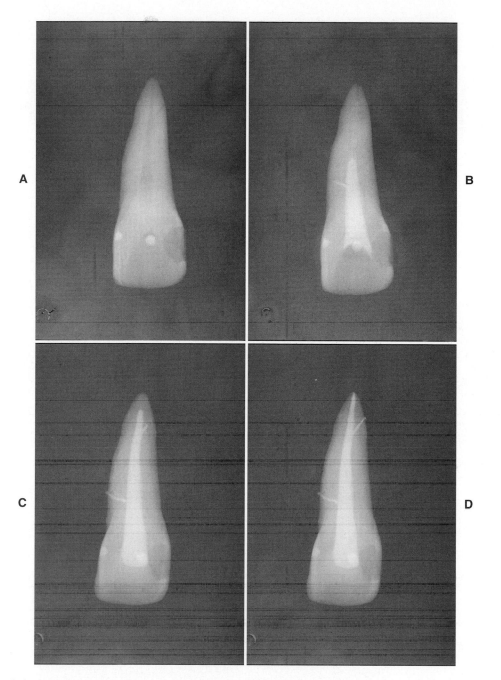

Fig. 8-15 **A,** Pretreatment radiograph of a maxillary central incisor. **B,** Radiopaque and water soluble "solution" is irrigated into the canal after initial preenlargement procedures. The solution is entering a lateral canal. **C,** The visualization solution circulates and penetrates deeper into the anatomy during progressive shaping procedures. **D,** The endogram roadmaps the anatomy, confirms the shape, and verifies the residual root wall thickness.

estingly, root canals have been prepared in vivo, voluminously irrigated with sodium hypochlorite, and reirrigated using a water-soluble radiopaque contrast solution. Radiographs taken periodically during canal-shaping procedures demonstrated that as NaOCl dissolved organic materials, the radiopaque solution progressively penetrated into all aspects of the root canal system (Fig. 8-16).[71] Radiopaque contrast solutions or *endograms* provide visual evidence that irrigating solutions can dynamically circulate along the pathways of the pulp[80] (see "Visualization Endogram" section later in this chapter).

Although endograms and postoperative films provide radiographic evidence suggesting a thoroughly cleaned and disinfected root canal system three-dimensionally, some doubt remains regarding the cleanliness of a root canal system when it is examined histologically. However, an abundance of studies published in refereed dental journals support the conclusion that root canal systems can be

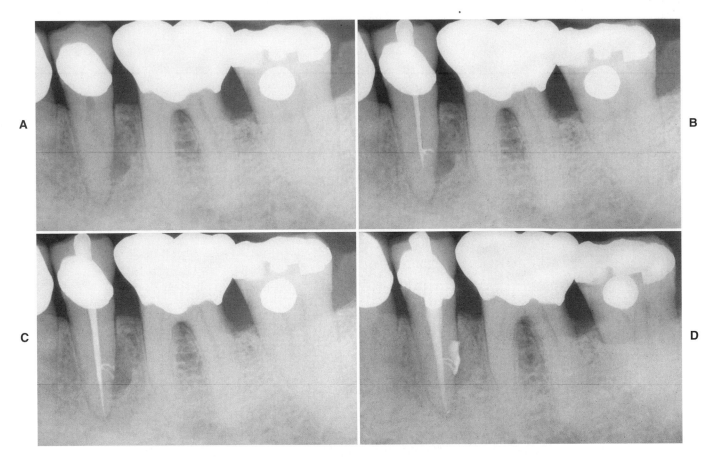

Fig. 8-16 **A,** A lesion of endodontic origin on the lateral aspect of a mandibular second premolar. **B,** After access and preenlargement procedures, a film taken with the rubber dam off demonstrates the radiopaque irrigant moving partially into two lateral canals. **C,** Another working film taken with the rubber dam off shows that although shaping is incomplete, the water-soluble solution has moved completely through the root canal system. **D,** Ten-year recall demonstrates that healing is predictable after three-dimensional cleaning, shaping, and obturation.

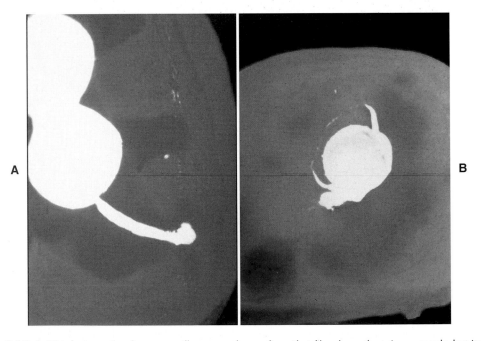

Fig. 8-17 **A,** Histologic section from a maxillary premolar confirms that files shape the primary canals, but it was the NaOCl that cleaned-out the lateral canal. **B,** Histologic section through an MB root demonstrates that shaped canals allow NaOCl to move into and clean out very fine ramifications. (Courtesy Dr. Gery Grey.)

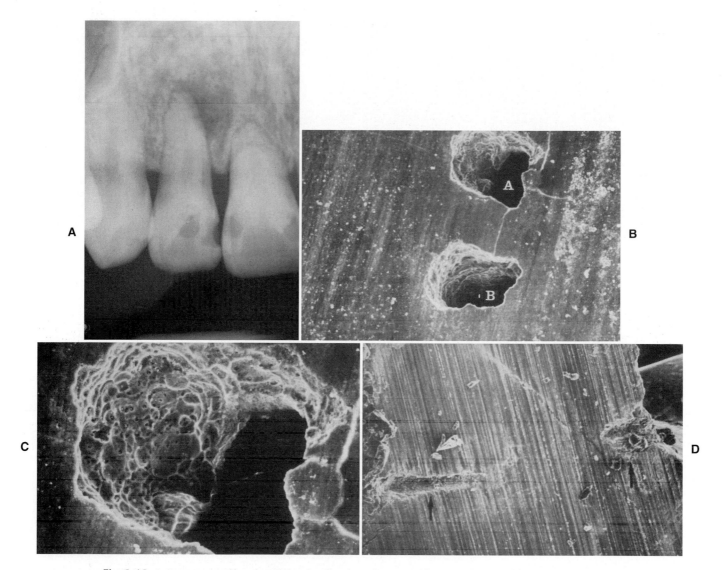

Fig. 8-18 **A,** Pretreatment film of a pulpless maxillary lateral incisor reaffirms that lesions of endodontic origin form adjacent to the portals of exit. **B,** After cleaning, shaping, and tooth extraction for prosthetic reasons, an SEM photograph (160×) shows a cleaned preparation wall containing two labeled accessory canals free of organic tissue. **C,** An SEM close-up photograph (470×) of accessory canal "A" shows open dentinal tubules lining the walls and confirms they are free of organic tissue. **D,** An SEM longitudinal section through a portion of accessory canal "A" demonstrates that it is free of organic debris within its internal and external ends. (Courtesy Dr. Jeffery A. Daughenbaugh.)

three-dimensionally cleaned and filled. As early as 1941, Dr. Louis Grossman demonstrated in vitro that pulp tissue will dissolve in 20 to 30 minutes while soaking in a 5.25% NaOCl solution. Then, in 1971, Dr. Gery Grey demonstrated in clear section analysis that a 5.25% solution of NaOCl routinely dissolved organic tissue and cleaned both large and extremely fine ramifications (Fig. 8-17).[52]

Later, Dr. Jeff Daughenbaugh performed canal preparation procedures in vivo on teeth that were subsequently extracted for prosthetic reasons (Fig. 8-18, *A*). He demonstrated that a 5.25% solution of NaOCl is able to penetrate, dissolve, and flush out organic tissue and related debris from inaccessible aspects of the root canal system where files cannot reach.[33] One specimen in his study exhibited two lat-

eral canals in close proximity (Fig. 8-18, *B*). Looking into the entrance of the more coronally positioned lateral canal revealed open, patent dentinal tubules lining the circumferential walls of this ramification (Fig. 8-18, *C*). Fortuitously, a longitudinal section through a portion of this lateral canal demonstrated that no organic tissue or debris was present (Fig. 8-18, *D*).[33] Investigators have definitively shown that shaped root canal systems can be cleaned when a 5.25% solution of NaOCl and 17% solution of EDTA are used.[10,22,134] Dr. Elio Berutti and his team in the 1990s (and this author in 1976) demonstrated that NaOCl cleans a root canal system after shaping, and it can penetrate deep into the dentinal tubules when used at the correct temperature and concentration for an appropriate amount of time (Fig. 8-19).[14,15,111]

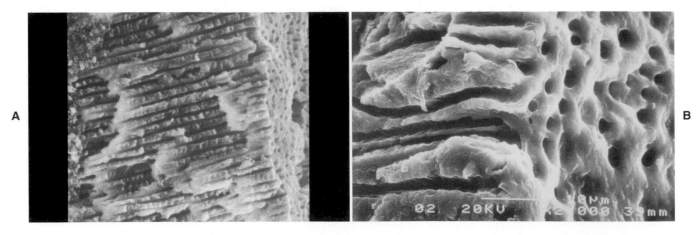

Fig. 8-19 **A,** An SEM photograph (750×) demonstrates that two lateral canals and the dentinal tubules were cleaned with NaOCl and are free of organic debris. **B,** An SEM photograph (2000×) demonstrates that canals prepared with heated full-strength NaOCl are clean, including open tubules that are free of organic debris. (**B** courtesy Dr. Elio Berutti.)

TRADITIONAL CLEANING AND SHAPING BREAKDOWNS

Failure to respect and appreciate the *biologic* and *mechanical* objectives of cleaning and shaping increases frustration and predisposes the patient to needless complications, such as blocks, ledges, apical transportations, and perforations (Fig. 8-20).[21,115,144] These iatrogenic mishaps can be attributable to inappropriate cleaning and shaping concepts, the sequencing of instruments used, and the method in which instruments are used.[13,141]

Working Short

Generations of dentists have been trained to work short of the radiographic terminus (RT). The extent of shortness, although well-intentioned, has been arbitrary and based on misinformation, misconception, and myth.[20] Every dentist who has worked short has experienced the frustration of apical "blockage," ending up even shorter than was intended. A loss of working length occurs because of the compaction of collagenous tissue apically or the accumulation of dentin mud or both.[148] Apically blocked canals frequently hold combinations of pulp, bacteria, and their endotoxins and dentin mud. In the instance of *the lost foramen*, many clinicians become frustrated and aggressively attack the obstacle, which serves to inadvertently compact debris apically. Therefore significant numbers of root canals have residual tissue and byproducts left in their terminal extents. Leaving pulp remnants or necrotic debris in the avascular root canal system is one of the major factors in persistent attachment apparatus disease.[145]

Researchers, academicians, and clinicians are well aware that there is a discrepancy between the anatomic position of the foramen on the external root surface and the root apex observed radiographically.[50,51] Traditional wisdom states that the canal terminates apically at the cementodentinal junction (CDJ) and that the working length should extend to this anatomic landmark. Histologically, the CDJ varies significantly from tooth to tooth, from root to root, and from wall to wall within each canal; it can never be located precisely by radiographs during clinical procedures. Electronic apex locators, although still imperfect, represent a significant improvement over radiographs because they more accurately identify the position of the foramen.[62,86] Working arbitrarily short of the RT (based on statistical averages) encourages the accumulation and retention of debris, which may result in apical blocks that predispose the patient to ledges and perforations. Working short has led to many frustrations, interappointment flare-ups, unexplained failures, surgical procedures, and even extractions.[106,108]

Apical Preparation First

The traditional approach to canal preparation was to negotiate and prepare the apical one third of the root canal first, followed by a coronal flaring technique to facilitate obturation.[48,49,54] In this technique the clinician selects a small diagnostic file, places an appropriate curve on the instrument, then eagerly works the file to length. When a file cannot be carried to the terminus, it is removed and the root canal space is reirrigated. The file is then recurved and reinserted, and a more focused effort is made to move it to length. The breakdown is the failure to recognize that frequently the rate of taper of the instrument exceeds the rate of taper of the canal that prevents the file's apical movement. When an instrument binds on its more shank side cutting blades, the clinician loses apical file control.

Attempting to negotiate and prepare the apical one third of the canal first is challenging in the most delicate part of the

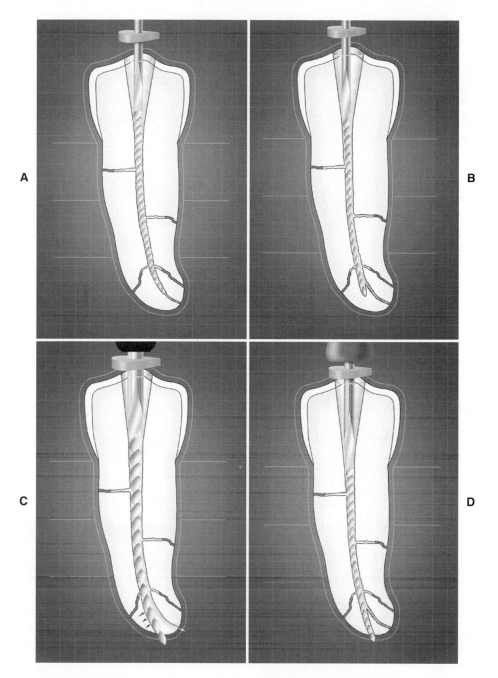

Fig. 8-20 **A,** Grinding files through canyons of restrictive dentin invites an apically blocked canal. Note the instrument is binding over length. **B,** An apically blocked canal, in conjunction with instrument selection and method of use, predisposes to an apical ledge. **C,** A transportation of the foramen results when larger, stiffer, and less flexible files are forced to length. **D,** A blocked canal apically predisposes to a ledge; if apical file grinding continues, a perforation results.

microanatomy. Often a straight root holds a curved canal. Clinicians need to recognize that most canals move through multiple planes of curvature over length. Mesial and distal curvatures are best visualized radiographically. However, hidden buccal and lingual curvatures also need to be appreciated.[95] Additionally, canals typically exhibit their greatest curvatures and deep divisions in their apical extents. The

degree, length, and abruptness of a canal curvature, in conjunction with its propensity to divide, should be factored into the preparation sequence. Specifically, passing a precurved negotiating file through a coronally tight and underprepared canal straightens the instrument.[131] Unknowingly attempting to work straighter files to length in curved canals first invites the block, then predisposes the patient to the formation of a ledge.[78] Further contributing to breakdowns in the *apical preparation–first* sequence is the fact that nonflared canals hold a minimal volume of irrigating solution that, in turn, invites the accumulation of dentin mud.[6,19,87] Working short, in conjunction with attempting to prepare the apical one third first, has contributed to blocked foramens. In other instances it has led to canals that have been ledged, externally transported, or apically perforated (see Fig. 8-20).[109,120]

Instruments and Methods of Use

Traditionally, most dentists use files, reamers, and hedstroems in conjunction with rotary driven instruments to perform root canal-shaping procedures. Until recently all hand instruments were end cutting, tapered .32 mm over 16 mm of cutting flutes, and twisted or machined from stainless steel stock.[124] In practice, increasing stiffness was clinically noted when progressing through any type of instrument series. In fact, the stiffness problem was compounded by the nonlinear increase in apical diameters between successively larger files.[119] Specifically, there is a significant percentage change in the diameters of the smaller instruments (see "Instruments and Geometries" section of this chapter and see Chapter 14).

In addition to imperfect file designs, a major contributor to cleaning and shaping breakdowns has been *method of use*.[12,144] Techniques advocating getting to length early have encouraged aggressive cutting action. Screwing larger, less flexible files into canals is the primary reason for iatrogenic mishaps. Preparation breakdowns continue to drive the growing field of endodontic retreatment (see Chapter 25).[79,109,120] Understanding the limitations of instruments is important, but knowing *how* they are used is critical.

The best technique to overcome iatrogenic problems is prevention. Having knowledge, respect, and appreciation for root canal system anatomy, coupled with a clear plan on how to select, sequence, and use shaping instruments, goes a long way toward eliminating avoidable problems when performing root canal preparation procedures.[26]

CLEANING AND SHAPING: OBJECTIVES AND STRATEGIES

Just as Michelangelo was said to have "freed" his statues from the stone, the *biologic* objectives for cleaning and shaping are to "free" the root canal system from the pulp, bacteria, and their endotoxins. The *mechanical* objectives for cleaning and shaping are to carve away restrictive dentin and sculpt a preparation that is thoroughly cleaned and prepared for obturation in three dimensions.[112,118,146]

Mechanical Objectives

Fulfilling the *mechanical objectives* of cleaning and shaping also achieves the biologic objectives and promotes predictable success. During canal preparation, there is no preconceived depth as to where any instrument must go; however, at the conclusion of treatment, all of the objectives of cleaning and shaping will have been met with greater ease, efficiency, and predictability.[90,146] The mechanical objectives for cleaning and shaping are:

1. A continuously tapering preparation–The canal preparation must flow and progressively narrow in an apical

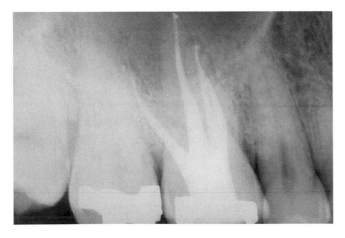

Fig. 8-21 Posttreatment film of a maxillary molar demonstrates that each system exhibits flow and fulfills the mechanical objectives of canal preparation.

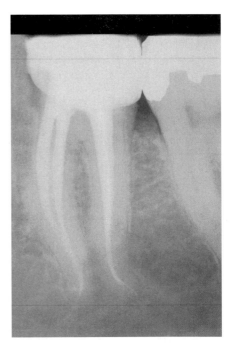

Fig. 8-22 Posttreatment film of a packed mandibular first molar demonstrates that in spite of long roots and canal recurvatures, the mechanical objectives for canal preparation were observed.

direction.[6] Starting at the orifice and moving apically, every cross-sectional diameter of the finished preparation should decrease with the smallest cross-sectional diameter at the apical terminus of the canal (Fig. 8-21). Coronally, the access cavity would represent the largest dimensions of the preparation. In the instance of a narrow root or a root that exhibits a significant external concavity or both, the preparation may approach parallelism in its coronal two thirds. However, it should exhibit a continuous taper in the apical third (i.e., *deep shape*), thus creating a resistance form to hold gutta-percha within the canal and eliminate the potential for packing overextensions.[27,117]

2. Original anatomy maintained—Canal systems move through multiple geometric planes and curve significantly more than the roots that harbor them. Additionally, external root concavities must always be considered so that the clinician can sculpt (i.e., file) away from danger, removing necessary amounts of dentin to ensure cleaning but with an eye toward maximizing residual circumferential dentin, especially on the furcal side of multirooted teeth.[1,70,84] The economy of the preparation is always a conscious balance between a canal that is three-dimensionally cleaned, shaped, and obturated and conserving maximum root structure (Fig. 8-22).

3. Position of the foramen maintained—Gently and minutely enlarging the apical foramen (or foramina) without relocating or losing its (their) position represents excellent mechanical shaping skills.[36,117,144] A lost or relocated foramen represents one of the greatest causes of endodontic failure. To maintain the position of the foramen during treatment, small "clearing" files are gently passed slightly beyond the apical terminus to prevent the accumulation of dentin mud and to maintain patency (Fig. 8-23).

4. Foramen as small as is practical—Keeping the apical foramen as small as is practical requires discipline. Doing this improves canal-shaping results and promotes confidence during three-dimensional obturation.[118] Needlessly overenlarging the foramen contributes to a number of iatrogenic mishaps. The mathematic expression for the area of a circle is πr^2; doubling the file size apically increases the surface area to seal fourfold.[51,145] In preenlarged and properly shaped canals, irrigants can reach the terminus when it is enlarged to a size no. 15 file or greater.[71] Warm gutta-percha can be readily compacted into tapered canals with apical cross-sectional diameters equal to or greater than 0.20 mm.[118] In other words, because thermosoftened and compacted gutta-percha will fit the preparation, there is no need to overenlarge the preparation to accommodate unheated gutta-percha. Some preparations, however, may require that the apical foramen be finished to exceed this diameter, especially in younger or pathologically involved teeth. The clinician should keep the foramen as small as practical and enjoy control when packing in three dimensions (Fig. 8-24).

Concepts and Strategies for Canal Preparation

Endodontic treatment can be simplified by dividing the entire procedure into a series of smaller steps. With few exceptions, the majority of teeth range from 19 to 25 mm in length. Most clinical crowns are about 10 mm, and most roots range from 9 to 15 mm in length. If we divide the root into coronal, middle, and apical thirds, then each third is from 3 to 5 mm in length (Fig. 8-25). The power of this strategy is best appreciated in longer roots that hold more complicated canals that exhibit significant calcification, challenging curvatures, or

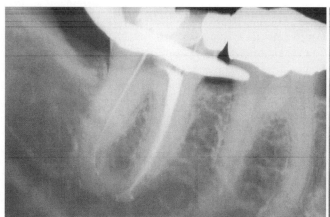
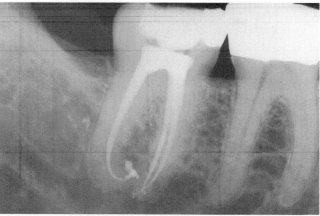

Fig. 8-23 **A,** Working film of a mandibular second molar demonstrates that the objectives for canal preparation were achieved in the MB and ML systems. A scouter file is following a difficult curvature in the distal system. **B,** Post-treatment film demonstrates the mechanical objectives for cleaning and shaping root canal systems were achieved.

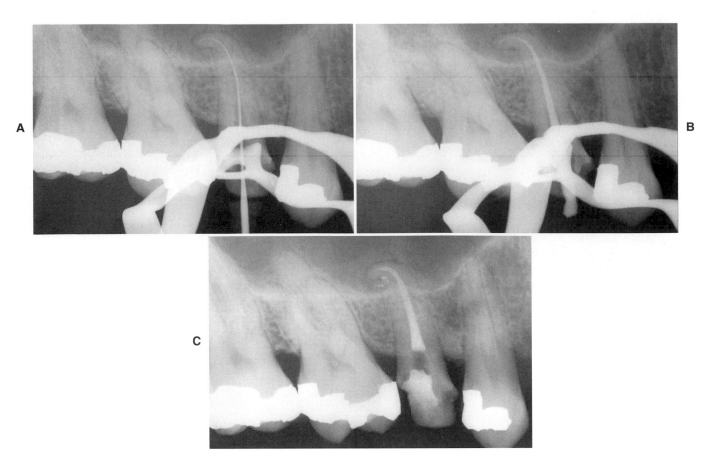

Fig. 8-24 A, Working film of a maxillary second premolar shows a diagnostic file following the pathway of canal curvature and approaching the terminus. **B,** Working film demonstrates that a smooth flowing preparation facilitates fitting the master gutta-percha cone. **C,** Posttreatment film emphasizes that keeping the foramen as small as practical serves to significantly reduce the potential for iatrogenic mishaps.

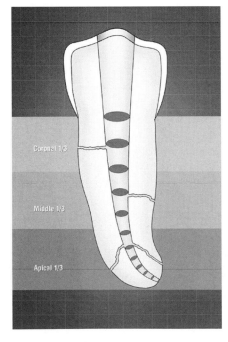

Fig. 8-25 This graphic illustrates the concept of dividing the roots into thirds, and that each cross-sectional diameter of the canal narrows toward the foramen.

deep divisions. In general more calcification is encountered within the pulp chamber. Calcification may also extend into the coronal and, to a lesser extent, into the middle thirds of canals. Fortunately the apical thirds of canals, although more narrow, are typically open and free of calcification. Preenlarged canals allow for a greater volume of irrigant, which promotes the elimination of debris and provides better access and control when preparing the apical third of the micro-anatomy.[19,137] The concept of first preenlarging a canal followed by finishing its apical one third is analogous to a crown preparation procedure in which the tooth is first reduced before finishing the margins.

Coronal Two-Thirds Preenlargement   Cleaning and shaping outcomes are significantly improved when the coronal two thirds of a canal is first scouted and then preenlarged (Fig. 8-26).[137] As discussed later in the chapter, the preenlargement of a canal can be accomplished with a variety of hand or rotary-shaping instruments. The benefits of first preenlarging the coronal two thirds of the canal are:

1. Preenlargement gives the clinician better *tactile control* when directing small, precurved negotiating files into the delicate apical third microanatomy. Early coronal

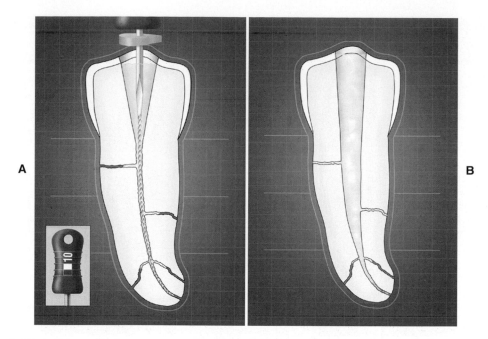

Fig. 8-26 **A,** This graphic demonstrates a scouter file gathering reconnaissance information from the coronal two thirds of the canal. **B,** Once the coronal two thirds of a canal has been scouted, it can be preenlarged to facilitate access into the apical third.

two-thirds enlargement removes restrictive dentin and reduces significant pressure from the more coronal cutting flutes of *any* file type. Preenlarging the coronal two thirds of a canal allows a precurved file to be more easily inserted, freely passed through areas once occupied by canyons of restrictive dentin, and gently finessed around pathways of curvature common to the apical third.

2. Preenlarged canals hold a greater volume of irrigant that serves to *enhance cleaning.* Narrow, more restrictive preparations are dangerous as files work in virtually dry canals. A preflared canal exhibits shape and holds a greater volume of warm irrigant, which accelerates the apical and lateral dissolution of *pulp* tissue. Early coronal enlargement increases the working time for the penetration and circulation of irrigant through all aspects of the root canal system.

3. Preenlarged and tapered canals dramatically promote the *removal of dentin mud.* A preflared canal increases the volume of irrigant and provides an improved pathway for liberating dentin mud.

4. Preenlargement *decreases posttreatment problems,* because the bulk of the pulp tissue and bacteria and their endotoxins (when present) have been removed. Passing files through a cleaned, preenlarged preparation equates to less debris inadvertently inoculated periapically. Passing files through debris-laden and infected canals has the potential to push more irritants into the periapical area, thereby causing more postoperative exacerbations.[39,99]

5. Preenlargement procedures *improve identifying the foramen.* A preenlarged canal passively accepts a larger file into the apical one third where its terminal extent is easier to visualize radiographically. Electronic apex locators are more reliable when used in preenlarged canals because instruments are more likely to contact dentin as they approach the apical foramen.[75,125] When the clinician does establish a working length, it will be more accurate as it occurs after a more direct path to the terminus has been established. Files, gates-gliddens (GG), and rotary-shaping files confined to the coronal two thirds generally require no working films.

Apical Third Finishing   When the coronal two thirds of a canal has been optimally preenlarged, access is available to more predictably address the apical third of the root canal system.[89] As the canal often exhibits its most dramatic curvatures and divisions in this zone, small, flexible, disposable, stainless steel files are used to scout and gather important information. When initiating apical third finishing procedures, the clinician should adhere to the following steps:

1. Scout to terminus—Small scouting files provide information regarding the apical third of root canals. Preenlarged canals generally accommodate small precurved hand files that can be used to gather specific information regarding the canal's apical third cross-sectional diameter and anatomy (Fig. 8-27).[21] The commonly encountered anatomical forms are canals that merge, curve, recurve, dilacerate, or divide (see Chapter 7). Even within each category, a considerable range of variation is normal.

2. Establish patency—Canal patency is performed by gently pushing small, highly flexible files to the RT (Fig. 8-28).[117] To ensure patency the file tip is intentionally

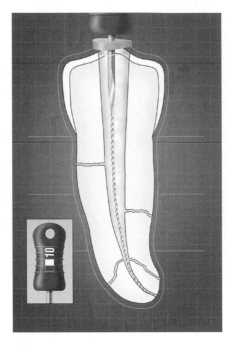

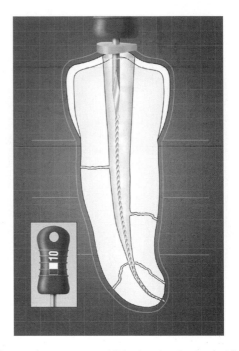

Fig. 8-27 A preenlarged canal improves the volume of irrigant and enhances moving a no. 10 file to length.

Fig. 8-28 Apical patency is established and maintained with a no. 10 file.

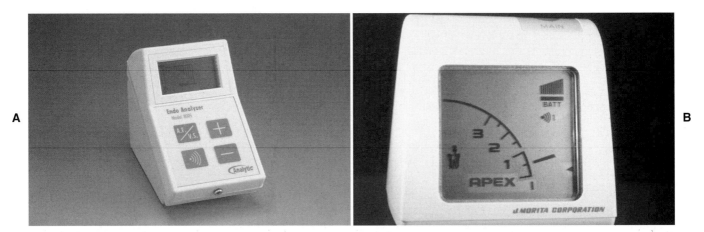

Fig. 8-29 A, The dual-use Endo Analyzer provides the clinician a state-of-the-art unit that performs electric pulp testing for determining working length. **B,** The Root ZX has a large backlit screen, an easy-to-read digital read-out, and provides an accurate method for determining working length.

inserted minutely (1.0 mm) through the foramen to prevent accumulated debris from blocking clear passage to the apical foramen. Working a small, flexible file to the RT will encourage the elimination of pulp remnants, related irritants, and dentin mud. Keeping the canal terminus patent helps avoid blocks, ledges, and perforations.[21] Considering the rich collateral circulation and healing potential of the attachment apparatus, it is illogical to assume that passing a small file passively and minutely through the apical foramen is going to com-

promise the result or predispose the patient to any irreversible conditions.

3. Working length—Clinicians who perform many endodontic procedures can generally estimate the working length with uncanny accuracy. Nevertheless, certain electronic apex locators are still necessary to ensure predictable, accurate, and reliable information about the working length. The latest generation of apex locators provides greater accuracy in length determination, even in canals that contain exudates or electrolytes (Fig.

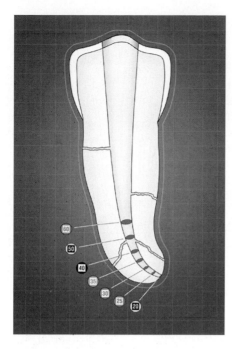

Fig. 8-30 Gauging and tuning procedures verify deep shape and confirm a finished preparation.

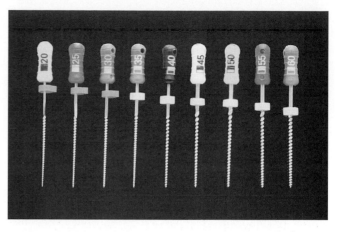

Fig. 8-31 If the no. 20 file is at length, consecutively larger instruments uniformly step out of the canal.

8-29).[93,125] Apex locators do not replace films, however, they are used in conjunction with radiographs.[37,46] When a smooth and predictable glide path is established to the RT and working length is confirmed, the apical one third of the canal can be finished in a variety of ways.[123]

4. Finishing—Creating a canal preparation with a cross-sectional diameter that progressively narrows apically allows for controlled, three-dimensional obturation to a consistent drying point.[110] Consistently finishing the root canal preparation is the *sine qua non* of excellence, and it is confirmed by gauging and tuning.

Gauging and *tuning* with ISO 0.02 tapered instruments is a technique directed toward confirming a uniform taper in the apical one third of the root canal preparation (Fig. 8-30).[21] The clinician begins to gauge the most apical cross-sectional diameter of the canal when a hand or rotary instrument feels snug at the terminus and resists further apical travel. To prove that the diameter of this file at length represents the true size of the foramen, the clinician must *tune*. Tuning is the clinical activity of recapitulating through a series of successively larger instruments and working them until they are observed to back out of the canal in a uniform way. The interval of back-out between successively larger files should not be greater than 0.5 mm (Fig. 8-31).[117] The file that begins to feel snug at length represents the true, most apical, cross-sectional diameter of the canal *if* each progressively larger instrument uniformly backs out of the canal in 0.5 mm intervals. Gauging and tuning *verify* deep shaping of the apical third of the canal.[107]

ARMAMENTARIUM FOR CANAL PREPARATION

Instruments and Geometries

The variety of instruments available for root canal preparation is staggering. Endodontic instruments vary according to metals, taper, length of cutting blades, and tip design. Software simulation models predict how the tapers, helical angles, and pitch influence the clinical behavior of any given instrument. Mathematic models can optimize file design and predict the stress, strain, and displacement behavior at all locations along the active part of a given file. Finite element analysis accurately prognosticates most efficient file sizes, preferred geometries, ideal depth and shape of the cutting blades, best materials, recommended method of use, and guidelines for safety.[122] Additionally, clinicians can select instruments that have cutting versus noncutting tips, and they can choose between single-file and multiple-file use.[88]

Today, computer-assisted machining delivers optimal instruments with the best features. Although science, technology, and marketing may proclaim a great instrument, its ultimate success will be measured by its clinical performance. The following discussion is intended to identify specific instruments and describe their geometries. Note that the *sequencing* of instruments and their method of use will be covered following this section. (See Chapter 14 for further discussion of all of the following instruments.)

Broaches   Barbed broaches (Moyco Union Broach, York, PA) come in a variety of sizes, and each instrument's shaft is essentially a parallel cylinder that contains an effective number of short, sharp, coronally angulated, semiflexible barbs. Although barbed broaches are used with decreasing frequency, they are still used to remove objects such as cotton pellets and paper points. With proper technique an appropriately selected barbed broach is most useful for rapidly and effectively extricating a significant amount of vital, inflamed, hemorrhagic pulp tissue (Fig. 8-32). Even with the advent of NiTi rotary-shaping instruments, it is still occasionally useful to perform broaching procedures. Broaching is a technique that may allow the clinician to extirpate an intact pulp *en toto.*

Hand Instruments

Traditionally, hand files were manufactured by twisting square or triangular shafts of metal on their long axis, thus converting the vertical edges into partially horizontal cutting blades. However, recently computer-assisted machining has enabled manufacturers to modify existing file geometries.[122,132] These new hybrid instruments have evolved to promote safety, predictability, and efficiency in clinical use. Purported advantages of these instruments are noncutting tips, parallel versus tapered cores that enhance flexibility, and a change of cross-sectional geometry from square to rhomboid that decreases core diameter and improves flexibility. Additionally, decreasing the helical angle and increasing the distance between the cutting blades have improved instrument efficiency. By making the interblade groove deeper, there is more space to accommodate dentinal shavings. Another method to improve results during canal shaping is the introduction of NiTi hand instruments.[140] At times the smaller NiTi files are too flexible, but the sizes (no. 35 to no. 60) provide extraordinary improvements when performing deep shaping procedures around pathways of curvature.[55,105]

The principle endodontic *hand instruments* used for root canal preparation procedures are files, reamers, hedstroems, and more recently, Greater Taper (GT) hand files (Dentsply Tulsa Dental, Tulsa, Okla.). These instruments can be used in a variety of ways to cut dentin. The following section will discuss the most important and relevant files and describe their geometries.

ISO Instruments

ISO-sized instruments (Dentsply Maillefer, Tulsa, Okla.) are available in different lengths but all have 16 mm of cutting flutes.[142] The cross-sectional diameter at the first rake angle of any file is termed D_0. One millimeter coronal to D_0 is termed D_1, although 2 mm coronal to D_0 is called D_2, and so forth. The most shank side cutting flute is 16 mm coronal to D_0. Identified as D_{16}, it represents the largest diameter and most active aspect of the instrument. Each instrument receives its numeric designation, or file name, from its diameter at D_0. This universal nomenclature is useful and allows machinists and dentists to specifically discuss various aspects of a file at specific locations. Because ISO files have a standard taper of 0.32 mm over 16 mm of cutting blades, the taper of any specific instrument is 0.02 mm per millimeter (Fig. 8-33).

Although the file name represents the size at its D_0 diameter, any given instrument has multiple cross-sectional diameters over its active blades. The no. 10 file is 0.10 mm in diameter at D_0, tapers 0.32 mm over 16 mm, and has a diameter of 0.42 mm at D_{16}. ISO file sizes no. 10 through no. 60 have diameters at D_0 that increase by 0.05 mm (i.e., 0.10, 0.15, 0.20, 0.25, 0.30, 0.35, 0.40, 0.45, 0.50, 0.55, and 0.60). From the size no. 60 file to the 140 file, the D_0 diameter increases by 0.10 mm (i.e., 0.60, 0.70, 0.80, 0.90, 1.00, 1.10, 1.20, 1.30, and 1.40). The no. 0.08 file is 0.02 mm larger at D_0 than the no. 0.06 file, and it is 0.02 mm smaller than the no. 10 file at the same point.

An enduring problem that has critically affected cleaning and shaping results is the innocent oversimplification that the D_0 diameters progressively increase by 0.05 mm between the sizes no. 10 and no. 60 files. Dr. Pierre Machtou and Dr. Herb Schilder were the first to caution that the D_0 diameter of a file from instrument to instrument did not have a *constant percentage change.*[79,119] The percentage change between consecutive instruments is calculated by taking the difference between their D_0 diameters, dividing this number by the D_0 diameter of the smaller file, and then multiplying that result by 100. As an example, the percent of increase in D_0 diameters between the no. 10 and no. 15 files is 50%. Note further

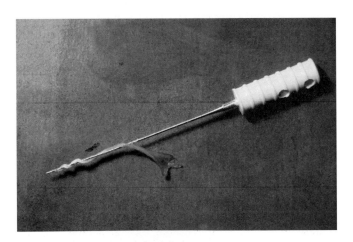

Fig. 8-32 A correctly sized barbed broach, in conjunction with proper technique, can remove an intact vital pulp.

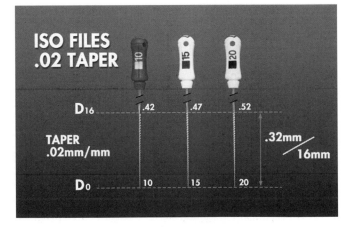

Fig. 8-33 Photograph showing ISO 0.02 no. 10, no. 15, and no. 20 files. Each instrument tapers 0.32 mm over its 16 mm of cutting blades.

that the no. 20 file is 33% larger than the no. 15 file at D_0, and the no. 55 file is 10% larger than the no. 50 file at D_0. This information is best illustrated in a graph that plots and compares the percentage change between files (Fig. 8-34).

The ISO specifications for instrument design inadvertently discourage the mechanical objectives for cleaning and shaping canals.[142] In fact, it would be more helpful to have lower percentage changes between successive D_0 diameters in the smaller file sizes.[119] The large percentage change between the smaller instruments can be dangerous, because these files typically work in the most delicate part of the microanatomy where most curvatures and canal divisions exist (see Chapter 7). To reduce the large percentage change between the smaller-sized files, the Golden Medium instrument series (Dentsply Maillefer, Tulsa, Okla.) was introduced. Golden Mediums provide half sizes between traditional instruments. Although Golden Medium instruments were intended to eliminate the significant percentage jumps between successive files, their use is not that important clinically, because machining tolerances of ±0.02 mm negates their intended advantage. Clinicians need to appreciate the nonlinear percentage change between instruments and use them accordingly.

Another product line of instruments, the ProFile Series 29 (Dentsply Tulsa Dental, Tulsa, Okla.), was developed in part to address the large percentage change at D_0 between the successive smaller-sized ISO instruments.[81,119] In this instrument series, each consecutively larger file increases at D_0 by a uniform 29%. There is logic to this system because it creates more useful instruments in the low end of the series. However, this intended advantage is offset and may even be counterproductive as the file sizes increase. At these larger diameters, the 29% increase between successive files is actually greater than the percentage change found in the ISO-file series. This large percentage increase between the larger

sizes of the Series 29 files can cause difficulties when creating deep shape around a curvature.

Clinically, when using ISO instruments, the 50% increase in diameter between the no. 10 and no. 15 files can be reduced by gently inserting the no. 10 file 1 mm through the foramen and establishing apical patency. A 0.02 tapered no. 10 file has a diameter of 0.12 mm at D_1. Inserting a no. 10 file 1 mm through the foramen dramatically reduces the percentage change between the no. 10 and no. 15 files, from 50% to 25% (see Fig. 8-28). Placing a no. 10 file minutely through the foramen paves the way for the passive insertion of the no. 15 file to length. Patency files promote *Mechanical Objective no. 3* of the cleaning and shaping guidelines.

Greater Taper Hand Files Recently a new series of hand files became available, providing clinicians with instruments with tapers that exceed the ISO guidelines of 0.02 mm/mm. This set of four Greater Taper (GT) files is made of NiTi. Each hand instrument is designed to be active in a counterclockwise direction and has a D_0 diameter of 0.20 mm. The GT files have increasing tapers of 0.06, 0.08, 0.10, and 0.12 mm/mm that correspond to fine, fine-medium, medium and medium-large gutta-percha master cones. Unlike ISO numerology, each GT instrument receives its numeric designation based on its rate of taper. To promote more flexibility, these instruments have a maximum flute diameter (MFD) of 1.00 mm. As such, the length of blades varies from file to file, depending on the taper (Fig. 8-35). These instruments have variably pitched flutes, providing the efficient cutting action of a reamer on the more shank side blades, then transitioning into the clinical attributes of a file toward D_0. GT files are designed to cut more toward their shank-side cutting blades. The most apical extent of a GT file should never engage dentin; rather it should passively follow a canal that is confirmed to be open at least to a diameter of 0.15 mm at its terminus.

GG Drills GG drills (Dentsply Maillefer, Tulsa, Okla.) are important carving instruments that may be used for preenlarging the coronal two thirds of most root canals.[79] Six instruments are in the series, and the number of marked rings on their proximal surfaces identify the specific GG drill. GGs are made of either stainless steel or NiTi and are available in various lengths. Each instrument has a long, thin shaft with an attached "flame-shaped" cutting head. The maximum cross-sectional diameter of the cutting blades is shown in Fig. 8-36. GGs are side-cutting, safe-ended instruments, and ideally used to cut dentin as it is withdrawn from the canal (i.e., cut on the outstroke). Their cutting action is generally circumferential in rounder-shaped roots, and they are used to cut deliberately away from external root concavities in single-rooted and furcated teeth.[1,63] GGs are confined to the straightaway portions of the canal and are used serially, passively, and so that each successively larger drill is worked shorter than the preceding smaller one.[117] GGs may also be used to open the canal orifices. Opening the orifices simpli-

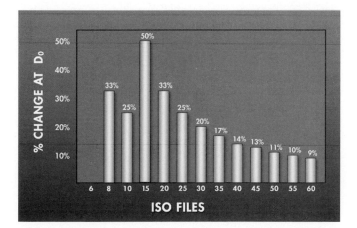

Fig. 8-34 The percentage change at D_0 among successively larger files. Note the largest percentage change occurs among the smaller instruments.

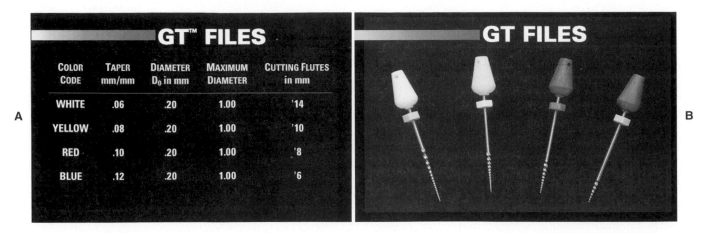

Fig. 8-35 A, Summary of each GT file's color code, taper, D_0 diameter, maximum flute diameter, and the approximate length of cutting blades. **B,** 0.06, 0.08, 0.10, and 0.12 tapered GT files.

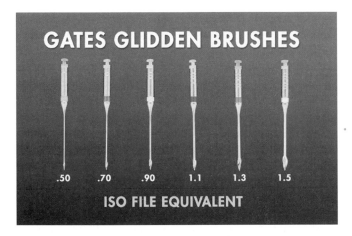

Fig. 8-36 Six Gates-Glidden drills that should be thought of as brushes. The maximum diameter of each cutting head is given in millimeters.

fies subsequent cleaning and shaping procedures and quickly establishes a smooth glide path through the access chamber into the root canal system (Fig. 8-37).[123]

Used properly, GGs are inexpensive, safe, and clinically beneficial. However, their improper use has contributed to "coke bottle" preparations, root thinning, and strip perforations.[70] Unfortunately, GGs have been called "drills," which tends to suggest a method of use. High RPM, excessive pressure, and the use of the GGs to drill into canals have created mishaps during canal preparation. Drilling into canals generates torsional loads on the GG head and dangerously ensures its complete circumferential contact, causing overzealous enlargements, perforations, and broken heads. These instruments may be used safely and to their fullest potential from 750 to 1000 RPM. The attributes of GG instruments are best appreciated using a gear reduction, slow-speed, high-torque hand piece. The GG should be thought of as a *"brush."* Just as the painter *brushes paint on the canvas*, the dentist can *"brush"* and carve away restrictive dentin.[107]

NiTi Rotary Shaping Instruments Many variables and interrelationships influence the clinical performance of the new generation of superelastic NiTi rotary-shaping instruments.[34,104] Much of what is known about NiTi rotary-shaping instruments has been learned in clinical practice on patients of record. Rotary instruments are here to stay; they will continue to improve, but they are *not* a panacea. However, they are an important adjunct for canal-shaping procedures.

NiTi rotary instruments have sharply reduced clinical mishaps, such as blocks, ledges, transportations, and perforations. However, these instruments also have an unpredictable, increased incidence of file breakage.[73,126,140] File breakage can be dramatically reduced by strictly following rotary *method-of-use* protocols.[97] Deviations from protocols increase the potential for breakage.[42,127] Besides method of use, the multiple use of what should really be considered a disposable file is another major cause of instrument separation.[67] Therefore *these instruments should be discarded after a single use* because of metal fatigue, loss of cutting efficiency, and the great variation in the length, diameter, and curvature of any given canal.[40,107]

The following discussion describes the most important and most widely selected instruments currently used for canal preparation. The concepts, strategies, and techniques for successful use are not unique to any one system; they generally apply to all NiTi instruments, regardless of geometries or brand.

ProFile Rotary Instruments The ProFile NiTi rotary instrument line includes orifice shapers, ProFile 0.04 and 0.06 Tapers, and Greater Taper (GT) files. These instruments all share the same cross-sectional geometries and have three radial lands that each contains bidirectional cutting edges. The radial lands keep the instrument centered in the canal; their cutting edges are intended to scrape rather than actively engage and screw into dentin.[18,87] The radial lands are separated by three U-shaped flutes that provide space for the accumulation of debris (Fig. 8-38). The U-shaped configura-

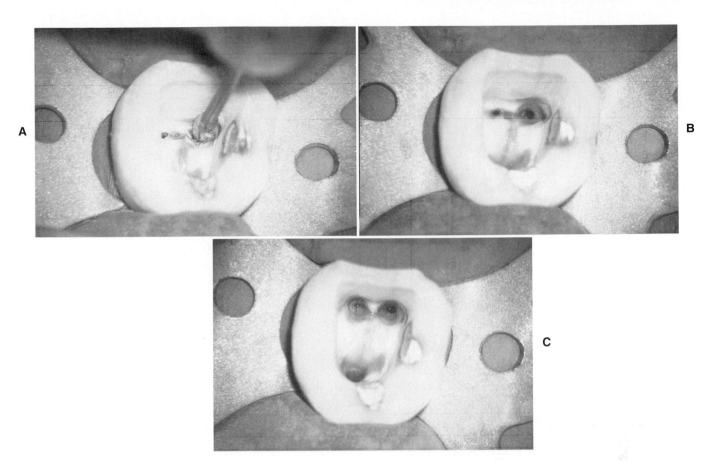

Fig. 8-37 **A,** Photograph (9×) of a mandibular molar access cavity demonstrates a GG opening the MB orifice. **B,** Photograph (9×) illustrates that a funneled orifice simplifies inserting instruments into this system. **C,** Photograph (9×) shows the orifices have been opened to facilitate cleaning and shaping procedures.

tion effectively augers debris coronally and out of the canal during clinical use.[81] These files have a parallel core to enhance flexibility; their noncutting tips are designed to follow a pilot hole and guide the instrument through the canal during preparation procedures (Fig. 8-39).[38,88,123] The recommended rotational speed for these instruments, regardless of the product line, is 150 to 300 RPM.[42]

ProFile 0.04 and 0.06 tapers.   The ProFile 0.04 and 0.06 instrument lines (Dentsply Tulsa Dental, Tulsa, Okla.) are the benchmark against which all other rotary-shaping files are measured.[73] These rotary-shaping instruments are machined with safe-ended noncutting tips, increasing D_0 diameters, and 16 mm of cutting blades. The ProFile 0.04 series was initially the instrument line of choice for those colleagues who filled root canal systems using a carrier-based obturation technique. ProFile 0.06 tapered instruments were developed for those clinicians who wanted a fuller shape over the length of the canal than the 0.04 tapered files alone could provide.[66] A few of the smaller ProFile 0.06 tapered series instruments and their geometries are reviewed in Fig. 8-40.

Orifice shapers.   Orifice shapers (Dentsply Tulsa Dental, Tulsa, Okla.) extend 19 mm below the head of the hand piece and have 10 mm of cutting blades. The series is

comprised of six instruments that are safe ended and have increasing D_0 diameters. If the clinician wants more continuous coronal shape than provided by the ProFile 0.04 and 0.06 systems, an appropriate orifice shaper can be selected based on the root dimensions. Two or three orifice shapers can generally prepare the coronal two thirds of a root canal system; in shorter teeth, they can prepare the entire length of the canal. (The most useful instruments and their geometries are reviewed in Fig. 8-41.) These instruments are designed to provide continuous shape in the coronal two thirds of root canals.

GT rotary files.   GT rotary files (Dentsply Tulsa Dental, Tulsa, Okla.) are made up of a series of four safe-ended instruments designed for canal preparation. Several features, such as the variably pitched flutes and the fixed minimal and maximal flute diameters, are intended to encourage the mechanical objectives for root canal preparation. Each instrument has a different linear length of cutting blades, because the tapers vary between a fixed D_0 diameter of 0.20 mm and a maximal flute diameter of 1.0 mm. The GT series instruments and their geometries are reviewed in Fig. 8-42.

Accessory GT files.   Accessory GT files (Dentsply Tulsa Dental, Tulsa Okla.) are designed to preenlarge the

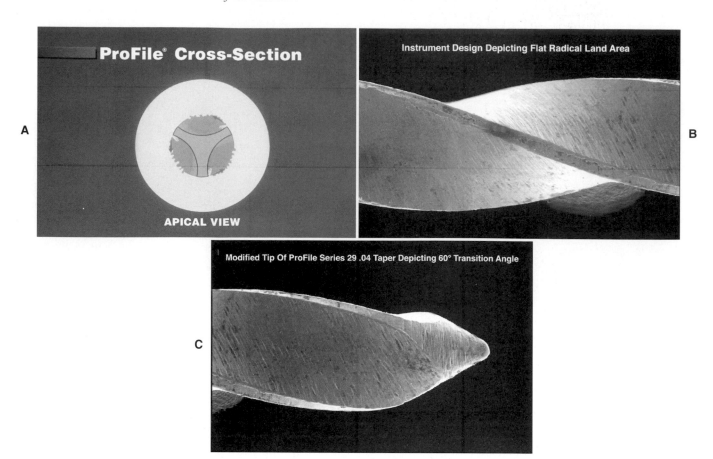

Fig. 8-38 **A,** Graphic cross section through a ProFile illustrates the radial lands cutting dentin and the U-shaped flutes providing space for the accumulation of debris. **B,** An SEM photograph (150×) of a ProFile Series 29 instrument depicts a flat radial land area. **C,** An SEM photograph (150×) of a ProFile Series 29 instrument depicts a safe-ended tip with a 60-degree transition angle. (**B** and **C** courtesy Dr. Edward J. McGreevey.)

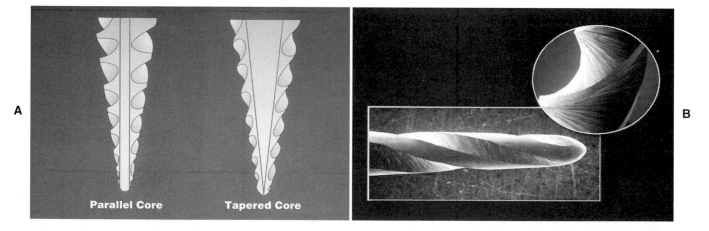

Fig. 8-39 **A,** The flexibility of a ProFile is significantly increased when the instrument's core is parallel versus tapered. **B,** An SEM photograph of a ProFile demonstrates its noncutting tip and intrablade space to accommodate debris.

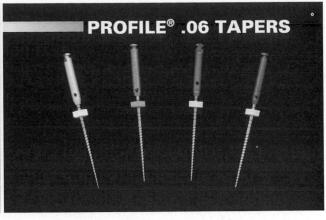

PROFILE® .06 TAPERS

COLOR CODE	TAPER mm/mm	DIAMETER D_0 in mm	DIAMETER D_{16} in mm
GOLD	.06	.20	1.16
RED	.06	.25	1.21
BLUE	.06	.30	1.26
GREEN	.06	.35	1.31

Fig. 8-40 **A,** Four of the instruments from the set of ProFile no. 0.06 tapered files. **B,** 0.20, 0.25, 0.30, and 0.35, 0.06 tapered ProFiles.

PROFILE® ORIFICE SHAPERS™

COLOR CODE	TAPER mm/mm	DIAMETER D_0 in mm	DIAMETER D_{10} in mm
GOLD	.05	.20	0.70
BLUE	.06	.30	0.90
BLACK	.06	.40	1.00
GOLD	.07	.50	1.20
BLUE	.08	.60	1.40

Fig. 8-41 **A,** Summary of five ProFile orifice shapers. **B,** 0.20, 0.30, 0.40, 0.50, and 0.60 orifice shapers. Note their various tapers.

GT™ FILES

COLOR CODE	TAPER mm/mm	DIAMETER D_0 in mm	MAXIMUM DIAMETER	CUTTING FLUTES in mm
WHITE	.06	.20	1.00	'14
YELLOW	.08	.20	1.00	'10
RED	.10	.20	1.00	'8
BLUE	.12	.20	1.00	'6

Fig. 8-42 **A,** Summary of the rotary GT files. **B,** 0.06, 0.08, 0.10, and 0.12 tapered rotary GT files.

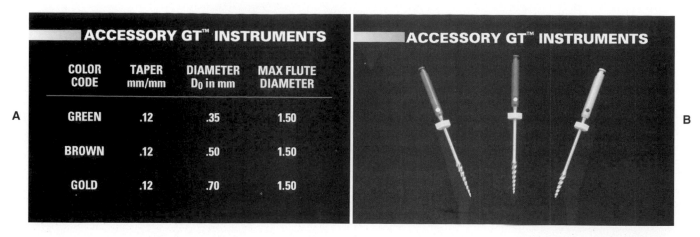

COLOR CODE	TAPER mm/mm	DIAMETER D_0 in mm	MAX FLUTE DIAMETER
GREEN	.12	.35	1.50
BROWN	.12	.50	1.50
GOLD	.12	.70	1.50

A
B

Fig. 8-43 **A,** Summary of the three Accessory GT files. **B,** The three Accessory GT files.

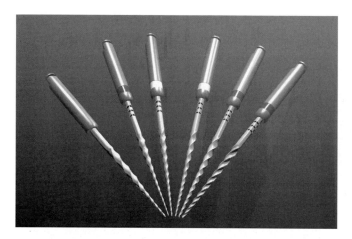

Fig. 8-44 The ProTaper rotary file series.

coronal portion of a canal or to prepare the apical one third of large root canal systems. The set consists of three NiTi instruments with tapers that are 0.12 mm/mm, MFDs are 1.5 mm, and D_0 diameters are either 0.35, 0.50, or 0.70 mm (Fig. 8-43). The use of Accessory GTs in posterior canals is limited to the coronal third because of their shank side cutting flutes equating to the same size as a GG no. 6.

ProTaper Instruments
The new ProTaper instruments (Dentsply Maillefer, Tulsa, Okla.) represent a significant development in root canal preparation procedures. The "basic" series is comprised of three "shaping" and three "finishing" instruments (Fig. 8-44).

The auxiliary shaping file, or shaper X, has an overall length of 19 mm, a D_0 diameter 0.19 mm, a partially active tip, 14 mm of cutting blades, and a D_{14} diameter of 1.2 mm. Shaper X has a much faster rate of taper from D_0 to D_9 as compared to the other two shaping files. Shaper X is used to optimally shape canals in shorter roots, relocate canals away

from external root concavities, and to produce more shape, as desired, in the coronal aspects of canals in longer roots.

Shaping files no. 1 and 2 have D_0 diameters of 0.185 mm and 0.20 mm, 14 mm of cutting blades, partially active tips, and their D_{14} diameters are 1.2 mm and 1.1 mm. The shaping files have increasingly larger tapers over the length of their cutting blades, allowing each instrument to engage, cut, and prepare a specific area of the canal. Shaping file no. 1 is designed to prepare the coronal one third of a canal, whereas shaping file no. 2 enlarges and prepares the middle one third. Although both instruments optimally prepare the coronal two thirds of a canal, they do progressively enlarge its apical one third.

Three finishing files have been developed to address the obvious variations in cross-sectional diameters that canals exhibit in their apical one thirds. The finishing instruments have D_0 diameters of 0.20, 0.25, and 0.30 mm and between D_0 and D_3, they taper 0.07%, 0.08%, and 0.09%, respectively. From D_4–D_{16}, each instrument has a decreasing taper, which increases flexibility and reduces the potential for dangerous taper-lock. Although these instruments have been designed to optimally finish the apical one third, they do subtly and progressively expand the shape in the middle one third of the canal. Generally, only one finishing instrument is required to prepare the apical one third of a canal, and the one selected is based on the specific canal's curvature and cross-sectional diameter.

A unique feature of the shaping files is their progressively tapered design, which clinically serves to significantly improve flexibility and cutting efficiency; it typically reduces the number of recapitulations needed to achieve length, especially in tight or more curved canals. Additionally, a progressively tapered file engages a smaller zone of dentin, which reduces torsional loads, file fatigue, and the potential for breakage.

Another unique feature of ProTaper instruments relates to their convex triangular cross section, which reduces the contact area between the file and dentin. This greater cutting

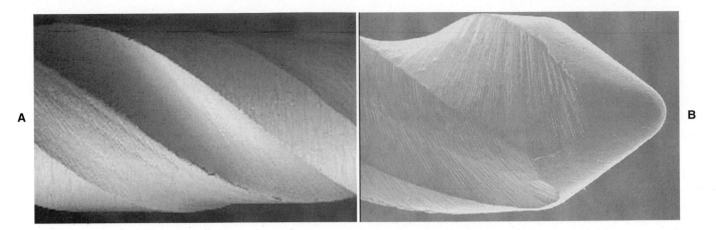

Fig. 8-45 **A,** An SEM photograph of a Quantec file shows the relieved radial lands. **B,** An SEM photograph shows the noncutting tip of a Quantec file.

efficiency has been safely improved by balancing the pitch and helical angle, which in combination prevents the instruments from inadvertently screwing into the canal. All the ProTaper instruments effectively auger debris out of the canal. Generally, only three instruments are required to produce a fully tapered canal that exhibits uniform shape over length.

The ProTaper instruments may be utilized in gear reduction electric handpieces at 300 RPM in accordance with universally recognized guidelines. Advancements in electric motors provide clinicians with the ability to choose the desired RPM and the recommended torque control for each specific instrument. The features and advantages of this type of electric motor (Tecnika/ATR, Dentsply Tulsa Dental, Tulsa, Okla.) promise to take rotary canal shaping to the next level.

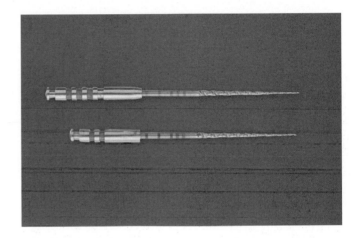

Fig. 8-46 Quantec's Axxess handles are 30% shorter than competitive files.

Quantec Files

The Quantec file series (Analytic Endodontics, Orange, Calif.) is a set of NiTi instruments available in tapers of 0.12, 0.10, 0.08, 0.06, 0.05, 0.04, 0.03, and 0.02 mm/mm. All of these instruments have D_0 diameters of 0.25 mm. The Quantec file has reduced radial lands to minimize surface tension, contact area, and stress on the instrument. Theoretically a relieved radial land improves irrigation flow apically and the movement of debris coronally.

The Quantec file is a two-fluted instrument that allows for a greater depth of flute, as compared with three-fluted instruments of the same tip, size, and diameter. Increasing the flute depth provides greater space for debris accumulation and subsequent travel out of the canal; it also potentially reduces file breakage. The variable helical angle of the Quantec flute design reduces the tendency of the file to screw into the canal (Fig. 8-45).

Quantec files vary in taper and rate of taper along their lengths. This feature is designed to balance the file's strength with flexibility. The Quantec file series offers the clinician a choice of a noncutting tip or a safe-cutting tip; the recommended rotational speed for all instruments is 340 RPM.

These instruments are available with Axxess handles that are 30% shorter than those of competitive files. When placed into the minihead, contra-angle handpiece (Analytic Endodontics, Orange, Calif.), these instruments provide 5 mm of additional interocclusal clearance (Fig. 8-46).

Canal Shape Versus File Taper

With the large variety of tapered instruments to choose from, it is easy to lose focus on the proper percentage for the tapered shape of a canal that ensures the root canal system is disinfected, and can be obturated in three dimensions. Research evaluating canal cleanliness (compared with canal shape in the respective thirds of roots) has clearly shown that preparations need to taper at least 0.08 mm/mm to ideally 0.10 mm/mm to ensure that a sufficient volume of irrigant can efficaciously circulate into the canal anatomy.[6,80,87] Even though instruments are available in tapers ranging from 0.02 mm/mm to 0.12 mm/mm, any tapered canal shape can be created given the appropriate techniques are used during root canal preparation (Fig. 8-47).

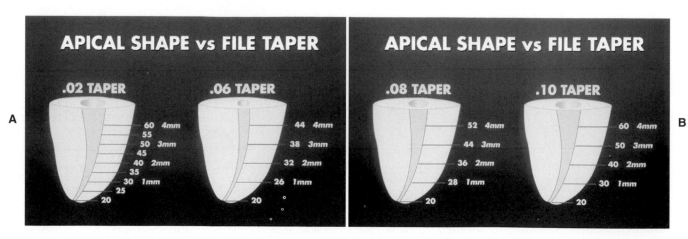

Fig. 8-47 Comparison of apical shape and file taper. **A,** Note that 0.02 tapered instruments used in a step-back manner can create a 10% taper. **B,** Note the differences in diameters at similar levels between preparations.

Cleaning Reagents, Devices, and Indicators

The concentration, ideal temperature, frequency of application, and delivery methods for irrigants, along with the time required for these solutions to thoroughly clean a shaped root canal system is continuously being investigated.[9,10,56] In fact, alternating between specific types of intracanal solutions or using them in combination has been shown to improve the potential for cleaning.[136] Furthermore, an enhancement in the area of irrigation is the use of radiopaque contrast solutions in conjunction with efficient and continuous delivery technologies.[71,114,147]

Sodium Hypochlorite The use of sodium hypochlorite (NaOCl) for treating wounds was introduced during World War I by a physician named Dakin.[32] Because antibiotics were not available until the bacteriologist, Alexander Flemming, discovered penicillin, lavaging large flesh wounds with "Dakin's solution" saved many lives that may have been otherwise lost to gangrenous infection.[41] Clorox or Purex are the sources for obtaining full-strength, 5.25% NaOCl. NaOCl is a powerful and inexpensive irrigant that has been shown to readily dissolve pulp tissue.[52,58] NaOCl should be used clinically in concentrations of 3% to 5% to take advantage of its ability to destroy all microorganisms upon direct contact and its unique ability to dissolve pulp tissue from all aspects of the root canal system.[71,128,147]

For example, as Grossman demonstrated 60 years ago, place a freshly broached pulp in a dappen dish filled with 5.25% NaOCl, and observe that it will dissolve within 20 to 30 minutes.[22] Studies have shown that in preflared canals where the coronal two thirds is first preenlarged, warming NaOCl to approximately 60°C (140°F) significantly increases the rate and effectiveness of tissue dissolution.[15,28,44] Clinically, a 60°C warm-water bath is prepared by placing a beaker of water on a hot plate. Preloaded syringes of NaOCl may be warmed by placing them into this warm-

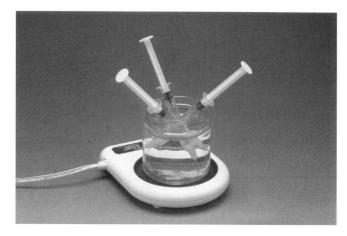

Fig. 8-48 Preloaded syringes of NaOCl are warmed by placing them in a 140°F water bath.

water bath (Fig. 8-48). Solutions of NaOCl should be prepared fresh daily to obtain optimal clinical results.[96] To maximize tissue dissolution, access cavities must be filled brimful with NaOCl (Fig. 8-49). In fact, one of the important advantages of pretreatment is to build teeth up so they have pulp chambers that can retain irrigants. The potential for an irrigant is maximized when it is *heated*, flooded into *shaped canals*, and given ample *time* to work.[15,19,107]

The frequency of irrigation is dictated by the amount of work that a particular instrument performs. As a rule, a clinician should irrigate copiously, recapitulate, and reirrigate at least after every two to three instruments. Generally, this cycle should be repeated more frequently in tighter, longer, and more curved canals, and especially if the system exhibits unusual anatomy.[21] Files potentially carry irrigant progressively deeper into the canal by surface tension. However, when an instrument is placed into a relatively small canal, the file tends to displace the irrigant. When the instrument is

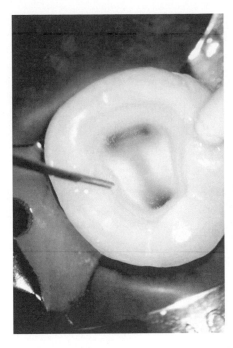

Fig. 8-49 The access cavity of a mandibular molar is filled brimful with heated, full-strength NaOCl.

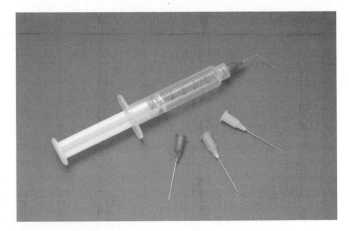

Fig. 8-50 Max-I-Probe irrigation system consisting of 25, 28, and 30 gauged closed ended side port–delivery irrigating canuli.

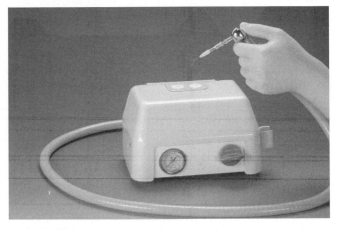

Fig. 8-51 The Endo Irrigator. This unit allows clinicians to conveniently choose and dispense various irrigants with the push of a button.

withdrawn, the irrigant usually flows back into the space the file occupied, unless there is an air pocket. This phenomenon must be appreciated to integrate the most efficacious irrigation method clinically.[107]

Clinicians can choose their preferred method for transporting irrigant from a variety of irrigating devices. Irrigation can be delivered in a variety of syringes and passively injected manually. Additionally, various gauged canuli can be chosen to achieve deeper and safer placement. Certain canuli dispense irrigant through a closed ended side port delivery system (Fig. 8-50).[65] Regardless of the method of introduction, it is essential to have a pulp chamber filled brimful with a reservoir of NaOCl to promote tissue dissolution, flushing-out of debris, and three-dimensional cleaning of the preparation. The hand that holds the irrigating syringe is *always kept in motion* when dispensing irrigant to prevent the needle from inadvertently wedging in the canal. Slowly injecting irrigant in combination with continuous hand movement will virtually eliminate NaOCl accidents.[11,107,113] It is important to irrigate frequently and voluminously to introduce fresh solution and potentiate its circulation into all aspects of the root canal system. Recently new technologies have been developed that deliver various types of "on-line" irrigants from in-office air-pressurized bottles (Vista Dental Products, Racine, WI). In this method of irrigation, clinicians can select among several solutions with a push of a button. Various gauged canuli can then be selected and attached onto the irrigating hand piece. New irrigation technology allows clinicians to conveniently choose, dispense, and more effectively irrigate root canal systems (Fig. 8-51).

Chelating Agents   Chelating agents containing ethylenediaminetetracitic acid (EDTA) may be used clinically to eliminate many cleaning and shaping frustrations.[47,61,135] The purpose of a chelator is for lubrication, emulsification, and holding debris in suspension. Chelators are formulated for clinical use and can be selected in either a viscous suspension or an aqueous solution. Viscous suspensions have several ingredients typically suspended in a water-soluble vehicle.

RC Prep (Premier Dental Products, King of Prussia, PA) is a viscous chelator; its principle ingredients are EDTA, urea peroxide, and propylene glycol. Glycol is the lubricant that coats instruments and facilitates their movement in open canals containing calcific material or in restricted canals that exhibit various degrees of calcification.[59,133] RC Prep can be obtained in a large preloaded syringe and an appropriate amount is then expressed into a small disposable syringe for single patient use. When indicated, the pulp chamber is filled brimful with chelator (Fig. 8-52). Precurved files are gently

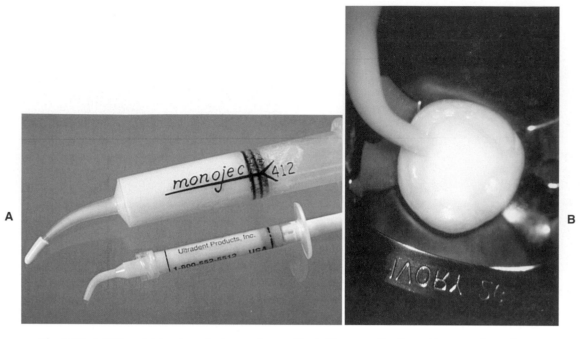

Fig. 8-52 **A,** RC Prep is taken from the large syringe and loaded into a smaller disposable syringe for single-patient use. **B,** A mandibular molar filled brimful with RC Prep after opening the orifices.

inserted through the pulp chamber and carry chelator into the canal by surface tension. The lubricant encourages the file to *slip* and *slide* by intracanal calcifications, such as pulp stones or sheaths of fibrotic tissue.[107] In tighter and more restrictive canals, chelators are very important to use during initial coronal enlargement, because these suspensions emulsify tissue, soften dentin, minimize blockages, and hold debris in suspension where it can be subsequently aspirated from the preparation.

A viscous suspension of a chelator advantageously promotes the emulsification of organic tissue and facilitates the negotiation of the canal. Collagen is a major constituent of vital pulp tissue and can be inadvertently packed into a glue-like mass that contributes to iatrogenic blocks. In vital cases, attempting to negotiate any portion of a canal with a no. 10 file without the aid of a chelator can be risky. When the instrument is withdrawn, the vital tissue tends to collapse and readhere to itself. A chelator discourages this tissue phenomenon and accelerates emulsification by leaving a favorable pilot hole that facilitates the introduction of the sequentially larger instrument. Viscous suspensions of chelating containing reagents are important adjuncts to overcome pockets of resistance within a canal and to assist in the development of a smooth glide path to the terminus. Chelators should be used for short periods, because their protracted use can soften dentin and predispose the patient to iatrogenic mishaps.[47]

A *viscous* chelator is best used for holding debris in liquid suspension. As an example, RC Prep encourages the flotation of pulpal remnants and dentinal mud that reduces the proba-bility of blocking the canal. Irrigation with NaOCl follows the use of RC Prep; it should be used passively, frequently, and voluminously. Using RC Prep in concert with NaOCl causes a nascent release of oxygen that kills anaerobic bacteria. Furthermore, RC Prep and NaOCl produce significant effervescence, creating an elevator action to evacuate debris that was dislodged from the root canal system (Fig. 8-53).[25,134]

An *aqueous* solution of chelator is best reserved for finishing the preparation; it removes the smear layer that is an organic or inorganic film or both formed on the walls of the canal by the cutting action of instruments (Fig. 8-54).[75,82,85] Although rotary NiTi instruments are known to effectively auger debris out of a canal, they simultaneously burnish dentinal mud and organic debris into the dentinal tubules.[87] Therefore after optimal canal preparation, a 17% solution of aqueous EDTA (Roth International, Chicago, IL) is irrigated into the canal.[61] Research has shown that rinsing for 1 minute with EDTA eliminates the smear layer, opens up the dentinal tubules, and provides a cleaner surface against which gutta-percha and sealer will adapt.[69,139]

"Visualization" Endogram   Central to successful endodontic treatment has been the use of chemicals to penetrate, circulate, and clean all aspects of the root canal system. The most important chemicals used to actively clean the root canal system, NaOCl and chelating agents, are radiolucent. Therefore these reagents do not help the dentist radiographically visualize the anatomy of the root canal system. Conventional radiographs and digital radiography (Schick Technologies, New York, NY) do not have sufficient resolution to

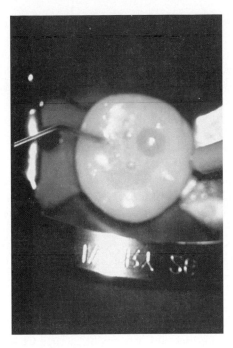

Fig. 8-53 Note the vigorous effervescence that results when NaOCl is irrigated into a chamber filled with RC Prep.

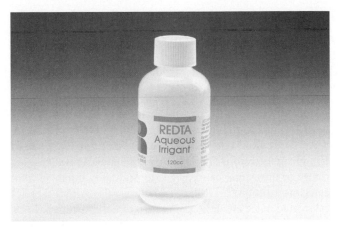

Fig. 8-54 A bottle containing an aqueous solution of 17% EDTA.

completely reveal the intricacies and microanatomy of the root canal systems.

Recently a new experimental irrigating solution, the Ruddle Solution, has been formulated to provide a breakthrough in clinical endodontics.[80,114,147] This experimental irrigant contains 5% NaOCl, hypaque, and 17% EDTA. Medicine has clinically used hypaque, high-contrast, and injectable dye for angiography, arteriography, urography, and nephrotomography. Hypaque is an aqueous solution of two iodine salts, diatrizoate meglumine and sodium iodine. The solution has the same specific gravity as NaOCl, is water soluble, has a pH of 6.7 to 7.7, and is stable at room temperature. Until now, dentistry has not used radiopaque contrast solutions to radiographically visualize root canal systems under clinical conditions. This composition simultaneously provides the *solvent action* of full-strength NaOCl, *visualization* (because its radiodensity is similar to gutta-percha), and improved *penetration* (because the tensioactive agent lowers surface tension).[12] Clinicians can use an endogram to visualize the microanatomy, verify the shape, and monitor the remaining root wall thickness during preparation procedures.[147]

Clinically, the solution is flushed into the root canal system of a tooth once sufficient access to the pulp chamber has been made. The sodium hypochlorite portion of the composition will dissolve the pulp and eliminate the bacteria, along with endotoxins that are harbored within the root canal system. The solvent action of this solution progressively clears out the contents of the root canal system, thus enabling the iodine portion of the composition to flow into this vacated space.[71] Endograms are useful in visualizing pathologic events, such as caries, certain fractures, missed canals, and leaking restorations. Additionally, endograms can assist the clinician in managing internal resorption, because the solution will map its location, size, and extent. In endodontic nonsurgical retreatment, the endogram has shown promise for improving diagnostics, treatment planning, and management of iatrogenic mishaps. This method of visualization assists dentists in determining the best course of action and in deciding whether to salvage or extract a particular tooth.

Ultrasonics and Microbrushes   Ultrasonic devices have been advocated and used with the hope that they will optimally clean the root canal system, either during or after canal preparation techniques.[8,29,30] However, ultrasonic instrumentation never fulfilled clinical expectations as a primary method to prepare root canals.[48,84] Further, ultrasonic techniques for canal preparation have not been clearly demonstrated to be as predictable, effective, or efficient as more conventional methods.[78,94]

However, the use of ultrasonic energy to activate irrigating solutions in optimally prepared canals continues to be intriguing.[8,49,64] Root canals prepared and tapered according to *Mechanical Objective no. 1* are good candidates for ultrasonic fluid activation. Traditionally, a small file would be placed passively in the canal and ultrasonically activated. The energized file produces a fluid movement called *acoustic streaming*. This mechanical energy warmed the NaOCl and dislodged residual debris from the preparation.[2,3,4] The combination of activating and heating the irrigating solution is a potent adjunct for cleaning into all aspects of the root canal system.[15,28] The clinical concern regarding the use of ultrasonically activated files is the potential for these instruments to gouge and mar the walls of the finished preparation.[31] Recently a noncutting NiTi instrument, designed to activate irrigant and enhance cleaning, has been field tested. This ultrasonically energized instrument is an improvement over an energized file with cutting blades, yet it cannot intimately contact the irregular walls that comprise the root canal system. These shortcomings have driven new armamentarium refinements.

Advancements in small-wire technology, injection-molding processes, bristle materials, and bristle-attaching techniques have enabled the creation of an endodontic microbrush for clinical field testing (Fig. 8-55, *A*). The best diameter, length, stiffness, and material of each bristle have been identified, and the optimal configuration studied (Fig. 8-55, *B*). Bristles can be attached to either braided wires or flexible, plastic cores, and the brushes can be activated using rotary or ultrasonic hand pieces to optimally finish the root canal preparation.[64,68] Rotary and ultrasonic endobrushes are fabricated in ISO lengths, contain 16 mm of bristles, have D_0 bristle diameters of 0.40, 0.50, 0.60, and 0.80 mm; they are the tapered equivalent of nonstandardized gutta-percha master cone sizes fine-medium, medium, medium-large and large, respectively (Fig. 8-55, *C, D*). Rotary activated micro-brushes turn at about 300 RPM, and the helical bristle pattern effectively augers residual debris out of the canal in a coronal direction. Microbrushes designed for ultrasonic use effectively brush the walls of the preparation and activate solutions of NaOCl and 17% EDTA to produce cleaned canals.[64,134,149] Research is being conducted to ascertain which method of microbrush activation, solution, or irriga-

tion sequence most predictably, effectively, and efficiently produces cleaned root canal walls with open dentinal tubules. Regardless of rotary versus ultrasonic activation, microbrushes can finish the preparation and should be used in the presence of 17% EDTA for 1 minute to optimally clean the root canal system.

CANAL PREPARATION TECHNIQUES

The mechanical objectives for canal preparation can be fulfilled using a variety of instruments. The concepts for canal preparation *endure,* whereas the instruments, strategies, and techniques used for cleaning and shaping root canals constantly *evolve.* Clinical performance is enhanced when there is use of the best technologies in conjunction with a high level of teamwork and organization (Fig. 8-56). In tennis, the best players shut out all distractions and enter a zone where they strive to be one with the ball. Just as in tennis, clinicians need to eliminate all distractions and delegate tasks so they too can enter a zone and be one with the root. Clinicians who are in the root mentally and physically can focus on doing small things well; this will improve predictability and results.

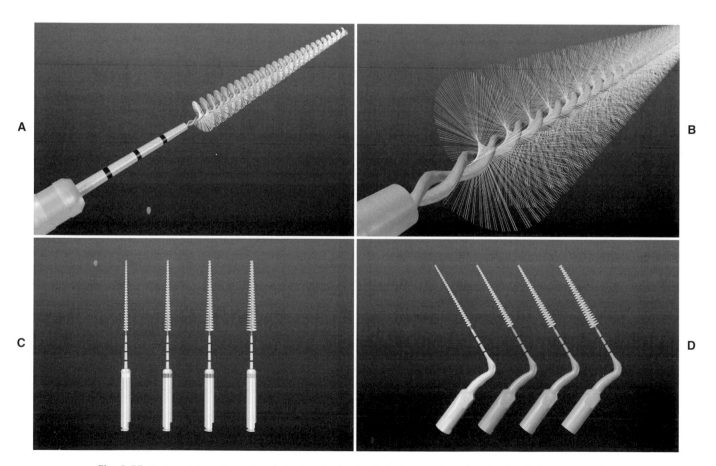

Fig. 8-55 **A,** A prototype tapered endodontic microbrush. **B,** A close-up view of a microbrush demonstrates the braided wires used to secure the bristles and their configuration. **C,** Four variably tapered–rotary driven microbrushes. **D,** Four variably tapered–ultrasonically driven microbrushes.

Root Canal Preparation Sequence

When straight-line access has been completed and all the orifices have been identified, attention is directed toward preparing the root canal. If the pulp is vital and bleeding, the chamber is filled brimful with a viscous chelator. When the pulp is necrotic, the chamber is irrigated and filled with a 5.25% solution of warm NaOCl. Based on the preoperative radiographs, the smaller stainless steel files are measured and precurved to conform to the anticipated full length and curvature of the root canal. Stainless steel, 0.02 tapered, no. 10 and no. 15 hand files are then used to scout the coronal two thirds of the root canal system. After scouting the coronal two thirds, the canal is flushed with NaOCl and preenlarged using hand instruments or rotary-shaping files. With the coronal two thirds optimally prepared and filled with irrigant, the apical third is then scouted and information is gathered. Scouter files are used to negotiate the rest of the canal, confirm a smooth glide path to the terminus, and establish patency. Typically working length is confirmed with an electronic apex locator or by exposing a radiograph. Even with the advantages of electronic apex locators, occasionally it is valuable to radiographically confirm the position of a file within a root canal. With the root canal negotiated and the anatomy fully appreciated, a decision can be made whether to finish the apical third with hand or rotary instruments. The following canal preparation methods will describe how to choose, use, and sequence instruments for preparing root canals.

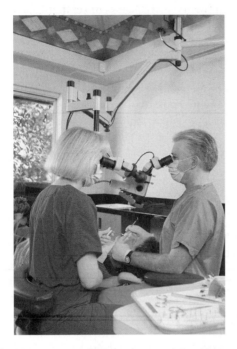

Fig. 8-56 Patient care emphasizing the use of the microscope, teamwork, and organization.

Scouting the Coronal Two Thirds

Disposable, stainless steel, ISO 0.02, tapered no. 10 and no. 15 hand files are used to scout the coronal two thirds. Scouting files are not just measuring wires; they provide the following important pieces of information (Fig. 8-57)[107]:

1. They reveal the cross-sectional diameter of a canal and provide information as to whether the canal is open, partially restricted, or calcified.

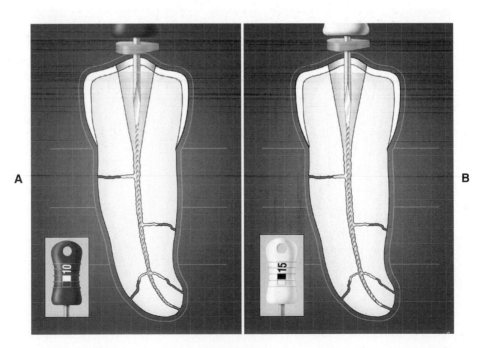

Fig. 8-57 **A,** A scouter file may be used to confirm straight-line access, verify the diameter of a canal, and reveal root canal system anatomy. **B,** The no. 15 file follows the path of the no. 10 file, improves the glide path, and dictates the next clinical step.

2. They confirm the presence or absence of straight-line access. Clinicians can observe the handle position of an instrument to see if it is upright and paralleling the long axis of the tooth or skewed off-axis. When the roots are under the circumferential dimensions of the clinical crown and the file handle is upright, the clinician is able to confirm both coronal and radicular straight-line access. However, when the handle of the initial scouting instrument is off the long axis of the tooth, then pre-enlargement procedures should be directed toward uprighting the file handle. This clinical activity often involves refining and expanding the access preparation and selectively removing restrictive dentin from the coronal third of the canal. This procedural nuance is critical, simplifies all subsequent instrumentation procedures, and eliminates many cleaning and shaping frustrations (Fig. 8-58).

3. They provide important information regarding root canal system anatomy. Clinicians need to appreciate the five commonly encountered anatomic forms (i.e., canals that merge, curve, recurve, dilacerate, or divide).

Most canals exhibit enough space to accommodate a no. 10 file. This instrument is inserted into the canal and passively pushed apically as its handle is gently rocked back and forth. A 15-degree clockwise (CW) rotation is followed by a 15-degree counterclockwise (CCW) rotation of the file handle. Repeating this reciprocating handle motion produces apical file movement, thus allowing the instrument to be automatically drawn down into the canal. Clinically, only two possibilities exist when attempting to negotiate a root canal:

1. In canals that are more straightforward, a reciprocating handle motion will passively pull the file into the canal; it may even slide to length.

2. In canals that are more narrow, curved, or exhibit intra-radicular divisions, the rate of taper of the instrument often exceeds the rate of taper of the canal. Consequently, apical file movement is limited.

In either instance, no attempt should be made to reach the terminus during the early phases of scouting the canal. If the no. 10 file moves with ease through the canal and feels as if it could go to length, the clinician should move to the next larger instrument. Scouting procedures are performed to create or verify that there is a predictable pathway in the coronal two thirds of the canal. Additionally, scouting files are used to explore any given third of a canal.

In the instance where the canal is more restrictive, the no. 10 file often will not go to length. This should not be a concern, because in this method of canal preparation there is no preconceived depth to which any file should advance. When the handle of the file feels snug, the clinician should bounce off resistance by pulling the file coronally 1 to 2 mm. The pull stroke ensures that the instrument is cutting *away from the terminus* toward the increasingly larger cross-sectional diameters of the canal. Again, the file should be passed into the canal until the handle feels snug; a short coronal pull stroke completes another cutting cycle. The clinician should passively take what the canal will give up and continue this motion and movement for five to six cutting cycles. Each cutting cycle removes restrictive dentin, carries more irrigant or chelator deeper, puts more debris into suspension, and

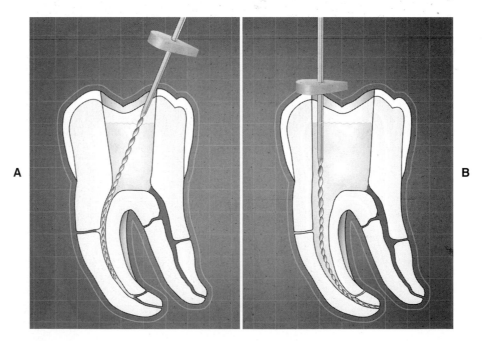

Fig. 8-58 A, Attempting to negotiate the canal when the handle of the file is off-axis because an inadequate access opening predisposes to iatrogenic mishaps. **B,** Expanding the access cavity in conjunction with preenlarging the coronal two thirds of the canal uprights the file and encourages it to slide to length.

improves the glide path into the canal. In the instance where a no. 10 scouting file moves easily through the canal and to within 2 to 3 mm of the working length, the clinician should proceed directly to the no. 15 file. Preenlargement procedures are directed toward creating space for more efficient rotary instruments; thus it is desirable at this stage of treatment for the scouting files to cut short of length, laterally cutting dentin while being drawn *out of the canal*.

The clinician should now proceed to a no. 15 file, which is 50% wider at D_0 than a no. 10 file. This instrument should be passively worked into the canal until the handle feels snug. Again, if the file approaches tentative working length, it should be withdrawn and the clinician should proceed to the next sequential instrument: a no. 20 file. If the file feels like it is binding in the canal short of the estimated working length, it can be worked reciprocally up-and-down to generate lateral space, expand the volume of irrigant, and improve the glide path. If the cutting flutes of the no. 15 file are lightly tapped into dentin and short of length, the clinician should cut away from the foramen (i.e., out of the canal) and toward the greater cross-sectional diameters. Each light push-and-pull repetition generates another cutting cycle that creates more coronal taper, which increases space for irrigation and promotes the removal of debris.

After the use of the no. 15 file, when the canal is *straightforward*, generally enough space exists to accommodate rotary-shaping files. The clinician should irrigate voluminously and passively with NaOCl. If RC Prep was in the pulp chamber, vigorous effervescence will effectively lift debris out of the pulpal space to the occlusal surface where it can be aspirated away. The clinician should then recapitulate with the no. 10 clearing file to carry fresh irrigant deeper and move debris into the irrigant solution. Generally, the no. 10 file will now move more easily through areas of the canal that were previously restrictive and, even if the canal was somewhat calcified, the file will move deeper. Once this clearing file extends apical from its original depth, the clinician should use several gentle, 1 to 2 mm amplitude push-and-pull strokes. This subtle and repeated movement breaks up debris and allows the instrument to *slip and slide*. Next, the push-and-pull stroke should be increased to an amplitude of 2 to 3 mm. If the file *slides and glides* along the length of the canal, the clinician should reirrigate to flush out the debris that was moved into solution (Fig. 8-59).

After using two 0.02 tapered files, enough space should have been created coronally to receive more efficient rotary-shaping instruments. However, if the canal is not yet large enough to accommodate a rotary-shaping instrument, no. 20, no. 25, and no. 30 files should be used to widen the canal space (as previously described). This will improve the glide path and create sufficient space to passively accommodate rotary-shaping instruments (Fig. 8-60).

Coronal Two-Thirds Preparation

Coronal two-thirds preenlargement of a canal may be accomplished in either a step-back or crown-down manner; the differences between these techniques must be appreciated. A step-back technique is the sequential use of instruments, starting with the smaller sizes and progressing toward the

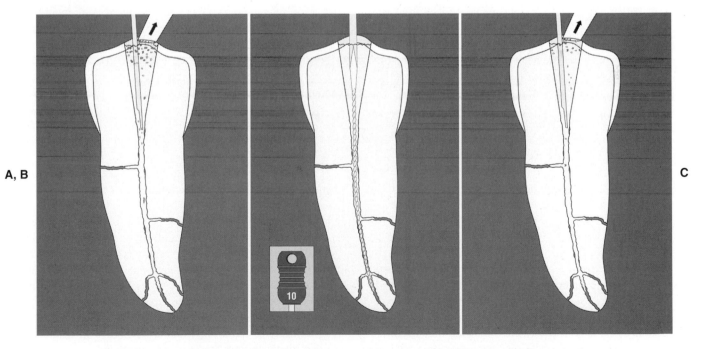

A, B   **C**

Fig. 8-59 **A,** The clinician should passively and voluminously irrigate to flush debris coronally where it can be suctioned out of the tooth. **B,** The no. 10 file is recapitulated and moved up and down in short amplitude strokes to break up pockets of debris and move it into solution. **C,** After the use of the clearing file, the clinician should irrigate passively to dislodge debris from the preparation.

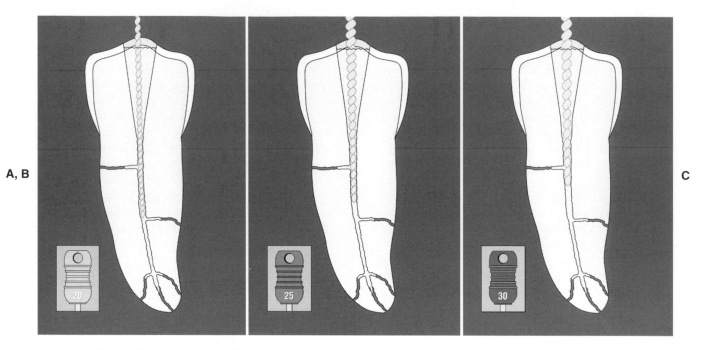

Fig. 8-60 A, A no. 20 flexofile is carried into the canal and, if short of length, is worked passively to extend the preparation. **B,** A no. 25 flexofile can be worked to progressively improve radicular access to the apical third. **C,** A no. 30 flexofile is used to eliminate more restrictive dentin, improve the volume of irrigant, and promote the preparation objectives.

larger sizes, regardless of the type of instrument series used.[27,49,100] A crown-down technique is the serial use of instruments, starting with the larger sizes and progressing toward the smaller sizes.[83,90] There is virtual consensus that NiTi rotary-shaping files are best used in a crown-down technique, whereas ISO hand files and GGs are best used in a step-back technique.[81] The advantages of preenlarging a canal using files and GGs in a step-back technique are two-fold:

1. Smaller instruments can initially be placed more easily and more deeply within a root canal space, where they can be used to *cut on the pull stroke.* In a crown-down technique, instruments *cut on the push stroke,* which tends to inadvertently drive pulp stones, fibrotic tissue, and debris deeper into the root canal space.

2. The coronal two thirds of canals can easily be moved and relocated away from furcal danger and toward the greatest bulk of dentin when GGs are used in a step-back technique.[63,79,107] This is especially important in the clinical situation where the handle of the scouter file is initially off the long axis of a furcated tooth (see Fig. 8-58). The clinical importance of moving the coronal aspect of a canal away from furcal danger is significant when we reflect on the anatomy of furcated teeth (Fig. 8-61, *A*).[70,84,98] Cross sections through the coronal third of furcated roots reveal that canals are not typically centered anatomically within their roots. Instead, they are often skewed toward the furcal-side concavities (Fig. 8-61, *B*) (see Chapter 7). GGs are used to cut and remove dentin on just one or two of the *outer* walls of the canal and

away from furcal danger (Fig. 8-61, *C*). Often the access cavity must be refined, expanded, and the axial wall moved mesially to create straight-line access into the apical one third of a preparation (Fig. 8-61, *D*). Using GGs in a step-back technique can preserve root structure, relocate a canal away from furcal danger, and fulfill the mechanical objectives of cleaning and shaping (Fig. 8-61, *E*). When there is not straight-line radicular access, experience has shown that any rotary instrument (used *large to small*) results in a final preparation that is not centered within the dimensions of the root. Preparations tend to move toward external root concavities because crown-down techniques circumferentially machine dentin uniformly around the existing long axis of a canal (Fig. 8-61, *F*).

A variety of techniques can be used to perform coronal two-thirds preenlargement techniques.

Hand Instruments   If the clinician chooses to prepare the coronal two thirds with hand instruments, an excellent method to remove dentin in this region is to use the balanced-force technique.[57,102,105] Modifications to the balanced-force technique that take advantage of its best attributes while eliminating certain undesirable aspects include:

- Use safe-ended NiTi file sizes no. 35 to no. 60.[104]
- Limit use to the straightforward portions in canals that exhibit abrupt curvatures or dilacerations.
- Use with caution in the apical 2 to 3 mm of canals exhibiting complex anatomy.

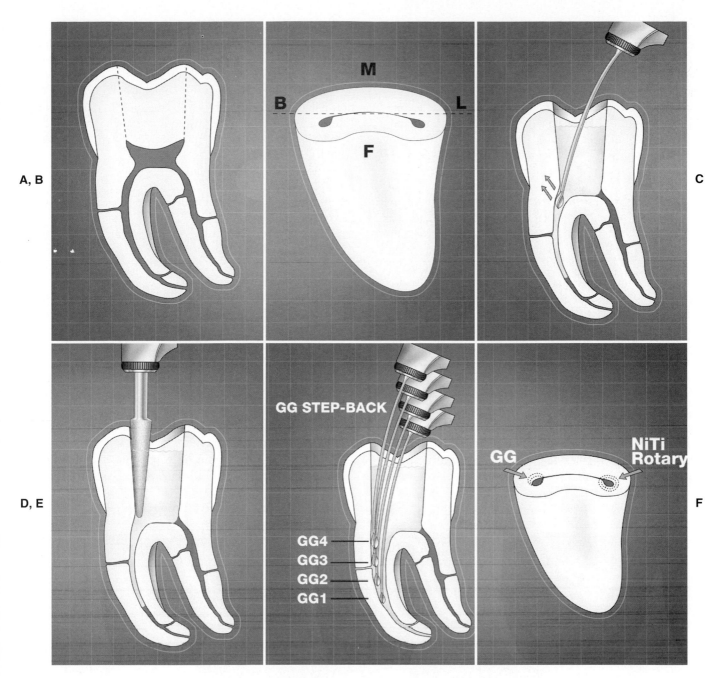

Fig. 8-61 **A,** The anticipated access path shows the mesial systems typically turn abruptly into the pulp chamber and emphasizes the mesial root–furcal side concavity. **B,** A cross section through the mesial root illustrates that the canals and related isthmus are skewed toward the furcation side of the root. **C,** GGs are ideally one- or two-walled cutting instruments. Their shafts are arced so the head will cut and move the canal away from the furca. **D,** A surgical length tapered diamond is used to refine and move the mesial wall of the access preparation mesially. **E,** GGs are used to relocate the canal away from furcal danger and are stepped out of the canal. **F,** A cross section through the mesial root illustrates that GGs provide a more centered canal. By contrast, NiTi rotary instruments cut all walls equally circumferentially around the canal axis.

The *balanced-force technique* uses instruments in a step-back manner to initiate preenlargement procedures and to rapidly gain access to the apical third. The following description represents the three distinct phases that comprise one "balanced-force" instrument cycle.

Phase I—file insertion. File insertion is accomplished by reciprocating the handle of the file in a back-and-forth motion until it feels snug. The handle of the file should then be turned in a 45- to 90-degree, CW rotation to draw the instrument down, move its cutting blades deeper into the canal, and engage dentin (Fig. 8-62, *A*).

Phase II—file cutting. During this phase, the clinician applies two *simultaneous* forces on the file handle. The file handle is rotated CCW while simultaneously pushed apically (Fig. 8-62, *B*). When rotated CCW, the tendency of the file to back out of the canal is balanced by the force of the file being pushed into the canal.[23,101,102] During file cutting, it is normal to hear clicking or popping as dentin is sheared, cut, and carved off the canal wall. After the first cutting cycle, the instrument is extended slightly deeper into the canal in the manner described in Phase I; another Phase II cutting cycle is then repeated. Phase I and Phase II can be repeated between two and four times; they are ultimately limited by the diameter of the file or the amount of accumulating debris or both that potentially prevents the cutting blades from engaging dentin.

Phase III—flute loading. The dentin cut in the manner described in phase II lies partially in the interblade spaces of the file and partially in the canal just apical to the instrument. This debris can then be removed from the canal by rotating the file handle CW, while simultaneously pulling the instrument coronally (Fig. 8-62, *C*). When flute loading is performed properly, the position of the file tip never advances apically, because the tendency of the file to be drawn into the canal is balanced by the force of the file being lifted out of the canal. After two or three rotations, the file is withdrawn from the canal; its apical flutes will be loaded with dentin mud.

The balanced-force technique is most efficient and affords three significant advantages when compared with other manual-shaping techniques used to pre-enlarge the coronal two thirds of a canal.[107] These three steps are:

1. File cutting occurs essentially at the apical extent of the NiTi file and not along its length. As such, the clinician gains better control of the file and can selectively cut and remove dentin within a specific region of the canal.

2. The safe-ended NiTi file tip stays centered in the root when activated in Phase II file cutting. Therefore dentin is safely cut and removed uniformly about the long axis of the canal and not at the expense of the furcal wall in multirooted teeth.

3. It is *not* necessary to precurve NiTi files to simulate canal anatomy; they should be used straight as manufactured. Because of its metallurgy and method of use, the file stays centered in the canal; thus the canal effectively guides the hand files in most curvatures.

The clinician may continue preenlargement procedures by selecting the no. 35, no. 40, and no. 45 NiTi files that will

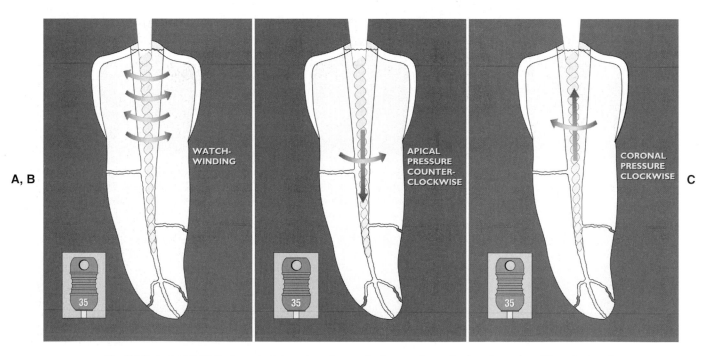

Fig. 8-62 **A,** A NiTi 35 file is worked down into the canal using a reciprocating handle motion. When the handle is begins to feel snug, it is rotated 45 to 90 degrees CW, so the file will engage dentin. **B,** To cut dentin the handle of the file is rotated CCW, while the instrument is simultaneously pushed apically to prevent it from backing out of the canal. **C,** Debris is removed by rotating the handle of the file CW, while the instrument is simultaneously pulled coronally to prevent it from screwing into the canal.

cut dentin and perform canal shaping with either a gentle, reciprocating push-and-pull or balanced-force technique (Fig. 8-63). In this approach, no preconceived depth exists to which any particular file must go. Each instrument is worked repeatedly, deliberately, and passively to whatever level the canal dictates to the clinician. If a given file does not engage dentin, it is usually because the rate of taper of the file exceeds the rate of taper of the canal, or because its cutting blades have been pushed off the canal wall because the instrument's flutes are full of dentin mud.

At this stage of the enlarging process, the clinician should irrigate, recapitulate with a no. 10 clearing file to break up pockets of resistance and move debris into solution, and reirrigate to flush out the canal (Fig. 8-64). After more body work the clinician should be able to place the no. 10 file deeper into the root canal system (often to the RT). Shaping can then continue with the no. 50, no. 55, and no. 60 files (Fig. 8-65). Again, the clinician can choose the particular handle motion or file movement desired for progressively enlarging, blending, and cleaning the coronal two thirds of the canal system. After every three files, the clinician should irrigate, recapitulate, and reirrigate (Fig. 8-66). During shaping procedures, the irrigating needle can be introduced progressively deeper into the canal space. Passive irrigation flushes and removes dentin mud. Fresh solution may then penetrate deeper into the dentinal tubules and lateral ramifications to further enhance cleaning.

The clinician can recapitulate through the file series to carry another wave of shaping progressively deeper into the root canal space. Two, three, or even more recapitulations (through a series of files passively and progressively) allow each instrument to automatically work deeper. Each pass through a series of files produces a more continuous canal taper, evidenced by observing successively larger instruments uniformly backing out of the canal. In this method of canal preparation, hand files, although not as efficient as rotary instruments, can be used partially or completely to prepare the coronal two thirds of a canal.

GG Drills   An excellent way to rapidly remove restrictive dentin in the coronal two thirds of a canal is to use a series of GG drills.[117] Experience suggests that the coronal two thirds of most canals can be preenlarged with GGs. GGs are only placed into canals that have been previously scouted with no. 10 and no. 15 files. The no. 10 and no. 15 files have diameters equivalent to 0.42 and 0.47 mm, respectively, at D_{16}. The maximum head diameter of a GG-1 is equivalent to an ISO size no. 50 file at D_0 (0.50 mm). After scouting files, if the canal is still too small to passively accommodate a GG-1, the clinician should continue progressive canal enlargement with hand instruments until adequate space is created. If RC Prep was used during scouting procedures, it is important to irrigate and fill the access cavity brimful with NaOCl before using the GGs.

Preenlargement techniques using GGs begins by placing a nonrotating GG-1 in a canal until it lightly contacts restrictive dentin. The clinician should bounce off resistance by lifting the GG coronally (about 1 mm) so that it is loose

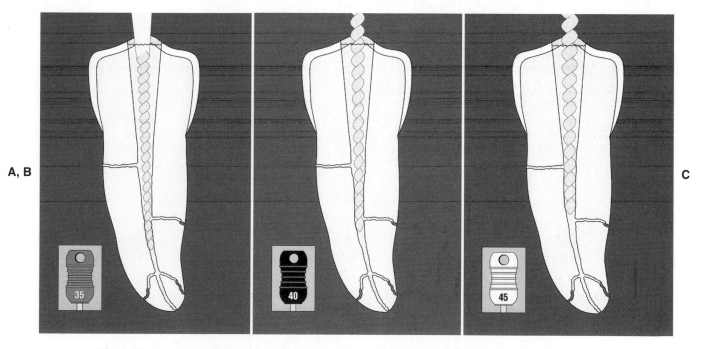

A, B

C

Fig. 8-63 **A,** A 35 NiTi file can be used in a variety of ways to generate more shape in the body of the canal. **B,** A 40 NiTi file typically works shorter and progressively enlarges the canal. **C,** A 45 NiTi file works even more coronally and improves access into the apical one third of the canal.

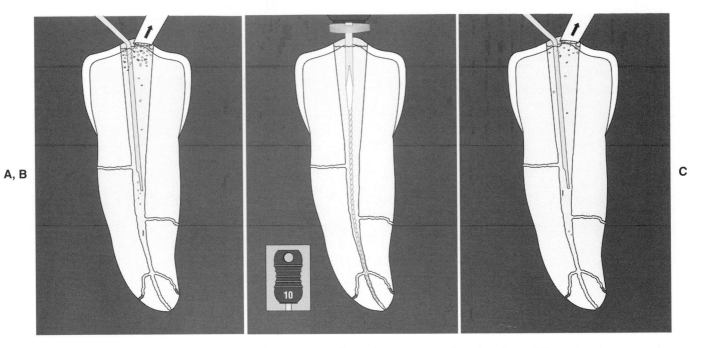

Fig. 8-64 **A,** After progressive preenlargement procedures, the irrigating canuli can be advanced deeper into the canal to passively deliver fresh irrigant. **B,** A clearing file is used in small amplitude strokes and short of length to break up debris and move it into solution. **C,** Reirrigating after using the clearing file to dislodge more debris; this allows fresh irrigant into the root canal system.

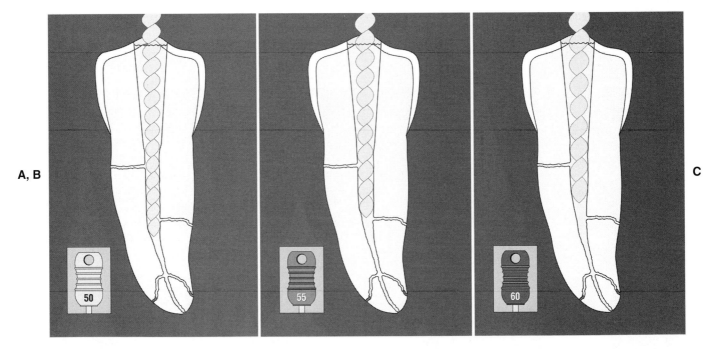

Fig. 8-65 **A,** A 50 NiTi file can be used to cut and remove restrictive dentin in the body of the canal. **B,** A 55 NiTi file, although only 10% bigger at D_0 than the 50 file, can be used (if desired) to create more canal shape. **C,** A 60 NiTi file progressively enlarges and refines the coronal two thirds of a canal and improves access into the apical third.

A, B

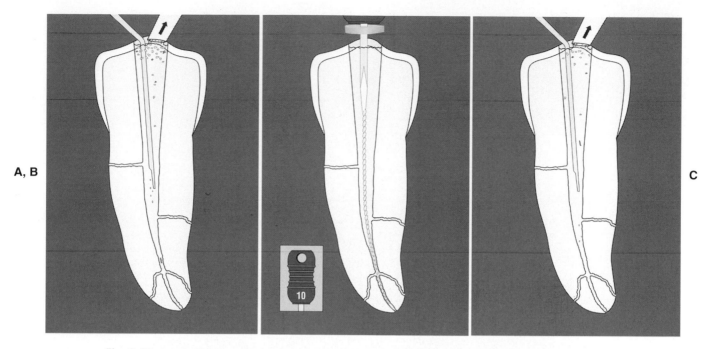

C

Fig. 8-66 **A,** Irrigating procedures are directed toward flushing debris out of the canal and replenishing the root canal system with fresh solution. **B,** A no. 10 file is used in short amplitude strokes to break up pockets of debris and move it into solution. **C,** Reirrigation after recapitulation with a no. 10 file eliminates more debris and ensures a reservoir of fresh irrigant.

within the canal. The loose flame-shaped cutting head of the GG is then placed on the dentinal wall of choice and brushed out of the canal in a coronal direction. The shaft of the GG should be arced, which will proportionally increase the pressure of the GG head on the selected wall and relocate the canal away from external root concavities and furcal danger. Next, the clinician should slowly, deliberately, and methodically sweep the GG head out of the canal to promote *Mechanical Objective no. 1.* It is good technique to arc the shafts of the smaller GGs, recognizing that an occasional instrument will break but that it is easily retrievable. Preenlargement procedures with GGs improve radicular access, enhance irrigation, and promote the removal of debris.

Once some coronal flaring and space have been created over a range of a few millimeters, the GG can be carried a little deeper into the root canal space. To accomplish deeper penetration, the rotating GG is gently tapped into the canal using a pressure similar to that used when writing lightly with a sharp lead pencil. This light tapping or "pecking action" will carry the GG a few millimeters deeper into the canal. The extent the GG should move apically is guided by the information provided from viewing three preoperative films that will suggest the root dimensions in terms of its mass, concavities, and curvature.

When the GGs cease to advance passively down the canal, the clinician should bounce off resistance and lift the GG coronally (about 1 mm). Next, the clinician should repeat the brush-cutting action and progressively expand the shape and flare of the canal from this more restricted apical level to the

ever expanding orifice. In rounder-shaped roots the cutting action is on the pull stroke out of the canal, circumferentially brushing one or two dentinal walls at a time. In single-rooted and furcated teeth exhibiting external concavities, the clinician should *always* brush-cut coronally, arcing the shaft of the GG so its head will cut *away* from furcal danger and toward the greatest bulk of dentin. When using GGs in furcated teeth, a helpful rule to remember is the *name* of the canal you are in is the *wall* to brush-cut.[107]

The secret to preparing the coronal two thirds of a canal with GGs is to first flare a particular region, then lightly tap further down into the canal using a pecking action. Repeating this cycle safely and progressively expands the preparation into a predefined shape. After the use of the GG-1 in straighter canals, it is normal to have the head of the hand piece nearly resting on the occlusal table with the instrument's cutting blades extending deep into the root canal space (Fig. 8-67, *A*). After each GG, the clinician should irrigate with NaOCl, recapitulate with a no. 10 clearing file to break up pockets of resistance, and then reirrigate to remove debris.

With the root canal system filled to capacity with NaOCl, the clinician should proceed to the next larger GGs. The nonrotating GG-2 is carried into the canal until the head engages the dentin walls. As before, the clinician should bounce off resistance and lift the GG coronal until just loose. The GG is then activated and used in the manner previously described. The GG-2, GG-3, and GG-4 are then used consecutively, with each larger GG working further away from the canal terminus than the previous GG (Fig. 8-67 *B-D*).

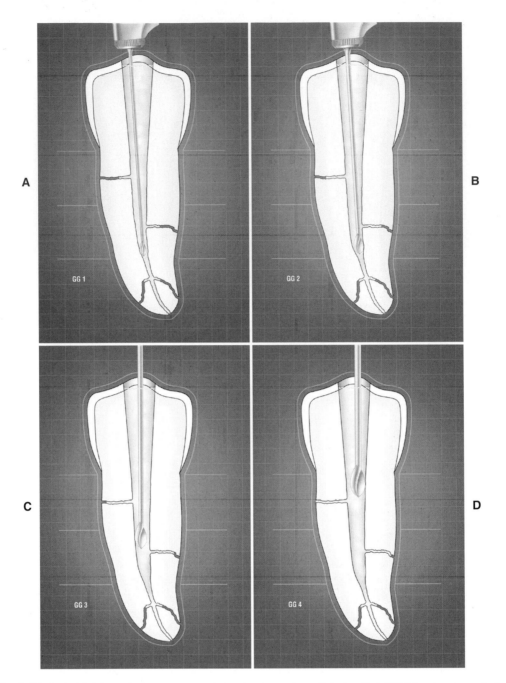

Fig. 8-67 A, A GG-1 is used to cut away restrictive dentin on the pull stroke. **B,** A GG-2 brush cuts a selected dentinal wall and improves radicular shape. **C,** A GG-3 is stepped-back and continues to expand the coronal two thirds of the preparation. **D,** A GG-4 blends the most coronal aspect of the canal into the axial walls of the access cavity.

Generally, the GG-1 is often carried 16 to 17 mm below the reference point. Each larger GG is uniformly stepped out of the canal about 2 to 3 mm so that the GG-4 is carried to about 1 head depth below the orifice in furcated teeth. The GG-5 and GG-6 are used above the orifice to expand the access cavity coronally, thus making a smooth transition between the pulp chamber and the canal. Carrying many or all of the GGs to essentially the same level within the preparation

excessively removes dentin, needlessly weakens roots, and appears on the posttreatment radiograph as a "coke bottle" preparation.

When shaping with GGs, common sense and tactile sense must prevail; their depth of use is dictated by root morphology and canal curvature. Ultimately clinicians must learn to develop a logical root canal preparation that is specific for each root.[98,107,117] GGs smooth, refine, and blend the

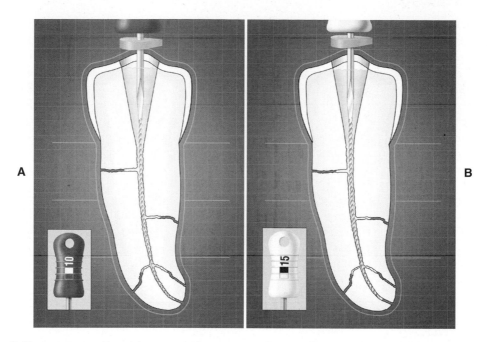

Fig. 8-68 **A,** A scouter file confirms straight-line access, verifies the diameter of a canal, and reveals root canal system anatomy. **B,** The no. 15 file follows the path of the no. 10 file, improves the glide path, and dictates the next clinical step.

coronal two thirds of the canal and generate considerable debris (i.e., dentin mud). After using each GG, or at most two, it is wise to irrigate, recapitulate with a no. 10 clearing file to break up pockets of debris, and reirrigate to flush out the canal. If the no. 10 file meets resistance, the clinician should gently pick through it and, once apical to this nuisance block, *gently and repeatedly* move the clearing file in short amplitude strokes (i.e., 1 to 2 mm) until the file moves freely. The no. 10 file will stir debris into solution, so it is necessary to reirrigate. Straighter and larger canals can generally be shaped in their coronal two thirds with a single pass through the GG series. However, more difficult canals may require two recapitulations through the GG series to create a uniform taper, and complex systems may require several recapitulations to carve the desired shape.

Rotary NiTi Shaping Instruments NiTi rotary-shaping files represent a significant improvement in optimally preparing the coronal two thirds of virtually all root canals. The clinician may choose among ProFile 0.04 or 0.06 tapers, orifice shapers, GT rotary files, ProTapers, the Quantec file series, or combinations of instruments within any of these or other name brand series.

Rotary shaping guidelines.   There are a few established rules regarding the use of NiTi rotary-shaping instruments. It is essential to prepare the access cavity so that straight-line access to the canal orifices exists. Further, rotary instruments should only be placed in portions of the canal that have first been scouted with hand instruments (Fig. 8-68). Small flexible, stainless steel, ISO 0.02 tapered

hand files confirm straight-line access, cross-sectional diameter, and canal anatomy; thus giving the clinician insight as to the propriety of introducing rotary instrumentation. In addition, certain standards have been established for rotary files regarding their specific speed, sequencing, and method of use. The following summarizes the rotary-shaping guidelines:

1. Straight-line access. Straight-line access is best determined by observing whether the handle position of the file is "on" or "off" the long axis of the tooth (see Fig. 8-58). When the roots are underneath the clinical crown and the file handle is off axis, proceeding with rotary-shaping procedures will potentially thin the root, predispose the root to fracture, or create a strip perforation along the lateral wall of the root. GGs may be advantageously used to upright the file so that it parallels the long axis of the tooth. Once the handles of the files appear parallel to the long axis of the root, rotary-shaping techniques may commence.

2. Cross-sectional diameter. The cross-sectional diameter of a canal needs to be confirmed with hand instruments before introducing a rotary-shaping file. Sufficient space must exist to accommodate and guide the noncutting or partially active tip of a rotary instrument. For example, if a canal has been scouted to within 2 to 3 mm of anticipated working length with no. 10 and no. 15 0.02 tapered files, then more space exists coronal to their tips than the files' numeric names suggest. A no. 10 file and no. 15 file have 16 mm of cutting flutes, and their D_{16} diameters are 0.42 and 0.47 mm, respectively. These

small instruments provide an opening for the use of rotary instruments.

3. Root canal system anatomy. Root canal system anatomy may be categorized into five commonly encountered anatomic forms. Scouter files provide critical information regarding the *curvature*, *recurvature*, or *dilaceration* of a canal. Further, before introducing rotary instruments, clinicians need to know if a single canal *divides* or if two canals within a root *merge* along their length. Generally, canals exhibiting these anatomic forms are not appropriate for NiTi rotary use. Scouter files are not just measuring wires; rather, they need to be thought of as providing essential reconnaissance information before initiating shaping procedures.

4. Speed and sequencing. All rotary instruments perform optimally with less breakage when used in gear reduction electric motors that automatically adjust the torque specific for any given file used (Fig. 8-69). Rotary instruments need to be used according to the guidelines gathered from market experience. To reduce the potential for breakage, rotary-shaping files are best used starting with the larger D_0 diameters or tapers and then proceeding to the smaller sized instruments. By using the instruments in a crown-down fashion, the area of the file engaging the canal is minimized, thereby reducing the torsional stress exerted on the instrument. NiTi rotary-shaping files with variable D_0 diameters tend to engage and cut dentin toward their terminal cutting blades. However, NiTi rotary-shaping files that have fixed D_0 diameters cut dentin toward their more shank side cutting flutes (i.e., toward the strongest portion of the instrument). Using files serially from large to small avoids dangerous taper lock that results when an instrument engages dentin over its full length of cutting blades.[16-18]

5. Lubrication and the "light touch." To reduce the risk of breakage, rotary-shaping instruments are always used in the presence of a lubricating irrigant.[21] Pulp chambers should be filled brimful with sodium hypochlorite or a chelator to reduce friction between the instrument and the wall of the canal. Rotary instruments should be used passively within the canal, and their use should be continued as long as they move easily. As stated previously, the desired pressure on an instrument should be equivalent to the pressure used when writing with a sharp lead pencil.

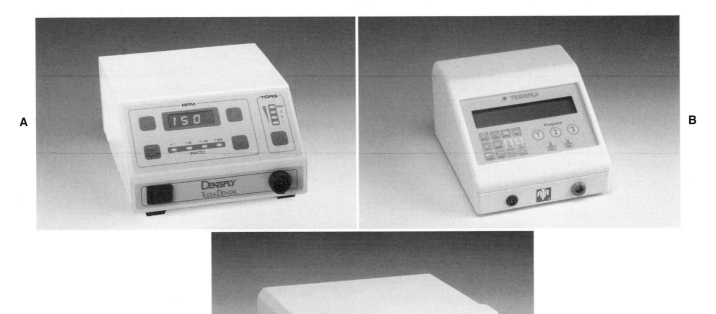

Fig. 8-69 **A,** The Aseptico electric motor offers the clinician a choice of RPM and torque control. **B,** The Tecnika electric motor offers the clinician a choice of RPM, torque control, and reciprocation features. **C,** The Quantec electric motor offers the clinician a choice of RPM.

Two possibilities exist when a NiTi rotary instrument passively resists apical movement. In this situation the file should be withdrawn because the diameter of the instrument's tip may not be able to follow the glide path previously established with scouter files. In these instances the clinician should irrigate and recapitulate with the smallest files to confirm available cross-sectional diameter and verify the anatomic configuration of the canal. Another possibility that limits the easy apical movement of an instrument is the accumulation of debris within the depth between the cutting blades. Interblade debris tends to deactivate an instrument because it pushes the active part of the file off the wall of the canal. If this happens the clinician should withdraw the instrument and clear its blades, irrigate the canal, recapitulate with a small hand file to confirm the existence of the previously established glide path, and then reirrigate to flush out debris.

Coronal two-thirds rotary shaping technique. With the root canal system scouted in the coronal two thirds and filled brimful with NaOCl, the clinician should select a rotary-shaping instrument that will just fit passively within the canal's orifice. Regardless of name brand or instrument line, the instrument should be used in a crown-down manner (Fig. 8-70). When used properly, the instrument will passively and progressively move into the canal. The extent an instrument will move depends on the canal's cross-sectional diameter, curvature, and anatomic form. The clinician should *never* try to move a rotary instrument deeper into a canal that has not been scouted.

When a rotary file ceases to move into a canal, it should be removed and the clinician should note where the debris is positioned along the length of its cutting blades. If the correct instrument was selected, the debris will be limited to a few millimeters of cutting blades. If debris is noted over a longer length of cutting blades, then more torsional loads have been generated within the instrument. In this instance the clinician should either select a larger or a smaller instrument to reduce dangerous taper lock. Clearing debris from the instrument allows close inspection of the cutting blades for evidence of stress, strain, or frank deformation. Depending on the specific geometry of the file used, debris should ideally be positioned on its more shank side cutting blades where it has a stronger cross-sectional diameter. Additionally, shank side debris implies the smaller and weaker portion of the instrument toward D_0 is loose and able to follow the preexisting pathway. After each NiTi rotary instrument, the clinician should passively irrigate, recapitulate with a small clearing file to move debris into solution, and then reirrigate to flush out debris and clear the canal.

With a confirmed glide path through the coronal two thirds of a canal, the clinician should either reintroduce the same rotary instrument to see if it will passively move deeper into the canal or proceed to the next smaller file. In either event the clinician should *"take what the canal will give,"* not force the instruments, and let the preparation evolve to its optimal shape.[107,117] After *each* rotary instrument, the clini-

cian should irrigate, recapitulate to break up pockets of debris and confirm the glide path, reirrigate, and continue through any given instrument series in a crown-down manner from large to small. In more calcified or anatomically difficult canals, it may be necessary to recapitulate through a portion or the entire instrument series a second or third time to create a clean, smooth, flowing coronal two thirds of a canal.

Apical One-Third Preparation

With the coronal two thirds preenlarged, excellent access exists to negotiate and prepare the apical one third of the root canal system.[89,107,137] The clinician should always obtain an accurate working length from radiographs or an electronic apex locator before introducing a file to the terminus.[46] Following inspection of mesial, distal, and straight-on angulated films allows the clinician to mentally begin building a more three-dimensional model of the tooth than any one angle alone.[95] If using conventional radiographic films, the clinician should position unidirectional silicone stops on the scouting files and superimpose a no. 10 file over the radiograph of the root to be treated; this allows precurvature of the apical extent of the file to simulate the curvature of the canal. Only the smaller files are precurved to conform to the anticipated full curvature of the root canal. Larger instruments require *less* curvature because they are typically working further away from the apical third where most canal curvatures exist. The unidirectional silicone stop is then set at the estimated working length and additionally turned to correspond to the apical curve of the instrument.

Scouting the Apical One Third
With the pulp chamber brimful with a chelator or NaOCl, the clinician should introduce the precurved and measured no. 10 file. In a tooth that radiographically exhibits an apical pathologic condition, it is helpful to direct the file toward the radiolucency (because a LEO forms adjacent to a POE). The handle of the instrument is reciprocated back and forth in an overall 30-degree arc. This handle motion will activate the file, drawing it down into the canal (Fig. 8-71, *A*). When the silicone stop is approximately 1 to 2 mm short of the coronal reference point, the reciprocating handle motion should cease and the file should be gently pushed to length.

In some instances the file can be placed easily to within a few millimeters of the RT, but then it suddenly meets resistance. This is known as *loose resistance* and may indicate the narrowing canal divides into multiple POEs or makes a sudden change in direction before terminating. In this case the clinician should remove the file, place a sharper curve closer to its tip, and reenter the canal. With the coronal two thirds previously enlarged, the clinician will have greater control of the file when gently exploring for the POEs. Once the file has been carried to the full length of the canal, the clinician should pull the handle in a coronal direction. This ensures that the file moves and cuts away from the foramen on the out stroke.

mechanical objectives of cleaning and shaping, the clinician should place the *smallest*, most flexible file to the RT (recognizing the instrument is minutely long). Cleaning canals to the RT promotes the biologic objectives of removing all the pulp, bacteria, and their endotoxins. Keeping the canal terminus patent at all times greatly reduces the potential for blocks, ledges, and perforations. Creating a canal preparation with a cross-sectional diameter that progressively narrows and is smallest apically allows for controlled three-dimensional obturation to the consistent drying point.

Once the no. 10 file has confirmed a smooth glide path to the preestablished length, the clinician should proceed to the no. 15 file. If the canal is narrow, the clinician should repeat the push-and-pull handle motion until the no. 15 file moves easily to the desired working length. The no. 15 file is confirmed at the RT (Fig. 8-71, *D*). Digital radiography (as discussed in Chapters 5 and 26) gives clinicians more options to interpret the position of the file, because the image can be adjusted for contrast and enlarged to visualize the terminal extent of the instrument more accurately. Electronic apex locators represent an important alternative to radiographs when determining working length. The Endo Analyzer (Analytic Endodontics, Orange, CA) and Root ZX (J. Morita Corporation, Tustin, CA) have advanced electronics that provide accurate, predictable, and time-saving information regarding the position of the apical foramen (see Fig. 8-29). These electronic apex locators are not limited by the presence of intracanal exudates or electrolytes. False readings can be avoided when the shaft of the working instrument is not touching metal restorations. The tip of the file contacts dentin at the estimated length, and the irrigants are restricted to the canal in multirooted teeth; if the chamber is filled with a conductive liquid, a false reading is likely.

Finishing the Apical One Third

The apical third of a root canal can be finished once it has been negotiated to length and the foramen has been enlarged to a size no. 15 file. The *sine qua non* of excellence in canal preparation is consistently finishing the apical third. The ideal finished preparation will always exhibit deep shape that tapers toward the canal terminus. The classic apical third preparation that can be cleaned and packed is a tapered shape that has been enlarged to at least a no. 20 file at the terminus; each successively larger instrument should uniformly move away from the foramen by ½ mm increments.

The clinician will have full confidence the apical third of the preparation has been optimally finished when the canal is "gauged and tuned" with ISO 0.02 hand files. The actual diameter of a foramen is *gauged* and equals the D_0 diameter of the file that is snug at length, if the clinician is able to visualize the silicone stop on each consecutively larger instrument uniformly moving away from the reference point. The apical third is *tuned* and deep shape is confirmed if the clinician is able to observe consecutively larger instruments uniformly moving away from the terminus. Recapitulating through a series of instruments once, twice, and perhaps a third time will progressively adjust and tune the canal and confirm the final shape of the apical third. Tuning provides the resistance form that is necessary for packing root canal systems in three dimensions.

Hand versus rotary finishing. When a no. 15 or larger file is confirmed at length, a decision on how to best finish the apical third must be made between hand and rotary instruments. *It is wise to finish root canal systems that exhibit difficult anatomy with hand instruments.* Small flexible files that scout the apical third provide information regarding canals that abruptly merge, excessively curve, significantly recurve, dilacerate, or divide. In general, if a no. 15 file can be gently pushed over a few millimeters and passively slid to length, then rotary NiTi instruments can generally be used to finish the apical third of the canal. However, certain canals exhibit anatomic challenges that require a back-and-forth handle motion to move a precurved no. 15 file to length. In these instances the apical third of a canal should be finished with hand instruments. At times difficult canals can be progressively enlarged with hand files until a smooth and predictable glide path to the terminus can be established; then rotary instruments may become suitable for finishing.

Finishing with ISO 0.02 tapered instruments. When the length of the canal has been carefully scouted and fully negotiated to its RT with sizes no. 10 and no. 15 files, then the apical third can be finished with ISO 0.02, no. 20 to no. 60 hand files. Sizes no. 20, no. 25, and no. 30 flexofiles (Dentsply Maillefer, Tulsa, Okla.) may be selected to initiate apical third finishing procedures because their flexibility and noncutting tips allow them to follow an existing pilot hole easily and safely.[138] All stainless steel instruments that will be carried into the apical third must be precurved to simulate the anticipated curvature of the canal based on well-angulated preoperative radiographs. NiTi hand files (sizes no. 35 to no. 60) are selected because their unmatched flexibility provides safety and control in finishing the apical third of a canal.[105]

With the pulp chamber brimful with NaOCl, the clinician should select and precurve the no. 20 file. Depending on the diameter and anatomic configuration of the canal, the no. 20 file will either move to full working length or will begin to snug into the canal some distance short of the RT. If any particular file passively moves to the full working length, the clinician should proceed directly to the next larger file. The handle of the no. 20 file is activated by using a 15-degree CW and then a 15-degree CCW back-and-forth motion, which will produce apical file movement. An overall 30-degree arc of reciprocating motion on the file handle is appropriate in the body of the canal. In general the degree of reciprocating handle motion decreases as the instrument's working end arrives in the apical third of the canal and converts to a straight push-and-pull motion as its tip approaches the foramen. A push-and-pull motion on the handle of a file encourages the flexible, precurved instrument to follow the canal's curvature precisely.

In the instance where the no. 20 file is greater than 2 mm away from the terminus, the clinician should gently rotate the handle of the instrument back and forth between the thumb and index finger. This motion activates the file and draws it down into the canal; its movement is complete when the handle feels snug. Once seated the file is pulled coronal approximately 1 to 2 mm, with its engaged blades cutting on the outstroke. Feeding the instrument into the canal and removing dentin on the pull stroke completes the first cutting cycle. With the same file in place again, the clinician should passively rock the handle back and forth in a reciprocating motion. Again, handle motion produces file movement; this works the instrument deeper into the canal. The clinician should take what the canal will give; when the file handle feels snug, the clinician should bounce off resistance by pulling the instrument coronally until just loose. The handle motion of the no. 20 file (i.e., *feed it in—then pull*) continues for five to six cutting cycles, until the instrument reaches the terminus (Fig. 8-72, *A*). All instruments are used passively (i.e., never forced) and the apical third of canals are never attacked. There should be no misguided fear of getting blocked if these preparation guidelines are followed. With this technique there is no preconceived concept regarding where any file in any root should go; the file's depth of placement is dictated by the canal's anatomy. When the canal anatomy is complicated or its contents are fibrotic, the clinician should remove the NaOCl and fill the chamber with RC Prep to promote the objectives of cleaning and shaping.

The next file selected should be the precurved no. 25 file. The same reciprocating motion used with the no. 20 file is used to work this larger instrument down into the canal; its

movement is continued apically until the handle feels snug. The clinician should pull the handle of the instrument coronally and cut away from the foramen. Apical movement of each larger instrument should be limited so that each file works ½ mm shorter than the previously used, smaller file (Fig. 8-72, *B*). At times instruments are not worked because they passively extend to just short of the previous file. Other times five to six cutting cycles are necessary to move a particular instrument progressively deeper to ensure a uniformly tapered preparation.

The clinician should now proceed to the precurved no. 30 file. In general, larger files require less curvature toward their working ends because these instruments do not extend as deeply into the canal. Again, a reciprocating back-and-forth motion works the instrument down into the canal; its movement is continued apically until it begins to feel snug. The clinician should pull the no. 30 file coronal 1 to 2 mm and (again) cut coronally away from resistance on the out stroke. A few cutting cycles will usually draw the no. 30 file down to within 0.5 mm of where the no. 25 file extended (Fig. 8-72, *C*). Larger instruments will generally begin to feel snug in the canal at a distance shorter than the previously used smaller files.

After every two to three files, it is essential to irrigate, recapitulate, and reirrigate to eliminate debris from the preparation. At this time a small patency file should move easily through the canal to the terminus. However, on occasion the instrument may encounter a pocket of resistance. When this occurs, the clinician should use gentle, pecking strokes until

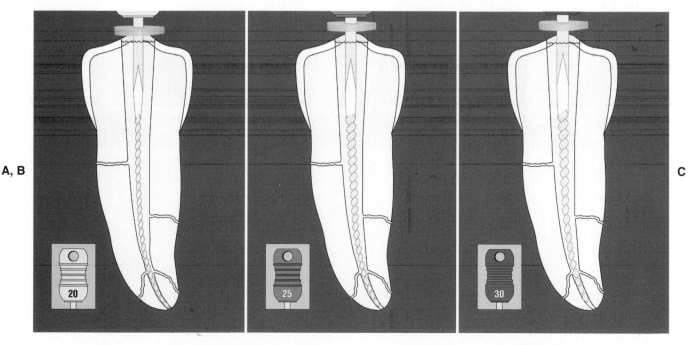

A, B   **C**

Fig. 8-72 **A,** With restrictive dentin removed, the precurved no. 20 flexofile can be gently negotiated into the apical foramen. **B,** When the 20 file feels snug at length, then the no. 25 flexofile ideally moves away from the terminus 0.5 mm. **C,** After a few cutting cycles, the no. 30 flexofile generally moves deeper into the canal and within 1 mm of the foramen.

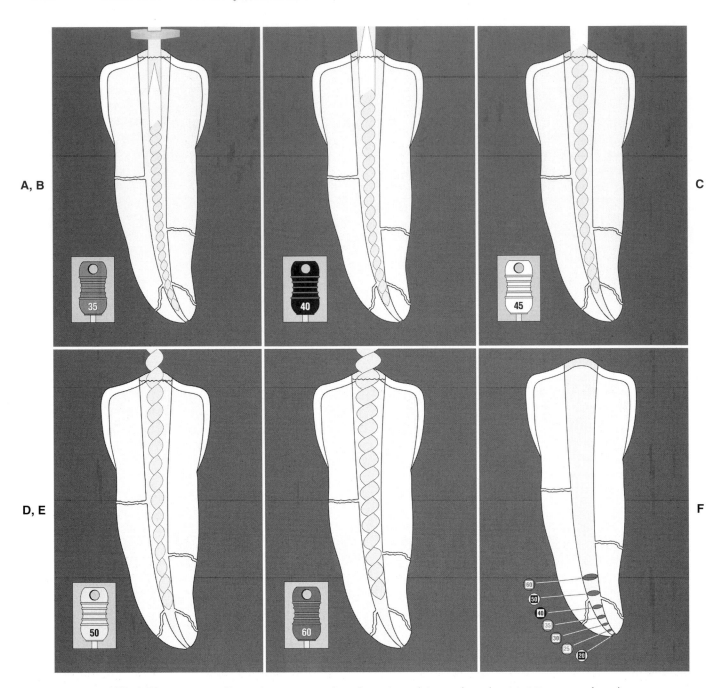

Fig. 8-73 **A,** A NiTi 35 file continues to create deep shape; its work is complete when it is 1.5 mm away from the terminus. **B,** A NiTi 40 file can be carried deep into the root canal system and worked until it is 2.0 mm short of working length. **C,** A NiTi 45 file continues the wave of shaping and its use is completed when it is 2.5 mm short of the foramen. **D,** A NiTi 50 file begins to blend the canal between the junction of the middle and apical thirds; it is worked until it is 3.0 mm short of length. **E,** Depending on the curvature and length of a canal, a 60 NiTi file generally concludes its work 4.0 mm short of the terminus. **F,** When each consecutively larger instrument uniformly steps back out of the canal, then deep shape is confirmed.

the instrument extends apical to the debris; then work the clearing file repeatedly in short 1 to 2 mm vertical strokes to break up and move the debris into solution. When the patency file can easily slip and slide along the glide path to the terminus, the clinician should reirrigate to flush out debris.

The clinician should then proceed to the NiTi no. 35 to no. 60 hand files to progressively blend, enlarge, and create uniform rate of taper over the length of the canal (Fig. 8-73, *A-E*). The no. 55 file is usually not needed, because it is only 10% larger than the no. 50 file at D_0. These NiTi hand instruments may be used with the motion described for the no. 20

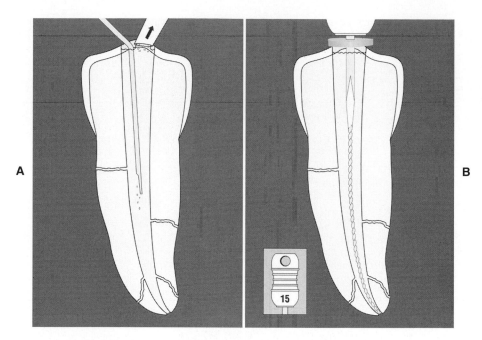

Fig. 8-74 **A,** Soaking the root canal systems with full-strength, heated NaOCl and 17% EDTA enhances cleaning. **B,** A no. 15 file is used to verify the glide path and confirm apical patency.

to no. 30 flexofiles, or they can be used in conjunction with the balanced-force technique. NiTi hand files can effectively, safely, and efficiently perform shaping procedures, especially around pathways of canal curvature.[121,122,140] The clinician should proceed through the instrument series and periodically irrigate, recapitulate, confirm apical patency, and reirrigate to eliminate dentin mud. Each larger file should work approximately 0.5 mm shorter than the smaller file; at this point the rate of taper of the preparation is becoming uniform. At the conclusion of canal preparation, it is common to have a no. 60 file or an equivalently sized instrument to within 3 to 5 mm from the terminus, depending on the case (Fig. 8-73, *F*). A no. 60 file positioned at approximately the junction of the middle and apical one thirds of a canal ensures sufficient space for effective irrigation and cleaning; it also creates the best shape for packing the root canal system in three dimensions.

An excellent method to verify a preparation has a uniform rate of taper is to clinically observe the silicone stops on each larger file moving away from the reference point by 0.5 mm intervals. Frequently after initial preparation efforts, increasingly larger instruments do not uniformly step back and out of the canal. *Finishing* requires repeating through any given instrument series until *uniform* taper is created. If the canal does not have uniform taper, the clinician should repeat the finishing sequence until a uniform taper is confirmed. Frequent irrigation and patency confirmation are essential (Fig. 8-74). In more difficult cases the clinician should recapitulate through the entire series again (and perhaps yet again) to create an extraordinarily clean, smooth, flowing, and evenly tapered preparation (Fig. 8-75). Many times when performing cleaning and shaping procedures, the clinician is just one recapitulation away from excellence.

Finishing with hand GT files.   GT NiTi hand files are another set of instruments available for enlarging and finishing the apical one thirds of root canals (see "Armamentarium for Canal Preparation" section in this chapter). These files are best used after coronal two-thirds preenlargement, when the apical third of a canal has been negotiated; the patent foramen is enlarged to at least a no. 15 (or a no. 20), ISO 0.02 hand file (Fig. 8-76, *A*). GT files are used serially, beginning with the largest and ending with the smallest tapered files. This order of use encourages each instrument to cut on its more shank side flutes, removing dentin in a crown-down manner. The terminal extents of these instruments should never engage and cut dentin. Instead, they should passively follow a preexisting and confirmed glide path. GT files are very effective in producing canal preparations that have uniform taper in their apical extents.

GT hand files are machined with a reverse screw and, consequently, engage dentin by turning counterclockwise. When hand instruments are indicated, the GT 0.08 and 0.10 tapered files are the most useful in providing a specific predefined shape in the apical third of a canal. In clinical use, a GT 0.10 tapered hand file is inserted into the canal using a reciprocating motion until the handle feels snug. The handle of this file is then rotated CCW between 45 and 90 degrees to pull the instrument down into the canal. This CCW rotation will activate the variably pitched shank side blades to form threads in the dentin. To cut dentin the clinician must push the handle of the file in an apical direction and simultaneously rotate the file clockwise. During this handle motion,

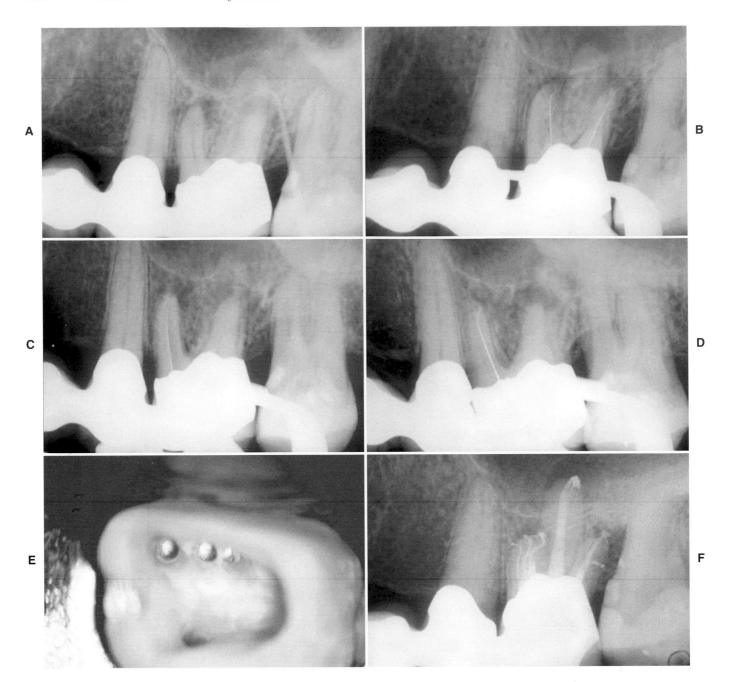

Fig. 8-75 **A,** An endodontically involved maxillary molar bridge abutment. A gutta-percha point traces along a sinus tract. **B,** Working film taken straight on after preenlargement procedures demonstrates that no. 10 files are at the foramina of the MB^I and DB systems. **C,** A distoblique film shows the no. 10 file abruptly recurving and at length in the MB^{II} system. **D,** An exaggerated, more distoblique film reveals the MB root's furcal side concavity and a no. 10 file recurving and at the terminus of the MB^{III} system. **E,** A photograph with the splint off shows the isolated tooth and the level of the down-packed MB^I, MB^{II}, and MB^{III} systems. **F,** A posttreatment radiograph emphasizes that endodontics can be the foundation of restorative and reconstructive dentistry.

torsional loads build up primarily along the file's engaged cutting blades. When the elastic limit of dentin is exceeded, it will be cut with an audible click. At this point the clinician should keep the file in the canal, repeat the preceding steps, and work the file down to engage dentin by turning the handle CCW between 45 and 90 degrees. The clinician should exert apically directed pressure on the handle of the file, while balancing this inward force with equal CW rotational force. Again the clinician will hear an audible click as dentin is cut; this completes another cutting cycle. The clinician should repeat the steps for three to four cutting cycles or until the 0.10 tapered file cannot move deeper into the

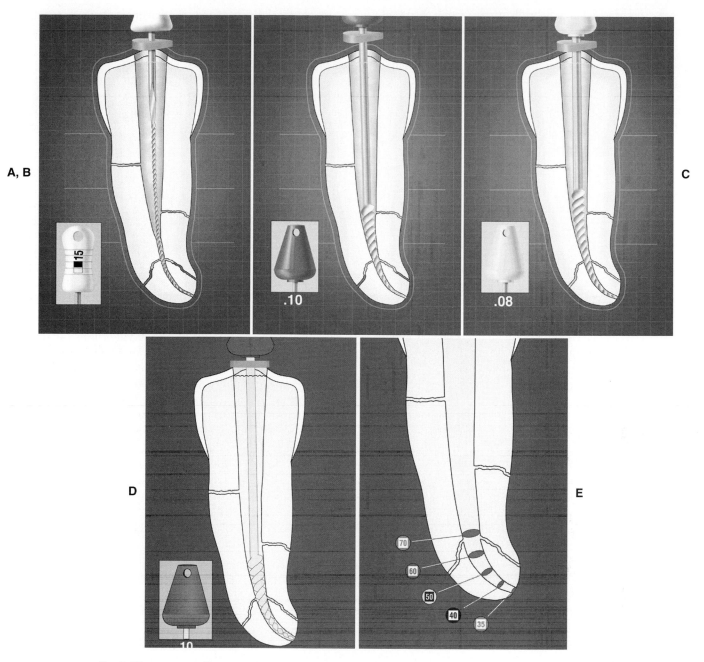

Fig. 8-76 **A,** A no. 15 file passing through a preenlarged canal, negotiating the apical one third, and going to length. **B,** A 0.10 tapered GT file creating deep shape short of the terminus of the canal. **C,** A 0.08 tapered GT file creating deep shape to the terminus of the canal. **D,** A GT file may bind in a canal on its more shank side cutting flutes, be at length, yet be deceptively loose apically. **E,** Illustration of the importance of using gauging and tuning procedures to verify the size of the foramen and confirm deep shape.

canal during the CCW rotation (Fig. 8-76, *B*). In this technique the GT files are used in a *reverse* balanced-force technique.

When the instrument does not advance apically, it is usually because of the accumulation of dentin debris pushing the cutting blades off the canal wall. Other reasons the instrument may not advance include the taper of the file exceeding the taper of the canal, or the last few millimeters of the file being too stiff to bend around the curvature of the canal. Regardless, dentin mud must be removed frequently by pulling the handle of the file coronally, while simultaneously turning the instrument CCW. The pull force prevents the instrument from screwing into the canal during the CCW rotation. The net effect is that the instrument stays at the same level, spins, and loads debris onto the file between its cutting blades.

After the removal of the GT file, the clinician should inspect the instrument to confirm where the debris is located on the cutting blades. Ideally, dentin mud will be positioned on the more shank side cutting blades. The clinician should clear the debris from the instrument, irrigate the canal, recapitulate with a no. 10 or no. 15 file, and reirrigate to flush out debris. This same GT file may be reinserted into the canal, and its method of use continued. In the event the GT file will not easily engage dentin and work down into the canal, the clinician should proceed to the next smaller 0.08 tapered GT file. Typically, only a few cutting cycles will move this instrument to length (Fig. 8-76, *C*). In general, most roots can accommodate a 0.10 tapered GT file to the foramen. However, roots that are more narrow or have deep concavities are best managed with an 0.08 tapered GT file to length.

The red-handled, 0.10 GT file creates the exact root canal shape as do nine ISO 0.02 files (sizes no. 20 to no. 60). For example, if a no. 20 file feels snug at length, then the preferred shape would have the no. 30 to no. 60 files uniformly moving away from the RT 1, 2, 3, and 4 mm. Although the GT files provide an economy of instruments and create uniform deep shape, these advantages are offset by the files' fixed flute diameters. In fact, many canals exhibit apical cross-sectional diameters exceeding the GT files' fixed D_0 diameters of 0.20 mm. Even when a GT file is confirmed to be at length and cannot be displaced periapically, it may actually be binding in the canal on its more shank side cutting flutes, giving a false impression of the canal's true apical diameter (Fig. 8-76, *D*).

To overcome this uncertainty, clinicians need to confirm the size of the apical foramen by first introducing an ISO no. 20 file. If the no. 20 file feels snug at length, then the diameter of the foramen is confirmed to be 0.20 mm. In the event the no. 20 file is loose at length, the clinician should proceed sequentially through the ISO 0.02 file series until the foramen is *gauged*, then *tune* to verify the shape (Fig. 8-76, *E*). After the use of GT hand files, ISO 0.02 files are frequently used simply as *"feeler gauges"* to rapidly verify the true diameter of the foramen and confirm deep shape.

The fixed maximum flute diameter of the GT file is another drawback, because it tends to produce canal preparations that are parallel in the coronal portion. Parallel canals limit irrigation and reduce the potential for three dimensional cleaning and obturation. To overcome this and flare a canal that is parallel in its coronal two thirds requires the use of *more* instruments, negating some of the simplicity of the GT file series.

Finishing the apical one third with NiTi rotary instruments. Rotary NiTi instruments can be used to finish the apical third of a root canal if a no. 15 file can be gently and predictably pushed over a range of a few millimeters to the terminus. NiTi rotary files include the ProFile instrument lines, the ProTaper finishing files, and the Quantec instrument series. Any of these instrument lines or combination of lines may be selected and used to finish the apical third of a canal (Fig. 8-77). Orifice shapers are 19 mm long, so they

can only reach the terminus and finish canals that are equal to or less than this length. Ultimately, the instruments chosen to finish the root canal preparation should be based on the same factors described earlier the chapter.

Any given series of files, regardless of the difference in geometries among various instrument lines, can create a variety of apical-third tapers based on its method of use. For example, ISO 0.02 hand files, when stepped out of the canal by 0.5 mm intervals, can create a canal taper of 0.10 mm/mm, or 10%.[117] Similarly, if an 0.04 tapered file is carried to length and is the only instrument used in the apical third, then the taper of the canal in this zone is 0.04 mm/mm, or 4%. A canal with a taper of 4% is clearly too narrow and too parallel to ensure effective cleaning and obturation. However, if a series of 0.04-tapered instruments are used to finish the apical third so that each successively larger file is uniformly stepped out of the canal, then a canal taper of 0.10 mm/mm, or 10%, can be achieved (see Fig. 8-47).[87]

Any rotary file series with instruments that have a fixed D_0 diameter will additionally require that the canal be *gauged* and *tuned* with ISO 0.02 hand files to confirm the diameter of the foramen (Fig. 8-78). It is unwise to pass any rotary-shaping file through a foramen that is larger than 0.20 mm with the hope of capturing its true diameter on the D_1, D_2, or D_3 aspects of a specific instrument. Theoretically a rotary NiTi file is designed to follow a canal to length as its noncutting, most flexible working end is guided by a pilot hole of circumferential dentin. If a portion of a rotary file extends beyond the foramen, especially in a curved canal, then there is no pilot hole to guide the instrument that, in conjunction with its rapidly increasing taper and stiffness, increases the probability for iatrogenic mishaps.

Whether rotary NiTi shaping files have fixed or variable D_0 diameters, they are best used starting with the larger instruments and working toward the smaller instruments in a crown-down manner. Each instrument is rotated at the recommended RPM and passively directed apically. In a preenlarged canal, smaller tapered instruments tend to engage dentin closer to their working ends. As such, clinicians should exert light pressure on the file equal to the pressure used to write with a *sharp lead pencil*. When the rotating instrument passively resists apical movement, the clinician should irrigate, recapitulate, and reirrigate to confirm the glide path and canal patency. Then the clinician should return to the canal preparation with the same rotary instrument or proceed with a smaller file.

Even in the presence of a smooth apical-third glide path, caution must be exercised in the terminal 1 to 2 mm of a canal to prevent instrument breakage. If rotary files will not float to length, the clinician should finish with hand instruments or recapitulate through the rotary instruments again (and perhaps again) to achieve length. The potential for file breakage increases when clinicians lose patience, when guidelines for safe use are not strictly adhered to, and when instruments are used multiple times. The best anecdote for a broken file is prevention, and this is largely accomplished by

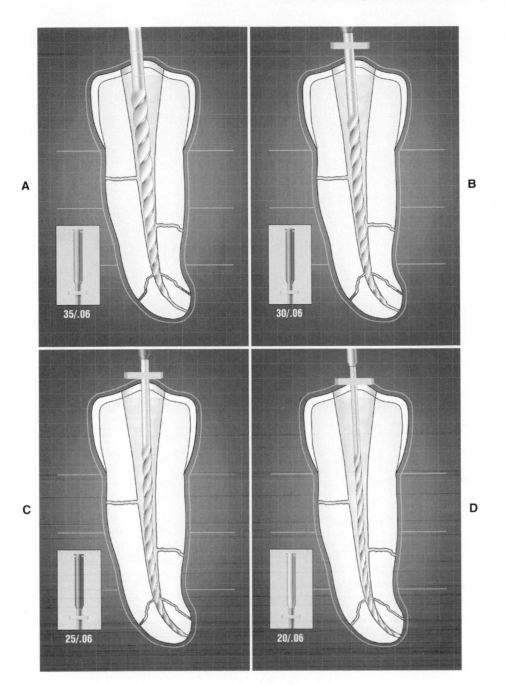

Fig. 8-77 **A,** A no. 35, 0.06 tapered NiTi rotary ProFile in a preenlarged canal and following the glide path into the curvature of the canal. **B,** A no. 30, 0.06 tapered NiTi rotary ProFile avoiding taper lock, working progressively deeper, and approaching the terminus of the canal. **C,** A no. 25, 0.06 tapered NiTi rotary ProFile loose over length, only cutting on its terminal flutes and nearly to length. **D,** A no. 20, 0.06 tapered NiTi rotary ProFile at the terminus of the canal.

thinking of shaping instruments as disposable items.[40,67] A benefit of using brand new files for each new case is that sharp instruments cut dentin more effectively and improve efficiency.

If the rotary-shaping instruments used to finish the apical third of a canal have sufficient taper and variable D_0 diameters, then the preparation is automatically gauged, tuned, and ready to pack. When the taper of a rotary-shaping instrument is deemed inadequate to achieve the cleaning, shaping, and packing objectives, then the desired canal taper can be achieved by uniformly stepping each successively larger instrument out of the canal.

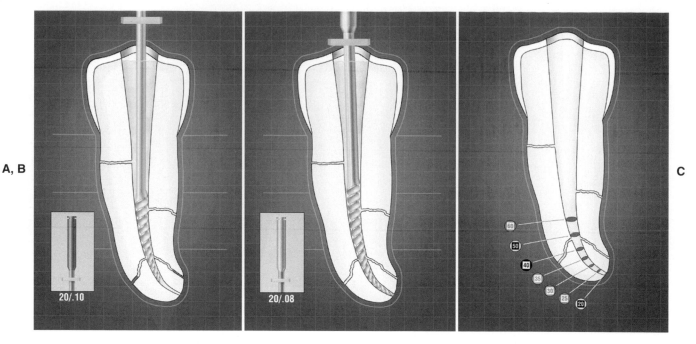

Fig. 8-78 **A,** A 0.10 tapered NiTi GT file working in a relatively parallel preenlarged canal and well short of length. **B,** A 0.08 tapered NiTi GT file at length. Note the canal is parallel in its coronal one half. **C,** An orifice shaper may be used to create a fully tapered canal over length; gauging and tuning are essential when using any instrument line with a fixed D_0 diameter.

FINALIZING THE PREPARATION

Smear Layer Management

When the blades of any file engage and cut dentin, a smear layer of organic and inorganic debris forms on the walls of the preparation.[48,82] Voluminous and frequent irrigation, in conjunction with clearing and patency files, reduce but *do not* eliminate the smear layer. The smear layer represents dentin debris, including pulp remnants, bacteria, endotoxins and, at times, restorative materials. The choice of whether to remove the smear layer or leave it intact has generated lively discussion and is still debated. If the smear layer is removed, then a tighter interface between the obturation materials and the dentin walls is possible.[69,139] If the smear layer is left, then the root canal system is thus incompletely sealed, and the potential for microleakage and subsequent failure increases significantly.

EDTA and Ultrasonics
Aqueous 17% EDTA flooded into well-shaped preparations for 1 minute has been shown to remove and eliminate the smear layer (Fig. 8-79).[61,149] Many clinicians have been interested in enhancing débridement and debris removal using piezoelectric ultrasonic energy.[24,53] The clinical intrigue of increasing the temperature, circulation, and activity of an intracanal irrigant is well founded.[14,15] However, the desirable attributes of acoustic streaming resulting from the ultrasonic activation of intracanal irrigant must be balanced by the potential damage to the walls of the preparation caused by ultrasonic instruments.[31]

EDTA and Microbrushes
Recently microbrushes have been introduced to optimally finish root canal preparations. Microbrushes can be used in either rotary or ultrasonic hand pieces (see Fig. 8-55). Finishing an irrigant-filled, shaped canal with a microbrush has been shown to significantly enhance the cleanliness of the preparation (Fig. 8-80).[68] Ongoing research is directed toward comparing the overall cleanliness of the finished preparation when using a rotary activated brush versus an ultrasonically energized brush. In any event, tapered microbrushes enhance cleaning as bristles deform into the irregularities of the preparation and move debris into solution where it can be removed from the root canal system.

Medicaments and Provisionalization
When one-visit, complete endodontic treatment cannot be provided, calcium hydroxide is an intracanal medicament often used between visits. Although its mechanisms of action are not well understood, its interappointment attributes have been thoroughly studied. During the subsequent appointment, irrigating with NaOCl in calcium hydroxide–filled canals has been shown to enhance the removal of intracanal tissue and related irritants.[24] Because calcium hydroxide is an excellent interappointment dressing, the vast majority of other medicaments has generally been discontinued. When an interap-

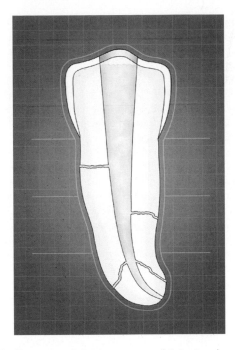

Fig. 8-79 Illustration of the importance of irrigating the completed preparation with 17% EDTA to remove the smear layer.

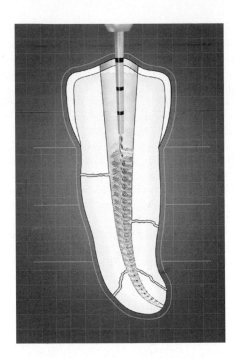

Fig. 8-80 An ultrasonically or rotary activated endodontic microbrush may be used in the presence of 17% EDTA to finish the preparation.

pointment dressing is needed, the canals can be filled with a calcium hydroxide medication (e.g., Vitapex). Then the clinician can place a cotton pellet moistened with chlorhexidine into the pulp chamber and seal the access with a durable restoration that prevents microleakage.

Postoperative Instructions   When practical, teeth that are undergoing endodontic treatment should be taken out of occlusion. Occlusally reduced teeth are generally more comfortable interappointment.[103] Postoperative instructions should be given orally and in written format to maximize patient retention and cooperation. Patients should be advised to anticipate soreness to biting pressure for 2 to 3 days and to discontinue chewing on the tooth in question during this period.

Often cleaning and shaping canals using the concepts, strategies, and techniques discussed in this chapter will lead to satisfied patients who do not require pharmaceuticals. Generally, mild, over-the-counter antiinflammatory analgesics are excellent and address the transient inflammatory symptoms observed clinically. (Prescribing antiinflammatory analgesics, narcotics, and antibiotics is discussed in Chapter 18.)

Root canal preparation techniques will significantly improve in the future because of technologically driven advancements. Rotary-shaping files of the future will exhibit dramatic improvements in materials and better geometries; they will improve safety and efficiency. The motors of the future will promote greater file efficiency and safety; electronic feedback features will automatically regulate RPM, torque control, and reciprocating movements. Intracanal irrigants will appear radiopaque on working films, and the future endogram will significantly enhance diagnostics. Further, irrigating devices and canuli will remarkably improve. Although the future holds great promise, clinicians must always remain alert to the fundamental concepts of cleaning and shaping that provide success.

It could be said that cleaning and shaping is a game and, as such, can be played at various skill levels to produce a range of endodontic results. Excellence in canal preparation provides the foundation for packing the root canal system in three dimensions. Visualizing and executing successful treatment allows the clinician to master and win the game of endodontics.

References

1. Abou-Rass M, Frank A, Glick D: The anticurvature filing method to prepare the curved root canal, *J Am Dent Assoc* 101:792, 1980.
2. Ahmad M et al: Ultrasonic débridement of root canals: acoustic cavitation and its relevance, *J Endod* 14:486, 1989.
3. Ahmad M, Pit-Ford TR, Crum LA: Ultrasonic débridement of root canals: acoustic streaming and its possible role, *J Endod* 13:490, 1987.

4. Ahmad M, Pitt-Ford TR, Crum LA: Ultrasonic débridement of root canals: an insight into the mechanisms involved, *J Endod* 13:93, 1987.

5. Albers H: *Tooth-colored restoratives,* ed. 8, Santa Rosa, Calif., 1996, Alto Books.

6. Allison CA, Weber CR, Walton RE: The influence of the method of canal preparation on the quality of the apical and coronal obturation, *J Endod* 5:298, 1979.

7. Alves J, Walton R, Drake D: Coronal leakage: endotoxin penetration from mixed bacterial communities through obturated, post-prepared root canals, *J Endod* 24(9):587, 1998.

8. Archer R et al: An in vivo evaluation of the efficacy of ultrasound after step-back preparation in mandibular molars, *J Endod* 18 (11):549, 1992.

9. Baker NA et al: Scanning electron microscopic study of the efficacy of various irrigating solutions, *J Endod* 1:127, 1975.

10. Baumgartner JC, Mader CL: A scanning electron microscopic evaluation of four root canal irrigation regiments, *J Endod* 13: 147, 1987.

11. Becker GL, Cohen S, Borer R: The sequelae of accidentally injecting sodium hypochlorite beyond the root apex, *Oral Surg* 38:633, 1974.

12. Bergenhotz G, Lekholm U, Milthon R, Engström B: Influence of apical overinstrumentation and overfilling on retreated root canals, *J Endod* 5:310, 1979.

13. Berutti E: Computerized analysis of the instrumentation of the root canal system, *J Endod* 19(5):236, 1993.

14. Berutti E, Marini R, Angeretti A: Penetration ability of different irrigants into dentinal tubules, *J Endod* 23(12):725, 1997.

15. Berutti E, Marini R: A scanning electron microscopic evaluation of the débridement capability of sodium hypochlorite at different temperatures, *J Endod* 22(9):467, 1996.

16. Blum JY, Cohen AG, Machtou P, Micallef JP: Analysis of forces developed during mechanical preparation of extracted teeth using Profile NiTi rotary instruments, *Int Endod J* 32(1): 24, 1999.

17. Blum JY, Machtou P, Esber S, Micallef JP: Analysis of forces developed during endodontic preparations: balanced force technique, *Int Endod J* 30:386, 1997.

18. Blum JY, Machtou P, Micallef JP: Location of contact areas of Profile NiTi rotary instruments in relation to the forces developed during mechanical preparation of extracted teeth, *Int Endod J* 32(2):108, 1999.

19. Brown DC, Moore BK, Brown CE Jr, Newton CW: An in vitro study of apical extrusion of sodium hypochlorite during endodontic canal preparation, *J Endod* 21(12): 587, 1995.

20. Brynolf I: A histological and roentgenological study of the periapical region of human upper incisors, *Odontol Revy* 18 (suppl 11), 1967.

21. Buchanan LS: Management of the curved root canal: predictably treating the most common endodontic complexity, *J Calif Dent Assoc* 17:40, 1989.

22. Bystrom A, Sundqvist G: The antibacterial action of sodium hypochlorite and EDTA in 60 cases of endodontic therapy, *Int Endod J* 18(1):35, 1985.

23. Calhoun G, Montgomery S: The effects of four instrumentation techniques on root canal shape, *J Endod* 14(6):273, 1988.

24. Cameron JA: The synergistic relationship between ultrasound and sodium hypochlorite: a scanning electron microscope evaluation, *J Endod* 13:541, 1987.

25. Chow TW: Mechanical effectiveness of root canal irrigation, *J Endod* 9:475, 1983.

26. Cimis GM, Boyer TJ, Pelleu GB: Effect of three file types on the apical preparation of moderately curved canals, *J Endod* 14:441, 1988.

27. Coffae KP, Brilliant JD: The effect of serial preparation versus nonserial preparation on tissue removal in the root canals of extracted mandibular human molars, *J Endod* 1(6):211, 1975.

28. Cunningham W, Balekjion A: Effect of temperature on collagen-dissolving ability of sodium hypochlorite irrigating solution, *Oral Surg* 49:175, 1980.

29. Cunningham W, Martin H: A scanning electron microscope evaluation of root canal débridement with the endosonic ultrasonic synergistic system, *Oral Surg* 53:527, 1982.

30. Cunningham WT, Martin H, Pelleu GB, Stoops DE: A comparison of antimicrobial effectiveness of endosonic and hand root canal therapy, *Oral Surg* 54(2):238, 1982.

31. Cymerman JJ, Jerome LA, Moodnik RM: A scanning electron microscope study comparing the efficacy of hand instrumentation with ultrasonic instrumentation of the root canal, *J Endod* 9(8):327, 1983.

32. Dakin D II: On the use of certain antiseptic substances in the treatment of infected wounds, *Br Med J* 2:318, 1915.

33. Daughenbaugh, JA: A scanning electron microscopic evaluation of NaOCl in the cleaning and shaping of human root canal systems, Boston, 1980, master's thesis, Boston University, 1980.

34. Dietz DB, Di Fiore PM, Bahcall JK, Lautenschlager EP: The effect of rotational speed on the breakage of nickel-titanium rotary files, *J Endod* 24:273, 1998.

35. Dow PR, Ingle JI: Isotope determination of root canal failure, *Oral Surg* 8:1100, 1955.

36. Dummer PMH, McGinn JH, Rees DG: The position and topography of the apical canal constriction and apical foramen, *Int End J* 17:192, 1984.

37. Ellingsen MA, Harrington GW, Hollender LG: Radiovisiography versus conventional radiography for detection of small instruments in endodontic length determination. I. In vitro evaluation, *J Endod* 21(6):326, 1995.

38. Esposito PT, Cunningham CJ: A comparison of canal preparation with nickel-titanium and stainless steel instruments, *J Endod* 21(4):173, 1995.

39. Fairbourn DR, McWalter GM, Montgomery S: The effect of four preparation techniques on the amount of apically extruded debris, *J Endod* 13:102, 1987.

40. Filho IB, Esberard RM, Leonardo R, del Rio CE: Microscopic evaluation of three endodontic files pre- and postinstrumentation, *J Endod* 24(7):461, 1998.

41. Fleming A: History and development of penicillin. *Penicillin: its practical application,* Philadelphia, 1946, The Blakiston Co.

42. Gabel WP et al: Effect of rotational speed on nickel-titanium file distortion, *J Endod* 25(11):752, 1999.

43. Gambarini G: Shaping and cleaning the root canal system: a scanning electron microscopic evaluation of a new instrumentation and irrigation technique, *J Endod* 25(12):800, 1999.

44. Gambarini G, De Luca M, Gerosa R: Chemical stability of heated sodium hypochlorite endodontic irrigants, *J Endod* 24(6):432, 1998.

45. Ganzberg S: Analgesics: Opioids and Nonopioids. In Ciancio SG, editor, *ADA Guide to Dental Therapeutics,* Chicago, 1998, ADA Publishing Co.

46. García AA, Navarro LF, Castelló VU, Laliga RM: Evaluation of a digital radiography to estimate working length, *J Endod* 23(6):363, 1997.

47. Goldberg F, Speilberg C: The effect of EDTAC and the variations of its working time analyzed with scanning electron microscopy, *Oral Surg* 53:74, 1982.

48. Goldman M, White RR, Moser CR, Tenca JI: A comparison of three methods of cleaning and shaping the root canal in vitro, *J Endod* 14(1):7, 1988.

49. Goodman A et al: An in vitro comparison of the efficacy of the step-back technique versus a step-back/ultrasonic technique in human mandibular molars, *J Endod* 11(6):249, 1985.

50. Green D: Stereomicroscopic study of the root apices of 400 maxillary and mandibular anterior teeth, *Oral Surg* 9:1224, 1956.

51. Green D: Stereomicroscopic study of the root apices of 700 maxillary and mandibular posterior teeth, *Oral Surg* 13:728, 1960.

52. Grey GC: The capabilities of sodium hypochlorite to digest organic debris from root canals with emphasis on accessory canals, master's thesis, Boston, 1990, Boston University.

53. Guignes P, Faure J, Maurette A: Relationship between endodontic preparations and human dentin permeability measured in situ, *J Endod* 22(2):60, 1996.

54. Haider J et al: An in vivo comparison of the step-back technique versus a step-back/ultrasonic technique in human mandibular molars, *J Endod* 15:195, 1989.

55. Haïkel Y et al: Mechanical properties of nickel-titanium endodontic instruments and the effect of sodium hypochlorite treatment, *J Endod* 24(11):731, 1998.

56. Hand RE, Smith ML, Harrison JW: Analysis of the effect of dilution on the necrotic tissue dissolution property of sodium hypochlorite, *J Endod* 4:60, 1978.

57. Hankins PJ, El Deeb ME: An evaluation of the Canal Master, balanced-force, and step-back techniques, *J Endod* 22(3):123, 1996.

58. Hasselgren G, Olsson B, Cvek M: Effects of calcium hydroxide and sodium hypochlorite on the dissolution of necrotic porcine muscle tissue, *J Endod* 14:125, 1988.

59. Heling I, Irani E, Karni S, Steinberg D: In vitro antimicrobial effect of RC-Prep within dentinal tubules, *J Endod* 25(12):782, 1999.

60. Hess W: *Anatomy of the root canals of the teeth of the permanent dentition,* New York, 1925, William Wood & Co.

61. Hottel TL, El-Refai NY, Jones JJ: A comparison of the effects of three chelating agents on the root canals of extracted human teeth, *J Endod* 25(11):716, 1999.

62. Huang L: An experimental study of the principle of electronic root canal measurement, *J Endod* 13:60, 1987.

63. Isom TL, Marshall JG, Baumgartner JC: Evaluation of root thickness in curved canals after flaring, *J Endod* 21(7):368, 1995.

64. Jensen SA, Walker TL, Hutter JW, Nicoll BK: Comparison of the cleaning efficacy of passive sonic activation and passive ultrasonic activation after hand instrumentation in molar root canals, *J Endod* 25(11):735, 1999.

65. Kahn FH, Rosenberg PA, Gliksberg J: An in vitro evaluation of the irrigating characteristics of ultrasonic and subsonic handpieces and irrigating needles and probes, *J Endod* 21(5):277, 1995.

66. Kavanagh D, Lumley PJ: An *in vitro* evaluation of canal preparation using Profile .04 and .06 taper instruments, *Endod Dent Traumatol* 14:16, 1998.

67. Kazemi RB, Stenman E, Spangberg LSW: The endodontic file is a disposable instrument, *J Endod* 21(9):451, 1995.

68. Keir DM, Senia SE, Montgomery S: Effectiveness of a brush in removing post-instrumentation canal debris, *J Endod* 16(7):323, 1990.

69. Kennedy WA, Walker WA III, Gough RW: Smear layer removal effects on apical leakage, *J Endod* 12:21, 1986.

70. Kessler JR, Peters DD, Lorton L: Comparison of the relative risk of molar root perforations using various endodontic instrumentation techniques, *J Endod* 9:439, 1983.

71. Klinghofer A: An in vivo study of penetration of sodium hypochlorite during the cleaning and shaping (Schilder technique) on necrotic pulp teeth, master's thesis, Boston, 1990, Boston University.

72. Kois J, Spear FM: Periodontal prosthesis: creating successful restorations, *J Am Dent Assoc* 10:123, 1992.

73. Kosa DA, Marshall G, Baumgartner JC: An analysis of canal centering using mechanical instrumentation techniques, *J Endod* 25(6):441, 1999.

74. Koskinen KP, Meurman JH, Stenvall LH: Appearance of chemically treated root canal walls in the scanning electron microscope, *Scand J Dent Res* 88:397, 1980.

75. Kovacevic M, Tamarut T: Influence of the concentration of ions and foramen diameter on the accuracy of electronic root canal length measurement — an experimental study, *J Endod* 24(5):346, 1998.

76. Lenchner NH: Restoring endodontically treated teeth: ferrule effect and biologic width, *Pract Periodontics Aesthet Dent* 1:19, 1989.

77. Levin H: Access cavities, *Dent Clin North Am* 701, November, 1967.

78. Luiten DJ, Morgan LA, Baumgartner JC, Marshall JG: A comparison of four instrumentation techniques on apical canal transportation, *J Endod* 21(1):26, 1995.

79. Machtou P: *Endodontie - guide clinique,* ed CDP, Paris 1993, CDP.

80. Machtou P: Irrigation investigation in endodontics, master's thesis, Paris, France, 1980, Paris VII.

81. Machtou P, Martin D: Utilisation raisonnee des ProFile, *Clinic* 18:253, 1997.

82. Mandel E, Machtou P, Friedman S: Scanning electron microscope observation of canal cleanliness, *J Endod* 16(6):279, 1990.

83. Marshall FJ, Pappin J: A crown-down pressureless preparation root canal enlargement technique, technique manual, Portland, 1980, Oregon Health Sciences University.

84. McCann JT, Keller DL, LaBounty GL: Remaining dentin/cementum thickness after hand or ultrasonic instrumentation, *J Endod* 16(3):109, 1990.

85. McComb D, Smith DC: A preliminary scanning electron microscopic study of root canals after endodontic procedures, *J Endod* 1:238, 1975.

86. McDonald NJ: The electronic determination of working length, *Dent Clin North Am* 36:293, 1992.

87. McGreevey, E: Investigation of profile series 29 .04 taper rotary instruments, Boston, 1995, master's thesis, Boston University.

88. Miserendino LJ, Moser JB, Heuer MA, Osetek EM: Cutting efficiency of endodontic instruments. II. Analysis of tip design, *J Endod* 12(1):8, 1986.

89. Montgomery S: Root canal wall thickness of mandibular molars after biomechanical preparation, *J Endod* 11(6):257, 1988.

90. Morgan LF, Montgomery S: An evaluation of the crown-down pressureless technique, *J Endod* 10(10):491, 1984.

91. Nevins M, Mellonig JT, editors: *Periodontal Therapy, Clinical Approaches and Evidence of Success*, Chicago, 1998, Quintessence Publishing Co.

92. Newman MG, Goodman AD: Antibiotics in endodontic therapy. In Smith J, editor: *Guide to antibiotic use in dental practice*, Chicago, 1984, Quintessence Publishing Co.

93. Pagavino G, Pace R, Baccetti T: A SEM study of in vivo accuracy of the Root ZX electronic apex locator, *J Endod* 24(6): 438, 1998.

94. Pedicord D, El Deeb ME, Messer HH: Hand versus ultrasonic instrumentation: its effect on canal shape and instrumentation time, *J Endod* 12(9):375, 1986.

95. Pineda F, Kuttler Y: Mesiodistal and buccolingual roentgeno-graphic investigation of 7275 root canals, *Oral Surg* 33:101, 1972.

96. Piskin B, Turkun M: Stability of various sodium hypochlorite solutions, *J Endod* 21(5):253, 1995.

97. Pruett JP, Clement DJ, Carnes DL Jr: Cyclic fatigue testing of nickel-titanium endodontic instruments, *J Endod* 23(2):77, 1997.

98. Raiden G et al: Residual thickness of root in first maxillary premolars with post space preparation, *J Endod* 25(7):502, 1998.

99. Reddy SA, Hicks ML: Apical extrusion of debris using two hand and two rotary instrumentation techniques, *J Endod* 24:180, 1998.

100. Reynolds MA et al: An in vitro histological comparison of the step-back, sonic, and ultrasonic instrumentation techniques in small, curved root canals, *J Endod* 13(7):307, 1987.

101. Roane JB, Sabala CL: Clockwise or counterclockwise, *J Endod* 10:349, 1984.

102. Roane JB, Sabala CL, Duncanson MG: The "balanced force" concept for instrumentation of curved canals, *J Endod* 11(5):203, 1985.

103. Rosenberg PA, Babick PJ, Schertzer L, Leung A: The effect of occlusal reduction on pain after endodontic instrumentation, *J Endod* 24(7):492, 1998.

104. Rowan MB, Nicholls JI, Steiner J: Torsional properties of stainless steel and nickel-titanium endodontic files, *J Endod* 22(7):341, 1996.

105. Royal JR, Donnelly JC: A comparison of maintenance of canal curvature using balanced-force instrumentation with three different file types, *J Endod* 21(6):300, 1995.

106. Ruddle CJ: Endodontic failures: the rationale and application of surgical retreatment, *Revue d'Odonto Stomatologia* 17(6): 511, 1988.

107. Ruddle CJ: Erfolreiche strategien bei der preparation des wurzelkanals, *Endodontie* 3:217, 1994.

108. Ruddle CJ: Microendodontic nonsurgical retreatment, Micro-scopes in Endodontics, *Dent Clin of North Am* 41(3):429, WB Saunders, Philadelphia, PA, July 1997.

109. Ruddle CJ: Nonsurgical endodontic retreatment, *J Calif Dent Assoc* 25:11, 1997.

110. Ruddle CJ: Obturation of the root canal system; Three-dimensional obturation: the rationale and application of warm gutta-percha with vertical condensation. In Cohen S, Burns RC, editors: *Pathways of the pulp*, ed 6, St Louis, 1994, Mosby.

111. Ruddle CJ: Scanning electron microscopic analysis of the warm gutta-percha vertical condensation technique, master's thesis, Boston, 1976, Harvard University.

112. Ruddle CJ: Three-dimensional obturation: The rationale and application of warm gutta-percha with vertical condensation, *J Mass Dent Soc* 43:3, 1994.

113. Sabala CL, Powell SE: Sodium hypochlorite injection into periapical tissues, *J Endod* 15:490, 1989.

114. Scarfe WC, Fana CR Jr, Farman AG: Radiographic detection of accessory/lateral canals: Use of RadioVisioGraphy and Hypaque, *J Endod* 21(4):185, 1995.

115. Schäfer E, Tepel J, Hoppe W: Properties of endodontic hand instruments used in rotary motion. II. Instrumentation of curved canals, *J Endod* 21(10):493, 1995.

116. Schilder H: Canal débridement and disinfection. In Cohen S, Burns RC, editors: *Pathways of the pulp*, ed 1, St Louis, 1976, Mosby.

117. Schilder H: Cleaning and shaping the root canal system, *Dent Clin North Am* 18(2):269, 1974.

118. Schilder H: Filling root canals in three dimensions, *Dent Clin North Am* 723, Nov. 1967.

119. Schilder H: Instruments, materials, and devices: a new concept in instrument design. In Cohen S and Burns RC, editors: *Pathways of the Pulp,* ed 6, St Louis, 1994, Mosby.

120. Scianamblo MJ: Principales causes d'echecs endodontiques, *Rev Odontoestomatol* 17:409, 1988.

121. Sepic AO, Pantera EA, Neaverth EJ, Anderson RW: A comparison of Flex-O-Files and K-type files for enlargement of severely curved molar root canals, *J Endod* 15(6):240, 1989.

122. Serene TP, Adams JD, Saxena A: *Nickel-titanium instruments: applications in endodontics*, St Louis, 1995, Ishiyaku EuroAmerica.

123. Serota KS, Glassman GD: Root canal preparation using engine-driven nickel-titanium rotary instruments, *Pract Periodontics Aesthet Dent* 11(9):1117, 1999.

124. Seto BG, Nicholls JI, Harrington GW: Torsional properties of twisted and machined endodontic files, *J Endod* 18(8):355, 1990.

125. Shabahang S, Goon WWY, Gluskin AH: An in vitro evaluation of Root ZX electronic apex locator, *J Endod* 22(11):616, 1996.

126. Short JA, Morgan LA, Baumgartner JC: A comparison of canal centering ability of four instrumentation techniques, *J Endod* 23:503, 1997.

127. Silvaggio J, Hicks ML: Effect of heat sterilization on the torsional properties of rotary nickel-titanium endodontic files, *J Endod* 23:731, 1997.

128. Siqueira JF Jr, Batista M, Fraga RC, de Uzeda M: Antibacterial effects of endodontic irrigants on black-pigmented gram-negative anaerobes and facultative bacteria, *J Endod* 24(6): 414, 1998.

129. Sorensen JA, Engelman MJ: Ferrule design and fracture resistance of endodontically treated teeth, *J Prosthet Dent* 63:529, 1990.

130. Southard DW: Immediate core build up of endodontically treated teeth: the rest of the seal, *Pract Periodontics Aesthet Dent* 11(4):519, 1999.

131. Southard DW, Oswald RJ, Natkin E: Instrumentation of curved molar root canals with the Roane technique, *J Endod* 13(10):479, 1987.

132. Stenman E, Spangberg LSW: Machining efficiency of endodontic files: a new methodology, *J Endod* 16(4):151, 1990.

133. Stewart GG: The importance of chemomechanical preparation of the root canal, *Oral Surg* 8:993, 1955.

134. Stewart GG: A scanning electron microscopic study of the cleansing effectiveness of three irrigating modalities on the tubular structure of dentin, *J Endod* 24(7):485, 1998.

135. Stewart G, Cobe H, Rappaport H: A study of a new medicament in the chemomechanical preparation of infected root canals, *J Am Dent Assoc* 63:33, 1961.

136. Svec TA, Hanson JW: The effect of effervescence on débridement of the apical regions of root canals in single-rooted teeth, *J Endod* 7:335, 1981.

137. Swindle RB, Neaverth EJ, Pantera EA, Ringle RD: Effect of coronal-radicular flaring on apical transportation, *J Endod* 17(4):147,1991.

138. Tepel J, Schafer E, Hoppe W: Properties of endodontic hand instruments used in rotary motion. I. Cutting efficiency, *J Endod* 21(8):418, 1995.

139. Wade AK, Walker WA, Gough RW: Smear layer removal effects on apical leakage, *J Endod* 12:21, 1986.

140. Walia H, Brantley WA, Gerstein H: An initial investigation of the bending and torsional properties of Nitinol root canal files, *J Endod* 14(7):346, 1988.

141. Walton RE: Histologic evaluation of different methods of enlarging the pulp canal space, *J Endod* 2:304, 1976.

142. Weine FS: The use of non-ISO tapered instruments for canal flaring, *Compend Contin Educ Dent* 17:651, 1996.

143. Weine FS, Buchanan LS: Controversies in clinical endodontics: filling from the open position, *Compendium* 18(9):906, 1997.

144. Weine FS, Kelly RF, Lio PJ: The effect of preparation procedures on original canal shape and on apical foramen shape, *J Endod* 1(8):255, 1975.

145. West JD: The relation between the three-dimensional endodontic seal and endodontic failure, master's thesis, Boston, 1975, Boston University.

146. West JD, Roane JB: Cleaning and shaping the root canal system. In Cohen S, Burns RC, editors: *Pathways of the Pulp*, ed 7, St Louis, 1998, Mosby.

147. Yana Y: An in vivo comparative study of the penetration of sodium hypochlorite in root canal systems during cleaning and shaping procedures using the B.U. technique and sonic instrumentation, master's thesis, Boston, 1989, Boston University.

148. Yee RDJ et al: The effect of canal preparation on the formation and leakage characteristics of the apical dentin plug, *J Endod* 10:308, 1984.

149. Yoshida T et al: Clinical evaluation of the efficacy of EDTA solution as an endodontic irrigant, *J Endod* 21(12): 592, 1995.

Chapter 9

Obturation of the Cleaned and Shaped Root Canal System

James L. Gutmann, David E. Witherspoon

Chapter Outline

HISTORIC PERSPECTIVES

In 1924 Hatton indicated, "Perhaps there is no technical operation in dentistry or surgery where so much depends on the conscientious adherence to high ideals as that of pulp canal filling."[76] The essence of this statement had been significantly influenced by years of trial and error in both the techniques and materials used to obturate the prepared root canal system. Much of the frustration and challenge that emanated from this concern, however, was due to the lack of development in root canal preparation techniques, coupled with indictments of the "focal infection" craze of that era.[84]

Before 1800 root canal filling, when done, was limited to gold. Subsequent obturations with various metals, oxychloride of zinc, paraffin, and amalgam resulted in varying degrees of success and satisfaction.[96] In 1847 Hill developed the first gutta-percha root canal filling material known as "Hill's stopping."[96] The preparation, which consisted principally of bleached gutta-percha and carbonate of lime and quartz, was patented in 1848 and introduced to the dental profession. In 1867 Bowman made claim (before the St Louis Dental Society) of the first use of gutta-percha for canal filling in an extracted first molar.[79]

References to the use of gutta-percha for root canal obturation before the turn of the twentieth century were few and vague. In 1883 Perry claimed that he had been using a pointed gold wire, wrapped with some soft gutta-percha (the roots of the present-day core carrier technique?).[129] He also began using gutta-percha rolled into points and packed into the canal. The points were prepared by cutting base plate gutta-percha into slender strips, warming them with a lamp, laying them on his operating case, and rolling them with another flat surface (a contemporary technique used to custom roll a large cone?). Perry then used shellac warmed over a lamp and rolled the cones into a point of desired size, based on canal shape and length. Before placing the final gutta-percha point, he saturated the tooth cavity with alcohol; capillary attraction let the alcohol run into the canal, softening the shellac so that the gutta-percha could be packed (the forerunner of a chemical-softening technique?).

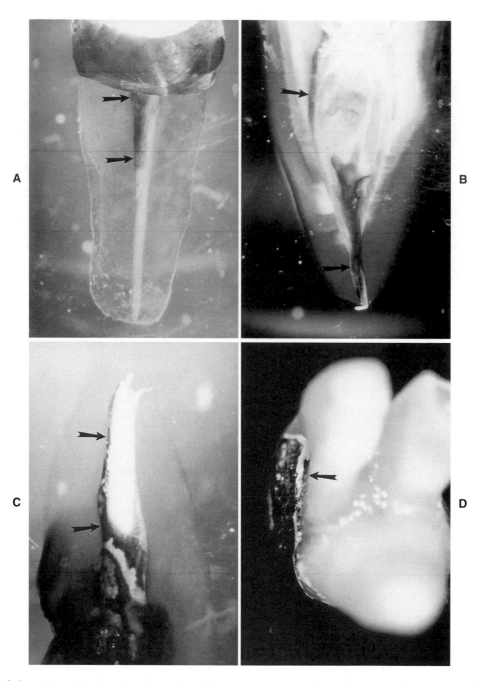

Fig. 9-1 **A**, Coronal leakage from beneath a full crown, moving apically *(arrows)* along the root canal filling. **B**, Coronal leakage *(arrows)* to the apical foramen in the mesial root of a mandibular molar. **C**, Coronal leakage under a crown on a maxillary molar. Viewed is the palatal root, which shows evidence of leakage down its entire surface *(arrows)*. Teeth in **A** through **C** were demineralized, dehydrated, and cleared for viewing. **D**, Artificial crown margins that are conducive to leakage *(arrow)*. These avenues must either be prevented or removed if root canal treatment is to be successful.

In 1887 the S.S. White Company began to manufacture gutta-percha points.[92] In 1893 Rollins introduced a new type of gutta-percha to which he added vermilion.[182] Because vermilion is pure oxide of mercury and therefore dangerous in the quantities suggested by Rollins, there were many critics of this technique.

With the introduction of radiographs into the assessment of root canal obturations, it became painfully obvious that the canal was not cylindric, as earlier imagined, and that additional filling material was necessary to fill the observed voids. At first hard-setting dental cements were used, but these proved unsatisfactory. It was also thought that the cement used should possess strong antiseptic action, hence the development of many phenolic- or formalin-type of paste cements. The softening and dissolution of the gutta-percha to serve as the cementing agent, through the use of rosins, was introduced by Callahan in 1914.[26] Subsequently a multitude of various pastes, sealers, and cements were created in an attempt to discover the best possible sealing agent for use with gutta-percha.

Over the past 70 to 80 years the dental community has seen attempts to improve on the nature of root canal obturation with these cements and with variations in the delivery of gutta-percha to the prepared canal system. During this era the impetus for these developments was based heavily on the continued belief in the concept of focal infection, elective localization, the hollow-tube theory, and the concept that the primary cause for failure of root canal treatment was the apical percolation of fluids, and (potentially) microorganisms, into a poorly obturated root canal system.[32,133,140] It is from this chronologic perspective of technical and scientific thought that this chapter clarifies and codifies contemporary concepts in the obturation of the cleaned and shaped root canal system.

PURPOSE, RATIONALE, AND IMPORTANCE OF OBTURATION: STANDARD OF CARE

The purposes of obturating the prepared root canal space are well-founded in the contemporary art and science of endodontology and, simply stated, are as follows: (1) to eliminate all avenues of leakage from the oral cavity or the periradicular tissues into the root canal system, and (2) to seal within the system any irritants that cannot be fully removed during canal cleaning and shaping procedures. The rationale for these objectives recognizes that microbial irritants (e.g., microorganisms, toxins, metabolites) and products of pulp tissue degeneration are the prime causes for pulpal demise and its subsequent extension into the periradicular tissue. Failure to eliminate these etiologic factors and to prevent further irritation via continued contamination of the root canal system are the prime causes for failure of nonsurgical and surgical root canal treatment.[25,57,142,160]

The importance of three-dimensional (3-D) obturation of the root canal system cannot be overstated. However, the ability to achieve this goal is primarily dependent on the quality of the canal cleaning and shaping and the skill of the clinician. Even with the most skilled clinician, however, many other factors (e.g., what materials are used, how materials are used, and radiographic interpretation of process and product) help to determine the ultimate success or failure of each case. What may loom as the most important attainment is the ultimate coronal restoration of the tooth after canal obturation. Reasonable evidence suggests that coronal leakage through improperly placed restorations after root canal treatment[136,148] and failure of the restorative treatment or lack of health of the supporting periodontium are the final determinants of success or failure in treatment[180] (Fig. 9-1).

Contemporary perspectives on the assessment of the quality of root canal obturation have placed an undue reliance on apical leakage studies[188] in addition to two-dimensional radiographic evaluation[95] (Fig. 9-2). This tends to create a false sense of security within the clinician, because there is no contemporary root canal obturation technique or material that is impervious to leakage[57] (Fig. 9-3, *A* and *B*), and there is a poor correlation between the quality of the root canal obturation (especially an impervious seal) and what is viewed on a buccal radiograph.[34,95] Likewise, when the radiographic appearance of the root canal filling is unacceptable, the likelihood of leakage is high. Additionally, when the root filling is radiographically acceptable, the likelihood of leakage is still rather high and failure may occur more than 14% of the time.[25,95] Therefore the clinician must choose a path of treatment that will result in the best possible cleaning and shaping of the root canal system, coupled with an obturation technique that will provide a 3-D seal, apically, laterally, and coronally within the confines of the root canal system. If these technical parameters are achieved, there is a high likelihood that the biologic parameters of ultimate periradicular tissue regeneration will be achieved. These parameters are highlighted by the formation of cementum that forms over and seals the apical foramen and evidences the presence of the insertion of Sharpey's fibers (Fig. 9-4, *A* and *B*).

CHARACTERISTICS OF AN IDEAL ROOT CANAL FILLING: STANDARD OF CARE

The American Association of Endodontists (AAE) has published *Appropriateness of Care and Quality Assurance Guidelines*[5] regarding all aspects of contemporary endodontic treatment. In that publication, root canal obturation is defined and characterized as "the three-dimensional filling of the entire root canal system as close to the cementodentinal junction as possible. Minimal amounts of root canal sealers, which have been demonstrated to be biologically compatible, are used in conjunction with the core filling material to establish an adequate seal." Additionally, "use of paraformaldehyde-containing materials for root canal obturation is below the standard for endodontic therapy." Finally, with regard to the radiographic assessment of root canal obturation, there

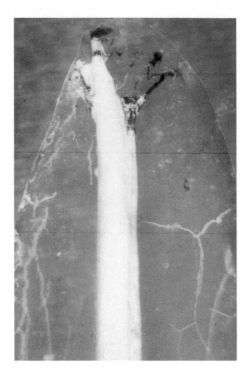

Fig. 9-2 Although the gutta-percha and sealer are well adapted in the apical portion of the canal, there is evidence of leakage into accessory canals. Apical portion of the gutta-percha was softened with chloroform before obturation.

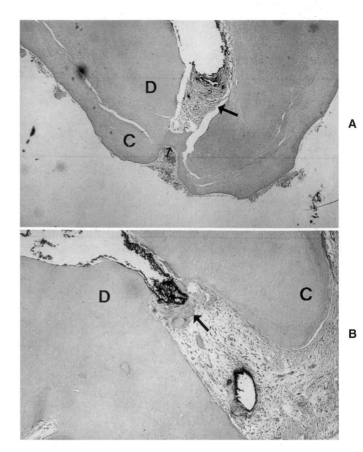

Fig. 9-4 **A**, Histologic evidence of complete cemental repair and sealing *(small arrow)* of the root canal system, regardless of the presence of apical debris *(large arrow)*. Note that the position of the filling material was short of the apical foramen. Stain H and E. **B**, Further evidence for apical repair with hard tissue *(arrow)* when the root filling is short of the apical foramen and the apical tissues (i.e., periodontal tissues) are protected from damage during instrumentation and obturation. C, Cementum; *D*, Dentin. Original magnification × 40.

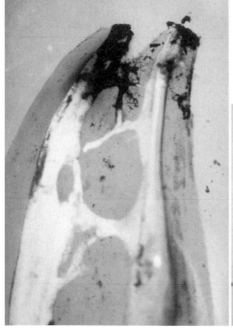

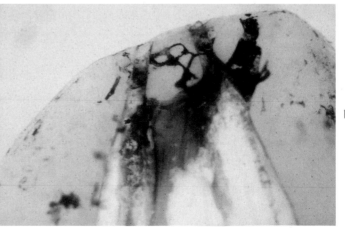

Fig. 9-3 **A**, Extensive apical leakage into canal anastomosis located between the mesiobuccal and mesiolingual canals of a mandibular molar. **B**, Delta formation at the apex of a mesial root of a mandibular molar. Note the extensive leakage into the apical irregularities, regardless of the canal obturation.

should be a "radiographic appearance of a dense, three-dimensional filling which extends as close as possible to the cementodentinal junction, *i.e.*, without gross overextension or underfilling in the presence of a patent canal." These standards, as stated, should serve as the benchmark for all clinicians who perform root canal treatment, and achievements below these standards must be considered as unacceptable. However, it is only through a cognizant "problem-solving" approach to root canal treatment, that quality assurance can be continually demonstrated in the obturation of the root canal system.[63] This approach demands inspection of the process and elimination of all variables that cause a departure from the standard of care.

Although there is a tremendous variance in the anatomy of the root canal system, the obturated root canal should reflect a shape that is approximately the same shape as the root morphology. Therefore proper cleaning and shaping within the confines of the root canal and in conjunction with the external anatomy of the root is essential. Additionally, the shape of the obturated canal should reflect a continuously tapering funnel preparation without excessive removal of tooth structure at any level of the canal system (Fig. 9-5). Techniques of preparation that encourage excessive removal of coronal root dentin with rotary instruments should be discouraged for three reasons[58] (Fig. 9-6, *A* and *B*): (1) the root walls will be weakened, (2) there is a greater likelihood for a lateral or strip perforation in posterior teeth, and (3) the gutta-percha and sealer root canal filling, although dense and well compacted in the coronal third, will not strengthen the root or compensate for lost dentin. Placement of a post in these teeth will not strengthen the root and may predispose to root fracture.[58]

Because of the high degree of variability in radiographic interpretation among clinicians, subtle characteristics of the obturated root canal may go unnoticed. In addition, because of differences in radiopacity in root canal sealer/cements, constituents in specific brands of gutta-percha, interpretation of voids in vivo versus in vitro,[195] the overlying bony anatomy, radiographic angulation, and the limited two-dimensional view of the obturated canal or canals, the quality of the obturation may not undergo sufficient assessment as to levels of achievement and quality assurance. For example, one of the most often overlooked aspects in the assessment of root canal

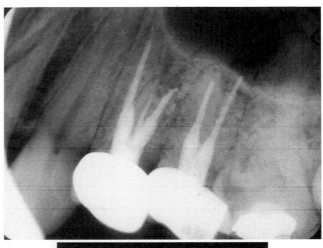

A

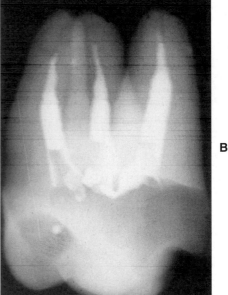

B

Fig. 9-6 Improper canal shaping that reflects an excessive use of rotary instruments in the coronal two thirds of the canal. The root walls of both teeth have been weakened, and the apical fillings may only be single cones with sealer in the premolar (**A**). Additionally, there has been the failure to achieve proper depth of penetration of the gutta-percha filling in the molar because of the irregular canal preparation (**B**).

Fig. 9-5 Well-shaped and obturated root canals using gutta-percha, sealer, and lateral compaction.

obturations is the density of the apical portion of the fill.[61] In essence the apical third of the canal is filled with a sea of root canal cement and a single, uncompacted master cone or poorly condensed mass of previously softened gutta-percha. Radiographically, the apical third of the canal appears less radiodense. An ill-defined outline to the canal wall is evident, along with obvious gaps or voids in the filling material or its adaptation to the confines of the canal (Fig. 9-7). In the case of highly radiopaque root canal sealers/cements, the apical portion may only be filled with sealer, giving the clinician the false impression of a dense, 3-D obturation with gutta-percha. Therefore it is necessary that the clinician master multiple techniques and become competent in the use of various sealers and cements to ensure the proper management of the wide diversity of anatomic scenarios encountered.

CHARACTERISTICS OF IDEAL ROOT CANAL FILLING MATERIALS

Although a plethora of materials have been advocated over the past 150 years for root canal obturation, gutta-percha has proven to be the material of choice for the successful filling of the canal from its coronal to apical extent. Although not the ideal filling material, it has satisfied the majority of tenets for an ideal root filling material highlighted by Brownlee in 1900 and reiterated by Grossman in 1940 (Table 9-1); its cited disadvantages (i.e., lack of rigidity and adhesiveness, ease of displacement under pressure)[115] do not overshadow its advantages. Sealer/cement is always used with the gutta-percha. Therefore contemporary materials of choice are gutta-percha in conjunction with sealer/cement. Neither sub-

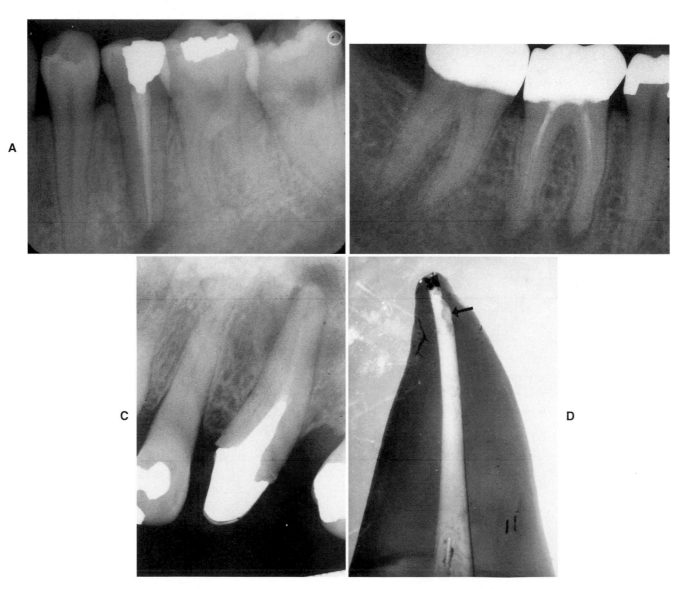

Fig. 9-7 **A** to **C**, Examples of root canal obturations that lack proper canal shape, in addition to a poorly compacted root canal filling. Voids are seen (apically and laterally) the length of the fillings. The treatment rendered in each case is below the standard of care, yet was allowed by each clinician that performed the treatment. Each case exhibits periradicular pathosis. **D**, Type of void *(arrow)* not always discernible on a dental radiograph. Over time this may contribute to treatment failure.

stance alone enables canal obturation up to the standard of care, regardless of the delivery system or compaction technique. This chapter focuses solely on the use of these materials, highlighting their contemporary use and achievement of success. Neither the materials used nor the techniques detailed will be successful without proper cleaning and shaping of the canal (as described in Chapter 8). Likewise, the materials and techniques described do not provide an impervious seal of the canal system; all canals leak to a greater or lesser extent.[57] Therefore it is necessary that the clinician master multiple obturation techniques and become competent with various root canal sealer/cements to manage the diversity of anatomic scenarios encountered.

Gutta-Percha

Gutta-percha is the preferred choice as a solid, core-filling material for canal obturation. It demonstrates minimal toxicity, minimal tissue irritability, and is the least allergenic material available when retained within the canal system.[115] In cases of inadvertent gutta-percha cone overextension into the periradicular tissues, it is considered as being well tolerated as long as the canal is clean and sealed. However, gutta-percha has been shown to produce an intense localized, tissue response in subcutaneous tissues when placed in fine particle form or when it has been altered with softening agents (e.g., rosin-chloroform).[161] This potential may impact on some advocated obturation techniques.

Chemically pure gutta-percha exists in two distinct, different crystalline forms, alpha and beta.[51] These forms are interchangeable, depending on the temperature of the material. Whereas most commercially available forms are the beta structure, newer products have adopted the alpha crystalline structure for compatibility with the thermosoftening of the material during obturation. This change has been made

because heating of the beta phase (98.6° F, 37° C) causes the crystalline structure to change to the alpha phase (107.6° to 111.2° F, 42° to 44° C) and ultimately into an amorphous melt (132.8° to 147.2° F, 56° to 64° C).[51] Subsequently, the gutta-percha undergoes significant shrinkage during its phase retransformation to the beta state, thereby necessitating thorough compaction during cooling. Produced in the alpha phase, however, the gutta-percha undergoes less shrinkage, and compaction pressures and techniques can better compensate for any shrinkage that may occur.

Gutta-percha can also be softened with chemical solvents to enhance adaptation to the irregularities of the prepared root canal system. However, shrinkage may occur because of solvent evaporation, or the periradicular tissues may be irritated if the solvent is expressed beyond the canal or significant amounts of softened gutta-percha are inadvertently placed into the periradicular tissues.[161]

For root canal obturation, gutta-percha is manufactured in the form of cones in both standardized and nonstandardized sizes. The standardized sizes coordinate with the ISO sizes of the root canal file sizes 15 through 140 and are used primarily as the main core material for obturation (Fig. 9-8). The nonstandardized sizes are more tapered from the tip or point to the top, and they are usually designated as *extra-fine, fine-fine, medium-fine, fine, fine-medium, medium, medium-large, large,* and *extra-large.* With some obturation techniques these cones are used as accessory or auxiliary cones during compaction, being matched with the shape of the prepared canal space or the compaction instrument. Although the standardized cones have been popular for years (since the standardization of the file system),[85] nonstandardized cones have assumed a greater role as the primary core material in the more contemporary obturation techniques. With the development of these techniques, in particular those of vertical compaction with heat softening of gutta-percha, there has been a resurgent interest in the nonstandardized cones. For injectable thermoplastic obturation techniques, gutta-percha may come in either pellet form or in cannulas. For some thermomechanical techniques, it is available in heatable syringes (Fig. 9-9).

The composition of the available gutta-percha cones is approximately 19% to 22% gutta-percha, 59% to 75% zinc oxide, with the remaining small percentages a combination of various waxes, coloring agents, antioxidants, and metallic salts. The particular percentages of the components vary by manufacturer, with resultant variations in the brittleness, stiffness, tensile strength, and radiopacity of the individual cones primarily because of the gutta-percha and zinc oxide percentages.[38,39] Primarily because of their content of zinc oxide, gutta-percha cones demonstrate definite antimicrobial activity.[112,113] At the very least, however, they should not support microbial growth. Most recently gutta-percha cones have become available containing an iodoform component called medicated gutta-percha (MGP) (Lone Star Technologies, Westport, Conn.) to enhance their antimicrobial properties.[106] However, long-term data on the clinical efficacy of these cones are lacking (see Chapter 14 for more information on gutta-percha).

TABLE 9-1   REQUIREMENTS FOR AN IDEAL ROOT CANAL FILLING MATERIAL

Brownlee 1900[23]	Grossman 1940[55]
Easily inserted	Easily introduced
Pliable or moldable	Liquid or semisolid and become solid
Completely fill and seal apex	Seal laterally and apically
Neither expand or contract	Not shrink
Impermeable to fluids	Impervious to moisture
Antiseptic	Bacteriostatic
Not discolor tooth	Not stain tooth
Chemically neutral	Not irritate periapical tissues
Easily removed	Easily removed
Tasteless and odorless	Sterile or sterilizable
Durable	Radiopaque

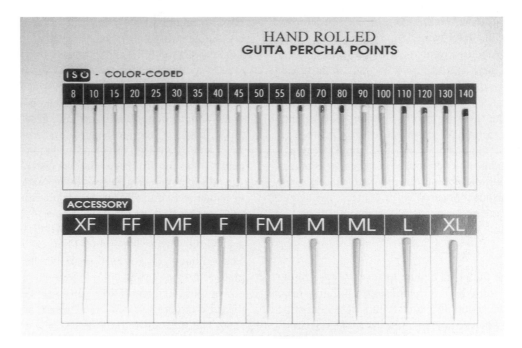

Fig. 9-8 Comparison of standardized gutta-percha cones *(top)* and nonstandardized cones *(bottom).*

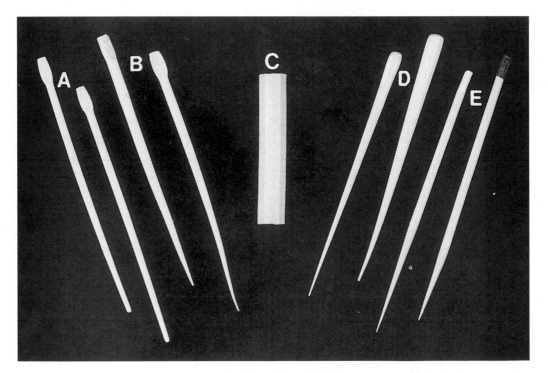

Fig. 9-9 Assortment of gutta-percha cones. *A,* Standardized ISO-sized gutta-percha that has a taper of .02; *B,* Non-standardized accessory cones with a variable taper; *C,* Pellet of gutta-percha for injectible thermoplasticized gutta-percha; *D,* .04 and .06 tapered gutta-percha; *E,* .08 and .12 tapered gutta-percha.

Sealers/Cements

The use of a sealer during root canal obturation is essential for success. It enhances the possible attainment of an impervious seal and serves as filler for canal irregularities and minor discrepancies between the root canal wall and core filling material. Sealers are often expressed through lateral or accessory canals, and they can assist in microbial control should there be microorganisms left on the root canal walls or in the tubules.[3,78,130] Sealers can also serve as lubricants to assist in the thorough seating of the core filling material during compaction. In canals in which the smear layer has been removed, many sealers demonstrate increased adhesive properties to dentin (in addition to flowing into the patent tubules).[59,100,119,157,185]

A good sealer should be biocompatible and well tolerated by the periradicular tissues.[167,168] All sealers exhibit toxicity when freshly mixed; however, their toxicity is greatly reduced on setting.[99] All sealers are resorbable when exposed to tissues and tissue fluids.[99] Subsequent tissue healing or repair generally appears unaffected by most sealers, provided their are no adverse breakdown products of the sealer over time.[16,19,20-22] In particular, the breakdown products may have an adverse action on the proliferative capability of periradicular cell populations.[54] Therefore sealers should not be placed routinely in the periradicular tissues as part of an obturation technique.[99]

Sealers can be grouped based on their prime constituent or structure, such as zinc oxide-eugenol, calcium hydroxide, resins, glass ionomers, or silicones. A listing of commonly used sealers/cements is found in Table 9-2. However, within this type of grouping, many of the sealers/cements are combinations of components, such as zinc oxide-eugenol and calcium hydroxide (e.g., Sealapex). The addition of the calcium hydroxide to the sealers, thereby increasing the pH of the material, is claimed to create a therapeutic material that can be inductive of hard-tissue formation. Although an osteogenic response has been observed,[82,164] the solubility of the calcium hydroxide sealers[172,177,178] and the ability of these sealers to sustain a high pH over time[97] have been questioned.

Globally, the listings in Table 9-2 are incomplete. However, all effective and safe root canal sealers/cements are of the types listed with minor variations in their constituents. Each clinician must read the product insert and material safety data sheet (MSDS) for each product purchased before use.

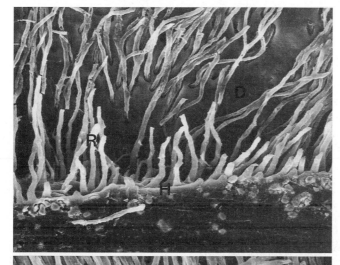

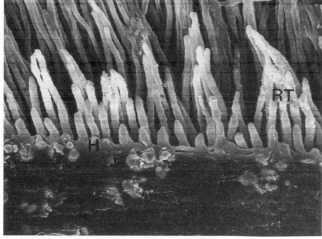

Fig. 9-10 **A**, Cross-sectional scanning electron microscopic view of the dentine adhesive interface. The hybrid layer *(H)*, resin filling material *(R)*, and demineralized dentin *(D)* are visible with resin tags extending deep into the demineralized tubules. Original magnification × 940. **B**, Cross-sectional scanning electron microscopic view displaying resin tags entering dentine tubules and contiguous with the hybrid layer *(H)*. Original magnification × 660. (From Leonard JE, Gutmann JL, Guo IY: Apical and coronal seal of roots obturated with a dentine bonding agent and resin, *Int Endod J* 29:76, 1996.)

New Directions

With the increased amount of root canal treatment being performed by both the generalist and specialist, there have been renewed efforts to develop better sealer and core obturation materials and techniques. In particular this has focused on the use of glass ionomers,[135] dentin-bonded composite resins[41,100] (Fig. 9-10, *A* and *B*), dentin-bonded apical dentinal plugs,[74] Super EBA and gutta-percha,[40] ultrasonic compaction of gutta-percha, and canal filling under a vacuum with gutta-percha and sealer.[132] To date none of these materials and techniques have safely reached the highest biologic and technical level. Ideally, future directions should focus on materials that (1) penetrate the patent dentinal tubules, (2) bind intimately to both the organic and inorganic phases of dentin, (3) neutralize or destroy microorganisms and their products, (4) predictably induce a cemental regenerative response over the apical foramen, and (5) strengthen the root system. The delivery system of such materials requires ease of placement with a rapid and thorough set once in the canal system. Within this futuristic framework, all previous requirements of a root canal sealer and filling material may be inadequate, along with presently used materials.

TABLE 9-2   COMMONLY USED ROOT CANAL SEALER/CEMENTS

Name	Manufacturer	Form	ZOE	Ca(OH)$_2$	Resin	GI	Silicone	Work	Set	Specific Indications: Usage Concerns
AH-26 (Thermaseal)	Dentsply, USA/Maillefer, Switzerland	P/L			X			L	L	Allergenic/mutagenic potential; adhesive; formaldehyde release (?); silver containing
AH-Plus*(Topseal)	Dentsply, USA/Maillefer, Switzerland	P/P			X			L	L	Nonmutagenic; no release of formaldehyde; radiopaque; all techniques; low solubility
Sealapex	Kerr Sybron, USA	P/P		X				L	L	Osteogenic (?); possible dissolution; expands on setting
Apexit	Ivoclar-Vivadent, Liechtenstein			X						
CRCS (Caleiobiotic)	Hygenic, USA	P/L		X				L	L	Softens gutta-percha; good for lateral compaction; viscous; adhesive
Pulp Canal Sealer	Kerr Sybron, USA	P/L	X					S/M	M/S	Silver containing, radiopaque; all techniques
Wach's Sealex-Extra	Balas Dental Supply	P/L	X					S/M	M	Adhesive; good for lateral compaction especially in small canals; softens gutta-percha; good if overextension possible
Grossman-type Stainless										
Roth 801	Roth International, USA	P/L	X					L	L	All techniques; expansion
Roth 811	Roth International, USA	P/L	X					M	M	All techniques
Roth 601	Roth International, USA	P/L	X					S	S	No vertical compaction
Procosal	Procosol Chemical, USA	P/L	X					L/M	L/M	All techniques
Endoseal	Centric Inc. USA	P/L	X					L/M	L/M	All techniques
Tubliseal	Kerr Sybron, USA	P/P	X					S	S	No vertical compaction
Tubliseal-EWT	Kerr Sybron, USA	P/P	X					M	M	All techniques
Grossman-Type Silver										
Roth 511	Roth International, USA	P/L	X					L	L	Avoid anterior teeth
Roth 515	Roth International, USA	P/L	X					M	M	Avoid anterior teeth
Ketac-Endo	ESPE-Premier, Germany/USA	Cap				X		S/M	M/S	No compaction; releases fluoride; tubule penetration; bond to dentin?
Lee Endo Fill	Lee Pharmaceuticals, USA	P/L					X			Strengthen root (?); polymerization shrinkage; Shrinkage (?); very dry canal necessary; Penetrates tubules

Cap, Capsule; GI, glass ionomer; L, long; M, moderate; P/L, powder/liquid; P/P, paste/paste; S, short; ZOE, zinc oxide-eugenol.
*No published reports on biocompability or clinical performance. Data obtainable, however, from studies done at the Universities of Berlin and Munich, Germany.

CONTROVERSIAL CONTEMPORARY ISSUES IN OBTURATION

A multitude of empiric opinions or ideas exists regarding various aspects of root canal obturation. Some are well-founded in years of clinical success. Others reflect the entrepreneurial spirit of both generalists and specialists. Some are based on an integration of fact and fiction, whereas other are based on merely a philosophy of "it works well for me!" Before discussing the specific root canal obturation techniques in detail, it is necessary that these ideas be addressed based on a blend of scientific evidence and clinical achievement. This discussion is designed to serve as the basis for the techniques cited and espoused.

Hermetic Seal: Myth or Misconception

Often cited as a major goal of root canal treatment is the achievement of a "hermetic seal." According to accepted dictionary definitions, the word *hermetic* means "sealed against the escape or entry of air or made airtight by fusion or sealing." Yet root canal seals are commonly evaluated for fluid leakage: a parameter used to praise or condemn obturation materials and techniques. This occurs both apically and coronally. The term *hermetic* has crept into endodontic nomenclature in a manner probably quite similar as did the invention of an airtight seal. An ancient god of wisdom, learning, and magic in ancient Egypt, Thoth, better known as Hermes Trismegistus (i.e., Hermes thrice greatest) is credited with this invention.[134] His significant contribution to civilization allowed the preservation of oils, spices, aromatics, grains, and other necessities in previously porous, earthenware vessels. A simple wax seal of the vessel walls helped to create the "hermetic seal." Endodontically speaking, the term *hermetic* is inappropriate, and terms such as a *fluid-tight, fluid-impervious*, or *bacteria-tight* seal should be adopted.

Compaction Versus Condensation

Traditionally, obturation methods were referred to as the *condensation* (vertical or lateral) of gutta-percha within the root canal space. A closer look at the word condensation provides a very different connotation than the process, which occurs during root canal obturation. Although its overwhelming meaning is to make more dense, its prime focus is that of compression, concentration, or reduction or a liquid or gas. Therefore in both the strictest sense and in the clinical sense, gutta-percha cannot be compressed, concentrated, or reduced. The word *compact*, which means to put firmly together, more readily reflects what occurs during root canal obturation. This concept, with regard to gutta-percha, was extensively researched and clearly detailed more than 20 years ago.[152] The sixth edition of *The Glossary—Contemporary Terminology for Endodontics* by the AAE has recognized the importance of that concept and has emphasized the use of the word *compaction* with reference to obturation

techniques.[6] This is the word of choice throughout this chapter.

Lateral Versus Vertical Techniques

The literature is replete with studies comparing lateral compaction with vertical compaction, and personal preferences abound. Likewise, endodontic programs have aligned themselves solely with one technique or another, with both authorities claiming superiority. When viewed objectively, many interesting facts emerge regarding this controversy. First, girded with the knowledge of force vectors, pure lateral or vertical compaction rarely occurs. The vectors of force applied during obturation techniques are an integrated blend of forces and result in a composite of forces that are neither true vertical or lateral. Even with the use of differing instruments, such as a spreader with a pointed tip or a plugger with a flattened tip, the vectors of force applied are still a composite. The use of engineering models,[46,150] photoelastic stress models,[73,105] and 3-D finite elemental analysis[137,174,191] to determine the nature and location of forces placed during obturation techniques indicates the complexity of this pattern. Second, if there is so much of a difference between the two obturation techniques and specific forces do make a difference, why is lateral compaction chosen as the comparative standard in almost all obturation studies? Third, apparently increases in the compaction pressures do not result in significant differences in apical leakage patterns.[77] Fourth, whether lateral or vertical compaction is performed, obturation can still fall below the standard of care for the same reasons (i.e., improper canal shaping, lack of competence in the obturation technique chosen). What appears important is the shape of the prepared canal,[46,73,137,174] the recognition that neither obturation technique is a pure technique, and the recognition that excellence with either technique is operator dependent. With proper execution, either manner of canal obturation can be highly successful; the clinician must be able to recognize when the application of either technique (or both techniques), in a pure or modified form, will enable the attainment of success on a predictable basis.

Softened Versus Solid Materials

Both Brownlee[23] and Grossman[55] indicated that a softened, pliable, or semisolid filling material would be ideal. Contemporary practices of obturation favor some type of material softening to enable the movement of the material into the canal intricacies, including the dentinal tubules[42,59] (Fig. 9-11, *A-E*). However, even these achievements do not guarantee that an impervious seal of the root canal system will be established.[36,40,163] Likewise, the dental advertising media are filled with the promotion of techniques via clinical "how to" articles that enhance the movement of softened obturation materials into accessory communications. Here too, there is no substantiation as to the levels of success or failure when these accessory channels are filled or unfilled.[183] More importantly, however, is the fact that with softened gutta-percha obturation techniques there has been a greater incidence of material extrusion beyond the confines of the canal[36] (see Fig. 9-11, *B*). Clinically, many cases have been shown to be successful when this occurs. However, long-term success with root canal treatment is highly predicated on retaining the root filling material within the root.[53,155,161,170] Although softening of gutta-percha may be viewed as highly desirable, the selective use of this technique

(solely or in combination with a solid core of gutta-percha) must be at the discretion of the competent clinician when anatomic dictates require this approach.

Use of Solvents for Material Adaptation

Chemical solvents have been used for almost 100 years to soften gutta-percha,[26] and a multitude of variations exist. Uses have ranged from merely dipping the gutta-percha

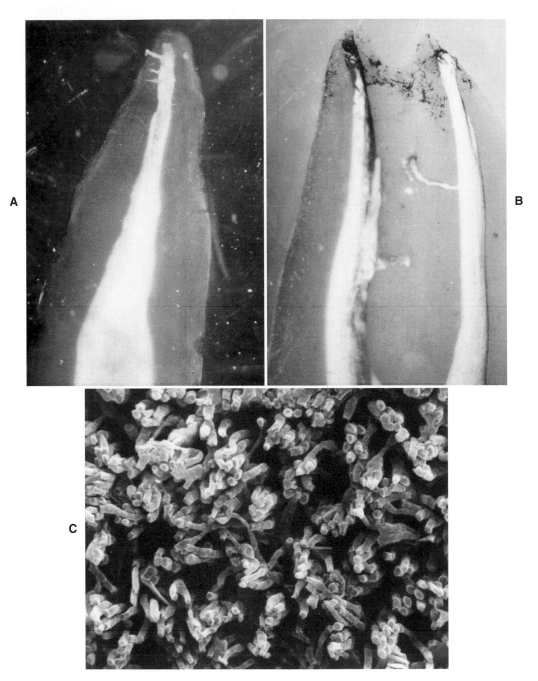

Fig. 9-11 **A** and **B**, ThermaFil technique. **C**, Scanning electron microscopic view of gutta-percha penetration into the dental tubules during compaction using thermoplasticized gutta-percha. Original magnification × 640 (see Fig. 9-63). Smear layer removed with all techniques.

cones into the solvent (1 second) for better canal adaptation to creating a completely softened paste of gutta-percha with the solvent (see Fig. 9-2). What appears to be crucial in the achievement of success with these techniques is the need to allow for dissipation of the chemical solvent, if volatile, or the removal of the excess solvent with alcohol. Failure to do this can result in significant dimensional change in the filling and possible loss of the apical seal.[93] This is possible in the "dip" techniques[71]; however, failure to compact the gutta-percha within a short period after dipping (i.e., 15 to 30 seconds) may result in loss of the desired plasticity of the material.[110] What influences the success of these techniques may actually be the shape of the canal, as opposed to the presence of residual solvent.[109] Even with softened gutta-percha, the quality of compaction is dependent on the movement of material into canal irregularities.

Small amounts of gutta-percha have also been dissolved in various solvents, such as chloroform (i.e., chloropercha), chloroform mixed with Canada balsam and zinc oxide (i.e.,

kloropercha), or eucalyptol (i.e., eucapercha), to enhance gutta-percha's adaptation within the canal. However, the efficacy and achievement of these approaches have been both praised[48] and questioned.[68,187] With the advent of thermoplasticized gutta-percha and its availability in the alpha phase, the need to consider the use of solvents at any time must be questioned. This is not to negate the achievement of success with this approach, but rather to bring about an enhanced focus on the contemporary techniques and the quality of achievement attainable without the use of potentially irritating chemical solvents.[7] The use of solvents, however, may still be considered for a number of challenges the clinician may face in daily practice,[108] such as the custom fitting of master cones in irregular apical preparations or after apexification.[60] Solvents commonly used are chloroform, methychloroformate, halothane, rectified white turpentine, and eucalyptol.[61,90]

Smear Layer Removal Versus Smear Layer Retention

The smear layer is a combination of organic and inorganic debris present on the root canal walls after instrumentation[107] (Fig. 9-12, *A* and *B*). When viewed under scanning electron microscope, the smear layer has an amorphous, irregular, and granular appearance[17,128,190] that represents dentinal shavings, tissue debris, odontoblastic processes, and (in previously infected root canals) microbial elements.[107] The appearance of the smear layer is formed by translocating and burnishing the superficial components of the dentinal wall during canal preparation.[9] During the early stages of canal preparation or in irregular anatomic variations of the canal, the smear layer would be predominantly organic in nature before any extensive dentin removal.[27]

The smear layer has been described as being (1) superficial on the dentinal surface and (2) packed into the dentinal tubules. The phenomenon of tubular packing with smear layer debris has been concluded to be the result of using endodontic instruments during canal preparation, although fluid dynamics and capillary action have also been identified as causative agents.[2,103]

Because the smear layer remaining on the root canal walls has been characterized, there is a controversy over whether or not to remove this layer before obturation. Biologically, the presence of the smear layer has been postulated to be an avenue for leakage and a source of substrate for bacterial growth and ingress.[127] The frequency of bacterial penetration in the presence of a smear layer, when canals were obturated with thermoplasticized gutta-percha and sealer, has been shown to be significantly higher than with smear layer removal and obturation.[11] On the other hand, although sophisticated models have demonstrated fluid movement through obturated root canals, bacterial penetration was slight to nonexistent.[189] A further concern is the presence of viable bacteria that may remain in the dentinal tubules and use the smear layer for sustained growth and activity.[17,120]

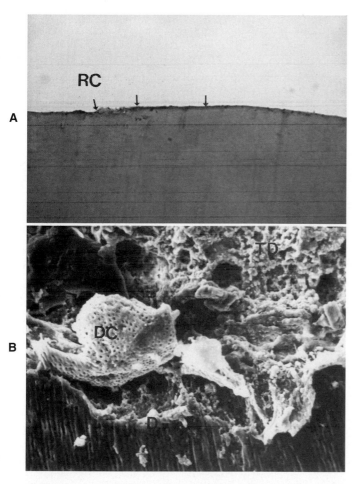

Fig. 9-12 A, Histologic identification of the smear layer on the surface of the cut dentin *(arrows)* in the root canal *(RC)*. Original magnification × 40. Stain H and E. **B,** Scanning electron micrograph of the smear layer (DC: dentin chips; TD: tissue debris; D: dentin). Original magnification × 480.

The presence of the smear layer may also prevent or delay the action of disinfectants on bacteria harbored in the dentinal tubules.[122] When the smear layer is not removed, it may slowly disintegrate and dissolve around leaking canal filling materials, or it may be removed by bacterial by-products, such as acids and enzymes.[158] Likewise, if the smear layer is removed, there is always the risk of reinfecting the dentinal tubules if the seal does fail.[101]

Technically, the smear layer may interfere with the penetration of gutta-percha into the tubules and the adhesion and penetration of root canal sealers into the dentinal tubules. Significant tubular penetration of gutta-percha and sealers has been shown with thermoplasticized obturations[59] (see Fig. 9-11, *E*) and experimentally with dentin-bonded composite resins with smear layer removal[100] (see Fig. 9-10, *A* and *B*). Studies have also shown a decreased incidence of microleakage with gutta-percha and sealer obturations when the smear layer was removed and the gutta-percha was chemically or thermally softened before obturation.[43,91] Similar findings were shown with dentin-bonded composite resins.[100] Thus the retention or removal of the smear layer before obturation may influence the quality of the obturation.

Methods for the removal of the smear layer before obturation have primarily focused on the alternating use of a chelating agent (i.e., disodium ethylenediaminetetraacetic acid [EDTA]) or weak acid (i.e., 10% citric acid), followed by thorough canal rinsing with 3% to 5% sodium hypochlorite (NaOCl) (Table 9-3; Fig. 9-13). The routine use of these techniques, however, has not been universally advocated, and the long-term value of smear layer removal has not been elucidated. The value of this procedure before obturation, however, is dependent on the canal cleaning and shaping and the chemical delivery system used (see Chapter 8).

Depth of Instrument Placement During Obturation

The need to compact the gutta-percha and sealer at the apical dentin matrix or constriction of the canal is essential for success. When applying vertical compaction forces or techniques with softened gutta-percha, placement of the compacting instrument short of the apical terminus of canal preparation is advocated. The softened filling material is compacted into the apical preparation in a 3-D manner. However, when using the lateral compaction technique, the master gutta-percha cone is already fit into the apical preparation, and compaction of this cone, or adaptation of this cone within the walls of the apical preparation, is essential for a proper seal. This implies the placement of the lateral compaction instrument (i.e., spreader) into the apical aspect of the canal. Many authors, however, do not define the parameters of this placement, and many master gutta-percha cones are not compacted in the apical aspect of the canal, which predisposes to leakage.[4] The importance of placing the spreader to within 1 to 2 mm of the prepared apical matrix or constriction has been vividly demonstrated, especially as it relates to canal shape.[4] Even these parameters may fall short of ideal in that failure to place the spreader to the full canal working length may still result in the lack of adaptation and compaction of the master gutta-percha cone in the apical portion of the canal[61] (Fig. 9-14). This results in a master cone surrounded by a sea of root canal cement that looks acceptable on the radiograph but does not seal the canal.

TABLE 9-3 SUGGESTED METHODS FOR REMOVING THE SMEAR LAYER

Author	Solution		Amount
Goldman et al. (1981)[47]	REDTA*	17%	20 ml
Goldman et al. (1982)[49]	REDTA*	17%	10 ml
	NaOCl	5.25%	10 ml
Yamada et al. (1983)[190]	REDTA*	17%	10 ml
	NaOCl	5.25%	10 ml
White et al. (1984)[186]	REDTA*	17%	10 ml
	NaOCl	5.25%	10 ml
Ciucchi et al. (189)[29]	NaOCl	3%	1 ml
	EDTA†	15%	2 ml
Gettleman et al. (1991)[45]	EDTA‡	17%	—
	NaOCl	5.25%	—

* Reprinted from Gutmann JL. Adaptation of injected thermoplasticized gutta-percha in the absence of the dentinal smear layer, *Int Endod J* 26:87, 1993, by permission.
EDTA, Disodium ethylenediaminetetraacetic acid; *NaOCl,* sodium hypochlorite; *REDTA,* disodium ethylenediaminetetraacetic acid, sodium hydroxide cetyltrimethylammonium bromide, and water mixture.
*Roth International, Chicago, Ill.
†Largal-Ultra, Septodent, Paris, France.
‡Unknown Source.

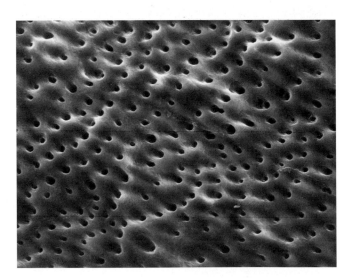

Fig. 9-13 Dentinal tubules after the removal of the smear layer. Note absence of debris seen in Fig. 9-12, *B*. Original magnification × 720.

An argument could be raised that placement of the spreader to the working length may result in unnecessarily placed apical forces, with the possibility for root fracture.[80] Likewise, it may result in the movement of the master cone beyond the confines of the root. In both cases, however, these undesirable outcomes are due to improper canal shaping or the lack of a good apical matrix or constriction in sound dentin. Contemporary canal shapes that favor funnel-type preparations from the apical matrix to the coronal orifice allow for proper placement of the compacting instrument and proper adaptation of the master gutta-percha cone (see Chapter 8).

Stainless Steel Versus NiTi Compactors

Historically, carbon steel or stainless steel compacting instruments were used routinely in the compaction of root canal filling materials. However, potential problems existed in the depth of penetration (especially in curved canals), the potential for wedging and root fractures, and the amount of stress focused on sections of the root walls during compaction. With the advent of NiTi metallic instruments, it is possible that many of these problems may be solved and that clinicians can achieve root canal fills with greater density of filling material.[168] Specifically, NiTi compactors (i.e., finger spreaders) create significantly less stress in curved canals than similar stainless steel compactors[33] and are able to penetrate further in curved canals than stainless steel compactors[13] (Fig. 9-15, *A* and *B*). Potential disadvantages include the buckling of the instrument under compaction pressure and the inability to precurve the instrument for ease of canal access. A combination of uses in canals has also been suggested,[168] with apical penetration using the NiTi instrument and coronal compaction using a stainless steel instrument in the more flared portion of the canal. Present studies have been limited, however, and long-term patterns of use are nonexistent. Clinician use of these new instruments also varies, and contemporary academic programs are only beginning to incorporate them into their teaching programs.

Homogeneity of the Canal Filling: Voids in the Root Canal Filling

The root canal filling should be a complete, homogenous mass that fills the prepared root canal in three dimensions. Often the achievement of this goal cannot be ascertained properly on a postobturation radiograph. Failure to achieve this ideal has been the focus of criticism of the lateral compaction technique, unless sealers are used that soften the material and allow for a chemical welding of the gutta-percha cones in the canal. Advocates of vertical compaction techniques with heat-softened gutta-percha use this parameter as a claim for technique superiority. However, even in the vertical compaction of thermoplasticized gutta-percha, voids are common and can occur for a number of reasons[61] (Fig. 9-16, *A*).

The prime source of voids in the final root canal obturation is the lack of skill and execution in the obturation technique chosen for a particular canal anatomy, coupled with improper canal shaping. In some cases highly radiopaque root canal sealers mask (radiographically) the presence of a void in the homogeneity of the root canal filling; in reality this detracts from the quality of the canal obturation. Voids may also be due to the pooling of large amounts of root canal sealers or the improper application of the compaction instrument into the cold or softened gutta-percha (Fig. 9-16, *B*). Voids may exist along the perimeters of the root canal filling or internally within the mass of the gutta-percha. Failure to place additional gutta-percha filling material into spaces created by the compacting instrument is also a prime reason for voids (Fig. 9-16, *C-E*). However, it is still unclear how important the presence of a void or voids is to the success or failure of final root canal obturation.

The presence of voids in both the apical and coronal portion of the root canal filling may provide avenues for leakage or for fluids to stagnate, if leakage should occur. Voids, evidenced as partly or improperly filled root canals, can give way to bacterial regrowth or reinfection, leading to failures.[130] Voids also detract from the clinician's assessment of the aesthetics of the treatment provided. The importance of this factor, however, is dubious. Voids observed in the root canal fillings may actually stimulate clinicians to seek further experience or alternative techniques in hopes of eliminating the routine presence of voids. If the canal system is cleaned and shaped properly, any of the gutta-percha obturation techniques may be used to achieve a well-filled, 3-D root filling. The two-dimensional radiographic determination of this ideal, however, must always be suspect.[95]

Pastes as Root Canal Fillings

The use of paste-type root canal obturation techniques is not advocated in contemporary endodontics for the following reasons.[61,99,115] The components of some pastes may leach into the periradicular tissues, resulting in chronic tissue inflammation or cellular toxicity. Because of porosities in paste fills, most pastes absorb in time, resulting in apical leakage, percolation, and the strong possibility of ultimate treatment failure. Systemically, components of some paste filling materials have been shown to be recovered in both blood samples and various vital organs.[15] In addition, chemical components of the paste have been shown to be antigenic, causing immunologic responses.[14] Finally, the apical control of paste fills is all but impossible, especially when no apical matrix is present or a root perforation exists.

Highly Radiopaque Sealers

Some root canal sealers contain significant amounts of radiopacifiers, such as barium sulfate or silver particles. These additives enhance the radiographic appearance of the root canal obturation, especially when the sealer is expressed

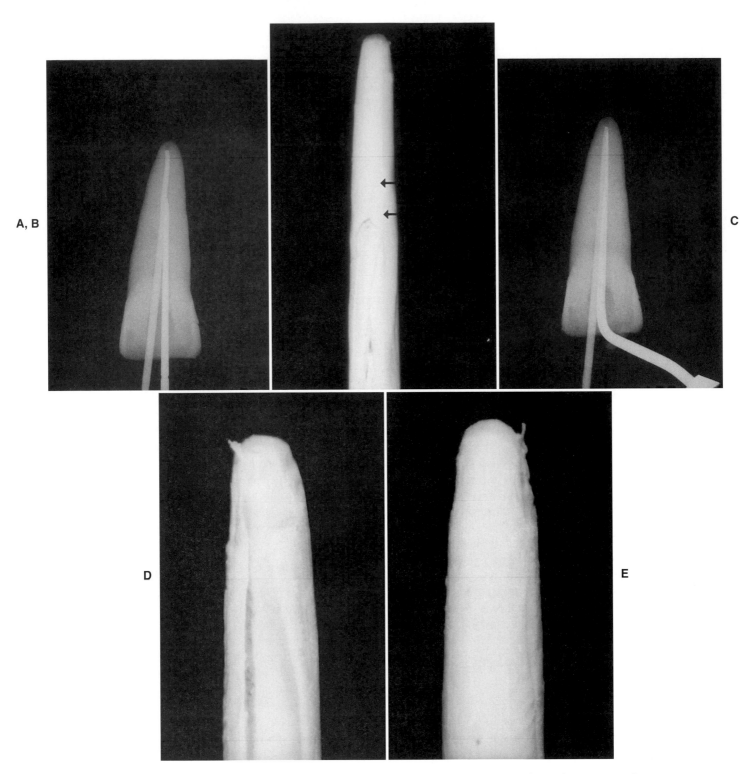

Fig. 9-14 **A**, Failure to achieve full penetration of a no. 50 spreader. **B**, Note position of spreader in gutta-percha cone *(arrows)* without evidence of apical compaction. **C**, Full penetration of a D11T spreader adjacent to a master cone. **D**, Facial view of compacted gutta-percha cone. **E**, Lingual view of compacted gutta-percha cone. Note adaptation to irregularities of the prepared canal at the apical matrix.

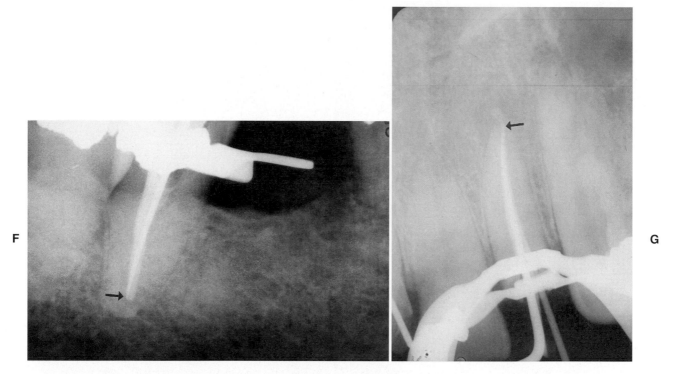

Fig. 9-14, cont'd **F**, Apical penetration *(arrow)* of a D11T spreader to the apical matrix adjacent to the master cone in a mandibular molar. Depth of penetration is essential for thorough apical compaction. **G**, Similar penetration *(arrow)* of a D11T spreader in a maxillary lateral incisor adjacent to both a master cone and one accessory cone.

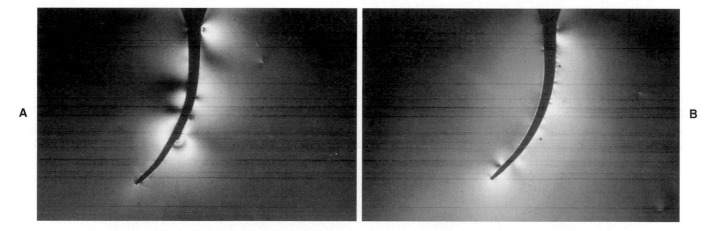

Fig. 9-15 **A**, Photoelastic stress patterns for a stainless steel finger spreader. Model with a master gutta-percha cone, two accessory cones, and finger spreader under load. Areas of point stress and uneven stress distribution are evident. **B**, Photoelastic stress patterns for a NiTi finger spreader. Model with a master gutta-percha cone, two accessory cones, and finger spreader under load. Areas of point stress are minimal, with an even distribution of stress evident. (Courtesy Dr. Gerald N. Glickman.)

through accessory or lateral communications. The routine use of these sealers may, however, detract from the quality of the compaction of the solid, core material and give a false sense of obturation radiodensity. Likewise, erroneous empiric claims have been made that obturations with highly radiopaque sealers are better than those made with less radiopaque materials (based on radiographic appearance).

This type of comparison and claim to superiority is both unfounded and unwarranted, and it has created divisions among many clinicians. Therefore undue importance is being placed on the radiographic appearance and "aesthetics" of the obturated canal system, as opposed to the necessary attention to detail required during canal cleaning, shaping, and obturation. Although the assessment of the root canal obturation is

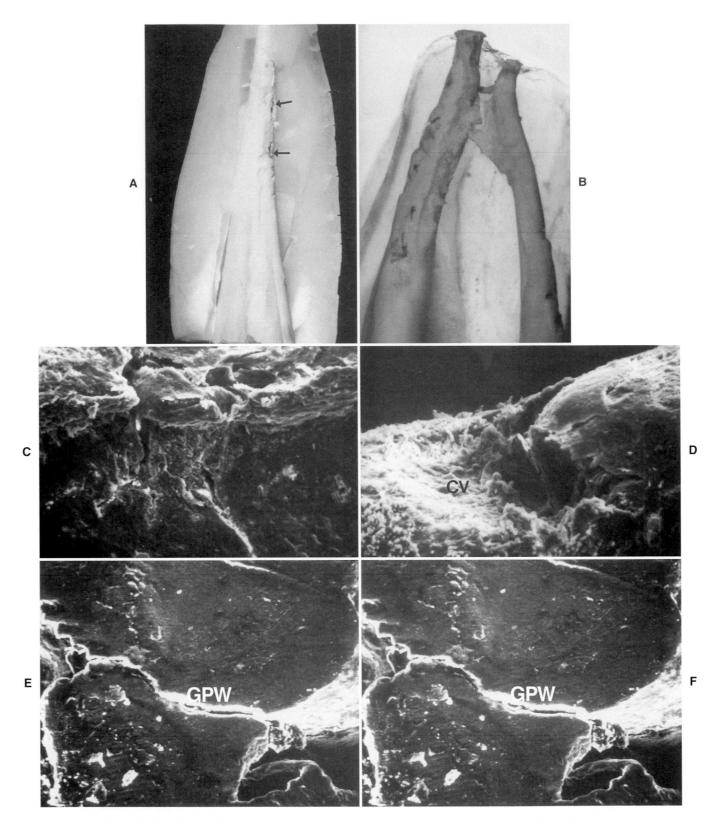

Fig. 9-16 **A**, Evidence of lateral voids *(arrows)* after vertical compaction with softened gutta-percha. **B**, Further evidence of voids attributed to lack of material softness, flow, and proper compactor penetration. **C**, Scanning electron microscopic evidence of voids and gaps during the vertical compaction of heat-softened gutta-percha. Compactor voids *(CV)* and gutta-percha welds *(GPW)* are visible. These are not discernible radiographically. Magnifications range from × 200 to × 380. **D-F**, Scanning electron microscopic evidence of voids and gaps during the vertical compaction of heat-softened gutta-percha. CVs and GPWs are visible; these are not discernible radiographically. Magnifications range from × 200 to × 380.

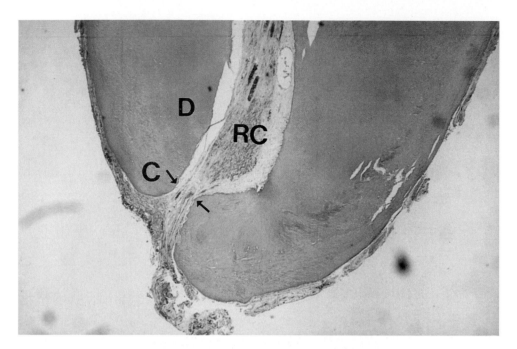

Fig. 9-17 Histologic appearance of the root apex (*C*: cementum; *D*: dentin; *RC*: root canal). Arrows indicate the narrowest constriction that is not specifically at the cementodentinal junction. Original magnification × 25. Stain H and E.

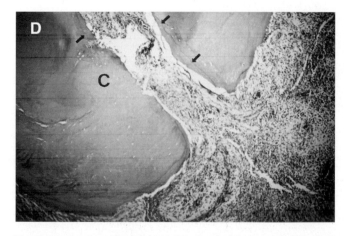

Fig. 9-18 Histologic appearance of a typical root apex. Note the thick layering of the cementum (*C*) in relation to the dentin (*D*). Also note the lack of a discrete cementodentinal junction because of to deposition of cementum *(arrows)* along the dentinal wall in the root canal. Original magnification × 40. Stain H and E.

primarily based on radiographic findings, root canal sealers do not have to be highly radiopaque to be effective.

Apical Position of the Obturation Material

Although filling the entire root canal system is the major goal of canal obturation, a major controversy exists as to what constitutes the apical termination of the root canal filling material. Working length determination guidelines often cite the cementodentinal junction or apical constriction as the ideal position for terminating canal cleaning and shaping procedures and the position to which the filling material should be placed[62] (Fig. 9-17). First, the cementodentinal junction is a histologic position, not a clinical position in the root canal system. Second, the cementodentinal junction is not always the most constricted portion of the canal in the apical portion of the root. Third, the distance from the apical foramen to the constricture depends on a multitude of factors, such as increased cemental deposition or radicular resorption. Both processes are strongly influenced by age, trauma, orthodontic movement, periradicular pathology, or periodontal disease. Especially in periodontal disease states, the cementodentinal junction location has no predictable anatomic appearance or location because of resorptive processes or cemental depositions that may extend well into the root canal[154] (Fig. 9-18). Therefore the foramen and position of the cementodentinal junction on the root is highly variable, and it can exist anywhere from the direct radiographic apex up to 3 mm or more coronal to the radiographic apex (depending on a particular root morphology).

These potential anatomic variances have had a major impact on the precise region or location for determining the working length and termination of root canal instrumentation and obturation. These clinical concerns, along with the integrity of the periradicular tissues, have formed the basis for success in prognostic studies that have identified that the optimal result is to end instrumentation and obturation inside the radiographic apex (approximating the cementodentinal junction) (Fig. 9-19, *A* and *B*). When instrumentation and

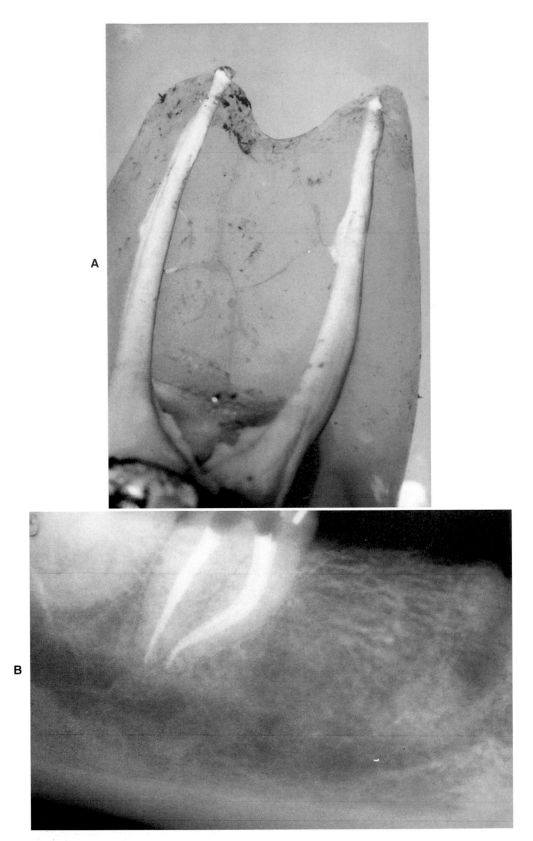

Fig. 9-19 **A**, Cleared tooth specimen with two canals; the left canal is filled beyond the root end, whereas the right one is filled within the confines of the root. Ideal location is within the root. **B**, Clinical case demonstrating this attainment using vertical compaction of heat-softened gutta-percha. (B courtesy Dr. Constantinos Laghios.)

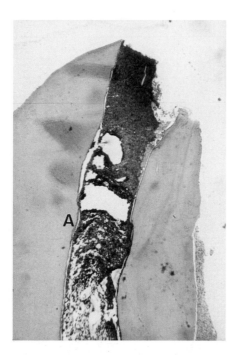

Fig. 9-20 Histologic picture of the damage that is done to the apical constriction when instrumentation is beyond the end of the canal and root. Canal is filled with gutta-percha to level *A*, and the remainder of the canal is filled with a blood clot. This environment is not biologically conducive to healing and tissue regeneration. Original magnification × 25, Stain H and E.

obturation are shorter than this, the success rates drop. When longer than this, especially with filling materials beyond the radiographic apex, an even poorer result is noted[75] (Fig. 9-20). From a realistic viewpoint, however, it is often impossible to know exactly where the apical foramen and apical constriction are located until after the canal has been obturated.

Many of the more contemporary obturation techniques advocate canal obturation to within 0.5 mm of the radiographic apex, to the radiographic apex, or beyond, which is confirmed by the presence of a "puff" of filling material. Empiric observations support a high degree of success with these techniques (Fig. 9-21). *However, no long-term prognostic studies have supported this position for the termination of root canal obturations.* Likewise, canals with filling material beyond the confines of the root canal system tend to cause more postoperative discomfort.[72,156]

If a major goal of root canal treatment is to create an environment conducive to the regeneration of cementum over the apical foramen, the periodontium that enters the apical foramen in teeth with vital, yet compromised, pulps should not be challenged with the extrusion of root canal filling materials beyond the end of the canal (Fig. 9-22, *A* and *B*). This concept has been scientifically valid for over 65 years[56,121,162] and is supported by numerous retrospective studies.[53,155,160,170] Even in those cases with periradicular radiolucencies, filling beyond the confines of the canal is less desirable,[155] although filling the root canal as close as pos-

sible to its terminus is desirable (Figs. 9-23 and 9-24). Most recently the most favorable histologic responses to canal cleaning, shaping, and obturation were noted when they were kept at or short of the apical constriction.[138] These findings were consistent in the presence of vital or necrotic pulps, when bacteria had penetrated the foramen and when they were present in the periradicular tissues. When sealer or gutta-percha or both were extruded in the periradicular tissues through the main foramen, lateral canals, or accessory canals, there was always a severe inflammatory reaction, including a foreign body reaction. *Contemporary endodontic practices and long-term evaluative studies favor and support obturation within the confines of the root canal system in all cases in an attempt to prevent further challenge to the already compromised and challenged periradicular tissues.*

Apical Seal Versus Coronal Seal: Which Is More Important?

Although historically the lack of an apical seal of the root canal system received the most attention as being the prime reason for failure of root canal treatment,[32] contemporary thought and literature documentation emphasize the need to address the thorough seal of the root canal system, both apically and coronally (Fig. 9-25). All techniques used during root canal treatment and the subsequent restoration of the tooth must favor both goals. This implies that compaction of gutta-percha into the root canal system must be complete in all dimensions from the orifice to the apical termination of the filling.

Use of Apical Barriers

A method often used to create an apical stop or matrix for the purpose of obtaining a biologic apical seal supports the placement of dentin chips or other artificial barriers (i.e., calcium hydroxide, demineralized dentin, lyophilized bone, tricalcium phosphate, hydroxyapatite, collagen) before canal obturation.[30,141] This technique is not new, and favorable results were obtained with dentin chips more than 60 years ago.[50] More contemporary studies have supported these findings, provided the dentin chips were uncontaminated by bacteria or their by-products.[83,176,178] Ironically, the packing of chips may occur inadvertently during cleaning and shaping,[194] especially if a patency file is not used routinely.[126] When intentionally placed, the chips are obtained from the coronal dentin using rotary instruments (e.g., GG burs, Peeso reamers) after the canal has been cleaned and shaped. Subsequently, the chips are packed in the apical 1 to 3 mm followed by standard canal obturation with gutta-percha and sealer.

In addition to possibly creating a biologic seal, the packed chips may assist in confining irrigating solutions to the canal and preventing overfilling, especially when a canal has been overinstrumented.[35] However, they may or may not enhance the seal of the canal apically.[1,194] Regardless, favorable periradicular tissue responses have been noted with enhanced

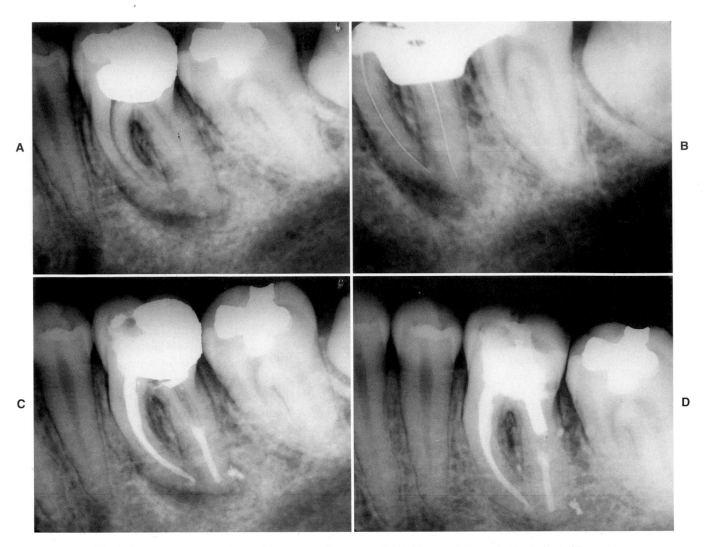

Fig. 9-21 **A**, Mandibular molar requiring root canal treatment. **B**, Working length determination is short of the root apex. Canals were prepared within the confines of the root. **C**, Root canal fill with "puffs" of sealer out both roots. Gutta-percha, however, was retained within the root canal during obturation. **D**, Fifteen-month recall examination shows repair is almost complete, yet the sealer is still present in the periradicular tissues. (Courtesy Dr. David Rossiter.)

healing, minimal inflammation, and apical cementum deposition.[123]

The use of calcium compounds, in particular calcium hydroxide, as an apical barrier has also been extensively investigated. Calcium hydroxide (in either a moist or dry state) is carried to or compacted into the apical 1 to 3 mm of the prepared canal before canal obturation. This process is facilitated with an amalgam carrier, lentula, or syringe with premixed calcium hydroxide. Significant calcifications have been noted at the apical foramen,[131] and the periradicular tissue response (in comparison to dentin chips) is indistinguishable.[81] Additionally, teeth with apical calcium hydroxide plugs have demonstrated significantly less leakage than teeth without plugs.[184]

Even with promising data that support the potential use of an artificial barrier in the apical portion of the prepared canal, the routine clinical use of this technique does not appear to be the standard of care. If this approach to treatment is to be adopted, a material with predictable inductive capabilities is necessary; one that seals the canal, negates any bacterial influences, and predictably stimulates cementum regeneration across the apical foramen. In the future, contemporary directives may favor the use of mineral trioxide aggregate (MTA)[175] (ProRoot, Tulsa Dental Co., Tulsa, Okla.) or similar material for this purpose.

Timing of Root Canal Obturation

Historically, root canal treatment was performed in multiple visits to accommodate the need for negative microbial cultures and to ensure the cessation of signs or symptoms. Although the need for cultures is rare, the presence of acute

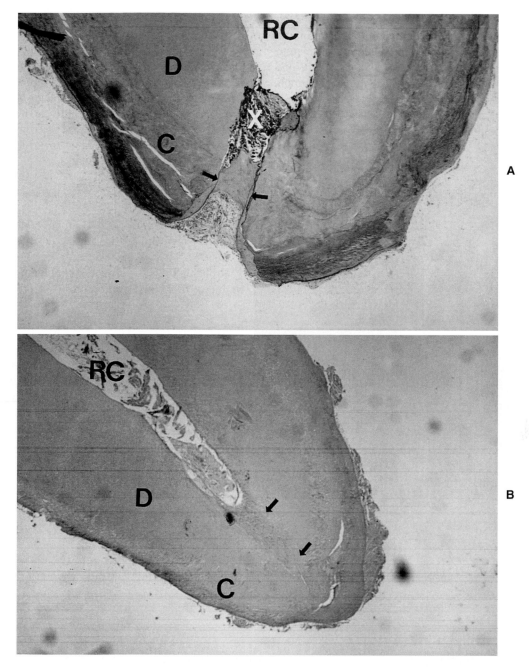

Fig. 9-22 A, Evidence of cemental regeneration *(arrows)* over the obturated root canal when the filling is retained within the root. This is even possible in the presence of debris that was packed apically (*C:* cementum, *D:* dentin, *X:* debris, *RC:* root canal). Original magnification × 25. Stain H and E. **B,** Repair of the end of the root canal with cementum occupying 3 to 4 mm of the apical portion of the canal adjacent to a short root filling *(arrows)* (*C:* cementum, *D:* dentin, *RC:* root canal). Original magnification × 25. Stain H and E.

signs or symptoms still exists as a contemporary rationale for not obturating the root canal at the time of cleaning and shaping. Even this dictate has its empiric challenges, although some data exist that support the single-visit management of an acute periradicular abscess.[165] On the other hand, filling of canals that are infected may result in an increase in postoperative discomfort.[86] In fact, the argument for potential

postoperative pain after root canal treatment in one visit has been used as a rationale for not obturating at the time of canal cleaning and shaping. Studies have shown however, that postoperative pain is not increased after complete root canal treatment in one visit.[44,114,117,139]

In the absence of significant signs or symptoms, root canal treatment can be completed in one visit. Patients with necrotic

canal contamination after cleaning and shaping. Often poorly placed temporary restorations fail within hours, and the canal systems are contaminated with oral bacteria. Inter-appointment endodontic emergencies are often due to the demise of the temporary restoration. Even the use of intra-canal medicaments, such as calcium hydroxide, is no guarantee that bacteria will not gain or regain a foothold in the cleaned canal. Therefore, in concert with the considerations stated above, the cleaned root canal should be obturated as expediently as possible to avoid further contamination.

Criteria for Determining the Adequacy of Canal Preparation Before Obturation

Although the timing of canal obturation has been discussed in the previous section, seven final issues regarding the technical adequacy of the canal preparation require attention, clarification, and emphasis:

1. The tooth must be isolated properly to eliminate all risks of canal contamination during obturation. This is an extremely important aspect of successful treatment that cannot be overlooked or regarded lightly.
2. Clean, white dentin chips are not a criterion for obturation. The appearance of the dentin chips does not guarantee they are free of bacteria or bacterial products. Likewise, it is all but impossible to sample the entire root canal system on this basis.
3. Preparing the apical portion of the canal three to four times larger than the first file to bind at the apical extent of the canal is not a criterion for obturation. It is highly unlikely that the canal is cleaned and shaped properly using this criterion. It is difficult to get irrigants into the apical portion of small canals (e.g., size no. 20 or no. 25) without proper canal shaping.
4. Preparing all canals to the same size apically (i.e., size no. 20), as is advocated when using some of the newer canal preparation techniques that provide enhanced canal flaring, does not guarantee the removal of all tissue debris in this area.
5. All compacting instruments must be prefit in the canal to determine their depth of penetration, their fit without binding, the location of binding (if any), and their appropriateness for a particular portion of the canal, especially in curved canals.
6. No type of fluid should be present in the canal before obturation. If fluids are present and they are hemorrhagic or purulent in nature, the canal may be unclean or have been overinstrumented. The clinician should also consider that another canal may exist; a residual infection may be present; or the canals may have become contaminated between appointments. In any of the above situations, the source of the problem must be identified and addressed before canal obturation.
7. In multirooted teeth, all efforts must be expended to ensure that the entire canal system has been cleaned and shaped.

METHODS AND TECHNIQUES OF ROOT CANAL OBTURATION

Over the years numerous methods have been advocated to obturate the prepared root canal system, each with their own claims of ease, efficiency, or superiority. Contemporary obturation techniques are no different. Although they do reflect a certain degree of sophistication and technologic advancement, contemporary techniques still rely on gutta-percha and sealer to achieve their goal—a 3-D filling of the cleaned and shaped root canal space. Therefore this discussion focuses on the basics of root canal obturation, with an emphasis on techniques and variations thereof that have proven successful and easy to master.

Four basic techniques exist for the obturation of the root canal system with gutta-percha and sealer:

1. The cold compaction of gutta-percha
2. The compaction of gutta-percha that has been heat softened in the canal and cold compacted
3. The compaction of gutta-percha that has been thermoplasticized, injected into the system, and cold compacted
4. The compaction of gutta-percha that has been placed in the canal and softened through mechanical means

A multitude of variations on these four basic themes exists, and some of the creative contemporary approaches are highlighted.

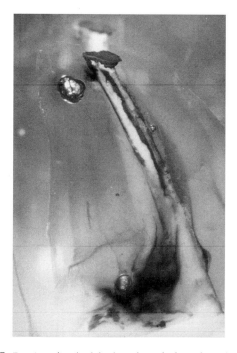

Fig. 9-25 Demineralized, dehydrated, and cleared tooth specimen from a maxillary first molar. There is significant coronal leakage through both the root canal fill and the root end filling; the latter was placed in an attempt to resolve the patient's continued discomfort after the nonsurgical root canal treatment. Even the root end filling could not stop the leakage and continued symptoms.

Cold Compaction

Most readers identify cold compaction as being synonymous with the lateral compaction of gutta-percha. This technique is applicable to most root canals and requires a continuously tapered funnel canal preparation with an apical matrix in sound dentin.

Brief Overview   In this technique a master gutta-percha cone is chosen that corresponds to the final root canal enlarging instrument that went to the apical extent of the canal (working length). The common compacting instrument is the spreader, which comes in various sizes and is chosen based on the canal size, length, and curvature (Table 9-4). The spreader can be a hand or finger instrument (Figs. 9-26 and 9-27). A root canal sealer that can be mixed to a creamy consistency and has ample working time (i.e., 15 to 30 minutes) is selected. The master cone is placed along with sealer in the canal, and both are compacted with the tapered metallic spreader in a lateral and vertical direction. The space created by the metallic spreader is filled with additional smaller or accessory cones that are also compacted until the canal is filled.

Detailed Technique

Master cone selection.   A master gutta-percha cone is selected based on the final prepared apical size of the root canal system. If standardized K-type and Hedström files are used for canal preparation and the canal is free of debris to the prepared apical matrix, the master cone should fit to the working length or slightly short of it (i.e., 0.5 mm) (Fig. 9-28). The cone is grasped with cotton pliers at a coronal position that approximates the working length. When placed in the canal, the cone should begin to contact the canals walls in the apical 1 to 3 mm, fit snugly at the designated length, resist movement beyond the apical matrix with coronal pressure, and demonstrate a slight resistance to removal from this position when a withdrawal pressure is applied coronally. If this does not occur, the cone may be carefully trimmed with a sharp scissors, however, a scalpel is preferable.[61,87] Portions of the cone should be removed in 0.5 to 1 mm increments, until the proper length and snugness are obtained. Sizing gauges for this purpose (Maillefer Instruments SA, Ballaigues, Switzerland) are available to assist in the preparation of the master cone, if necessary[104] (Fig. 9-29). The final position of the cone within the tooth can be recorded by scoring the cone at the incisal or occlusal reference point with a pointed instrument or by pinching the cone with cotton pliers. Subsequently, the position of the cone is verified radiographically and evaluated as follows:

I. If the cone fits to or within 0.5 mm of the working length, if the cone demonstrates a snugness of fit in the apical 1 to 3 mm, and if there is space visible on the radiograph lat-

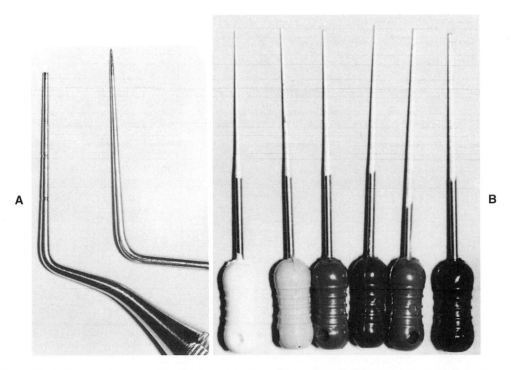

Fig. 9-26 **A**, Root canal plugger with a flat tip and depth markings at 10 and 15 mm from the tip *(left)*. Root canal spreader with a pointed tip *(right)* (see Tables 9-4 and 9-5). Rubber stops may be placed on the spreader at the proper length for compaction. **B**, Finger spreaders *(left)* and pluggers *(right)* on plastic handles are available from many manufacturers in both stainless steel and NiTi.

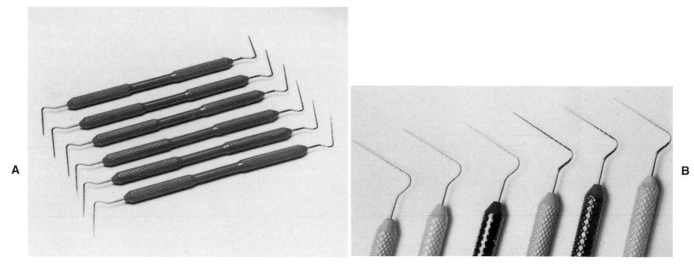

A

B

Fig. 9-27 Calibrated color-coded plugger spreaders with sizes and tapers matching the ISO standardization of root canal files. These are referred to as the "M" series according to Dr. Howard Martin. **A,** Sizes no. 20, 25, 30, 40, 50, and 60. One end is a spreader for lateral compaction; the other end is a plugger for vertical compaction. **B,** Close-up of the spreader end of the instrument (see Tables 9-4 and 9-5). (Courtesy Caulk/Dentsply, Milford, Del.)

TABLE 9-4 ROOT CANAL SPREADERS

Root Canal Spreader (RCS) Code	Diameter 1 mm from the Tip (mm)	Diameter 16 mm from the Tip (mm)	Distance from the Tip to the Bend (mm)
RCS3*	0.35	0.88	24.43
RCSD11*	0.50	1.01	22.46
RCSD11S*	0.28	0.80	23.18
RCSD11T*	0.34	1.01	21.50
RCSD11TS*	0.25	1.01	20.40
RCSGP1*	0.24	0.75	20.86\
RCSGP2*	0.24	0.82	23.69
RCSGP3*	0.30	0.68	28.35
RCSMA57*	0.22	0.79	26.25
RCSW1S*	0.36	0.91	19.85
RCSW2S*	0.39	0.97	18.92
RCS30*	0.30	0.70	28.10
RCS40*	0.45	0.77	28.10
RCS50*	0.50	0.85	28.10
RCS60*	0.55	0.92	28.10
S20†	0.23	0.52	28.82
S25†	0.30	0.60	28.60
S30†	0.33	0.63	28.76
S40†	0.44	0.73	28.88
S50†	0.42	0.82	28.79
S60†	0.55	0.90	28.72

*Hu-Friedy Co.
†Caulk M-series.

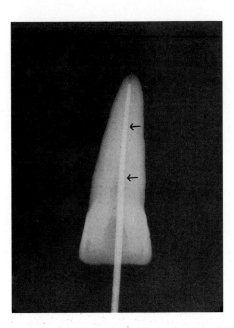

Fig. 9-28 Placement of the master gutta-percha cone to the proper depth for lateral compaction. Note also the space visible along the lateral aspects of the cone *(arrows)*. This is essential for proper depth of the compacting instrument.

eral to the master cone from the junction of the apical and middle third of the canal to the coronal orifice, compaction may proceed.

II. If the cone fits short of the desired length, the following conditions may exist:

A. Dentin chips may be packed in the apical portion of the canal; this represents inadequate cleaning. These chips must be removed with small files[126] and copious irrigation before refitting the master cone (as described in Chapter 8).

B. The canal may be ledged at a position short of the working length. If this is the case, efforts should be made to renegotiate the canal to the full distance.

C. There may be a curve in the canal that is not visible on the two-dimensional radiograph. The anatomy of the canal must be verified, and the placement of a curved gutta-percha cone may assist in full canal penetration.

D. The master cone selected may be too large, and a smaller cone must be selected. Sometimes cones taken from the same container may have different tapers or altered shapes. The use of the sizing instrument is helpful in this situation.

E. The most probable reason for failure to seat the cone to the prepared canal length is improper 3-D canal shaping in the apical to middle third of the tooth.[61] Under these circumstances the canal must be reshaped to receive the master cone to the desired length and with the desired snugness of fit.

III. If the cone fits to the proper working length, exhibits snugness of fit, but does not have space lateral to it in the coronal two thirds of the canal, the canal must be reshaped before obturation. Failure to see this space on the radiograph usually indicates that the canal is not properly shaped for adequate spreader penetration during obturation.[61] This usually results in failure to seat and compact the cone properly in the prepared apical seat.

IV. If the master cone goes beyond the working length, the cone can either be cut (as previously described) or a new, larger cone can be selected (Fig. 9-30). However, with a larger cone also comes a larger taper that may minimize the amount of lateral space available for spreader penetration in a given canal. Also, with the selection of a larger cone in a curved canal, the cone tends to bind too far coronally because of the constricted canal shape at the bend.

V. If the cone goes to length and exhibits snugness of fit clinically, yet there is space visible alongside the cone in the apical third but not in the coronal two thirds, the cone is improperly shaped and sized for the preparation or the canal is not properly shaped in the coronal two thirds of the canal.

VI. If the cone goes to length and radiographically exhibits a wiggly or S-shaped appearance, the cone is too small for the canal and a larger cone must be selected (Fig. 9-31).

Canal preparation.   Once the master cone has been fit, it is removed from the canal and placed in a sterilizing solution of 70% isopropyl alcohol or 2.5% to 5% NaOCl. The canal system is then dried with paper points. If the smear layer is to be removed, appropriate solutions are used at this time (refer to *Smear Layer Removal Versus Smear Layer Retention* in this chapter). Some authors recommend the removal of all residual moisture by rinsing the canal with 95% ethyl alcohol or 99% isopropyl alcohol.[115] The alcohol is left in the canal for 2 to 3 minutes and then removed with additional sterile paper points.

Compactor selection.   Before sealer placement, the compacting instruments are chosen. Sterile (or thoroughly disinfected) compacting instruments are used during the cleaning and shaping phase to determine if the proper shape has been prepared for depth of instrument placement.

Lateral compaction is achieved with a hand spreader or finger spreader (see Table 9-4). The instrument chosen should reach the canal working length without binding in an empty canal (Fig. 9-32). This implies the need for both proper length and taper of the compacting instrument relative to canal shape, size, and curvature (Table 9-5). In curved canals a stainless steel instrument can be curved before placement in the canal (Fig. 9-33), or a NiTi instrument can be used (see Fig. 9-15). Whenever possible a rubber stop is placed on the instrument at the working length. This is not necessary when the metallic instrument is already scored with specific length markers.

Sealer placement.   After the selection of the compacting instrument and the drying of the canal, the root canal sealer is placed in the canal. The effective distribution of root canal sealers throughout the root canal system has been suggested as essential to obtain the best possible root canal seal.[36] Various methods of sealer placement have been identified or evaluated for this purpose, including lentula spirals,

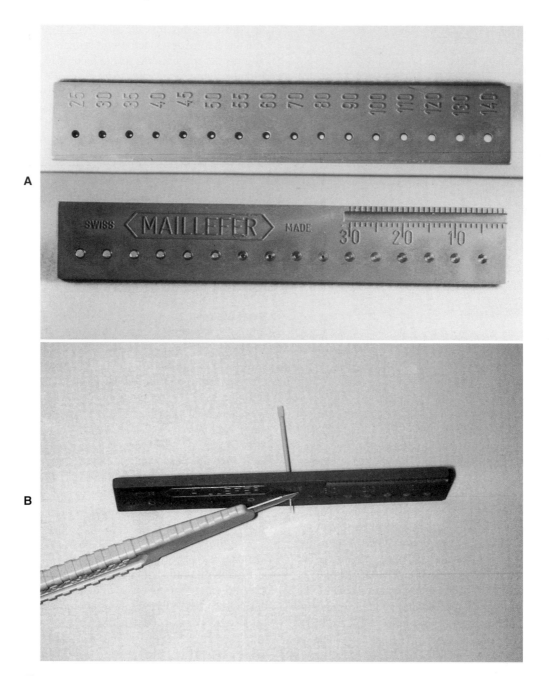

Fig. 9-29 A, Sizing instrument for gutta-percha cones. **B,** Placement of a cone through the hole that represents the properly sized gutta-percha point for the canal. Excess and improperly tapered tips can be removed carefully with a scalpel blade.

files or reamers, master gutta-percha cones, and ultrasonic instruments. Evaluation of the efficacy of these techniques has occurred on extracted teeth, using serial sectioning, radiographs, specimen clearing, and direct observation, in the clinical setting. Parameters of sealer distribution used for evaluation have included percentages of dentin walls covered, sealer extrusion beyond the apical foramen, demonstration of accessory canals, and voids in the sealer coverage. Clinician expertise in using a particular placement technique must also be considered.

With cold lateral compaction the use of the master cone, a file, or a lentula to place the sealer is acceptable (Fig. 9-34). For the best distribution of sealer, however, placement with an ultrasonic instrument may be considered.[169] Whatever vehicle is chosen, it is lightly coated with the sealer and placed in the canal, distributing the sealer evenly over the prepared walls. In larger canals this may have to be done more than once. For lateral compaction the sealer is to be placed to the working length of the canal. The complete filling of the canal with sealer should be avoided, as addi-

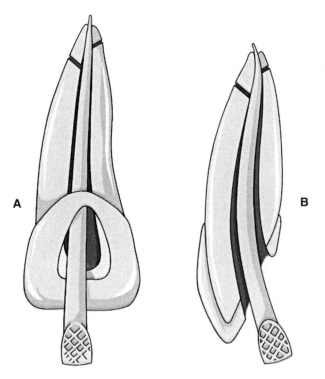

Fig. 9-30 Diagram of a master gutta-percha cone that is too long and must be trimmed or exchanged for a proper fitting cone. This can be accomplished with a scalpel and the sizing instrument.

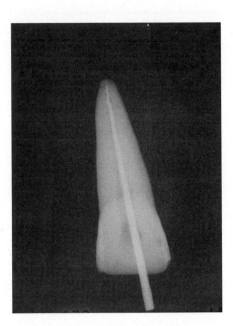

Fig. 9-31 Improperly fit cone that is too small apically. When the irregular appearance is obvious radiographically or clinically, a differently sized and shaped cone must be chosen.

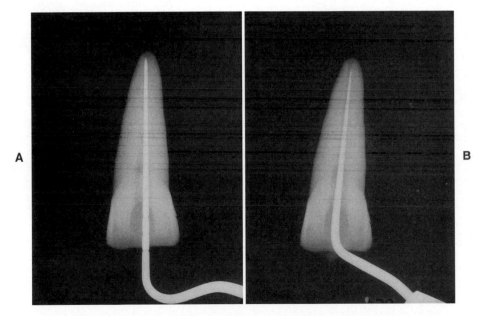

Fig. 9-32 **A,** Improperly fit spreader. Note the instrument occupies the entire canal space and may more than likely wedge between the canal walls. **B,** Properly fit spreader, demonstrating looseness of fit and proper depth of placement.

TABLE 9-5 **SUGGESTED SPREADERS AND PLUGGERS CORRESPONDING TO MASTER GUTTA-PERCHA CONES**

Final Apical Size	Recommended Spreader (Hand or Corresponding Finger Spreader)	Recommended Plugger (Hand or Corresponding Finger Plugger)
25	D11S, D11TS, GP1, GP2, W1S, S20, S25 (depending on canal taper and length)	P30, 8, 8A ⅓ (depending on canal taper, length and desired depth penetration)
30	Same as for No. 25 except use S30; MA57 or GP3 can be used in long canals >25 mm	P30, 8, 8A, ⅓
35	Same as for No. 25 except use D11T or S35	P30, 8, 8A, ⅓
40	D11T, GP2, W2S, S40	P30, 8, 8A, ⅓
45	D11T, GP2 or GP3, S40	P40, 8½, 8½A, ⅓
50	D11, D11T, GP2 or GP3, S50	P50, 9, 9A, or 9½, 9½A, PL1
55	D11, S3, S50	P50, 9, 9A, or 9½, 9½A, PL2
60	D11, S3, S60	P60, 9, 9A, or 9½, 9½A
70	D11, S3, S70	P70, 9½, 9½A, 10, 10A, 10½, 10½A, 5/7
80	D11, S3, S80	P80, 10, 10A, 10½, 10½A, PL3, 5/7
90	D11, S3, S80	P80, 10, 10A, 10½, 10½A, PL3, 5/7
100	D11, S3, S80	P80, 10, 10A, 10½, 10½A, PL3, 9/11
110	D11, MA 57, S3, S80	PL3 or PL4, 9/11, 11, 11½, 11A, 11½A, or higher

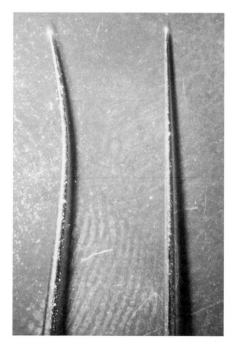

Fig. 9-33 Spreader shapes can be easily changed before entry into curved canals. This facilitates depth of penetration and gutta-percha compaction.

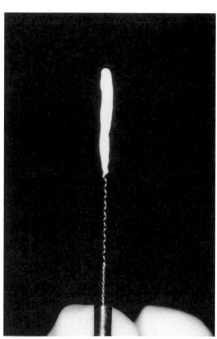

Fig. 9-34 The use of a lentula for the placement of the root canal sealer. Do not use excessive amounts in the canal system with any technique.

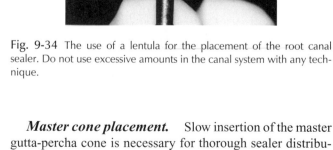

tional sealer is generally carried to the canal during compaction on the accessory gutta-percha cones. If an ultrasonic file is used, the instrument is lightly coated with the sealer, placed in the canal, and energized for 5 seconds while moving the file in a circumferential motion.[169] Subsequently, a master cone, lightly coated with sealer, is placed directly to the apical matrix (Fig. 9-35).

Master cone placement. Slow insertion of the master gutta-percha cone is necessary for thorough sealer distribution, the dissipation of trapped air, the lateral and coronal movement of the sealer, and the minimization of sealer extrusion beyond the apical foramen. Once in place, as evidenced by the relationship of the scored master cone to the occlusal or incisal reference point, the cone is held in place

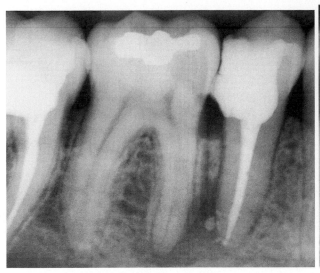
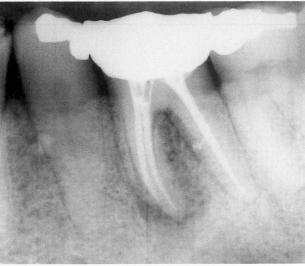

Fig. 9-35 Two examples of root canal obturation in which the smear layer was removed, the sealer was placed with an ultrasonic device, and the canals were obturated using the lateral compaction of gutta-percha. Both cases are filled within the confines of the canal with significant dispersal of sealer into accessory channels. This result can occur with any technique that encourages smear layer removal and the proper dispersion of sealer. (Courtesy Dr. David Stamos.)

for 20 to 30 seconds to secure its position apically. If the patient has not been anesthetized, the movement of trapped air or sealer apically may cause momentary discomfort. Advising the patient ahead of time of the possibility of discomfort is essential. If there is any doubt as to the position of the master cone and sealer (and a slow-setting sealer has been used), radiographic verification can be done at this time. If necessary, the cone can be removed and repositioned according to its desired position.

Master cone compaction. Subsequent to master cone placement, the spreader is slowly inserted alongside the master cone, either to the working length marked on the spreader or to within 0.5 to 1 mm of this length (Fig. 9-36). As previously discussed, failure to achieve this depth may result in lack of adaptation of the master gutta-percha cone to the prepared apical seat. Although the master gutta-percha cones can be elongated and moved apically with compaction, there is no technique that can consistently provide for this occurrence because of variations in the shaping of the canal system and the nature of the gutta-percha cones used. The potential of root fracture with this approach has been previously discussed,[92,134,151] and with proper canal shaping and choice of tapered spreader before canal obturation, the wedging forces are insignificant.

As the spreader reaches the desired depth, the master gutta-percha cone is laterally and vertically compacted, moving the instrument in a 180-degree arc. In curved canals this arc is reduced relative to the degree of canal curvature.[71] During this movement the cone is compacted against a particular canal wall while, at the same time, space is created lateral to the master cone for additional accessory gutta-percha cones (Fig. 9-37).

Placement of accessory cones. Accessory cones are chosen based on the size of the spreader used, the size of the canal, and the position of the space created in the canal (Table 9-6). For example, to the depth of the first spreader penetration, an accessory cone in the range of *extra-fine* to *fine-fine* is used. Both of these cone sizes match well with a D11T or D11TS hand spreader or a no. 25 or no. 30 finger spreader. Other combinations of spreaders and specific cone sizes also exist and are seen in Table 9-6. The accessory cone is lightly coated with sealer and placed to the same length that the compacting instrument was placed (Fig. 9-38). If this is not possible, the following conditions may be present:

- The accessory cone is too large or is improperly tapered for the space provided.
- The spreader is too small and does not match well with the accessory cone.
- The compaction of the master cone was insufficient to create usable space for an accessory.
- The canal lacks the necessary taper for proper penetration of both the spreader and accessory cone.
- The master cone may have been dislodged during the initial compaction.
- The small end of the accessory cone may have curled up or become bent in the canal, preventing full penetration of the cone.
- The sealer may have begun to harden, which prevents placement of the accessory cone.

Each of these potential problems with the placement of accessory cones must be assessed, and corrective action must be taken when appropriate. Failure to place the accessory cones to the proper depth results in significant voids throughout the canal. These may be discrete radiolucencies or longi-

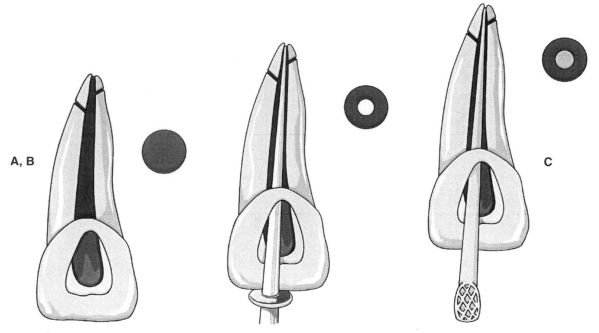

Fig. 9-36 **A**, Diagram of prepared canal system in the shape of a funnel. **B**, Spreader fit to the proper depth. Note the space available adjacent to the spreader. This instrument must reach the proper apical depth without binding. **C**, Fit of master gutta-percha cone. Note how this cone binds only in the apical portion of the prepared root.

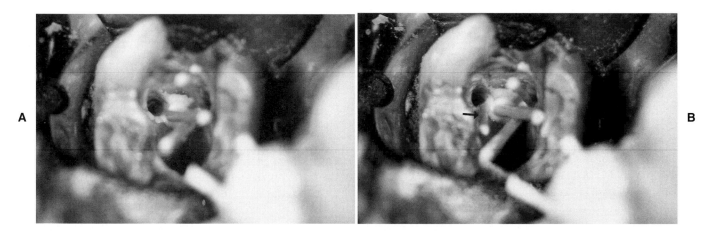

Fig. 9-37 **A**, Mesiobuccal canal of a mandibular first molar. Master gutta-percha cone has been laterally compacted with sealer. Note how the cone has been moved against the wall of the canal, making room for additional accessory cones. **B**, After compaction with one accessory cone *(arrow)*. Note again the space available for additional cones because of the true lateral movement of the gutta-percha during compaction. Failure to do this results in a poorly filled canal.

tudinal voids (i.e., spreader tracks). In either case the obturation is below the standard of care outlined earlier in this chapter. If necessary, corrections can be made in most situations by removing the already compacted gutta-percha, recleaning the canal, determining the causative agent for the problem, eliminating the causative agent, and refilling the canal.

As the canal becomes obturated with accessory gutta-percha cones apically, the space that is created in the canal moves more coronally (Fig. 9-39). Generally this space is more tapered, and larger accessory cones (i.e., *medium fine* or *fine*) may be used, depending on the prepared anatomy of the canal. Accessory cones often have very fine tips that may be easily bent, either in their original container or during manipulation. Some clinicians prefer to remove the very fine tip before obturation. Likewise, some clinicians prefer to remove the coronal aspect of the accessory cone before compaction, creating custom accessory cones with lengths

TABLE 9-6   **RECOMMENDED ACCESSORY CONE SIZES CORRESPONDING TO THE CHOSEN SPREADER**

Spreader	Recommended Accessory Cones
D11TS, GP1 and GP2, S20 MA57	Extra fine or size No. 20
D11TS, D11T, GP3, S25	Fine or sizes No. 20 or 25
D11T, S3, W1S, W2S, S30	Fine or size No. 25
D11, S40, S50	Medium fine
Not recommended as accessory cones for lateral compaction	Fine medium, medium, large medium, and large

appropriate for the canal to be obturated. This is especially helpful in posterior teeth or when access to canals and their orifices are limited.

When removing the spreader from a canal during compaction, the instrument again should be moved in a 180-degree arc,[61] only without compacting pressure. During the movement a light-but-steady coronal pressure should be applied to loosen the spreader without dislodging the compacted cones. Here also (if the canal is curved) the arc of movement should be limited to approximately 90 degrees or less. The use of finger spreaders may prevent the dislodging of the gutta-percha, because a greater rotation can be used during removal without detriment to the already compacted mass.

Completion of obturation and management of the pulp chamber. The canal is filled with accessory cones until the spreader can penetrate only 2 to 3 mm into the canal orifice (Fig. 9-40). At this point a heated instrument (e.g., Glick no. 1 or heater-plugger) or special heating device (e.g., Touch n' Heat, EIE/Analytic Technology, San Diego, Calif.) is used to sear off the extended ends of the accessory cones and soften the gutta-percha in the coronal portion of the canal. This is followed by vertical compaction with root canal pluggers (Table 9-7) to adapt the coronal gutta-percha to the canal walls and to enhance the coronal seal of the canal. Pluggers used in this manner must not be wedged between the canal walls. This requires the careful fitting of a plugger into the coronal portion of the canal before obturation. Spreaders are not to be heated and used to remove the gutta-percha because no effective contemporary spreader made of metal is designed to be heated while, at the same time, used as a spreader. Likewise, the use of endodontic spoon excavators has also been advocated for this purpose, but these also are not designed to be heated (their prime purpose is to excavate caries and remove pulp tissue efficiently).

Once the gutta-percha has been compacted coronally, the pulp chamber is cleaned thoroughly with cotton pellets soaked in alcohol to remove remnants of unset sealer and particles of gutta-percha. A substantial temporary restoration

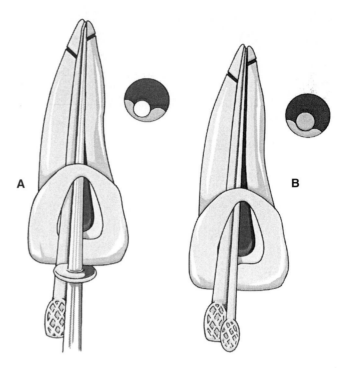

Fig. 9-38 **A,** Spreader is placed alongside the master cone to the proper apical depth. **B,** After careful removal of the spreader, an accessory cone lightly coated with sealer is placed to the apical depth created by the spreader.

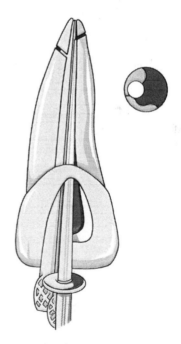

Fig. 9-39 As the obturation process continues, the depth of apical penetration of the spreader is lessened and the accessory cones gradually obturate the canal.

TABLE 9-7 ROOT CANAL PLUGGERS

Root Canal Spreader (RCS) Code	Diameter at the Tip (mm)	Diameter 16 mm from the Tip (mm)	Distance from the Tip to the Bend (mm)
RCP30*	0.33	0.66	27.96
RCP40*	0.41	0.70	27.82
RCP50*	0.53	0.82	27.78
RCP60*	0.63	0.94	27.72
RCP8A*	0.44	1.10	22.50
RCP8½A*	0.48	1.12	21.40
RCP9A*	0.55	1.11	22.00
RCP9½A*	0.66	1.11	22.10
RCP10A*	0.78	1.11	22.50
RCP10½A*	0.91	1.18	22.60
RCP11A*	1.04	1.27	22.60
RCP11½A*	1.18	1.35	22.90
RCP12A*	1.32	1.40	22.40
RCP8*	0.40	1.09	21.38
RCP8½*	0.50	1.20	21.49
RCP9*	0.55	1.18	21.45
RCP9½*	0.65	1.25	22.40
RCP10	0.82	1.22	22.60
RCP10½*	0.90	1.20	22.30
RCP11*	1.05	1.33	21.75
RCP11½*	1.25	1.30	21.80
RCP12	1.40	1.40	22.90
RCP*1*/3*	0.42	0.98	21.20
RCP1/*3*	0.52	1.02	21.13
RCP*5*/7*	0.56	1.05	21.21
RCP5/*7*	0.79	1.13	21.13
RCP*9*/11*	1.05	1.33	21.24
RCP9/*11*	1.17	1.32	21.09
RCPL1*	0.51	1.19	18.76
RCPL2*	0.53	1.05	18.80
RCPL3*	0.80	1.29	18.33
RCPL4*	1.07	1.37	16.94
P30†	0.33	0.66	27.39
P40†	0.39	0.72	28.69
P50†	0.52	0.84	28.74
P60†	0.62	0.92	27.59
P70†	0.73	1.02	28.42
P80†	0.80	1.12	28.60

Heat Transfer Instrument Code	Diameter 1 mm from the Tip (mm)	Diameter 16 mm from the Tip (mm)	Distance from the Tip to the Bend (mm)
RCS00P*	0.42	1.03	24.66
RCS0P*	0.38	0.87	22.65

*Hu-Friedy Co.
†Caulk M-series.
Italics and bold indicate end being measured.
RCP8A to RCP12A and RCP8 to RCP12 represent the Schilder-type pluggers. The "A" designation refers to pluggers for anterior teeth; the others are designated for posterior teeth. RCS00P and RCS0P represent the Schilder-type heat transfer instrument.

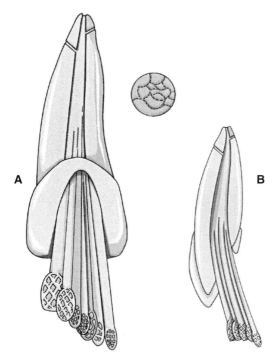

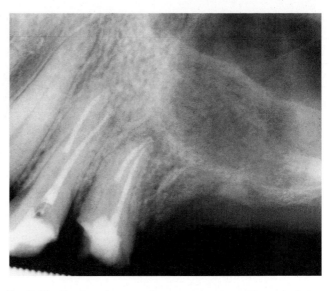

Fig. 9-41 After lateral compaction, post space is readily made. Immediate restoration of root canal–treated teeth is recommended to prevent coronal leakage and to protect the weakened tooth structure.

Fig. 9-40 **A**, Complete canal obturation as viewed facially and, **B**, proximally.

is placed; in some situations an immediate post space is created (Fig. 9-41) (see Chapter 21), and a permanent restoration is initiated. A final radiograph, without the rubber dam in position, is taken from an angle that demonstrates adequately the obturation of each canal (Figs. 9-42 and 9-43).

Variations in the cold lateral compaction technique. Variations within the previous description are common and are usually based on anatomic irregularities, clinician-induced errors, or personal choices. Because of the variations used, many of these techniques have become known as "hybrid techniques." Some of the more common variations include the following:

- Apical adaptation techniques for the master cone with solvents. This concept has been discussed previously, and the technique is often referred to as the "direct impression technique." This technique has many variations, some of which are dictated by the size of the apical preparation or canal curvature.[18]
- Canal obturation with lateral compaction in the apical one third only, followed by the searing off of the extended cones and obturation of the coronal portion of the canal with either segments of warmed gutta-percha (vertically compacted) or the injection of thermally softened gutta-percha (vertically compacted) (see subsequent sections).
- Canal obturation with lateral compaction to the canal orifice, followed by a segmental removal of gutta-percha with concomitant vertical compaction to the apical third of the canal. The coronal two thirds is then refilled with either lateral or vertical compaction.

- Placement of artificial barriers (as previously discussed) that may also include collagen-based sponges, such as CollaCote or CollaPlug (CollaTec Inc., Plainsboro, N.J.). This is more common in cases of apexification or when the apical matrix has been destroyed through overinstrumentation.
- Canal obturation with lateral compaction in the apical one third only, followed by the thermomechanical compaction of the accessory cones that extend from the canal.[173]
- Seating of the master cone and removal of the coronal portion of the cone with heat, followed by a vertical compaction of the apical segment. The remainder of the canal is obturated with the standard lateral compaction.[52]
- Placement of the compacting spreader to length adjacent to the master cone and waiting for approximately 1 minute for the master cone to adapt to the apical portion of the canal.[162] This technique is especially advocated when a sealer that contains a gutta-percha softening agent (e.g., eucalyptol) is used (see Table 9-2). During the softening of the gutta-percha, the pressure applied by the compacting instrument adapts the cone to the canal walls.

Anatomic considerations. The anatomic complexities that may demand variations in the delivery of cold, laterally compacted gutta-percha deserve a brief mention. These include **C**-shaped canals that have a wide variation of canal anastomoses, webbings, and irregular communications. Commonly found in second molars, these canal systems are much better obturated using techniques that heat soften the gutta-percha and enhance its movement into the canal irregularities (Fig. 9-44). Hybrid techniques may also be better suited for S-shaped canals (see Fig. 9-19, *B*) because of the double curvature and limited safe penetration with stainless steel compactors. Primarily found in maxillary second pre-

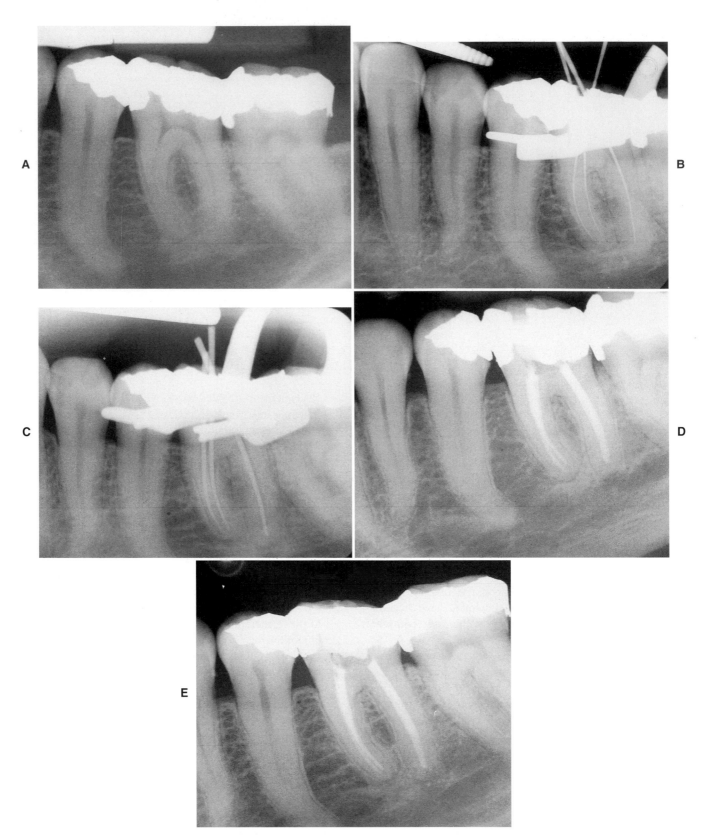

Fig. 9-42 **A,** Mandibular molar diagnosis: irreversible pulpitis with acute apical periodontitis. **B,** Working length determination within the confines of the root. **C,** Fitting of master cones in all three roots. Note the space adjacent to the length of the cones for the compaction instrument. **D,** Root canal obturation with lateral compaction and a zinc oxide-eugenol–based sealer; filling material retained within the canal. **E,** Twelve-month recall examination indicating good periradicular healing; patient is clinically symptom free.

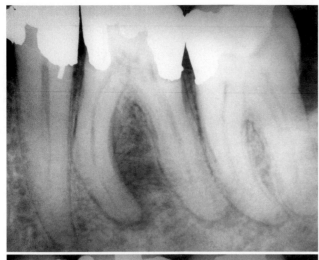

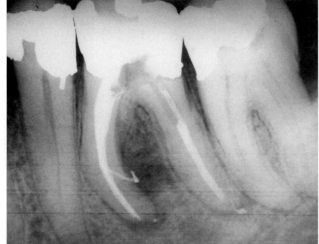

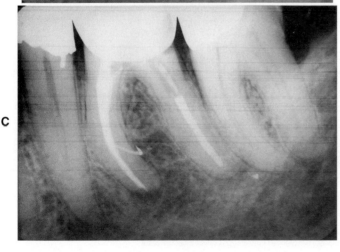

Fig. 9-43 **A**, Mandibular molar exhibiting significant bone destruction in the periradicular tissues. **B**, Canals were cleaned, shaped, and obturated using lateral compaction, gutta-percha, and a zinc oxide–eugenol–based sealer. Major lateral canal is obturated using this technique. **C**, Twelve-month recall indicates that repair is almost complete. (Courtesy Dr. David P. Rossiter.)

molars, one solution may be to use NiTi spreaders with these anatomic variations or consider a hybrid technique. The NiTi spreaders are also highly recommended with severely curved root canal systems. Internal resorption also poses a challenge for strictly cold lateral compaction. Here again, variations are necessary based on the extent of the defect and often require a segmental, warm or injectable, warm gutta-percha technique (see subsequent sections) (Fig. 9-45).

Root ends with resorptive defects, delta formations, or numerous apical openings may benefit through the use of apical impression techniques in conjunction with cold, lateral compaction of gutta-percha. Finally, obturation of canals after apexification requires a modification of the master gutta-percha cone to better adapt to the irregularly formed apical matrix or barrier. This may be accomplished by heat or chemical softening of commercially available, large cones or the creation of a large, custom cone. The details of each technique are as follows:

Chemical softening and adaptation.   The apical 2 to 3 mm of a slightly oversized master cone is placed in a solvent (e.g., chloroform, methylchloroform, rectified white turpentine, eucalyptol) for about 3 to 5 seconds, removed, and placed into the canal until the working length is achieved with a good apical fit (Fig. 9-46, *A* and *B*). The position of the cone in the canal is marked with regard to depth of placement and orientation to curves. This can be done by scoring the cone with either a cotton forceps or an explorer. The cone is fit into the canal when an irrigant is present to prevent the adherence of the softened gutta-percha to the canal walls and to moderate the action of the solvent. Once fit, the cone is checked radiographically (see Fig. 9-46, *B*), removed, and thoroughly irrigated with sterile water to eliminate any residual solvent. Alcohol can also be used to remove the solvents, and the master cone should be allowed to dry for 1 or 2 minutes before cementation and compaction.

Heat softening and adaptation.   In place of a chemical solvent, heated water can be used to soften the apical portion of the master cone before it is placed in the canal.[61] The cone is dipped into the water (100° to 120° F, 37.8° to 48.8° C) for 2 to 4 seconds to soften only the outer layers of the apical portion of the cone. The coronal portion of the cone remains firm and serves as a mechanical plunger to seat the softened cone into the prepared apical matrix (Fig. 9-47, *A-C*). Radiographic verification of the position of the cone and scoring of the cone for orientation are necessary before the cone is removed from the canal (see Fig. 9-47, *B*). Normal compaction procedures are then instituted, which may be cold, lateral compaction (see Fig. 9-47, *C*) or a variation of this technique.

Development of custom cone.   Two or more cones (either standardized, nonstandardized, or a combination of the two) are chosen, depending on the shape of the canal (Fig. 9-48, *A*). The cones are softened with a light amount of heat until they become tacky and adhere to each other (Fig. 9-48, *B*). The cones are rolled and fused together between two glass slabs to the desired shape and taper[60,61] (Fig. 9-48, *C* and *D*). Finally, the apical portion of the cone is softened,

Text continued on p. 336

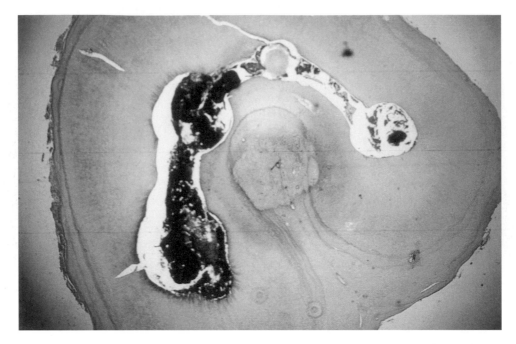

Fig. 9-44 Histologic view of a C-shaped canal. Note the irregularities. It would be difficult to obturate this type of system with lateral compaction.

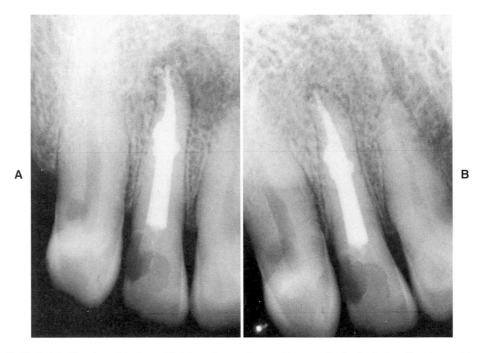

Fig. 9-45 A, Maxillary lateral incisor with internal resorption and large periradicular lesion. Canal was obturated with gutta-percha and sealer using primarily lateral compaction. Heat softening of the filling material in the middle third helps to achieve a 3-D fill of the resorptive defect. **B,** Eighteen-month recall shows almost complete osseous repair; patient is symptom free. (Courtesy Dr. Paul Lovdahl.)

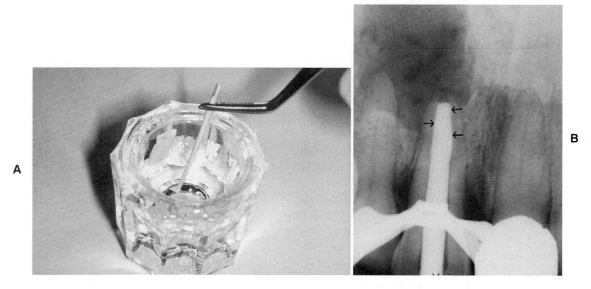

Fig. 9-46 **A,** Master gutta-percha cone is placed in a solvent for 2 to 3 seconds to soften the external surface of the cone. **B,** Radiographic appearance of the softened cone as it has adapted to the large, irregular canal space *(arrows).*

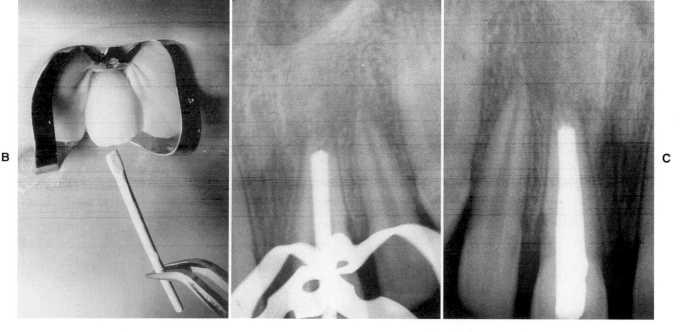

Fig. 9-47 **A,** Master gutta-percha cone has been reversed and the coronal end has been softened in hot water before placement into a maxillary central incisor that has undergone apexification. Larger end of the cone was chosen because of the size of the root canal. **B,** Radiograph shows the position of the reversed cone in the tooth adjacent to the apical bridge that has formed. **C,** Canal has been obturated with lateral compaction. Note small amounts of sealer have been expressed apically through the porous openings in the apical bridge.

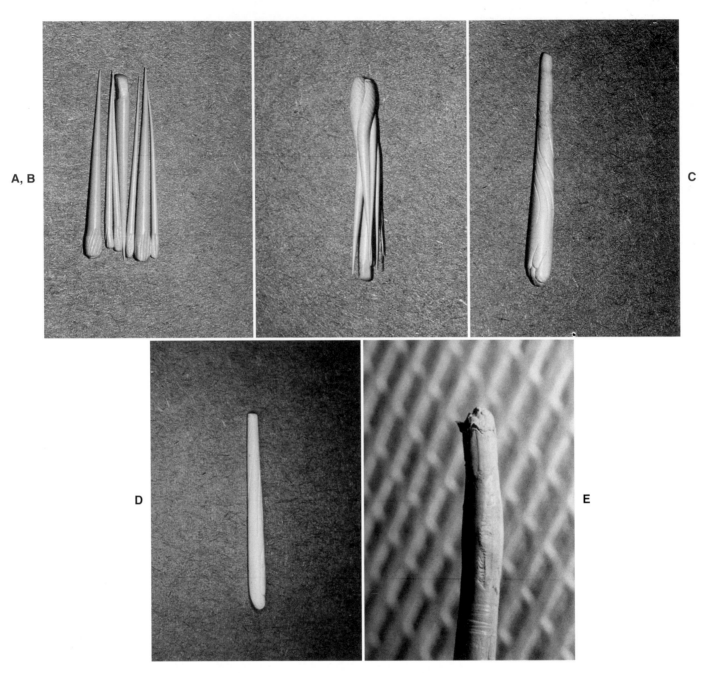

Fig. 9-48 **A**, Custom cones can be fabricated by fusing multiple cones together, softening the mass, and shaping the newly formed cone to fit the root canal to be obturated. Size and shape of the canal determine the type of cones to be fused. In this case nonstandardized cones have been selected. **B**, Cones are softened with heat and the fusion begins. With continued warming the mass is rolled between two sterile glass slabs. Angle of the top slab to the bottom slab determines the shape or taper of the canal, whereas the amount of pressure on the slab determines the thickness of the cone at any point along its length. **C**, Example of variably shaped cones. **D**, Example of variably shaped cones. **E**, Once shaped, the apical portion of the cone is softened with heat or chemicals and placed to the apical position within the root canal. Note this cone has been adapted to the canal irregularities, both apically and laterally.

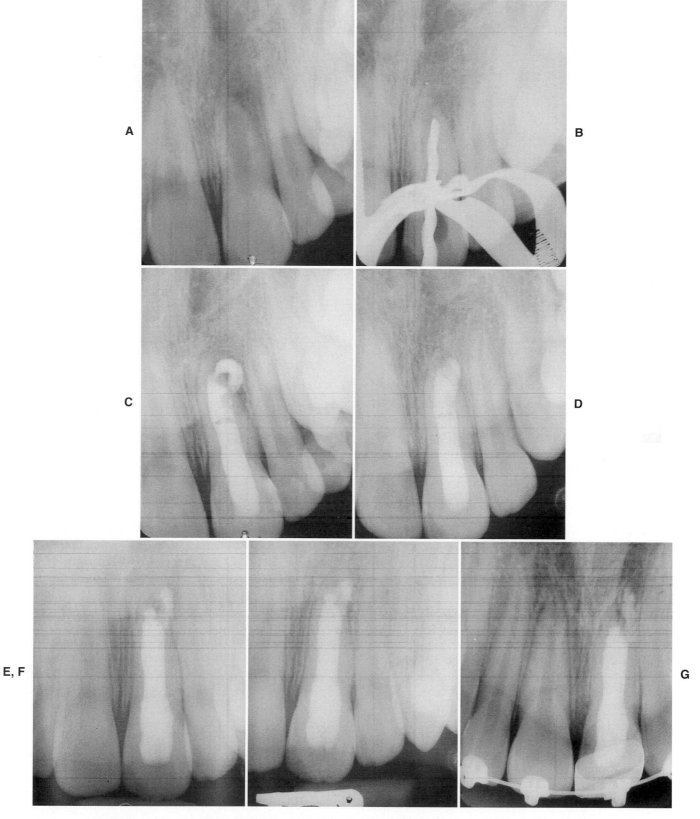

Fig. 9-49 **A**, Traumatized maxillary central incisor. Pulp became necrotic before root closure. **B**, Root canal system is accessed and cleaned. Working length is maintained within the canal space. **C**, Calcium hydroxide (mixed 4 parts to 10) with barium sulfate is placed in and beyond the canal system. Placement beyond gives the clinician important information regarding the nature of the apical bridge that has formed. **D**, Six-month recall examination shows the beginning of osseous repair. **E**, Custom cone was prepared, and the canal was obturated with a calcium hydroxide sealer using a combination of lateral and vertical compaction. Some sealer is extruded beyond the root-end barrier. **F**, Six months after obturation there is further evidence of apical repair. **G**, Twelve months after obturation the extruded sealer and calcium hydroxide-barium sulfate is being absorbed. Patient has been banded for orthodontic tooth movement.

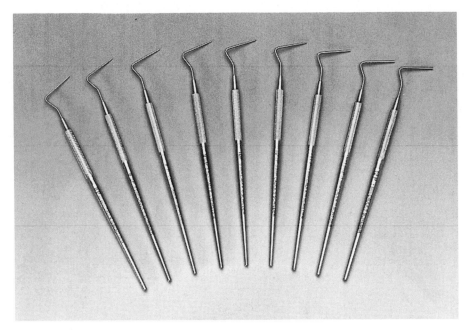

Fig. 9-50 Root canal pluggers used for the vertical compaction of heat softened gutta-percha. These pluggers are often referred to as Schilder pluggers and come in lengths for anterior and posterior teeth (see Table 9-7).

either with chemicals or heat, and adapted to the irregular shape of the apical portion of the canal (Fig. 9-48, *E*). Subsequent canal obturation can be with either lateral or vertical compaction (Fig. 9-49).

Compaction of Heat-Softened Gutta-Percha

The concept of thermoplasticized compaction is not new and covers any technique that is based entirely on the heat softening of gutta-percha combined primarily with vertical compaction. In its purest form it is similar to lateral compaction, only the material is heated and adapted to the prepared root canal with vertical compaction. In some circles it is called a warm, sectional technique; vertical compaction with warmed gutta-percha; or the Schilder technique.[151] The essential elements of the technique have been with us for almost a century,[181] with entrepreneurial efforts shaping its contemporary evolution and form.[12,151]

Brief Overview   A master gutta-percha cone is chosen that approximates the length and shape of the prepared canal. The cone is fit snugly to within 1 to 2 mm of the apical extent of the preparation, depending on the nature of the canal anatomy and shape. The common compacting instrument is the plugger, which is chosen based on canal size, length, and curvature (Fig. 9-50) (see Figs. 9-26 and 9-27 and Table 9-7). The plugger can be a hand or finger instrument, and the selected instruments are prefitted into the canal to determine the proper depth of penetration without binding against the canal walls. A root canal sealer that can be mixed to a creamy consistency and has ample working time (i.e., 15 to 30 min-

utes) is selected. The sealer is placed into the canal to the depth of the master cone position; the master cone is lightly coated on its apical half and placed in the canal. A heated instrument is used to sear off and remove coronal segments of gutta-percha and to transfer heat to the remaining portion of the master cone. A cold plugger is used to compact the softened portion of the cone apically and laterally. This process of heating, removing, and compacting are continued until softened gutta-percha is delivered into the apical 1 to 2 mm of the prepared canal. Subsequently, softened segments are added and compacted to obturate the canal from the apical segment to the canal orifice.

Detailed Technique   *Master cone selection.* A master gutta-percha cone is selected, based on the approximate length and shape of the canal. With this technique the shape of the cone chosen is most important. The choice of cone is a nonstandardized cone, such as *fine, fine medium, medium large,* and so forth. The shape of these cones provides the necessary bulk of gutta-percha for the vertical compaction technique.

The master cone is fit to within 1 to 2 mm of the prepared apical matrix or constriction (Fig. 9-51). The premise for this choice is based on the fact that the softened material moves apically into the prepared canal in a softened state, thereby adapting more intimately to the canal walls. Care must be exercised to ensure that the cone binds only at its most apical extent and not higher in the canal. This is a function of both proper canal shaping and cone selection. Once the cone is fit to clinical expectations, its position in the canal is verified radiographically and evaluated as follows:

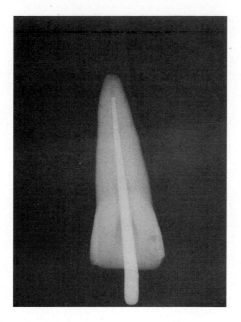

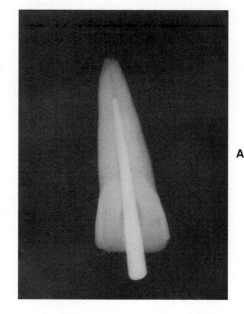

Fig. 9-51   Nonstandardized master cone fit to the correct length for vertical compaction. Note shape of the cone approximates the shape of the prepared canal space.

I. If the cone fits to or within 1 to 2 mm of the working length, if the cone demonstrates a snugness of fit at that point, and if the shape of the cone approximates the shape of the canal throughout the canal length, compaction may proceed.

II. If the cone fits short of the desired length, the following conditions may exist (Fig. 9-52):

A. The cone is binding higher in the canal.

B. An improperly tapered cone has been chosen.

C. Dentin chips may be packed in the apical portion of the canal.

D. Clinician errors, such as a ledge, block, or zip, may be present.

E. There may be a curve in the canal that is not visible on the two-dimensional radiograph, and the canal preparation narrows rapidly at the curve.

III. If the cone fits beyond the desired length, the following conditions may exist (Fig. 9-53):

A. The taper of the cone is insufficient or incorrect.

B. The apical matrix or constriction has been destroyed through overinstrumentation.

In either case, if the cone is too short or too long, the problem must be assessed and the causative factors removed. This can be done by selecting a new cone, cutting segments from the apical portion of a cone with a scalpel, custom fitting a cone with chemical or heat softening, or reshaping the canal for a more desirable fit of the cone selected.

Canal preparation.   Once the master cone has been properly fitted, it is removed from the canal and placed in a sterilizing solution, such as NaOCl. The canal system is then dried with paper points. If the smear layer is to be removed, appropriate solutions are used at this time (see *Smear Layer*

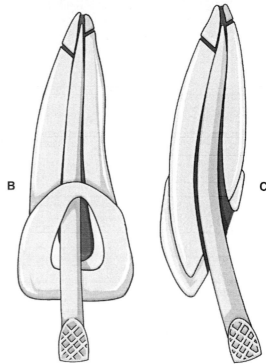

Fig. 9-52   **A,** Nonstandardized master cone is too large and improperly shaped for the prepared canal. Depth of penetration is insufficient. **B** and **C,** Diagrammatic illustration of this clinical problem.

Removal Versus Smear Layer Retention in this chapter). If desired all residual moisture in the canal may be removed by rinsing the canal with 95% ethyl alcohol or 99% isopropyl alcohol. The alcohol is left in the canal for 2 to 3 minutes and then removed with additional sterile paper points.

Compactor selection.   The careful fitting and selection of the compactors used for vertical compaction is crucial to the success of this technique (see Tables 9-5 and 9-7). For

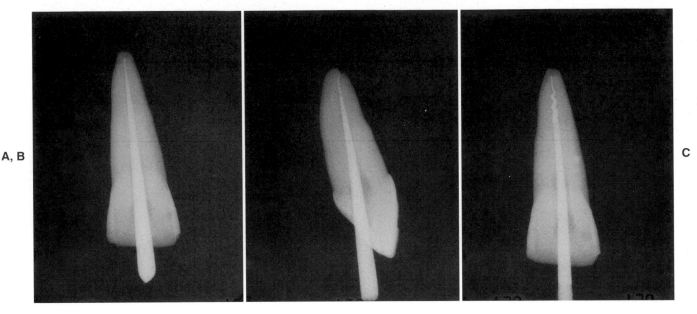

Fig. 9-53 **A** and **B**, Nonstandardized master cone is too long and is not properly adapted to the prepared canal. Note views from the facial and proximal views. **C**, Master cone is too small apically and curls up when apical pressure is applied. This usually indicates the taper of the cone and the prepared views do not match; another cone must be chosen.

many canals two to three different sizes are necessary to match the tapered, flared canal. One plugger should fit to within a few millimeters of the end of the canal, whereas other pluggers fit at variable distances into the canal (Fig. 9-54). Under no circumstances should any plugger contact the walls of the canal in a wedging manner. This may readily dispose to a vertical root fracture.[152] Therefore the pluggers must be fit to a point where maximal depth is achieved without binding. Pluggers that have markings or are scored at 5 mm increments are desirable. Likewise, rubber stops can be placed on the plugger to help control the depth of penetration into the canal, if necessary.

In addition to selecting pluggers for vertical compaction, a heat transfer instrument (e.g., 0 or 00, Caulk/Dentsply, Milford, Del.; Hu-Friedy Co., Chicago, Ill.) or a heating instrument (e.g., Touch n' Heat, EIE/Analytic Technology, San Diego, Calif.) is chosen to remove segments of the gutta-percha during the compaction apically or to heat and add segments of gutta-percha during the compaction of the coronal portion of the canal.

Sealer placement.   As opposed to lateral compaction, the placement of sealer for vertical compaction is minimized in the apical segment of the canal. This prevents excessive movement of the sealer beyond the canal, if the foramen is patent; it also prevents the filling of the apical portion of the canal with sealer only, if the foramen is not patent. Therefore using instruments similar to those suggested for cold, lateral compaction, a light coating of sealer is placed circumferentially on the canal walls to the approximate depth of the master cone placement. Vertical compaction of the heat-softened gutta-percha provides for a thin coating of the filling material as it is moved apically and laterally. Likewise, some of the sealer moves coronally in a hydraulic fashion during compaction.

Master cone placement.   A disinfected master cone is coated lightly with sealer over its apical one third and slowly placed into the canal so as not to force large amounts of the sealer apically. At this point some clinicians choose to expose a radiograph and evaluate the position of the cone before compaction.

Master cone compaction: coronal to apical obturation.   The coronal end of the master gutta-percha cone is removed above the canal orifice with a heated instrument (i.e., heat transfer instrument or heating device), and the warmed end of the master cone that remains in the canal is compacted, folding it into the coronal portion of the canal (Fig. 9-55, *A*). This is accomplished with the largest plugger that was prefit in the canal. The blunted end of the plugger creates a deep depression in the center of the master cone. The outer walls of the softened gutta-percha are then folded inward to fill the central void, while at the same time the mass of softened gutta-percha is moved laterally and apically (Fig. 9-55, *B*). Subsequently, the heated instrument is used to remove additional 2 to 3 mm segments of gutta-percha, followed by the compaction of the softened gutta-percha remaining in the canal (Fig. 9-55, *C*). This sequence is repeated until the apical 3- to 4-mm segment of gutta-percha is softened and compacted into the apical preparation. Often it is advisable to expose radiographs during this procedure to monitor the movement of the filling material (Fig. 9-55, *D-F*).

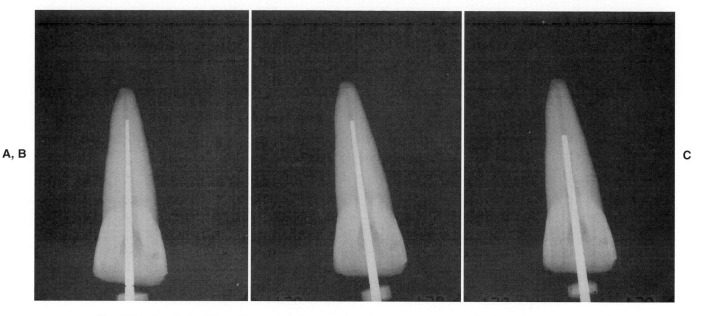

Fig. 9-54 **A** to **C**, Prefitting of increasingly larger vertical pluggers to appropriate depths in the canal is essential before obturation (A: RCP 9; B: RCP 10; C: RCP 10). (See Table 9-7.)

Success with the heat softening and apical compaction is predicated on a number of factors that are within the clinician's control. Therefore adherence to the following guidelines is very important:

- Use the plugger that has been prefit in each portion or segment of the canal. Larger pluggers are generally applied in the coronal portion, with decreasing sizes used as the compaction proceeds apically. The last plugger used should fit freely in the apical 2 to 3 mm of the canal without contacting the walls.
- The pluggers should be wiped with alcohol or possibly a dry dental cement powder (as a separating medium) to prevent their sticking to the warmed gutta-percha.
- The clinician should not be aggressive and compact the entire remaining segment of the gutta-percha at one time. The heat applied during the removal of the segments only travels 3 to 4 mm into the remaining gutta-percha. Therefore only the coronal most material is softened sufficiently to obtain quality compaction. Additionally, small incremental heating and compacting provide a fluid movement and adaptation of the gutta-percha to the canal walls and irregularities.
- Controlled application of apical pressure usually results in the best obturation, as opposed to rapid and irregular poking at the gutta-percha.
- Once the plugger has reached the depth of 1 to 3 mm into the softened gutta-percha, the plugger is carefully removed and the material on either side of the depression made with the plugger is compacted into the central portion of the canal. Failure to compact this material evenly results in voids in the softened material. This is not a

major concern during the coronal to apical compaction, but it is during the apical-to-coronal compaction to follow.
- In curved canals it is necessary to curve the pluggers to the approximate shape of the canal before entry. Fortunately, most of the curves are in the apical one half to one third, and the small pluggers can be easily curved. The best instrument for this is orthodontic pliers or possibly the bending tool that comes with one of the contemporary thermoplasticized gutta-percha delivery units (Obtura II, Obtura Corp., Fenton, Mo.) (see following sections).
- Do not move the apical segment of gutta-percha into the prepared apical portion of the canal until the most apical gutta-percha can be thoroughly softened and carefully adapted to the canal walls, apical constriction, or matrix.

Placement of softened segments: apical to coronal obturation.   Once the final segment of gutta-percha has been compacted, a radiograph is exposed to assess the apical fill. If satisfactory, the root canal appears essentially empty, except at its most apical extent, where a dense apical plug of gutta-percha is located (see Fig. 9-55, *F*). The remaining portion of the canal is obturated with small segments (i.e., 2 to 4 mm in length) that have been previously prepared to conform to the shape of the pluggers and the canal, from the apical segment to the coronal orifice. The segments are speared with the heating instrument and carefully and lightly warmed over a flame to reach a firm, yet tacky, consistency (Fig. 9-55, *G* and *H*). Subsequently, they are carried to the depth of the gutta-percha in the canal where the tacky segment is lightly touched to the filling material already in place. This results in an adherence of the segment to the apical gutta-percha. This is followed by compaction with the

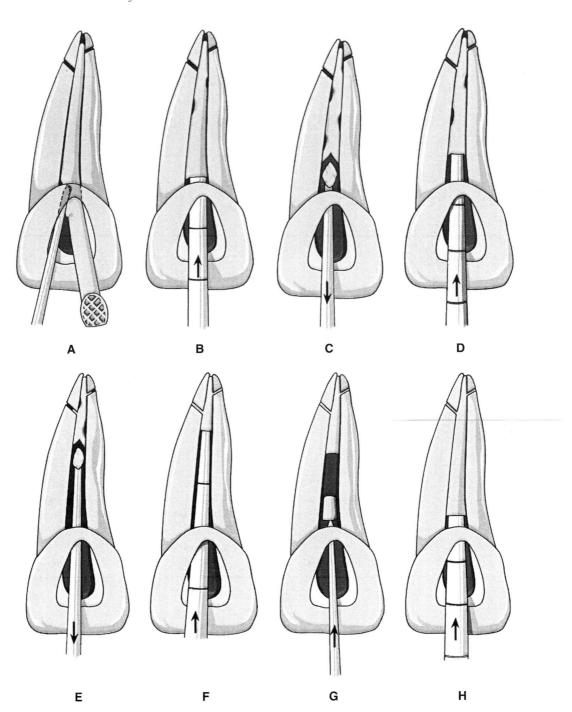

Fig. 9-55 **A,** Removal of the coronal portion of the master cone with a heated instrument. Note the apical position of the cone is short of the working length. **B,** Initial compaction of the coronal portion of the softened gutta-percha. Note the plugger must be of sufficient size to move the material without merely penetrating the softened mass. **C,** Segment of gutta-percha is removed with a heat transfer instrument. **D,** Continued compaction of the softened gutta percha in the middle third of the canal with a properly sized plugger. **E,** Removal of additional gutta-percha segment, followed by apical compaction (**F**). **G,** Small segment of gutta-percha is heated on the heated transfer instrument, carried to the canal, and compacted until the canal is filled to the desired level (**H**).

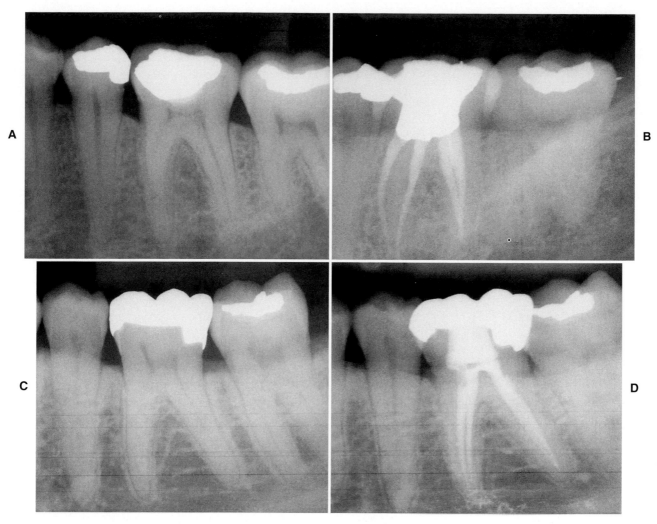

Fig. 9-56 **A** to **D**, Preoperative and postoperative views of two mandibular molars with four canals, each obturated using vertical compaction with heat-softened gutta-percha. (Courtesy Dr. James C. Douthitt.)

prefit pluggers as previously described. The clinician should compact the material in all dimensions by folding the gutta-percha in on itself to create a dense mass that fully adheres to, and is homogeneous with, the previously compacted material. This prevents voids. This entire process is continued until the canal is fully obturated to the canal orifice or to a specific depth if a postcore restoration is planned.

Consider the following guidelines:

- The segments of gutta-percha should not be overheated, because they will become too soft to apply, they will compact, or they will easily burn. This aspect of the technique requires practice to achieve a consistent result. Suggestions to enhance heating consistency in the delivery of the segments have been made through the use of controlled heating devices, such as the Touch n' Heat.[88]
- Sealer should not be applied to the softened segments, because it will prevent their adherence to the body of gutta-percha in the canal.

- The material should be compacted with a light-but-firm, controlled force.
- The segments used should be no larger than 2 to 4 mm in length.
- The pluggers used should be appropriately sized and prefit.

On a final note with this technique, the filling of the canal with softened gutta-percha from the apical plug to the coronal orifice has been enhanced significantly with newer, injection gutta-percha systems (see *Technique Variations* later in this chapter). However, the technique as presented still provides high-quality obturation, and it is the technique of choice of many clinicians (Figs. 9-56 and 9-57).

Completion of obturation and management of the pulp chamber.   Once the gutta-percha has been compacted coronally, the pulp chamber is cleaned thoroughly with cotton pellets soaked in alcohol to remove remnants of unset sealer and particles of gutta-percha. A substantial tem-

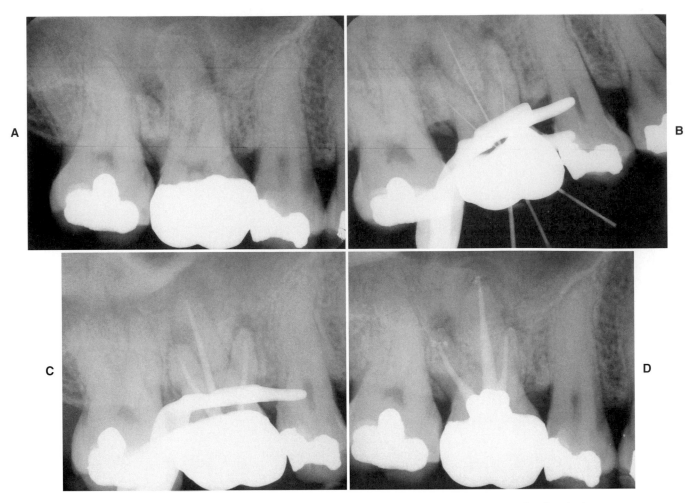

Fig. 9-57 **A,** Maxillary molar with a necrotic pulp and chronic periradicular periodontitis. **B,** Working lengths determined. **C,** Nonstandardized master cones fit to the appropriate lengths for vertical compaction. **D,** Canals obturated with extrusion of small amounts of sealer through accessory foramina. (Courtesy Dr. Constantinos Laghios.)

porary restoration is placed; in some situations, immediate post space is created (see Chapter 21), and a permanent restoration is initiated. A final radiograph, without the rubber dam in position, is taken from an angle that adequately demonstrates the obturation of each canal.

Technique Variations

Since the inception of the vertical compaction with warm gutta-percha technique in its contemporary format,[12,151] multiple attempts have been made to simplify the approach to heat softening and compaction of gutta-percha. These innovations have focused primarily on enhanced heating systems for intracanal softening of gutta-percha (System B, EIE/Analytic Technology, San Diego, Calif.) before compaction[24]; injectable, thermoplasticized gutta-percha (Obtura II, Obtura Corp., Fenton, Mo.)[64,193]; core carrier techniques in which the gutta-percha is coated on a carrier before heating and delivery to the canal (ThermaFil, Tulsa Dental Products, Tulsa, Okla.; Densfil, Caulk/Dentsply, Milford, Del.; Soft-

Core, Soft-Core Systems Inc., North Richland Hills, Tex.)[89]; and thermocompaction techniques with rotary instruments (JS Quick-fill, JS Dental, Ridgefield, Conn.).[125,147] Variations and combinations of these innovations are available (Inject-R-Fill, UBECO, York, Pa.; SimpliFill, Lightspeed Technology Inc., San Antonio, Tex.; EZ-Fill, Essential Dental Systems, Hackensack, N.J.). The most popular techniques are discussed in subsequent sections.

Enhanced heated systems.   A major improvement in the vertical compaction with warm, softened gutta-percha was the development of the System B heat source. This device can monitor the temperature at the tip of its heat carrier devices and can deliver a precise amount of heat for an indefinite period of time. When the heat carrier is also designed as a plugger, simultaneous heating and compacting can occur; this approach has been referred to as a continuous-wave technique.[24] With this system the pluggers have also been designed to match the taper of nonstandardized gutta-percha cones. Therefore, when a master cone has been

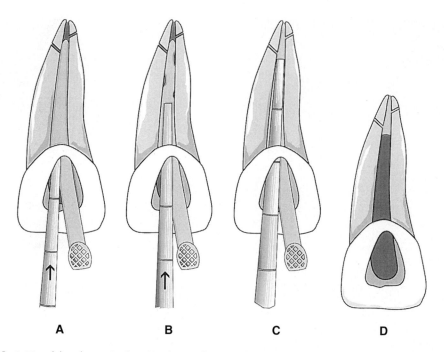

Fig 9-58 A, Tip of the plugger is placed in the canal next to the gutta-percha and activated. **B,** Heated plugger is driven through the master cone. **C,** The plugger is continued to its most apical position, the heat is reduced, and the plugger is maintained with apical pressure. **D,** A short burst of heat is delivered to facilitate loosening and removal of the plugger.

properly fitted, the same size plugger can be chosen for heating and compaction. This combination allows compaction of the filling material at exactly the same instant it has been heat softened, and it creates a single wave of heating and compacting (as opposed to the multiple-phase approach previously described). An additional advantage includes the compacting of the filling materials at all levels simultaneously, throughout the movement of the heating and compacting instrument apically.

In this technique, pluggers are fitted to within 5 to 7 mm from the canal terminus. The heat source is set to 392° F ± 50° F (200° C ± 10° C), the canal is thoroughly dried, and the fitted master cone is placed (with sealer) into the canal. The tip of the plugger is placed into the canal orifice, and the switch on the System B is activated. The plugger is driven through the master cone, using a single motion, to a point about 3 mm short of its apical binding position (Fig. 9-58, *A-C*). While pressure on the plugger is maintained, the button on the heating system is released and the plugger is slowed in its apical movement as the its tip cools. When the pluggers stops short of its binding position, pressure is maintained on the plugger until the apical mass of the gutta-percha has set (5 to 10 seconds). This compensates for any material shrinkage during cooling. Then the switch is reactivated for a short burst of heat (1 second) to release the plugger and surplus gutta-percha (Fig. 9-58, *D*). During this short burst the System B is programmed to send a one half–second heat surge (572° F, 300° C) to the plugger, with a subsequent return to 392° F (200° C). These short bursts should be limited to allow only for removal of the plugger (as opposed to heating up the remaining gutta-percha).

The System B is also designed to maintain a stable 392° F (200° C) at the tip of the plugger to ensure constant temperature throughout the apical compaction procedure. If it is too hot, the plugger rapidly drives through the oversoftened gutta-percha and the backpressure necessary for 3-D obturation is lost.

Once the apical segment has been obturated, the coronal portion of the canal is backfilled. This can be done with the same system with modified temperatures (212° F, 100° C), or can be done with an injectable gutta-percha technique (see the following section). When the System B is used, the plugger is the same as that used for the initial apical compaction with another gutta-percha cone that has the same taper as the master cone and a tip diameter that matches the tip diameter of the plugger. The backfilling cone is prepared at the same time as the original master cone. Sealer is used with the backfilling cone, which is seated in the canal. The cone is warmed without pressure to soften it, followed by sustained pressure to allow the cone to adapt to the walls and "set" in the canal. Excessive temperatures applied too long must be avoided to prevent the plugger from deeply penetrating the cone and pulling it from the canal. The plugger should be rotated slightly during its removal from the compacted mass. This mass of gutta-percha that was added to the coronal portion can be reheated and compacted as necessary (Fig. 9-59).

Although minimal equipment is required to perform this technique, cost factors in equipment purchase must be con-

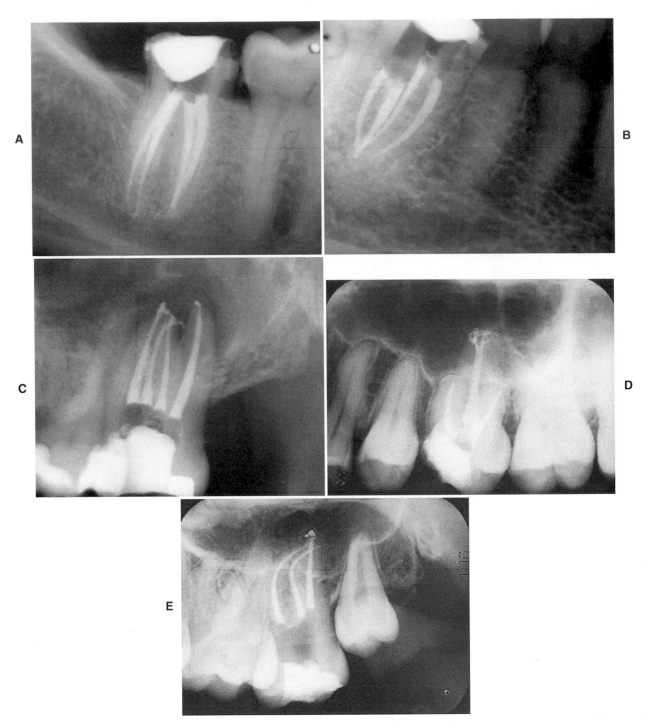

Fig. 9-59 **A** to **E**, Examples of root canal obturation in molars with vertical compaction using the System B – backfilled with Obtura. Note the canal shaping that is necessary and the movement of both sealer and (possibly) gutta-percha beyond the apical confines or through accessory foramina. (Courtesy Dr. Constantinos Laghios.)

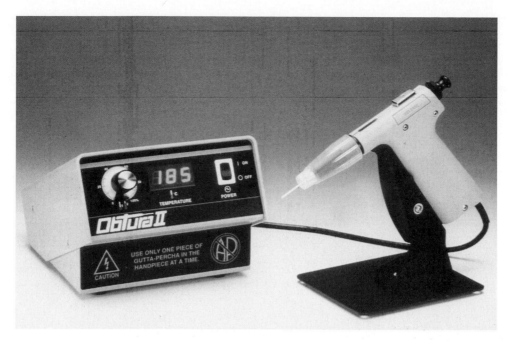

Fig. 9-60 Obtura II thermoplasticized gutta-percha system.

sidered. Likewise, adaptation of this technique to unusual circumstances and mastery of it with straightforward cases require practice. Presently there are no prospective or retrospective clinical studies to support the safety, efficacy, and long-term success of this technique, nor are there studies that have evaluated the potential effects of the heat generated on the supporting periodontium. Dye leakage and material adaptation studies have shown this technique to be comparable in quality to other contemporary obturation techniques.[31]

Injectable Gutta-percha Techniques The prime injectable gutta-percha technique available is the Obtura II (Obtura Corp., Fenton, Mo.) (Fig. 9-60). This technique has also been referred to as a "high-heat" technique. This is mainly because of the temperature required to soften the gutta-percha for delivery into the canal.

Obtura II technique. Canals to be obturated must have a continuously tapering funnel, from the apical matrix to the canal orifice.[64] Of significance is a properly shaped canal in the apical to middle transitional area, particularly in curved canals. The proper shaping is essential for the flow of the softened material. Also a definite apical matrix is essential to confine and retain the gutta-percha in the canal system, because filling beyond the end of the root may occur.[36]

Gutta-percha is available in pellets that are inserted into the heated delivery system, which looks like a caulking device (Fig. 9-61). The gutta-percha is heated to approximately 365° to 392° F (185° to 200° C). A needle or applicator tip (gauges 20 and 23) designed to deliver the softened gutta-percha is introduced into the canal to the junction of the

middle and apical third (Fig. 9-62). The applicator tip is prefit to ensure that it does not bind against the canal walls. Likewise, the pluggers are also prefit to determine the proper depth of placement for compaction (see Fig. 9-54). If necessary, pluggers can be curved, or newer NiTi pluggers can be used.

Even though the gutta-percha is softened and can be adapted to the intricacies of the prepared canal, root canal sealer is still essential with this technique.[36,163] However, sealer must be placed carefully in the canal to prevent its movement beyond the confines of the canal apically and to ensure the placement of gutta-percha at the terminus of the canal system. One to two drops of sealer are placed with an instrument of choice to the approximate depth of the prefit applicator tip or needle. The clinician should not fill the apical portion of the canal with sealer; a fast-setting sealer is not recommended.

With the needle in its proper position in the canal, the gutta-percha is injected passively into the root canal system, avoiding apical pressure on the needle. In 2 to 5 seconds the softened material fills the apical segment and begins to lift the needle out of the tooth (Fig. 9-63, *A-D*). During this lifting by the softened, flowing mass, the middle and coronal portions of the canal are filled until the needle reaches the canal orifice. Controlled compaction of the material follows with prefitted pluggers to adapt the gutta-percha to the prepared canal walls (see Fig. 9-63, *B-D*). If necessary, additional amounts of gutta-percha can be injected to achieve complete obturation. The clinician should not use excessive compaction pressure but fold the material in on itself (as previously described) for vertical compaction.

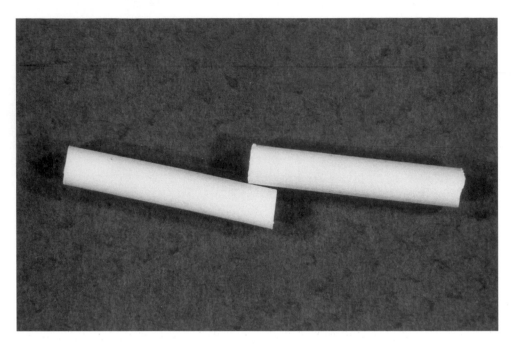

Fig. 9-61   Pellets of gutta-percha for use in the Obtura II system.

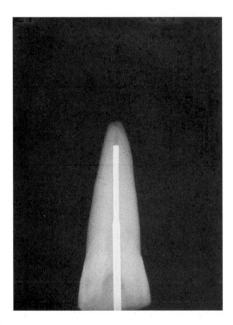

Fig. 9-62 Prefitting of the injection-applicator tip of the Obtura II system into the apical third of the prepared canal without binding is essential for proper delivery and flow of the softened material.

Multiple variations exist with this technique. The softened material can be placed in the apical 2 to 3 mm and compacted at that point (see Fig. 9-63, *E-G*). Subsequently, the remainder of the canal can be filled as previously described, or segmental additions can be added and compacted.[179] Control of the apical movement of gutta-percha and sealer appears to be better with this approach. Often this technique is used with the lateral or vertical compaction techniques. After the compaction of a master cone in the apical 2 to 3 mm, the cone is seared off with a heated instrument and the coronal portion compacted. The Obtura II is then used to backfill the remainder of the canal, either in segments or in toto.

With an increased demand for the use of this technique, variations in the consistency of the gutta-percha have become available (Schwed Co. Inc., Kew Gardens, N.Y.). These alterations are designed to improve flow and regulate viscosity. The *regular-flow gutta-percha* is a homogenized formulation with superior flow characteristics, whereas the *easy-flow gutta-percha* maintains its smooth flow consistency at lower temperatures and has a longer working time. The latter would favor the management of complex cases in which extensive compaction is necessary and cases with small curved canals (in addition to favoring the inexperienced clinician).

The use of the injected thermoplasticized gutta-percha is especially beneficial when managing canal irregularities, such as fins, webs, cul-de-sacs, internal resorption, C-shaped canals, accessory or lateral canals, and arborized foramina.[64] The adaptation of the softened gutta-percha to the canal walls has been shown to be significantly better than lateral compaction (Fig. 9-64, *A*), and the removal of the smear layer and obturation of canals with the injectable system result in the movement of gutta-percha and sealer into the dentinal tubules[59] (see Figs. 9-11, *E*, and 9-64, *B* and *C*). Initial evaluation of clinical success with this technique has also proven favorable[164] (Fig. 9-65). The effective use of this technique, however, is predicated on mastery of its demands and nuances, and application on extracted teeth or models is essential before patient use.[64]

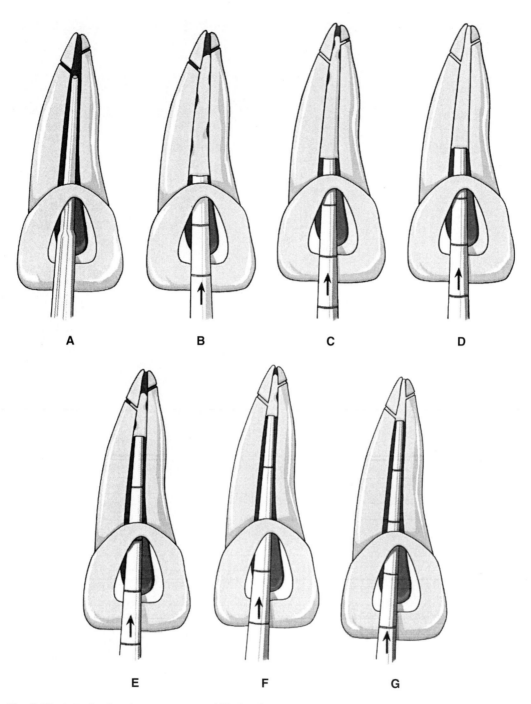

Fig. 9-63 **A**, Prefit of applicator tip. **B**, Canal filled in the coronal two thirds with softened gutta-percha. Properly sized plugger begins the apical movement of the material. **C**, As the plugger penetrates deeper into the canal, the material is folded on itself and compacted apically. **D**, Smaller pluggers are used in the apical portion. **E**, Variation of technique. Softened gutta-percha can be placed only in the apical third, followed by compaction with appropriately sized pluggers, which do not bind in the canal (**F** and **G**).

Both the potential for extrusion of the gutta-percha and sealer beyond the apical foramen (Fig. 9-66) and the possibility of heat damage to the periodontium have been identified as possible drawbacks to this technique. Temperature rises on the external lateral surface of the roots appear to be negligible, with minimal to no tissue damage.[8,64] Whereas the apical tissues may experience an inflammatory reaction, even to gutta-percha retained within the root canal system.[111] Of importance in these findings is the fact that this data came from an evaluation of the original Obtura system. Therefore it does not necessarily represent information applicable to the newer Obtura II system, especially with the availability of gutta-percha that can flow at lower temperatures.

Core Carrier Techniques   The prime core carrier techniques are the ThermaFil Plus (Tulsa Dental Products, Tulsa, Okla.), Densfil (Caulk/Dentsply, Milford, Del.) and Soft-Core (Soft-Core Systems Inc., North Richland Hills, Tex.). For business purposes, Densfil was created under a licensing agreement with the creators of ThermaFil and, subsequently, can be considered as the same product. Likewise, Soft-Core is used in a manner similar to ThermaFil; therefore, it will not be discussed further. Initially the core carrier delivery system was solely designed to use metallic cores on which the gutta-percha was coated. Contemporary technology has resulted in the development of a firm plastic carrier (Fig. 9-67). The discussion to follow focuses primarily on this type of carrier.

ThermaFil technique.   As with all other techniques, and this one is no exception, canal shaping is of utmost importance in achieving success. Unique to this technique is the availability of size verification, naked-plastic cores that are the exact size of the cores covered with gutta-percha (Fig. 9-68). Therefore the size and shape of the canal can be determined accurately before choosing the desired ThermaFil core carrier (Fig. 9-69).

The core carrier is placed in a specific oven (ThermaPrep Plus, Tulsa Dental Products, Tulsa, Okla.) and heated for the specific timeframe designated (Fig. 9-70). During this time the canal is rinsed and dried with paper points. The smear layer should be removed with a chelating agent or low-percentage acid (e.g., 10% citric acid). This will promote the movement of the softened material into the dentinal tubules and enhance the seal.[11] Removal of the smear layer, followed by the placement of a plastic ThermaFil, has been shown to decrease coronal bacterial penetration significantly.[100] This is presumably due to the ability of the filling materials to penetrate the patent dentinal tubules. After the canal is dried, a light coating of sealer is applied to all the walls in the middle and coronal third of the root canal.

When the ThermaFil carrier is heated, it is removed from the oven and placed into the canal to the predetermined depth marked with a rubber stop on the carrier. The carrier is not twisted during placement, and attempts to reposition the carrier may lead to a disruption of the gutta-percha position in the canal (Fig. 9-71, *A-D*) because the carrier serves to pro-

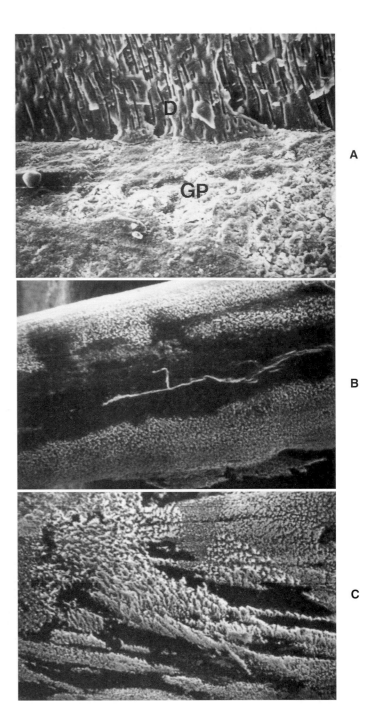

Fig. 9-64   **A,** Scanning electron microscopic view of the adaptation of thermoplasticized gutta-percha to the dentinal walls (*D:* **dentin;** *GP:* gutta-percha). **B** and **C,** Penetration of the dentinal tubules (scanning electron micrograph) with thermoplasticized gutta-percha after the removal of the smear layer. Original magnification range from × 76 to × 220.

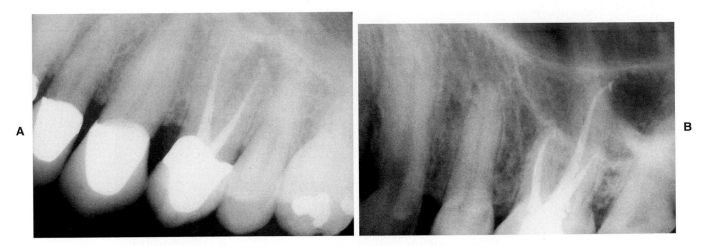

Fig. 9-65 Two maxillary teeth obturated using the original Obtura system of canal filling.

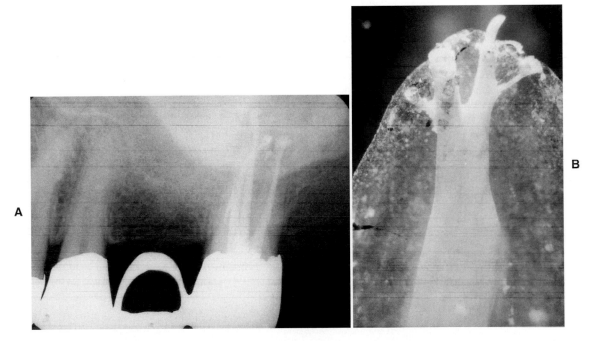

Fig. 9-66 **A,** Maxillary molar obturated with the Obtura system. Note the extrusion of material beyond the apical foramen in addition to the adaptation of the softened material to canal irregularities and accessory canals. **B,** Magnified view of apical obturation with the original Obtura system. Note the filling of the apical delta and the overfilling of the canal system.

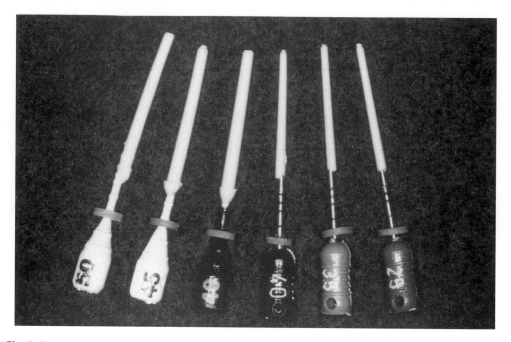

Fig. 9-67 ThermaFil carriers. Plastic core (*left*) and metal cores (*right*). Plastic core carriers are recommended.

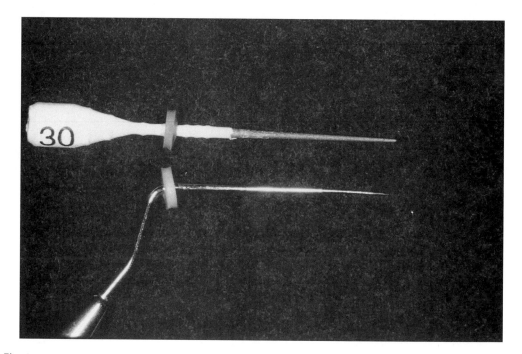

Fig. 9-68 Naked ThermaFil plastic carrier can be used to verify the size of the prepared canal (*top*). Comparison with a root canal spreader (*bottom*).

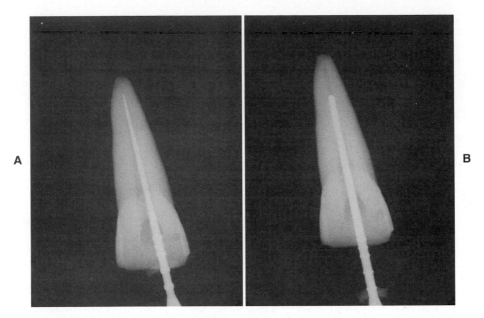

Fig. 9-69 **A**, Proper fit of the naked ThermaFil plastic carrier. **B**, Improper fit of a naked carrier. Carrier must fit loosely to the appropriate length (similarly to the fitting of a root canal spreader).

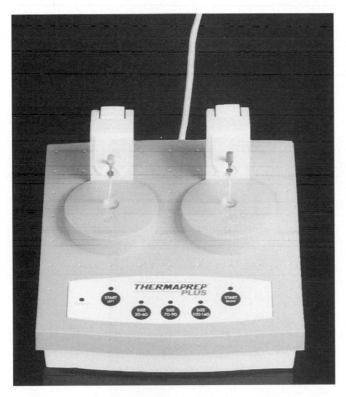

Fig. 9-70 ThermaPrep Plus heating system. (Courtesy Tulsa Dental Products, Tulsa, Okla.)

vide both lateral and vertical movement of the softened gutta-percha (Fig. 9-72). The position of the carrier and gutta-percha can be determined radiographically; if the position is satisfactory, the top of the carrier is cut off 1 to 2 mm above the orifice. This is done with a no. 35 or no. 37 inverted cone, while holding the handle with firm apical pressure. A no. 37 inverted-cone bur is used to trim off the shaft 2 mm above the coronal orifice. Specific burs have also been developed for this task (Prepost Preparation Instrument—Prepi Bur, Tulsa Dental Products, Tulsa, Okla.) (see Fig. 9-71, *D*).

If the obturated root canal is wide buccolingually, a spreader or plugger may be inserted alongside the core, compacting the entire mass and creating space for additional gutta-percha (Fig. 9-73). Accessory cones are added laterally, coupled with concomitant lateral or vertical compaction (Fig. 9-74). If sufficient space is present, an injectable technique can also be used along with appropriate compaction. The cold cones easily become embedded in the softened mass. The gutta-percha sets in about 2 to 4 minutes. The root strains associated with the compaction of gutta-percha delivered from the Obtura and ThermaFil with lateral compaction have been evaluated and compared.[150] The ThermaFil technique required only minimal compaction that was limited to the coronal end of the carrier. Therefore with this technique there was significantly less strain during delivery and compaction than the other filling techniques.

The precurving of ThermaFil obturators is not necessary if the canal is prepared properly, because the flexible carrier will easily move around curves. With this technique, gutta-percha will flow into canal irregularities, such as fins, anastomoses, lateral canals, and resorptive cavities.[67]

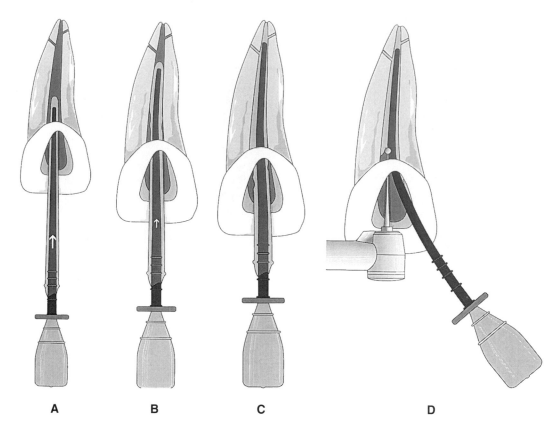

A   **B**   **C**   **D**

Fig. 9-71 **A,** Heated carrier is positioned in the canal orifice and placed slowly into the canal without twisting. **B,** As the carrier is placed deeper, the softened gutta-percha contacts the walls of the canal and begins to flow apically and laterally. **C,** As the core reaches the apical third, the softened gutta-percha reaches the canal constriction, slows the apical movement of the gutta-percha, and delivers a resistance to further apical movement of the core material. **D,** The core is cut at the canal orifice with a prepi bur or round bur; this is followed by further apical compaction.

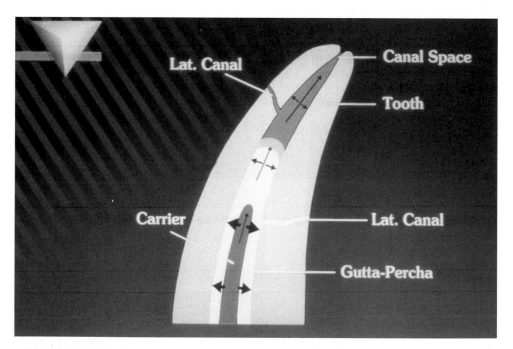

Fig. 9-72 Diagrammatic representation of gutta-percha movement in the root canal system during placement of a plastic ThermaFil core carrier. Note how the carrier can provide both lateral and vertical movement of the heat-softened material. (Courtesy Tulsa Dental Products, Tulsa, Okla.)

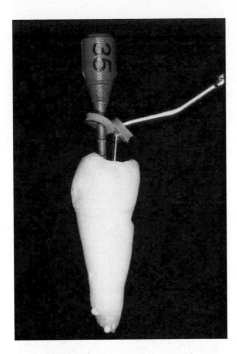

Fig. 9-73 Placement of a root canal spreader adjacent to a heated and positioned ThermaFil core gutta-percha carrier resulted in further compaction and movement of gutta-percha and sealer through root canal foramina. This approach is necessary in wide buccolingual canals and allows for a more 3-D obturation.

Radiographic assessment of this delivery technique has been shown to be quite favorable[66] (Fig. 9-75), and leakage studies have shown the sealability of the technique to be equal to, if not better than, lateral compaction.[42,67,153] Most recently both short- and long-term leakage was reported, when comparing ThermaFil with System B in the absence of the smear layer.[98] There were no significant differences in the short-term leakage patterns (10 and 24 days), but leakage at 67 days was greater in the ThermaFil group. Unlike other studies, however, these specimens were stored in Hanks Balanced Salt Solution to simulate the periradicular tissue fluid environment.

With this method of obturation, adaptation of gutta-percha to the prepared canal walls and irregularities has been determined to be excellent[67,116] (Fig. 9-76). Clinical parameters of application have also been favorable in its rapidity and efficiency of use[69,116] (Fig. 9-77).

Post space preparation with this technique has been evaluated and facilitated through the use of various instruments. The space necessary for an intraradicular post can be created immediately or on a delayed basis without altering the apical seal[149] (Fig. 9-78). Effective use of Peeso reamers, Prepi burs (Tulsa Dental Products, Tulsa, Okla.), or ThermaCut burs (Maillefer Instruments SA, Ballaigues, Switzerland) has resulted in rapid softening and removal of the coronal portion of the plastic carrier and gutta-percha (see Chapter 21 for further details).

Thermomechanical Compaction   The thermocompaction of gutta-percha, introduced in 1979, was an innovative approach to heat softening and canal obturation. Using a newly developed instrument called a *McSpadden Compactor,* gutta-percha was softened with the rotary action of the instrument in the canal and moved apically and laterally within the prepared system. Entrepreneurial efforts resulted in the further development of rotary compactors, such as the *Condenser* (Maillefer Instruments SA, Ballaigues, Switzerland) and the *Engine Plugger* (Zipperer, VDW, Munich, Germany). Recent developments have resulted in compactors precoated with gutta-percha, such as JS Quick-fill (JS Dental, Ridgefield, Conn.), and the injectable system of coating compactors, such as *Multi-Phase II Pac Mac Compactors* (NT Company, Chattanooga, Tenn.).

Initially there were numerous studies that evaluated the efficacy of this technique of canal obturation. Findings were highly variable but appeared positive. These techniques were rapid, the seal of the canal system appeared adequate, and adaptation of the material was acceptable.* Initial problems included vertical root fractures, cutting of dentin, and breakage of compactors.[118,124] Likewise, the potential for the generation of excessive and deleterious frictional heat levels on the external root surface has been identified.[10,37,70,145,146] Therefore, for the technique to be efficacious, slower speeds and low-temperature gutta-percha were identified as necessary to minimize both temperatures and stress on the root canal system during rotary compaction. Likewise, careful canal shaping and careful depth of penetration of the rotary compactor helps to prevent potential problems with this technique.

Because of the multiple variations with this technique, only the essence of the process is presented. The clinician is advised to learn the nuances involved with each technique on extracted teeth or tooth models before patient application.

Thermocompaction technique.   A master cone is fit in the canal (as discussed in previous techniques) and placed in the canal with sealer. Good adaptation to the canal length and shape is essential. The rotating compactor is placed in the canal and moved apically with gentle pressure to a point 3 to 4 mm short of the working length (or until resistance is met). The compactor is then removed, while still rotating and compacting the gutta-percha apically and laterally. If the canal is too wide, the master cone and additional cones may be added before compaction. After the initial rotary compaction, additional gutta-percha may be added in many different ways.

Variation 1.   The master cone in the apical portion of the canal may be laterally or vertically compacted. This is followed by the thermocompaction of the cones in the canal (i.e., lateral technique) or the fitting of an additional large cone followed by thermocompaction.

Variation 2.   An appropriately sized compactor (i.e., 0.02 or 0.04 taper) is coated with a beta phase gutta-percha (e.g., multiPhase I), which is then overcoated with an alpha phase gutta-percha (e.g., multiPhase II) (NT Company,

---

*References 28,71,94,102,144,171.

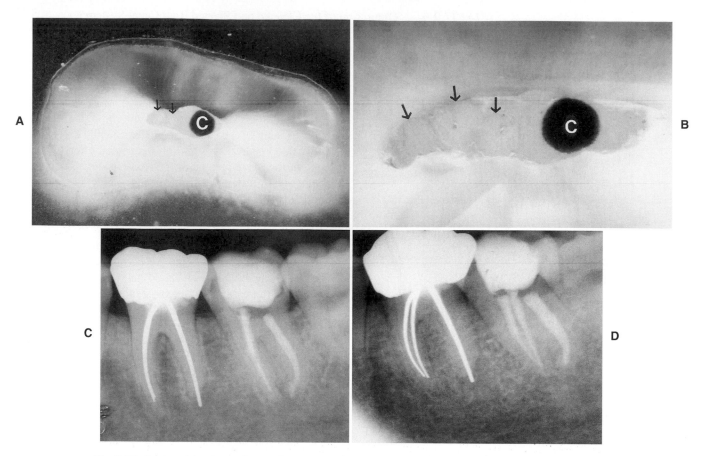

Fig. 9-74 Sectioned distal root of a mandibular first molar. **A**, Section at the junction of the apical and middle thirds after the placement of a plastic, ThermaFil carrier, and the use of lateral compaction with accessory cones. Arrows indicate position of the accessory cones. Gutta-percha surrounding the plastic core (C) is from the carrier. **B**, Section at the junction of the middle and coronal thirds. Three accessory canals *(arrows)* are visible and are embedded in the thermoplasticized gutta-percha of the core carrier (C). **C**, Mandibular molar with all canals obturated with the ThermaFil technique. Distal canal has had additional lateral compaction and the placement of accessory cones. **D**, Mesial view shows the obturation of the wide distal canal and why it is necessary to use additional cones to achieve a 3-D fill.

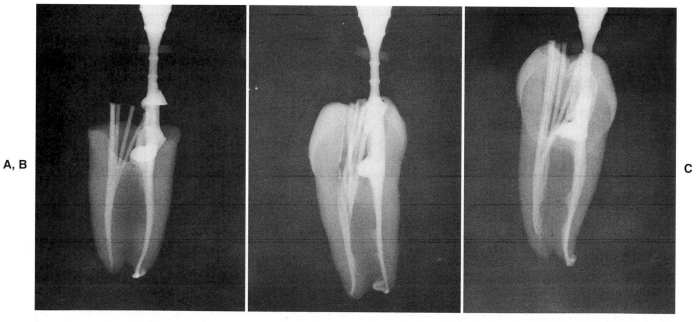

Fig. 9-75 **A** to **C**, Three mesial roots from mandibular molars from a proximal view. One canal was filled with gutta-percha and sealer using lateral compaction; the other canal in each root was filled using the ThermaFil technique. In **A**, the quality of the obturations is comparable; in **B**, the ThermaFil obturation is long but shows movement of material into canal eccentricities; in **C**, the quality of the ThermaFil obturation is superior to that of lateral compaction.

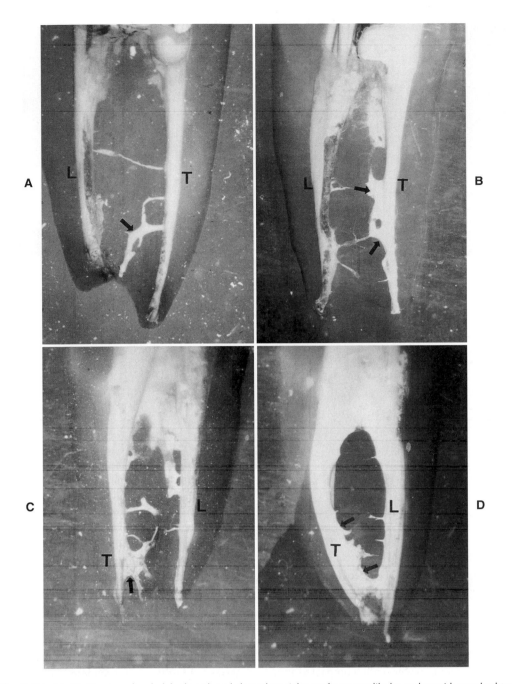

Fig. 9-76 **A** to **D**, Demineralized, dehydrated, and cleared mesial roots from mandibular molars with canals obturated with either lateral compaction (*L*) or ThermaFil (*T*). All roots are viewed from the proximal view. Generally speaking there is greater movement of both gutta-percha and sealer into the canal irregularities when filled using the ThermaFil technique. Note specifically the areas marked with arrows.

Chatanooga, Tenn.). Sealer is placed on the outer surface of the gutta-percha. The triple-coated compactor is inserted apically slightly short (i.e., 0.5 mm) of the working length as possible, without excessive force and without rotation. The force of placement is along the long axis of the compactor. The compactor is rotated at 4000 to 5000 RPM in a special reduction hand piece without exerting apical pressure and resisting backpressure. The compactor is then moved in a circular pattern for 2 seconds and withdrawn slowly while gentle pressure is applied on one side of the canal. Rotation continues until the compactor is fully withdrawn. The chamber may be cleaned of any sealer and gutta-percha as previously discussed.

Variation 3.   If the apical foramen is open because of resorption, overinstrumentation, or lack of growth, a bolus of beta phase gutta-percha may be deposited near the foramen and carefully compacted; or an artificial apical barrier may also be placed (refer to *Use of Apical Barriers* in this chapter), followed by the delivery of a thermocompacted cone or the presoftened injected-coated compactor obturation.

ferent clinician. This case can be used to identify subtle shortcomings based on the goals presented in this chapter. First, notice the voids in the fillings in the canals of the second molar, compared with the first molar. Notice also the length of the obturated space and the variations in the density of the fills from the orifice to the apex. The key determining factor in this case is not so much the shortcomings in the obturation technique but the lack of proper shaping of the canals in the second molar that, in all likelihood, prevented a more thorough obturation of the canals. Before any clinician begins to troubleshoot obturation techniques and outcomes, it is necessary to ensure that canal preparation techniques are at the standard of care necessary to achieve the goals cited for canal obturation.

Case 5

A patient had a maxillary premolar that had had root canal treatment and a crown. The patient wanted a new crown for aesthetic reasons, because the recently placed crown had come off. Radiographic examination of the case showed a poorly shaped and obturated root canal, with definite voids and unfilled canal space, both laterally and apically (Fig. 9-83, *A*). When advised that a new crown would not be made until the shortcomings in the root canal treatment were rectified, the patient stated that a root canal treatment had been performed 2 months ago and everything had been fine since that time. The patient could not understand why the root canal treatment needed revising and complained to his previous dentist, who felt that the root canal treatment was not only acceptable but was at the standard of care. Six weeks later the patient returned with severe pain to percussion and palpation on the maxillary premolar and agreed to have the root canal retreatment. A new working length was estab-

lished (Fig. 9-83, *B*), and the canal was properly cleaned, shaped, and obturated (Fig. 9-83, *C*). Comparison of the treatment rendered in this case demonstrates the levels of achievement that are necessary to ensure predictable outcomes with endodontic treatment or, as stated in the beginning of this chapter, quality assurance. Achievement of these levels of treatment on a regular basis ensures that the care provided for patients is at the standard of care.

The final case of this chapter is presented as a standard and a realistic goal that can be routinely achieved by all who choose to do root canal treatment for their patients. This achievement is predicated, however, on a triad of knowledge, application, and assessment, all integrated into a successful outcome.

Case 6

A female patient reported episodes of spontaneous pain over the past year. The mandibular first molar was tender to bite and often displayed sensitivity to hot and cold. The tooth was determined to have an irreversible pulpitis with acute periradicular periodontitis (Fig. 9-84, *A*). The root canal treatment was begun and completed in one visit. All canals were prepared using .04 and .06 rotary, NiTi rotary files to an approximate size 30 at the apical extent of the canal, which was determined to be slightly within the confines of the root. Four canals were obturated with warm, vertical compaction of a nonstandardized gutta-percha cone and pulp canal sealer, using the System B and Obtura II injectable techniques (Fig. 9-84, *B*). Technically, this case embodies the concepts of contemporary endodontics and sets a standard of achievement that should be emulated by all clinicians. (Case courtesy Dr. Myron S. Hilton.)

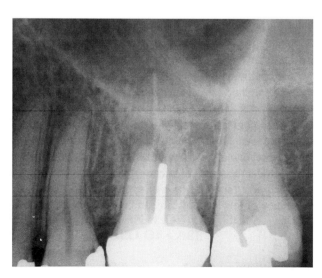

Fig. 9-81 Case 3.

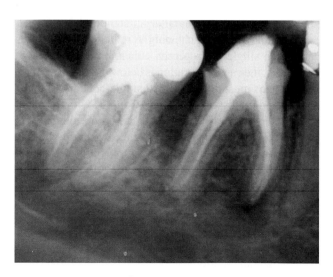

Fig. 9-82 Case 4.

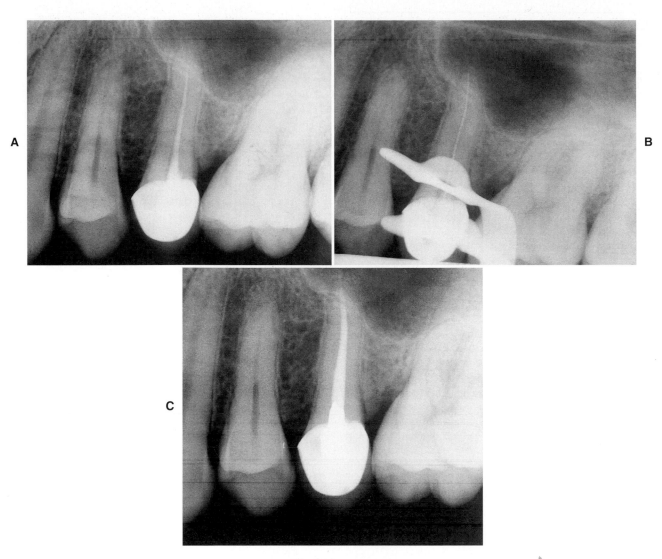

Fig. 9-83 Case 5.

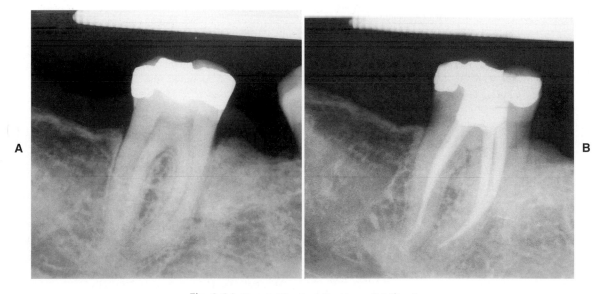

Fig. 9-84 Case 6. (Courtesy Dr. Myron S. Hilton.)

References

1. Adams WR, Patterson SS, Swartz ML: The effect of the apical dentinal plug on broken endodontic instruments, *J Endod* 5:121, 1979.
2. Aktener BO, Cengiz T, Piskin B: The penetration of smear material into dentinal tubules during instrumentation with surface active reagents: a scanning electron microscopic study, *J Endod* 15:588, 1989.
3. Al-Khatib ZZ et al: The antimicrobial affect of various endodontic sealers, *Oral Surg Oral Med Oral Pathol Oral Radiol Endod* 70:784, 1990.
4. Allison DA, Weber CR, Walton RE: The influence of the method of canal preparation on the quality of apical and coronal obturation, *J Endod* 5:298, 1979.
5. American Association of Endodontists: *Appropriateness of care and quality assurance guidelines,* Chicago, 1994, The Association.
6. American Association of Endodontists: *Glossary, contemporary terminology for endodontics,* ed 6, Chicago, 1998, The Association.
7. Barbosa SV, Burkard DH, Spångberg LSW: Cytotoxic effects of gutta-percha solvents, *J Endod* 20:6, 1994.
8. Barkhordar RA, Goodis HE, Wantanabe L, Koumdjian J: Evaluation of temperature rise on the outer surface of teeth during root canal obturation techniques, *Quintessence Int* 21: 585, 1990.
9. Baumgartner JC, Mader CL: A scanning electron microscopic evaluation of four root canal irrigations regimens, *J Endod* 13:147, 1987.
10. Beatty RG, Vertucci FJ, Hojjatie B: Thermomechanical compaction of gutta-percha: effect of speed and duration, *J Endod* 21:367, 1988.
11. Behrend GD, Cutler CW, Gutmann JL: An in vitro study of smear layer removal and microbial leakage along root canal fillings, *Int Endod J* 29:99, 1996.
12. Berg B: The endodontic management of multirooted teeth, *Oral Surg Oral Med Oral Pathol Oral Radiol Endod* 6:399, 1953.
13. Berry KA, Primack PD, Loushine RJ: Nickel-titanium versus stainless steel finger spreaders in curved canals, *J Endod* 21: 221, 1995.
14. Block RM et al: Antibody formation to dog pulp tissue altered by "N2" paste within the root canal, *J Endod* 3:309, 1977.
15. Block RM et al: Systemic distribution of N2 paste containing paraformaldehyde following root canal therapy in dogs, *Oral Surg Oral Med Oral Pathol Oral Radiol Endod* 50:350, 1980.
16. Boiesen J, Brodin P: Neurotoxic effect of two root canal sealers with calcium hydroxide on rat phrenic nerve in vitro, *Endod Dent Traumatol* 7:242, 1991.
17. Brannström M: Smear layer: pathological and treatment considerations, *Oper Dent Suppl* 3:35, 1984.
18. Brilliant JD, Christie WH: A taste of endodontics, *J Acad Gen Dent* 23:29, 1975.
19. Briseno BM, Willerhausen B: Root canal sealer cytotoxicity on human gingival fibroblasts. I. Zinc oxide-eugenol based sealers, *J Endod* 16:383, 1990.
20. Briseno BM, Willerhausen B: Root canal sealer cytotoxicity on human gingival fibroblasts. II. Silicone- and resin-based sealers, *J Endod* 17:537, 1991.
21. Briseno BM, Willerhausen B: Root canal sealer cytotoxicity on human gingival fibroblasts. III. Calcium hydroxide-n-based sealers, *J Endod* 18:110, 1992.
22. Brodin P, Roed A, Aars H, Ørstavik D: Neurotoxic effects of root filling materials on rat phrenic nerve in vitro, *J Dent Res* 61:1020, 1982.
23. Brownlee WA: Filling of root canals in recently devitalized teeth, *Dominion Dent J* 12(8):254, 1900.
24. Buchanan LS: The continuous wave of obturation technique: "centered" condensation of warm gutta-percha in 12 seconds, *Dent Today* 15:60, 1996.
25. Buckley M, Spångberg L: The prevalence and technical quality of endodontic treatment in an American subpopulation, *Oral Surg Oral Med Oral Pathol Oral Radiol Endod* 79:92, 1995.
26. Callahan JR: Rosin, solution for the sealing of the dental tubuli and as an adjuvant in the filling of root canals, *Allied Dent J* 9(53):110, 1914.
27. Cameron JA: The use of ultrasound for the removal of the smear layer: the effect of sodium hypochlorite concentrations: SEM study, *Aust Dent J* 33:193, 1988.
28. Chaisrisookumporn S, Rabinowitz JL: Evaluation of ionic leakage of lateral condensation and McSpadden methods by autoradiography, *J Endod* 8:493, 1982.
29. Ciucchi B, Khettabi M, Holz J: The effectiveness of different endodontic irrigation procedures on the removal of the smear layer: a scanning electron microscopic study, *Int Endod J* 22: 21, 1989.
30. Coviello J, Brilliant JD: A preliminary clinical study on the use of tricalcium phosphate as an apical barrier, *J Endod* 5:6, 1979.
31. Davalou S, Gutmann JL, Nunn MH: Assessment of apical and coronal root canal seals using contemporary endodontic obturation and restorative materials and techniques. *Int Endod J* 32:388, 1999.
32. Dow PR, Ingle JI: Isotope determination of root canal failures, *Oral Surg Oral Med Oral Pathol Oral Radiol Endod* 8:1100, 1955.
33. Dwan JJ, Glickman GN: 2-D photoelastic stress analysis of NiTi and stainless steel finger spreaders during lateral condensation, *J Endod* 21:221, 1995.
34. Ebert J, Pawlick H, Petschelt A: Relation between dye penetration and radiographic assessment of root canal fillings in vitro, *Int Endod J* 29:198, 1996.
35. ElDeeb ME, Nguyen TT-Q, Jensen JR: The dentinal plug: its effect on confining substances to the canal and on the apical seal, *J Endod* 9:355, 1983.
36. Evans JT, Simon JHS: Evaluation of the apical seal produced by injected thermoplasticized gutta-percha in the absence of smear layer and root canal sealer, *J Endod* 12:101, 1986.
37. Fors U, Jonasson E, Bergquist A, Berg J-O: Measurements of the root surface temperature during thermomechanical root canal filling in vitro, *Int Endod J* 18:199, 1985.
38. Friedman CE, Sandrik JL, Heuer MA, Rapp GW: Composition and physical properties of gutta-percha endodontic filling materials, *J Endod* 3:304, 1977.
39. Friedman CE, Sandrik JL, Heuer MA, Rapp GW: Composition and mechanical properties of gutta-percha endodontic points, *J Dent Res* 54:921, 1975.
40. Fulkerson MS, Czerw RJ, Donnelly JC: An in vitro evaluation of the sealing ability of Super-EBA cement used as a root canal sealer, *J Endod* 22:13, 1996.

41. Gee JY: A comparison of five methods of root canal obturation by means of dye penetration, *Aust Dent J* 32:279, 1987.
42. Gençoglu N, Samani S, Günday M: Dentinal wall adaptation of thermoplasticized gutta-percha in the absence or presence of smear layer: a scanning electron microscopic study, *J Endod* 19:558, 1993.
43. Gençoglu N, Samani S, Günday M: Evaluation of sealing properties of Thermafil and Ultrafil techniques in the absence or presence of smear layer, *J Endod* 19:599, 1993.
44. Genet JM, Hart AAM, Wesselink PR, Thoden van Velzen SK: Preoperative and operative factors associated with pain after the first endodontic visit, *Int Endod J* 20:53, 1987.
45. Gettleman BH, Messer HH, ElDeeb ME: Adhesion of sealer cements to dentin with and without the smear layer, *J Endod* 17:15, 1991.
46. Gimlin DR, Parr CH, Aguirre-Ramirez G: A comparison of stress produced during lateral and vertical condensation using engineering models, *J Endod* 12:235, 1986.
47. Goldman LB et al: The efficacy of several irrigating solutions for endodontics: a scanning electron microscopic study, *Oral Surg Oral Med Oral Pathol Oral Radiol Endod* 52:197, 1981.
48. Goldman M: Evaluation of two filling methods for root canals, *J Endod* 1:69, 1975.
49. Goldman M et al: The efficacy of several endodontic irrigating solutions: a scanning electron microscopic study: part 2, *J Endod* 8:487, 1982.
50. Göllmer L: Grund der reparativen Fahigkeit der Wurzelhaut (The use of dentin debris as a root canal filling), *Z Stomatol* 34:761, 1936.
51. Goodman A, Schilder H, Aldrich W: The thermomechanical properties of gutta-percha. II. The history and molecular structure of gutta-percha, *Oral Surg Oral Med Oral Pathol Oral Radiol Endod* 37:954, 1974.
52. Goon WWY: The apical push: hermetic seal enhancement using lateral condensation into warm gutta-percha, *Compend Contin Educ Dent* 6:499, 1985.
53. Grahnén H, Hansson L: The prognosis of pulp and root canal therapy: a clinical and radiographic follow-up examination, *Odontol Revy* 12:146, 1961.
54. Granche D et al: Endodontic cements induce alterations in the cell cycle of in vitro cultured osteoblasts, *Oral Surg Oral Med Oral Pathol Oral Radiol Endod* 79:359, 1995.
55. Grossman LI: *Root canal therapy,* Philadelphia, 1940, Lea & Febiger, p 189.
56. Grove CJ: Why root canals should be filled to the dentinocemental junction, *J Am Dent Assoc* 17:293, 1930.
57. Gutmann JL: Clinical, radiographic, and histologic perspectives on success and failure in endodontics, *Dent Clin North Am* 36:379, 1992.
58. Gutmann JL: The dentin-root complex: anatomic and biologic considerations in restoring endodontically treated teeth, *J Prosthet Dent* 67:458, 1992.
59. Gutmann JL: Adaptation of injected thermoplasticized gutta-percha in the absence of the dentinal smear layer, *Int Endod J* 26:87, 1993.
60. Gutmann JL, Heaton JF: Management of the open (immature) apex. II. Non-vital teeth, *Int Endod J* 14:173, 1981.
61. Gutmann JL, Hovland EJ: Problems in root canal obturation. In Gutmann JL, Dumsha TC, Lovdahl PE, Hovland EJ, editors: *Problem solving in endodontics,* ed 3, St Louis, 1997, Mosby.
62. Gutmann JL, Leonard JE: Problem solving in endodontic working length determination, *Compend Contin Educ Dent* 16:288, 1995.
63. Gutmann JL, Lovdahl PE: Problems in the assessment of success and failure, quality assurance and their integration into endodontic treatment planning. In Gutmann JL, Dumsha TC, Lovdahl PE, Hovland EJ, editors: *Problem solving in endodontics,* ed 3, St Louis, 1997, Mosby.
64. Gutmann JL, Rakusin H: Perspectives on root canal obturation with thermoplasticized injectable gutta-percha, *Int Endod J* 20:261, 1987.
65. Gutmann JL, Rakusin H, Powe R, Bowles WH: Evaluation of heat transfer during root canal obturation with thermoplasticized gutta-percha. II. In-vivo response to heat levels generated, *J Endod* 13:441, 1987.
66. Gutmann JL, Saunders WP, Saunders EM, Nguyen L: An assessment of the plastic Thermafil obturation technique. I. Radiographic evaluation of adaptation and placement, *Int Endod J* 26:173, 1993.
67. Gutmann JL, Saunders WP, Saunders EM, Nguyen L: An assessment of the plastic Thermafil obturation technique. II. Material adaptation and sealability, *Int Endod J* 26:179, 1993.
68. Haas SB et al: A comparison of four root canal filling techniques, *J Endod* 15:596, 1989.
69. Haddix JE, Jarrell M, Mattison GD, Pink FE: An in vitro investigation of the apical seal produced by a new thermoplasticized gutta-percha obturation technique, *Quintessence Int* 22:159, 1991.
70. Hardie EM: Heat transmission to the outer surface of the tooth during the thermomechanical compaction technique of root canal obturation, *Int Endod J* 19:73, 1986.
71. Harris GZ, Dickey DJ, Lemon RR, Luebke RG: Apical seal: McSpadden vs. lateral condensation, *J Endod* 8:273, 1982.
72. Harrison JW, Baumgartner JC, Svec TA: Incidence of pain associated with clinical factors during and after root canal therapy. II. Postobturation pain, *J Endod* 9:434, 1983.
73. Harvey TE, White JT, Leeb IJ: Lateral condensation stress in root canals, *J Endod* 7:151, 1981.
74. Hasegawa M et al: An experimental study of the sealing ability of a dentinal apical plug treated with bonding agent, *J Endod* 19:570, 1993.
75. Hasselgren G: Where shall the root filling end? *N Y State Dent J* 60(6):34, 1994.
76. Hatton EH: Changes produced in the pulp and periapical regions, and their relationship to pulp-canal treatment and to systemic disease, *Dent Cosmos* 66:1183, 1924.
77. Hatton JF, Ferrillo PJ, Wagner G, Stewart GP: The effect of condensation pressure on the apical seal, *J Endod* 14:305, 1988.
78. Heling I, Chandler NP: The antimicrobial effect within dentinal tubules of four root canal sealers, *J Endod* 22:257, 1996.
79. *History of dentistry in Missouri,* Fulton, Mo, 1938, The Ovid Press, Inc.
80. Holcomb J, Pitts D, Nicholls J: Further investigation of spreader loads required to cause vertical root fracture during lateral condensation, *J Endod* 13:277, 1987.
81. Holland GR: Periapical response to apical plugs of dentin and calcium hydroxide in ferret canines, *J Endod* 10:71, 1984.
82. Holland R, de Souza V: Ability of a new calcium hydroxide root canal filling material to induce hard tissue formation, *J Endod* 11:535, 1985.

83. Holland R et al: Tissue reactions following apical plugging of the root canal with infected dentin chips, *Oral Surg Oral Med Oral Pathol Oral Radiol Endod* 49:366, 1980.

84. Hunter W: The role of sepsis and of antisepsis in medicine, *Lancet* 1:79, 1911.

85. Ingle JI: A standardized endodontic technique using newly designed instruments and filling materials, *Oral Surg Oral Med Oral Pathol Oral Radiol Endod* 14:83, 1961.

86. Ingle JI, Zeldow BJ: An evaluation of mechanical instrumentation and the negative culture in endodontic therapy, *J Am Dent Assoc* 57:471, 1958.

87. Jacobsen EL: Clinical aid: adapting the master gutta-percha cone for apical snugness, *J Endod* 10:274, 1984.

88. Jerome CE: Warm vertical gutta-percha obturation: a technique update, *J Endod* 20:97, 1994.

89. Johnson WB: A new gutta-percha technique, *J Endod* 4:184, 1978.

90. Kaplowitz GJ: Evaluation of gutta-percha solvents, *J Endod* 16:539, 1990.

91. Karagöz-Kücükay I, Bayirli G: An apical leakage study in the presence and absence of the smear layer, *Int Endod J* 27:87, 1994.

92. Keane HC: A century of service to dentistry, Philadelphia, 1944, SS White Dental Manufacturing Co.

93. Keane K, Harrington GW: The use of a chloroform-softened gutta-percha master cone and its effect on the apical seal, *J Endod* 10:57, 1984.

94. Kersten HW, Fransman R, Thoden van Velzen SK: Thermomechanical compaction of gutta-percha. I. A comparison of several compaction procedures, *Int Endod J* 19:125, 1986.

95. Kersten HW, Wesselink PR, Thoden van Velzen SK: The diagnostic reliability of the buccal radiograph after root canal filling, *Int Endod J* 20:20, 1987.

96. Koch CRE, Thorpe BL: *A history of dental surgery,* vols 2 and 3, Fort Wayne, Ind., 1909, National Art Publishing Co.

97. Kontakiotis E, Panopoulos P: pH of root canal sealers containing calcium hydroxide, *Int Endod J* 29:202, 1996.

98. Kytridou V, Gutmann JL, Nunn MH: Adaptation and sealability of two contemporary obturation techniques in the absence of the dentinal smear layer, *Int Endod J* 32:464, 1999.

99. Langeland K: Root canal sealants and pastes, *Dent Clin North Am* 18:309, 1974.

100. Leonard JE, Gutmann JL, Guo IY: Apical and coronal seal of roots obturated with a dentine bonding agent and resin, *Int Endod J* 29:76, 1996.

101. Love RM, Chandler NP, Jenkinson HF: Penetration of smeared or nonsmeared dentine by *Streptococcus gordonii, Int Endod J* 29:2, 1996.

102. Lugassy AA, Yee F: Root canal obturation with gutta-percha: a scanning electron microscope comparison of vertical compaction and automated thermatic condensation, *J Endod* 8:120, 1982.

103. Mader CL, Baumgartner JC, Peters DD: Scanning electron microscopic investigation of the smeared layer on root canal walls, *J Endod* 10:477, 1984.

104. Marais JT, van der Vyver PJ: Sizing gutta-percha points with a gauge to ensure optimal lateral condensation, *J Dent Assoc South Afr* 51:403, 1996.

105. Martin H, Fischer E: Photoelastic stress comparison of warm (Endotec) versus cold lateral condensation techniques, *Oral Surg Oral Med Oral Pathol Oral Radiol Endod* 70:325, 1990.

106. Martin H, Martin TR: Iodoform gutta-percha: MGP, a new endodontic paradigm. *Dent Today* 18(4):76, 1999.

107. McComb D, Smith DC: A preliminary scanning electron microscopic study of root canals after endodontic procedures, *J Endod* 7:238, 1975.

108. McDonald NM, Vire DE: Chloroform in the endodontic operatory, *J Endod* 18:301, 1992.

109. Metzger Z et al: Apical seal by customized versus standardized master cones: a comparative study in flat and round canals, *J Endod* 14:381, 1988.

110. Metzger Z et al: Residual chloroform and plasticity in customized gutta-percha master cones, *J Endod* 14:546, 1988.

111. Molyvdas I, Zervas P, Lanbrianidis T, Veis A: Periodontal tissue reactions following root canal obturation with an injection-thermoplasticized gutta-percha technique, *Endod Dent Traumatol* 5:32, 1989.

112. Moorer WR, Genet JM: Antibacterial activity of gutta-percha cones attributed to the zinc oxide component, *Oral Surg Oral Med Oral Pathol Oral Radiol Endod* 53:508, 1982.

113. Moorer WR, Genet JM: Evidence for antibacterial activity of endodontic gutta-percha cones, *Oral Surg Oral Med Oral Pathol Oral Radiol Endod* 53:503, 1982.

114. Mulhern JM, Patterson SS, Newton CW, Ringel AM: Incidence of postoperative pain after one-appointment endodontic treatment of a symptomatic pulpal necrosis in single-rooted teeth, *J Endod* 2:370, 1982.

115. Nguyen NT: Obturation of the root canal system. In Cohen S, Burns RC, editors: *Pathways of the pulp,* ed 6, St Louis, 1994, Mosby, pp. 219-271.

116. Nykaza R, Wong M: Heat-softened gutta-percha: an update, *Gen Dent* 39:196, 1991.

117. O'Keefe EM: Pain in endodontic therapy: a preliminary clinical study, *J Endod* 2:315, 1976.

118. O'Neill KJ, Pitts DL, Harrington GW: Evaluation of the apical seal produced by the McSpadden compactor and by lateral condensation with a chloroform-softened primary cone, *J Endod* 9:190, 1983.

119. Oksan T, Aktener BO, Sen BH, Tezel H: The penetration of root canal sealers into dentinal tubules: a scanning electron microscopic study, *Int Endod J* 26:301, 1993.

120. Olgart L, Brannström M, Johnson G: Invasion of bacteria into dentinal tubules: experiments in-vivo and in-vitro, *Acta Odontol Scand* 32:61, 1974.

121. Orban B: Why root canals should be filled to the dentinocemental junction, *J Am Dent Assoc* 17:1086, 1930.

122. Orstavik D, Haapasalo M: Disinfection by endodontic irrigants and dressings or experimentally infected dentinal tubules, *Endod Dent Traumatol* 6:142, 1990.

123. Oswald RJ, Friedman CE: Periapical response to dentin filings, *Oral Surg Oral Med Oral Pathol Oral Radiol Endod* 49: 344, 1980.

124. Page ML, Hargreaves KM, ElDeeb M: Comparison of concentric condensation technique with laterally condensed gutta-percha, *J Endod* 21:308, 1995.

125. Pallarés A, Faus V, Glickman GN: The adaptation of mechanically softened gutta-percha to the canal walls in the presence or absence of smear layer: a scanning electron microscopic study, *Int Endod J* 28:266, 1995.

126. Parris J, Wilcox L, Walton R: Effectiveness of apical clearing: histological and radiographic evaluation, *J Endod* 20: 219, 1994.

127. Pashley DH: Smear layer: physiological considerations, *Oper Dent* (suppl) 3:13, 1984.

128. Pashley DH et al: Scanning electron microscopy of the substructure of smear layers in human dentine, *Arch Oral Biol* 33:265, 1988.

129. Perry SG: Preparing and filling the roots of teeth, *Dent Cosmos* 25:185, 1883.

130. Peters LB, Wesselink PR, Moorer WR: The fate and role of bacteria left in root dentinal tubules, *Int Endod J* 28:95, 1995.

131. Pitts DL, Jones JE, Oswald RJ: A histological comparison of calcium hydroxide plugs and dentin plugs used for the control of gutta-percha root canal filling material, *J Endod* 10:283, 1984.

132. Portmann P, Lussi A: A comparison between a new vacuum obturation technique and lateral condensation: an in vitro study, *J Endod* 20:292, 1994.

133. Prinz H: Filling root canals with an improved paraffin compound. Paper delivered to the St Louis Dental Society, St Louis, Sept 2, 1912.

134. Ramsey WO: Hermetic sealing of root canals: the Greeks had a name for it, *J Endod* 8:100, 1982.

135. Ray H, Seltzer S: A new glass ionomer root canal sealer, *J Endod* 17:598, 1991.

136. Ray HA, Trope M: Periapical status of endodontically treated teeth in relation to the technical quality of the root filling and the coronal restoration, *Int Endod J* 28:12, 1995.

137. Ricks-Williamson LJ et al: A three-dimensional finite-element stress analysis of an endodontically prepared maxillary central incisor, *J Endod* 21:362, 1995.

138. Ricucci D, Langeland K: Apical limit of root canal instrumentation and obturation. II. A histological study, *Int Endod J* 31:394, 1998.

139. Roane JB, Dryden JA, Grimes EW: Incidence of postoperative pain after single- and multiple-visit endodontic procedures, *Oral Surg Oral Med Oral Pathol Oral Radiol Endod* 55:68, 1983.

140. Rosenow EC: Studies on elective localization: focal infection with special reference to oral sepsis, *J Dent Res* 1:205, 1919.

141. Rossmeisl R, Reader A, Melfi R, Marquard J: A study of freeze-dried (lyophilized) cortical bone used as an apical barrier in adult monkey teeth, *Oral Surg Oral Med Oral Pathol Oral Radiol Endod* 53:303, 1982.

142. Rud J, Andreasen JO: A study of failures after endodontic surgery by radiographic, histologic, and stereomicroscopic methods, *Int J Oral Surg* 1:311, 1972.

143. Sakkal S, Weine FS, Lemian L: Lateral condensation: inside view, *Compend Contin Educ Dent* 12:796, 1991.

144. Saunders EM: The effect of variation in thermomechanical compaction techniques upon the quality of the apical seal, *Int Endod J* 22:163, 1989.

145. Saunders EM: In vivo findings associated with heat generation during thermomechanical compaction of gutta-percha. I. Temperature levels at the external surface of the root, *Int Endod J* 23:263, 1990.

146. Saunders EM: In vivo findings associated with heat generation during thermomechanical compaction of gutta-percha. II. Histological response to temperature elevation on the external surface of the root, *Int Endod J* 23:268, 1990.

147. Saunders EM, Saunders WP: Long-term coronal leakage of JS Quickfill root fillings with Sealapex and Apexit sealers, *Endod Dent Traumatol* 11:181, 1995.

148. Saunders WP, Saunders EM: Coronal leakage as a cause of failure in root canal therapy: a review, *Endod Dent Traumatol* 10:105, 1994.

149. Saunders WP, Saunders EM, Gutmann JL, Gutmann ML: An assessment of the plastic Thermafil obturation technique. III. The effect of post space preparation on the apical seal, *Int Endod J* 26:184, 1993.

150. Saw L-P, Messer HH: Root strains associated with different obturation techniques, *J Endod* 21:314, 1995.

151. Schilder H: Filling root canals in three dimensions, *Dent Clin North Am* 11:723, 1967.

152. Schilder H, Goodman A, Aldrich W: The thermomechanical properties of gutta-percha. I. The compressibility of gutta-percha, *Oral Surg Oral Med Oral Pathol Oral Radiol Endod* 37:946, 1974.

153. Scott AC, Vire DE: An evaluation of the ability of a dentin plug to control extrusion of thermoplasticized gutta-percha, *J Endod* 18:52-57, 1992.

154. Seltzer S: *Endodontology: biologic considerations in endodontic procedures,* ed 2, Philadelphia, 1988, Lea & Febiger.

155. Seltzer S, Bender IB, Turkenkopf S: Factors affecting successful repair after root canal therapy, *J Am Dent Assoc* 67: 651, 1963.

156. Seltzer S, Naidorf I: Flare-ups in endodontics. II. Therapeutic measures, *J Endod* 11:559, 1985.

157. Sen BH, Piskin B, Baran N: The effect of tubular penetration of root canal sealers on dye microleakage, *Int Endod J* 29:23, 1996.

158. Sen BH, Wesselink PR, Türkün M: The smear layer: a phenomenon in root canal therapy, *Int Endod J* 28:141, 1995.

159. Sjögren U, Figdor D, Persson S, Sundqvist G: Influence of infection at the time of root filling in the outcome of endodontic treatment of teeth with apical periodontitis. *Int Endod J* 30: 297, 1997.

160. Sjögren U, Hägglund B, Sundqvist G, Wing K: Factors affecting the long-term results of endodontic treatment, *J Endod* 16: 498, 1990.

161. Sjögren U, Sundqvist G, Nair PNR: Tissue reaction to gutta-percha particles of various sizes when implanted subcutaneously in guinea pigs, *Eur J Oral Sci* 103:313, 1995.

162. Skillen WG: Why root canals should be filled to the dentino-cemental junction, *J Am Dent Assoc* 17:2082, 1930.

163. Skinner RL, Himel VT: The sealing ability of injection-molded thermoplasticized gutta-percha with and without the use of sealers, *J Endod* 13:315, 1987.

164. Sonat B, Dalat D, Günhan O: Periapical tissue reaction to root fillings with Sealapex, *Int Endod J* 23:46, 1990.

165. Southard D, Rooney T: Effective one-visit therapy for the acute apical abscess, *J Endod* 10:580, 1984.

166. Spångberg L: Biologic effect of root canal filling materials, *Odont Tidskr* 77:502, 1969.

167. Spångberg L: Biologic effects of root canal filling materials, *Odontol Revy* 20:133, 1969.

168. Speier MB, Glickman GN: Volumetric and densitometric comparison between nickel-titanium and stainless steel condensation, *J Endod* 22:195, 1996.

169. Stamos DE, Gutmann JL, Gettleman BH: In-vivo evaluation of root canal sealer placement and distribution, *J Endod* 21: 177, 1995.

170. Swartz DB, Skidmore AE, Griffin JA: Twenty years of endodontic success and failure, *J Endod* 9:198, 1983.

171. Tagger M, Katz A, Tamse A: Apical seal using the GPII method in straight canals compared with lateral condensation, with or without sealer, *Oral Surg Oral Med Oral Pathol Oral Radiol Endod* 78:225, 1994.

172. Tagger M, Taffer E, Kfir A: Release of calcium and hydroxyl ions from set endodontic sealers containing calcium hydroxide, *J Endod* 14:588, 1988.

173. Tagger M, Tanse A, Katz A, Korzen BH: Evaluation of the apical seal produced by a hybrid root canal filling method, combining lateral condensation and thermatic compaction, *J Endod* 10:299, 1984.

174. Telli C, Gülkan P, Günel H: A critical reevaluation of stresses generated during vertical and lateral condensation of gutta-percha in the root canal, *Endod Dent Traumatol* 10:1, 1994.

175. Torabinejad M, Chivian N. Clinical applications of mineral trioxide aggregate, *J Endod* 25:197, 1999.

176. Torneck CD, Smith JS, Grindall P: Biologic effects of procedures on developing incisor teeth. II. Effect of pulp injury and oral contamination, *Oral Surg Oral Med Oral Pathol Oral Radiol Endod* 35:378, 1973.

177. Tronstad L: Tissue reactions following apical plugging of the root canal with dentin chips in monkey teeth subjected to pulpectomy, *Oral Surg Oral Med Oral Pathol Oral Radiol Endod* 45:297, 1978.

178. Tronstad L, Barnett R, Flax M: Solubility and biocompatibility of calcium hydroxide-n-containing root canal sealers, *Endod Dent Traumatol* 4:152, 1988.

179. Veis A, Lambrianidis T, Molyvdas I, Zervas P: Sealing ability of sectional injection thermoplasticized gutta-percha technique with varying distance between needle tip and apical foramen, *Endod Dent Traumatol* 8:63, 1992.

180. Vire DE: Failure of endodontically treated teeth, *J Endod* 17:338, 1991.

181. Webster AE: Some experimental root canal fillings, *Dominion Dent J* 12:109, 1900.

182. Weinberger BW: *An introduction to the history of dentistry*, St Louis, 1948, Mosby.

183. Weine FS: The enigma of the lateral canal, *Dent Clin North Am* 28:833, 1984.

184. Weisenseel JA Jr, Hicks ML, Pelleu GB Jr: Calcium hydroxide as an apical barrier, *J Endod* 13:1, 1987.

185. Wennberg A, Ørstavik D: Adhesion of root canal sealers to bovine dentine and gutta-percha, *Int Endod J* 23:13, 1990.

186. White RR, Goldman M, Sun Lin P: The influence of the smeared layer upon dentinal tubule penetration by plastic filling materials, *J Endod* 10:558, 1984.

187. Wong M, Peters DB, Lorton L: Comparison of gutta-percha filling techniques: three chloroform gutta-percha filling techniques: part 2, *J Endod* 8:4, 1982.

188. Wu M-K, Wesselink PR: Endodontic leakage studies reconsidered. I. Methodology, application and relevance, *Int Endod J* 26:37, 1993.

189. Wu M-K et al: Fluid transport and bacterial penetration along root canal fillings, *Int Endod J* 26:203, 1993.

190. Yamada RS et al: A scanning electron microscopic comparison of a high volume final flush with several irrigating solutions: part III, *J Endod* 9:137, 1983.

191. Yaman SD, Alacam T, Yaman Y: Analysis of stress distribution in a vertically condensed maxillary central incisor root canal, *J Endod* 21:321, 1995.

192. Yared GM, Bou Dagher FE: Elongation and movement of the gutta-percha master cone during initial lateral condensation, *J Endod* 19:395, 1993.

193. Yee FA, Marlin J, Krakow AA, Grøn P: Three-dimensional obturation of the root canal using injection-molded, thermoplasticized dental gutta-percha, *J Endod* 3:168, 1977.

194. Yee RDJ, Newton CW, Patterson SS, Swartz M: The effect of canal preparation on the formation and leakage characteristics of the apical dentin plug, *J Endod* 10:308, 1984.

195. Youngson CC, Nattress BR, Manogue M, Speirs AF: In vitro radiographic representation of the extent of voids within obturated root canals, *Int Endod J* 28:77, 1995.

196. Zmener O et al: Biocompatibility of a thermoplasticized gutta-percha in the subcutaneous connective tissue of the rat, *J Dent Res* 67:616, 1988.

Chapter **10**

❖ **Records and Legal Responsibilities**

Edwin J. Zinman

Chapter Outline

ENDODONTIC RECORD EXCELLENCE

Importance

Endodontic therapy records serve as an important map to guide the clinician down the correct diagnostic and treatment path. Documentation is essential to attaining endodontic excellence.

Content

Endodontic treatment records should include the following information:

1. Name of patient
2. Date of visit
3. Medical and dental history (periodically updated)
4. Chief complaints
5. Radiographs of diagnostic quality
6. Clinical examination findings
7. Differential and final diagnosis
8. Treatment plan
9. Prognosis
10. Referral, including patient refusals (if any)
11. Communications with any other health care providers
12. Progress notes (including complications)
13. Completion notes
14. Canceled or missed appointments and stated reasons
15. Emergency treatment
16. Patient concerns and dissatisfactions
17. Planned follow ups
18. Drug and laboratory prescriptions
19. Patient noncompliance
20. Consent forms
21. Accounting
22. Recall notifications
23. Name or initial of entry author

Function

Dental records should document the following information:

1. Course of therapy by recorded diagnosis, informed consent, treatment, and prognosis
2. Communications among the treating dentist and other health care providers, consultants, subsequent treating practitioners, and third-party carriers
3. Necessity and reasonableness of diagnosis and treatment capable of peer review and insurance carrier evaluation
4. Standard of care compliance

Patient Information Form

A patient information form provides essential data for patient identification and office communication. The patient's name; home, business, and e-mail addresses; and telephone and fax numbers are needed to contact the patient for scheduling purposes and to inquire about postoperative sequelae.[35] Location information about the patient's spouse, relative, or a close friend who can be notified in an emergency is also suggested. In the event the patient is a minor, the responsible parent or guardian should provide the information. Questions about dental insurance and financial responsibility are included on the form to avoid any later misunderstandings and to help fulfill federal requirements of the Truth in Lending Law, applicable if four or more installment pay-

ments are arranged (whether or not there are interest or late-payment charges).[21b] Patient information and history forms should be updated periodically (Fig. 10-1).

Medical Health History

Past and present health status should be thoroughly reviewed by the dentist before proceeding with treatment so that dental treatment can be safely initiated. Health questionnaires open avenues for discussion about problems of major organ systems and important biochemical mechanisms, such as blood coagulation, allergy, immunocompromised status, and disease susceptibility. The dentist may request that the patient be examined by a physician or tested by a laboratory under medical supervision to determine whether a suspected medical problem may require attention before endodontic therapy proceeds or if drug sensitivity or allergy mandate treatment modifications.[37,70] Current medications, medical therapy, and the name and location of the treating physician to be contacted in the event of emergency is essential.

Medical histories must be updated periodically (or at least annually) as the need arises. The patient should be asked to view and review the history (see Fig. 10-5). If no changes are necessary, the patient should date and sign the history form. If any, the patient should identify each updated medical change and date and sign the form where indicated for medical update information. Periodically the patient should provide an entirely new updated form, rather than changing data on the old form. Earlier medical histories should be retained in the chart for future reference. If physician communication for treatment occurs, the clinician should record such contacts. In addition, the clinician should verify physician approvals by fax or letter or both, with copies retained in the chart.

Updating the medical history requires the practitioner to be apprised of changes in the patient's medical condition and any new medications that the patient is taking. A patient untrained in medical science may not appreciate the fact that new medication may suggest new diseases or changes in existing disease status. For instance, certain valvular heart diseases may require antibiotic prophylaxis. New medications may also cause a synergistic effect with other medications that the patient is using or the treating dentist is prescribing.

Dental History

The dental history should include past dental difficulties, name and address of current or most recent dentist, chief complaint (including duration and intensity of any pain), relevant prior dental treatment, and attitude regarding tooth retention. Positive responses suggest further patient consultation and consideration for obtaining records (by written release) for elucidation from the patient's previous dentist.[46]

PATIENT ACCOUNT INFORMATION

Name: _____ Social Security No.: _____ Today's Date: _____

Birth date: _____ Responsible Parent or Guardian's Name: _____

Marital Status: ____ Single   ____ Married   ____ Widowed   ____ Divorced

Address: _____ City: _____ State: _____ Zip Code: _____

E-mail Address: _____ Phone: _____ Fax: _____

REFERRED BY: _____ Patient Driver's License No.: _____

Occupation: _____ Employer: _____ How long: _____

Business Address: _____ City: _____ State: _____ Zip Code: _____

E-mail Address: _____ Phone: _____ Fax: _____

Spouse's Name: _____

Occupation: _____ Employer: _____ How long: _____

Business Address: _____ City: _____ State: _____ Zip Code: _____

E-mail Address: _____ Phone: _____ Fax: _____

PERSON FINANCIALLY RESPONSIBLE FOR ACCOUNT: _____

Address (if different from patient): _____

City: _____ State: _____ Zip Code: _____ Phone: _____

Relationship to patient: _____

DENTAL INSURANCE CARRIERS:

_____ Group No.: _____ Local No.: _____

Name of Insured Person: _____ Social Security No.: _____

Relationship to patient: _____

SECOND DENTAL INSURANCE CARRIER (if dual coverage):

_____ Group No.: _____ Local No.: _____

Name of Insured Person: _____ Social Security No.: _____

Relationship to patient: _____

Date: _____   Signature: _____

Fig. 10-1 Patient information form.

After receiving positive responses, the clinician may also wish to obtain prior radiographs for current comparison and notes of any progressive changes[63] (Fig. 10-2).

Diagnostic and Progress Records

Diagnostic and progress records often combine the "fill-in" and "check-off" types of forms. Fill-in or essay-type forms allow greater latitude of response to a question, resulting in a more detailed description. However, one drawback to these forms is that they are open to oversights unless a dentist is very conscientious in following up with further clinical information.

Using only an essay-type health history is insufficient. Often a patient may not appreciate the significance of important symptoms. Also, a check-off format is efficient and more practical. Forms with questions that reveal pertinent data alert the clinician to medical or dental conditions that warrant further consideration or consultation.[11] Moreover, such records can document any missing medical information that the patient failed to provide orally. At the end of the check-off portion of the medical history, an essay question allows the patient to provide any omitted pertinent medical information.

Radiographs

Radiographs are essential for diagnosis and also serve as additional documentation of the patient's pretreatment condition. A panographic radiograph is not diagnostically accurate for endodontics and therefore should be used only as a screening device (see Chapter 5).[53,74] Diagnostic quality periapical plain film or digital radiographs are essential aids for diagnosis, for working films (e.g., measuring the length of root canals, fitting gutta-percha cones), to verify the final fill, and for follow-up comparisons at recall examinations. Therefore the clinician should retain all radiographs and retake any radiographs that are not of diagnostic quality.

Digital radiography is recommended because it increases endodontic efficiency. No developing time is needed; thus procedural radiographs can be viewed instantly and approved or retaken with little time in between (no down time is required to wait for a film to exit the film processor).

Evaluation and Differential Diagnosis

Diagnosis includes evaluating pertinent history of the current problem, clinical examination, pulpal testing, periodontal probe charting, and recorded radiographic results. If therapy is indicated, the reasons should be discussed with the patient in an organized way. When other factors affect the prognosis (e.g., strategic importance or restorability of the tooth), the clinician should consider further consultation with the referring dentist or specialists, including prosthodontist or periodontist or both, before initiating any treatment.

Diagnostic Tests

Sound endodontics begins with a proper diagnosis. Otherwise, unnecessary or risky treatment with compromised prognosis follows. Generally the following endodontic tests should be performed to arrive at a correct and accurate diagnosis:
1. Percussion
2. Thermal testing
3. Electrical testing (optional)
4. Palpation
5. Mobility
6. Periodontal assessment (pockets and furcation)

Both positive and negative pulpal testing results should be recorded. Juries, peer review committees, and insurance consultants often disbelieve unrecorded test results. Uncharted tests may be regarded as not ever having been done because reasonable dentists should record all testing results.

Treatment Plan

Treatment records should contain a written plan that includes all aspects of the patient's oral health. Treatment plans should be coordinated, preferably in writing, with other concurrent or jointly treating dentists. If an aspect of the patient's care not under direct supervision is not proceeding properly, the clinician should initiate contact with the other treating dentist. The patient should also be advised of the problem. For instance, endodontic treatment will probably fail if underlying periodontal pathology is ignored and untreated. Therefore the clinician should assess the patient's entire dentition, not just a single root canal system. The clinician should also recommend a periodontal consultation if periodontal therapy is required.

If the scope of the examination or treatment is intentionally limited, such as a screening examination or emergency endodontic therapy, the limited scope of the visit should be recorded. Otherwise, the chart appears as if the examination was superficial and treatment incomplete. If a suspicious apical lesion requires subsequent reevaluation, the clinician should record the future reevaluation date and differential diagnosis (e.g., "Small apical lesion on no. 28 to be evaluated for any changes in two months. Also to check for any root fractures"). If this is not done it appears (on the chart) as if the dentist ignored a potentially pathologic condition, such as suspected root fracture. General soft tissue examination (including cancer check) is a standard part of any complete dental examination.

Consent Form

After endodontic diagnosis, the benefits, risks, treatment plan, and alternatives to endodontic treatment, including any patient refusal of recommended treatment, should be presented to the patient (or patient's guardian) to document acceptance or rejection of the consultation recommendations. The patient (or guardian) should sign and date the con-

TELL US ABOUT YOUR DENTAL SYMPTOMS

First Name: _____   Last Name: _____

1. Are you experiencing any pain at this time? If not, please go to Question 5.   Yes ____ No ____

2. If yes, can you locate the pain?   Yes ____ No ____

3. When did you first notice the symptoms? _____

4. Did symptoms occur suddenly or gradually? _____

Please check the frequency and quality of the discomfort, and the number that most closely reflects the intensity of your pain:

LEVEL OF INTENSITY   FREQUENCY   QUALITY

(On a scale of 1 to 10)
1 = Mild, 10 = Severe

1 __ 2 __ 3 __ 4 __ 5 __ 6 __ 7 __ 8 __ 9 __ 10 __   __ Constant   __ Sharp
                                                                 __ Intermittent   __ Dull
                                                                 __ Momentary   __ Throbbing
                                                                 __ Occasional

Is there anything you can do to relieve the pain?   Yes ____ No ____

If yes, what? _____

Is there anything you can do to cause the pain to increase?   Yes ____ No ____

If yes, what? _____

When eating or drinking, is your tooth sensitive to: Heat ____ Cold ____ Sweets ____

Does your tooth hurt when you bite down or chew?   Yes ____ No ____

Does it hurt if you press the gum tissue around this tooth?   Yes ____ No ____

Does a change in posture (lying down or bending over) cause your tooth to hurt?   Yes ____ No ____

5. Do you grind or clench your teeth?   Yes ____ No ____

6. If so, do you wear a night guard?   Yes ____ No ____

7. Has a restoration (filling or crown) been placed on this tooth recently?   Yes ____ No ____

8. Prior to this appointment, has root canal therapy been started on this tooth?   Yes ____ No ____

9. Any past trauma or injury to this tooth?   Yes ____ No ____

10. If the answer to the preceding question is yes, describe past trauma and state the occurrence date.

    _____

11. Is there anything else we should know about your teeth, gums or sinuses that would assist us in our diagnosis? _____

Signature of Patient (or Parent) _____   Date _____

Fig. 10-2 Endodontic treatment record.

sent form, including viewing any informed consent video. Subsequent changes in the proposed treatment plan should also be discussed and initialed by the patient to indicate continued acceptance and to acknowledge understanding of any newly disclosed risks, alternatives, or referrals.

Despite a patient's confirmed signature on an informed consent form, a jury is free to believe that the patient never understood the informed consent form's content before signing. If this is the case, the patient was uninformed and consent legally voidable. For instance, the patient may claim it was impossible to have read the consent form because the patient did not have reading glasses when signing (or that no one ever explained the form contents). Another scenario is that the patient was told it was a standard consent form, which was a mere procedural formality requiring patient signature. For these reasons numerous legal cases have been lost on the issue of informed consent, despite signed consent forms.

To obviate a patient's claim that no explanation existed upon which patient understanding could be based, a patient questionnaire can be used in addition to any video consent, written consent, and chart recording. Patients can be instructed that unless they score 100%, proposed procedures will not be done (because patient understanding is imperative and essential for cooperation, including postoperative care). To be effective the patient questionnaire should be relatively short and simple (Fig. 10-3), and the patient should be given an opportunity to correct any questions missed after the dentist reviews with the patient any incorrect answers. Note that the majority of answers are false, which precludes a patient from guessing the correct answer by assuming that all test information is necessarily true.

Treatment Record: Endodontic Chart

A suggested chart is presented herein to facilitate recording of information pertinent to the diagnosis, recommendations, and treatment of the endodontic patient (Fig. 10-4). Systematic acquisition and arrangement of data from the patient questionnaire, along with clinical and radiographic examinations and careful recording of treatment information, expedite accurate diagnosis and maximize clinician efficiency. Suggested chart format and use are described in the following sections.

General Patient Data   Patient name, address, phone numbers, referring dentist, and chief complaint are printed or typed in the corresponding space at the patient's initial office visit.

The patient's appointment and financial record is divided into two parts:
1. The treating dentist or staff completes the first portion after the diagnosis and treatment plan have been formulated and presented to the patient. Tooth number and quoted fee are posted. Treatment plan is recorded by circling the appropriate description. Under "Special

Instructions," specific treatment requests by the referring dentist are circled. Details of planned adjunctive procedures (e.g., hemisection, root resection) may be written in the adjacent space, along with information from the patient data section. The dentist can then use this for general reference during future treatment. The dental secretary can also use this information when scheduling appointments and establishing financial arrangements.
2. Business personnel complete the second portion. Financial agreements, third-party coverage, account status, and appointment data, including the day, date, and scheduled procedure are recorded.

Either the dentist or the assistant may complete portions of the following diagnosis and treatment sections. However, the dentist should review and approve all entries.

Dental History   Chief complaint should note if the patient is symptomatic at the time of examination. Narrative facts regarding the presenting problem are then recorded. Additional details of the chief complaint obtained during successive questioning are recorded by circling the applicable word within each symptom parameter. The pain intensity index (i.e., 0 to 10) or pain classification (i.e., mild +, moderate + +, severe + + +) should be registered alongside the appropriate description. For accurate assessment of the effects of prior dental treatment pertaining to the examination site, a summarized account of such procedures should be documented. In addition, all pretreatment signs and symptoms should be described.

Medical History   More medical history information is obtained from a patient-administered questionnaire than from the dentist obtaining an oral history from the patient.[58] Maximum information is obtained if the dentist reviews (with the patient) the written health history form that the patient has completed.

Reference information (e.g., personal physician's name, address, and phone number; patient's age; date of last physical examination) are recorded. The clinician can obtain a detailed medical history by completing a survey of the common diseases and disorders significant to dentistry, along with a comprehensive review of corresponding organ systems and assorted pathologic conditions. Specific entities that have affected the patient are circled. Essential remarks regarding these entries (e.g., details of consultations with the patient's physician) should be documented on an attached blank sheet with dated treatment notes, or they should be attached to the back of the chart (Fig. 10-5). A review of the patient's medical status (including recent or current conditions, treatments, and medications) completes the medical history. Medical histories should be updated at least annually and at reevaluation visits, particularly if evidence of failing endodontic procedures necessitates retreatment.

A current medical status will alert the practitioner to the potential for interaction between any newly prescribed drugs and drugs the patient is already taking. Older patients are

ENDODONTIC INFORMED CONSENT QUESTIONNAIRE

In order to help your understanding of endodontic benefits, risks, and alternatives, please answer the following questions by checking the true box if the statement is correct and the false box if the statement is incorrect. In the event that your answers suggest the need for further explanation, Dr. Cohen will review root canal information with you and answer any questions.

Please feel free to ask questions so that you may feel comfortable with our understanding of the surgical endodontic procedure on tooth number __19__ and your consent to endodontic surgery.

	True	False
1. Endodontic surgical success is guaranteed.	☐	☐
2. Since endodontic surgery is carefully done, there is no chance of any infection occurring after surgery.	☐	☐
3. As with any surgical procedure involving the human body, there are associated risks. One of these risks is numbness of the lower lip or chin on the side that the surgery is done. Any numbness is usually temporary but, on rare occasions, it can be permanent.	☐	☐
4. Daily oral hygiene care after endodontic surgery is unnecessary.	☐	☐
5. Dr. Cohen is unavailable for emergency calls after business hours.	☐	☐

I understand that I may ask Dr. Cohen any question I may have regarding endodontics at any time. Dr. Cohen has answered all of my questions, if any, to my satisfaction.

Date: _____   _____

Patient's signature   Witness

Fig. 10-3 True-or-false endodontic informed consent form.

FIRST NAME	LAST NAME	AGE

DENTAL HISTORY: CHIEF COMPLAINT   SYMPTOMATIC   ASYMPTOMATIC

SYMPTOMS	Location	Chronology	Quality		Affected By		Prior Tx			Initials: Dr._____ Asst._____
		Inception	sharp	intensity	hot	palpation	Tx: restorative	Yes	No	**TOOTH**
			dull	+ ++ +++	cold	manipulation	emergency	Yes	No	
		Clinical Course:		spontaneous			RCT	Yes	No	R ————————— L
			pulsating	provoked	biting	head position				
localized	referred	constant momentary	steady	reproducible	chewing	activity	Sx Pre-Tx:	Yes	No	
diffuse	radiating	intermittent lingering	enlarging	occasional	percussion	time of day	Sx Post-Tx:	Yes	No	

MEDICAL HISTORY

Heart Condition	Anemia / Bleeding	Epilepsy / Fainting	Allergies:	Major Medical Prob:	CONSULTATION:
angina	Diabetes / Kidney	Sinusitis / ENT	penicillin / antibiotics	Females:	Date: Dr.:
coronary	Hepatitis / Liver	Glaucoma / Visual	aspirin / Tylenol	Pregnant _____ mo	Recommendation:
surgery	Herpes	Mental / Neural	codeine / narcotics	Recent Hosp. Operation:	
pacemaker	Thyroid / Hormonal	Tumor / Neoplasms	local anesthetic	Current Medical TX:	
Rheumatic Fever / Murmur	Asthma / Respiratory	Alcoholism / Addictions	N_2O/O_2	Medications:	
Hypertension / Circulatory	Ulcers / Digestive	Infectious Diseases	Latex	Pre-meds:	
Immunosuppression	Migraine / Headaches	Venereal Disease	other:		Initials: Dr._____ Asst._____

CLINICAL FINDINGS

EXAMINATION	RADIOGRAPHIC		CLINICAL		DIAGNOSTIC TESTS						
Tooth		Attachment Apparatus	Tooth	Soft Tissues	Tooth #						
WNL		PDL normal	WNL	WNL	perio						
caries		PDL thickened	discoloration	extra-oral swelling	mobility						
restoration		alveolar bone, WNL	caries	intra-oral swelling	percussion						
calcification		diffuse lucency	pulp exposure	sinus tract	palpation						
resorption		circumscribed lucency	prior access	lymphadenopathy	cold						
fracture		resorption	attrition / abrasion	TMJ TMD	hot						
perforation / deviation		apical	fracture	perio B	EPT						
prior RCTx/RCF		lateral	restoration		bite / chewing						
separated instrument		hypercementosis	amalgam	M ——————— D	date:						
canal obstruction		osteosclerosis	composite		bruxism: yes_____ no_____						
post / build-up		perio	glass ionomer								
open apex			inlay / onlay	L							
			temporary		nightguard: yes_____ no_____ Initials: Dr._____ Asst._____						
			crown								
			abutment								

DIAGNOSIS

PULPAL	PERIAPICAL	ETIOLOGY		PROGNOSIS		
				ENDODONTIC	PERIODONTAL	RESTORATIVE
WNL	WNL	idiopathic	trauma	favorable	favorable	favorable
reversible pulpitis	acute apical periodontitis	caries	periodontal	questionable	questionable	questionable
irreversible pulpitis	acute apical abscess	restoration	orthodontic	poor	poor	poor
necrosis	chronic periapical inflammation	attrition / abrasion	prior RCTx	hopeless	hopeless	hopeless
prior RCTx/RCF	phoenix abscess	developmental	intentional			
	osteosclerosis	sinusitis	systemic			

PT. CONSULT	___ Examination Findings ___ Periodontal Status ___ Fracture ___ Surgery ___ Prognosis Referral:
	___ Treatment Plan ___ Restoration ___ Discoloration ___ Recall ___ Consent Form Initials: Dr._____ Asst._____

TREATMENT			CONS		PRE-TREATMENT				CLEANING / SHAPING							OBTURATION							SURG						Rx								
DATE			pt.	Dr.	local	R.D.	rel oc.	O.D.	access	pulpec.	canal	test	final	G.G.B.	s. file	cotton	temp	G.P.	sealer	tech.	post	post space	B-U	temp	I&D	hemisection	bicuspidization	root resect	S. R.	microsurg. retro.	analgesic	Antibiotic	Ca(OH)2	X-Ray	crown lengthening	bleach	retreatment	doctor initial	chairside init.
mo	day	yr																																					

CANAL	REF	Elec.	X-Ray	Adj.	Final	Size	Rx Date	MEDICATION	DOSE	DISP		INSTR.	
B F									x			q	h
L P									x			q	h
MB									x			q	h
ML									x			q	h
DB									x			q	h
DL									x			q	h

Fig. 10-4 Dental history form.

TELL US ABOUT YOUR MEDICAL HISTORY

First Name: _____   Last Name: _____

How would you describe your health? Please circle one.   Excellent   Good   Fair   Poor

When did you have your last physical examination? _____

Are you currently being treated for any illness or medical condition?   Yes _____   No _____

If yes, please describe: _____

_____

Who is treating you for this condition? _____

Have you ever had any kind of surgery?   Yes _____   No _____

When did you have this surgery? _____

What type of surgery did you have? _____

Have you ever had any trouble with prolonged bleeding after surgery?   Yes _____   No _____
Do you wear a pacemaker or any other kind of prosthetic device?   Yes _____   No _____
Are you taking any medication or drugs at this time?   Yes _____   No _____
Have you ever taken Fen-phen and/or Redux (diet drugs)?   Yes _____   No _____
What medications, drugs, or herbs are you taking?

_____

Why are you taking these medications? _____

_____

Have you ever had an unusual reaction to an anesthetic or drug (like penicillin)?   Yes _____   No _____

If yes, please explain: _____

Please circle any present or past illness you now have or had in the past:

Alcoholism	Blood Pressure	Epilepsy	Hepatitis	Kidney or Liver	Rheumatic Fever
Allergies	Cancer	Glaucoma	Herpes	Mental	Sinusitis
Anemia	Diabetes	Head/Neck Injuries	Immunodeficiency	Migraine	Ulcers
Asthma	Drug Dependency	Heart/Valve Disease	Infectious Diseases	Respiratory	Venereal Disease

Are you allergic to Latex or any other substances or materials?   Yes _____   No _____

If so, please explain. _____

If female, are you pregnant?   Yes _____   No _____

Is there any other information that should be known about your health? _____

_____

Signature of Patient (or Parent) _____   Date _____

Fig. 10-5 Medical history form.

more likely to be taking drugs for medical conditions concomitant with dental treatment. Recent Federal Drug Administration (FDA) approval of newly marketed drugs risks drug interactions not discovered in premarket research–controlled drug trials. Currently, pharmaceutical manufacturers budget more for marketing than research and development.[64] Some drug manufacturers have suppressed publication of adverse research.[14]

The small number of premarket patients studied may lack sufficient statistical power to expose serious side effects that occur infrequently but are, nonetheless, life threatening. For instance, mibefradil (Posicor) was withdrawn from the market after 1 year because it increased plasma concentrations of 25 other coadministered drugs, including erythromycin.[45] In another example the popular prescription nighttime heartburn drug Propulsid (cisapride) was linked to 70 deaths and more than 270 significant negative reactions since 1993. In 2000 the FDA office of Post-Marketing Drug Risk Assessment changed the label warnings. The new Propulsid label highlights risks to patients taking a wide range of other medications, including antibiotics such as erythromycin, all protease inhibitors prescribed for patients with acquired immunodeficiency syndrome (AIDS), and the class of antidepressants including Elavil or Serzone. In previous, less stringent FDA warnings, taking Propulsid with grapefruit juice was labeled as dangerous.[69]

Current medication history should include over-the-counter herbal and illicit drugs, because many have the potential for synergistic or antagonistic interaction with dentist- prescribed drugs. Ephedra (ma-huang) has been associated with 54 deaths, primarily involving cranial hemorrhage or stroke.[10,10a] Echinacea increases potential for liver damage when used with steroids. Gingko biloba and fenerfew interfere with anticoagulants, such as Coumadin.[18] In 1998 California investigators found about one third of 260 imported Asian drugs were either spiked with unlisted drugs or contained mercury, lead, or arsenic.

Newly marketed drugs may not list all drug interactions. Therefore the FDA's MedWatch program encourages dentists to report suspected drug interactions. Dentist reporting to the FDA is confidential. Interested clinicians can contact the FDA by telephone at (800) FDA-1088 or fax at (800) FDA-0178 to obtain the FDA Medical Products Reporting Program (MedWatch) form (FDA form #3500). The back portion of the Physicians' Desk Reference (PDR) contains a MedWatch form. Clinicians can also report suspected drug interactions by modem at (800) FDA-7737. Other electronic drug databases are available to report and access important drug interaction information.[72] For FDA approved safety-related drug labeling on line, see http://www.fda.gov/medwatch.

Dentists who pass the buck by claiming, "Oh it was my secretary or my assistant. I could do nothing about it," are nonetheless legally liable for their staff's actions or inactions. A dentist exclusively relying on staff members to obtain medical histories in a waiting room full of patients is making a mistake, because the accuracy of the histories must first be checked and then followed up by the dentist. Training and monitoring staff are duties that dentists cannot afford to ignore. President Harry Truman's sage advice, "The buck stops here," applies to treating dentists who overdelegate to unlicensed staff members who lack the requisite education for adequate medical history follow-up.

Abbreviations

Abbreviated records can be frustrating if the practitioner is unable to decipher his or her own handwritten entries. Therefore the clinician should use standard or easily understood abbreviations. Pencil entries are legally valid, but ink entries are less vulnerable to a plaintiff's claim of erasure or alteration. A short pencil is better than a long memory; records remember but patients and dentists may forget.

A sample of a completed endodontic chart (Fig. 10-6) illustrates its proper use. An explanatory key listing the standard abbreviations used in the chart is provided in Fig. 10-7.

Computerized Treatment Records

Increasingly, dentists are using computerized record storage as described in Chapter 26. To avoid a claim of record falsification, whatever computer system is used should be able to demonstrate that records indicating earlier treatment were not recently falsified. Software technology, such as the "write only read memory" (WORM) system, used to identify computer data tampering is not foolproof because it cannot detect tampering where an entire disk of recent origin has been substituted for an earlier version. Periodically a hard copy of computer data should be printed out, hand-initialed, and dated in ink to provide written verification of the computer records.

Department of Health and Human Services' Security and Electronic Signature Standards rule is part of the Health Insurance Portability and Accountability Act of 1996. This act emphasizes the safeguarding of healthcare information by healthcare providers. Some states have begun authorizing digital electronic signatures as binding for most contracts and orders.* Digital signatures with electronic transactions are authorized by the Third Millennium Electronic Commerce Act (also called Electronic Signature in Global and National Commerce Act) (15 U.S.C.A. §§ 7001 et seq.)

Record Size

Clinicians who keep brief records risk creating incomplete documentation. While there is little harm in recording too much information, there is great danger in recording too

---

*California adopted the Uniform Electronics Transactions Act (effective January 1, 2000) that authorizes, but does not require, an electronic signature; California Civil Code § 1633.1 et seq.; California Financial Code § 18608, as amended 2000.

little. Standard 8½ × 11 inch or larger clinical records possess the advantage of providing the treating dentist adequate space for clinical notes.

Identity of Entry Author

Either a dentist or an auxiliary can chart clinical entries unless state law indicates otherwise.* What is important is that the correct clinical information is recorded. Each person who makes an entry should record the date and initial the entry. Otherwise, the author's identity may be forgotten, should the individual who recorded the entry be needed in a legal proceeding. For instance, initialing the entry makes it easier to identify the particular dentist or auxiliary who, since the original recording, is now employed elsewhere.

Patient Record Request

Patient requests for record transfers or copies must be honored. It is unethical to refuse to transfer patient records, on patient request, to another treating dentist.†

Moreover, it is illegal in some states, subjecting the dentist to discipline and fines should the records not be provided to the patient on written request, even if an outstanding balance is owed.‡

Patient Education Pamphlets

Patient education pamphlets may be used in litigation as evidence that a patient was properly informed and given endodontic alternatives but instead chose extraction. Such pamphlets include the American Dental Association's (ADA's) *Your Teeth Can Be Saved by Endodontic Root Canal Treatment* or the American Association of Endodontists (AAE's) *Your Guide to Endodontic Treatment* and *Your Guide to Endodontic Surgery.* The clinician should indicate in the patient's chart which pamphlets the patient was provided.

Postoperative Instructions

It is unlikely a patient will remember oral postoperative instructions unless accompanied with written instructions. After endodontic procedures the patient may be sedated or affected by analgesic drugs; therefore written postoperative instructions are beneficial. Emergency phone numbers to contact the treating dentist should be included on the form. Written instructions reduce postoperative morbidity and pain and improve patient compliance.[4] The clinician should document that postoperative instructions were provided.

Recording Referrals

Every dentist, including the endodontic specialist, has a duty to refer under appropriate circumstances. If consultations with additional experts or specialists become necessary, referrals should be recorded, lest they be forgotten or refused. Carbonless, two-part referral cards allow the clinician to provide an original referral slip to the patient while retaining a copy for the patient's chart. The clinician or staff member should document the fact that the original referral card was given to the patient and record the name of the person who provided card and the date on which it was provided. If it is mailed to the patient, that fact should also be recorded. A copy of the card should also be sent to the referred doctor. If the patient fails to keep the referral appointment, this copy will provide proof that a referral was made. The clinician should request that the patient and the referred doctor report back if the referral appointment is cancelled; staff should verify that the referral consultation occurred.

Record Falsification

Records must be complete, accurate, legible, and dated. All diagnosis, treatments, and referrals should be recorded. Chart additions may expand, correct, define, modify, or clarify (as long as they are currently dated to indicate the belated entry).

To correct an entry, the clinician should make a line through (but not erase or obscure) the erroneous entry. The correction should then be written on the next available line and dated. Handwriting and ink experts use ink chemical tags, age dating, and infrared technology to prove falsified additions, deletions, or substitutions. If records are proven to be falsified, the dentist may be subject to punitive damages in civil litigation. In addition, the dentist may be subject to license revocation for intentional misconduct.* In most cases professional liability insurance policies will not cover punitive damages if the dentist is found to have committed fraud or deceit.† In addition, insurance carriers may deny renewal of professional liability coverage to a dentist who has been proven to have fraudulently altered dental records.

When patient records have been requested or subpoenaed, it is wise to refrain from examining them to avoid anxiety and the temptation to clarify an entry. Alteration of records is a cause of large settlements. Dental records are business documents; the clinician should not be cavalier about making undisclosed, belated record changes. Instead, late entries should be dated with the late entry date.

Records are (1) subject to audits by insurance carriers for documentation that treatment was performed, (2) reviewed by peer review committees, and (3) subject to subpoena by state licensing boards or agencies for disciplinary proceed-

---

*California Business and Professions Code § 1683.

†American Dental Association: *Principles of Ethics and Code of Professional Conduct* § I.B.

‡See, e.g., California Health and Safety Code § 123110(g).

*California Business and Professions Code, § 1680(s).

†*PPF Industries Inc. v Transamerica Insurance Co,* 20 Cal. 4th 310, 1999; *Stone v The Regents of the University of California,* 77 Cal. App 4th 736, 2000.

LAST NAME		FIRST NAME		DR MR. MISS MRS.	ADDRESS			HOME PHONE BUSINESS PHONE		

REF. DR.			REF. DR. ADDRESS			REF. DR. PHONE	

TOOTH — R 30 L   FEE   TREATMENT PLAN — (CONSULT) EET   (RCT) AE PE (ME)   SURGERY Ca(OH)$_2$ SPECIAL INSTRUCTIONS — POST SPACE (PREFORMED POST/B.U.) COMP (AMAL) TEMP. CR.   *Distal Canal*

INSURANCE S D	AMT DUE	REC'D	DATE	DAY	TIME	PRO- CEDURE	X-RAY	REMARKS:
PRE-AUTH Y N								
% COVERED								
VERIFIED								
FORM SIGNED								
PT. INFORMED								
PT. PORTION								
INS SENT								

MO	DAY	YR	REMARKS	SIGNATURE
2	14	01	Pt. urged to have a cast metal crown made as soon as possible. Confirming letter sent to referring doctor.	EZ

(MIDDLE INITIAL, FIRST NAME, LAST NAME labels appear along the left margin.)

Fig. 10-6 Progress notes.

FIRST NAME	LAST NAME	AGE
May	Sui	40

DENTAL HISTORY: CHIEF COMPLAINT (SYMPTOMATIC) ASYMPTOMATIC

Crown placed one week ago. Diffuse pain began the next day. Pt. cannot localize the pain. Heat, cold and chewing increase the pain.

SYMPTOMS	Location	Chronology	Quality	Affected By	Prior Tx	Initials: Dr. SC Asst. EZ

Left side
V1 – V3

Inception 6 days

- (sharp)
- dull
- (pulsating)
- steady
- enlarging

intensity
+ (++) +++
spontaneous
provoked
(reproducible)
occasional

- (hot) ✗
- (cold) ++
- palpation
- manipulation
- biting
- (chewing)
- percussion
- head position
- activity
- time of day

Clinical Course:

localized   referred   (constant)   momentary
(diffuse)   (radiating)   (intermittent) (lingering)

Tx: restorative (Yes) No Crown
emergency Yes (No)
RCT Yes (No)

Sx Pre-Tx: Yes (No)
Sx Post-Tx: (Yes) No

TOOTH
R —————— L
(19)

MEDICAL HISTORY

Heart Condition
- angina
- coronary
- surgery
- pacemaker
- Rheumatic Fever / Murmur
- Hypertension / Circulatory
- Immunosuppression

Anemia / Bleeding
(Diabetes) / Kidney
Hepatitis / Liver
Herpes
Thyroid / Hormonal
Asthma / Respiratory
Ulcers / Digestive
(Migraine) / Headaches

Epilepsy / Fainting
(Sinusitis) / ENT
Glaucoma / Visual
Mental / Neural
Tumor / Neoplasms
Alcoholism / Addictions
Infectious Diseases
Venereal Disease

Allergies:
- penicillin / antibiotics
- aspirin / Tylenol
- codeine / narcotics
- local anesthetic
- N.O.O.
- (Latex)
- other:

Major Medical Prob:
Females:
Pregnant _____ mo
Recent Hosp. Operation:
Current Medical TX:
Medications:

Initials: Dr. SC Asst. EZ

CLINICAL FINDINGS

EXAMINATION	RADIOGRAPHIC	CLINICAL		DIAGNOSTIC TESTS

Tooth

- WNL
- caries
- (restoration)
- (calcification) mesial
- resorption
- fracture
- perforation / deviation
- prior RCTx/RCF
- separated instrument
- canal obstruction
- post / build-up
- open apex

Attachment Apparatus
- PDL normal
- (PDL thickened)
- alveolar bone, WNL
- diffuse lucency
- circumscribed lucency
- resorption
  - apical
  - lateral
- hypercementosis
- osteosclerosis
- perio

Tooth
- WNL
- discoloration
- caries
- pulp exposure
- prior access
- attrition / abrasion
- fracture
- (restoration)
- amalgam
- composite
- glass ionomer
- inlay / onlay
- temporary
- (crown)
- abutment

Soft Tissues
- (WNL)
- extra-oral swelling
- intra-oral swelling
- sinus tract
- lymphadenopathy
- TMJ
- perio

B 2
M 3 — D 3
L 2

Tooth #	18	19	20			
perio	wnl	wnl	wnl			
mobility	wnl	wnl	wnl			
percussion	wnl	+	wnl			
palpation	wnl	wnl	wnl			
cold	wnl	+++	wnl			
hot	wnl	++	wnl			
EPT						
bite / chewing	wnl	++	wnl			
date:	2/14/01					

bruxism: yes ✓ no _____
nightguard: yes ✓ no _____ Initials: Dr. SC Asst. EZ

DIAGNOSIS   PULPAL   PERIAPICAL   ETIOLOGY   PROGNOSIS

PULPAL
- WNL
- reversible pulpitis
- (irreversible pulpitis)
- necrosis
- prior RCTx/RCF

PERIAPICAL
- WNL
- (acute apical periodontitis)
- acute apical abscess
- chronic periapical inflammation
- phoenix abscess
- osteosclerosis

ETIOLOGY
- idiopathic
- caries
- (restoration)
- attrition / abrasion
- developmental
- sinusitis
- trauma
- periodontal
- orthodontic
- prior RCTx
- intentional
- systemic

PROGNOSIS

ENDODONTIC	PERIODONTAL	RESTORATIVE
(favorable)	(favorable)	(favorable)
questionable	questionable	questionable
poor	poor	poor
hopeless	hopeless	hopeless

PT. CONSULT
- ✓ Examination Findings
- ✓ Treatment Plan
- ✓ Periodontal Status
- ✓ Restoration
- ✓ Fracture
- ___ Discoloration
- ✓ Surgery
- ✓ Recall
- ✓ Prognosis
- ✓ Consent Form

Referral:
Initials: Dr. SC Asst. EZ

TREATMENT	CONS	PRE-TREATMENT	CLEANING / SHAPING	OBTURATION	SURG	Rx												

DATE			pt.	Dr.	local	R.D.	rel oc.	O.D.	access	pulpec.	canal	test	final	G.G.B.	s. file	cotton	temp	G.P.	sealer	tech.	post	post space	B-U	temp	I&D	REF	hemisection	bicuspidization	root resect	S.R.	analgesic	Antibiotic	Ca(OH)2	X-Ray	crown lengthening	bleach	retreatment	doctor initial	chairside init.
mo	day	yr																																					
2	14	01	✓	✓	✓				✓	✓	✓	✓	✓					✓	✓	w(T) + glass ionomer core																		SC	EZ

CANAL	REF	Elec.	X-Ray	Adj.	Final	Size	Rx Date	MEDICATION	DOSE DISP	INSTR.
B F							2/14/01	Ibuprofen	600 mg 12	1 q 6 h
L P									x	q h
MB		21.0				25			x	q h
ML		20.5				25			x	q h
DB		21.0				30			x	q h
DL		21.0				30			x	q h

Fig. 10-6, cont'd Medical history form.

Ab	=	Antibiotic
ABS	=	Abscess
access	=	Access cavity
analg.	=	Analgesic
apico	=	Apicoectomy
B-U	=	Buildup of tooth
canal	=	Identify canal that has been cleaned and shaped
cotton	=	Placed in pulp chamber between treatments
ENDO	=	Endodontics
EPT	=	Electric pulp test
epin	=	Epinepherine
final	=	Final file
G.G.B.	=	Gates-Glidden bur
G.P.	=	Gutta-percha
I & D	=	Incision and drainage
L.A. or local	=	Local anesthetic
O.D.	=	Open and drain
perio	=	Periodontal
post	=	Preformed, custom, or transilluminated post
pt	=	Patient
pulpec	=	Pulpectomy
R.D.	=	Rubber dam
Rel occ	=	Relieved occlusion
resorp.	=	Resorption
retro	=	Retrograde procedure
S/R	=	Suture removal
s.file	=	Serial filing
S/D	=	Single insurance or dual coverage
sealer	=	Type of sealer used
tech.	=	Technique for canal obturation
temp	=	Temporary restoration
test	=	Test file
WNL	=	Within normal limits
Y/N	=	Insurance preauthorized? Yes or No

Fig. 10-7 Standard abbreviation key.

ings. Accordingly, incomplete or missing records expose the dentist not only to civil liability for professional negligence but also to criminal penalties for criminal offenses, such as insurance fraud.[66]

False Claims

Performing or billing for unnecessary endodontic therapy, such as prophylactic endodontic therapy with every crown preparation, subjects the practitioner to fraud. In nonpulpal exposure crown preparation, the likely incidence of subsequent endodontic therapy is approximately 3%. Therefore performing prophylactic endodontics on the other 97% of patients represents unnecessary and therefore fraudulent treatment. Excessive treatment also ethically violates the Hippocratic oath of "Primum non nocere" (i.e., "first, do no harm").

The Federal False Claims Act* carries both civil and general penalties of treble damages, fines, and attorney's fees for fraudulently billing government programs, such as the

Champus (Civilian Health and Medical Program of the Uniformed Services) or Medicare. Fines between $5,000 and $10,000 per claim form apply if the U.S. Mail was used for a false-claim submission. If any portion of the claimed treatment was fraudulently misrepresented, even if a small minority, a violation results.* Fraudulent intent need not be conclusively proven. Reckless disregard for the accuracy of submitted data is all that is necessary to obtain a federal criminal conviction or prove civil wrongdoing.

Spoliation

Spoliation is a tort in which the wrongdoer alters, changes, or substitutes dental records in an attempt to defeat a civil lawsuit.† It is better to defend a dental negligence lawsuit with poor records than with altered (i.e., falsified) records. Otherwise, the jury may conclude the dentist acted with consciousness of guilt rather than with clerical oversight in maintaining adequate records.

Record alteration may subject the dentist to licensing,‡ ethical discipline, or punitive damages for deceitful misconduct. Texaco paid a record settlement of $176 million dollars when tape recordings of company executives revealed a plan to destroy documents evidencing discriminatory employment practices.[29] Additionally, the Texaco executives were criminally prosecuted for obstruction of justice.[67]

Digital radiography may have dental advantages, but because the digital images may be computer manipulated, they may be legally unreliable.[34,65] Therefore hard copies of the digital images should be printed and dated with ink to show the informational baseline on which the practitioner based diagnostic or therapeutic decisions. This also protects against computer glitches, such as disk drive crashes, electrical power surges, computer viruses, and operator delete errors.

Record alteration may be detected by questioned document experts who determine ink dates, examine watermarks, or use infrared techniques to discover (or ascertain) additions or deletions in records, including prior erasures, whiteouts, and indentations made when one page is overwritten on another page.

If an erroneous entry occurs, the clinician should add another late entry dated as such, to demonstrate later corrected information. For example:

- 10-12-01—Hot, cold, and percussion tests negative

---

*31 U.S.C. § 3279 et. seq. See also, 18 U.S.C. § 287 (false claims), 18 U.S.C. § 1001 (false statements), and Health Insurance Portability and Accountability Act (HIPAA). See, "$486 million health care settlement," (including $101 million fine against National Medical Care, Inc. for medical fraud), *San Francisco Daily Journal* p 7, January 20, 2000.

U.S. ex rel Pogue v American Health Corp. Inc., 914 F. Suppl. 1507, 1996.
†*Gomez v Acquistapace,* 50 Cal. App. 4th 740, 57 Cal. Rptr. 821, 1996; *Thor v Boska* 38 Cal. App. 3d 558, 113 Cal. Rptr. 296, 1974; *Cedars-Sinai Medical Center v Superior Court* 18 Cal. 4th 1, 1998; *Temple Community Hospital v Superior Court* 20 Cal. 4th 464, 1999; *Holmes v. Amerex Rent-A-Car,* A. 2d, No. 97-SP, 943,1998 WL 162147 CDC, Apr 9, 1998.†*U.S. ex rel Pogue v American Health Corp. Inc.,* 914 F. Suppl. 1507, 1996.
‡California Business and Professions Code § 1680 (s).

- 10-13-01—Corrected entry for 10-12-01. Should have been recorded:

Hot, cold, and percussion tests slightly positive. Recommend reevaluation in 24 hours and repeat pulpal tests. Appointment scheduled 10/13/01 at 9 AM.

LEGAL RESPONSIBILITIES

Malpractice Prophylaxis

Good dentists keep good records. Records represent the single most critical evidence a dentist can present in court as confirmation of accurate diagnosis and proper treatment.

Prevention is the goal of modern dental care. Competent endodontic treatment performed within the requisite standard of care not only saves endodontically treated teeth but also helps prevent a lawsuit for professional negligence. Thus sound endodontic principles, when carefully applied, protect both dentist and patient. Prudent care reduces avoidable and unreasonable risks associated with careless endodontic therapy.

Standard of Care

Good endodontic practice, as defined by the courts, is the standard of reasonable care legally required to be performed by the treating dentist. The standard of care does not require perfection; instead, the legal standard is that *reasonable* degree of skill, knowledge, or care ordinarily possessed and exercised by dentists under similar circumstances.

Although the standard of care is a flexible standard that accommodates individual variations in treatment, it is objectively tested based on what a reasonable dentist should do. Reasonable conduct represents a minimum required for legal due care. Additional precautionary steps that rise above this minimal floor of reasonableness and approach the ceiling of ideal care are laudable, but they are not legally mandated. Nevertheless, prudent practices should always strive to achieve a higher level of care than barely or minimally adequate. Excellent clinicians always strive to do their best and practice endodontics at the highest standard.

Health Maintenance Organization Care Versus Standard of Care
Prudent practitioners (not insurance carriers) set the standard of care. Third-party payers may limit reimbursement but should not limit access to the quality of care. Practitioners have an affirmative duty on behalf of the patient to appeal insurance carrier care denial decisions.* Practitioners have an affirmative duty on behalf of the patient to appeal insurance carrier care denial deci-

sions and, in some states, are protected against retaliation.* The dentist who complies (without protest) with the limitations imposed by a third-party payer when dental judgment dictates otherwise, cannot avoid ultimate responsibility for the patient's care.

Although they do not set the standard of care, insurance carriers may contractually limit dental benefits. Therefore a dentist is obligated to inform patients of their dental needs, irrespective of carrier reimbursement. Patients may then elect to pay out of pocket or decline uninsured services. Informed choice is uninformed if the dentist fails to provide patients with all reasonable options and alternatives.

If an insurance carrier denies endodontic therapy or limits endodontics to only certain clinical conditions, a prudent practitioner must provide informed consent to the patient both legally[16] and ethically, if a tooth may be endodontically treated and retained, rather than extracted. The California Dental Association's *Dental Patient Bill of Rights* advises patients that "You have the right to ask your dentist to explain all treatment options regardless of coverage or cost."[32]

Dentists may agree to a discounted fee with a health maintenance organization (HMO) carrier but must not ever discount the quality of care provided. Peer review and the courts recognize only one standard of care; they do not lower the standard or create a double standard for reduced-fee HMO plans. Improved efficiency should not be accomplished at the expense of quality care.

An Illinois appellate court held that a physician may be sued for injuries that a patient suffers as a result of the doctor's failure to disclose a contractual arrangement with the patient's HMO that creates financial incentives to minimize diagnostic tests and referrals to specialists. The court recognized a distinct cause of action for breach of fiduciary duty for failure to disclose these types of financial incentives.† In reaching its conclusion the court cited an American Medical Association (AMA) ethics opinion that stated that a physician must ensure that a patient is aware of financial incentives through which health insurers limit diagnostic tests and treatment options.

Managed care organizations use a variety of strategies to influence the practice styles of providers. One of the most controversial of these methods is the use of financial incentives designed to limit referrals to specialists. Such financial incentives usually take the form of bonus payments drawn from surpluses in risk pools funded by "withholds." These funds are deducted from the primary care provider's base payments or otherwise reserved under contracts in which the care provider bears financial risk. Thus bonuses are based on referral limitations.[26]

Plans that delay treatment approval resulting in endodontic complications or tooth nontreatability may be subject to

---

Wickline v State of California, 192 Cal. App. 3d 1630, 1645, 239 Cal. Rptr. 810, 1986. See also, Pear R: *HMOs loophole to prevent litigation, San Francisco Examiner* p A-6, November 17, 1996.

---

*California Business and Professional Code, Sec 2056.
†*Neade v Portes*, 710 N.E. 2d 418, 1999.

liability*[62] However, HMO carriers usually argue that the 1974 Employee Retirement Income Security Act (ERISA) preempts state law dental negligence claims against entities who administrate health care benefits to an ERISA plan and shift any blame entirely to the dentist or provider. Case law has produced mixed results regarding carrier liability, but Congress may intervene if the courts continue to exempt ERISA carriers.[39,54]

Capitation systems have a built-in incentive to undertreat, to delay, or to discourage treatment and access to care. For the dentist who is paid by capitation, the patient may be perceived as a threat to profits. Thus capitation creates incentives that can transform dentists from the patient's advocate to the patient's adversary.

Although dentists seem like double agents serving two masters (i.e., managed care carriers and patients), the law is clear that the dentist must always consider the patient's best interests. Should the carrier deny requested care, the dentist is legally obligated to appeal the decision to protect the patient's health.†

Welcome to the Twenty-First Century   Although profitable to insurance carriers, the success of denying or limiting benefits has created an era of angry patients and frustrated dentists. Therefore the clinician must guard against patient disappointment with limited insurance benefits by explaining that while insurance carriers determine coverage under their patient's insurance policy, they do not set the standard of care. Regardless of the how much or how little is covered by the patient's insurance carrier, it is the prudent dentist who sets the standard of care.

Dental Negligence Defined

Dental negligence is defined as a violation of the standard of care (i.e., an act or omission that a reasonably prudent dentist under similar circumstances would not have done).‡ Negligence is equated with carelessness or inattentiveness.[42] Malpractice is a lay term for such professional negligence. Dental negligence occurs for two possible reasons:

1. If a dentist either fails to possess a reasonable degree of education and training to act prudently, or
2. Despite reasonable schooling, training, and continuing education, acts unreasonably, or imprudently fails to act.

One simple test to determine if a particular treatment outcome results from negligence is to ask the following question: Was the treatment result reasonably avoidable? If the answer is "yes," it is probably malpractice. If the answer is

"no," it is probably an unfortunate incident that resulted despite the best of reasonable care.

Note: All examples of negligent endodontic treatment are not included in this chapter because the myriad of malpractice incidents far exceed its scope. Rather, select examples are elucidated for educational purposes.

Locality Rule

The locality rule, which provides for a different standard of care in different communities, is rapidly becoming outdated. Originating in the nineteenth century, the rule was designed to acknowledge differences in facilities, training, and equipment between rural and urban communities.*

The trend across the country is to move from a locally-based standard to a statewide standard, at least for generalists. For endodontists, a national standard of care is applied, considering that the AAE Board is national in scope.† Because of nationally published endodontic literature, advances in Internet communication, continuing education courses, and reasonably available transportation for patients no disparity generally exists between small town and urban endodontic standards.

A dentist should provide proper endodontic care to a patient regardless of treatment locality. Rather than focusing on different standards for different communities, other more important considerations include knowledge of endodontic advances in the field gained with continuing education and using improved diagnostics and instrumentation.

The locality rule has two major drawbacks. In areas with small populations, dentists may be reluctant to testify as expert witnesses against other local dentists. Also, the locality rule allows a small group of dentists in an area to establish a local standard of care inferior to what the law requires of larger urban areas. Publications are available to all dentists, in print and on the Internet. In addition, dentists travel great distances to attend courses. Therefore there is little excuse to blame ignorance on the fact that the dentist is working in a rural location.

Standards of Care: Generalist Versus Endodontist

A general practitioner performing treatment ordinarily performed exclusively by specialists, such as apical endodontic surgery, periodontal surgical grafting, or full bony impaction surgery, will be held to the specialist's standard of care.[24,25] A generalist should refer to a specialist rather than perform procedures that are beyond the general practitioner's training or competency to avoid performing treatment that is below the specialist's standard. The three levels of clinical skill are (1) competency or beginning level, (2) proficiency, and (3)

Nealy v U.S. Healthcare HMO, 711 N.E. 2d 621, 1999; Studdert DM, Brennan TA: The problems with punitive damages in lawsuits against managed-care organizations, *N Engl J Med* 342(4):280, 2000.
†*Wickline v State of California*, 192 Cal. App. 3d 1630, 239 Cal. Rptr. 810, 1986.
‡*California Book of Approved Jury Instructions*, no. 6.00.1 (ed 8).

---

*A.L.R. 4th 603.
†*Sheeley v Memorial Hospital*, 710 A 2d 161, 1998.

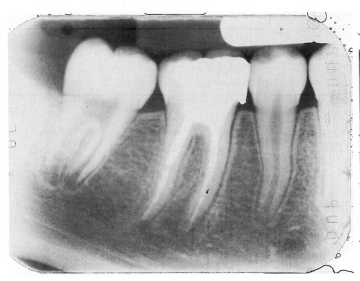

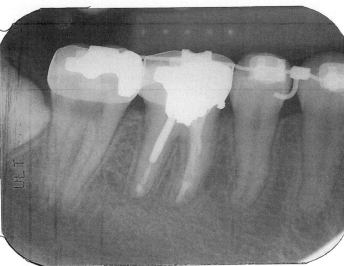

Fig. 10-8 A general dentist's radiograph that ostensibly shows a complete endodontic fill within the root canal space.

Fig. 10-9 Endodontist's radiograph demonstrating a transported canal.

mastery. The ability to "know what we don't know" is an important feature of any competent, ethical practice.[36]

Approximately 80% of general practitioners in the United States provide some endodontic therapy. Endodontic expansion into the realm of the generalist can be linked to (1) refinements in root canal preparation and improved filling (i.e., packing) techniques currently taught in dental schools; (2) continuing education courses; and (3) significant improvements in the armamentarium of instruments, equipment, and materials available to dentists.

Higher Standard of Care for Endodontists: Extended Diagnostic and Treatment Responsibilities

Endodontists, as specialists, may be held to a higher standard of skill, knowledge, and care than general practitioners.* Endodontists set the standard for routine endodontics. Therefore if the same standard of care cannot be met, the generalist must refer the patient to an endodontist.[24,25]

Endodontists should not forget their general dentistry training. Even though a patient may be referred for a specific procedure or undertaking, the endodontist should not overlook sound biologic principles inherent in the overall treatment. A specialist may also be held liable for relying solely on the information referral card or radiographs of the referring dentist, should the diagnosis or therapeutic recommendations prove incorrect or the referral card list the wrong tooth for treatment. Fig. 10-8 demonstrates a general dentist's radiograph showing apparent complete endodontic fill within the

canal space, whereas Fig. 10-9 demonstrates an endodontist's radiograph showing a transported canal. The difference is explained by radiographic quality and angulation.

Without performing an independent examination, the endodontist risks misdiagnosis and resulting incorrect treatment. Prevention of misdiagnosis or incorrect treatment requires an accurate medical and dental history and a clinical examination (not only of the specific tooth, or teeth, involved but also the general oral condition). Obvious problems, such as oral lesions, periodontitis, or gross decay, should be noted in the chart and the patient advised regarding a referral for further examination, testing, or consultation.

Radiographs from the referring dentist should be reviewed for completeness, clarity, and diagnostic accuracy. An endodontist should expose a new radiograph to verify current status before treatment and only use the referring dentist's radiograph for historical comparison. Unfortunately, the referring dentist may surreptitiously send a pretreatment film with the referred patient, rather than the generalist's own posttreatment film depicting a perforation or broken file. This may occur because the generalist is attempting to conceal negligently performed endodontic treatment or attempting to shift blame for bungled treatment to the endodontist. In such cases the endodontist learns a valuable lesson about exposing independent pretreatment radiographs, rather than relying exclusively on the generalist's pretreatment radiographs.

Poor oral hygiene may contribute to periodontal disease. In such cases endodontic treatment may be compromised unless the associated periodontal condition, along with the tooth being tested endodontically, is brought under periodontal disease control. Referral to a periodontist may be necessary before or contemporaneous with completion of endodontic treatment.

---

*Carmichael v. Reitz, 17 Cal. App. 3d 958, 1971; *California Book of Approved Jury Instructions*, (ed 8).

In summary, it is necessary for the endodontist to do the following:

1. Be alert to any contributory medical or dental condition within the operative area of endodontic treatment.
2. Undertake an independent examination of the treatment area and treatment plan without relying solely on the referring dentist.
3. Perform a general dental examination (at least a screening) of the patient's mouth.
4. Evaluate status and prognosis of adjacent and opposing teeth.
5. Advise the referring dentist and patient of pertinent findings.

Ordinary Care Equals Prudent Care

Ordinary is commonly understood (outside its legal context) to mean "lacking in excellence" or "being of poor or mediocre quality."[42] As expressed in the context of actions for negligence, however, ordinary care has assumed a technical legal definition somewhat different from its common meaning. *Black's Law Dictionary*, 4th edition, describes ordinary care as "that degree which persons of ordinary care and prudence are accustomed to use or employ . . . that is, reasonable care."

In adopting this distinction the courts have defined ordinary care as "that degree of care which people ordinarily prudent could be reasonably expected to exercise under circumstances of a given case."* It has been equated with the reasonable care and prudence exercised by ordinarily prudent persons under similar circumstances.† It is not extraordinary or ideal care.

Although the standard required of a professional cannot be only that of the most highly skilled practitioner, neither can it be limited to the average member of the profession, because those who have less-than-median skill may still be competent and qualify.‡ By such an illogical definition of average, half of all dentists in a community would automatically fall short of the mark and be negligent as a matter of law. As one case held: "We are not permitted to aggregate into a common class the quacks, the young men who have not practiced, the old ones who have dropped out of practice, the good, and the very best, and then strike an average between them."§

Customary Practice versus Negligence

Customary practice may constitute evidence of the standard of care, but it is not the only determinant. Moreover, if the customary practice constitutes negligence, it is not consid-

ered reasonable (although customarily practiced by a majority of dentists).* Rather, the reasonably prudent dentist *is* the standard of care and not an average or mediocre practitioner. For instance, the majority of dentists are not performing biological testing of the dental unit waterlines despite ADA recommendations to do so.[2,44] However, cautious clinicians still follow this procedure.

Typical examples of negligent behavior by dentists and hygienists include the following:

- Failing to probe and record periodontal pockets[5]
- Failing to take diagnostic-quality radiographs[53,74]
- Failing to refer patients for complicated procedures†
- Failing to use aseptic practices, such as rubber gloves and face masks[49]
- Failing to use rubber dams for endodontics‡
- Failing to install or periodically check valves in dental units to prevent water retraction suck-back cross-contamination§
- Failing to do thermal pulp to aid before diagnosing pulpal disease (see Chapter 1).[18a]
- Failing to discontinue quarternary ammonium chloride-based products for pre-cleaning and/or disinfection of environmental surfaces

Merely because a majority of clinicians in a community practice a particular method does not establish it as the standard of care if it is unreasonable or imprudent.‖ Ultimately, the courts determine what is or is not reasonable dental practice by considering available dental knowledge and evaluating the risks and benefits of a particular procedure.

The law does not require dental perfection.# Instead, the legal yardstick by which such conduct is measured is what a reasonably prudent practitioner would do under the same or similar circumstances, regardless of how many or how few practitioners conform to such a standard.

In one case it was shown that it was not customary practice in the state of Washington for ophthalmologists to test patients under 40 for glaucoma, because the incidence was only one in 25,000 patients. Nevertheless, the Supreme Court of Washington State held that the defendant ophthalmologist was negligent as a matter of law, irrespective of customary medical practice.**

Little excuse exists for failing to routinely probe and chart periodontal pockets before rendering endodontic therapy, no matter how many other dentists in the community fail to do so. The benefit of pulp testing and probing for periodontal disease substantially outweighs the virtually nonexistent risks of conducting these diagnostic procedures. A legal defense likely to

Fraijo v Hartland Hospital, 99 Cal. App. 3d 331 (1979); *California Book of Approved Jury Instructions*, no. 3.16 (ed 8); *Switzer v Atchison, Topeka & Santa Fe Railroad Co.*, 7, Cal. App. 2d 661, 47 P 2d 353, 1935; see 57 Am. Jur. 2d (rev.), Negligence § 144 et seq.
†Restatement Second of Torts, §§ 283, 289.
‡Restatement Second of Torts, § 299A (comment [e]).
§61 Am. Jur. 2d (rev.), Physicians and surgeons and other healers § 110; *Scarano v Schnoor*, 158 Cal. App. 2d 618, 323 P. 2d 178, 1958.

Barton v Owen, 71 Cal. App. 3d 484, 139 Cal. Rptr. 494, 1977.
†*Seneris v Hass*, 45 Cal. 2d 811, 291 P. 2d 915, 1955; 53 A.L.R. 2d 124.
‡*Simpson v Davis*, 219 Kan. 584, 549 P. 2d 950, 1976.
§*Hughes v Blue Cross of Northern California*, 215 Cal. App. 3d 832 (1998).
‖*Barton v Owen*, 71 Cal. App. 3d 484, 139 Cal. Rptr. 494, 1977.
Gurdin v Dongieux, 468 So. 2d 1241, 1985.
**Helling v Carrey*, 83 Wn. 2d 514, 519 P. 2d 981; but see *Meeks v Marx*, 15 Wn. App. 571, 556 P. 2d 1158, 1974.

invoke a jury's wrath is to claim that a necessary diagnostic or prophylactic procedure is "too time consuming," when the dental and medical health of the patient are at risk.

Scientific Research Evaluation

In evaluating scientific research the clinician should remember epidemiological data of risk factors is not always equivalent to etiology. Thus epidemiology is not a synonym for etiology. The scientific community has never exclusively relied upon epidemiology as the accepted method of evaluating cause-and-effect relationships in an effort to make clinical, medical, or dental decisions. Therefore clinicians should not consider only one class of data to supply ultimate proof when conducting an evaluation. Instead, clinicians should consider the strength of any study to be related to the presence and contributing cause of other cofactors.[50,71] This means that the unusual characteristics of a particular patient's case can place the patient at higher or lower risk than the average patient.

New products, intermediate products, and procedures are often introduced faster than epidemiologic and toxicologic studies implemented to evaluate their potential risks. Academic medical centers are facing severe pressure on their reimbursement for health care services and graduate medical education. This creates the need to examine additional sources of revenue to fund their tripartite mission of education, research, and patient care delivery. Reduced government spending for research has resulted in proprietary interests (with proprietary goals) funding more research.[28] Since 1984 the *New England Journal of Medicine*'s policy is to refuse publication of research done by those with financial ties to drug makers. However, in 1999 the journal admitted conflicts in nearly half of the drug studies published since 1997.[6a] The next year, the retiring editor of the *New England Journal of Medicine* concluded that despite tax-supported privileges and extraordinary profits, the best interests of society are not always served. A public trust more accountable to science is needed.

Although much emphasis is currently placed on evidence-based medicine and dentistry, most of the decisions made in clinical practice are not based on data derived from randomized clinical trials.[51] It is virtually impossible to conduct a trial to test the validity of every possible patient management option. Many therapeutic choices are so compelling that a test would be unethical; others are so trivial that a test might not be worth the time or effort. Physicians and dentists do not always practice evidence-based medicine or dentistry, even when evidence is available from randomized clinical trials. This is because knowing the right answer is only the first step in the process of adopting a new treatment methodology. Many practitioners will not use a new drug simply because supporting research data indicates that it works. Instead, identification of the probable mechanism of action is often a prerequisite before adopting a new treatment.

However, clinicians should not avoid using certain drugs if the data supporting their use is overwhelming. When the results of a clinical trial conflict with a widely held mechanistic model, many clinicians doubt the evidence from the study.[41] However, when the results from well-researched clinical trials become so convincing that they can no longer be ignored, prudent practice embraces the new model and discards previously held concepts. Endodontics advances as disproven old ideas retreat. For example, delaying extractions until after several days of antibiotic use to reduce infection is no longer the accepted practice. Rather, immediate extraction, along with any necessary antibiotics, is the preferred current therapy.[4]

Proceed cautiously with new devices, which lack definitive research studies. For instance, high-intensity wireless, fast-curing lights may generate heat at the wand tip and cause pulpal pathology. First-generation halogen bulbs require longer composite curing time to achieve polymerization but generate only 400 to 800 mW/cm. Plasma arc bulbs reduce curing time but generate 2000 mW/cm.

Examination   After gathering the dental and medical history, findings obtained from the various phases of the clinical and radiographic examinations are recorded. Lists in each category afford the clinician a systematic format for recording details pertinent to a proper diagnosis. Appropriate descriptions are circled, followed by the necessary notations in the accompanying spaces. Tabular arrangement allows easier recording and comparison of diagnostic test data acquired from one tooth on different dates or from different teeth on the same visit. A pain intensity index (i.e., 0 to 10) or pain classification (i.e., mild +, moderate + +, severe + + +) should be used whenever possible to differentiate diagnostic test results.

Diagnosis   Careful analysis of accumulated examination data should result in the determination of an accurate pulpal and periapical diagnosis. Clinical conditions and the probable etiologic factors for the presenting problem are circled. Alternative modalities of therapy are considered and analyzed. The recommended treatment plan is circled, followed by a prognostic assessment of the intended therapeutic course.

Patient Consultation   Patients should be advised of each diagnosis and should consent to the treatment plan before therapy is instituted. Consultation should include an explanation of reasonable alternative treatment approaches and rationales, treatment consequences, including risks from nontreatment or delayed treatment that may affect the outcome of intended therapy. Such discussion is documented by simply completing and endorsing the checklist.

Treatment   All treatment provided on a given date is documented by placing a check mark (✓) within the designated procedural category. Only the most frequent retreatment procedures are included for tabulation. Descriptions of occasional procedures or explanatory treatment remarks should be entered in writing. A separate dated entry should be made for each patient visit, phone call, e-mail message, and fax communication (e.g., consultations with the patient or other doctors) or correspondence (e.g., biopsy report, treatment completion letters).

Individual root canal lengths are recorded by (1) circling the corresponding anatomic designation and the method of length determination (e.g., radiograph or electronic measuring device), (2) writing the measurement (in millimeters), and (3) indicating the reference point. For any medication prescribed, refilled, or dispensed, the treatment record should show the date and type of drug (including dose, quantity, and instructions for use) in the treatment table under the heading of *Rx*. Periodic recall intervals, dates, and findings are entered in the spaces provided.

Negligence Per Se

Compliance with a safety statute does not conclusively establish due care, because regulations require only minimal care and not (necessarily) prudent care or what the law regards as due care.* A civil liability duty of care may be imposed by statutes and safety ordinances. For example, violation of a health safety statute may create a presumption of negligence on the part of the dentist.† Although at trial the plaintiff ordinarily has the burden of proving negligence, a refutable presumption of negligence shifts the burden of proof to the defendant, if the following conditions are met:
1. Violation of a health safety statute, ordinance, or regulation of a public entity occurs
2. Violation caused injury
3. Injury resulted from an occurrence that the statute, ordinance, or regulation was designed to prevent
4. Person suffering injury was one of the persons for whose protection the statute, ordinance, or regulation was adopted‡

Ability to Foresee Unreasonable Risk

Each endodontic procedure has some degree of inherent risk. The standard of care requires that the dentist avoid unreasonable risks that may harm the patient. Treatment is deemed negligent when a reasonable dentist would have foreseen some unreasonable risk of harm to the patient. Failure to follow the dictates of sound endodontic practice increases the risk of negligently induced deleterious results. Accordingly, prophylactic endodontic practice is designed to prevent foreseeable or reasonably avoidable injury risks.

It is not necessary that the exact injuries that occur be foreseeable. Nor is it necessary to foresee the precise manner or circumstances under which injuries are inflicted. It is enough that a reasonably prudent dentist would foresee that injuries of the same general type would be likely to occur in the absence of adequate safeguards.*

Informed Consent Principles

In General   The legal doctrine of informed consent requires that the patient be advised of reasonably foreseeable material risks of endodontic therapy, the nature of the treatment, reasonable alternatives, and the consequences of nontreatment.[75]† This doctrine is based on the legal principle that individual patients have the right to do with their own bodies as they see fit, including the right to prematurely lose teeth, regardless of recommended dental treatment. Thus once the dentist has informed the patient of the diagnosis, the prognosis and risks faced with treatment, the prognosis and risks faced without treatment, as well as recommendations for corrective treatment or alternative therapy, the patient must make the decision of how to proceed. An adult of sound mind is entitled to elect to do nothing about existing endodontic disease, rather than elect corrective treatment.

To be effective a patient's consent to treatment must be legally informed consent. Accordingly, a dentist has a fiduciary duty to disclose all material information necessary for the patient to make a decision.‡ The scope of a dentist's duty to disclose information is measured by the amount of knowledge a patient needs to make an informed choice. Material information is that disclosure a dentist knows (or should know) that would be regarded as significant by a reasonable person in the patient's position who must decide whether to accept or reject a recommended endodontic procedure.

If a dentist fails to reasonably disclose information and a reasonable person in the patient's position would have declined the procedure if provided with that disclosure, the dentist may be liable should an undisclosed risk manifest. Beyond the foregoing minimal disclosure, a dentist must also reveal such additional information as a skilled practitioner of good standing would provide under similar circumstances.

The personal bond between dentist and patient has long been considered an essential element of the therapeutic environment. Information is empowering; laws requiring informed consent put patients on a closer footing with their dentists. In addition to the transfer of information in both directions, bonding takes place when the doctor and patient engage in a conversation of length and substance. Canned disclosure displaces this human interaction. *The surest safeguard dentists can have against malpractice litigation is the bond of personal relationship forged with their patients.*[55]

Texas & Pacific Railway Co. v Behymer, 189 U.S. 468, 47 L. Ed. 905, 23 S. Ct. 622, 1903; Daum v. Spinecare Medical Group, Inc., 52 Cal. App. 4th 1285; 61 Cal. Rptr. Sd 260, 1997.
†*McGee v Cessna Aircraft Co.*, 139 Cal. App. 3d 179, 188 Cal. Rptr. 542, 1983.
‡California Evidence Code, § 669.

*Restatement Second of Torts, § 282 et seq.; Witkin: *Summary of California law* (Torts, § 751), ed 9, San Francisco, 1988, Bancroft Whitney.
†*Johnson v Kokemoor*, 545 N.W. 2d 495, 1996.
‡*Cobbs v Grant*, 8 Cal. 3d 229, 104 Cal. Rptr. 505, 502 P. 2d 1, 1972; *California Book of Approved Jury Instructions*, no. 6.11 (ed 8); Miller FH: Health care information technology and informed consent: computer and doctor-patient relationship, *Ind L Rev.* 31:1019, 1998.

Application of Standard   Informed consent is a flexible standard that considers reasonably foreseeable consequences, depending on the clinical situation present both before and during treatment. For instance, a fractured or separated endodontic instrument left in the root canal creates the possibility of root canal failure or impaired success (depending on whether the fracture occurred in the coronal, middle [least favorable], or apical third of the root canal). Therefore the dentist must advise the patient of the relative risk of future failure and suggest treatment alternatives to correct the problem. This way the patient can make an intelligent choice among apicoectomy, referral to an endodontist for attempted retrieval, or close radiographic observation at recall visits. In Fig. 10-10 the dentist overinstrumented and perforated the inferior alveolar nerve, causing both a permanent dysesthesia and parasthesia. The dentist should have immediately referred the patient to an endodontist for attempted gutta-percha retrieval before the endodontic sealant eugenol-containing set and caused more deleterious chemical injury to the inferior alveolar nerve. If retrieval was unsuccessful, the patient should have been referred to a microsurgeon within 36 hours.

Adequate disclosure includes clinical judgment and experience, which assesses current research and applies it to the clinical needs of each patient. Today's advance may be tomorrow's retreat, if materials, devices, or instruments lacking adequate, long-term study of safety and efficacy are used but fail. For instance, one- component bonding agent is more technique sensitive than its two-component predecessor. This is because the one-component agent contains acetone that desiccates the tooth surface and requires a moist surface to avoid postoperative sensitivity. Long-term testing before marketing would have revealed that the two-step system is more reliable and forgiving.[61] Reasonable dentists do not sacrifice patient safety for speed and profit and then compensate with desensitizing agents.

Material disclosure concerns whether the patient was provided sufficient information for a reasonable patient to achieve a general understanding of the proposed treatment or procedure. This disclosure includes information concerning any dentally acceptable alternatives, any predictable risks of serious injury, and any likely consequences should the patient refuse the proposed therapy. The standard to be applied is whether a reasonable person in the patient's position would have consented to the procedure or treatment in question if adequately informed of all significant perils.[16]* Informed consent applies only to inherent risks of nonnegligent treatment, because a patient's consent to negligent treatment is voidable as being contrary to public policy.† For instance, a patient who refuses necessary diagnostic radiographs should be refused treatment.

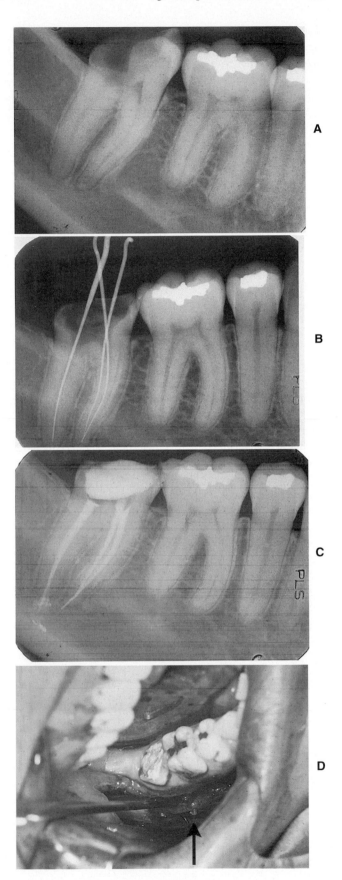

Fig. 10-10 **A**, Preoperative radiograph. **B**, Measuring film without a rubber dam. **C**, Postoperative radiograph. **D**, Decompression microsurgery showing protruding "dagger" of bone to the right of the retractor at the inferior border of the inferior alveolar nerve resulting from prior perforation of the mandibular canal. This is probably due to file overinstrumentation. **C** courtesy Dr. Tony Pogrell.

---

*See *Ashe v Radiation Oncology Associations*, M1997-00036-SC-R11-CV, 1999.

†*Tunkl v Regents of University of California*, 60 Cal. 2d 92, 32 Cal. Rptr. 33, 383 P. 2d 441, 1963.

Advice Regarding Different Schools of Thought

After advising treatment, if other reasonable dentists would disagree or if there are other respectable schools of thought on the correct treatment, this material information should be disclosed to the patient.* For example, assume that there are two schools of thought concerning the optimal treatment for retrofilling and apicoectomy. One school posits that a retrograde with intermediate restorative material (IRM) is the appropriate procedure, whereas the minority review asserts that retrograde with Super EBA is the preferred treatment.[73] Assume further that an explanation of these two different methods of treatment constitutes material information for the purposes of informed consent. The mere fact that there is a disagreement within the relevant endodontic community does not establish that the selection of one procedure as opposed to the other constitutes negligent endodontic therapy. Because competent endodontists regularly use both procedures, a patient would have a difficult time proving dental negligence (i.e., that the endodontist failed "to have the knowledge and skill ordinarily possessed, and to use the care and skill ordinarily used, by reputable specialists practicing in the same field and in the same or a similar locality and under similar circumstances"). Moreover, neither school of thought possesses long-term clinical research results to prognosticate apical sealant insolubility rates in an 18-year-old patient with an additional 60-year life expectancy.[7] Long-term durability depends upon an insoluble seal to reduce the risk of bacterial leakage. Fig. 10-11 represents a preoperative and postoperative radiograph of a successful apicoectomy and retrograde in a 14-year-old adolescent.

On the other hand, the specialist would have a duty under such hypothetical circumstances to disclose the two recognized schools of treatment so that the patient could be sufficiently informed to make the final, personal decision. An endodontist, being the expert, appreciates the risks inherent in the procedure prescribed, the risks of a decision not to undergo the treatment, and the probability of a successful outcome of the treatment. Once this information has been disclosed, this aspect of the endodontist's expert function has been performed. The weighing of these risks against the individual subjective fears and hopes of the patient is not an expert skill. Such evaluation and decision is a nondental judgment reserved for the patient alone.† In this hypothetical situation, failure to disclose such material information would deprive the patient of the opportunity to weigh the risks. Consequently, the dentist would have failed in the duty of disclosure, which the doctrine of informed consent requires.

When improved technology offers clearly superior results, it no longer becomes a patient choice issue but, rather, a requisite requirement to fulfill the standard of care.

Apical microsurgery with ultrasonic tips for retrofilling exemplifies improved technology and the current standard of practice. Likewise, apical retrogrades should be done with mineral trioxide aggregate (MTA) and not amalgam.[21]

Avoiding Patient Claims

If a dentist fails to obtain adequate informed consent, a plaintiff can recover damages (even in the absence of any negligent treatment) should the patient testify that performed treatment would have been refused if the clinician had provided information concerning possible risks. Therefore discussions of treatment risks with the patient must be documented. Informed consent forms are very helpful, although not legally mandated, because a jury may believe that the patient was informed orally. Equally, if not more important than consent forms, is a chart notation indicating that the dentist discussed informed consent risks and alternatives (and that the patient understood and accepted this information). Patients may mentally block out frightening information. Trauma and a potent anesthetic can create retrograde amnesia. Therefore clinicians must document (in the patient's chart) any risks, benefits, alternatives, and consequences of nontreatment provided to the patient.

Clinicians should follow only the patient-authorized and consented to treatment plan. If an emergency precludes advising treatment risks to the minor patient, lack of informed consent may be defensible as implied consent (because no reasonable person would refuse necessary, nonelective emergency treatment).

The following example shows how a clinician should record any recommended treatment that the patient has refused and the reason for that refusal:

"Patient refused endodontic referral for consultation with endodontist (Dr. Gudguy) because husband was laid off work last month and cannot afford treatment. After explanation, patient understands detrimental delay risks."

Patients may initial any referral refusal on the chart. Although not mandatory, it will enhance the clinician's credibility should the patient later dispute the referral.

Reasonable familiarity with a new product or technique is required before it is used. In addition, a patient is entitled to know the dentist's personal experience with a particular modality, because the patient has a right to chose between reasonable alternatives or to seek care from a dentist who has more experience with a particular modality or product. A dentist who fails to obtain informed consent may be liable for injury caused by a product or instrument. The fact that the dentist followed the manufacturer's instructions is no defense if the dentist did not provide adequate information concerning a product or instrument risk (to permit the patient to intelligently weigh the disclosed information and choose among treatment options).

Endodontic Informed Consent

If the practitioner's own statistical experience varies significantly from national statistics, using statistics presented in

---

Vandi v Permanente Medical Group, 7 Cal. App. 4th 1064, 9 Cal. Rptr. 2d 463, 1992; Weisman G: Direct restorations. *Dental Products Report* p 21, Jan 2000.
†*Cobbs v Grant*, 8 Cal. 3d 229, 104 Cal. Rptr. 505, 502 P. 2d 1, 1972; *California Book of Approved Jury Instructions*, no. 6.11 (ed 8).

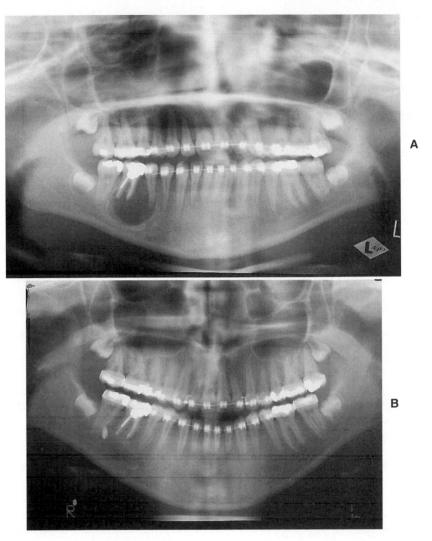

Fig. 10-11 Preoperative (**A**) and postoperative (**B**) panoramic radiographs showing a successful apicoectomy and retrograde. (Courtesy Dr. Edmond Bedrossian.)

national literature regarding success rates for endodontic procedures is considered insufficient disclosure and does not fulfill the legal requirements of informed consent (Fig. 10-12).*

Among specialists the reported incidence of treatment complications in endodontics is relatively low. Based on a Southwest Endodontic Society retrospective study, a reasonable endodontist or a practitioner with similar abilities should disclose the following facts to patients[59]:

1. Endodontic therapy cannot be guaranteed.
2. Although endodontic therapy is usually successful, a small percentage of teeth are lost despite competent endodontic care, owing to complications or treatment failure.

3. Slight overextending or underfilling root canals occurs in 2% to 4% of cases, which may contribute to treatment failure.
4. Slight to moderate transient postoperative pain may occur; severe postoperative pain rarely occurs.
5. Irreparable damage to the existing crown or restoration secondary to endodontic treatment is uncommon.

Video-Informed Consent   Animated video-informed consent shown to the patient is a dynamic method of providing informed consent. Because the video-informed consent is considered part of the dentist's records, in the event the patient disputes having ever been advised of (1) the nature of endodontic disease, (2) the availability of endodontic specialists, or (3) the relative indications for nonsurgical versus surgical endodontic care, the videotape can be played back to the jury as proof that the patient was informed. It is doubtful a jury would believe a forgetful patient who admits having

---

*Hales v Pittman, 118 Ariz. 305, 576 P. 2d 493, 1978; Shelter v Rochelle, 2 Ariz. App. 370, 409 P. 2d 86, 1965.

INFORMED CONSENT

We are concerned not only about your dental health and endodontic treatment needs, but also about your right as a patient to make the treatment decision that you feel is best for you. Our commitment to you is to provide you with detailed and complete information about your dental needs as we diagnose them. We will share our diagnostic processes with you, and we invite and welcome all of your questions regarding our treatment.

Towards this aim of a mutual sharing of information, we feel it is important to advise you of the reasonably foreseeable risks of endodontic therapy. The following is important information you should consider to aid your treatment decision.

■ Root canal therapy is a procedure designed to retain a tooth that may otherwise require extraction. Root canal therapy has a very high degree of success. However, it is a biological procedure, and results cannot therefore be guaranteed.

■ Approximately 5% to 10% of teeth that have undergone nonsurgical root canal therapy may require retreatment or root-end surgery.

■ Despite our best efforts, approximately 5% of endodontically treated teeth may fail and require extraction.

■ Final restoration (crown) of the tooth that has undergone root canal therapy is essential to root canal success and retention of the tooth. A final restoration should be completed within 30 days of root canal therapy. This restoration should be done by your restorative dentist.

Signature of Patient (or Parent) _____ Date _____

Witness _____ Date _____

Fig. 10-12 Informed consent form.

previously viewed the videotape, because the videotape refreshes the stream of memories that may have otherwise faded away into the unconscious.

A patient viewing the videotape is more likely to understand the informed consent disclosure. After viewing the videotape and discussing its contents with the dentist, the patient should sign a video consent form to verify that the video was viewed and all of the patient's questions were answered.

Alternative Technique Choice

Filling the root canal with the lateral compaction method or using vertical warm gutta-percha delivery systems, including heat-transfer units for warm gutta-percha, are currently taught, and there are zealous advocates for each technique. Both methods are reasonable and acceptable choices and conform to the standard of care. The choice of techniques changes as new products are introduced and scientific research is conducted. However, the vertical warm gutta-percha technique promising to deliver improved flow to fill lateral canals is likely to predominate in the twenty-first century.

Ethics

Endodontics is one of eight ADA recognized dental specialties. Although any licensed dentist may legally practice endodontics, it is unethical to announce that one specializes in endodontics without specialty training or being "grandfathered" into endodontic practice. It is ethically impermissible for a general practitioner to characterize a general practice as "limited to endodontics."* However, the general practitioner is permitted to emphasize endodontics by advertising as a "general practitioner of endodontics."

Referrals to Other Dentists

Every dental practitioner, including specialists, will at some time need to refer a patient to a specialist for treatment to comply with the standard of care required of a reasonable and prudent dentist. †

Generally if the referral takes place within the same dental practice, the legal doctrine of *respondeat superior* ("let the master answer") may be applicable. Under this rule, a dentist is liable for the dental negligence of a person acting as his agent, employee, or partner.‡ This is determined by whether the principal dentist controls the agent dentist's methodology, regardless of whether such control is actually exercised.

If the referral is made (even within the same physical environment) to an "independent contractor" endodontist who does not diagnose or treat under the direction or supervision of the referring dentist and that referring dentist has no right of control as to the mode of performing the treatment, the principle of agency and responsibility for the acts of another does not apply.* The legal test for agency is the principal's right to control, regardless if the control is exercise over the agent.

To ensure that the referred dentist is not considered the agent of the referring dentist within the same facility, fees for the referred dentist should not be set by the referring dentist. Nor should the fees be divided equally or shared based on some other arrangement. Also the referred dentist should bill separately and exercise independent diagnostic and therapeutic judgment. Advise the patient that the referred dentist is independent of the referring dentist. Otherwise, the referred dentist or specialist may be regarded or inferred to be the ostensible agent of the referring dentist in the same office (although this is not the case). The legal test for agency is how the facts or circumstances appear to a reasonable patient, regardless of the dentist's understanding or intent that the other treating dentist be considered an independent contractor. Thus agency may be actual in fact or, alternatively, ostensible (i.e., implied by circumstantial conduct).†

Surgical Versus Nonsurgical Endodontics

Litigation to determine whether nonsurgical or surgical endodontics was the proper treatment choice will not be decided by any one clinician, the ADA, AAE, or the ablest of judges. Rather, after considering all of the evidence and the opinions of experts, a jury of the patient's peers will decide the disputed matter. Depending on the individual case, the jury may decide that either a combination of nonsurgical and surgical endodontic therapy, rather than one method exclusively, should have been attempted. The jury may also decide that the patient should have been advised of the availability of such alternative therapy. Similarly, the jury may determine that apical surgery should have been done microscopically, rather than macroscopically, depending upon expert testimony regarding the relative advantages of each method or upon presenting clinical circumstances (e.g., suspected calcification, viewing a separated instrument).

Failing endodontics that necessitate endodontic disassembly should first be considered for a nonsurgical option because it is less invasive and therefore represents risk reduction. The clinician should first evaluate for coronal leakage, fractures, missed canals, silver point corrosion, and incomplete fills. Root canal systems can then be recleaned or cor-

*American Dental Association: *Principles of ethics and code of professional conduct*, §§ 5-C and 5-D; California Dental Association: *Principle of ethics*, §§ 8 and 9.
†*Simone v Sabo*, 37 Cal. 2d 253, 231 P. 2d 19, 1951.
‡*Restatement Second of Agency*, §§ 228-237.

Mission Insurance Co. v Worker's Comp Appeals Board, 123 Cal. App. 3d 211, 1981.
†*California book of approved jury instructions*, no. 13.20.5 (ed 8).

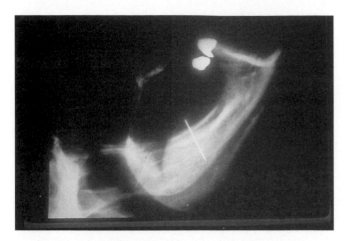

Fig. 10-13   Needle became lodged in this patient's soft tissue.

rectly transported, then reshaped and packed in three dimensions, thereby often avoiding apical surgery, with its attendant risks and reduced potential for long-term success.

Product Liability

Today's dentist exploring ways to improve the quality and success of endodontic therapy is constantly presented with new dental products and techniques. For prescribing and using drugs or other agents, the ADA's *Principles of Ethics*, Section 10, provides this guideline:

"The dentist has an obligation not to prescribe, dispense, or promote the use of drugs or other agents whose complete formulas are not available to the dental profession. He also has the obligation not to prescribe or dispense, except for limited investigative purposes, any therapeutic agent, the value of which is not supported by scientific evidence. The dentist has the further obligation of not holding out as exclusive any agent, method, or technique."

Ethical dentists should not indiscriminately use every new product but, instead, review the supporting research rather than risk the patient's welfare with inadequately tested or research products only tested in vivo.

Separated Instruments   Risk reduction of broken files can be accomplished if all hand and rotary nickel and titanium (NiTi) cleaning and shaping files are not resterilized and reused. Efficiency is also increased because approximately 50% of cutting efficiency is lost after initial use. Episodes of broken instruments will be dramatically reduced and nearly eliminated when files are used correctly and *discarded after single-tooth use*. Breakage increases sharply when hand or rotary shaping files are reused. Therefore the clinician should *discard rotary instruments after a single-use visit.* Chair and staff time efficiency, along with improved safety, dictate single-visit use of files. The clinician should save broken or defective instruments (e.g., the remaining portion from a needle that has broken and become lodged in

a patient's soft tissue) (Fig. 10-13). The instrument manufacturer may be liable because the product was defective, rather than the dentist being liable for dental negligence.* Electron microscopy spectrographic analysis can determine if manufacturing defects with contaminants caused the break, rather than the dentist excessively bending the needle.

Equipment and Supplies   Keep equipment in good repair by checking and following the manufacturer's recommended maintenance schedule. The clinician should carefully read the manufacturer's instruction warnings on instruments and inform staff of any important points. Infection control in operating dental equipment is mandatory, such as updating and maintaining dental units with check valves to prevent water retraction or suck back. The clinician should inspect check valves monthly and change clogged valves immediately.[43] Water retraction testers, at no charge to the dentist, are available from some manufacturers.† The dentist or a staff member should also disassemble the unit's hand piece, run water through the line for a few seconds, then stop. If a bubble of water is visible at the end of the water hose holes, the check valve is operating properly. If the bubble of water is not visible, water may be sucked back because of an absent or clogged check valve. An absent or clogged check valve is a source of cross-contamination. Therefore it is important for the clinician or staff to perform weekly spore testing of sterilizer and monthly bacteriologic testing of water lines.[2] The clinician or staff should consider filters, and flush daily with FDA-approved chemical disinfectants of dental unit water lines to reduce water tubing biofilm. Some chemical disinfectants claim improved cost effectiveness by increasing hand piece and bur longevity concomitant with water line purging or with continual use during treatment. Fig. 10-14 shows a student who was burned because of an inadequately maintained hand piece that overheated. This case settled for $280,000.00.

Drugs   Clinicians should exercise extreme caution when administering or prescribing dangerous drugs. For sedative or narcotic drugs, cautionary directions should be written on prescriptions, and the pharmacist should place these directions on the prescription container as a patient reminder. For example, for the appropriate drugs, the clinician should prepare a prescription rubber stamp or obtain preprinted prescriptions that state the following:

"Do not drive or operate dangerous machinery after taking medication because drowsiness is likely to occur. Alcohol, sedative, or tranquilizing drugs will cause drowsiness if taken in combination with this prescribed drug."

The ADA and AMA provide prescription drug warning pads. Clinicians should document each drug information form provided with the prescription in the patient's chart.

---

*Restatement Second of Torts, § 402A. (see Fig. 10-14)
†A-Dec, for instance.

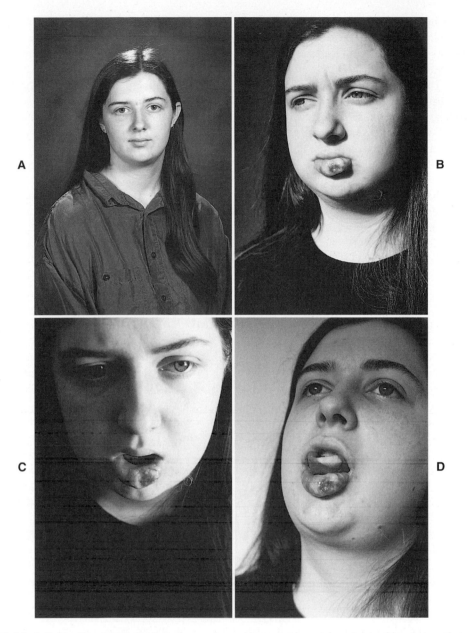

Fig. 10-14 **A,** Before injury. **B-D,** Student who was burned by an inadequately maintained hand piece that overheated. This lawsuit settled for $280,000.

Overuse of antibiotics risks resistant-strain development and side effects. Studies demonstrate generally no increased therapeutic efficiency of endodontic therapy with antibiotics when performed in the absence of facial swelling.[68] Unless persistent infections occur or compelling systemic reasons exist (e.g., uncontrolled diabetes, antibiotic prophylaxis necessary because of mitral valve regurgitation), antibiotics should not be prescribed prophylactically.[21a] Neither pain nor localized swelling justify antibiotics. However, extraoral swelling, cellulitis, or lymphadenopathy may require surgical drainage or antibiotics or both. The Centers for Disease Control and Prevention (CDC) estimates about one third of all antibiotic outpatient prescriptions are unnecessary.[6]

Dentist's Liability for Staffs' Acts or Omissions

A dentist is liable for the acts or omissions of the dentist's staff under the doctrine of *respondeat superior* ("let the master answer"). This is termed *vicarious liability*, which means that the dentist is responsible, not because he or she did anything wrong personally, but because the dentist assumes legal responsibility for the conduct of employees and agents who act in the course and scope of their employment.

The dentist should instruct the staff in advising patients regarding posttreatment complaints. For example, if the staff ignores signs of infection, such as difficulty in swallowing or breathing or elevated temperature, and dismisses the patient's complaints as normal postoperative swelling, the dentist may be held liable for injury to the patient, such as delayed cellulitis, diagnosis or treatment of Ludwig's angina, brain abscess, or other serious complications.

A clinician must be cautious when delegating responsibilities and give clear instructions to ensure that staff properly represent the clinician and the chosen practice methods. Auxiliaries should not be allowed to practice beyond their competency level or license. For example, in states where legally permissible, the dentist should check an assistant-placed restoration before patient dismissal. Staff members should not make final diagnoses or handle patient clinical complaints without the dentist's involvement. Staff should be instructed to ask appropriate questions and to relay the patient's answers to the dentist so that the dentist can determine what should be done.

Abandonment

Once endodontic treatment is initiated, the dentist is legally obligated to complete the treatment regardless of the patient's payment of any outstanding balance. This requirement is posited on the legal premise that any person who attempts to rescue another from harm must reasonably complete the rescue with beneficial intervention, unless another rescuer (i.e., dentist) is willing to assume the undertaking.* Another view is that should a patient be placed in a position of danger unless further treatment is performed, the dentist must institute reasonable therapeutic measures to ensure that adverse consequences do not result.†

A dentist performing endodontic therapy should have reasonable means of communicating with patients after regular office hours to avoid a claim for abandonment. A recorded message is inadequate if the dentist fails to check for recorded messages frequently. Therefore answering services, pagers, and cell phones are required by the standard of care.

If the dentist providing endodontic therapy is away from the office for an extended period, a substitute on-call dentist should be available for any endodontic emergency and to answer patients' emergency calls. The endodontic treating dentist should arrange in advance for emergency service with a covering dentist. Leaving a name on the office answering machine or with the answering service without first determining the availability of the covering dentist is a mistake.

To avoid an abandonment claim, several prophylactic measures apply:
1. No legal duty requires a dentist to accept all patients for treatment. A private practice dentist may legally refuse to treat a new patient, despite severe pain or infection, except on the grounds of race or disability.* If treatment is limited to emergency measures only, the clinician must advise the patient that only temporary emergency endodontic therapy is being provided and that endodontic treatment is incomplete. The clinician should record this information in the patient's chart. For example:

"Emergency palliative treatment only. Patient advised endodontic treatment of tooth no. 8 needs to be completed, either here or with another dentist. Explained complications likely if not soon completed, including infection recurrence or tooth loss or both."

The patient should also be asked to acknowledge that treatment is limited to the existing emergency by endorsing an informed consent to emergency endodontics statement as follows:

"I agree to emergency endodontic treatment of my tooth no. 8 and have been advised that (1) emergency treatment is for temporary relief of pain and (2) further root canal treatment of tooth no. 8 after emergency treatment is necessary to avoid further complications, including, but not limited to, pain, infection, fracture, abscess, or tooth loss."

2. No legal duty requires a dentist to continue treating former patients on recalls or subsequent emergency care once treatment is complete. Thus completion of endodontic treatment for tooth no. 19 does not legally obligate the dentist to initiate endodontic therapy for tooth no. 3, if endodontic disease began months after the clinician completed treatment of tooth no. 19.

3. Any patient may be discharged from a practice for any arbitrary reason, except on the grounds of race or disability, so long as all initiated treatment is completed. Accordingly, a former patient who evokes memories of a "frictional" relationship, who is financially irresponsible, or who arrives at the office after an absence of several years with an acute apical abscess in a site where previous care was not rendered may legally be refused treatment.

4. It is not considered abandonment if a patient is given reasonable notice to seek endodontic treatment with another dentist and the patient is willing to seek endodontic services elsewhere.† Thus if rapport with the patient dissolves, the clinician should not hesitate to suggest that the patient would be better served if any remaining endodontic treatment were performed by a different dentist.

*Lee v Deubre, 362 S.W. 2d 900, 1962; Clark v Hoek, 219 Cal. Rptr. 845, 1985.
†McNamara v Emmons, 36 Cal. App. 2d 199, 97 P. 2d 503, 1939; Small v Wegner, 267 S.W. 2d 26, 1954; 50 A.L.R. 2d 170.

*Bragdon v Abbott 118 S. Ct. 2196, 1998; McNamara v Emmons, 36 Cal. App. 2d 199, 1939; 97 P. 2d 503; Small v Wegner, 267 S.W. 2d 26, 1954; 50 A.L.R. 2d 1970. The Americans With Disabilities Act (Publ. No. 101-336); Americans with Disabilities Act, Title III, Regulations, 28 C.F.R., Part 36, Nondiscrimination on the basis of disability by public accommodations and in commercial facilities, U.S. Department of Justice, Office of the Attorney General and Americans with Disabilities Act, Title I Regulations, 29 C.F.R., Part 1630, Equal employment opportunity for individuals with disabilities, U.S. Equal Employment Opportunity Commission.
†Murray v U.S., 4th Cir., 329 F. 2d 270, 1964.

The clinician may discontinue treatment, provided it is not done at a time when the patient's dental health will be jeopardized (e.g., in the middle of treatment). To discontinue treatment, the clinician should do the following:

1. Notify the patient of the plan to discontinue treatment after a certain date.
2. Allow enough time for the patient to obtain care with another dentist, usually 30 days.
3. Offer to make emergency service available during the interim 30 days until a new dentist is obtained.
4. Provide diagnostic quality records, copies of radiographs, and other pertinent clinical information in transfer records to the new treating dentist.
5. Allow the patient to select a new practitioner or suggest referral by the local dental society if a referral service exists.
6. Document all of the above in the patient's records, including a copy of a certified letter sent to the patient proposing discontinuance of treatment.

Expert Testimony

The standard of care that a dentist must possess and exercise is particularly within the knowledge of dental experts. However, there are occasional exceptions where the conduct involved is within the common knowledge of laypersons, in which case expert testimony is not required. In determining whether expert testimony is required to establish negligence, one California court commented: "The correct rule on the necessity of expert testimony has been summarized by Bob Dylan: 'You don't need a weatherman to know which way the wind blows.'"*

Incorrectly operating on the contralateral side because of mismounted radiographs or marking the wrong tooth on an endodontic referral card are examples of negligent conduct within the common knowledge of laypersons for which expert testimony is not required.

Increasingly, courts act as gatekeepers regarding the admissibility of scientific expert testimony. Anecdotal comparisons appear compelling, but such evidence may be judicially excluded in the courtroom. Some experts rely solely on their skill for experience-based observation, rather than research testing of risk factors, such as occurs with epidemiological research.

The U.S. Supreme Court (in the *Daubert* four factors checklist†) advises that an expert's testimony may be reliably admitted into evidence based upon the following:

1. Whether the expert's technique or theory may be tested or refuted

2. Whether the technique or theory has been the subject of peer review or publication
3. Known or potential rate of technique error
4. Degree of acceptance of a theory or technique within the relevant scientific community

Courts determine whether testimony is based upon the application of scientific principle or clinical experience. In general, courts are flexible and adaptable in determining whether there is a bright line separating scientific and unsupported nonscientific evidence. Often technical and specialized knowledge gained though continuing education and scientific journals, rather than an expert performing the research, is considered sufficient as long as the expert's opinion complies with the *Daubert* principle.

States are not bound to follow the Federal Rules of Evidence in state court trials.* Nonetheless, U.S. Supreme Court decisions influence state courts that consider placing limitations upon expert testimony. State court trial judges may either be more liberal or more restrictive in admitting expert witness testimony. If the trial court judge denies admission of scientific evidence as unreliable, untrustworthy, or irrelevant, the end result may be to preclude an expert offering any opinion. On the other hand, the court may admit such evidence and instruct the jury that they may consider the scientific basis for the expert opinions and give such evidence the evidentiary weight it deserves.

Recently, the Court held in *Weisgram v. Marley Co.* that appellate courts have the power, under Federal Rule of Civil Procedure 50(a), to direct a district court to enter judgment notwithstanding the verdict against a winning plaintiff if the appellate court determines that admitted expert testimony was unreliable and inadmissible under *Daubert v. Merrell Dow Pharmaceuticals, Inc.*

MALPRACTICE INCIDENTS

Screw Posts

Screw posts represent a restorative anachronism. The risk of root fracture is too great compared with the benefit, particularly when reasonable and superior passive alternatives exist (see Chapter 21). Even if the screw post is initially placed passively, the temptation to turn the screw is too great, considering human nature. Therefore screw posts are not a reasonable and prudent treatment choice.

Paresthesia

Endodontic surgery in the vicinity of the mandibular canal or mental foramen carries with it the significant risk of irreversible injury to the inferior alveolar or mental nerve,

---

*Jorgensen v Beach 'N' Bay Realty, Inc., 125 Cal. App. 3d 155, 177 Cal. Rptr. 882, 1981 (quoting "Subterranean Homesick Blues" from "Bringing It All Back Home.") Accord: Easton v Strassburger, 152 Cal. App. 3d 90, 199 Cal. Rptr. 383, 1984; 46 A.L.R. 4th 521.
†Daubert v Merrell Dow Pharmaceuticals, Inc., 509 U.S. 579 (1993).

*Wisconsin Supreme Court and 23 states have agreed to follow the federal standard in Daubert, supra. Bunting v Jamieson, 984 P. 2d 467, 1999.

respectively. Consequently, the clinician must advise the patient in lay terms of the risk of temporary or permanent anesthesia or paresthesia before any surgery near these structures is performed. To document that adequate informed consent was provided, the clinician should have the patient execute a written informed consent form confirming that the patient was so advised. Informed consent is inapposite if the surgery was negligently chosen or negligently performed, because informed consent only applies to nonnegligent treatment risks.

Failure of Treatment

A dentist should not guarantee treatment success. It is foolish to assure the patient of a perfect result.* Endodontic failures may occur despite the best endodontic care.[33]† Negligent contributing factors to failure include perforation, missed or transported canal, uninstrumented portion of a root canal, infiltrate via a leaky coronal restoration contaminating the root canal filling,[17] overextension errors, and inadequate isolation of the tooth from contaminants during instrumentation because of lack of a rubber dam.

To avoid claims based on failed endodontics, the patient should be advised in advance of treatment of the inherent (but relatively small) risk of failure (i.e., about 5% to 10%). It may be adequate to advise the patient of the high statistical probability of success in endodontics as long as the clinical condition of the tooth and the clinician's past success rate warrant such representation.‡ Clinicians should avoid quoting the national success rate of endodontics when (1) the patient's tooth is of questionable periodontal status and (2) the clinician is known to have an unusually high endodontic failure rate (i.e., a rate that varies markedly from national statistics).

An endodontic treating dentist is also liable for failure to disclose evident pathology in the quadrant being treated. The patient should be advised of any periodontal disease that adversely affects the prognosis of abutment teeth for partial dentures or bridges. A dentist should also advise of cysts, fractures, or lesions of suspected neoplasms. In addition, the clinician must be careful not to ignore any evident pathology which, if untreated, may adversely affect the dental or medical health of the patient. A dentist who fails to plan treatment properly is planning for treatment failure.

The doctrine of informed consent protects both the dentist and the patient so that there will be no surprises or patient disappointment if an adverse result occurs. Should nonnegligent failure or complication occur, the availability of a signed informed consent form can serve as a reminder to the patient that the risk of complications, including failure, was discussed in advance of treatment and that, unfortunately, the patient's endodontic treatment fell outside of the usual 90% or greater success rate.

Slips of the Drill

A slip of the drill, like a slip of the tongue, may be unintentional; nevertheless, it can cause harm. When a cut tongue or lip occurs, it is usually the result of operator error. To paraphrase Alexander Pope, to err is human, but to forebear divine. To increase the likelihood that a patient will forebear from filing suit because of a cut lip or tongue, the clinician should follow these steps:

1. Inform the patient that the clinician regrets having injured the patient. This is not a legal admission of guilt, but rather an admission that the clinician is a compassionate human being.
2. Repair the injured tissue or refer the patient to an oral or plastic surgeon, depending on the extent of the injury and whether a plastic revision in necessary because scarring is likely.
3. Advise the patient that the clinician will pay the bill for the referred treatment of the oral or plastic surgeon. Request the oral or plastic surgeon send the bill directly to the clinician for payment. Send the oral or plastic surgeon's bill to the clinician's professional liability carrier. Most carriers will pay the claim under the medical payments provisions of the general liability policy for an "accident," rather than as a malpractice incident compensable under the professional liability policy. Call the patient periodically to check on healing, recovery, and follow-up plastic surgery.

Electrosurgery

Electrosurgery can cause problems if mishandled. Damage to the oral cavity caused by poor use of electrosurgical devices consists primarily of gingival and osseous necrosis, sloughing distal to the surgical field, and pulpal necrosis of affected teeth.

All equipment should be properly maintained and certified to meet the American National Standard (ADA specification no. 44 on electrical safety standards). Check current equipment to see that units meet these standards and that electrical cords and other components are in good repair. Electrical receptacles should meet the requirements of the National Electrical Code for circuit grounding and ground fault protection. During use, the dispersive electrode plate should be well away from metal parts of the dental chair and the patient's clothing, because skin contact can cause burns. Therefore use of plastic mirrors, saliva ejectors, and evacuator tips is strongly recommended.

The most frequent cause of failure in endodontic apical resection is the incomplete apical sealing between the root canal system and adjacent periradicular tissues. Achieving an adequate seal with apical surgery requires use of an ultra-

---

Christ v Lipsitz, 99 Cal. App. 3d 894; 160 Cal. Rptr. 498, 1979.
†Endodontic failures do not equal malpractice: see *Gurdin v Dongieux*, 468 So. 2d 1241, 1985 [L.A. App. 4 Cir.].
‡*Hales v Pittman*, 118 Ariz. 305, 576 P. 2d 493 (1978).

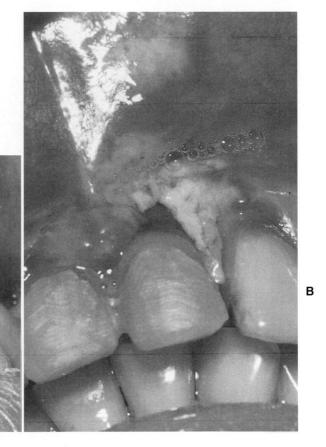

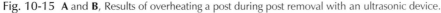

Fig. 10-15 **A** and **B**, Results of overheating a post during post removal with an ultrasonic device.

sonic rotary root end cavity preparation of at least 3 mm in vertical length.[23]

Reasonable Versus Unreasonable Errors in Judgment

Although a dentist is legally responsible for unreasonable errors in judgment, mistakes occasionally happen despite adherence to the standards of reasonable care. However, a mistake does not prove malpractice, unless the mistake is caused by a malpractice error or omission.*

For example, accessory or fourth canals on molar teeth are frequently difficult to locate and tax the best of operators. Failure to locate an accessory or fourth canal does not conclusively constitute an unreasonable error of judgment. Rather, this may represent a reasonable error of judgment in the performance of endodontics. Nevertheless, if the additional canal was readily apparent radiographically, the existence of a fourth canal should have been considered and treatment should have extended to instrument and seal it. Also if symptoms persist, consideration for retreatment to locate a fourth or accessory canal should be considered.

Gurdin v Dongieux, 468 So. 2d 1241, 1985; *Trapani v Holzer*, 158 Cal. App. 2d 1, 321 P. 2d 803, 1958.

Treatment of the Incorrect Tooth   A reasonable, nonnegligent mistake in judgment may occur because the clinician has difficulty localizing the source of endodontic pain. Vital pulps may, on occasion, be sacrificed in an attempt to diagnose the pain source. Nevertheless, it is unreasonable and therefore inexcusable to treat the wrong tooth because it is not adequately tested with pulp tests, because it has been recorded incorrectly on the referral slip, or because the radiographs are mounted incorrectly. Also, treating large numbers of teeth endodontically (e.g., an entire quadrant) when attempting to localize chronic pain suggests pain is of nonendodontic origin.

If the wrong tooth is treated because of an unreasonable mistake in judgment, the dentist should be compassionate, waive payment for all endodontic treatment, and offer to pay the fee for crowning the unnecessarily treated tooth.

Post Retrieval   Ultrasonic instruments will vibrate loose the cement around posts. The clinician can avoid overheating the post by proceeding slowly and checking the post temperature periodically to be certain overheating is not occurring. The use of a medical temperature probe is also helpful. Fig. 10-15 demonstrates what happened when an endodontist negligently overheated the post during attempted removal, causing tissue necrosis, bone loss, need for augmentation

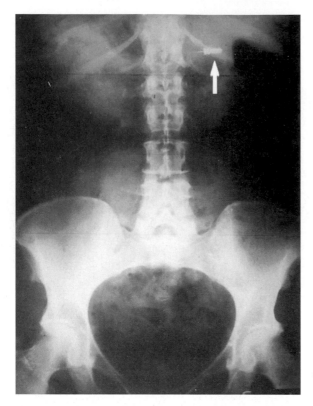

Fig. 10-16 Swallowed endodontic instrument demonstrates the wisdom of using a rubber dam.

procedures, and irreversible pulpitis in an adjacent tooth, as well as the loss of two teeth.*

Swallowing or Aspirating an Endodontic Instrument

Use of a rubber dam in endodontics is mandatory.† Even if the endodontically treated tooth is broken down and cannot be clamped, a rubber dam, regardless of required modification, should be used in all instances (see Chapter 5). Not only is microbial contamination reduced with the use of a rubber dam, the risk of a patient's aspirating or swallowing an endodontic instrument is also eliminated (Fig. 10-16). Accordingly, if a patient swallows or aspirates a file, it is likely because of the dentist's failure to observe the standard of care. If a swallowing or inhalation incident does occur, the clinician should do the following:

1. Advise the patient that the clinician regrets what occurred
2. Refer the patient for immediate medical care, including radiographic imaging, to determine if the instrument is lodged in the bronchus or stomach so that appropriate medical measures are taken promptly to remove it
3. Offer to pay for the patient's out-of-pocket medical expenses and wage loss. Most professional liability poli-

---

*He v Michaelian, San Francisco Superior Court, Docket No. 315630, 2000.
†Simpson v Davis, 219 Kan. 584; 549 P. 2d 950, 1976.

cies will cover the incident as medical payment for an "accident" and not as a malpractice claim

Overextensions A very slight overextension of a root canal filling with conventional packing or sealants can occur without violating the standard of care (see Chapter 9). Gross overextension usually indicates faulty technique. Nevertheless, so long as the overextension is not in contact with vital structures, such as the inferior alveolar nerve or sinuses, permanent harm is unlikely, unless the root canal is filled with a paraformaldehyde-containing sealant (causing neurotoxic chemical burn type of injury).

If, however, severe postoperative pain is foreseeable as a result of overextension, the patient should be advised of the likelihood of postoperative discomfort because of contact of the sealant material with the surrounding tissue. Similarly, if the overextension is very slight and increased postoperative pain is unlikely, the patient need not be advised, lest it cause unnecessary alarm. However, a note should be made on the patient's chart of the overextension and of the reason for not informing the patient, lest symptoms later manifest. Fortunately, slight-to-moderate overextensions with inert conventional endodontic sealers, such as gutta-percha with Grossman's sealant, often repair themselves and produce no irreversible changes without direct contact into the sinus or inferior alveolar nerve.

Overextending the root canal filling material risks permanent consequences if the underlying inferior alveolar nerve is initially penetrated with files. Portal of entry into the nerve canal results from overinstrumentation penetration and not packing material alone. Flexible gutta-percha alone does not penetrate beyond the mature root into the mandibular canal without prior instrument perforation.

Paraformaldehyde-containing sealants can create cytotoxic chemical destruction of the inferior alveolar nerve if placed in close proximity to, although not directly contacting, the underlying inferior alveolar nerve. On the other hand, conventional packing and sealants usually require direct contact with the inferior alveolar nerve before permanent anesthesia or paresthesia results (Fig. 10-17). Consequently, the incidence of permanent sequelae with conventional filling materials is extremely low compared with the greater cytotoxic potential with paraformaldehyde-containing sealants.[60] Because of the higher risks associated with paraformaldehyde-containing endodontic materials, use of N2 is contraindicated and violates the standard of care because permanent injury risk is substantially less with traditional eugenol-containing filling materials. When safer, less risky alternative therapy exists, it is unreasonable (and substandard) to elect an unsafe alternative methodology. Also, the doctrine of informed consent is inapposite because it is contrary to public policy to request a patient to assume inherently dangerous treatment risks that are reasonably avoidable.

Any significant overextension should be considered for immediate retreatment by attempted retrieval of the overextended gutta-percha. The clinician also has the option of

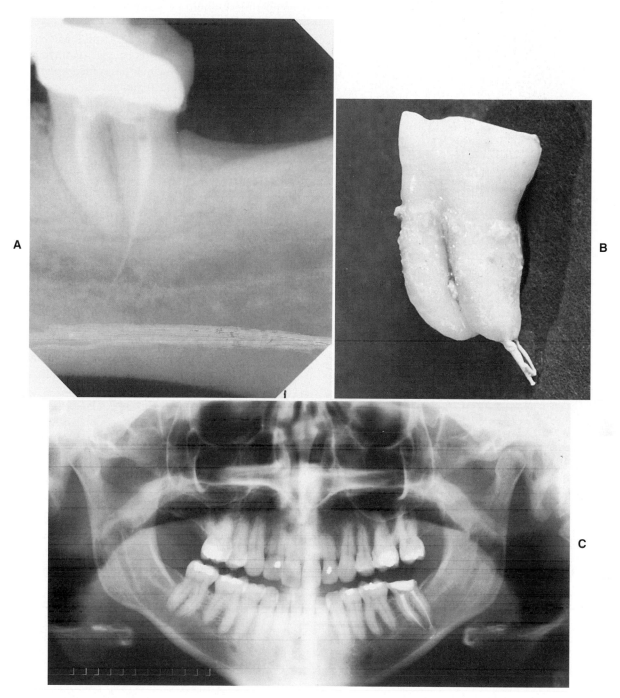

Fig. 10-17 **A-C**, Overextended gutta-percha and extracted tooth with gutta-percha intact.

immediately referring the patient to an endodontist for retrieval before the sealant sets. Conventional filling agents, such as gutta-percha, do not penetrate the cortical walls of the mandibular canal unless preceded by prior penetration with overinstrumentation (this is also true for sinus perforation). If the patient feels an electrical shock during mandibular molar or premolar instrumentation, despite local anesthesia, this may be a warning sign that the inferior alveolar nerve was pierced with endodontic files. If this occurs, the root canal should not be filled; instead, a periapical radiograph should be exposed with instruments in place to confirm or deny inferior alveolar nerve penetration. Removal of gutta-percha and sealants that have entered the mandibular inferior alveolar nerve canal should be attempted as soon as possible (preferably within the first 24 to 36 hours). The eugenol component of the sealant causes an inflammatory reaction in a constricted space; this reaction is best relieved by retrieval. If retrieval fails, a decortication procedure with

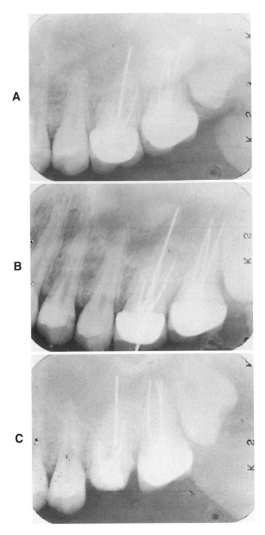

Fig. 10-18 **A-C**, Gross overfill into sinus with a silver point, which ultimately caused sinusitis and loss of tooth no. 14 as a result of endodontic failure.

compartment syndrome is a consequence of closure of small vessels. Increased compartment pressure increases the pressure on the walls of arterioles within the compartment. Increased local pressure also occludes small veins, resulting in venous hypertension within the compartment. The arteriovenous gradient in the region of the pressurized tissue becomes insufficient for tissue perfusion. The clinician should have a high index of suspicion whenever a closed compartment has the potential for bleeding or swelling. Compartment syndromes are characterized by pain beyond what should be experienced from the initial injury. Also, diminished sensation may be noted in the distribution of the nerve with a compartment that is being compressed. Elevation of compartment pressure to more than 30 mm/Hg for over 8 hours can cause irreversible tissue death.

Current Use of Silver Points Based on what has been known for over two decades, use of silver points in lieu of gutta-percha or other conventional endodontic filling materials represents a departure from the current standard of care. This is because silver points corrode in time and a tight three-dimensional apical seal is lost. Fig. 10-18 represents gross overextension with a silver point that ultimately caused the loss of tooth no. 14 as a result of endodontic failure.

Use of N-2 (Sargenti Paste) Dental literature reports that permanent paresthesias are associated with gross overfilling with paraformaldehyde sealant (N-2) that are not usually associated or reported with conventional sealants (Fig. 10-19).[38,48] Current use of paraformaldehyde-containing endodontic sealants is not merely the result of a philosophic difference between two respectable schools of thought. Rather, the distinction is between the reasonable and prudent school of thought that advocates conservative conventional endodontics, and the imprudent, radical school of paraformaldehyde providers who unreasonably risk permanent, deleterious injury with N-2 overextensions. Regardless of the number of practitioners using this latter technique and cytotoxic material, it is unsafe and should be avoided.

Dentists may be liable for fraudulent concealment, intentional misrepresentation, or co-conspiracy if they discover that a previous dentist's negligence is the cause of dental disease and they fail to advise their patient. For instance, if a gross overextension of a paraformaldehyde packing or sealant is evident radiographically and the patient reports that another dentist caused the overextension (that resulted in permanent lip anesthesia), subsequent treating dentists may be liable for fraudulent or negligent concealment if they tell the patient that the anesthesia will probably disappear shortly and that using N-2 merely reflects a philosophic difference, rather than substandard practice. Likewise, if the radiographs indicate sealant is inside the mandibular canal and the patient complains of persistent anesthesia, the patient should not be told to wait for return of sensation. Rather, the clinician should refer the patient immediately for microsurgical consultation regarding decortication and decompression surgery.

an oral surgeon is indicated at the earliest possible time (preferably within the first 24 to 36 hours).

By analogy, inflammatory edema, which compresses and compromises blood supply to soft tissues and nerves in limited spaces, is termed *compartment syndrome*.[8,57] Compartment syndromes are a group of conditions that result from increased pressure within a limited anatomic space, acutely compromising the circulation and ultimately threatening the function of the tissue within that space. Compartment syndrome results from an elevation of the interstitial pressure in a closed osseofascial compartment that results in microvascular compromise. The pathophysiology of compartment syndrome is an insult to normal local tissue homeostasis that results in increased tissue pressure, decreased capillary blood flow, and local tissue necrosis caused by oxygen deprivation. Compartment syndrome is caused by localized hemorrhage or postischemic swelling. The pathophysiology of

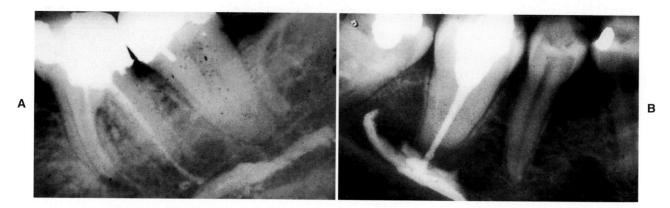

Fig. 10-19 **A** and **B**, Overextensions of Sargenti paste filling the inferior alveolar nerve canal. Both cases could have been avoided if the practitioners had selected a conventional sealing material and used a technique that emphasizes length control.

The Federal Food, Drug, and Cosmetic Act of 1938 (amended in 1962), prohibits interstate shipment of an unapproved drug or individual components used to compound the drug.* On February 12, 1993, the FDA dental advisory panel confirmed that N-2's safety and effectiveness remain unproven. N-2 may not be shipped interstate or distributed intrastate if any of the N-2 ingredients were acquired interstate. Mail order shipments of N-2 from out-of-state pharmacies in quantities greater than for single-patient use are considered a bulk sales order rather than a prescription, thus violating FDA regulations.† A San Francisco jury awarded punitive damages against the N-2-distributing New York pharmacy for knowingly shipping N-2 in violation of FDA regulations done with deliberate disregard for patient safety.‡

Defective Restorations   Marginal gaps greater than 50 micrometers lead to cement dissolution and cause 10% of crown failures within 7 years postcementation. Dull or worn explorers substantially increase the likelihood of nondetection of open margins. A sharp explorer can detect margin defects as small as 35-micrometer opening.[9] Accordingly, a sharp clinician utilizes a sharp explorer to detect open margins. Open margins contribute to endodontic failure and should be avoided (see Chapter 22).

PROPHYLACTIC ENDODONTIC PRACTICE

Periodontal Examination

Competent endodontic treatment begins with adequate diagnostic procedures, as discussed in Chapters 1 and 2. An adequate periodontal evaluation must accompany each endodontic diagnosis, which requires a diagnostic radiograph, clinical visualization, evaluation of the periodontal tissues, and probing for periodontal pockets with a calibrated periodontal probe, particularly in furcation areas.[40]

Although endodontic treatment may be successful, tooth loss may result from progression of any residual, untreated periodontitis. Consequently, periodontal evaluation and prognosis are mandatory so that the patient and dentist can make an informed and intelligent choice about whether to proceed with endodontics, a combination of periodontal and endodontic treatment, or extraction.

Each tooth undergoing endodontic therapy (and adjacent teeth) should be probed with a calibrated periodontal instrument to obtain six measurements per tooth. Pockets of 4 mm or greater should be recorded on the patient's chart. If no pockets exist, WNL (within normal limits) or a similar abbreviation should be noted. Mobility should also be charted and designated class I, II, or III. Gingival recession, furcations, and mucogingival deficiencies should also be recorded.*

A dentist who treats with endodontic success but ignores loss of periodontal attachment may misdiagnose or fail to appreciate the risk of failure because of poor periodontal prognosis. The endodontic treating dentist should not assume that an adequate periodontal evaluation has been performed by another dentist, even the referring dentist. Instead, an independent periodontal evaluation should be done with a calibrated periodontal probe.

If clinically significant periodontal disease is present, the endodontic treating dentist should consult with the restorative dentist to determine whether the periodontal disease will be properly treated or referred to a periodontist in conjunction with endodontic treatment. A patient should be advised of any

---

*U.S.C.A. § 301 et seq.

†*Cedars N Towers Pharm. Inc. v U.S.A.* (August 18, 1978) (Fla. Fed. Dist. Ct. No. 77-4965, summary judgment).

‡*Irsheid v Elbee Chemists and Available Products Inc.*, San Francisco Superior Court, Docket No. 908373 (1992).

---

*American Academy of Periodontology: *Guidelines for periodontal therapy*. See also AAP insurance policy statement: *Periodontal Charting and Third Parties*.

compromise of the endodontically treated tooth's periodontal status to comply with required informed consent disclosure.

Preoperative and Postoperative Radiographs

Pretreatment, midtreatment, and posttreatment radiographs or digital images are essential for endodontic diagnosis and treatment.

1. A current, preoperational diagnostic periapical radiograph is mandatory.
2. Measurement films or digital images are necessary to verify canal length (if an electronic canal-measuring

device is not used) and the apical extent of the gutta-percha fill to the radiographic apex.

3. Posttreatment radiographs are essential for determining the adequacy of the endodontic seal or if further treatment is necessary (see Chapter 9).

Digital radiography endodontic applications are ever increasing. The standard of care does not currently require digital imaging, because traditional silver halide radiographic film is a reasonable alternative. When there is more than one reasonably acceptable practice modality, a practitioner who chooses either modality meets the standard of care. Fig. 10-20 represents a distal open margin on tooth no. 30 (shown digitally) that is not evident in Fig. 10-21 with plain-film radiography.

Digital Radiography

Advertised claims of 80% reduction in radiation with direct digital radiography (rather than film) assumes the following[13,27]:

1. Ultra speed D-speed film is used. (Ektaspeed "E" and the new "F" speed film reduces radiation 50% and 60%, respectively, while producing images of comparable quality to D speed.)[1]
2. No rectangular collimation is used, which reduces exposure another 30%.
3. No extra radiographs are taken to compensate for a smaller area. For instance, a 2 charged-coupling device (CCD) sensor has an active area smaller than size 1 film and may require an extra image with additional radiation exposure. In sum, caveat emptor applies to claims of

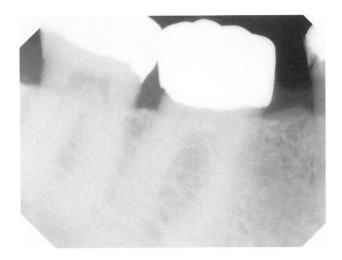

Fig. 10-20 Distal open margin on tooth no. 30 (shown digitally).

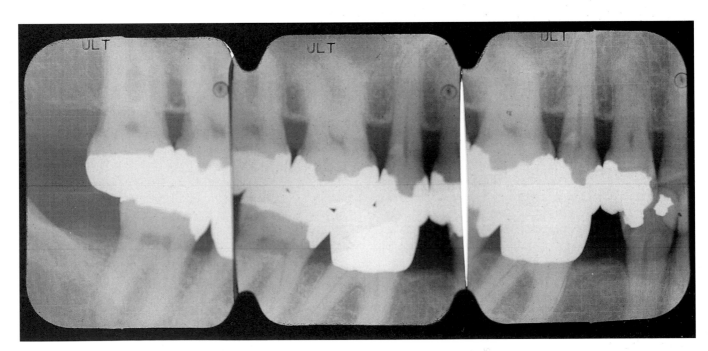

Fig. 10-21 Distal open margin on tooth no. 30 not evident with plain-film radiography.

superior safety made by equipment manufactures. Improved radiation safety of "F" speed film, which is also more environmentally friendly, will likely sustain the 550 million units of dental films sold annually.

Dental Fear

Dental fear may result in patients delaying or avoiding dental care. Frequent cancellations and missed appointments are characteristically associated with fearful dental patients. Although it is ordinarily a defense of contributory negligence, if patients do not follow a dentist's treatment recommendations, the patient's advocate may contend that the defendant dentist negligently failed to diagnose a fearful patient. Fearful patients tend to avoid dental treatment, because the patient believes it may exacerbate a prior traumatic dental experience. Referral to practitioners who specialize in treating fearful patients should be considered to facilitate comprehensive dental treatment and to avoid future emergency endodontic care because of repeated cancelled treatment visits.

Dental anxiety and finances are the two most important barriers to patients obtaining regular dental care. Fearful dental patients avoid necessary treatment, delay recalls, and are reluctant to undergo painful procedures. Therefore it is essential that such patients be identified for proper management or referral for fear-reduction therapy. A patient who experiences a high intensity of anxiety in the dental chair, together with a history of avoiding dental care, indicates a diagnosis of dental phobia. Fearful dental patients fear loss of control during clinical treatment and require reassurance and reaffirmation that they have the power to halt the procedure by a raise of hand or other appropriate gesture. After trust is gained, additional procedures may be performed.

In addition to desensitizing techniques, the use of proven topical-anesthesia delivery systems help ensure a relatively painless injection of local anesthetics. Topical-anesthetic patches and oral-anesthetic rinses may prove a valuable aid for pain management of the fearful patient.

The use of psychological questionnaires, such as the *Dental Anxiety Scale*[30] or the *Modified Dental Anxiety Scale*,[22] may be helpful in identifying such individuals. These simple questionnaires are short, quick, easy to complete, and users are provided with cut-off scores that help the dentist to identify patients who have psychologic special needs. In this way the dentist will be in a position to assist the dentally anxious or dentally phobic patient in accessing dental health care.

Patient Rapport

Good patient relations are 15% dependent on the clinician's competency to cure and 85% dependent on the clinician's ability to demonstrate the fact that the treatment being given will be the best possible.

Rapport between dentist and patient reduces the likelihood the patient will sue despite an adverse result. The clinician can develop rapport by demonstrating genuine interest in the patient and making the patient feel valued. Patients feel important if they are seated in the operatory within a reasonable time after arriving. The longer a patient is kept waiting, the more frustration and animosity build. If the patient cannot be seen within a reasonable time, a staff member should communicate the reason and, if appropriate, offer to reschedule the appointment. Staff or doctor should telephone the patient at the end of the day after any difficult procedure or surgery to check on the patient's status and remind the patient to follow postoperative instructions. The clinician should record any patient complaints, symptoms, and noncompliance with instructions. The latter can be used as evidence of patient contributory negligence, should litigation occur.

The clinician should remember that the patient lacks the information and expertise to evaluate quality and performance. Patients have their own experiences and perceptions and often rely on lay information when gathering facts about dental procedures and treatment options. However, clinicians should expect some patients (especially those with access to the Internet) to ask technical questions and expect sophisticated responses.

Rapport Building Blocks

Sir William Osler advised, "Listen to the patient. He is trying to tell you what's wrong with him." The best communicators listen more than they speak. When they do speak, it is mostly to clarify what the patient has said. Difficult doctor and patient relationships create poor communications. Improved understanding of the patient's complaints fosters better rapport, aids treatment, and reduces the likelihood of litigation.

In discussing the patient's complaints the clinician should ask, "What do you think is causing the problem?" Otherwise, the clinician may solve the patient's dental problem, while failing to solve the patient's perceived problem. Failing to clarify the patient's expectations about diagnoses and recommended treatment leaves the patient with unresolved worries and concerns. For instance, a patient may fear that a retained endodontic file is carcinogenic, unless this fear is allayed with a careful explanation that it is not.

Do Not Rush the Visit

Full attention to the patient's complaints, good eye contact, and respectful addressing of the patient gain rapport, improve communication, and prevent lawsuits. The clinician should avoid questions that require a yes-or-no answer. Instead, the clinician should ask what the patient perceives as the problem, rephrase the patient's complaints to prevent miscommunication, and ask if the patient's complaints have been summarized accurately. Summarizing clarifies understanding by repeating important points. The clinician should also inquire if there are any remaining questions. Nonverbal communication is a powerful tool; therefore the clinician should shake hands initially or comfort with an outstretched hand if pain is provoked.

Emotions are the dominant force behind most malpractice claims. Patients who feel misled, betrayed, or abandoned become angry and may seek vindication instead of simply seeking financial compensation. Thus the clinician should maintain a tactful and courteous approach and be attentive to the patient's needs and complaints. In addition the clinician should always make sure that communications with the patient are clear, even to the point of being repetitious, by asking if the patient has any questions. The patient should never be abandoned in the middle of a course of treatment, and the clinician should always be available to provide follow-up care. Clinicians should avoid making a diagnosis over the telephone; instead, they should suggest office initial or follow-up care.

Good telephone communication is a matter of asking the right questions, such as asking a patient complaining of postoperative swelling if there is difficulty breathing or swallowing, as well as the degree and location of swelling. In cases of suspected infection, clinicians should ask the patient or family member to call back with a temperature reading to verify the patient is afebrile.

Do Not Make Off-the-Cuff Diagnoses

One dentist misdiagnosed a patient's party guest's endodontic problem as "sensitivity due to gum recession" and recommended a desensitizing toothpaste. Although the conversation took place in a social setting, a lawsuit resulted based on an inadequate diagnosis.

Keep Conversations Professional

Making light of a minor occurrence, such as the dropping of an instrument, with a quip about your "one drink too many" at lunch, may seem funny at the time. However, it may not sound so funny if the patient soberly reiterates your quip to the jury.

Do not let a patient's flattery of your abilities undermine your best professional judgment. Heroic measures usually result in treatment failures, dissatisfied patients, and, ultimately, lawsuits for uninformed consent.

A patient dissatisfied with prior treatment, which appears adequately performed, should signal the clinician to stop treatment. Young practitioners are more apt to walk into traps involving a patient's request for unreasonable treatment. A compassionate and concerned dentist who is able to demonstrate that the patient is cared about and cared for, avoids many malpractice actions. Thus when an iatrogenic mishap occurs, it behooves the clinician to be frank and forthright with the patient. Moreover, concealment of negligence may extend the statute of limitations, because most states with discovery statutes construe discovery as the date on which the patient discovered the negligent cause of the injury and not the date of the injury itself.* Furthermore, belated discovery of injury from another dentist evokes a

feeling of betrayal in the patient and destroys rapport that would otherwise dissuade the patient from instituting litigation. Beginning July 2001, the Joint Commission on Accreditation of Health Care will require hospitals to provide an honest explanation to patients regarding medical mishaps. These standard are designed to prevent errors and to reduce medical negligence claim payouts. In 1999, the Annals of Internal Medicine concluded that "extreme honesty may be the best policy." A full-disclosure policy in a study involving a hospital in Lexington, Kentucky showed that this hospital was in the top 25% of claim incidence, but it was also in the bottom 25% of claim payouts ($1.3 million over 7 years).

Fees

Clinicians should clarify fees and payment procedures *before* initiating treatment. If the dental treatment becomes more extensive than originally planned, the clinician should discuss any increased charges and reasons for those charges with the patient before continuing treatment. Charging for untoward complications, such as extended postoperative visits or retrieving broken instruments, should be resisted.

An overzealous receptionist who places payment pressure on a dissatisfied patient, or the dentist who sues to collect a fee from an already displeased patient, may invite a countersuit for malpractice. Refunding fees or paying for the treatment fee of the subsequent treating dentist is usually much less expensive than a week in court and a jury award for a patient's pain and suffering. If clinicians must sue for a fee, they should do so only if treatment is beyond reproach and records substantiate proper diagnosis, treatment, and informed consent options.

Suing for unpaid fees continues to be a proven method for getting counter-sued for dental malpractice. The client who has paid fees in the past, but who stops at some point, is either unhappy with the dental service received or short of funds. Dealing with a patient's countersuit takes time, and collection of unpaid fees may prove difficult. The patient being sued may seek an attorney, who will scrutinize the clinician's handling of the patient and use 20/20 hindsight to second-guess the clinician's treatment.

Some cross-complaints for dental malpractice lack merit, while others have genuine merit. Whenever possible, clinicians should avoid suing patients for unpaid fees. Before ever considering suing, the clinician should discuss the fee situation with the patient and consider a payment schedule or fee reduction.

The amount of money being awarded by juries is increasing. In 1999 a New York City jury awarded three and one-half million dollars against a general dentist who had replaced three amalgams with composites. To relieve postoperative sensitivity, endodontics was performed and subsequently failed. Chronic temporomandibular disorder (TMD) followed the extraction, from which the patient was likely to suffer lifetime pain.

---

*Dolan v Borelli, 13 Cal. App. 4th 816 (1993); *Franklin v Albert*, 411 N.E. 2d 458 (1980) (Mass); 38 *Mont. L. Rev.* 399, 1977; Annot. (1961) 80 A.L.R. 2d 368, § 7b.

Post Perforation

Post selection is important for avoiding perforations. Generally posts should not exceed one third of the mesiodistal width of a tooth, should follow the canal anatomy, and should leave 3 to 5 mm of sealant in the opened post space. Excessively large posts violate these guidelines and unreasonably increase the risk of perforation or tooth fracture.

Ordinarily, a prudent practitioner performing endodontic therapy should be able to avoid post perforations. If post perforation occurs, early diagnosis and treatment is important, because belated diagnosis and treatment substantially increase the risk of endodontic failure. If perforation is relatively small in size (i.e., 1 mm or less) and promptly diagnosed at the time of the post perforation, immediate treatment with intracanal sealants in the area of the perforation will probably succeed. However, delayed diagnosis and treatment (beyond 24 hours) results in bacterial contamination in the area surrounding the perforation. Delayed perforation repair therapy can cause periodontal and/or endodontic lesions or lateral periodontal abscesses occurring secondary to delayed diagnosis, which usually prognosticates a high failure risk.

Cores

Incorrect choice of cores can contribute to failure, including fractures. For instance, some manufacturers (e.g., ESPE Premier for Ketac silver) recommend against use of their core material unless at least two thirds of the tooth remains before buildup. Failure to follow the manufacturer's directions can be considered by an expert when determining whether the standard of care was met.

Resin-reinforced post-and-core systems show promise for structurally weakened incisors, but long-term longevity has not been reported. A ferrule or other counter-rotational core design is an important consideration for fracture resistance and retention,[31] although not proven as statistically significant for the resin-reinforced dowel systems.[56]

Posttrauma Therapy

The reader is referred to Chapter 16 for a full discussion of how to treat and manage patients who have sustained a traumatic injury.

Continuing Education

A dentist is legally obligated to maintain current knowledge in the field of endodontics. If not, the dentist may have only 1 year of knowledge (repeated thirty times) during the span of a 30-year career.

Examples of recent endodontic advancements include improved cleansing, shaping, filling, and packing techniques. Microscopes, variable tapered file systems, heat plugers, non-eugenol resin cements, and NiTi instruments are but some examples of improved technologic advancements.

By not maintaining continuing education knowledge and updating clinical skills, a practitioner may unreasonably condemn otherwise salvageable teeth because of inadequate diagnosis or treatment.

Millennium Management of Endodontic Advances

Technologic advances are touted as ideal endodontics. However, the standard of care is a minimal standard of reasonably acceptable practice, rather than the perfect ideal. Thus the reasonable and prudent practitioner is not required to know and use all of the latest technologic advances in endodontics. On the other hand, the reasonable and prudent practitioner must keep current with available advances that are generally accepted and research proven. Microsurgical endodontics is an example of improved endodontics technology; use of magnifying loupes or similar devices may prove inadequate. Therefore the clinician should be willing to adopt proven improvements in the endodontic field.

If studies demonstrate significantly superior results for some alternative to surgical endodontics, the informed consent standard of care may require that the patient be advised of the alternative technique, even if it is more expensive. There may be more than one path to success. So long as the dentist uses reasonably acceptable techniques and informs the patient of reasonable alternatives, the standard of care is met. However, clinicians should remember that today's surgical advance may be tomorrow's retreat, such as breast and temporomandibular joint (TMJ) implants in which inadequately tested technology proved disastrous.*,[52] Microscopic apical surgery has gained general acceptance, is performed by the majority of endodontists, and represents the current standard of care.

Clinicians should evaluate the quality of peer-reviewed research articles for new products rather than accepting them at face value. For instance, a case report amounts to no more than the author's personal experience with one patient. Some authors report a series of patients if there are only two patients. Finally, a brash conclusion is to state something has occurred time and time again if similar findings were observed with only three patients. Valid scientific principles mandate a test result can be replicated by other competent scientists duplicating a particular research protocol. If research cannot be duplicated, sweeping conclusions should not be made.

Prudent practitioners do not adopt every new technology. Before adoption, such technology must have demonstrated benefits with acceptable levels of risk. It must also be adequately tested, with sufficient numbers of test subjects, over a significant length of time. Because manufacturers' rush their products to market, few technologies exist that meet this criterion. Therefore except for breakthrough technological changes, a practitioner will not likely be judged negligent for failure to adopt the latest gadget or technique. How-

---

Federal Register 58:43442-43445, August 16, 1993.

ever, clinicians must keep in mind that in the information technology industry, 1 year is considered several generations, if not an eternity.[12,47]

The standard of care usually does not mandate incorporation of every new technology. However, in those states with informed consent laws that are based upon what a prudent patient would want to know, rather than what prudent practitioners do, the patient may argue that an alternative technology or technique used by a different practitioner would have been chosen had the dentist provided the patient with such information. For instance, even if the majority of practitioners have not yet adopted microsurgery to aid grafting gingival recession areas, should graft failure occur, the patient may claim that the dentist failed to provide the option of microsurgical periodontal grafting before obtaining the patient's informed consent.

Thorough instrumentation and obturation of the entire root canal system, using generally accepted instruments, materials, and devices, are the best means of ensuring endodontic success.

Other Dentists' Substandard Treatment

Clinicians should not be overly protective of blatant examples of another dentist's substandard dental treatment. Upon discovery of possible negligent treatment by a previous dentist, the clinician should obtain the patient's written authorization for transfer of a copy of the previous dentist's records, including radiographs. If the negligence is still suspected after reviewing the records, the clinician should consider discussing with the previous dentist to learn what occurred during the patient's past treatment (after obtaining the patient's consent).

On discovery of a gross violation of the minimal standard of dental care, a dentist has an ethical responsibility to report the matter to the local dental society, peer review, or dental licensing board or agency.[3] If this is not done and the patient later discovers negligent treatment, which is patently obvious, the clinician could be sued as a coconspirator to fraudulent concealment of another practitioner's neglect.

Peer Review

If despite good rapport, candid disclosure, and an offer to pay corrective medical or surgical bills the patient is still unsatisfied, the clinician should consider referring the patient to peer review. Peer review committees award damages for out-of-pocket losses, not for pain and suffering or lost wages. Consequently, even if the committee's decision is adverse to the dentist, the damage award will probably be less than a jury's verdict. If peer review finds for the dentist, the patient may be discouraged from proceeding further with litigation. Peer review proceedings, including the committee's decision, are not admissible in court.*

*California Evidence Code § 1157.

Insurance carriers usually honor and pay a peer review committee award, because a fair adjudication of the merits has been determined. The award is usually less than a jury would award. Also, defense costs, including attorney's fees, are saved.

Human Immunodeficiency Virus and Endodontics

A dentist may not ethically refuse to treat an HIV-seropositive patient solely because of such diagnosis.[20] Although in the 1980s no federal law had clearly extended the protection of the handicapped laws to patients with AIDS, federal congressional action in 1990 extended this protection to the dental office setting with the passage of the Americans with Disabilities Act.* Many states already offer additional protection under state law.[15]†

Confidentiality for patients disclosing their HIV status is important, because an inadvertent disclosure to an insurance carrier or to other third parties, without any need to know, may result in cancellation of the patient's health, disability, or life insurance.

This cancellation could result in a claim against the dentist whose office disclosed such information without authorization. Therefore employees should sign the confidentiality agreement shown in Fig. 10-22. In signing this agreement the staff may be alerted to the seriousness and importance of maintaining the confidentiality of patient health histories, because these histories may document AIDS, venereal disease, or other socially stigmatizing diseases.

If a patient requests that the dentist not inform the staff of the patient's HIV status, the dentist should refuse to treat that patient; this information is essential to staff members who could come in contact with the infection. For example, an accidental needle stick with HIV-infected blood, which carries a risk of approximately one chance in 250 of seroconversion, may occur. Current medical protocol includes prophylactic administration of zidovudine (AZT), either to prevent or to slow the manifestation of AIDS from a deep, penetrating, accidental needle stick exposure.

Although a treating dentist risks devastating a dental practice by informing patients that the dentist has contracted AIDS, the legal risk of not informing patients is much greater. The health care provider may be required to advise patients of positive HIV test results under the doctrine of informed consent (i.e., advising of a known risk of harm from accidental exposure).‡ Even if an uninformed patient never contracts AIDS, in those states that use a reasonable patient standard for disclosure of material risks of treatment (which could include accidental direct contact such as an

*Americans with Disabilities Act, Pub. L. 101-336.
†Decision and Order of the New York City Commission on Human Rights, *Whitmore v The Northern Dispensary*, August 17, 1988.
‡*Doe v U.S. Attorney General*, (N.D. CA December 28, 1992) No. C-88-3820.

unintended cut or needle stick), the patient may decide to bring an action for intentional concealment as a variant of informed consent and seek to recover emotional distress and punitive damages. Conversely, patients may be legally liable for lying on their health history regarding their HIV status.*

Infective Endocarditis

If a patient's medical history shows infective endocarditis, the clinician should consult with the patient's physician to determine the necessity of antibiotic prophylaxis against infective endocarditis in accordance with current American Heart Association (AHA) Guidelines.[19] If the physician does not appear knowledgeable about those guidelines, the clinician should provide a copy of the guidelines to the physician. If the physician advises deviation from AHA guidelines, the clinician should discover why the physician feels that this is appropriate. The clinician should also record any discussions with the physician in the patient's chart and confirm the discussion and the physician's recommendation in writing (by letter to the physician).

Communications with the physician should be specific, because the physician may not appreciate dental treatment risks, such as overextension of files or filling material sealants that occur nonsurgically and may enter the bloodstream. The following format might be used:

Dear Doctor:
Your patient requires potentially invasive dental treatment that will likely result in a transient bacteremia. Does the patient have a heart valve defect that increases the risk of infective endocarditis? If so, please advise of the diagnosed defect and recommended prophylactic antibiotics and dose for nonsurgical endodontic treatment or periapical surgery. If you require the patient to have a current cardiac evaluation or echocardiogram to provide an answer, please so advise me and the patient.

Please also advise if your recommendation is in accordance with the enclosed American Heart Association current guidelines concerning bacterial endocarditis relating to dental treatment.

Thank you for your anticipated cooperation.
Enclosure: 1997 American Heart Association guidelines

Individuals who have undergone total-joint replacement surgery may also be at increased risk for bacterial infection to the artificial joint. Late joint infections (i.e., less than 6 months) may occur as the result of bacteria introduced into the oral cavity. Antibiotic prophylaxis is recommended for certain individuals with total joint replacements before specific dental procedures (they are identical to those recommended by the AHA). The drugs (e.g., cephalexin, cephradine, amoxicillin) used to prevent the late infection of

---

DENTAL AUXILIARY CONFIDENTIALITY AGREEMENT

I, _____, have been informed by
(Dental Assistant)

_____, DDS, that all dental, medical,and
(Dentist Name)

financial information concerning patients is confidential.

As a condition of employment, I agree to maintain the confidentiality of all oral and written information, including treatment charts, and to not disclose such information to any unauthorized outside persons, including any family members, except upon request and authorization by the patient, the patient's agent, or supervising dentist.

I understand and agree that breach of this employment agreement shall constitute good cause for my discharge from employment. I acknowledge that I may by personally liable for any violation of a patient's privacy or civil rights committed by me without consent of the patient, or the patient's agent, or approval by above-named dentist.

Date: _____   _____

Witness: _____   Signature of Dental Assistant

Fig. 10-22 Dental auxiliary confidentiality agreement.

prosthetic joints differ slightly from those recommended by the AHA.[1a]

CONCLUSION

If the dentist performs endodontics within the standard of care as described in this chapter, there should be little concern that a lawsuit for professional negligence will be successful. Prophylactic measures suggested in this chapter should help lessen the likelihood of litigation by reducing avoidable risks associated with endodontic care.

Both the patient and dentist benefit from risk reduction. To do it wrong does not take long: it is far better for the dentist to take the extra precautionary minute to do it right. We are a profession that deserves the public's trust, but only if that trust is earned. Clinicians can earn public trust by providing safe, excellent, quality patient care. The best defense against being sued is to do it right the first time rather than repeatedly defending your wrongs to the patient or jury.[21c]

References

1. Ackers S: Personal correspondence with Kodak, Jan. 4, 2001.
1a. ADA American Academy of Orthopeadic Surgeons: Advisory statement, antibiotic prophylaxis for dental patients with total joint replacements, *JADA* 128:1004, 1997.
2. ADA Council on Scientific Affairs: Dental unit waterlines: approaching the year 2000, *JADA* 130:1653, 1999.
3. ADA principles of ethics and code of professional conduct, I-G: justifiable criticism, *J Am Dent Assoc* 123:102, 1992.
4. Alexander RE: Eleven myths of dentoalveolar surgery, *JADA* 129:1271, 1998.

Boulais v Lustig, Los Angeles Superior Court BC038105 ($102,500 jury verdict to an ungloved surgical technician).

5. American Academy of Periodontology: *Periodontal screening and recording,* Chicago, 1992, The Academy.

6. American Association of Endodontists: Endodontics—colleagues for excellence, prescription for the future—reasonable use of antibiotics in endodontic therapy, vol 2, Spring/Summer 1999.

6a. Angell M: The pharmaceutical industry–to whom is it accountable, *N Engl J Med* 342:1902, 2000.

7. Aqrabawi J: Sealing ability of a Super EBA & MTA when used as a retrograde filling material, *Br Dent J* 11:266, 2000.

8. Azar FM, Pickering RM: *Campbell's operative orthopaedics,* ed 9, vol 2, St Louis, 1998, Mosby.

9. Baldissara P, Baldissara S, Scotti R: Reliability of tactile perception using sharp and dull explorers in marginal opening identification, *Int J Prosthodont* 11:591, 1998.

10. Benovitz N, Haller C: New evidence of harm from herbal supplement: UCSF team cites 54 deaths since mid 90s, *San Francisco Chronicle,* Nov 7, 2000.

10a. Haller CA, Benovitz NL: Adverse cardiovascular and central nervous system events associated with dietary supplements containing ephedra alkaloids, *N Engl J Med* 343:1833, 2000.

11. Berhelsen CL, Stilley KR: Automated personal health inventory for dentistry: a pilot study, *JADA* 131:59, 2000.

12. Berry J: Physicians report boost in use of world wide web, *ADA News* 31(1): 3, January 10, 2000.

13. Brown R, Hadley JN, Chambers DW: An evaluation of Ektaspeed Plus film versus Ultraspeed film for endodontic working length determination, *J Endod* 24:54, 1998.

14. Burton TM: Unfavorable drug study sparks battle over publication of results, *Wall Street Journal* p B1, Nov 1, 2000.

15. California court upholds ban on AIDS discrimination, *ADA News* 21(3):8, February 5, 1990.

16. Carroll R: Risk management handbook for healthcare organizations, Chicago, 1997, American Hospital Publishing.

17. Cheung G: Endodontic failures, *Int Dent J* 146:131, 1996.

18. Colline W: Should I stop taking herbs before surgery? *WebMD,* Sep 16, 2000.

18a. CRA newsletter, 24:12, 2000.

19. Dajani AS et al: Prevention of bacterial endocarditis. Recommendations by the American Heart Association, *JADA* 128(8): 1142, 1997.

20. Davis M: Dentistry and AIDS: an ethical opinion, *J Am Dent Assoc* 119:(suppl 9-5) 95, 1989.

21. Dorn S, Gartner A: Retrograde filling materials: a retrospective study of amalgam, EBA, and IRM, *J Endod* 16:391, 1990.

21a. Epstein JB, Chong S, Le ND: A survey of antibiotic use in dentistry, *J Am Dent* 131, 1600, 2000.

21b. Federal Truth in Lending Act, 15 U.S.C. § 1601 et seq.

21c. Forkner-Dunn DJ: Commentary: to err is human—but not in health care, *Am J Med Qual* 15:263, 2000.

22. Freeman R: Barriers to accessing dental care: patient factors, *Br Dent J* 187:141, 1999.

23. Gagliani M, Taschieri S, Molinari R: Ultrasonic root end preparation: influence of cutting angle on the apical seal, *J Endod* 24:726, 1998.

24. Goldman RP, Brown JL: *The California dentist's legal handbook,* San Francisco, 1998, Law offices of Ronald Goldman.

25. Goldman RP: Your duty to refer, *ADA Legal Adviser* 2(9):6, 1998.

26. Grumbach K et al: Primary care physicians' experience of financial incentives in managed care systems, *New Engl J Med* 341:2008, 1999.

27. Hadley J: Dental radiology quality of care: the dentist makes the difference, *J Calif Dent Assoc* 23:17, 1995.

28. Hardison DC, Schnetzer T: Using information technology to improve the quality and efficiency of clinical trial research in academic medical centers, *Qual Manag Health Care* 7(3):37, 1999.

29. Holmes S: Texaco settlement could lead to more lawsuits, *San Francisco Examiner* p A-8, November 17, 1996.

30. Humphris GM, Morrison T, Lindsay SJ: The modified dental anxiety scale: validation and United Kingdom norms, *Comm Dent Health* 12:143, 1995.

31. Hunt P, Gogamoiu D: Evaluation of post and core systems, *J Esthet Dent* 8(2):74, 1996.

32. California Dental Association: *Improved patient bill of rights unveiled, California dental association update,* Sacramento, 1996, The Association.

33. Ingle J, Beveridge E: *Endodontics,* ed 2, Philadelphia, 1976, Lea & Febiger.

34. Jones G, Behrents R, Bailey G: Legal considerations for digitized images, *Gen Dent* 44(3):242, 1996.

35. Kane B, Sands D: Guidelines for clinical use of electronic mail with patients, *J Am Med Inform Assoc* 5:104, 1998.

36. Kasegawa TK, Matthews M Jr: Knowing when you don't know: the ethics of competency, *Prosthodontic Insights* 10(1): 5, 1998.

37. Keeling D: Malpractice claim prevention, *J Calif Dent Assoc* 3(8):55, 1975.

38. Kleirer D, Averbach R: Painful dysesthesia on the inferior alveolar nerve following use of a paraformaldehyde-containing root canal sealer, *Endod Dent Traumatol* 4:46, 1988.

39. Labor Secretary Robert Reich interview, *San Francisco Examiner,* p A-6, November 17, 1996.

40. McFall WT, Bader JD, Rozier RG, Ramsey D: Presence of periodontal data in patient records of general practices: patient records, *J Periodontol* 59:445, 1988.

41. McNeill C: Occlusion: what it is and what it is not, *J Calif Dent Assoc* 28:748, 2000.

42. *Merriam Webster's Collegiate Dictionary,* Miami, 1994, PSI Associates, p. 777.

43. Miller C: Cleaning, sterilization and disinfection: basics of microbial killing for infection control, *J Am Dent Assoc* 124: 48, 1993.

44. Mills S: The dental unit waterline controversy: defusing the myths, defining the solutions, *JADA* 131:1427, 2000.

45. Moore PA et al: Adverse drug interactions in dental practice: professional and educational implications, *JADA* 130:47, 1999.

46. Morris WO: *Dental litigation,* ed 2, Charlottesville, Va., 1977, The Michie Co.

47. *The National Law Journal,* p. B7, January 17, 2000.

48. Neaverth E: Disabling complications following inadvertent overextension of a root canal filling material, *J Endod* 15:135, 1989.

49. OSHA: Occupational Safety and Health Administration Directive, Washington, DC, 1999, WWW.OSHA.90V (on-line).

50. Oxman AD, Thomson MA, Davis DA, Haynes RB: No magic bullets: a systematic review of 102 trials of interventions to

improve professional practice, *Can Med Assoc J* 153:423, 1995.

51. Packer M, Miller AB: A symposium: can physicians always explain the results of clinical trials? A case study of amlodipine in heart failure, *Am J Cardiol* p. 1L-2L, August 19, 1999.

52. Randall T: Antibodies to silicone detected in patients with severe inflammatory reactions, *JAMA* 268:14, 1992.

53. Rohlin M, Kullendorff B, Ahlqwist M, Stenstrom B: Observer performance in the assessment of periapical pathology: a comparison of panoramic with periapical radiography, *Dentomaxillofac Radiol* 20(3):127, 1991.

54. Rosenbaum S, Frankford DM, Moore B: Who should determine medical care necessity? *N Engl J Med* 340:229, 1999.

55. Roter DL: Patient participation in the patient-provider interactions: the effects of patient question asking on the quality of interaction, satisfaction, and compliance, *Health Educ Monogr* 50:281, 1977.

56. Saupe W, Gluskin A, Radke R: A comparative study of fracture resistance between morphologic dowel and cores and resin-reinforced dowel system in the intraradicular restoration of structurally compromised roots, *Quintessence Int* 27:483, 1996.

57. Schwartz SI, Shires GT, Spencer FC: *Principles of Surgery*, ed 7, New York, 1999, McGraw-Hill.

58. Scully C, Boyle P: Reliability of a self-administered questionnaire for screening for medical problems in dentistry, *Comm Dent Oral Epiderm* 11(2):105, 1983.

59. Selbst A: Understanding informed consent and its relationship to the incidence of adverse treatment events in conventional endodontic therapy, *J Endod* 16:387, 1990.

60. Serper A, Ucer O, Onur R, Etikan I: Comparative neurotoxic effects of root canal filling material on root sciatic nerve, *J Endod* 24:592, 1998.

61. Simonsen R: Greed and gravy train: is this success? *J Esthetic Dent* 11:287, 1999.

62. Studdert DM, Brennan TA: The problems with punitive damages in lawsuits against managed-care organizations, *N Eng J Med* 342(4):280, 2000.

63. Terezhalmy G, Bottomley W: General legal aspects of diagnostic dental radiography, *Oral Surg* 48:486, 1979.

64. Trust me – I'm a drug salesman, *Financial Times* p 6, October 24, 2000.

65. Tsang A, Sweet D, Wood RE: Potential for fraudulent use of dental radiography, *JADA* 130:1325, 1999.

66. Tulsa dentist found guilty of mail fraud, conspiracy, *Tulsa World* p 1, January 12, 1993.

67. *Wall Street Journal* p. A3, November 20, 1996.

68. Walton RE: News: antibiotics not always necessary, *JADA* 130:782, 1999.

69. Warning on popular heartburn drug, FDA says Propulsid linked to 70 deaths, should be a last resort, *San Francisco Chronicle* p. A3, January 25, 2000.

70. Weichman J: Malpractice prevention and defense, *J Calif Dent Assoc* 3(8):58, 1975.

71. Wensing M, Van der Weijden T, Grol R: Implementing guidelines and innovations in general practice: which interventions are effective? *Br J Gen Pract* 48:991, 1998.

72. Wynn RL: Internet web sites for drug information, *Gen. Dent* 46(1):12, 1998.

73. Yatsushiro JD, Baumgartner JC, Tinkle JS: Longitudinal study of microleakage of two root end filling materials using a fluid conductive system, *J Endod* 24:716, 1998.

74. Zeider S, Ruttimann U, Webber R: Efficacy in the assessment of intraosseous lesions of the face and jaws in asymptomatic patients, *Radiology* 162:691, 1987.

75. Zinman E: Informed consent to periodontal surgery: advise before you incise, *J West Soc Periodontol* 24:101, 1976.

PART TWO

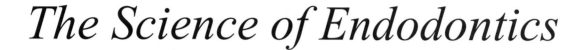

The Science of Endodontics

Chapter 11

Structure and Functions of the Dentin and Pulp Complex

Henry Trowbridge, Syngcuk Kim, Hideaki Suda

The pulp is a soft tissue of mesenchymal origin with specialized cells, the odontoblasts, arranged peripherally in direct contact with dentin matrix. The close relationship between odontoblasts and dentin, sometimes referred to as the *pulp-dentin complex*, is one of several reasons why dentin and pulp should be considered as a functional entity. Certain peculiarities are imposed on the pulp by the rigid mineralized dentin in which it is enclosed. Thus it is situated within a low-compliance environment that limits its ability to increase in volume during episodes of vasodilation and increased tissue pressure. Because the pulp is relatively incompressible, the total volume of blood within the pulp chamber cannot be greatly increased (although reciprocal volume changes can occur between arterioles, venules, lymphatics, and extravascular tissue). In the pulp, therefore, careful regulation of blood flow is of critical importance.

The dental pulp is in many ways similar to other connective tissues of the body, but its special characteristics deserve serious consideration. Even the mature pulp bears a resemblance to embryonic connective tissue. The pulp houses a number of tissue elements, including nerves, vascular tissue, connective tissue fibers, ground substance, interstitial fluid, odontoblasts, fibroblasts, immunocompetent cells, and other cellular components.

The pulp is actually a microcirculatory system, and its largest vascular components are arterioles and venules. No true arteries or veins enter or leave the pulp. Unlike most tissues the pulp lacks a true collateral system and is dependent on the relatively few arterioles entering through the root foramina. The vascular system of the pulp decreases progressively with age.

The tooth pulp is a unique sensory organ. Being encased in a protective layer of dentin, which in turn is covered with enamel, it might be expected to be quite unresponsive to stimulation. However, despite the low thermal conductivity of dentin, the pulp is undeniably sensitive to thermal stimuli, such as ice cream and hot drinks. The unusual mechanism that allows the *pulp-dentin complex* to function as such an exquisitely responsive sensory system is discussed later in the chapter.

After tooth development the pulp retains its ability to form dentin throughout life. This enables the vital pulp to partially compensate for the loss of enamel or dentin caused by mechanical trauma or disease. How well it serves this function depends on many factors, but the potential for regeneration and repair is as much a reality in the pulp as in other connective tissues of the body.

It is the purpose of this chapter to bring together what is known about the development, structure, and function of the pulp-dentin complex in the hope that this knowledge will provide a firm biologic basis for clinical decision making.

DEVELOPMENT

Embryologic studies have shown that the pulp is derived from the cephalic neural crest. Neural crest cells arise from the ectoderm along the lateral margins of the neural plate and migrate extensively. Those that travel down the sides of the head into the maxilla and mandible contribute to the formation of the tooth germs. The dental papilla, from which the mature pulp arises, develops as ectomesenchymal cells proliferate and condense adjacent to the dental lamina at the sites where teeth will develop (Fig. 11-1). It is important to remember the migratory potential of ectomesenchymal cells when the ability of pulp cells to move into areas of injury and

replace destroyed odontoblasts are considered later in the chapter.

During the sixth week of embryonic life, tooth formation begins as a localized proliferation of ectoderm associated with the maxillary and mandibular processes. This proliferative activity results in the formation of two horseshoe-shaped structures, one on each process. These structures are termed the *primary dental laminae*. Each primary dental lamina splits into a vestibular and a dental lamina (Fig. 11-2).

Numerous studies have indicated that the embryonic development of any tissue is promoted by interaction with an adjacent tissue. The complex epithelial and mesenchymal interactions during tooth development have been studied extensively. Cell-to-cell and cell-to-extracellular matrix (ECM) interactions direct the differentiation of ameloblasts and odontoblasts by causing these cells to change gene expression.

The timing and position of epithelium and mesenchyme are thought to reside in the sequential expression of cell transmembrane linkage molecules, such as integrin, cell adhesion molecules (CAMs), and substrate adhesion molecules (SAMs). CAMs mediate morphogenesis through controlled cell proliferation, specific cell-to-cell adhesion, and migration. Cells contain membrane proteins called *integrins*, which are specific receptors for CAMs. Laminin is the CAM of basement membranes. It contains binding domains for heparin sulfate, type IV collagen, and cells. SAMs carry out cell-to-ECM interactions. The best-studied SAMs of the ECM are the fibronectins, a family of glycoproteins that bind to fibrin, collagen, heparin sulfate, and cell surfaces.

Growth factors are polypeptides produced by cells that initiate proliferation, migration, and differentiation of a variety of cells. It can be assumed that growth factors are involved in signaling during epithelial and mesenchymal interactions that regulates tooth morphogenesis and cell differentiation. For example, epidermal growth factor (EGF) has been shown to play a role in tooth development by stim-

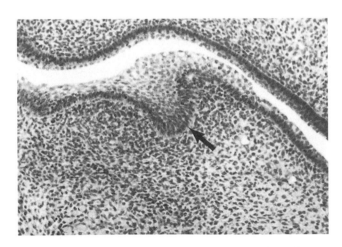

Fig. 11-1 Dental lamina (*arrow*) arising from the oral ectoderm.

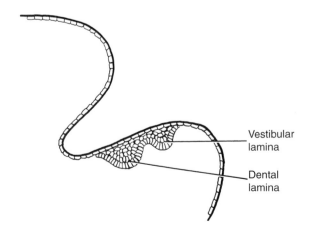

Fig. 11-2 Diagram showing formation of the vestibular and dental lamina from oral ectoderm.

Vestibular lamina

Dental lamina

ulating proliferation of cells in the enamel organ and pre-odontoblasts.[111] It has been hypothesized that transforming growth factor-b$_1$ (TGF-b$_1$) may regulate changes in the composition and structure of ECM.[114] A fibroblast growth factor may also be involved in the determination and differentiation of odontoblasts.

From the onset of tooth formation, a dental basement membrane (DBM) exists between the inner dental epithelium and the dental mesenchyme. The DBM consists of a thin basal lamina, which is formed by the epithelial cells, and a layer of ECM derived from the dental mesenchyme. The basal lamina is composed of an elastic network composed of type IV collagen, which has binding sites for other basement membrane constituents, such as laminin, fibronectin, and heparan sulfate proteoglycans. Laminin binds to type IV collagen and also to receptors on the surface of preameloblasts and ameloblasts. The DBM also contains mesenchyme-derived type I and type III collagen, hyaluronate, heparan sulfate, and chondroitin 4- and 6-sulfates. Odontoblast cell surface proteoglycans function as receptors for matrix molecules. Signals from components of the matrix influence the migration and differentiation of odontoblasts. The composition of the DBM changes during tooth development, and these alterations appear to modulate the successive steps in odontogenesis. With the differentiation of odontoblasts, type III collagen disappears from the predentin matrix, and fibronectin, which surrounds preodontoblasts, is restricted to the apical pole of mature odontoblasts.[71]

The initial stage of development of the dental papilla is characterized by proliferative activity beneath the dental lamina at sites corresponding to the positions of the prospective primary teeth. Even before the dental lamina begins to form the enamel organ, a capillary vascular network develops within the ectomesenchyme, presumably to support the increased metabolic activity to the presumptive tooth buds. This primordial vascularization is thought to play a key role in induction of odontogenesis.

Stages of Development

Although formation of the tooth is a continuous process, as a matter of convenience the process has been divided into three stages: (1) bud, (2) cap, and (3) bell (Fig. 11-3). The *bud stage* is the initial stage of tooth development, wherein the epithelial cells of the dental lamina proliferate and produce a budlike projection into the adjacent ectomesenchyme. The *cap stage* is reached when the cells of the dental lamina have proliferated to form a concavity that produces a caplike appearance. The outer cells of the "cap" are cuboidal and constitute the outer enamel epithelium. The cells on the inner or concave aspect of the "cap" are somewhat elongated and represent the inner enamel epithelium. Between the outer and inner epithelia is a network of cells termed the stellate reticulum because of the branched reticular arrangement of the cellular elements. The rim of the enamel organ (i.e., where the outer and inner enamel epithelia are joined) is termed the *cervical loop*. As the cells forming the loop continue to proliferate, there is further invagination of the enamel organ into the mesenchyme. The organ assumes a bell shape, and tooth development enters the *bell stage* (Fig. 11-4). During the bell stage the ectomesenchyme of the dental papilla becomes partially enclosed by the invaginating epithelium. Also during this stage the blood vessels become established in the dental papilla.

The condensed ectomesenchyme surrounding the enamel organ and dental papilla complex forms the dental sac and ultimately develops into the periodontal ligament (see Fig. 11-4). As the tooth bud continues to grow, it carries

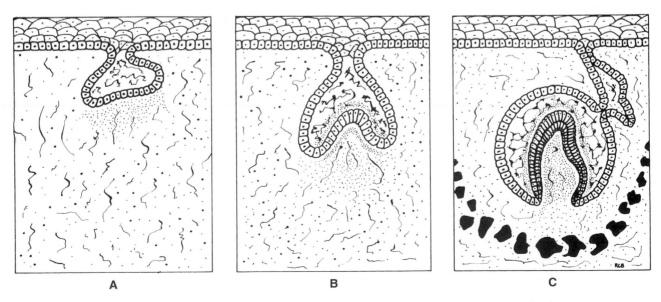

Fig. 11-3 Diagrammatic representation of the bud (**A**), the cap (**B**), and the bell stages (**C**) of tooth development.

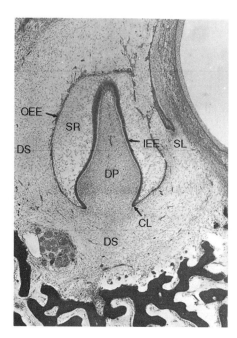

Fig. 11-4 Bell stage of tooth development showing the outer enamel epithelium (*OEE*), stellate reticulum (*SR*), inner enamel epithelium (*IEE*), dental papilla (*DP*), cervical loop (*CL*), successional lamina (*SL*), and dental sac (*DS*).

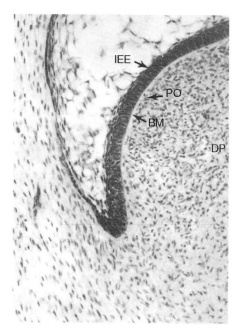

Fig. 11-5 Bell stage shows preodontoblasts (*PO*) aligned along the basement membrane (*BM*) separating the inner enamel epithelium (*IEE*) from the dental papilla (*DP*).

a portion of the dental lamina with it. This extension is referred to as the *lateral lamina*. During the bell stage the lateral lamina degenerates and is invaded and replaced by mesenchymal tissue. In this way the epithelial connection between the enamel organ and the oral epithelium is severed. The free end of the dental lamina associated with each of the primary teeth continues to grow and form the successional lamina. It is from this structure that the tooth germ of the succedaneous tooth arises. As the maxillary and mandibular processes increase in length, the permanent first molar arises from posterior extensions of the dental lamina. After birth the second and third molar primordia appear as the dental laminae proliferate into the underlying mesenchyme.

Differentiation of Odontoblasts

Differentiation of epithelial and mesenchymal cells into ameloblasts and odontoblasts, respectively, occurs during the bell stage of tooth development. This differentiation is always more advanced in the apex of the "bell" (i.e., the region where the cusp tip will develop) than in the area of the cervical loop. From the loop upward toward the apex, the cells appear progressively more differentiated. The preameloblasts differentiate at a faster rate than the corresponding odontoblasts, so at any given level mature ameloblasts appear before the odontoblasts have fully matured. In spite of this difference in rate of maturation, dentin matrix is formed before enamel matrix.

During the bell stage of development there is still mitotic activity among the relatively immature cells of the inner enamel epithelium in the region of the cervical loop. As they commence to mature into ameloblasts, mitotic activity ceases and the cells elongate and display the characteristics of active protein synthesis (i.e., an abundance of rough endoplasmic reticulum [RER], a well-developed Golgi complex, and numerous mitochondria).

As the ameloblasts undergo differentiation, changes are taking place across the basement membrane in the adjacent dental papilla. Before differentiation of odontoblasts, the dental papilla consists of sparsely distributed polymorphic mesenchymal cells with wide intercellular spaces (Fig. 11-5). With the onset of differentiation a single layer of cells, the presumptive odontoblasts (i.e., preodontoblasts), align themselves along the basement membrane separating the inner enamel epithelium from the dental papilla. These cells stop dividing and elongate into short columnar cells with basally situated nuclei (Fig. 11-6). Several cytoplasmic projections from each of these cells extend toward the basal lamina. At this stage the preodontoblasts are still relatively undifferentiated.

As the odontoblasts continue to differentiate, they become progressively more elongated and take on the ultrastructural characteristics of protein-secreting cells. Cytoplasmic processes from these cells extend through the DBM toward the basal lamina, and more and more collagen fibrils appear within the ECM. The first formed collagen fibers pass between the preodontoblasts and extend toward the basal

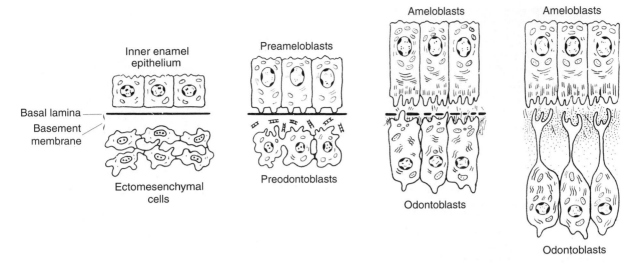

Fig. 11-6 Diagrammatic representation of the stages of odontoblast differentiation.

lamina to form large, fan-shaped bundles 1000 to 2000 Å in diameter, often referred to as von Korff fibers. These fibers stain with silver stains and are associated with a high content of proteoglycans. Some smaller collagen fibers approximately 500 Å in diameter also pass between the odontoblasts and are thought to arise in the dental papilla subjacent to the odontoblasts.[10]

A study on collagen gene expression during rat molar tooth development found both types I and III collagen mRNA in developing odontoblasts.[23] Levels of type I collagen mRNA increased with the progression of odontoblast differentiation, whereas type III collagen gene expression decreased as dentinogenesis proceeded. Both type I and type III collagen mRNA was detected in dental pulp mesenchyme.

Dentinogenesis first occurs in the developing tooth at sites where the cusp tips or incisal edge will be formed. It is in this region that odontoblasts reach full maturity and become tall columnar cells, at times attaining a height of 50 mm or more (see Fig. 11-6). The width of these cells remains fairly constant at approximately 7 mm. Production of the first dentin matrix involves the formation, organization, and maturation of collagen fibrils and proteoglycans. As more collagen fibrils accumulate subjacent to the basal lamina, the lamina becomes discontinuous and eventually disappears. This occurs as the collagen fibers become organized and extend into the spaces between the ameloblast processes. Concurrently the odontoblasts extend several small processes toward the ameloblasts. Some of these become interposed between the processes of ameloblasts, resulting in the formation of enamel spindles (i.e., dentinal tubules that extend into the enamel). Membrane-bound vesicles bud off from the odontoblast processes and become interspersed among the collagen fibers of the dentin matrix. These vesicles subsequently play an important role in the initiation of mineralization (this subject is discussed later in the chapter). With the

onset of dentinogenesis, the dental papilla becomes the dental pulp.

As predentin matrix is formed, the odontoblasts commence to move toward the central pulp, depositing matrix at a rate of approximately 4 to 8 mm per day in their wake. Within this matrix a process from each odontoblast becomes accentuated and remains to form the primary odontoblast process. It is around these processes that the dentinal tubules are formed.

Root Development

Root development commences after the completion of enamel formation. The cells of the inner and outer enamel epithelia, which comprise the cervical loop, begin to proliferate and form a structure known as the Hertwig epithelial root sheath (Fig. 11-7). This sheath determines the size and shape of the root or roots of the tooth. As in the formation of the crown, the cells of the inner enamel epithelium appear to influence the adjacent mesenchymal cells to differentiate into preodontoblasts and odontoblasts. As soon as the first layer of dentin matrix mineralizes, gaps appear in the root sheath, allowing mesenchymal cells from the dental sac to move into contact with the newly formed dentin. These cells then differentiate into cementoblasts and deposit cementum matrix on the root dentin.

Epithelial Rests of Malassez

The epithelial root sheath does not entirely disappear with the onset of dentinogenesis. Some cells persist within the periodontal ligament and are known as epithelial rests of Malassez. Although the number of these rests gradually decreases with age, it has been shown that at least some of them retain the ability to undergo cell division[127] (Fig. 11-8). *In later life if a*

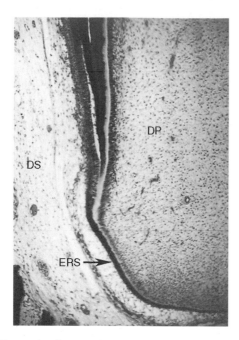

Fig. 11-7 Root development showing dental pulp (*DP*), dental sac (*DS*), and epithelial root sheath (*ERS*).

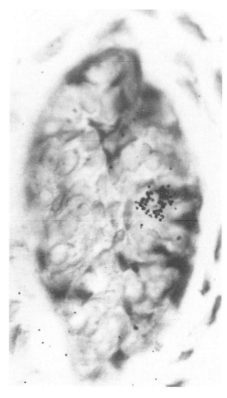

Fig. 11-8 Radioautograph of an epithelial rest cell showing ³H-thymidine labeling of the nucleus, indicating that the cell is preparing to divide. (From Trowbridge HO, Shibata F: *Periodontics* 5:109, 1967.)

chronic inflammatory lesion develops within the periapical tissues as a result of pulp disease, proliferation of the epithelial rests may produce a periapical (radicular) cyst.

Accessory Canals

Occasionally during formation of the root sheath a break develops in the continuity of the sheath, producing a small gap. When this occurs, dentinogenesis does not take place opposite the defect. The result is a small "accessory" canal between the dental sac and the pulp. An accessory canal can become established anywhere along the root, thus creating a periodontal-endodontic pathway of communication and a possible portal of entry into the pulp if the periodontal tissues lose their integrity. *In periodontal disease the development of a periodontal pocket may expose an accessory canal and allow microorganisms or their metabolic products to gain access to the pulp.*

DENTIN

Fully mature dentin is composed of approximately 70% inorganic material and 10% water. The principal inorganic component consists of $Ca_{10}(PO_4)_6(OH)_2$ (i.e., hydroxyapatite). Organic matrix accounts for 20% of dentin, of which about 91% is collagen. Most of the collagen is type I, but there is a minor component of type V. Noncollagenous matrix components include phosphoproteins, proteoglycans, g-carboxyglutamate-n-containing proteins (i.e., gla-proteins), acidic

glycoproteins, growth factors, and lipids. The elasticity of dentin provides flexibility for the overlying brittle enamel.

Dentin and enamel are closely bound together at the dentinoenamel junction (DEJ), and dentin joins cementum at the cementodentinal junction (CDJ). Electron microscopy has revealed that the hydroxyapatite crystals of dentin and enamel are intermixed in the area formerly occupied by the basal lamina of the inner enamel epithelium. Because the basal lamina is dissolved before the onset of dentinogenesis, no organic membrane separates the crystals of enamel from those of dentin.

Types

Developmental dentin is that which forms during tooth development. Dentin formed physiologically after the root is fully developed is referred to as *secondary dentin*. Developmental dentin is classified as *orthodentin*, the tubular form of dentin found in the teeth of all dentate mammals. Mantle dentin is the first formed dentin and is situated immediately subjacent to the enamel or cementum. It is typified by its content of the thick fan-shaped collagen fibers deposited immediately subjacent to the basal lamina during the initial stages of dentinogenesis. These fibers run roughly perpendicular to the DEJ. Spaces between the fibers are occupied by smaller collagen fibrils lying more or less parallel with the DEJ or CDJ.

Circumpulpal dentin is formed after the layer of mantle dentin has been deposited, and it constitutes the major part of developmental dentin. The organic matrix is composed mainly of collagen fibrils, approximately 500 Å in diameter, that are oriented at right angles to the long axis of the dentinal tubules. These fibrils are closely packed together and form an interwoven network.

Predentin

Predentin is the unmineralized organic matrix of dentin situated between the odontoblast layer and the mineralized dentin. Its macromolecular constituents include type I and type II trimer collagens. Noncollagenous elements consist of several proteoglycans (i.e., dermatan sulfate, heparan sulfate, hyaluronate, keratin sulfate, chondroitin 4-sulfate, chondroitin 6-sulfate), glycoproteins, glycosaminoglycans (GAGs), gla-proteins, and *phosphophoryn* (i.e., dentin phosphoprotein). Phosphophoryn is a highly phosphorylated, tissue-specific molecule that is unique to the odontoblast cell lineage.[15] It is produced by the odontoblast and transported to the mineralization front. It is thought to bind to calcium and play a role in mineralization. In addition, growth factors such as TGF-b, insulin-like growth factors, and platelet-derived growth factor have been identified in dentin.

Mineralization

Mineralization of dentin matrix commences within the initial increment of mantle dentin. Calcium phosphate crystals begin to accumulate in matrix vesicles within the predentin. Presumably these vesicles bud off from the cytoplasmic processes of odontoblasts. Although matrix vesicles are distributed throughout the predentin, they are most numerous near the basal lamina. The hydroxyapatite crystals grow rapidly within the vesicles, and in time the vesicles rupture. The crystals released mix with crystals from adjoining vesicles to form advancing crystal fronts that merge to form small globules. As the globules expand, they fuse with adjacent globules until the matrix is completely mineralized.

Apparently matrix vesicles are involved only in mineralization of the initial layer of dentin. As the process of mineralization progresses, the advancing front projects along the collagen fibrils of the predentin matrix. Hydroxyapatite crystals appear on the surface and within the fibrils and continue to grow as mineralization progresses, resulting in an increased mineral content of the dentin.

Dentinal Tubules

A characteristic of human dentin is the presence of tubules that occupy from 20% to 30% of the volume of intact dentin. These tubules house the major cell processes of odontoblasts. Tubules form around the odontoblast processes and, thus, traverse the entire width of the dentin from the DEJ or CDJ to the pulp. They are slightly tapered, with the wider portion situated toward the pulp. This tapering is the result of the progressive formation of peritubular dentin, which leads to a continuous decrease in the diameter of the tubules toward the enamel.

In coronal dentin the tubules have a gentle *S* shape as they extend from the DEJ to the pulp. The *S*-shaped curvature is presumably a result of the crowding of odontoblasts as they migrate toward the center of the pulp. As they approach the pulp, the tubules converge because the surface of the pulp chamber has a much smaller area than the surface of dentin along the DEJ.

The number and diameter of the tubules at various distances from the pulp have been determined (Table 11-1).[38] Investigators[2] found the number and diameter of dentinal tubules to be similar in rats, cats, dogs, monkeys, and humans, indicating that mammalian orthodentin has evolved constantly.

Lateral tubules containing branches of the main odontoblastic processes have been demonstrated by other researchers,[61] who suggested that they form pathways for the movement of materials between the main processes and the more distant matrix. It is also possible that the direction of the branches influences the orientation of the collagen fibrils in the intertubular dentin.

Near the DEJ the dentinal tubules ramify into one or more terminal branches (Fig. 11-9). This is because during the initial stage of dentinogenesis the differentiating odontoblasts extended several cytoplasmic processes toward the DEJ, but as the odontoblasts withdrew, their processes converged into one major process (see Fig. 11-6).

Peritubular Dentin

Dentin lining the tubules is termed *peritubular dentin*, whereas that between the tubules is known as *intertubular dentin* (Fig. 11-10). Presumably precursors of the dentin matrix that is deposited around each odontoblast process are synthesized by the odontoblast, transported in secretory vesicles out into the process, and released by reverse pinocytosis. With the formation of peritubular dentin, there is a corresponding reduction in the diameter of the process.

Peritubular dentin represents a specialized form of orthodentin not common to all mammals. The matrix of peritubular dentin differs from that of intertubular dentin in having relatively fewer collagen fibrils and a higher proportion of sulfated proteoglycans. Because of its lower content of collagen, peritubular dentin is more quickly dissolved in acid than is intertubular dentin. By preferentially removing peritubular dentin, acid-etching agents used during dental restorative procedures enlarge the openings of the dentinal tubules, thus making the dentin more permeable.

Peritubular dentin is more highly mineralized and, therefore, harder than intertubular dentin. The hardness of peritubular dentin may provide added structural support for the intertubular dentin, thus strengthening the tooth.

Intertubular Dentin

Intertubular dentin is located between the rings of peritubular dentin and constitutes the bulk of dentin (see Fig. 11-10). Its organic matrix consists mainly of collagen fibrils having diameters of 500 to 1000 Å. These fibrils are oriented approximately at right angles to the dentinal tubules.

Dentinal Sclerosis

Partial or complete obturation of dentinal tubules may occur as a result of aging or develop in response to stimuli, such as attrition of the tooth surface or dental caries. When tubules become filled with mineral deposits, the dentin becomes sclerotic. Dentinal sclerosis is easily recognized in histologic ground sections because of its translucency (because of the homogeneity of the dentin). This translucency is caused by the mineralization of both matrix and tubules. Studies using dyes, solvents, and radioactive ions have shown that sclerosis

Table 11-1 **MEAN NUMBER AND DIAMETER PER SQUARE MILLIMETER OF DENTINAL TUBULES AT VARIOUS DISTANCES FROM THE PULP IN HUMAN TEETH**

Distance from Pulp (mm)	Number of Tubules (1000/mm²)		Tubule Diameter (µm)	
	Mean	Range	Mean	Range
Pulpal wall	45	30-52	2.5	2.0-3.2
0.1-0.5	43	22-59	1.9	1.0-2.3
0.6-1.0	38	16-47	1.6	1.0-1.6
1.1-1.5	35	21-47	1.2	0.9-1.5
1.6-2.0	30	12-47	1.1	0.8-1.6
2.1-2.5	23	11-36	0.9	0.6-1.3
2.6-3.0	20	7-40	0.8	0.5-1.4
3.1-3.5	19	10-25	0.8	0.5-1.2

(From Garberoglio R, Brännström M: Scanning electron microscopic investigation of human dentinal tubules, *Arch Oral Biol* 21:355, 1976.)

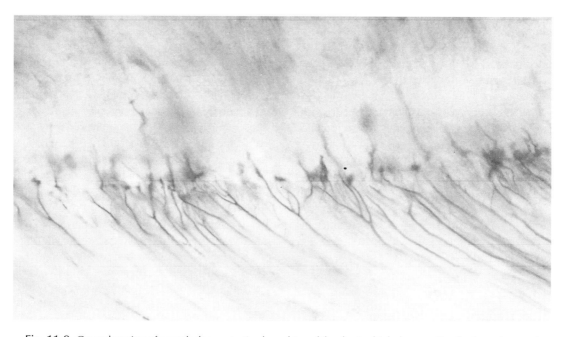

Fig. 11-9 Ground section of a tooth demonstrating branching of the dentinal tubules near the dentin and enamel junction (DEJ). This branching may account for the increased clinical sensitivity at the DEJ.

results in decreased permeability of dentin. Thus dentinal sclerosis, by limiting the diffusion of noxious substances through the dentin, helps to shield the pulp from irritation.

One form of dentinal sclerosis is thought to represent an acceleration of peritubular dentin formation. This form appears to be a physiologic process, and in the apical third of the root it develops as a function of age.[109] Dentinal tubules can also become blocked by the precipitation of hydroxyapatite and whitlockite crystals within the tubules. This type occurs in the translucent zone of carious dentin and in attrited dentin and has been termed *pathologic sclerosis*.[135]

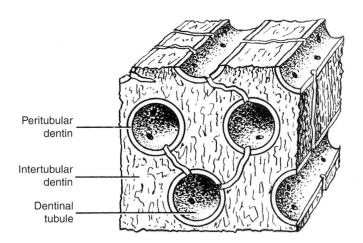

Peritubular dentin

Intertubular dentin

Dentinal tubule

Fig. 11-10 Diagram illustrating peritubular and intertubular dentin. (From Trowbridge HO: *Dentistry* 2[4]:22-29, 1982.)

Interglobular Dentin

The term *interglobular dentin* refers to organic matrix that remains unmineralized because the mineralizing globules fail to coalesce. This occurs most often in the circumpulpal dentin just below the mantle dentin where the pattern of mineralization is more likely to be globular than appositional. In certain dental anomalies (e.g., vitamin D-resistant rickets and hypophosphatasia) large areas of interglobular dentin are a characteristic feature (Fig. 11-11).

Dentinal Fluid

Free fluid occupies about 22% of the total volume of dentin. This fluid is an ultrafiltrate of blood in the pulp capillaries, and its composition resembles plasma in many respects. The fluid flows outward between the odontoblasts into the dentinal tubules and eventually escapes through small pores in the enamel. It has been shown that the tissue pressure of the pulp is approximately 14 cm H_2O (10.3 mm Hg).[21] Consequently, there is a pressure gradient between the pulp and the oral cavity that accounts for the outward flow of fluid. Exposure of the tubules by tooth fracture or during cavity preparation often results in the outward movement of fluid to the exposed dentin surface in the form of tiny droplets. Dehydrating the surface of the dentin with compressed air, dry heat, or the application of absorbent paper can accelerate this outward movement of fluid. Rapid flow of fluid through the tubules is thought to be a cause of dentin sensitivity.

Bacterial products or other contaminants may be introduced into the dentinal fluid as a result of dental caries, restorative procedures, or growth of bacteria beneath restora-

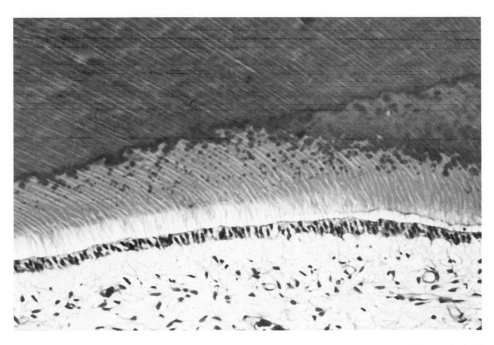

Fig. 11-11 Section showing interglobular dentin (ID) in a deciduous incisor from a 3-year-old boy with childhood hypophosphatasia.

tions.[11,12] Dentinal fluid may thus serve as a sump from which injurious agents can percolate into the pulp, producing an inflammatory response.

Dentin Permeability

The permeability of dentin has been well characterized.[94-96] Dentinal tubules are the major channels for fluid diffusion across dentin. Because fluid permeation is proportional to tubule diameter and number, dentin permeability increases as the tubules converge on the pulp (Fig. 11-12). The total tubular surface near the DEJ is approximately 1% of the total surface area of dentin,[94] whereas close to the pulp chamber the total tubular surface may be nearly 45%. Thus from a clinical standpoint, it should be recognized that dentin beneath a deep cavity preparation is much more permeable than dentin underlying a shallow cavity when the formation of sclerotic or reparative dentin is negligible.

One study[34] found that the permeability of radicular dentin is much lower than that of coronal dentin. This was attributed to a decrease in the density of the dentinal tubules from approximately 42,000/mm^2 in cervical dentin to about 8000/mm^2 in radicular dentin. These investigators found that fluid movement through outer radicular dentin was only approximately 2% that of coronal dentin. The low permeability of outer radicular dentin should make it relatively impermeable to toxic substances, such as bacterial products emanating from plaque.

Factors modifying dentin permeability include the presence of odontoblast processes in the tubules and the sheath-like lamina limitans that lines the tubules. Collagen fibers have also been observed in some tubules. Thus the functional or physiologic diameter of the tubules is only about 5% to 10% of the anatomic diameter (i.e., the diameter seen in microscopic sections).[81]

In dental caries an inflammatory reaction develops in the pulp long before the pulp actually becomes infected.[125] This indicates that bacterial products reach the pulp in advance of the bacteria themselves. Dentinal sclerosis (i.e., reparative dentin formation) beneath a carious lesion reduces the permeation by obstructing the tubules, thus decreasing the concentration of irritants that are introduced into the pulp.

The cutting of dentin during cavity preparation produces microcrystalline grinding debris that coats the dentin and clogs the orifices of the dentinal tubules. This layer of debris is termed the *smear layer*. Because of the small size of the particles, the smear layer is capable of preventing bacteria from penetrating dentin.[83] Removal of the grinding debris by acid etching greatly increases the permeability of the dentin by decreasing the surface resistance and widening the orifices of the tubules. Consequently, the incidence of pulpal inflammation may be increased significantly if cavities are treated with an acid cleanser, unless a cavity liner, base, or dentin-bonding agent is used.

When researchers exposed the dentin surface of vital and nonvital teeth to the oral environment for 150 days, bacterial invasion of dentinal tubules occurred more rapidly in the

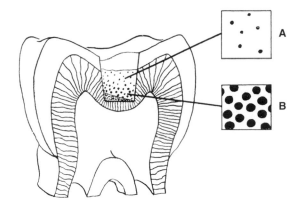

Fig. 11-12 Diagram illustrating the difference in size and density of tubules in the dentinal floor between a shallow (A) and a deep (B) cavity preparation. (From Trowbridge HO: *Dentistry* 22[4]:22-29, 1982.)

nonvital teeth.[83] Presumably this was due to the resistance offered by the outward movement of dentinal fluid and the presence of odontoblast processes in the tubules of vital teeth. It is also possible that antibodies or other antimicrobial components may be present within the dentinal fluid of teeth with vital pulps.

MORPHOLOGIC ZONES OF THE PULP

Odontoblast Layer

The outermost stratum of cells of the healthy pulp is the odontoblast layer (Figs. 11-13 and 11-14). This layer is located immediately subjacent to the predentin; the odontoblast processes, however, pass on through the predentin into the dentin. Consequently, the odontoblast layer is actually composed of the cell bodies of odontoblasts. Additionally, capillaries, nerve fibers, and dendritic cells may be found among the odontoblasts.

In the coronal portion of a young pulp the odontoblasts assume a tall columnar form. The tight packing together of these tall, slender cells produces the appearance of a palisade. The odontoblasts vary in height; consequently, their nuclei are not all at the same level and are aligned in a staggered array. This often produces the appearance of a layer three to five cells in thickness. Between odontoblasts there are small intercellular spaces approximately 300 to 400 Å in width.

The odontoblast layer in the coronal pulp contains more cells per unit area than in the radicular pulp. Whereas the odontoblasts of the mature coronal pulp are usually columnar, those in the midportion of the radicular pulp are more cuboidal (Fig. 11-15). Near the apical foramen the odontoblasts appear as a flattened cell layer. Because there are fewer dentinal tubules per unit area in the root than in the crown of the tooth, the odontoblast cell bodies are less crowded and are able to spread out laterally.

Between adjacent odontoblasts there are a series of specialized cell-to-cell junctions (i.e., junctional complexes) including desmosomes (i.e., zonula adherens), gap junctions

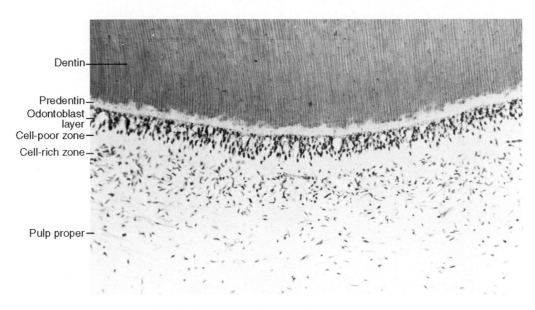

Fig. 11-13 Morphologic zones of the mature pulp.

(i.e., nexuses), and tight junctions (i.e., zonula occludens). Spot desmosomes located in the apical part of odontoblast cell bodies mechanically join odontoblasts together. Numerous gap junctions provide low-resistance pathways through which electrical excitation can pass between cells (Fig. 11-16). These junctions are most numerous during the formation of primary dentin. Gap junctions and desmosomes have also been observed joining odontoblasts to the processes of fibroblasts in the subodontoblastic area. Tight junctions are found mainly in the apical part of odontoblasts in young teeth. These structures consist of linear ridges and grooves that close off the intercellular space. It appears that tight junctions determine the permeability of the odontoblast layer by restricting the passage of molecules, ions, and fluid between the extracellular compartments of the pulp and predentin.[130]

Cell-Poor Zone

Immediately subjacent to the odontoblast layer in the coronal pulp, there is often a narrow zone approximately 40 mm in width that is relatively free of cells (see Fig. 11-13). It is traversed by blood capillaries, unmyelinated nerve fibers, and the slender cytoplasmic processes of fibroblasts (see Fig. 11-14). The presence or absence of the cell-poor zone depends on the functional status of the pulp. It may not be apparent in young pulps, where dentin forms rapidly, or in older pulps, where reparative dentin is being produced.

Cell-Rich Zone

Usually conspicuous in the subodontoblastic area is a stratum containing a relatively high proportion of fibroblasts, compared with the more central region of the pulp (see Fig. 11-13). It is much more prominent in the coronal pulp than in the radicular pulp. Besides fibroblasts, the cell-rich zone

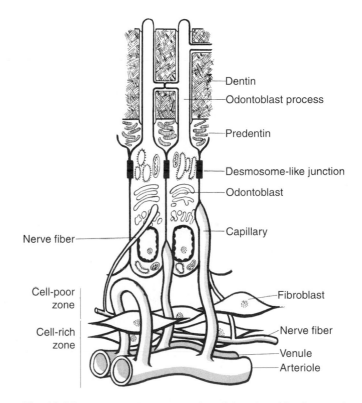

Fig. 11-14 Diagrammatic representation of the odontoblast layer and subodontoblastic region of the pulp.

may include a variable number of macrophages, dendritic cells, and lymphocytes.

On the basis of evidence obtained in rat molar teeth, it has been suggested[39] that the cell-rich zone forms as a result of peripheral migration of cells populating the central regions of the pulp, commencing at about the time of tooth eruption.

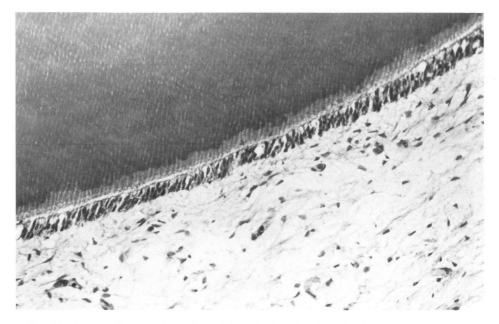

Fig. 11-15 Low columnar odontoblasts of the radicular pulp. The cell-rich zone is inconspicuous.

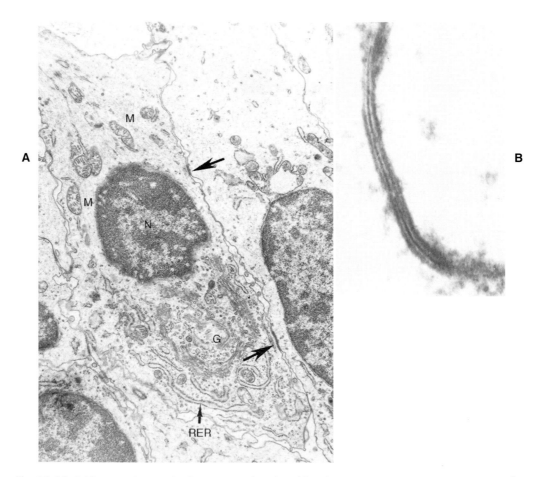

Fig. 11-16 **A,** Electron micrograph of a mouse molar odontoblast demonstrating gap junctions (*arrows*), nucleus (*N*), mitochondria (*M*), Golgi complex (*G*), and *RER*. **B,** High magnification of a section fixed and stained with lanthanum nitrate to demonstrate a typical gap junction. (Courtesy Dr. Charles F. Cox, School of Dentistry, University of Alabama.)

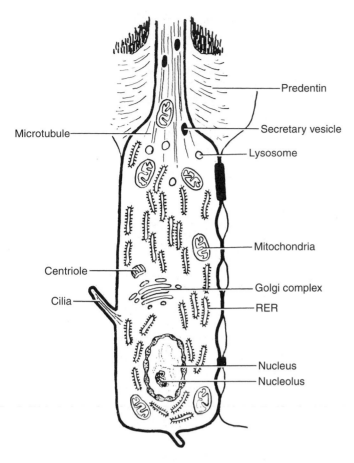

Fig. 11-17 Diagram of a fully differentiated odontoblast.

Although cell division within the cell-rich zone is a rare occurrence in normal pulps, death of odontoblasts causes a great increase in the rate of mitosis. Because irreversibly injured odontoblasts are replaced by cells that migrate from the cell-rich zone onto the inner surface of the dentin,[33] this mitotic activity is probably the first step in the formation of a new odontoblast layer.

Pulp Proper

The pulp proper is the central mass of the pulp (see Fig. 11-13). It contains the larger blood vessels and nerves. The connective tissue cells in this zone consist of fibroblasts or pulpal cells.

CELLS OF THE PULP

Odontoblast

Because it is responsible for dentinogenesis both during tooth development and in the mature tooth, the odontoblast is the most characteristic cell of the pulp-dentin complex. During dentinogenesis the odontoblasts form the dentinal

tubules, and their presence within the tubules makes dentin a living tissue.

Dentinogenesis, osteogenesis, and cementogenesis are in many respects quite similar. Therefore it is not surprising that odontoblasts, osteoblasts, and cementoblasts have many similar characteristics. Each of these cells produces a matrix composed of collagen fibers and proteoglycans that are capable of undergoing mineralization. The ultrastructural characteristics of odontoblasts, osteoblasts, and cementoblasts are likewise similar in that each exhibits a highly ordered RER, a prominent Golgi complex, secretory granules, and numerous mitochondria. In addition, these cells are rich in RNA, and their nuclei contain one or more prominent nucleoli. These are the general characteristics of protein-secreting cells.

Perhaps the most significant differences between odontoblasts, osteoblasts, and cementoblasts are their morphologic characteristics and the anatomic relationship between the cells and the structures they produce. Whereas osteoblasts and cementoblasts are polygonal to cuboidal in form, the fully developed odontoblast of the coronal pulp is a tall columnar cell. In bone and cementum some of the osteoblasts and cementoblasts become entrapped in the matrix as osteocytes or cementocytes, respectively. The odontoblasts, on the other hand, leave behind cellular processes to form the dentinal tubules. Lateral branches between the major odontoblast processes interconnect the processes through canals, just as osteocytes and cementocytes are linked together through the canaliculi in bone and cementum. This provides for intercellular communication and circulation of fluid and metabolites through the mineralized matrix.

The ultrastructural features of the odontoblast have been the subject of numerous investigations. The cell body of the active odontoblast has a large nucleus that may contain up to four nucleoli (Fig. 11-17). The nucleus is situated at the basal end of the cell and is contained within a nuclear envelope. A well-developed Golgi complex, centrally located in the supranuclear cytoplasm, consists of an assembly of smooth-walled vesicles and cisternae. Numerous mitochondria are evenly distributed throughout the cell body. RER is particularly prominent, consisting of closely stacked cisternae forming parallel arrays that are dispersed diffusely within the cytoplasm. Numerous ribosomes closely associated with the membranes of the cisternae mark the sites of protein synthesis. Within the lumen of the cisternae filamentous material (probably representing newly synthesized protein) can be observed.

Apparently the odontoblast synthesizes mainly type I collagen, although small amounts of type V collagen have been found in the ECM. In addition to proteoglycans and collagen, the odontoblast secretes dentin sialoprotein and phosphophoryn, a highly phosphorylated phosphoprotein involved in extracellular mineralization. Phosphophoryn is unique to dentin and is not found in any other mesenchymal cell lines. The odontoblast also secretes alkaline phosphatase, an enzyme that is closely linked to mineralization. However, the precise role of alkaline phosphatase is yet to be illuminated.

The labels on the figure are: Predentin, Secretary vesicle, Lysosome, Mitochondria, Golgi complex, RER, Nucleus, Nucleolus, Microtubule, Centriole, Cilia.

In contrast to the active odontoblast, the resting or inactive odontoblast has a decreased number of organelles and may become progressively shorter. These changes can begin with the completion of root development.

Odontoblast Process

A dentinal tubule forms around each of the major processes of odontoblasts. The odontoblast process occupies most of the space within the tubule and somehow mediates the formation of peritubular dentin. Fine cytofilaments are the other structures found in the process.

Microtubules and microfilaments are the principal ultrastructural components of the odontoblast process and its lateral branches.[53] Microtubules extend from the cell body out into the process. These straight structures follow a course that is parallel with the long axis of the cell and impart the impression of rigidity. Although their precise role is unknown, theories as to their functional significance suggest that they may be involved in cytoplasmic extension, transport of materials, or the provision of a structural framework. Occasionally, mitochondria can be found in the process where it passes through the predentin.

The plasma membrane of the odontoblast process closely approximates the wall of the dentinal tubule. Localized constrictions in the process occasionally produce relatively large spaces between the tubule wall and the process. Such spaces may contain collagen fibrils and fine, granular material that presumably represents ground substance. The peritubular dentin matrix lining the tubule is circumscribed by an electron-dense limiting membrane.[107] A space separates the limiting membrane from the plasma membrane of the odontoblast process. This space is usually narrow, except in areas where (as mentioned previously) the process is constricted.

In restoring a tooth, preparation of a cavity or crown often disrupts odontoblasts. Consequently, it would be of considerable clinical importance to establish conclusively the extent of the odontoblast processes in human teeth. With this knowledge the clinician would be in a better position to estimate the impact of the restorative procedure on the underlying odontoblasts. The extent to which the process extends outward in the dentin has been a matter of considerable controversy. It has long been thought that the process is present throughout the full thickness of dentin. However, ultrastructural studies using transmission electron microscopy have described the process as being limited to the inner third of the dentin.[51,116] This could possibly be the result of shrinkage occurring during fixation and dehydration during histologic processing. Other studies employing scanning electron microscopy have described the process extending further into the tubule, often as far as the DEJ.[40,62,139] However, it has been suggested that what has been observed in scanning electron micrographs is actually an electron-dense structure, the lamina limitans, that lines the surface of the tubule.[106,107]

In an attempt to resolve this issue, monoclonal antibodies directed against microtubules were used to demonstrate tubulin in the microtubules of the process. Immunoreactivity was observed throughout the dentinal tubule, suggesting that the process extends throughout the entire thickness of dentin.[99,100] However, a more recent study employing fluorescent carbocyanine dye and confocal microscopy found that odontoblast processes in rat molars do not extend to the outer dentin or DEJ, except during the early stages of tooth development.[18] Obviously this problem warrants further study.

The odontoblast is considered to be a fixed postmitotic cell in that once it has fully differentiated, it apparently cannot undergo further cell division. If this is indeed the case, the life span of the odontoblast coincides with the life span of the viable pulp.

Relationship of Odontoblast Structure to Function

Isotope studies have shed a great deal of light on the functional significance of the cytoplasmic organelles of the active odontoblast.[127] In experimental animals the intraperitoneal injection of collagen precursors (e.g., ^{3}H-proline) is followed by autoradiographic labeling of the odontoblasts and predentin matrix (Fig. 11-18). Rapid incorporation of the isotope in the RER soon leads to labeling of the Golgi complex in the area where the procollagen is packed and concentrated into secretory vesicles. Labeled vesicles can then be followed along their migration pathway until they reach the base of the odontoblast process. Here they fuse with the cell membrane and release their tropocollagen molecules into the predentin matrix by the process of reverse pinocytosis.

It is now known that collagen fibrils precipitate from a solution of tropocollagen and that the aggregation of fibrils occurs on the outer surface of the odontoblast plasma membrane. Fibrils are released into the predentin and increase in thickness as they approach the mineralized matrix. Whereas fibrils at the base of the odontoblast process are approximately 150 Å in diameter, fibrils in the region of the calcification front have attained a diameter of about 500 Å.

Similar tracer studies[126] have elucidated the pathway of synthesis, transport, and secretion of the predentin proteoglycans. The protein moiety of these molecules is synthesized by the RER of the odontoblast, whereas sulfation and addition of the GAG moieties to the protein molecules take place in the Golgi complex. Secretory vesicles then transport the proteoglycans to the base of the odontoblast process, where they are secreted into the predentin matrix. Proteoglycans, principally chondroitin sulfate, accumulate near the calcification front. The role of the proteoglycans is speculative, but mounting evidence suggests that they act as inhibitors of calcification by binding calcium. It appears that just before calcification the proteoglycans are removed, probably by lysosomal enzymes secreted by the odontoblasts.[25]

Pulp Fibroblast

Fibroblasts are the most numerous cells of the pulp. They appear to be tissue-specific cells that are capable of giving rise to cells that are committed to differentiation (e.g., odon-

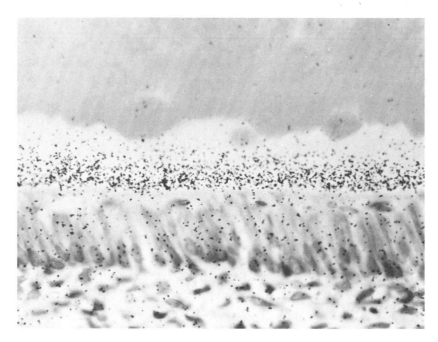

Fig. 11-18 Radioautograph demonstrating odontoblasts and predentin in a developing rat molar 1 hour after intraperitoneal injection of ³H-proline.

toblast-like cells), if given the proper signal. These cells synthesize types I and III collagen, as well as proteoglycans and GAGs. Thus they produce and maintain the matrix proteins of the ECM. Because they are also able to phagocytose and digest collagen, fibroblasts are responsible for collagen turnover in the pulp.

Although distributed throughout the pulp, fibroblasts are particularly abundant in the cell-rich zone. The early differentiating fibroblasts are polygonal and appear to be widely separated and evenly distributed within the ground substance. Cell-to-cell contacts are established between the multiple processes that extend out from each of the cells. Many of these contacts take the form of gap junctions, which provide for electronic coupling of one cell to another. Ultrastructurally the organelles of the immature fibroblasts are generally in a rudimentary stage of development, with an inconspicuous Golgi complex, numerous free ribosomes, and sparse RER. As they mature, the cells become stellate in form and the Golgi complex enlarges, the RER proliferates, secretory vesicles appear, and the fibroblasts take on the characteristic appearance of protein-secreting cells. Along the outer surface of the cell body, collagen fibrils commence to appear. With an increase in the number of blood vessels, nerves, and fibers, there is a relative decrease in the number of fibroblasts in the pulp.

A colleague once remarked that the fibroblasts of the pulp are very much like Peter Pan, because they "never grow up." There may be an element of truth in this statement, for these cells do seem to remain in a relatively undifferentiated modality (compared with fibroblasts of most other connective tissues[44]). This perception has been fortified by the observation of large numbers of reticulin-like fibers in the pulp. Reticulin fibers have an affinity for silver stains and are similar to the argyrophilic fibers of the pulp. However, in a careful review of the subject, Baume[5] concluded that because of distinct histochemical differences, reticulin fibers, such as those of gingiva and lymphoid organs, are not present in the pulp. He suggested that these pulpal fibers be termed *argyrophilic collagen fibers*. The fibers apparently acquire a GAG sheath, and it is this sheath that is impregnated by silver stains. In the young pulp the nonargyrophilic collagen fibers are sparse, but they progressively increase in number as the pulp ages.

Many experimental models have been developed to study wound healing in the pulp, particularly dentinal bridge formation after pulp exposure or pulpotomy. One study[33] demonstrated that mitotic activity preceding the differentiation of replacement odontoblasts appears to occur primarily among fibroblasts.

Macrophage

Macrophages are the monocytes that have left the bloodstream, entered the tissues, and differentiated into various subpopulations. Many are found in close proximity to blood vessels (Fig. 11-19). A major subpopulation of macrophages is quite active in endocytosis and phagocytosis (Fig. 11-20). Because of their mobility and phagocytic activity, they are able to act as scavengers, removing extravasated red blood cells, dead cells, and foreign bodies from the tissue. Ingested material is destroyed by the action of lysosomal enzymes. Another subset of macrophages participates in immune reac-

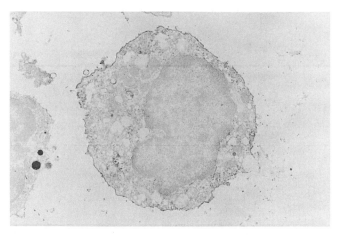

Fig. 11-19 Immunolectron micrograph of a HLA-DR+ young macrophage in the human pulp, showing reaction products along the cytoplasmic membrane.

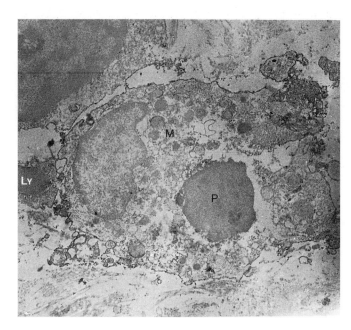

Fig. 11-20 Immunolectron micrograph of a HLA-DR+ matured macrophage (*M*) in the human pulp, showing a phagosome (*P*) (Ly: lymphocyte).

tions by processing antigen and presenting it to memory T cells. The processed antigen is bound to class II major histocompatibility complex (MHC) molecules on the macrophage, where it can interact with specific receptors present on naive or memory T cells. Such interaction is essential for T cell–dependent immunity. When activated by the appropriate inflammatory stimuli, macrophages are capable of producing a large variety of soluble factors, including interleukin-1, tumor necrosis factor, growth factors, and other cytokines.

Dendritic Cell

Dendritic cells are accessory cells of the immune system. Similar cells are found in the epidermis and mucous membranes, where they are called *Langerhans' cells*. Dendritic cells are primarily found in lymphoid tissues, but they are also widely distributed in connective tissues, including the pulp[60,70] (Fig. 11-21). These cells are termed *antigen-presenting cells* and are characterized by dendritic cytoplasmic processes and the presence of cell surface class II antigens (Fig. 11-22). They are known to play a central role in the induction of T cell–dependent immunity. Like antigen-presenting macrophages, they engulf protein antigens and then present an assembly of peptide fragments of the antigens and class II molecules. It is this assembly that T cells can recognize. Then, the assembly binds to T cell receptor and T cell activation occurs (Fig. 11-23). Fig. 11-24 shows a cell-to-cell contact between a dendritic-like cell and a lymphocyte.

Lymphocyte

Hahn[42] reported finding T lymphocytes in normal pulps from human teeth. T8 (suppressor) lymphocytes were the predominant T-lymphocyte subset present in these pulps. Lympho-

cytes have also been observed in the pulps of impacted teeth.[69] The presence of macrophages, dendritic cells, and T lymphocytes indicates that the pulp is well equipped with cells required for the initiation of immune responses. B lymphocytes are scarcely found in the normal pulp.

Mast Cell

Mast cells are widely distributed in connective tissues, where they occur in small groups in relation to blood vessels. Mast cells are seldom found in the normal pulp tissue, although they are routinely found in chronically inflamed pulps. This cell has been the subject of considerable attention because of its dramatic role in inflammatory reactions. The granules of mast cells contain heparin, an anticoagulant, and histamine, an important inflammatory mediator.

METABOLISM

The metabolic activity of the pulp has been studied by measuring the rate of oxygen consumption and the production of carbon dioxide or lactic acid by pulp tissue in vitro.[29,32,100] A later investigation[43] employed the radiospirometry method.

Because of the relatively sparse cellular composition of the pulp, the rate of oxygen consumption is low in comparison to that of most other tissues. During active dentinogenesis, metabolic activity is much higher than after the completion of crown development. As would be anticipated, the greatest metabolic activity is found in the region of the odontoblast layer.

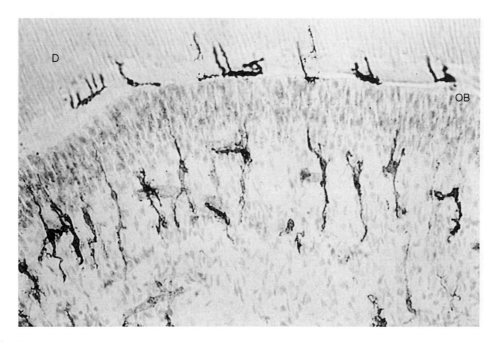

Fig. 11-21 Class II antigen-expressing dendritic cells in the pulp and dentin border zone in normal human pulp, as demonstrated by immunocytochemistry (*D*: dentin, *OB*: odontoblastic layer).

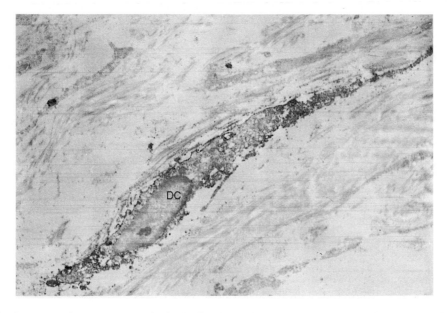

Fig. 11-22 Immunoelectron micrograph of a dendritic-like cell (*DC*) in the human pulp, showing a dendritic profile with a relatively small amount of lysosomal structures.

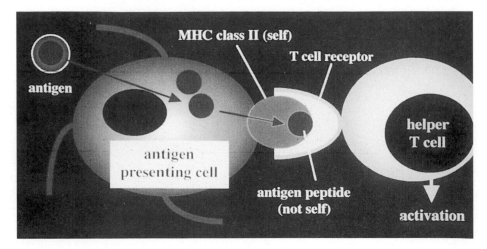

Fig. 11-23 Function of MHC class II molecule-expressing cells. They act as antigen-presenting cells that are essential for the induction of helper T cell–dependent immune responses. (Courtesy Dr. Takashi Okiji, Dental Hospital, Tokyo Medical and Dental University.)

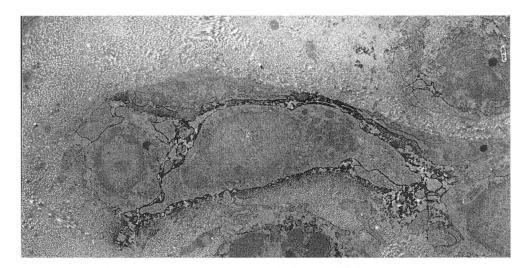

Fig. 11-24 Immunoelectron micrograph of a dendritic cell-like cell and a lymphocyte. They show a cell-to-cell contact.

In addition to the usual glycolytic pathway, the pulp has the ability to produce energy through a phosphogluconate (i.e., pentose phosphate) shunt type of carbohydrate metabolism,[30] suggesting that the pulp may be able to function under varying degrees of ischemia. This could explain how the pulp manages to withstand periods of vasoconstriction resulting from the use of infiltration anesthesia employing epinephrine-containing local anesthetic agents.[65]

Several commonly used dental materials (e.g., eugenol, zinc oxide and eugenol, calcium hydroxide, silver amalgam) have been shown to inhibit oxygen consumption by pulp tissue, indicating that these agents may be capable of depressing the metabolic activity of pulpal cells.[31,59] One study[43] found that application of orthodontic force to human premolars for 3 days resulted in a 27% reduction in respiratory activity in the pulp.

GROUND SUBSTANCE

Connective tissue is a system consisting of cells and fibers, both embedded in the pervading ground substance, or extracellular matrix (ECM). Cells that produce connective tissue fibers also synthesize the major constituents of the ECM. Whereas the fibers and cells have recognizable shapes, ECM is described as being amorphous. It is generally regarded as a gel rather than a sol and, therefore is considered to differ from tissue fluids. Because of its content of polyelectric polysaccharides, the ECM is responsible for the water-holding properties of connective tissues.

Nearly all proteins of the ECM are glycoproteins. Proteoglycans are an important subclass of glycoproteins. These molecules support cells, provide tissue turgor, and mediate a variety of cell interactions. They have in common the presence of GAG chains and a protein core to which the chains are linked. Except for heparan sulfate and heparin, the chains are composed of disaccharides. The primary function of GAG chains is to act as adhesive molecules that can bond to cell surfaces and other matrix molecules.

Fibronectin is a major surface glycoprotein that, together with collagen, forms an integrated fibrillary network that influences adhesion, motility, growth, and differentiation of cells. Laminin, an important component of basement membranes, binds to type IV collagen and cell surface receptors. Tenascin is another substrate adhesion glycoprotein.[1]

In the pulp the principal proteoglycans include hyaluronic acid*, dermatan sulfate, heparan sulfate, and chondroitin sulfate.[77] The proteoglycan content of pulp tissue decreases approximately 50% with tooth eruption.[74] During active dentinogenesis, chondroitin sulfate is the principal proteoglycan, particularly in the odontoblast and predentin layer, where it is somehow involved with mineralization; with tooth eruption, hyaluronic acid and dermatan sulfate increase and chondroitin sulfate decreases greatly.

The consistency of a connective tissue (e.g., the pulp) is largely determined by the proteoglycan components of the ground substance. The long GAG chains of the proteoglycan molecules form relatively rigid coils constituting a network that holds water, thus forming a characteristic gel. Hyaluronic acid, in particular, has a strong affinity for water and is a major component of ground substance in tissues with a large fluid content, such as Wharton's jelly of the umbilical cord. The water content of the pulp is very high (approximately 90%); thus the ground substance forms a cushion capable of protecting cells and vascular components of the tooth.

Ground substance also acts as a molecular sieve in that it excludes large proteins and urea. Cell metabolites, nutrients, and wastes pass through the ground substance between cells and blood vessels. In some ways, ground substance can be likened to an ion exchange resin, because the polyanionic chains of the GAGs bind cations. Additionally, osmotic pressures can be altered by excluding osmotically active molecules. Thus proteoglycans can regulate the dispersion of interstitial matrix solutes, colloids, and water, and (in large measure) determine the physical characteristics of a tissue, such as the pulp.

Degradation of ground substance can occur in certain inflammatory lesions in which there is a high concentration of lysosomal enzymes. Proteolytic enzymes, hyaluronidases, and chrondroitin sulfatases of lysosomal and bacterial origin are examples of the hydrolytic enzymes that can attack components of the ground substance. The pathways of inflammation and infection are strongly influenced by the state of polymerization of the ground substance components.

CONNECTIVE TISSUE FIBERS OF THE PULP

Two types of structural proteins are found in the pulp: (1) collagen and (2) elastin. Elastin fibers are confined to the walls of arterioles and, unlike collagen, are not a part of the ECM.

A single collagen molecule, referred to as tropocollagen, consists of three polypeptide chains, designated as either a1 or a2 depending on their amino acid composition and sequence. The different combinations and linkages of chains making up the tropocollagen molecule have allowed collagen fibers and fibrils to be classified into a number of types:

- Type I collagen is found in skin, tendon, bone, dentin, and pulp.
- Type II collagen is found in cartilage.
- Type III collagen is found in most unmineralized connective tissues. It is a fetal form found in the dental papilla and the mature pulp. In the bovine pulp it comprises 45% of the total pulp collagen during all stages of development.
- Types IV and VII collagen are components of basement membranes.
- Type V collagen is a constituent of interstitial tissues.

Type I collagen is synthesized by odontoblasts and osteoblasts; fibroblasts synthesize types I, III, V, and VII.

In collagen synthesis the protein portion of the molecule is formed by the polyribosomes of the RER of connective tissue cells. The proline and lysine residues of the polypeptide chains are hydroxylated in the cisternae of the RER, and the chains are assembled into a triple-helix configuration in the smooth endoplasmic reticulum. The product of this assembly is termed procollagen, and it has a terminal unit of amino acids known as the *telopeptide of the procollagen molecule*. When these molecules reach the Golgi complex, they are glycosylated and packaged in secretory vesicles. The vesicles are transported to the plasma membrane and secreted via exocytosis into the extracellular milieu, thus releasing the procollagen. Here the terminal telopeptide is cleaved by a hydrolytic enzyme, and the tropocollagen molecules begin aggregating to form collagen fibrils. It is believed that aggregation of tropocollagen is somehow mediated by the GAGs. The conversion of soluble collagen into insoluble fibers occurs as a result of cross-linking of tropocollagen molecules.

In the young pulp, small collagen fibers stain black with silver impregnation stains. Thus they are referred to as *argyrophilic fibers* (Fig. 11-25). They are very similar (if not identical) to reticular fibers in other loose connective tissues because they are not arranged in bundles and tend to form delicate networks. The presence of collagen fibers passing from the dentin matrix between odontoblasts into the dental

---

*Because there is still some doubt as to whether hyaluronic acid is linked to protein, it should probably be referred to as GAG rather than proteoglycan.

pulp has been reported in fully erupted teeth.[10] Larger collagen fiber bundles are not argyrophilic, but they can be demonstrated with special histochemical methods, such as the Masson trichrome stain or Mallory's triple connective tissue stain (Fig. 11-26). These fibers are much more numerous in the radicular pulp than in the coronal pulp. The highest concentration of these larger fiber bundles is usually found near the apex (Fig. 11-27). Thus Torneck[123] advised that during pulpectomy, if the pulp is engaged with a barbed broach in the region of the apex, this generally affords the best opportunity to remove it intact.

INNERVATION

Pain is a complex phenomenon that involves not only sensory response but also emotional, conceptual, and motivational aspects of behavior. Nevertheless, it is the evoked potentials in the tooth that initiate signals to the brain; therefore, control of dental pain should be based on an understanding of the origin of these pain signals.

The sensory system of the pulp appears to be well suited for signaling potential damage to the tooth. The tooth is innervated by a large number of myelinated and unmyelinated nerve fibers. (The number of axons entering a human premolar may reach 2000 or more.)

Regardless of the nature of the sensory stimulus (i.e., thermal change, mechanical deformation, injury to the tissues), almost all afferent impulses from the pulp result in the sensation of pain. However, when the pulp is weakly stimulated by an electric pulp tester, nonpainful sensation (i.e., prepain) could be evoked. The innervation of the pulp includes both *afferent neurons*, which conduct sensory impulses, and *autonomic fibers*, which provide neurogenic

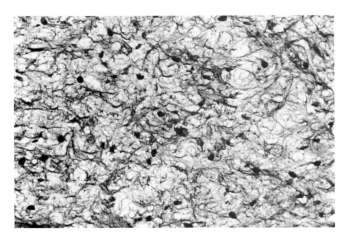

Fig. 11-25 Delicate network of pulpal collagen fibers as demonstrated by the Pearson silver impregnation method.

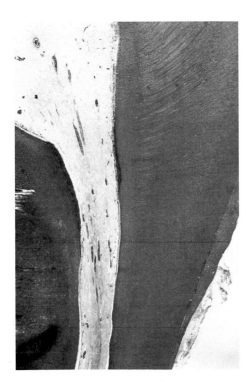

Fig. 11-26 Histologic section of pulp stained with Masson trichrome stain showing abundance of collagen fibers in the radicular pulp, as compared with the coronal pulp.

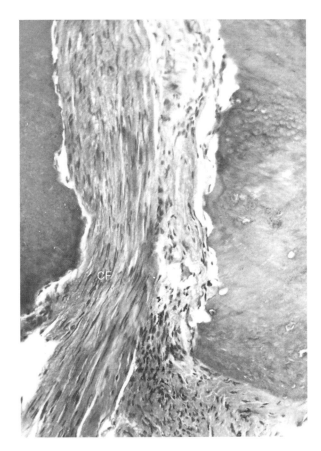

Fig. 11-27 Dense bundles of collagen fibers (*CF*) in the apical pulp.

modulation of the microcirculation and perhaps regulate dentinogenesis.

In addition to sensory nerves, sympathetic fibers from the superior cervical ganglion appear with blood vessels at the time the vascular system is established in the dental papilla. In the adult tooth sympathetic fibers form plexuses, usually around pulpal arterioles. Stimulation of these fibers results in constriction of the arterioles and a decrease in blood flow. Both adrenergic and cholinergic fibers have been found in close relation to odontoblasts.[55] It is thought that these nerve endings may be involved in the regulation of dentin formation.

Nerve fibers are usually classified according to their diameter, conduction velocity, and function as shown in Table 11-2. In the pulp there are two types of sensory nerve fibers: (1) myelinated (A fibers) and (2) *unmyelinated* (C fibers). Investigators showed that there is some functional overlapping between pulpal A and C fibers.[54] The A fibers include both A beta (Aβ) and A delta (Aδ) fibers. The Aβ fibers may be slightly more sensitive to stimulation than the Aδ fibers, but functionally these fibers are grouped together. Approximately 90% of the A fibers are Aδ fibers. The principal characteristics of these fibers are summarized in Table 11-3.

During the bell stage of tooth development, "pioneer" nerve fibers enter the dental papilla following the path of blood vessels. Although only unmyelinated fibers are observed in the dental papilla, a proportion of these fibers are probably A fibers that have not yet become myelinated. Myelinated fibers are the last major structures to appear in the developing human dental pulp. The number of nerve fibers gradually increases, and some branching occurs as the fibers near the dentin; during the bell stage very few fibers enter the predentin.

The sensory nerves of the pulp arise from the trigeminal nerve and pass into the radicular pulp in bundles via the foramen in close association with arterioles and venules (Fig. 11-28). Each of the nerves entering the pulp is invested within Schwann cells, and the A fibers acquire their myelin sheath from these cells. With the completion of root development the myelinated fibers appear grouped in bundles in the central region of the pulp (Fig. 11-29). Most of the unmyelinated C fibers entering the pulp are located within these fiber bundles; the remainder are situated toward the periphery of the pulp.[98] *It should be noticed that single pulpal nerve fibers have been reported to innervate multiple tooth pulps.*[49]

Investigators[56] found that in the human premolar the number of unmyelinated axons entering the tooth at the apex reached a maximal number shortly after tooth eruption. At this stage they observed an average of 1800 unmyelinated axons and more than 400 myelinated axons, although in some teeth fewer than 100 myelinated axons were present. Five years after eruption the number of A fibers gradually

Table 11-2 CLASSIFICATION OF NERVE FIBERS

Type of Fiber	Function	Diameter (μm)	Conduction Velocity (m/sec)
Aα	Motor, proprioception	12-20	70-120
Aβ	Pressure, touch	5-12	30-70
Aγ	Motor, to muscle spindles	3-6	15-30
Aδ	Pain, temperature, touch	1-5	6-30
B	Preganglionic autonomic	<3	3-15
C dorsal root	Pain	0.4-1.0	0.5-2.0
sympathetic	Postganglionic sympathetic	0.3-1.3	0.7-2.3

Table 11-3 CHARACTERISTICS OF SENSORY FIBERS

Fiber	Myelination	Location of Terminals	Pain Characteristics	Stimulation Threshold
Aδ	Yes	Principally in region of pulp-dentin junction	Sharp, pricking	Relatively low
C	No	Probably distributed throughout pulp	Burning, aching, less bearable than Aδ fiber sensations	Relatively high, usually associated with tissue injury

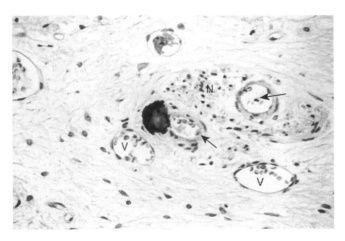

Fig. 11-28 Cross section of the apical pulp of a human premolar, demonstrating nerve fiber bundle (*N*), arterioles (*arrows*), and venules (*V*). Note presence of a small pulp stone projecting outward from the wall of an arteriole.

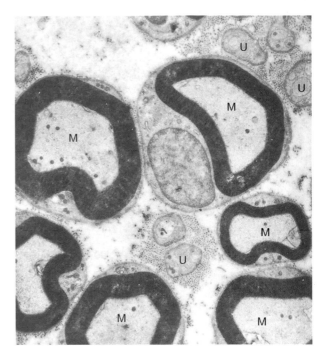

Fig. 11-29 Electron micrograph of the apical pulp of a young canine tooth, showing in cross section myelinated nerve axons (*M*) within Schwann cells. Smaller, unmyelinated axons (*U*) are enclosed singly and in groups by Schwann cells. (Courtesy Dr. David C. Johnsen, School of Dentistry, Case Western Reserve University.)

increased to more than 700. *The relatively late appearance of A fibers in the pulp may help to explain why the electric pulp test tends to be unreliable in young teeth.*[36]

A quantitative study of nerve axons 1 to 2 mm above the root apex of fully developed human canine and incisor teeth has been conducted.[57] It reported a mean of 361 and 359 myelinated axons in canines and incisors, respectively. The number of unmyelinated axons was much greater, with means of 2240 for canines and 1591 for incisors. Thus approximately 80% of the nerves were unmyelinated fibers. However, some myelinated fibers may lose their sheaths before entering the apex or, in young teeth, they may not yet have acquired a sheath. Consequently, it has been difficult to accurately assess the true proportion of myelinated and unmyelinated fibers entering the pulp.

The nerve bundles pass upward through the radicular pulp together with blood vessels. Once they reach the coronal pulp, they fan out beneath the cell-rich zone, branch into smaller bundles, and finally ramify into a plexus of single-nerve axons known as the *plexus of Raschkow* (Fig. 11-30). Full development of this plexus does not occur until the final stages of root formation.[27] It has been estimated that each fiber entering the pulp sends at least eight branches to the plexus of Raschkow. There is prolific branching of the fibers in the plexus, producing a tremendous overlap of receptor fields.[45] It is in the plexus that the A fibers emerge from their myelin sheaths and, while still within Schwann cells, branch repeatedly to form the subodontoblastic plexus. Finally, terminal axons exit from their Schwann cell investiture and pass between the odontoblasts as free nerve endings (Figs. 11-31 and 11-32).

The extent to which dentin is innervated has been the subject of numerous investigations. With the exception of the intratubular fibers discussed above, dentin is devoid of sensory nerve fibers. This offers an explanation as to why pain-producing agents (e.g., acetylcholine and potassium

chloride) do not elicit pain when applied to exposed dentin. Similarly, application of topical anesthetic solutions to dentin does not decrease its sensitivity. A very high concentration of lidocaine solution is needed to block the response of intradental nerves to mechanical stimulation of the dentin.[3]

One investigator[41] studied the distribution and organization of nerve fibers in the pulp-dentin border zone of human teeth. On the basis of their location and pattern of branching, this colleague described several types of nerve endings (Fig. 11-33) and found simple fibers that run from the subodontoblastic nerve plexus toward the odontoblast layer. However, these fibers do not reach the predentin; they terminate in extracellular spaces in the cell-rich zone, the cell-poor zone, or the odontoblast layer. Other fibers extend into the predentin and run straight or spiral through a dentinal tubule in close association with an odontoblast process. Most of these intratubular fibers extend into the dentinal tubules for only a few mm, but a few may penetrate as far as 100 mm. The area covered by a single such terminal complex often reach thousands of square microns.

Intratubular nerve endings are most numerous in the area of the pulp horns, where as many as up to 40% of the tubules contain fibers.[72] The number of intratubular fibers decreases in other parts of the dentin, and in root dentin only about one tubule in a hundred contains a fiber. The anatomic relationships between the odontoblast processes and sensory nerve

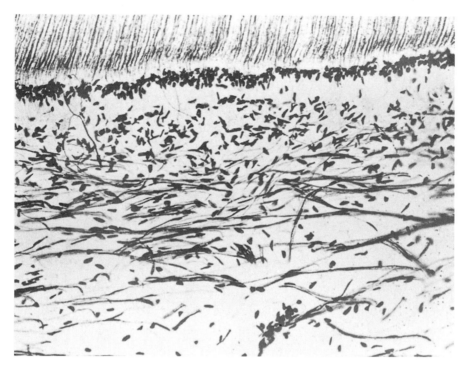

Fig. 11-30 Parietal layer of nerves (i.e., plexus of Raschkow) below the cell-rich zone. (From Avery JK: *J Endod* 7:205, 1981.)

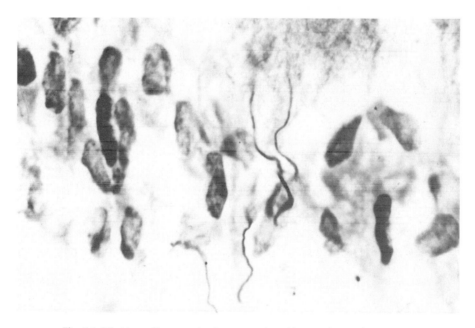

Fig. 11-31 Nerve fibers passing between odontoblasts to the predentin (PD).

endings have led to much speculation as to the functional relationships between these structures, if any. The nerve fibers lie in a groove or gutter along the surface of the odontoblast process, and toward their terminal ends they twist around the process like a corkscrew. The cell membranes of the odontoblast process and the nerve fiber are closely approximated and run closely parallel for the length of their proximity but are not synaptically linked.[52]

Although it may be tempting to speculate that the odontoblasts and their associated nerve axons are functionally interrelated and that together they play a role in dentin sensitivity, evidence for this is lacking. If the odontoblast were acting as

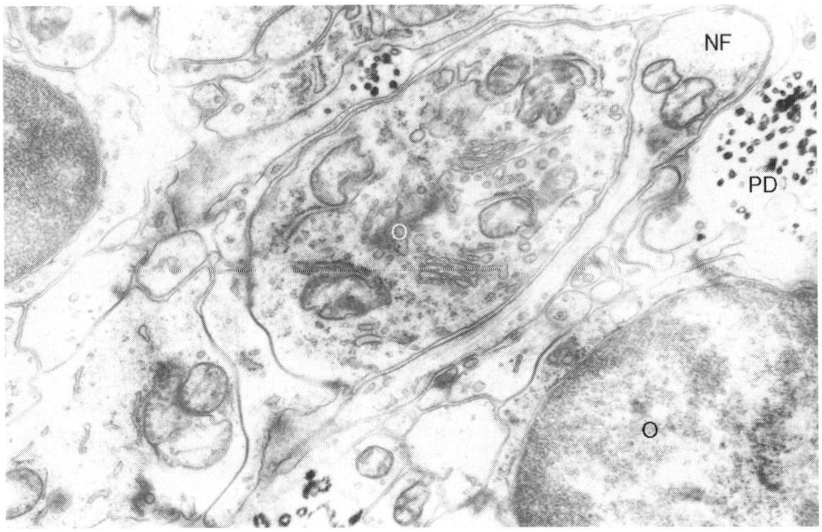

Fig. 11-32 Unmyelinated nerve fiber (*NF*) without a Schwann cell covering located between adjacent odontoblasts (*O*) overlying pulp horn of a mouse molar tooth. Predentin (*PD*) can be seen at upper right. Within the nerve there are longitudinally oriented fine neurofilaments, microvesicles, and mitochondria. (From Corpron RE, Avery JK: *Anat Rec* 175:585, 1973.)

a receptor cell*, it would synapse with the adjacent nerve fiber. However, researchers have been unable to find synaptic junctions that could functionally couple odontoblasts and nerve fibers together. With regard to the membrane properties of odontoblasts, it has been reported that the membrane potential of the odontoblast is low (around -30 mV) and that the cell does not respond to electrical stimulation.[68,138] Thus it would appear that the odontoblast does not possess the properties of an excitable cell. Furthermore, the sensitivity of dentin is not diminished after disruption of the odontoblast layer.[14,73]

Another study showed that a reduction in pulpal blood flow induced by stimulation of sympathetic fibers leading to the pulp results in depressed excitability of pulpal A fibers.[24] The excitability of C fibers is less affected than that of A fibers by a reduction in blood flow.[122]

Of considerable clinical interest is the evidence that nerve fibers of the pulp are relatively resistant to necrosis.[25,82] This is apparently because nerve bundles, in general, are more resistant to autolysis than other tissue elements. Even in degenerating pulps, C fibers might still be able to respond to stimulation. Furthermore, it may be that C fibers remain excitable even after blood flow has been compromised in the diseased pulp, for C fibers are often able to function in the presence of hypoxia.[122] This may offer an explanation as to why instrumentation of the root canals of apparently nonvital teeth sometimes elicits pain.

---

*A receptor cell is a nonnerve cell capable of exciting adjacent afferent nerve fibers. Synaptic junctions connect receptor cells to afferent nerves.

Pulp Testing

The electric pulp tester delivers a current sufficient to overcome the resistance of enamel and dentin and stimulate the sensory A fibers at the pulp-dentin border zone. C fibers of the pulp do not respond to the conventional pulp tester because significantly more current is needed to stimulate them.[86] Bender et al[6] found that in anterior teeth the optimal placement site of the electrode is the incisal edge of anterior teeth, as the response threshold is lowest at that location and increases as the electrode is moved toward the cervical region of the tooth.

Cold tests using carbon dioxide (CO_2) snow or liquid refrigerants and heat tests employing heated gutta-percha or hot water activate hydrodynamic forces within the dentinal tubules, which in turn excite the intradental A fibers. C fibers are not activated by these tests unless they produce injury to the pulp. It has been shown that cold tests do not injure the pulp.[36] Heat tests have a greater potential to produce injury; but if the tests are used properly, injury is not likely.

Sensitivity of Dentin

The mechanisms underlying dentin sensitivity have been the subject of keen interest in recent years. How are stimuli relayed from the peripheral dentin to the sensory receptors located in the region of the pulp-dentin border zone? Converging evidence indicates that *movement of fluid in the dentinal tubules is the basic event in the arousal of pain.*[124] It now appears that pain-producing stimuli, such as heat, cold, air blasts, and probing with the tip of an explorer, have in common the ability to displace fluid in the tubules.[11] This is referred to as the *hydrodynamic mechanism of dentin*

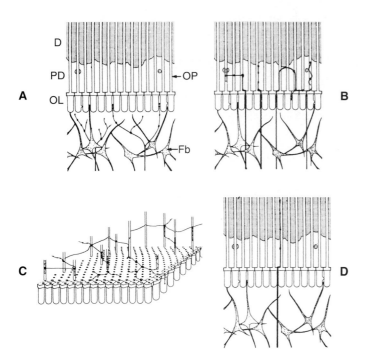

Fig. 11-33 Schematic drawing showing distribution of nerve fibers in the pulp-dentin border zone. **A,** Fibers running from the subodontoblastic plexus to the odontoblast layer (*D*: dentin, *Fb*: fibroblast, *OL*: odontoblast layer, *OP*: odontoblast process, *PD*: predentin). **B,** Fibers extending into the dentinal tubules in the predentin. **C,** Complex fibers that branch extensively in the predentin. **D,** Intratubular fibers extending into the dentin. (Courtesy T. Gunji, Niigata University, Japan.)

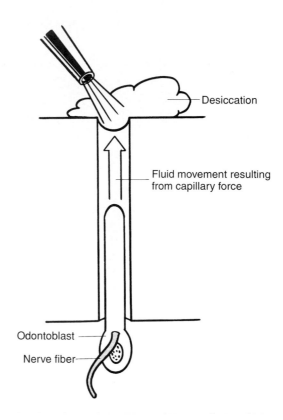

Fig. 11-34 Diagram illustrating movement of fluid in the dentinal tubules resulting from the dehydrating effect of a blast of air from an air syringe.

sensitivity. Thus fluid movement in the dentinal tubules is translated into electrical signals by sensory receptors located within the tubules or subjacent odontoblast layer. Researchers[79,132] were able to demonstrate a positive correlation between rate of fluid flow in the tubules and discharge evoked in intradental nerves. It was found that outward flow of fluid produced a much stronger nerve response than inward movement.

In experiments on humans, brief application of heat or cold to the outer surface of premolar teeth evoked a painful response before the heat or cold could have produced temperature changes capable of activating sensory receptors in the underlying pulp.[129] The evoked pain was of short duration: 1 or 2 seconds. The thermal diffusivity of dentin is relatively low; yet the response of the tooth to thermal stimulation is rapid, often less than a second. How best can this be explained? Evidence suggests that thermal stimulation of the tooth results in a rapid movement of fluid into the dentinal tubules. This results in activation of the sensory nerve terminal in the underlying pulp. Presumably heat expands the fluid within the tubules, causing it to flow toward the pulp, whereas cold causes the fluid to contract, producing an outward flow. The rapid movement of fluid across the cell membrane of the sensory receptor deforms the membrane and activates the receptor. All nerve cells have membrane channels through which charged ions pass, and this current flow,

if great enough, can stimulate the cell and cause it to transmit impulses to the brain. Some channels are activated by voltage, some by chemicals, and some by mechanical pressure. In the case of pulpal nerve fibers that are activated by hydrodynamic forces, pressure would increase the flow of sodium and potassium ions through pressure-activated channels, thus initiating generator potentials.

The dentinal tubule is a capillary tube having an exceedingly small diameter.* Therefore the effects of capillarity are significant, because the narrower the bore of a capillary tube, the greater the effect of capillarity. Thus if fluid is removed from the outer end of exposed dentinal tubules by dehydrating the dentinal surface with an air blast or absorbent paper, capillary forces produce a rapid outward movement of fluid in the tubule (Fig. 11-34). According to Brännström[12] desiccation of dentin can theoretically cause dentinal fluid to flow outward at a rate of 2 to 3 mm/sec. In addition to air blasts, dehydrating solutions containing hyperosmotic concentrations of sucrose or calcium chloride can produce pain if applied to exposed dentin.

---

*To appreciate fully the dimensions of dentin tubules, understand that the diameter of the tubules is much smaller than that of red blood cells.

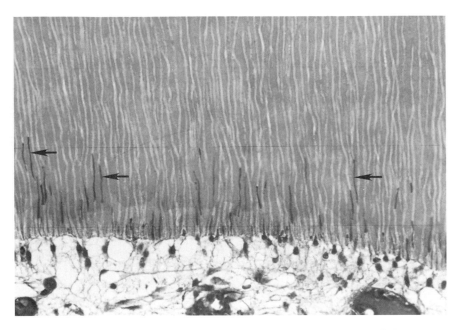

Fig. 11-35 Odontoblasts (*arrows*) displaced upward into the dentinal tubules.

Investigators have shown that it is the A fibers rather than the C fibers that are activated by stimuli (e.g., heat, cold, air blasts) applied to exposed dentin.[88] However, if heat is applied long enough to increase the temperature of the pulp-dentin border several degrees Celsius, the C fibers may respond, particularly if the heat produces injury. It seems that the A fibers are mainly activated by a rapid displacement of the tubular contents.[85] Slow heating of the tooth produced no response until the temperature reached 43.8° C, at which time C fibers were activated, presumably because of heat-induced injury to the pulp.

It has also been shown that pain-producing stimuli are more readily transmitted from the dentin surface when the exposed tubule apertures are wide and the fluid within the tubules is free to flow outward.[58] For example, other researchers found that acid treatment of exposed dentin to remove the smear layer opens the tubule orifices and makes the dentin much more responsive to stimuli, such as air blasts and probing.[50]

Perhaps the most difficult phenomenon to explain is pain associated with light probing of dentin. Even light pressure of an explorer tip can produce strong forces.* Presumably these forces mechanically compress the openings of the tubules and cause sufficient displacement of fluid to excite the sensory receptors in the underlying pulp. Considering the density of the tubules in which hydrodynamic forces would be generated by probing, thousands of nerve endings would be simultaneously stimulated, thus producing a cumulative effect.

Another example of the effect of strong hydraulic forces that are created within the dentinal tubules is the phenomenon of odontoblast displacement. In this reaction the cell bodies of odontoblasts are displaced upward in the dentinal tubules, presumably by a rapid movement of fluid in the tubules produced when exposed dentin is desiccated, as with the use of an air syringe or cavity-drying agents (Fig. 11-35). Such displacement results in the loss of odontoblasts, because cells thus affected soon undergo autolysis and disappear from the tubules. (Displaced odontoblasts may eventually be replaced by cells that migrate from the cell-rich zone of the pulp, as discussed later in the chapter.)

The hydrodynamic theory can also be applied to an understanding of the mechanism responsible for hypersensitive dentin. Hypersensitive dentin is associated with the exposure of dentin normally covered by cementum. The thin layer of cementum is frequently lost as gingival recession exposes cementum to the oral environment. Cementum is subsequently worn away by brushing, flossing, or the use of toothpicks. Once exposed, the dentin may respond to the same stimuli to which any exposed dentin surface responds (e.g., mechanical pressure, dehydrating agents). Although the dentin may at first be very sensitive, within a few weeks the sensitivity usually subsides. This desensitization is thought to occur as a result of gradual occlusion of the tubules by mineral deposits, thus reducing the hydrodynamic forces. Additionally, deposition of reparative dentin over the pulpal ends of the exposed tubules probably also reduces sensitivity.

Currently the treatment of hypersensitive teeth is directed toward reducing the functional diameter of the dentinal tubules to limit fluid movement. To accomplish this objective, there are four possible treatment modalities[126]:

---

*A force of 10 g (0.022 lb) applied to an explorer having a tip 0.002 inch in diameter would produce a pressure of 7000 psi on the dentin.

1. Formation of a smear layer on the sensitive dentin by burnishing the exposed root surface
2. Application of agents, such as oxalate compounds, that form insoluble precipitates within the tubules
3. Impregnation of the tubules with plastic resins
4. Application of dentin bonding agents to seal off the tubules

Dentin sensitivity can be modified by laser irradiation. However, clinicians must be concerned about its effect on the pulp.[112,118]

Neuropeptides

Of immense current interest is the presence of neuropeptides in sensory nerves. Pulpal nerve fibers contain neuropeptides, such as calcitonin gene-related peptide (CGRP), substance P (SP), neuropeptide Y, neurokinin A, and vasoactive intestinal polypeptide (VIP).[75,93,134] In rat molars the largest group of intradental sensory fibers contains CGRP. Some of these fibers also contain other peptides, such as SP and neurokinin A.[16] Release of these peptides can be triggered by such things as tissue injury, complement activation, antigen-antibody reactions, or antidromic stimulation of the inferior alveolar nerve. Once released, vasoactive peptides produce vascular changes that are similar to those evoked by histamine and bradykinin (i.e., vasodilation). In addition to their neurovascular properties, SP and CGRP contribute to hyperalgesia and promote wound healing.

It has been reported[79] that mechanical stimulation of dentin produces vasodilation within the pulp, presumably by causing the release of neuropeptides from intradental sensory fibers. Electrical stimulation of the tooth has a similar effect.[47]

Plasticity of Intradental Nerve Fibers

It has become apparent that the innervation of the tooth is a dynamic complex in which the number, size, and cytochemistry of nerve fibers can change because of aging, tooth injury,[17,35] and dental caries. For example, nerve fibers sprout into inflamed tissue surrounding sites of pulpal injury, and the content of CGRP and SP increases in these sprouting fibers.[19] When inflammation subsides there is a decrease in the number of sprouts. Fig. 11-36 compares the normal distribution of CGRP-immunoreactive sensory fibers in an adult rat molar with those beneath a shallow cavity preparation. Regulation of such change appears to be a function of nerve growth factor (NGF). NGF receptors are found on intradental sensory fibers and Schwann cells. Evidence indicates that NGF is synthesized by fibroblasts in the coronal subodontoblastic zone (i.e., cell-rich zone), particularly in the tip of the pulp horn.[20] Maximal sprouting of CGRP- and SP-containing nerves fibers corresponds to areas of the pulp where there is increased production of NGF. Fig. 11-37 (*top*) shows enormous nerve sprouting under a human dental caries lesion. Simultaneous increase in pulpal dendritic cells was also observed in the same region (Fig. 11-37 (*bottom*).

This coincrease of pulpal nerves and dendritic cells may imply neuroimmune interaction.[99]

Hyperalgesia

Three characteristics of hyperalgesia are (1) spontaneous pain, (2) a decreased pain threshold, or (3) an increased response to a painful stimulus. It is recognized that hyperalgesia can be produced by sustained inflammation, as in the case of sunburned skin. Clinically, it has been observed that the sensitivity of dentin is often increased when the underlying pulp becomes acutely inflamed, and the tooth may be more difficult to anesthetize. Although a precise explanation for hyperalgesia is lacking, apparently localized elevations in tissue pressure that accompany acute inflammation play an important role.[111] Clinically, we know that when a pulp chamber of a painful tooth with an abscessed pulp is opened, drainage of pus soon produces a reduction in the level of pain. This suggests that pressure may contribute to hyperalgesia.

In addition, certain mediators of inflammation (e.g., bradykinin, 5-hydroxytryptamine (5-HT), prostaglandin E_2) are capable of producing hyperalgesia. For example, 5-HT and CGRP are able to sensitize intradental fibers to hydrodynamic stimuli, such as cold, air blasts, and osmotic stimulation.[89] Unmyelinated fibers are activated by a number of inflammatory mediators. Bradykinin, for example, produces a dull, aching pain when placed in a deep cavity in a human tooth.

Leukotriene B_4 (LTB_4) was shown to have a long-lasting sensitizing effect on intradental nerves, suggesting that it may potentiate nociceptor activity during pulpal inflammation.[76] Both LTB_4 and complement component C5a stimulate neutrophils to secrete a pain-producing leukotriene, 8(R), 15(S)-diHETE.

It is known that there are many silent nerve fibers in the normal pulp. Usually they are not excited by ordinary external stimuli. However, once they are sensitized through pulpal inflammation, they begin to respond to hydrodynamic stimuli.[87] This phenomenon may be involved in dentin hypersensitivity.

Painful Pulpitis

From the foregoing it is apparent that pain associated with the stimulation of the A fibers does not necessarily signify that the pulp is inflamed or that tissue injury has occurred. A fibers have a relatively low threshold of excitability, and painful pulpitis is more likely to be associated with nociceptive C fiber activity. The clinician should carefully examine symptomatic teeth to rule out the possibility of hypersensitive dentin, cracked or leaky fillings, or tooth fracture, each of which may initiate hydrodynamic forces, before establishing a diagnosis of painful pulpitis.

Pain associated with an inflamed or degenerating pulp may be either provoked or spontaneous. The hyperalgesic pulp may respond to stimuli that usually do not evoke pain,

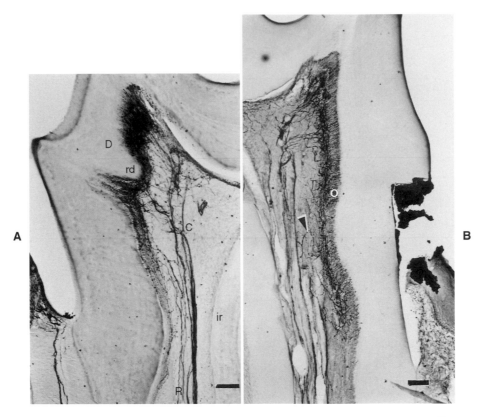

Fig. 11-36 **A,** Normal distribution of CGRP-immunoreactive sensory fibers in adult rat molar. Nerve fibers typically are unbranched in the root (*R*), they avoid interradicular dentin (*ir*), and form many branches in coronal pulp (*C*) and dentin (*D*). Nerve distribution is often asymmetric, with endings concentrated near the most columnar odontoblasts (in this case on the left side of the crown). When reparative dentin (*rd*) forms, it alters conditions so that dentinal innervation is reduced. **B,** Shallow class I cavity preparation on the cervical root of a rat molar was made 4 days earlier. Primary odontoblast (*O*) layer survived, and many new CGRP-n-immunoreactive terminal branches spread beneath and into the injured pulp and dentin. Terminal arbor can be seen branching (*arrowhead*) from a larger axon and growing into the injury site. Scale bar: 0.1 mm. **A,** × 75; **B,** × 45. (From Byers MR: Dynamic plasticity of dental sensory nerve structure and cytochemistry, *Arch Oral Biol* 39(suppl):13S, 1994.)

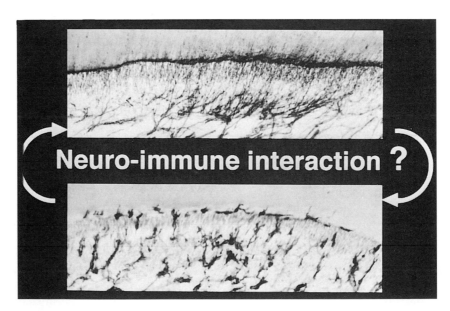

Fig. 11-37 Immunohistochemistry shows enormous nerve sprouting in the human pulp under a caries lesion (*top*) and simultaneous increase of pulpal dendritic cells (*bottom*) in the same region as *above*. This coincrease of pulpal nerves and dendritic cells may imply neuroimmune interaction. (Courtesy Dr. Kazuo Sakurai, Dental Hospital, Tokyo Medical and Dental University.)

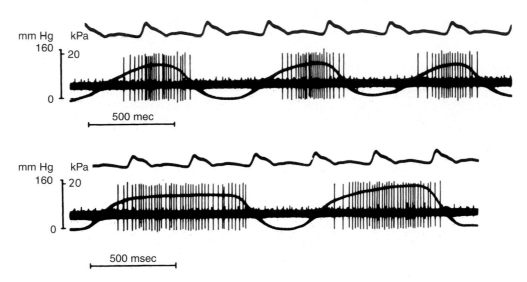

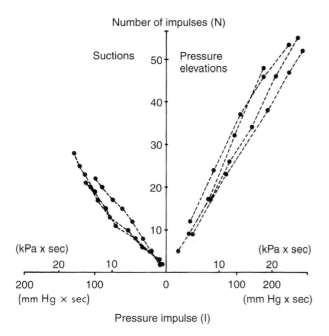

Fig. 11-38 Response of a single dog pulp nerve fiber to repeated hydrostatic pressure stimulation pulses. Lower solid wavy line of each recording indicates the stimulation pressure applied to the pulp. Upper line (kPa) is the femoral artery blood pressure curve recorded to indicate the relative changes in the pulse pressure and the heart cycle. (From Närhi M: Activation of dental pulp nerves of the cat and the dog with hydrostatic pressure, *Proc Finn Dent Soc* 74[suppl 5]:1, 1978.)

Fig. 11-39 Relationship between the number of nerve impulses (N) and the pressure impulse (I) of a small group of pulpal cat nerve fibers with three suction stimuli and four pressure elevations (pressure impulse is labeled as both mm Hg × sec and kPa × sec). (From Närhi M: Activation of dental pulp nerves of the cat and the dog with hydrostatic pressure, *Proc Finn Dent Soc* 74[suppl 5]:1, 1978.)

or the pain may be exaggerated and persist longer. On the other hand, the tooth may commence to ache spontaneously in the absence of any external stimulus. There is not a satisfactory explanation as to why a pulp that has been inflamed but asymptomatic for weeks or months suddenly begins to ache at 3 AM. Such unprovoked pain manifests itself as a dull, aching, poorly localized sensation qualitatively different from the brief, sharp, well-localized sensation associated with the hydrodynamic mechanism of dentin sensitivity.

Närhi[84] has done much to elucidate the role of hydrostatic pressure changes in the activation of pulpal nerve fibers. In his experiments involving cats and dogs, both positive and negative pressure changes were introduced into the pulp by means of a cannula inserted into the dentin. Using single-fiber recording techniques, he found a positive correlation between the degree of pressure change and the number of nerve impulses leaving the pulp. He theorized that the pressure changes produced local deformities in the pulp tissue, resulting in a stretching of the sensory nerve fibers (Figs. 11-38 and 11-39).

VASCULAR SUPPLY

Blood from the dental artery enters the tooth via arterioles having diameters of 100 mm or less. These vessels pass through the apical foramen or foramina with nerve bundles (see Fig. 11-28). Smaller vessels may enter the pulp via lateral or accessory canals. The arterioles course up through the central portion of the radicular pulp and give off branches that spread laterally toward the odontoblast layer, beneath which they ramify to form a capillary plexus (Fig. 11-40). As the

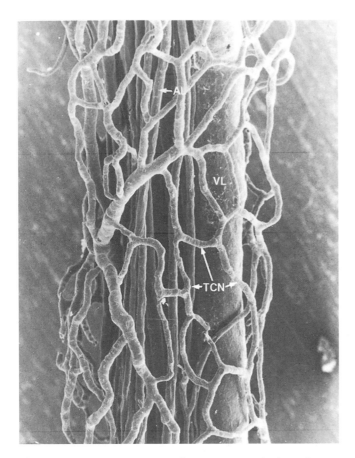

Fig. 11-40 High-power scanning electron micrograph of vascular network in the radicular pulp of a dog molar showing the configuration of the subodontoblastic terminal capillary network (*TCN*). Venules (*VL*) and arterioles (*AL*) are indicated. (Courtesy Dr. Y. Kishi, Kanagawa Dental College, Kanagawa, Japan.)

arterioles pass into the coronal pulp, they fan out toward the dentin, diminish in size, and give rise to a capillary network in the subodontoblastic region (Fig. 11-41). This network provides the odontoblasts with a rich source of metabolites.

Capillary blood flow in the coronal portion of the pulp is nearly twice that in the root portion.[64] Moreover, blood flow in the region of the pulp horns is greater than in other areas of the pulp.[80] In young teeth, capillaries commonly extend into the odontoblast layer, thus assuring an adequate supply of nutrients for the metabolically active odontoblasts (Fig. 11-42).

The subodontoblastic capillaries are surrounded by a basement membrane, and occasionally fenestrations (i.e., pores) are observed in capillary walls.[97] These fenestrations are thought to provide rapid transport of fluid and metabolites from the capillaries to the adjacent odontoblasts.

Blood passes from the capillary plexus, first into postcapillary venules (see Fig. 11-41) (Fig. 11-43) and then into larger venules. Venules in the pulp have unusually thin walls, which may facilitate the movement of fluid in or out of the vessel. The muscular coat of these venules is thin and dis-

continuous. The collecting venules become progressively larger as they course to the central region of the pulp. The largest venules have a diameter that may reach a maximum of 200 mm; thus they are considerably larger than the arterioles of the pulp. According to one study[67] the principal venous drainage in multirooted teeth sometimes flows down only one root canal or courses out through an accessory canal in the bifurcation or trifurcation area of the tooth.

Arteriovenous anastomoses (AVAs) may be present in both the coronal and radicular portions of the pulp, particularly in the latter.[113] Such vessels provide a direct communication between arterioles and venules, thus bypassing the capillary bed. The AVAs are relatively small venules, having a diameter of approximately 10 mm.[67] It is hypothesized that the AVAs play an important role in the regulation of the pulp circulation. Theoretically they could provide a mechanism for shunting blood away from areas of injury or inflammation, where damage to the microcirculation may result in thrombosis and hemorrhage.

It has been reported that the fraction of blood in the coronal pulp of cat canines is 14.4%.[133] The average capillary density was found to be 1404/mm², which is higher than in most other tissues of the body.

Among the oral tissues, the young and normal pulp has the highest volume of blood flow, but it is substantially lower than blood flow in the major visceral organs (Fig. 11-44). This reflects the fact that the respiratory rate of pulp cells is relatively low. As would be anticipated, pulpal blood flow is greater in the peripheral layer of the pulp (i.e., the subodontoblastic capillary plexus) than in the central area.[67]

Regulation of Pulpal Blood Flow

Several systems are involved in the regulation of pulpal blood flow, including sympathetic adrenergic vasoconstriction,[66] b-adrenergic vasodilation,[119] a sympathetic cholinergic vasoactive system,[1] and an antidromic vasodilation system involving sensory nerves, including axon reflex vasodilation.[103] It has been shown that a parasympathetic vasodilator mechanism is not present in cat dental pulp.[102] However, the presence of cholinergic nerve endings among odontoblasts in mouse and monkey pulps has been reported, along with the suggestion that these fibers may influence dentinogenesis.[4]

The walls of arterioles and venules are associated with smooth muscle that is innervated by unmyelinated sympathetic fibers. When stimulated, these fibers transmit impulses that cause the muscle fibers to contract, thus decreasing the diameter of the vessel (i.e., vasoconstriction). It has been shown experimentally that electrical stimulation of sympathetic fibers leading to the pulp results in a decrease in pulpal blood flow using laser Doppler technique.[24] Activation of a-adrenergic receptors by the administration of epinephrine-containing local anesthetic solutions may result in a marked decrease in pulpal blood flow.[63]

One investigation measured tissue and intravascular pressures in the pulps of cats.[121] The tissue pressure was esti-

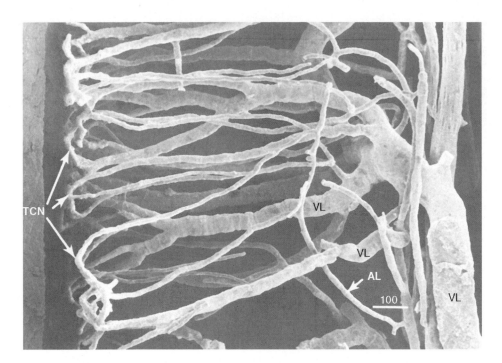

Fig. 11-41 Subodontoblastic terminal capillary network (TCN), arterioles (*AL*), and venules (*VL*) of young canine pulp. Dentin would be to the far left and the central pulp to the right. Scale bar: 100 ×m. (From Takahashi K, Kishi Y, Kim S: A scanning electron microscope study of the blood vessels of dog pulp using corrosion resin casts, *J Endod* 8:131, 1982.)

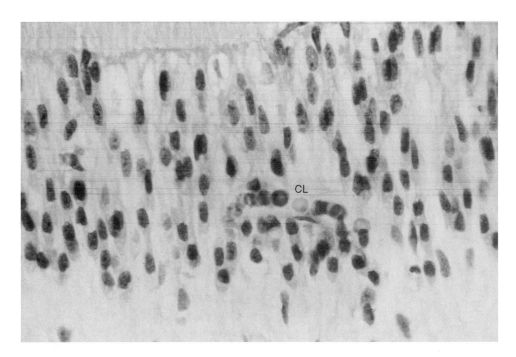

Fig. 11-42 Capillary loop (*CL*) extending into the odontoblast layer of a young pulp.

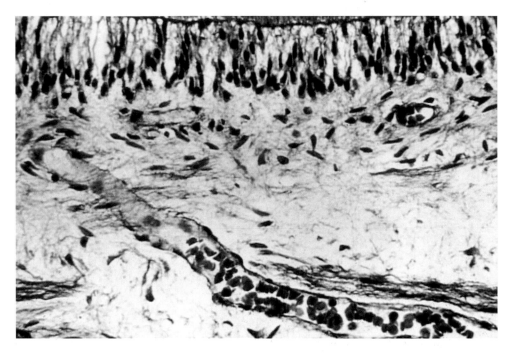

Fig. 11-43 Postcapillary venule draining blood from subodontoblastic capillary plexus.

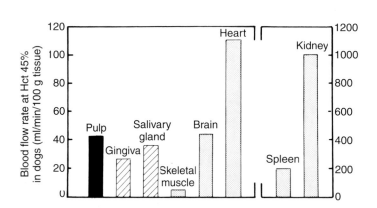

Fig. 11-44 Blood flow per 100 g tissue weight for various organs and tissues at 45% hematocrit (Hct) in dogs. (From Kim S: *J Endod* 11:465, 1985.)

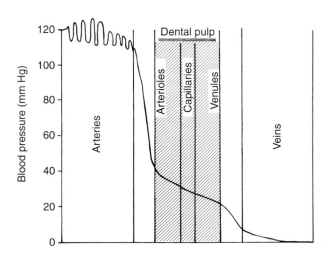

Fig. 11-45 Blood pressure fall along extrapulpal and intrapulpal blood vessels. (Modified from Heyeraas KJ: *J Dent Res* 64[special issue]:585, 1985.)

mated to be approximately 6 mm Hg. Pressure in the arterioles, capillaries, and venules was 43, 35, and 19 mm Hg, respectively (Fig. 11-45).

Blood circulation in an inflamed pulp involves very complex pathophysiologic reactions that have not been fully elucidated, in spite of numerous studies.[48,64] A unique feature of the pulp is that it is rigidly encased within dentin. This places it in a low-compliance environment, much like the brain, bone marrow, and nail bed. Thus pulp tissue has limited ability to expand, so vasodilation and increased vascular per-

meability evoked during an inflammatory reaction result in an increase in pulpal hydrostatic pressure.[131] Presumably any sudden rise in intrapulpal pressure would be distributed equally within the area of pressure increase, including the blood vessels. Theoretically if tissue pressure increases to the point that it equals the intravascular pressure, the thin-walled venules would be compressed, thereby increasing vascular resistance and reducing pulpal blood flow.[63] This could explain why injection of vasodilators (i.e., bradykinin) into an artery leading to the pulp results in a reduction rather than

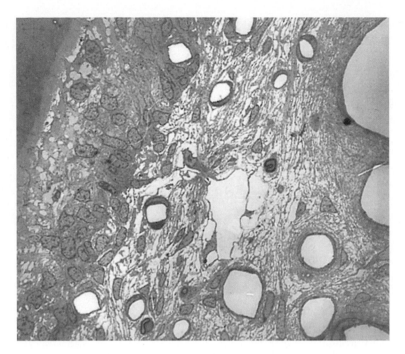

Fig. 11-46 Electron micrograph showing lymphatic vessel (*arrows*) in a cat dental pulp. (From Bishop MA, Malhotra MP: An investigation of lymphatic vessels in the feline dental pulp, *Am J Anat* 187:247, 1990.)

an increase in pulpal blood flow.[119,120] However, Heyeraas[47] observed that an increase in intrapulpal tissue pressure promoted absorption of tissue fluid back into the blood and lymphatic vessels, thereby reducing the pressure. Thus it would appear that blood flow can increase, in spite of an elevation in tissue pressure. Obviously a combined multidisciplinary approach is needed to better understand the intricate circulatory changes occurring during the development of pulpal inflammation.

Lymphatics

The existence of lymphatics in the pulp has been a matter of debate, because it is not easy to distinguish between venules and lymphatics by ordinary light microscopic techniques. However, studies using light and electron microscopy have described lymphatic capillaries in human and in cat dental pulps[9,78] (Fig. 11-46).

REPAIR

The inherent healing potential of the dental pulp is well recognized. As in all other connective tissues, repair of tissue injury commences with débridement by macrophages, followed by proliferation of fibroblasts, capillary buds, and the formation of collagen. Local circulation is of critical importance in wound healing and repair. An adequate supply of blood is essential to transport inflammatory elements into the area of pulpal injury and to provide the young fibroblasts

with nutrients from which to synthesize collagen. Unlike most tissues the pulp has essentially no collateral circulation; for this reason it is theoretically more vulnerable than most other tissues. Thus in the case of severe injury, healing would be impaired in teeth with a limited blood supply. It seems reasonable to assume that the highly cellular pulp of a young tooth, with a wide open apical foramen and rich blood supply, has a much better healing potential than does an older tooth with a narrow foramen and a restricted blood supply. Dentin that is produced in response to the death of primary odontoblasts has been known by several different names:

- Irregular secondary dentin
- Irritation dentin
- Tertiary dentin
- Reparative dentin

The term most commonly applied to irregularly formed dentin is reparative dentin, presumably because it so frequently forms in response to injury and appears to be a component of the reparative process. It must be recognized, however, that this type of dentin has also been observed in the pulps of normal, unerupted teeth without any obvious injury.[91]

It will be recalled that secondary dentin is deposited circumpulpally at a very slow rate throughout the life of the vital tooth. In contrast, the formation of reparative dentin occurs at the pulpal surface of primary or secondary dentin at sites corresponding to areas of irritation. For example, when a carious lesion has invaded dentin, the pulp usually responds by depositing a layer of reparative dentin over the dentinal tubules of the primary or secondary dentin that communicate with the carious lesion (Fig. 11-47). Similarly when occlusal wear removes the overlying enamel and exposes the dentin to the oral environment, reparative dentin is deposited on the pulpal surface of the exposed dentin. Thus the formation of reparative dentin allows the pulp to retreat behind a barrier of mineralized tissue.

Compared with primary dentin, reparative dentin is less tubular and the tubules tend to be more irregular with larger lumina. In some cases no tubules are formed. The cells that form reparative dentin are not as columnar as the primary odontoblasts of the coronal pulp and are often cuboidal (Fig. 11-48). The quality of reparative dentin (i.e., the extent to which it resembles primary dentin) is quite variable. If irritation to the pulp is relatively mild, as in the case of a superficial carious lesion, the reparative dentin formed may resemble primary dentin in terms of tubularity and degree of mineralization. On the other hand, reparative dentin deposited in response to a deep carious lesion may be relatively atubular and poorly mineralized with many areas of interglobular dentin. The degree of irregularity of reparative dentin is probably determined by factors, such as the amount of inflammation present, the extent of cellular injury, and the state of differentiation of the replacement odontoblasts.

The poorest quality of reparative dentin is usually observed in association with marked pulpal inflammation. In fact, the dentin may be so poorly organized that areas of soft tissue are entrapped within the dentinal matrix. In histologic sections these areas of soft tissue entrapment impart a Swiss cheese appearance to the dentin (Fig. 11-49). As the entrapped soft tissue degenerates, products of tissue degeneration further contribute to the inflammatory stimuli assailing the pulp.

It has been reported[22] that trauma caused by cavity preparation that is too mild to result in the loss of primary odontoblasts does not lead to reparative dentin formation, even if the cavity preparation is relatively deep. This evidence would suggest that reparative dentin is formed by new odontoblast-like cells. For many years it has been recognized that destruction of primary odontoblasts is soon followed by increased mitotic activity within fibroblasts of the subjacent cell-rich zone. It has been shown that the progeny of these dividing cells differentiate into functioning odontoblasts.[33] Other investigators[140] have studied dentin bridge formation in the teeth of dogs and found that pulpal fibroblasts appeared to undergo dedifferentiation and revert to undifferentiated mesenchymal cells (Fig. 11-50). These cells divided, and the new cells then redifferentiated in a new direction to become odontoblasts. Recalling the migratory potential of ectomesenchymal cells from which the pulpal fibroblasts are derived, it is not difficult to envision the differentiating odontoblasts moving from the subodontoblastic zone to the area of injury to constitute a new odontoblast layer.

The similarity of primary odontoblasts to replacement odontoblasts was established by D'Souza et al.[23] These researchers were able to show that cells forming reparative

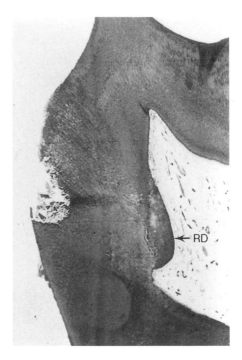

Fig. 11-47 Reparative dentin (*RD*) deposited in response to a carious lesion in the dentin. (From Trowbridge HO: Pathogenesis of pulpitis resulting from dental caries, *J Endod* 7:52, 1981.)

dentin synthesize type I (but not type III) collagen, and they are immunopositive for dentin sialoprotein.

Baume[5] has suggested that the formation of atubular "fibrodentin" results in the secondary induction of odontoblast differentiation, provided a capillary plexus develops beneath the fibrodentin. This is consistent with the observation made by other researchers[133] that the newly formed dentin bridge is composed first of a thin layer of atubular dentin on which a relatively thick layer of tubular dentin is deposited. The fibrodentin* was lined by cells resembling mesenchymal cells, whereas the tubular dentin was associated with cells closely resembling odontoblasts.

Still other researchers[108] studied reparative dentin formed in response to relatively traumatic experimental class V cavity preparations in human teeth. They found that seldom was reparative dentin formed until about the 30th postoperative day, although in one case dentin formation was observed on day 19. The rate of formation was 3.5 mm/day for the first 3 weeks after the onset of dentin formation; then it decreased markedly. By postoperative day 132, dentin formation had nearly ceased. Assuming that most of the odontoblasts were destroyed during cavity preparation, as was likely in this experiment, it is probably that the lag phase between cavity preparation and the onset of reparative dentin formation represented the time required for the proliferation and differentiation of new replacement odontoblasts.

---

*Actually, the term *osteodentin* was used rather than *fibrodentin*.

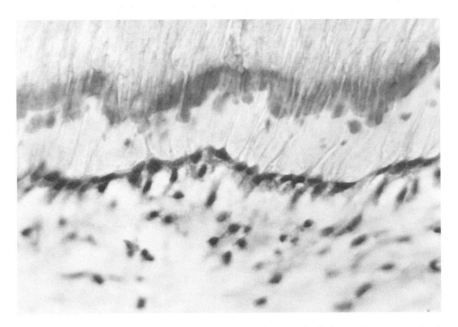

Fig. 11-48 Layer of cells forming reparative dentin. Note the decreased tubularity of reparative dentin as compared with the developmental dentin above it.

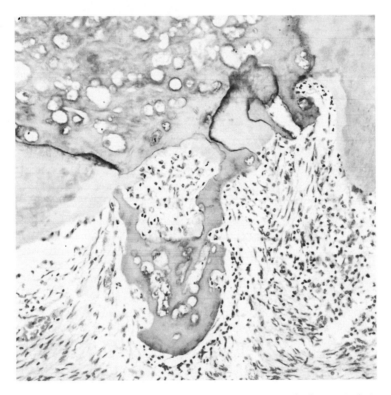

Fig. 11-49 Swiss cheese type of reparative dentin. Note the numerous areas of soft tissue inclusion and infiltration of inflammatory cells in the pulp.

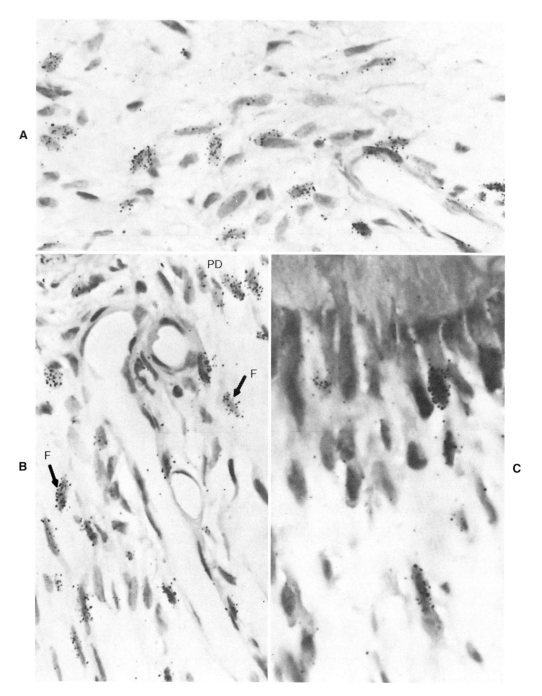

Fig. 11-50 Autoradiographs from dog molars illustrating uptake of ³H-thymidine by pulp cells preparing to undergo cell division after pulpotomy and pulp capping with calcium hydroxide. **A,** Two days after pulp capping. Fibroblasts, endothelial cells, and pericytes beneath the exposure site are labeled. **B,** By the fourth day fibroblasts (*F*) and pre-odontoblasts adjacent to the predentin (*PD*) are labeled, which suggests that differentiation of preodontoblasts occurred within 2 days. **C,** Six days after pulp capping, new odontoblasts are labeled and tubular dentin is being formed. (Tritiated thymidine was injected 2 days after the pulp capping procedures in **B** and **C**.) (From Yamamura T et al: *Bull Tokyo Dent Coll* 21:181, 1980.)

Does reparative dentin protect the pulp, or is it simply a form of scar tissue? To serve a protective function, it would have to provide a relatively impermeable barrier that would exclude irritants from the pulp and compensate for the loss of developmental dentin. The junction between developmental and reparative dentin has been studied. Using a dye diffusion technique, Fish[28] noted the presence of an atubular zone situated between primary dentin and reparative dentin (Fig. 11-51). Scott and Weber[104] found, in addition to a dramatic reduction in the number of tubules, that the walls of the tubules along the junction were thickened and often occluded with material similar to peritubular matrix. These

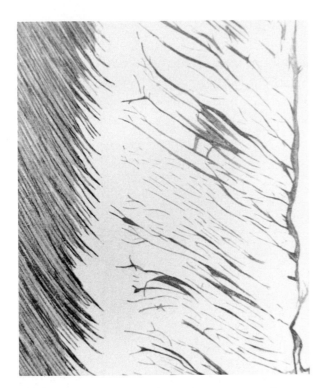

Fig. 11-51 Diffusion of dye from the pulp into reparative dentin. Note atubular zone between reparative dentin (*RD*) and primary dentin on the left. (From Fish EW: *Experimental investigation of the enamel, dentin, and dental pulp*, London, 1932, John Bale Sons & Danielson, Ltd.)

observations would indicate that the junctional zone between developmental and reparative dentin is an atubular zone of low permeability. Researchers reported that the accumulation of pulpal dendritic cells was reduced after reparative dentin formation, which may indicate the reduction of incoming bacterial antigens.

One group[117] studied the effect of gold foil placement on human pulp and found that this was better tolerated in teeth in which reparative dentin had previously been deposited beneath the cavity than in teeth that were lacking such a deposit. It would thus appear that reparative dentin can protect the pulp, but it must be emphasized that this is not always the case. It is well-known that reparative dentin can be deposited in a pulp that is irreversibly injured and that its presence does not necessarily signify a favorable prognosis (see Fig. 11-49). The quality of the dentin formed, and hence its ability to protect the pulp, to a large extent reflects the environment of the cells producing the matrix.

Periodontally diseased teeth have smaller root canal diameters than teeth that are periodontally healthy.[70] The root canals of such teeth are narrowed by the deposition of large quantities of reparative dentin along the dentinal walls.[105] The decrease in root canal diameter with increasing age, in the absence of periodontal disease, is more likely to be the result of secondary dentin formation.

In one study,[46] it was shown in a rat model that scaling and root-planing frequently result in reparative dentin formation along the pulpal wall subjacent to the instrumented root surface.

Fibrosis

Not uncommonly the cellular elements of the pulp are largely replaced by fibrous connective tissue. It appears that in some cases the pulp responds to noxious stimuli by accumulating large fiber bundles of collagen, rather than by elaborating reparative dentin (Fig. 11-52). However, fibrosis and reparative dentin formation often go hand in hand, indicating that both are expressions of a reparative potential.

PULPAL CALCIFICATIONS

Calcification of pulp tissue is a very common occurrence. Although estimates of the incidence of this phenomenon vary widely, it is safe to say that one or more pulp calcifications are present in at least 50% of all teeth. In the coronal pulp, calcification usually takes the form of discreet, concentric pulp stones (Fig. 11-53); whereas in the radicular pulp, calcification tends to be diffuse (Fig. 11-54). Some authors believe that pulp calcification is a pathologic process related to various forms of injury, whereas others regard it as a natural phenomenon. (Perhaps the greatest endodontic significance of pulp calcification is that it may hinder root canal shaping.)

Pulp stones range in size from small, microscopic particles to accretions that occupy almost the entire pulp chamber (Fig. 11-55). The mineral phase of pulp calcifications has been shown to consist of carbonated hydroxyapatite.[128] Histologically, two types of stones are recognized: (1) those that are round or ovoid, with smooth surfaces and concentric laminations (see Fig. 11-53), and (2) those that assume no particular shape, lack laminations, and have rough surfaces (Fig. 11-56). Laminated stones appear to grow by the addition of collagen fibrils to their surface, whereas unlaminated stones develop via the mineralization of preformed collagen fiber bundles. In the latter type the mineralization front seems to extend out along the coarse fibers, making the surface of the stones appear fuzzy (Fig. 11-57). Often these coarse fiber bundles appear to have undergone hyalinization, thus resembling old scar tissue.

Pulp stones may also be formed around epithelial cells (i.e., remnants of Hertwig's epithelial root sheath). Presumably the epithelial remnants induce adjacent mesenchymal cells to differentiate into odontoblasts. Characteristically these pulp stones are found near the root apex and contain dentinal tubules.

Quite frequently, small mineralizations are observed in association with the walls of arterioles, even in normal pulps of young teeth (see Fig. 11-28). Such deposits usually project outward from the vessel wall and do not encroach on the lumen.

The cause of pulpal calcification is largely unknown. Calcification may occur around a nidus of degenerating cells, blood thrombi, or collagen fibers. Many authors believe this

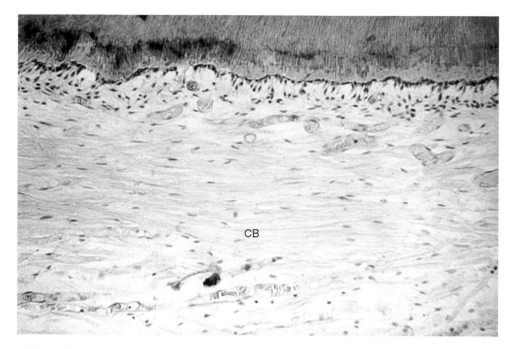

Fig. 11-52 Fibrosis of dental pulp showing replacement of pulp tissue by large collagen bundles (*CB*).

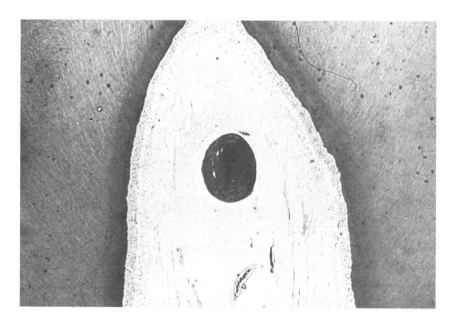

Fig. 11-53 Pulp stone with a smooth surface and concentric laminations in the pulp of a newly erupted premolar extracted in the course of orthodontic treatment.

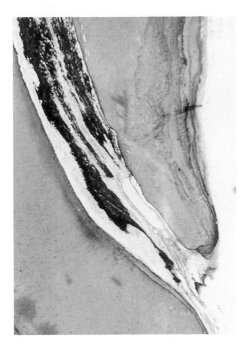

Fig. 11-54 Diffuse calcification near the apical foramen.

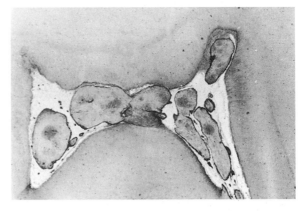

Fig. 11-55 Pulp stones occupying much of the pulp chamber.

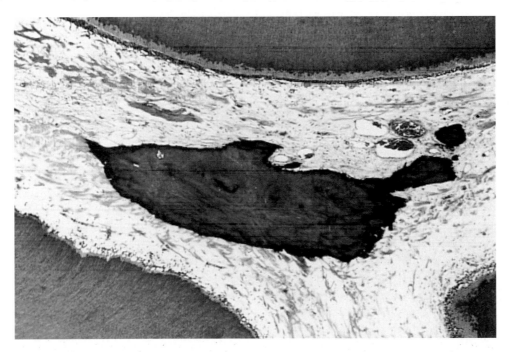

Fig. 11-56 Rough surface form of pulp stone. Note hyalinization of collagen fibers.

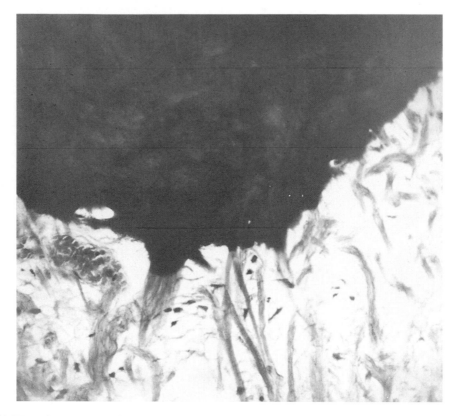

Fig. 11-57 High-power view of a pulp stone from Fig. 11-50 showing the relationship of mineralization fronts to collagen fibers.

represents a form of dystrophic calcification. In this type, calcium is deposited in tissues, which degenerate. Calcium phosphate crystals may be deposited within the cell. Initially this takes place within the mitochondria, because of the increased membrane permeability to calcium resulting from a failure to maintain active transport systems within the cell membranes. Thus degenerating cells serving as a nidus may initiate calcification of a tissue. In the absence of obvious tissue degeneration, the cause of pulpal calcification is enigmatic. It is often difficult to assign the term *dystrophic calcification* to pulp stones, because they so often occur in apparently healthy pulps, suggesting that functional stress need not be present for calcification to occur. Calcification in the mature pulp is often assumed to be related to the aging process. However, in a study involving 52 impacted canines from patients between 11 and 76 years of age, Nitzan et al[91] found that concentric denticles demonstrated a constant incidence for all age groups, indicating no relation to aging. Diffuse calcifications, on the other hand, increased in incidence to age 25 years; thereafter they remained constant in successive age groups.

At times, numerous concentric pulp stones with no apparent cause are seen in all the teeth of a young individual. In such cases the appearance of pulp stones may be ascribed to individual biologic characteristics (e.g., torus, cutaneous nevi).[91]

Although soft tissue collagen does not usually calcify, it is not at all uncommon to find calcification occurring in old hyalinized scar tissue in the skin. This may be due to the increase in the extent of cross-linking between collagen molecules (because increased cross-linkage is thought to enhance the tendency for collagen fibers to calcify). Thus there may be a relationship between pathologic alterations in collagen molecules within the pulp and pulpal calcification.

Calcification replaces the cellular components of the pulp and may possibly hinder the blood supply, although concrete evidence for this is lacking. Idiopathic pulpal pain has frequently been attributed to the presence of pulp stones; but because calcification so often occurs in pathologically involved pulps, it is difficult to establish a cause-and-effect relationship, particularly because pulp stones are so frequently observed in teeth lacking a history of pain.

Calcific Metamorphosis

Luxation of teeth as a result of trauma may result in calcific metamorphosis, a condition that can, in a matter of months or years, lead to partial or complete radiographic obliteration of the pulp chamber. The cause of radiographic obliteration is excessive deposition of mineralized tissue resembling cementum or, occasionally, bone on the dentin walls (Fig. 11-58). Histologic examination invariably reveals the pres-

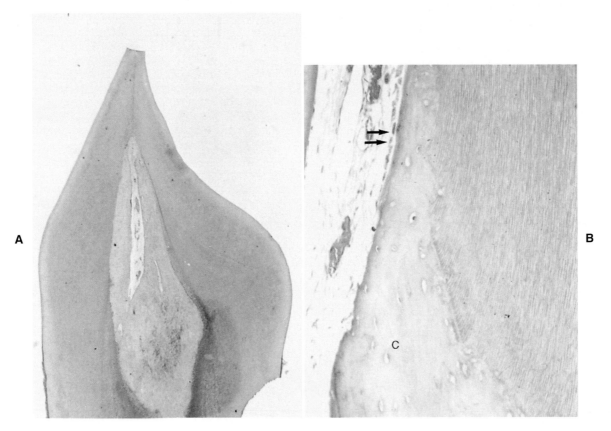

Fig. 11-58 **A,** Calcific metamorphosis of pulp tissue after luxation of tooth as a result of trauma. Note presence of soft tissue inclusion. **B,** High-power view showing cementoblasts (*arrows*) lining cementum (C), which has been deposited on the dentin walls.

ence of some soft tissue, and cells resembling cementoblasts can be observed lining the mineralized tissue. Such calcific metamorphosis of the pulp has also been reported in replanted teeth of the rat.[90]

Clinically, the crowns of teeth affected by calcific metamorphosis may show a yellowish hue compared with adjacent normal teeth. This condition usually occurs in teeth with incomplete root formation. Trauma results in disruption of blood vessels entering the tooth, thus producing pulpal infarction. The wide periapical foramen allows connective tissue from the periodontal ligament to proliferate and replace the infarcted tissue, bringing with it cementoprogenitor and osteoprogenitor cells capable of differentiating into either cementoblasts or osteoblasts or both.

AGE CHANGES

Continued formation of secondary dentin throughout life gradually reduces the size of the pulp chamber and root canals, although the width of the cementodentinal junction appears to stay relatively the same.[37,110] In addition, certain regressive changes in the pulp appear to be related to the aging process. There is a gradual decrease in the cellularity

and a concomitant increase in the number and thickness of collagen fibers, particularly in the radicular pulp. The thick collagen fibers may serve as foci for pulpal calcification (see Fig. 11-57). The odontoblasts decrease in size and number, and they may disappear altogether in certain areas of the pulp, particularly on the pulpal floor over the bifurcation or trifurcation areas of multirooted teeth.

With age there is a progressive reduction in the number of nerves and blood vessels.[7] There is also evidence that aging results in an increase in the resistance of pulp tissue to the action of proteolytic enzymes,[141] hyaluronidase, and sialidase,[8] suggesting an alteration of both collagen and proteoglycans in the pulps of older teeth.

The main changes in dentin associated with aging are an increase in peritubular dentin, dentinal sclerosis, and the number of dead tracts.[*] Dentinal sclerosis produces a gradual decrease in dentinal permeability as the dentinal tubules become progressively reduced in diameter.

---

[*]The term *dead tract* refers to a group of dentinal tubules in which odontoblast processes are absent. Dead tracts are easily recognized in ground sections, because the empty tubules refract transmitted light and the tract appears black in contrast to the light color of normal dentin.

References

1. Aars H, Brodin P, Anderson E: A study of cholinergic and b-adrenergic components in the regulation of blood flow in the tooth pulp and gingiva of man, *Acta Physiol Scand* 148:441, 1993.
2. Ahlberg K, Brännström M, Edwall L: The diameter and number of dentinal tubules in rat, cat, dog and monkey: a comparative scanning electronic microscopic study, *Acta Odontol Scand* 33:243, 1975.
3. Amess TR, Matthews B: *The effect of topical application of lidocaine to dentin in the cat on the response of intradental nerves to mechanical stimuli: proceedings of the International Conference on Dentin/Pulp Complex,* Tokyo, 1996, Quintessence pp 272-273.
4. Avery JK, Cox CF, Chiego DJ Jr: Presence and location of adrenergic nerve endings in the dental pulps of mouse molars, *Anat Rec* 198:59, 1980.
5. Baume LJ: The biology of pulp and dentine. In Myers HM, editor: *Monographs in oral science,* vol 8, Basel, 1980, S Karger AG.
6. Bender IB et al: The optimum placement-site of the electrode in electric pulp testing of the 12 anterior teeth, *J Am Dent Assoc* 118:305, 1989.
7. Bernick S, Nedelman C: Effect of aging on the human pulp, *J Endod* 1:88, 1975.
8. Bhussary BR: Modification of the dental pulp organ during development and aging. In Finn SB, editor: *Biology of the dental pulp organ: a symposium,* Birmingham, 1968, University of Alabama Press.
9. Bishop MA, Malhotra MP: A investigation of lymphatic vessels in the feline dental pulp, *Am J Anat* 187:247, 1990.
10. Bishop MA, Malhotra M, Yoshida S: Interodontoblastic collagen (von Korff fibers) and circumpulpal dentin formation: an ultrathin serial section study in the cat, *Am J Anat* 191:67, 1991.
11. Brännström M: Communication between the oral cavity and the dental pulp associated with restorative treatment, *Oper Dent* 9:57, 1984.
12. Brännström M: *Dentin and pulp in restorative dentistry,* Nacka, Sweden, 1981, Dental Therapeutics AB.
13. Brännström M: The transmission and control of dentinal pain. In Grossman LJ, editor: *Mechanisms and control of pain,* New York, 1979, Masson Publishing USA.
14. Brännström M, Astrom A: A study of the mechanism of pain elicited from the dentin, *J Dent Res* 43:619, 1964.
15. Butler WT et al: Recent investigations on dentin specific proteins, *Proc Finn Dent Soc* 88(suppl 1):369, 1992.
16. Byers MR: Dynamic plasticity of dental sensory nerve structure and cytochemistry, *Arch Oral Biol* 39(suppl):13S, 1994.
17. Byers MR, Schatteman GC, Bothwell MA: Multiple functions for NGF-receptor in developing, aging and injured rat teeth are suggested by epithelial, mesenchymal and neural immunoreactivity, *Development* 109:461, 1990.
18. Byers MR, Sugaya A: Odontoblast process in dentin revealed by fluorescent Di-I, *J Histochem Cytochem* 43:159, 1995.
19. Byers MR, Taylor PE: Effect of sensory denervation on the response of rat molar pulp to exposure injury, *J Dent Res* 72: 613, 1993.
20. Byers MR, Wheeler EF, Bothwell M: Altered expression of NGF and p75 NGF-receptor mRNA by fibroblasts of injured teeth precedes sensory nerve sprouting, *Growth Factors* 6:41, 1992.
21. Cuicchi B et al: Dentinal fluid dynamics in human teeth, in vivo, *J Endod* 21:191, 1995.
22. Diamond RD, Stanley HR, Swerdlow H: Reparative dentin formation resulting from cavity preparation, *J Prosthet Dent* 16:1127, 1966.
23. D'Souza RN et al: Characterization of cellular responses involved in reparative dentinogenesis in rat molars, *J Dent Res* 74:702, 1995.
24. Edwall L, Kindlová M: The effect of sympathetic nerve stimulation on the rate of disappearance of tracers from various oral tissues, *Acta Odontol Scand* 29:387, 1971.
25. England MC, Pellis EG, Michanowicz AE: Histopathologic study of the effect of pulpal disease upon nerve fibers of the human dental pulp, *Oral Surg* 38:783, 1974.
26. Engström C, Linde A, Persliden B: Acid hydrolases in the odontoblast-predentin region of dentinogenically active teeth, *Scand J Dent Res* 84:76, 1976.
27. Fearnhead RW: Innervation of dental tissues. In Miles AEW, editor: *Structure and chemical organization of teeth, vol 1,* New York, 1967, Academic Press.
28. Fish EW: *Experimental investigation of the enamel, dentin, and dental pulp,* London, 1932, John Bale Sons & Danielson, Ltd.
29. Fisher AK: Respiratory variations within the normal dental pulp, *J Dent Res* 46:24, 1967.
30. Fisher AK, Walters VE: Anaerobic glycolysis in bovine dental pulp, *J Dent Res* 47:717, 1968.
31. Fisher AK et al: Effects of dental drugs and materials on the rate of oxygen consumption in bovine dental pulp, *J Dent Res* 36:447, 1957.
32. Fisher AK et al: The influence of the stage of tooth development on the oxygen quotient of normal bovine dental pulp, *J Dent Res* 38:208, 1959.
33. Fitzgerald M, Chiego DJ, Heys DR: Autoradiographic analysis of odontoblast replacement following pulp exposure in primate teeth, *Arch Oral Biol* 35:707, 1990.
34. Fogel HM, Marshall FJ, Pashley DH: Effects of distance of the pulp and thickness on the hydraulic conductance of human radicular dentin, *J Dent Res* 67:1381, 1988.
35. Fried K: Changes in pulp nerves with aging, *Proc Finn Dental Soc* 88(suppl 1):517, 1992.
36. Fuss Z et al: Assessment of reliability of electrical and thermal pulp testing agents, *J Endod* 12:301, 1986.
37. Gani O, Visvisian C: Apical canal diameter in the first upper molar at various ages, *J Endod* 10:689, 1999.
38. Garberoglio R, Brännström M: Scanning electron microscopic investigation of human dentinal tubules, *Arch Oral Biol* 21:355, 1976.
39. Gotjamanos T: Cellular organization in the subodontoblastic zone of the dental pulp II. Period and mode of development of the cell-rich layer in rat molar pulps, *Arch Oral Biol* 14:1011, 1969.
40. Grossman ES, Austin JC: Scanning electron microscope observations on the tubule content of freeze-fractured peripheral vervet monkey dentine (Cercopithecus pygerythrus), *Arch Oral Biol* 28:279, 1983.
41. Gunji T: Morphological research on the sensitivity of dentin, *Arch Histol Jpn* 45:45, 1982.

42. Hahn C-L, Falkler WA Jr, Siegel MA: A study of T cells and B cells in pulpal pathosis, *J Endod* 15:20, 1989.

43. Hamersky PA, Weimer AD, Taintor JF: The effect of orthodontic force application on the pulpal tissue respiration rate in the human premolar, *Am J Orthod* 77:368, 1980.

44. Han SS: The fine structure of cells and intercellular substances of the dental pulp. In Finn SB, editor: *Biology of the dental pulp organ*, Birmingham, 1968, University of Alabama Press.

45. Harris R, Griffin CJ: Fine structure of nerve endings in the human dental pulp, *Arch Oral Biol* 13:773, 1968.

46. Hattler AB, Listgarten MA: Pulpal response to root planing in a rat model, *J Endod* 10:471, 1984.

47. Heyeraas KJ, Jacobsen EB, Fristad I: *Vascular and immunoreactive nerve fiber reactions in the pulp after stimulation and denervation: proceedings of the International Conference on Dentin/Pulp Complex*, Tokyo, 1996, Quintessence, pp 162-168.

48. Heyerass KJ, Kvinnsland I: Tissue pressure and blood flow in pulpal inflammation, *Proc Finn Dent Soc* 88(suppl 1):393, 1992.

49. Hikiji A et al: Increased blood flow and nerve firing in the cat canine tooth in response to stimulation of the second premolar pulp, *Arch Oral Biol* 45:53, 2000.

50. Hirvonen T, Närhi M: The excitability of dog pulp nerves in relation to the condition of dentine surface, *J Endod* 10:294, 1984.

51. Holland GR: The extent of the odontoblast process in the cat, *Am J Anat* 121:133, 1976.

52. Holland GR: Morphological features of dentine and pulp related to dentine sensitivity, *Arch Oral Biol* 39(suppl):3S, 1994.

53. Holland GR: The odontoblast process: form and function, *J Dent Res* 64(special issue):499, 1985.

54. Ikeda H, Tokita Y, Suda H: Capsaicin-sensitive A?fibers in cat tooth pulp, *J Dent Res* 76:1341, 1997.

55. Inoue H, Kurosaka Y, Abe K: Autonomic nerve endings in the odontoblast/predentin border and predentin of the canine teeth of dogs, *J Endod* 18:149, 1992.

56. Johnsen DC, Harshbarger J, Rymer HD: Quantitative assessment of neural development in human premolars, *Anat Rec* 205:421, 1983.

57. Johnsen D, Johns S: Quantitation of nerve fibers in the primary and permanent canine and incisor teeth in man, *Arch Oral Biol* 23:825, 1978.

58. Johnson G, Brännström M: The sensitivity of dentin: changes in relation to conditions at exposed tubule apertures, *Acta Odontol Scand* 32:29, 1974.

59. Jones PA, Taintor JF, Adams AB: Comparative dental material cytotoxicity measured by depression of rat incisor pulp respiration, *J Endod* 5:48, 1979.

60. Jontell M, Bergenholtz G: Accessory cells in the immune defense of the dental pulp, *Proc Finn Dent Soc* 88(suppl 1): 345, 1992.

61. Kaye H, Herold RC: Structure of human dentine. I. Phase contrast, polarization, interference, and bright field microscopic observations on the lateral branch system, *Arch Oral Biol* 11:355, 1966.

62. Kelley KW, Bergenholtz G, Cox CF: The extent of the odontoblast process in rhesus monkeys (Macaca mulatta) as observed by scanning electron microscopy, *Arch Oral Biol* 26:893, 1981.

63. Kim S: Neurovascular interactions in the dental pulp in health and inflammation, *J Endod* 14:48, 1990.

64. Kim S, Schuessler G, Chien S: Measurement of blood flow in the dental pulp of dogs with the ^{133}xenon washout method, *Arch Oral Biol* 28:501, 1983.

65. Kim S et al: Effects of local anesthetics on pulpal blood flow in dogs, *J Dent Res* 63:650, 1984.

66. Kim S et al: Effects of selected inflammatory mediators in blood flow and vascular permeability in the dental pulp, *Proc Finn Dent Soc* 88(suppl 1):387, 1992.

67. Kramer IRH: The distribution of blood vessels in the human dental pulp. In Finn SB, editor: *Biology of the dental pulp organ*, Birmingham, 1968, University of Alabama Press.

68. Kroeger DC, Gonzales F, Krivoy W: Transmembrane potentials of cultured mouse dental pulp cells, *Proc Soc Exp Biol Med* 108:134, 1961.

69. Langeland K, Langeland LK: Histologic study of 155 impacted teeth, *Odontol Tidskr* 73:527, 1965.

70. Lantelme RL, Handleman SL, Herbison RJ: Dentin formation in periodontally diseased teeth, *J Dent Res* 55:48, 1976.

71. Lesot H, Osman M, Ruch JV: Immunofluorescent localization of collagens, fibronectin and laminin during terminal differentiation of odontoblasts, *Dev Biol* 82:371, 1981.

72. Lilja J: Innervation of different parts of the predentin and dentin in a young human premolar, *Acta Odontol Scand* 37:339, 1979.

73. Lilja J, Noredenvall K-J, Brännström M: Dentin sensitivity, odontoblasts and nerves under desiccated or infected experimental cavities, *Swed Dent J* 6:93, 1982.

74. Linde A: The extracellular matrix of the dental pulp and dentin, *J Dent Res* 64(special issue):523, 1985.

75. Luthman J, Luthman D, Hökfelt T: Occurrence and distribution of different neurochemical markers in the human dental pulp, *Arch Oral Biol* 37:193, 1992.

76. Madison S et al: Effect of leukotriene B$_4$ on intradental nerves, *J Dent Res* 68(special issue)243:494, 1989.

77. Mangkornkarn C, Steiner JC: In vivo and in vitro glycosaminoglycans from human dental pulp, *J Endod* 18:327, 1992.

78. Marchetti C, Piacentini C: Examin au microscope photonique et au microscope electronique des capilaries lymphatiques de al pulpe dentaire humaine, *Bulletin du Groupement International Pour la Récherche Scientifque en Stomatologie et Odontologie* 33:19, 1990.

79. Matthews et al: *The functional properties of intradental nerves: proceedings of the International Conference on Dentin/Pulp Complex,* Tokyo, 1996, Quintessence pp 146-153.

80. Meyer MW, Path MG: Blood flow in the dental pulp of dogs determined by hydrogen polarography and radioactive microsphere methods, *Arch Oral Biol* 24:601, 1979.

81. Michelich V, Pashley DH, Whitford GM: Dentin permeability: a comparison of functional versus anatomical tubular radii, *J Dent Res* 57:1019, 1978.

82. Mullaney TP, Howell RM, Petrich JD: Resistance of nerve fibers to pulpal necrosis, *Oral Surg* 30:690, 1970.

83. Nagaoka S et al: Bacterial invasion into dentinal tubules of human vital and nonvital teeth, *J Endod* 21:70, 1995.

84. Närhi M: Activation of dental pulp nerves of the cat and the dog with hydrostatic pressure, *Proc Finn Dent Soc* 74(suppl 5):1, 1978.

85. Närhi M et al: Activation of heat-sensitive nerve fibers in the dental pulp of the cat, *Pain* 14:317, 1982.

86. Närhi M et al: Electrical stimulation of teeth with a pulp tester in the cat, *Scand J Dent Res* 87:32, 1979.

87. Närhi M et al: The neurophysiological basis and the role of inflammatory reactions in dentine hypersensitivity, *Arch Oral Biol* 39(suppl): 23, 1994.

88. Närhi M et al: Role of intradential A- and C-type nerve fibers in dental pain mechanisms, *Proc Finn Dent Soc* 88(suppl 1): 507, 1992.

89. Ngassapa D, Närhi M, Hirvonen T: The effect of serotonin (5-HT) and calcitonin gene-related peptide (CGRP) on the function of intradental nerves in the dog, *Proc Fin Dent Soc* 88(suppl 1):143, 1992.

90. Nishioka M et al: Tooth replantation in germ-free and conventional rats, *Endod Dent Traumatol* 14:163, 1998.

91. Nitzan DW et al: The effect of aging on tooth morphology: a study on impacted teeth, *Oral Surg* 61:54, 1986.

92. Okiji T et al: An immunohistochemical study of the distribution of immunocompetent cells, especially macrophages and Ia antigen-presenting cells of heterogeneous populations, in normal rat molar pulp, *J Dent Res* 71:1196, 1992.

93. Olgart L et al: Release of substance P-n-like immunoreactivity from the dental pulp, *Acta Physiol Scand* 101:510, 1977.

94. Pashley DH: Dentin conditions and disease. In Lazzari G, editor: *CRC handbook of experimental dentistry*, Boca Raton, FL, 1993, CRC Press.

95. Pashley DH: Dentin permeability and dentin sensitivity, *Proc Finn Dent Soc* 88(suppl 1):31, 1992.

96. Pashley DH: Dentin permeability: theory and practice. In Spangberg L, editor: *Experimental endodontics*, Boca Raton, FL, 1989, CRC Press.

97. Rapp R et al: Ultrastructure of fenestrated capillaries in human dental pulps, *Arch Oral Biol* 22:317, 1977.

98. Reader A, Foreman DW: An ultrastructural qualitative investigation of human intradental innervation, *J Endod* 7:161, 1981.

99. Sakurai K, Okiji T, Suda H: Co-increase of nerve fibers and HLA-DR- and/or factor XIIIa-expressing dendritic cells in dentinal caries-affected regions of the human dental pulp: an immunohistochemical study, *J Dent Res* 78:1596, 1999.

100. Sasaki S: Studies on the respiration of the dog tooth germ, *J Biochem* (Tokyo) 46:269, 1959.

101. Sasano T, Kuriwada S, Sanjo D: Arterial blood pressure regulation of pulpal blood flow as determined by laser Doppler, *J Dent Res* 68:791, 1989.

102. Sasano T et al: Absence of parasympathetic vasodilatation in cat dental pulp, *J Dent Res* 74:1665, 1995.

103. Sasano T et al: Axon reflex vasodilatation in cat dental pulp elicited by noxious stimulation of the gingiva, *J Dent Res* 73: 1797, 1994.

104. Scott JN, Weber DF: Microscopy of the junctional region between human coronal primary and secondary dentin, *J Morphol* 154:133, 1977.

105. Seltzer S, Bender IB, Ziontz M: The interrelationship of pulp and periodontal disease, *Oral Surg* 16:1474, 1963.

106. Sigal MJ et al: A combined scanning electron microscopy and immunofluorescence study demonstrating that the odontoblast process extends to the dentinoenamel junction in human teeth, *Anat Rec* 210:453, 1984.

107. Sigal MJ et al: The odontoblast process extends to the dentinoenamel junction: an immunocytochemical study of rat dentine, *J Histochem Cytochem* 32:872, 1984.

108. Stanley HR, White CL, McCray L: The rate of tertiary (reparative) dentin formation in the human tooth, *Oral Surg* 21:180, 1966.

109. Stanley HR et al: The detection and prevalence of reactive and physiologic sclerotic dentin, reparative dentin and dead tracts beneath various types of dental lesions according to tooth surface and age, *J Oral Pathol* 12:257, 1983.

110. Stein TJ, Corcoran JF: Anatomy of the root apex and its histologic changes with age, *Oral Surg* 69:238, 1990.

111. Stenvik A, Iverson J, Mjör IA: Tissue pressure and histology of normal and inflamed tooth pulps in Macaque monkeys, *Arch Oral Biol* 17:1501, 1972.

112. Sunakawa M, Tokita Y, Suda H: Pulsed Nd:YAG laser irradiation of the tooth pulp in the cat: II. Effect of scanning lasing, *Lasers Surg Med* (vol 26), 2000 (in press).

113. Takahashi K, Kishi Y, Kim S: A scanning electron microscope study of the blood vessels of dog pulp using corrosion resin casts, *J Endod* 8:131, 1982.

114. Thesleff I, Vaahtokari A: The role of growth factors in determination and differentiation of the odontoblast cell lineage, *Proc Finn Dent Soc* 88(suppl 1):357, 1992.

115. Thomas HF: The extent of the odontoblast process in human dentin, *J Dent Res* 58(D):2207, 1979.

116. Thomas HF, Payne RC: The ultrastructure of dentinal tubules from erupted human premolar teeth, *J Dent Res* 62:532, 1983.

117. Thomas JJ, Stanley HR, Gilmore HW: Effects of gold foil condensation on human dental pulp, *J Am Dent Assoc* 78:788, 1969.

118. Tokita Y, Sunakawa M, Suda H: Pulsed ND:YAG laser irradiation of the tooth pulp in the cat: I. Effect of spot lasing, *Lasers Surg Med* (vol 26), 2000 (in press).

119. Tönder KJH: Effect of vasodilating drugs on external carotid and pulpal blood flow in dogs: "stealing" of dental perfusion pressure, *Acta Physiol Scand* 97:75, 1976.

120. Tönder KJH, Naess G: Nervous control of blood flow in the dental pulp in dogs, *Acta Physiol Scand* 104:13, 1978.

121. Topham RT et al: Effects of epidermal growth factor on tooth differentiation and eruption. In Davidovitch Z, editor: *The biological mechanisms of tooth eruption and root resorption*, Birmingham, Ala., 1988, Ebsco Media.

122. Torebjörk HE, Hanin RG: Perceptual changes accompanying controlled preferential blocking of A and C fiber responses in intact human skin nerves, *Exp Brain Res* 16:321, 1973.

123. Torneck CD: Dentin-pulp complex. In Ten Cate AR, editor: *Oral histology: development, structure, and function*, ed 4, St Louis, 1994, Mosby.

124. Trowbridge HO: Intradental sensory units: physiological and clinical aspects, *J Endod* 11:489, 1985.

125. Trowbridge HO: Pathogenesis of pulpitis resulting from dental caries, *J Endod* 7:52, 1981.

126. Trowbridge HO: Review of current approaches to in-office management of tooth hypersensitivity, *Dent Clin North Am* 34:561, 1990.

127. Trowbridge HO, Shibata F: Mitotic activity in epithelial rests of Malassez, *Periodontics* 5:109, 1967.

128. Trowbridge HO, Stewart JCB, Shapiro IM: *Assessment of indurated, diffusely calcified human dental pulps: proceedings of the International Conference on Dentin/Pulp Complex,* Tokyo, 1996, Quintessence pp 297-300.

129. Trowbridge HO et al: Sensory response to thermal stimulation in human teeth, *J Endod* 6:6405, 1980.

130. Turner DF: Immediate physiological response of odontoblasts, *Proc Finn Dent Soc* 88(suppl 1):55, 1992.

131. van Hassel HJ: Physiology of the human dental pulp, *Oral Surg* 32:126, 1971.

132. Vongsavan N, Matthews B: The relation between fluid flow through dentine and the discharge of intradental nerves, *Arch Oral Biol* 39(suppl):140S, 1994.

133. Vongsavan N, Matthews B: The vascularity of dental pulp in cats, *J Dent Res* 71:1913, 1992.

134. Wakisaka S: Neuropeptides in the dental pulp: their distribution, origins and correlation, *J Endod* 16:67, 1990.

135. Weber DF: Human dentine sclerosis: a microradiographic study, *Arch Oral Biol* 19:163, 1974.

136. Weinstock A, Weinstock M, Leblond CP: Autoradiographic detection of ^{3}H-fucose incorporation into glycoprotein by odontoblasts and its deposition at the site of the calcification front in dentin, *Calcif Tiss Res* 8:181, 1972.

137. Weinstock M, Leblond CP: Synthesis, migration and release of precursor collagen by odontoblasts as visualized by radioautography after ^{3}H-proline administration, *J Cell Biol* 60:92, 1974.

138. Winter HF, Bishop JG, Dorman HL: Transmembrane potentials of odontoblasts, *J Dent Res* 42:594, 1963.

139. Yamada T et al: The extent of the odontoblast process in normal and carious human dentin, *J Dent Res* 62:798, 1983.

140. Yamamura T: Differentiation of pulpal wound healing, *J Dent Res* 64(special issue):530, 1985.

141. Zerlotti E: Histochemical study of the connective tissue of the dental pulp, *Arch Oral Biol* 9:149, 1964.

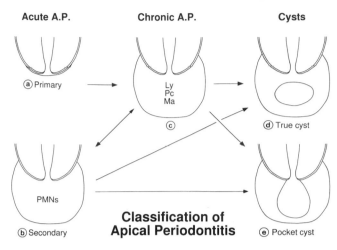

Acute A.P.   Chronic A.P.   Cysts

(a) Primary

Ly
Pc
Ma

(c)

(d) True cyst

PMNs

Classification of Apical Periodontitis

(b) Secondary   (e) Pocket cyst

Fig 12-1 Histopathologic classification of apical periodontitis (AP): acute (a,b), chronic (c), and cystic (d,e) lesions. The acute apical periodontitis may be primary (a) or secondary (b) and is characterized by the presence of a focus of neutrophils (PMNs). The major components of chronic lesions (c) are lymphocytes (Ly), plasma cells (Pc), and macrophages (Ma). Periapical cysts can be differentiated into true cysts (d) with completely enclosed lumina and pocket cysts (e) with cavities open to the root canal. Arrows indicate the direction in which the lesions can change. (Adapted from Nair PNR: Pathology of apical periodontitis. In Ørstavik D, Pitt-Ford TR, editors: *Essential endodontology*, Oxford, 1998, Blackwell.)

Table 12-1 **WHO (1995) CLASSIFICATION OF DISEASES OF PERIAPICAL TISSUES**

Code Number	Category
K04.4	Acute apical periodontitis
K04.5	Chronic apical periodontitis (Apical granuloma)
K04.6	Periapical abscess with sinus (Dentoalveolar abscess with sinus, Periodontal abscess of pulpal origin)
K04.60	Periapical abscess with sinus to maxillary antrum
K04.61	Periapical abscess with sinus to nasal cavity
K04.62	Periapical abscess with sinus to oral cavity
K04.63	Periapical abscess with sinus to skin
K04.7	Periapical abscess without sinus (Dental abscess without sinus, Dentoalveolar abscess without sinus, Periodontal abscess of pulpal origin without sinus)
K04.8	Radicular cyst (Apical periodontal cyst, Periapical cyst)
K04.80	Apical and lateral cyst
K04.81	Residual cyst
K04.82	Inflammatory paradental cyst

* Names in parentheses denote given synonyms and conditions that are included in the category.

their role in the destruction of the periapical tissues was not anticipated. Most of the early clues for that scenario came from research data on marginal periodontitis.[211] As more and more evidence accumulated for the major role of defense cells and immune reactions in the tissue destruction associated with marginal periodontitis (and by *de facto* in apical periodontitis), the immune system itself was regarded as the "culprit" for the disease process. This, to a certain extent, sidelined the central role of microorganisms in the development of apical periodontitis.[303]

The last decade has witnessed the arrival of several research papers of "periapical origins" that attempted to provide a molecular basis for the disease process at the tooth apex.* Currently apical periodontitis is viewed as the body's defense response to the destruction of the tooth pulp and the hostile "foreign occupation" of the root canal. The microbial and host-defense forces clash and destroy much of the periapex, resulting in the formation of various classes of apical periodontitis lesions.

NOMENCLATURE AND CLASSIFICATION

Apical periodontitis is inflammation of the periodontium caused by infection of the pulp canal system. It has been the subject of numerous terms and classifications. *Periapical lesions, apical granuloma and cysts, periapical osteitis,* and

*References 12,52,165,230,265,290,293,305,320.

periradicular lesions are frequently used synonyms. Although *periradicular* includes inflammation of the furcal and lateral locations, it does not etymologically distinguish the pulpally derived periodontitis from marginally spreading lesions. The limitations of the various terms and the arguments for the preferential retention of *apical periodontitis* have been discussed recently.[209]

Being an inflammatory disease, apical periodontitis can be classified on the basis of symptoms, cause, histopathology, and so on. The World Health Organization (WHO)[324] classified apical periodontitis under diseases of periapical tissues into several categories (Table 12-1) based on clinical signs. This useful classification, however, does not take into account the structural aspects of the diseased tissues. As the structural framework forms the basis of understanding of the disease process, a histopathologic classification is used here (Fig. 12-1). It is based on the distribution of inflammatory cells within the lesion, the presence or absence of epithelial cells, whether the lesion has been transformed into a cyst, and the relationship of the cyst-cavity to the root canal of the affected tooth.

Acute apical periodontitis is acute inflammation of the periodontium of endodontic origin that is characterized by the presence of a distinct focus of neutrophils within the lesion. It is said to be *primary* when the inflammation is of short duration and is initiated within a healthy periodontium

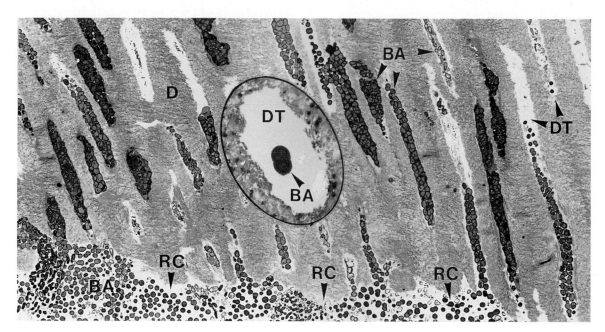

Fig. 12-2 Bacteria (*BA*) in dentinal tubules (*DT*) at the apical part of human root dentine. The tubules are invaded from the infected root canal (*RC*). The presence of dividing forms (*inset*) is a clear sign of vitality of the microorganisms at the time of fixation. (Magnification × 2'480, *inset* × 9'600.)

(see Fig. 12-1, *A*) in response to irritants. It is called *secondary* when the acute response occurs in an already existing chronic apical periodontitis lesion (see Fig. 12-1, *B*). The latter form is also referred to as *periapical flare-up, exacerbation, or "phoenix abscess."* The lesions may be nonepithelialized or epithelialized.

Chronic apical periodontitis is a long-standing inflammation of the periodontium of endodontic origin that is characterized by the presence of a granulomatous tissue, predominantly infiltrated with lymphocytes, plasma cells, and macrophages (see Fig. 12-1, *C*). The lesions may be nonepithelialized or epithelialized.

Periapical true cyst is an apical inflammatory cyst with a distinct pathologic cavity that is completely enclosed in an epithelial lining so that no communication to the root canal exists (see Fig. 12-1, *D*).

Periapical pocket cyst[192] is an apical inflammatory cyst containing a saclike, epithelium-lined cavity that is open to and continuous with the root canal (see Fig. 12-1, *E*).

MICROBIAL DISEASE

Pathways of Infection

There are several routes through which microorganisms can reach the dental pulp. Openings in the dental hard tissue wall, resulting from caries, clinical procedures, or trauma-induced fractures and cracks are the most frequent portals of pulpal infection. However, microbes have also been isolated from teeth with necrotic pulps and apparently intact

crowns.* Endodontic infections of such teeth are preceded by pulp necrosis. It has been suggested that bacteria from the gingival sulci or periodontal pockets might reach the root canals of these teeth through severed blood vessels of the periodontium.[89] However, it is very unlikely that microorganisms would survive the immunologic defenses between the marginal gingiva and the apical foramen. The teeth may clinically appear intact but reveal microcracks in hard tissues. The latter may provide portals of entry for bacteria. Pulpal infection can also occur through exposed dentinal tubules at the cervical root surface because of gaps in the cemental coating.

It has been proposed that bacteria remaining in infected dentinal tubules (Fig. 12-2) can be a potential reservoir for endodontic reinfection.† Microbial infection has also been claimed to reach and seed in the necrotic pulp via the general blood circulation by the "anachoresis."[5,42,86,223] However, bacteria could not be recovered from the root canals when the blood stream was experimentally infected unless the root canals were overinstrumented and, presumably, the apical periodontal blood vessels were injured during the period of bacteremia.[71] Evidence that further discredits anachoresis as a potential source of necrotic pulpal infection comes from the study of Möller et al[175] in which all experimentally devitalized pulps (n = 26) in monkeys remained sterile for more than 6 months. Therefore exposure of the dental pulp to the oral cavity is the most important route of endodontic infection.

---

*References 20,24,37,48,74,153,174,275,327.
†References 8,150,184,187,214,217,247,314.

Microflora of Infected and Untreated Necrotic Pulp

The endodontic microbiologic nature of teeth with infected necrotic pulps and apical periodontitis has been extensively researched. However, the results of most of the earlier endodontic microbial culture studies have become irrelevant because of the difficulty of avoiding bacterial contamination from the oral surroundings[28,174,325] and the absence of appropriate anaerobic methods for root canal sampling and cultivation of fastidious organisms. To recover such microorganisms from the necrotic pulp, stringent anaerobic sampling and cultivation techniques are necessary; these methods have been optimized only during the last 30 years.[108]

The two most significant advances in anaerobic technology have been (1) the innovative use of an anaerobic glove box[226,257] in which bacteria are protected from oxygen during isolation and cultivation, and (2) the development of prereduced, anaerobically sterilized culture media.[113,179] Obligate anaerobes were believed to be killed by brief exposure to atmospheric O_2, but they can survive for several hours in media supplemented with hemolysed blood.[47] The enzyme catalase, present in hemolysed blood, breaks down the toxic H_2O_2 in the O_2 and H_2O. These advances in anaerobic techniques have not only enabled the isolation and characterization of obligate anaerobes from the root canals of periapically affected teeth but also helped to study their pathogenic properties.*

In principle a sample of the vast oral microbiota[180] can infect the tooth pulp when the integrity of dental hard tissues is lost. However, the remarkable feature of the endodontic flora is the small number of species that are consistently isolated from such root canals. Application of advanced anaerobic techniques helped to establish that the root canal flora of teeth with clinically intact crowns but having necrotic pulps and diseased periapices is dominated (>90%) by obligate anaerobes[45,91,275,282] usually belonging to the genera *Fusobacterium*, *Porphyromonas* (formerly *Bacteroides*[242]), *Prevotella* (formerly *Bacteroides*[243]), *Eubacterium*, and *Peptostreptococcus*. On the other hand, the microbial composition, even in the apical third of the root canal of periapically affected teeth with pulp canals exposed to the oral cavity by caries (Fig. 12-3), is not only different but also less dominated (<70%) by strict anaerobes.[18] In addition, spirochetes have been found in necrotic root canals using microbiologic methods,[55,92,123] dark-field microscopy,[37,54,294] and transmission electron microscopy (TEM)[187] (Fig. 12-4). Spirochetes are motile, invasive pathogens that are associated with certain marginal periodontitis[147] and suggested causative agents of acute necrotizing ulcerative gingivitis (ANUG).[148] However, their role in apical periodontitis remains to be clarified.

Endodontic Flora in Previously Root-Filled Teeth

The microbiologic nature of root-filled canals is far less understood than that of untreated, infected, necrotic dental pulps. This is probably a consequence of searching for nonmicrobial causes of purely technical nature for the failure of root canal treatments.[60,280] The taxonomy of the endodontic flora of root canal–treated teeth depends on the quality of the treatment and obturation of the canals. As such, teeth with inadequate instrumentation, débridement, root canal medication, and poor obturation should be expected to harbor a flora that is similar to that found in untreated canals. On the other hand, only a very restricted number of species has been found in the root canals and periapices of teeth that have undergone proper, conventional endodontic treatment but that, on follow up, reveal persisting, asymptomatic periapical radiolucencies.

The bacteria found in these cases are predominantly gram-positive cocci, rods, and filaments. Using microbiologic techniques, species belonging to the genera *Actinomyces*, *Enterococcus,* and *Propionibacterium* (previously *Arachnia*) are the most frequently isolated and characterized microorganisms from such root canals.* The repeated recovery of *Enterococcus faecalis* deserves particular attention.[83,173,174,281] Although *E. faecalis* is an insignificant organism in infected but untreated root canals,[280] it is extremely resistant to most of the intracanal medicaments used, particularly to the calcium hydroxide–containing dressings.[43] It can also survive in root canals as monoinfection, without any synergistic support from other bacteria.[76] Thus *E. faecalis* is a recalcitrant candidate among the causative agents of failed endodontic treatments.

Earlier microbiologic[174] studies and more recent correlative electron microscopic[196] studies have shown the presence of yeastlike microorganisms (Fig. 12-5) in canals of root-filled teeth with unresolving apical periodontitis, so as to implicate fungi as potential therapy-resisting endodontic organisms. *Candida albicans* is the most frequently isolated fungus from root filled teeth with apical periodontitis.[73,281]

Pathogenicity of Endodontic Flora

Any microbe that infects the root canal has the potential to initiate a periapical inflammation. However, the virulence and pathogenicity of individual species vary considerably and can be affected in the presence of other microbes. Although the individual species in the endodontic flora are usually of low virulence, collectively they are pathogenic due to a combination of factors. These factors include (1) interactions with other microorganisms in the root canal, so as to develop synergistically beneficial partners; (2) the release of endotoxins; (3) the synthesis of enzymes that damage host tissues; and (4) the ability to interfere with and evade host defenses.

---

*References 58,59,75,76,77,123,174,175,275,284,327.

*References 83,93,173,174,252,281,283.

Text continued on p. 464

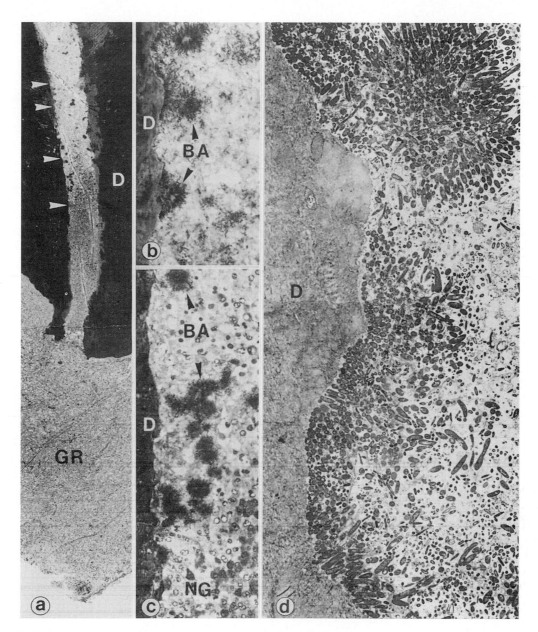

Fig 12-3 The root canal flora of a human tooth with apical periodontitis (GR). The areas in between the upper two and the lower two arrowheads in *A* are magnified in *B* and *C*, respectively. Note the dense bacterial aggregates (BA) sticking (*B*) to the dentinal (D) wall and also remaining suspended among neutrophilic granulocytes (NG) in the fluid phase of the root canal (*C*). The NGs form a defensive wall against the advancing bacterial front. A transmission electron microscopic view (*D*) of the pulpodentinal interface shows bacterial condensation on the surface of the dentinal wall forming thick, layered plaque. (Magnifications: *A* × 46, *B* × 600, *C* × 370, *D* × 2350.) (From Nair PNR: Apical periodontitis: a dynamic encounter between root canal infection and host response, *Periodontology 2000* 13:121, 1997.)

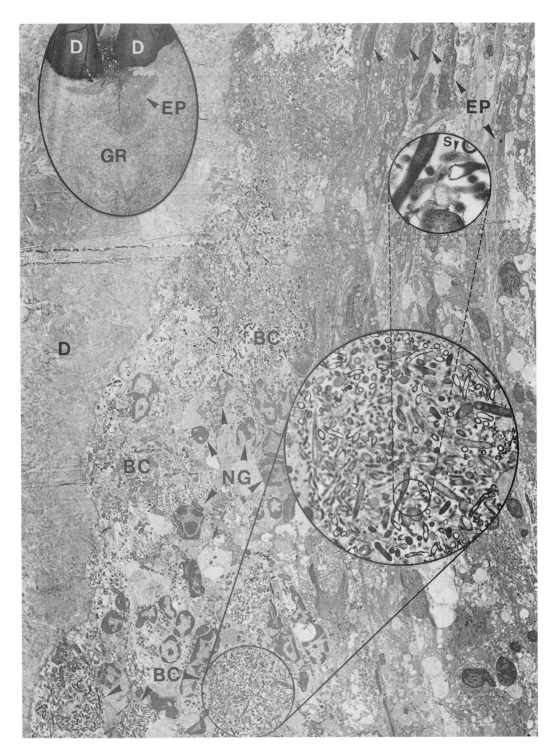

Fig. 12-4 Polymicrobial flora at the apical foramen of a human tooth with periapical granuloma (*GR* in *inset*). The microbial front appears to be blocked at the foramen by an epithelial plug (*EP* in *inset*). The transmission electron microscopic montage shows the dentinal wall (*D*), necrotic pulp with epithelial cells (*EP, arrowheads*), neutrophilic granulocytes (*NG*), and bacteria. The latter exist in numerous clusters, (*BC*) one of which is demarcated and magnified (*large inset*). The microbial clusters consist of cocci, rods, filaments, and spirochetes (*S in upper circular inset*). They appear to form complex microbial communities existing in a synergistic relationship. (Magnifications: × 2400, *oval inset* x 15, *large circular inset* × 6700, *upper small circular inset* × 59,800.) (From Nair PNR: Apical periodontitis: a dynamic encounter between root canal infection and host response, *Periodontology 2000* 13:121, 1997.)

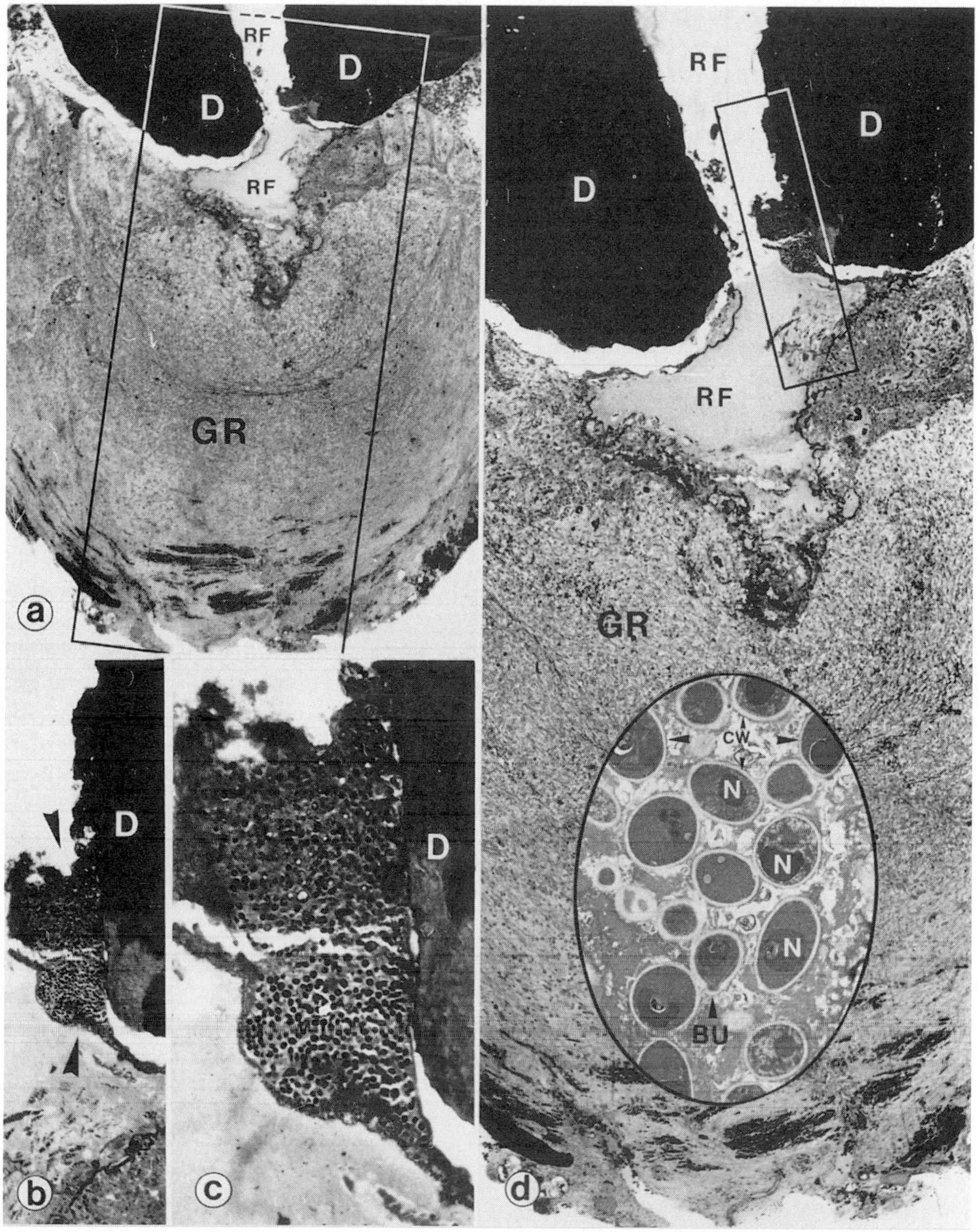

Fig. 12-5 Fungi as a potential causative agent of human apical periodontitis. *A,* Low-power overview of an axial section of a root-filled (*RF*) tooth with a persisting apical periodontitis lesion (*GR*). The rectangular demarcated areas in *A* and *D* are magnified in *D* and *B,* respectively. Note the two microbial clusters (*arrowheads* in *B*), further magnified in *C.* The oval inset in *D* is a transmission electron microscopic view of the organisms. Note the electron-lucent cell wall (*CW*), nuclei (*N*), and budding forms (*BU*). (Magnifications: *A* x 35, *B* x 130, *C* x 330, *D* x 60, oval inset x 3400.) (Adapted from Nair PNR et al: Intraradicular bacteria and fungi in root-filled, asymptomatic human teeth with therapy-resistant periapical lesions: A long-term light and electron microscopic follow-up study, *J Endod* 16:580, 1990.)

Microbial Interaction Overwhelming evidence suggests that microbial interaction plays a significant role in the ecologic regulation and eventual development of an endodontic habitat-adapted polymicrobial flora.[276,277] The importance of the mixed bacterial flora has been well exemplified in carefully planned animal studies.[76,77,284] Bacteria (*Prevotella oralis* and 11 other species) isolated from the root canals of periapically involved teeth of experimental monkeys were inoculated in various combinations or as separate species into the root canals of other monkeys.[76] When individual bacterial species were inoculated, only a mild apical periodontitis developed. However, in combinations, the same bacterial species induced more severe periapical reactions. Further, *Prevotella oralis* failed to establish in root canals as a monoinfection, whereas it survived and dominated the endodontic flora when introduced with the other bacterial species involved in the study.

Microbial interactions that influence the ecology of the endodontic flora may be positive (i.e., synergistic) or negative associations as a result of certain organisms influencing the respiratory and nutritional environments of the entire root canal flora. During early stages of pulpal infection, facultative anaerobes dominate the microflora[77] and use most of the available O_2, progressively lowering the endodontic O_2-partial pressure,[149] which favors the growth of obligate anaerobes.[77] Nutritionally, the metabolic end products of some species of microbes may form part of the food chain for other species.[46,143]

Endotoxin Richard Pfeiffer,[222] a student of Robert Koch, coined this misnomer for the highly pyrogenic, thermostable macromolecule, which has been later identified as lipopolysaccharide (LPS). LPS forms an integral part of the outer layer of gram-negative cell walls. It is released during disintegration of bacteria after death and is also shed in small quantities during multiplication and growth. The pathobiologic effects of LPS are because of its interaction with endothelial cells and macrophages. LPS of most gram-negative bacteria can signal the endothelial cells to express adhesion molecules and activate the latter to produce a number of molecular mediators, such as the tumor necrosis factor-α (TNF-α) and interleukins.[11] The former is the primary mediator of the damaging effects of LPS.

Exogenous TNF-α administered into experimental animals can induce a lethal shock that is indistinguishable from that induced by LPS. As endotoxins are primarily released after death of the bacteria, the lethal effects of LPS on host tissues cannot be beneficial to the bacteria in question. However, to the host defense cells LPS signals the presence of gram-negative microorganisms in the area, and they react violently. As Thomas[297] pointed out, "When we sense LPS, we are likely to turn on every defense at our disposal; we will bomb, defoliate, blockade, seal off, and destroy all tissues in the area." The presence of LPS has been reported in samples taken from the root canal[57,235] and the pulpal dentinal wall of periapically involved teeth.[110] As gram-negative organisms

dominate the endodontic flora, it is not surprising that they may multiply and die in the apical root canal, thereby releasing LPS that can egress through the apical foramen into the periapex[329] to initiate and sustain apical periodontitis.[56,61]

Exotoxin What is the role of exotoxins in the pathogenicity of endodontic flora? Exotoxins, unlike endotoxins, are highly antigenic, nonpyrogenic, thermolabile polypeptides actively secreted by living microorganisms that can be converted into toxoids. Leukotoxin is the most celebrated exotoxin known to be involved in the pathogenesis of certain types of marginal periodontitis. It produces small holes on leukocyte cell membranes that result in lysis of the cells.[287] Leukotoxin is known to be produced by species of *Fusobacterium necrophorum*[78,140] and *Actinobacillus actinomycetemcomitans*.[286] However, among the *Fusobacterium*, it is *F. nucleatum* that is the most frequently encountered endodontic pathogen, and it does not produce any exotoxins. *A. actinomycetemcomitans* is highly capnophilic and may not survive in the root canal environment. Therefore exotoxins do not seem to play any significant role in the pathogenicity of endodontic flora.

Enzymes Endodontic microbes produce a variety of enzymes, which are not directly toxic but may aid the spread of the organisms in host tissues. Microbial collagenase, hyaluronidase, fibrinolysins, and several proteases are some examples. Microbes are also known to produce enzymes that degrade various plasma proteins involved in blood coagulation and other body defenses. The ability of some *Porphyromonas* and *Prevotella* species to break down plasma proteins, particularly IgG, IgM,[126] and the complement factor C_3,[279] is of significance because these molecules happen to be opsonins necessary for both humoral and phagocytic host defenses.

Microbial Interference The ability of certain microbes to shirk the host defenses and to interfere with it has been well elaborated.[278] As has been mentioned before, LPS of many bacteria can signal the endothelial cells to express leukocyte adhesion molecules, thereby initiating extravasation of white blood cells into the area of the microbial presence. It has been reported that *Porphyromonas gingivalis*, an important endodontic and periodontal pathogen, and its LPS do not signal the endothelial cells to express E-selectin. *P. gingivalis*, therefore, has the ability to block the first important step of inflammatory response, "hide" from the host, and multiply. The antigenicity of LPS occurs in a multitude of variations and results in mitogenic stimulation of B-lymphocytes, so as to produce nonspecific antibodies. From the microorganism's point of view, it is a definite advantage to "cheat" the host this way. Gram-negative organisms release membrane particles (i.e., blebs) and soluble antigens that may "mop up" effective antibodies, making them unavailable to act against the organism itself.[170] Individual organisms of *Actinomyces israelii*, a recalcitrant, periapical pathogen, are easily killed by polymorphonuclear leukocytes (PMN) *in vitro*.[79] In tissues, however, *A. israelii* aggregate to form large, cohesive colonies that cannot be killed by host phagocytes.[79]

HOST DEFENSE

Apical periodontitis is viewed as body's defense response to the threat of microbial invasion from the root canal. The host tissue mounts a formidable array of defense that consists of cells, intercellular mediators, metabolites, effector molecules, and humoral antibodies.

Cells

Several classes of body cells participate in the periapical defense. The majority of them is recruited from the defense systems and includes neutrophils, lymphocytes, plasma cells, and macrophages. In addition, structural cells, such as fibroblasts, osteoblasts, and epithelial remnants of the enamel organ (rests of Malassez),[156] also play significant roles.

Polymorphonuclear Leukocytes   The PMN, or neutrophils, are the front line fighting force against microbes (and the hallmark of acute inflammation); their function is to locate and destroy microbes that intrude into the body. PMNs are nonspecific phagocytes and are well equipped to attack enemies with weapons already stored within (or quickly assembled by) them. Their ammunitions consist of various cytoplasmic granules that are classified into *primary*, *secondary*, and *tertiary* groups. The primary granules (i.e.,

azurophilic granules) contain lysosomes, myeloperoxidase, cationic proteins, and neutral proteinases. The secondary (i.e., specific) granules are marked by lactoferrin and vitamin B_{12} binding protein. The tertiary (i.e., secretory granules) are released into the tissues in response to stimuli.[315]

In response to tissue injury, PMN extravasate (Fig. 12-6) in great numbers to the site of injury where they seek the targets by chemotaxis. They move in the direction of an ascending gradient of the chemotactic molecules, so as to congregate at the site of maximum concentration that coincides with the site of microbial presence. By the time the PMN meet the microbes, the latter are generally opsonized. Opsonins are complement factors or antibodies that coat the surface of microbes that trigger and enhance phagocytosis. The microbes are ingested and isolated in membrane-bound phagosomes. Depending on the availability of oxygen (O_2) the PMN are equipped with two pathways for intracellular killing of the enemy.

During the initial phases of inflammation, there is generally plenty of oxygen in the tissues and the PMN follow an aerobic route (i.e., "respiratory burst") in which the enzyme NADPH oxidase (situated on the phagosome membrane) converts molecular O_2 into oxygen-derived free radicals. These are atoms or molecules with unpaired electrons. They are highly unstable, reactive, and literally "rob" electrons from other molecules, thereby damaging them. Speroxide (O_2-) is formed when NADPH oxidase acts on stable O_2. A pair of O_2- can interact to form a molecule of hydrogen peroxide (H_2O_2). Both the O_2- and H_2O_2 are mildly microbicidal. However, the latter (in the presence of the enzyme myleoperoxidase) oxidizes halides (CL-) to form hypochlorous acid (HOCL), which is highly bactericidal. This antimicrobial

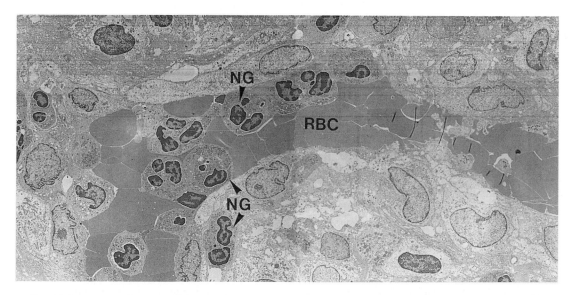

Fig. 12-6   Intravascular neutrophilic granulocytes (*NG*) marginating, adhering to the endothelial cells, and transmigrating across the blood vessel wall into the inflamed periapical tissues (*RBC*: red blood cells). (Magnification × 1650.) (From Nair PNR: Pathology of apical periodontitis. In Ørstavik D, Pitt-Ford TR, editors: *Essential endodontology*, Oxford, 1998, Blackwell.)

pathway is known as the *H_2O_2-halidemyeloperoxidase system*. Under hypoxic conditions (e.g., abscess), PMN shift the intracellular killing process to the anaerobic pathway in which the phagosomes fuse with primary or secondary granules containing powerful enzymes that can kill and digest the microbes.

The PMN are primarily mobilized to kill microorganisms (Fig. 12-7, *A*), but they also cause severe damage to the host tissues. Their cytoplasmic granules contain scores of enzymes that, on release, can degrade the structural elements of tissue cells and extracellular matrices. The zinc-dependent enzymes that are responsible for the breakdown of most of the extracellular matrices are now classified under the super family of enzymes, called the matrix metalloproteinases (MMP).[185] However, once launched or released, these enzymatic and chemical weapons (i.e., super oxide, hydrogen peroxide, hypochlorous acid) do not discriminate between hostile enemy and host tissues.[315] PMN are short-lived cells (i.e., about 3 days) that die in great numbers at acute inflammatory sites.[229] Therefore irrespective of the cause of PMN mobilization, the accumulation and local death of neutrophils is a major cause for tissue breakdown in acute phases of apical periodontitis.

Lymphocytes   Lymphocytes belong to the elite force of the defense system and are central to inflammation and immunity. They play several roles in apical periodontitis. There are three major classes of lymphocytes designated as T-lymphocytes, B-lymphocytes, and the natural killer (NK) cells. The primary function of NK cells is to monitor and destroy neoplastic and virus-infected cells. Therefore they may not be of significance in apical periodontitis. But the T- and B-lymphocytes are of particular importance. The three classes of lymphocytes originate from bone marrow stem cells but undergo different pathways of growth and differentiation. Nevertheless, they are morphologically identical (Fig. 12-7, *B*) and cannot be distinguished by conventional staining or microscopic examination. Today lymphocytes and other leukocytes are phenotyped on the basis of surface receptors using monoclonal antibodies against the latter. Cells so identified are given a *cluster of differentiation* (CD) number.

T-lymphocytes   T-lymphocytes are thymus-derived (T) cells. Originating from the bone marrow stem cells, the preT-cells migrate to the thymus and undergo further differentiation, immunologic specialization, and stringent selection before the "successful candidates" are released into general circulation. T-cells constitute about 60% to 70% of blood circulating lymphocytes. They also concentrate in the paracortic areas of lymph nodes and other lymphoid organs. T-cells are multifunctional, with certain division of labor, so that the various functions are performed by their subpopulations.

The nomenclature of T-cells can be confusing. Traditionally, they have been designated after their effect or functions. For instance, the T-cells working with B-cells have long been known as T-helper/inducer ($T_{h/i}$) cells, and those with direct

toxic and suppressive effects on other cells have been named T-cytotoxic/suppressive ($T_{c/s}$) cells. The $T_{h/i}$ cells are CD4+; and the $T_{c/s}$ cells are CD8+. The CD4+ cells differentiate further into two types known as T_{h1} and T_{h2} cells. The former produce IL-2 and interferon-γ (IF-γ) and control the cell-mediated arm of the immune system. The T_{h2} cells secrete IL-4, IL -5, IL -6, and IL-10 to control the humoral immune responses by regulating the production of antibodies by the plasma cells.

B-lymphocytes   The lymphocytes directly responsible for antibody production are the bursa-equivalent (B) cells. This is because B-cells were originally discovered in chicken (their early differentiation was found to take place in a gut-associated organ called the *bursa of Fabricius*). Humans do not have this structure; the origin and differentiation of B-cells in man occur in bone marrow itself.[225] The differentiated B-cells enter the blood circulation, where they constitute about 10% to 20% of the lymphocyte population. They also accumulate and proliferate in and around the germinal centers of extrathymic lymphoid tissues. On receiving signals from antigens and the T_{h2}-cells, some of the B-cells transform into large *plasma cells* (Fig. 12-7, *C*) with characteristic nuclei of cartwheel appearance and extensive rough endoplasmic reticulum. Plasma cells are the only cells that can manufacture and secrete antibodies, the specific chemical weapons of the immune system.

Cellular Composition   The presence of neutrophils, macrophages, lymphocytes, plasma cells, and epithelial cells has long been recognized in human apical periodontitis lesions. It seems reasonable to expect that high concentrations of neutrophils and some macrophages are present during the acute phase, and that lymphocytes, macrophages, and plasma cells accumulate during the chronic phase of the disease process. Most of the quantitative studies focus on chronic lesions.* However, the data on various classes of cells in human periapical lesions have been conflicting for several reasons. It should be emphasized that because of the great heterogeneity of the structural components of apical periodontitis lesions[188] and the resulting methodologic and tissue-sampling problems that were critically reviewed,[188,189] the available quantitative data on the cellular composition of apical periodontitis lesions are not representative of the lesions, particularly those of human origin.

Macrophages   The macrophage[167] is the prima donna of chronic inflammation and immunity. It is a large mononuclear phagocyte (Fig. 12-7, *D*) that represents the major differentiated element of the *mononuclear phagocytic system*,[212,316] previously known as the *reticuloendothelial system*. This system consists of closely related cells of bone marrow origin that comprise blood monocytes and tissue macrophages. The latter are diffusely distributed throughout

---

*References 14,25,53,130,151,202,215,268,269,270,306.

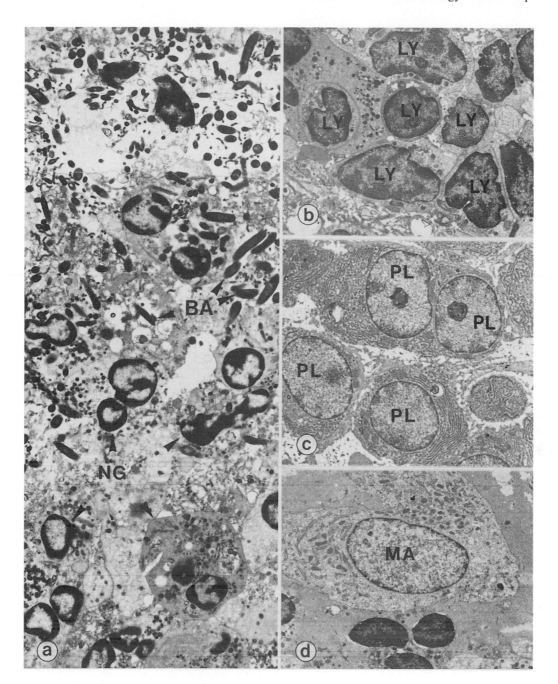

Fig. 12-7 Inflammatory cells in apical periodontitis lesions. Neutrophils (*NG* in *A*) in combat with bacteria (*BA*) in a secondary acute apical periodontitis. Lymphocytes (*LY* in *B*) are the major components of chronic apical periodontitis, but their subpopulations cannot be identified on a structural basis. Plasma cells (*PL* in *C*) form a significant component of chronic asymptomatic lesions. Note the highly developed rough endoplasmic reticulum of the cytoplasm and the localized condensation of heterochromatin subjacent to the nuclear membrane that gives the typical "cartwheel" appearance in light microscope. Macrophages (*MA* in *D*) are voluminous cells with elongated or U-forming nuclei and cytoplasm with rough endoplasmic reticulum. (Magnifications *A-D* × 3900.) (Adapted from Nair PNR: Pathology of apical periodontitis. In Ørstavik D, Pitt-Ford TR, editors: *Essential endodontology,* Oxford, 1998, Blackwell.)

the body. Depending on their location, they have been known by various names, such as the macrophages of connective and lymphoid tissues, alveolar macrophages of the lung, Kupffer's cells of the liver, Langerhans' cells of the integument, microglial cells of the brain, and fusion macrophages that produce various types of multinucleated giant cells (e.g., osteoclasts, dentoclasts, foreign-body giant cells).

Macrophages have several functions that include (1) phagocytic killing of microorganisms, (2) scavenging of dead cells and tissue components, (3) removal of small foreign particles, (4) immunologic surveillance by antigen capture, (5) processing and presentation of antigens to immune competent cells, and (6) secretion of wide variety of biologically active molecules and their regulation.

Monocytes begin to migrate relatively early in inflammation. Extravasation of monocytes is governed by the same factors that are involved in PMN emigration. On reaching the extravascular tissue, monocytes undergo transformation into large phagocytic cells: the macrophages (see Fig. 12-7, *D*). Unlike PMN, macrophages are long living (i.e., months), slow moving cells. Once they arrive the macrophages can stay at the inflammatory site for several months. If the first wave of PMN defense has failed to exterminate the enemy, the process becomes a chronic inflammation. Thus macrophages form a major component of the inflammatory cells in later stages of inflammation.

Macrophages move by chemotaxis and are activated by microorganisms, their products (i.e., LPS), chemical mediators, or foreign particles. Activated macrophages become larger, show numerous lysosomal and other cytoplasmic granules, and a greater affinity for phagocytosis and intracellular killing of microorganisms. They possess the same biochemical weapons for killing of microbes as the PMN do and can attach to foreign objects.[253] Among the various molecular mediators that are secreted by macrophages, the cytokines IL-1, TNF-α, interferons (IFN), and growth factors are of particular importance in apical periodontitis. They also contribute serum components and metabolites, such as prostaglandins and leukotrienes, which are important in inflammation.

Osteoclasts

One of the major pathologic events of apical periodontitis is the destruction of bone and dental hard tissues. Osteoclasts are the effector cells in this process. There are extensive reviews on the origin,[201] structure,[85] regulation,[102] and "coupling"[220] of these cells with osteoblasts. Bone marrow stem cells provide the progenitor cells of osteoclasts. The proosteoclasts migrate through blood as monocytes to the periradicular tissues and attach themselves to the surface of bone. They remain dormant until signaled for further changes and activity. In the physiologic state those signals, involving several cytokines and other mediators, are given by osteoblasts. During apical periodontitis these mediators are released not only by osteoblasts but also by several other cells that stimulate the proosteoclasts. As a result the latter begin to proliferate, and several daughter

cells fuse to form multinucleated osteoclasts that spread over injured and exposed bone surface. The cytoplasmic border of the osteoclasts facing the bony surface becomes ruffled as a result of multiple infolding of the plasma membrane. Bone resorption takes place beneath this ruffled border, known as the *subosteoclastic resorption compartment*. At the periphery, the cytoplasmic clear zone is a highly specialized area that regulates the biochemical activities involved in breaking down the bone.

Bone destruction occurs extracellularly (at the osteoclast-and-bone interface) and involves (1) demineralization of the bone by solubilizing the mineral phase in the resorption compartment as a result of ionic lowering of pH in the microenvironment and (2) enzymatic dissolution of the organic matrix. In the process the enzyme families cystineproteinases and MMP are involved. Root cementum and dentin are also resorbed in apical periodontitis by fusion macrophages designated as odontoclasts. However, they belong to the same cell population as osteoclasts (in view of their ultrastructural and histochemical similarities).[231]

Epithelial Cells

About 30% to 52% of all apical periodontitis lesions contain proliferating epithelium.* During periapical inflammation the dormant cell rests of Malassez[156] are believed to be stimulated by cytokines and growth factors to undergo division and proliferation, a process commonly described as inflammatory hyperplasia. These cells participate in the pathogenesis of radicular cysts by serving as the source of epithelium. However, ciliated epithelial cells are also found in periapical lesions,[245] particularly in lesions affecting maxillary molars. The maxillary sinus epithelium was suggested to be a source of those cells.[193]

Molecular Mediators

Cytokines

Cytokines[50] are intercellular mediators that are produced by a variety of haematopoietic and structural cells and have pleotropic effects on target cells in the regulation of immunologic defense, inflammatory response, cellular growth and differentiation, and tissue remodeling and repair. They are low molecular weight (i.e., < 30 kDa) polypeptides or glycoproteins, secreted transiently by activated source cells under various stimuli.[75] Cytokines act on multiple target cells with numerous effects (i.e., ambiguity), and structurally dissimilar cytokines may have overlapping spectrum of actions (i.e., redundancy). They function in a network fashion to increase or decrease the production of other cytokines. Most of the cytokines have short action radius, with synergistic or antagonistic effects on the source cell (i.e., autocrine) or other target cells (i.e., paracrine) in the neighborhood. Spillover into general circulation with affects on distant cells (i.e., endocrine) are exceptional. Cytokines are effective in very low concentrations (i.e., Pg/ml) because

---

*References 82,139,192,241,248,259,295,331.

they produce their actions by binding to high-affinity cell surface receptors.

Cytokine nomenclature.   The current body of knowledge on cytokines is evolved from various independent sources of research in the fields of immunology, virology, cell, and molecular biology. Consequently, a unifying concept of cytokines has been slow emerging and the nomenclature has been in a state of flux and confusion. In the 1960s when early evidence for the existence of intercellular mediators in supernatants of antigen-sensitized lymphocytes in culture were reported, they were designated on the basis of their biologic effects. The terms *lymphokines* and *monokines* have been used to denote the products of lymphocytes and macrophages, respectively. By late 1970s a plethora of eponyms existed for the monocyte- and lymphocyte-derived activities. It also became evident that a large number of designations existed for the same biochemical molecule. This motivated a group of investigators at the Second International Lymphokine Workshop to propose the term *interleukin* (IL) to describe the molecular messengers acting between leukocytes. The names IL-1 and IL-2 were introduced for the two important molecules, which until then had been known under various names. But IL is a restrictive term used to designate the signal molecules among leukocytes. A number of IL are, however, not only produced by nonhaematopoietic cells but also affect the functions of diverse somatic cells. Therefore after a long period of negligence, the term *cytokine*[50] has become the preferred, collective designation for the cell-regulatory proteins. Nevertheless, many cytokines continue to be designated as IL, and many others remain known by their old designations based on historic names (i.e., interferons) or biologic effects (i.e., cytotoxic factors, colony-stimulating factors, certain growth factors).

Interleukins.   Among the various IL described so far,[207] IL-1, IL-6, and IL-8 are of particular importance in the development of apical periodontitis. IL-1α and IL-1β are proinflammatory cytokines produced mainly by macrophages. Many of their systemic effects are identical to those observed in toxic shock. Local effects include enhancement of leukocyte adhesion to endothelial walls, stimulation of lymphocytes, potentiation of neutrophils, activation of the production of prostaglandins and proteolytic enzymes, enhancement of bone resorption, and inhibition of bone formation.

IL-1β is the predominant form found in human periapical lesions and their exudates,[15,144,161] and IL-1α is primarily involved in the pathogenesis of apical periodontitis in rats.[290,320] IL-6[105] is produced by both lymphoid and a variety of nonlymphoid cells under the influence of IL-1, TNF-α, and IFN-γ. It down regulates the production and also counters some of the effects of IL-1. The significance of IL-6 in apical periodontitis may be associated with its antiinflammatory properties. Although IL-6 has not yet been demonstrated in human periapical lesions, it has been shown to be present in inflamed gingiva[122] and adult marginal periodontitis.[330] IL-8 is a family of chemotactic cytokines[62]; they are produced by

macrophages and a variety of tissue cells, including fibroblasts under the influence of IL-1β and TNF-α. Massive infiltration of neutrophils is a characteristic feature of the acute phases of apical periodontitis. Therefore IL-8 may be active in apical periodontitis in concert with other chemoattractants, such as bacterial peptides, plasma-derived complement split-factor C_{5a}, and leukotriene B_4.

Tumor necrosis factors.   TNF are proinflammatory cytokines with direct cytotoxic effects on certain cells and general debilitating effects in chronic disease. In addition to the cytotoxic effects, the macrophage derived TNF-α[310] and the T-lymphocyte derived TNF-β,[228] formerly *lymphotoxin*, have numerous systemic and local effects similar to those previously described for IL-1. The presence of TNF has been reported in human apical periodontitis lesions and root canal exudates of teeth with apical periodontitis.[12,230]

Interferons.   IFN were originally described in 1957 as selective antiviral agents.[117] They have gradually become recognized as regulatory proteins produced by a variety of cells with wide range of actions on both immunologic and somatic cells. As a result, IFN are now classified as cytokines. There are three structurally distinct IFN: (1) -α molecules, (2) -β molecules, and (3) -γ molecules. The original antiviral protein is the IFN-γ, which is produced by a variety of virus-infected cells and normal T-lymphocytes under various stimuli. However, the IFN-α/β proteins are produced by a variety of normal cells, particularly macrophages and B-lymphocytes.

Colony-stimulating factors.   Another major group of cytokines that regulate the proliferation and differentiation of haematopoietic cells are the colony-stimulating factors (CSF). Their name originates from the early observation that certain polypeptide molecules promote the formation of granulocyte or monocyte colonies in semisolid medium. Three distinct proteins of this category have been isolated, characterized and designated as cytokines. They are (1) granulocyte-macrophage colony stimulating factor (G-MCF), (2) granulocyte colony stimulating factor (G-CSF), and (3) macrophage colony stimulating factor (M-CSF). In general, CSF stimulate the proliferation of neutrophil and osteoclast precursors in the bone marrow. They are also produced by osteoblasts,[220] thus providing one of the communication bridges between osteoblasts and osteoclasts in bone resorption.

Growth factors.   These are proteins that regulate the growth and differentiation on nonhaematopoietic cells. All growth factors are not included among cytokines, but many of them posses some cytokine-like actions. *Transforming growth factors* (TGF) are polypeptides produced by normal and neoplastic cells that were originally identified by their ability to induce nonneoplastic, surface-adherent colonies of fibroblasts in soft agar cultures. This process appears to be similar to neoplastic transformation of normal to malignant cells and, therefore, the name TGF.

Based on their structural relationship to the epidermal growth factor (EGF), TGF are classified into TGF-α and TGF-β. The former is closely related to EGF in structure and biologic effects but produced primarily by malignant cells. Therefore TGF-α is not of much significance in apical periodontitis. However, TGF-β is synthesized by a variety of normal cells and platelets and involved in the recruitment and activation of macrophages, proliferation of fibroblasts, synthesis of connectives tissue fibers and matrices, local angiogenesis, healing, and down regulation of numerous functions of T-lymphocytes. Therefore TGF-β may be an important mediator in countering the adverse effects of inflammatory host response. Based on what is known about its structure and biologic activities, TGF-β polypeptides qualify as cytokines.

Eicosanoids.   When body cells are activated by diverse stimuli, their membrane lipids are remodeled to generate biologically active compounds that serve as intracellular and intercellular signals. Arachidonic acid is a 20-carbon, polysaturated fatty acid that is abundantly present in all cell membranes. It does not occur free in cells but is released from membrane phospholipids by a variety of stimuli and rapidly metabolized to form several biologically active C_{20} compounds (known collectively as eicosanoides [Greek: *eicosi* = twenty]). The eicosanoides are best thought of as hormones with profound physiologic effects at extremely low concentrations. They mediate inflammatory response, regulate blood pressure, induce blood clotting, pain and fever, and control several reproductive functions, such as ovulation and induction of labor. Prostaglandins (PG) and leukotrienes (LT)[234] are two major groups of eicosanoides involved in inflammation.

Prostaglandins.   Prostaglandins were first identified in human semen and were thought to have originated from prostate gland (hence the name). They (e.g., PGE_2, PGD_2, PGF_{2a}, PGI_2) are formed when arachidonic acid is metabolized via the cyclooxygenase pathway. Among them, PGE_2 and PGI_2 are important in inflammation. They are potent activators of osteoclasts. Much of the rapid bone loss in both marginal and apical periodontitis happens during episodes of acute inflammation when the lesions are dominated by PMN, which are important source of PGE_2. High levels of PGE_2 have been shown to be present in acute apical periodontitis lesions.[165] Apical hard tissue resorption can be suppressed by parenteral administration of indomethacin, an inhibitor of cyclooxygenase.[304]

Leukotrienes.   Leukotrienes (e.g., LTA_4, LTB_4, LTC_4, LTD_4, LTE_4) are released when arachidonic acid is oxidized via the lipoxygenase pathway. Among them, LTB_4 is of particular interest because it is a powerful chemotactic agent for neutrophils[206] and causes adhesion of PMN to the endothelial walls. LTB_4[305] and LTC_4[52] have been detected in apical periodontitis, with a high concentration of the former in symptomatic lesions.[305]

Effecto Molecules   Degradation of extracellular matrices is one of the earliest histopathologic changes that takes place in both apical and marginal periodontitis. The destruction of the matrices is caused by enzymatic effector molecules.

At least four degradation pathways have been recognized: (1) osteoclastic pathways, (2) phagocytic pathways, (3) plasminogen-dependent pathways, and (4) MMP-dependent pathways.[30] The MMP are primarily responsible for the degradation of much of the tissue matrices built on collagen, fibronectin, laminin, gelatin, and proteoglycan core proteins. Their biologic activities have been extensively researched and reviewed[31,32]; their importance in the pathogenesis of apical periodontitis is obvious.

Antibodies   Antibodies are the specific chemical weapon system of the body and are produced solely by plasma cells, the progeny of B-lymphocytes. Various classes of immunoglobulins have been found in plasma cells* and extracellularly,[135,160,186,309] in chronic human apical periodontitis. The concentration of IgG in apical periodontitis was found to be nearly five times of that in noninflamed oral mucosa.[88] Immunoglobulins have also been shown in plasma cells residing in the periapical cyst wall[219,256,267,301] and in the cyst fluid.[237,254,301,334] Their concentration in the cyst fluid was found to be several times higher than that in samples of blood.[237,254]

The specificity of the antibodies present in apical periodontitis may be very low, because LPS may act as antigens or mitogens. The resulting antibodies may be a mixture of both monoclonal (i.e., specific) and polyclonal varieties. The latter are nonspecific to the microbial invader and, therefore, ineffective. However, the monoclonal component of the antibody mixture may participate in the antimicrobial response and intensify the pathogenic process by forming antigen and antibody complexes.[304] It has been shown that intracanal application of an antigen (against which the animal was immunized previously) resulted in the induction of a transient apical periodontitis.[307]

PATHOGENESIS AND HISTOPATHOLOGIC NATURE

The microbial and host factors outlined previously may allow clinicians to develop a cohesive view of the pathogenesis of apical periodontitis (Fig. 12-8) and to describe the shifting histopathologic nature of various classes of lesions. The structural components of the lesions depend on the balance between the microbial factors and the host defenses. As the dynamic equilibrium at the periapex tilts toward or away from the host defenses (because of local or unrelated systemic factors), the histologic picture of the lesions can vary considerably. Therefore, the morphologic description[271] of apical periodontitis based on a zonal pattern (originally described for inflammation induced in bone[80]) does not seem to represent the componental variation existing in the majority of periapical lesions. In fact, great structural hetero-

---

*References 120,135,182,219,255,267.

geneity is the "norm" of apical periodontitis, particularly among chronic lesions.[188]

Initially the tooth pulp is infected and becomes necrotic because of an autogenous oral microflora. The endodontic environment provides a selective habitat for the establishment of a mixed, predominantly anaerobic, microbial community in the apical part of the root canal (see Figs. 12-3 and 12-4). The products of such a polymicrobial flora residing in the apical root canal, collectively, have several biologic properties, such as antigenicity, mitogenic activity, vasoactivity, chemotaxis, enzymatic histolysis, and activation of the host defense. As the body defenses cannot exterminate the invaders (well entrenched in the necrotic root canal that is outside the body milieu[134]), apical periodontitis do not heal by themselves. However, the inflammatory response at the periapex prevents microbial invasion into the periradicular tissues, which explains why infectious organisms are only seldom encountered in the body of periapical lesions. Further, many of the endodontic microbial species may not have tissue-invasive properties.[56]

Acute Apical Periodontitis (Primary)

This is usually caused by microorganisms residing in or invading from the apical root canal into the periapical tissue, but it may also be induced by accidental trauma, injury from instrumentation, or irritation from chemicals and endodontic materials, each of which can provoke an intense host response of short duration. It is accompanied by clinical symptoms, such as pain, tooth elevation, and tenderness to pressure on the tooth.

Histopathologically the tissue changes are generally limited to the apical periodontal ligament and the neighboring spongiosa. They are characterized by hyperaemia, vascular congestion, oedema of the periodontal ligament, and extravasation of neutrophils. The latter are attracted to the area by chemotaxis, induced initially by tissue injury, bacterial products (e.g., LPS), and complement factor C_{5a}. As the integrity of the hard tissues (i.e., bone, cementum, dentin) has not yet been disturbed, the periapical changes are radiographically undetectable. If some noninfectious but irritating agents have induced inflammation, the lesion may subside and the structure of the apical periodontium will be restored by healing.

When infection is involved, the neutrophils not only attack and kill the microorganisms but also release leukotrienes and prostaglandins. The former (LTB$_4$) attracts more neutrophils and macrophages into the area, and the latter activate osteoclasts. In a few days the bone surrounding the periapex can be resorbed and a radiolucent area may be detectable at the periapex.[265] This initial rapid bone resorption can be prevented by indomethacin[304,307] that inhibits cyclooxygenase, thus suppressing prostaglandin synthesis. Neutrophils die in great numbers at the inflammatory site and release enzymes from their "suicidal bags," causing destruction of the extracellular matrices and cells. The self-induced destruction of the tissues in the "battle zone" is to

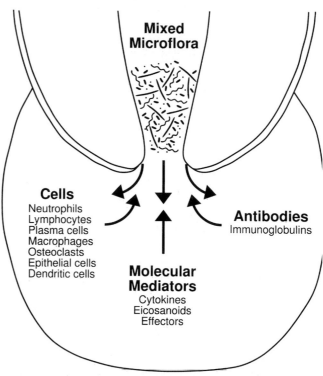

THE INVADERS

Mixed Microflora

Cells
Neutrophils
Lymphocytes
Plasma cells
Macrophages
Osteoclasts
Epithelial cells
Dendritic cells

Antibodies
Immunoglobulins

Molecular Mediators
Cytokines
Eicosanoids
Effectors

THE HOST DEFENSE

Fig. 12-8 A simplified schematic chart of apical periodontitis that is the body's defense response to the destruction of the tooth pulp and the hostile "foreign occupation" of the root canal. The microbial and host defense forces clash and destroy much of the periapical tissues, resulting in the formation of different categories of apical periodontitis lesions. (From Nair PNR: Apical periodontitis: a dynamic encounter between root canal infection and host response, *Periodontology 2000* 13:121, 1997.)

prevent the spread of infection to other parts of the body and also to provide space for the deployment of reinforcements arriving in the form of more specialized defense cells as the battle prolongs to a protracted war.

During the later stages of the acute response, macrophages begin to appear at the periapex. Activated macrophages produce a variety of mediators, among which the proinflammatory (i.e., IL-1, IL-6, TNF-α) and chemotactic (i.e., IL-8) cytokines are of particular importance. These cytokines intensify the local vascular response, osteoclastic bone resorption, effector-mediated degradation of the extracellular matrices, and they can place the body on general alert by endocrine action to sharply raise the output of acute-phase proteins and other serum factors by hepatocytes.[142] They also act in concert with IL-6 to up regulate the production of haematopoietic CSF, which rapidly mobilize the neutrophils and the promacrophages from bone marrow. The acute response can be intensified (particularly in later stages) by the formation of antigen and antibody complexes.[304,307] The acute early lesion may take several possible courses, such as spontaneous healing, further intensification and spreading into the bone (i.e., alveolar abscess), "point" and open to the exterior (i.e., fistulation or sinus tract formation), or the lesion may become chronic.

Chronic Apical Periodontitis

In the continual presence of irritants (e.g., bacteria or their products), the neutrophil-dominated early lesion gradually shifts to a macrophage, lymphocyte, and plasma cell–rich lesion that is encapsulated in a collagenous connective tissue. Such asymptomatic, radiolucent lesion can be visualized as a "lull phase," after the intense and "high casualty" battle in which neutrophils "fell" in great numbers but the foreign intruders into the periapex were temporarily beaten and the enemy held back in the root canal (see Fig. 12-3). The macrophage-derived proinflammatory cytokines (i.e., IL-1, -6, TNF-α) are powerful lymphocyte stimulators. Although the quantitative data on the various types of cells residing in chronic periapical lesions are probably far from representative, investigations based on monoclonal antibodies tend to suggest a predominant role for T-lymphocytes and macrophages.

Activated T-cells produce a variety of cytokines that down regulate the output of proinflammatory cytokines (i.e., IL-1, IL-6, TNF-α), leading to the suppression of osteoclastic activity and reduced bone resorption. On the other hand, the T cell–derived cytokines may concomitantly up-regulate the production of growth factors (i.e., TGF-β), with stimulatory and proliferative effects on fibroblasts and the microvasculature. T_{h1} and T_{h2} cell populations may participate in this process. The option to down regulate the destructive process explains the absence of (or slowed) bone resorption and rebuilding of the collagenous connective tissue during the chronic phase of the disease. Consequently, the chronic lesions can remain "dormant" and symptomless for long periods of time without major changes in the radiographic status. However, at any time the delicate equilibrium prevailing at the periapex can be disturbed by one or more factors that may favor the microbial enemy stationed within the root canal. The microbes may advance into the periapex (Figs. 12-9 and 12-10) and the lesion spontaneously becomes acute, with clinical manifestations (i.e., secondary acute apical periodontitis, periapical exacerbation, phoenix abscess). As a result, microorganisms can be found extraradicularly during these acute episodes (see Fig. 12-10), with possibly rapid enlargement of the radiolucent area. The presence of this characteristic radiographic feature is because of apical bone resorption occurring rapidly during the acute phases, with relative inactivity during the chronic periods. The progression of the disease, therefore, is not continuous, but happens in discrete leaps after periods of "stability."

Chronic apical periodontitis is commonly referred to as dental or periapical granuloma. Histopathologically it consists of a granulomatous tissue with infiltrate cells, fibroblasts (Fig. 12-11, *A*), and a well-developed fibrous capsule. Serial sectioning shows[192] that about 45% of all chronic periapical lesions are epithelialized (Fig. 12-11, *B*). When the epithelial cells begin to proliferate, they may do so in all directions at random, forming an irregular epithelial mass in which vascular and infiltrated connective tissue becomes enclosed. In some lesions the epithelium may grow into the entrance of the root canal, forming a pluglike seal at the apical foramen.[157,195,259] The epithelial cells generate an "epithelial attachment" to the root surface or canal wall, which in TEM reveals a basal lamina and hemidesmosomal structures.[195] In random histologic sections the epithelium in the lesion characteristically appears as arcades and rings (see Fig. 12-11, *B*). The extraepithelial tissue predominantly consists of small blood vessels, lymphocytes, plasma cells, and macrophages. Among the lymphocytes, T-cells are likely to be more numerous than B-cells[53,130,202,306] and CD4+ cells may outnumber CD8+ cells[15,151,159,215] in certain phases of the lesions. The connective tissue capsule of the lesion consists of dense collagenous fibers that are firmly attached to the root surface so that the lesion may be removed *in toto* with the extracted tooth.

Periapical or Radicular Cyst

Periapical or radicular cysts are generally considered to be a direct sequel to chronic apical periodontitis, but not every chronic lesion develops into a cyst. Although the reported incidence of cysts among apical periodontitis lesions varies from 6% to 55% (Table 12-2), investigations based on meticulous serial sectioning and strict histopathologic criteria[192,248,259] show that the actual incidence of the cysts may be well below 20%. As has been stated before, there are two distinct categories of radicular cysts: (1) those containing cavities completely enclosed in epithelial lining (Fig. 12-12), and (2) those containing epithelium-lined cavities that are open to the root canals (Fig. 12-13).[192,248] The latter was originally described as "bay cysts"[248] but has been newly designated as *periapical pocket cysts*.[192] More than half of the cystic lesions are apical true cysts, and the reminder are apical pocket cysts.[192,248] In view of the structural difference between the two categories of cysts, the pathogenic pathways leading to the formation of them may differ in certain respects.

Periapical True Cyst   There have been several attempts to explain the pathogenesis of apical true cysts.* The process of true cyst formation has been discussed as occurring in three stages.[245] During the first phase the dormant cell rests of Malassez[156,157] are believed to proliferate, probably under the influence of growth factors that are released by various cells residing in the lesion. During the second phase, an epithelium-lined cavity comes into existence.

---

*References 84,155,224,244,292,295,303.

Text continued on p. 476

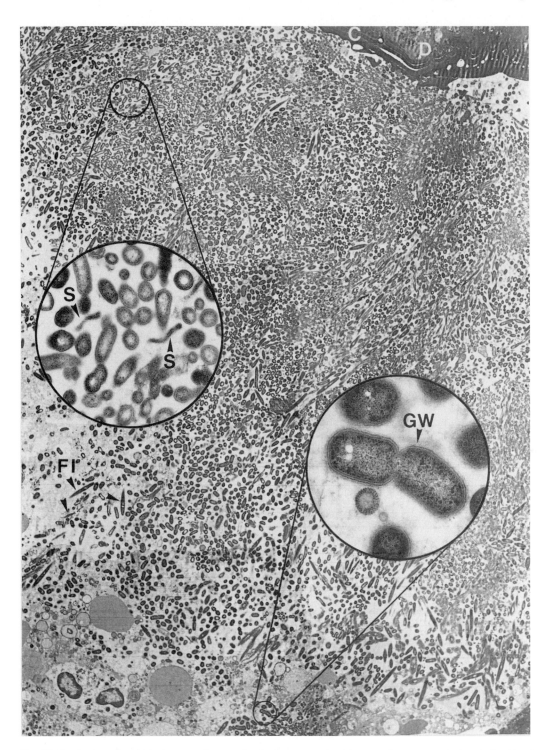

Fig. 12-9 Massive microbial plaque at the root tip of a human tooth with secondary acute apical periodontitis of endodontic origin. The mixed bacterial flora consists of numerous dividing cocci, rods (*lower inset*), filaments (*Fl*), and spirochetes (*S, upper inset*). Rods often reveal a gram-negative cell wall (*GW, lower inset*). (*C*: cementum, *D*: dentin.) (Magnifications: × 2' 680, *upper inset* × 19' 200, *lower inset* × 36' 400.) (Adapted from Nair PNR: Light and electron microscopic studies of root canal flora and periapical lesions, *J Endod* 13:29, 1987.)

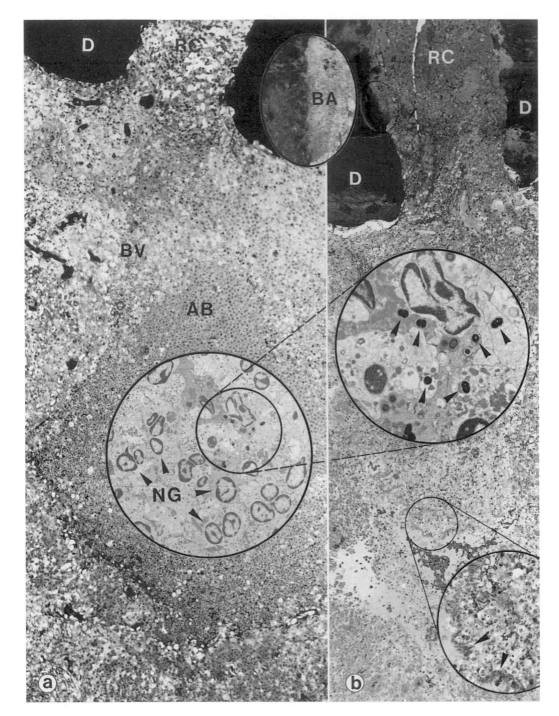

Fig. 12-10 Structure of secondary periapical abscess. **A**, An axial section of an abscessed apical periodontitis. The microabscess (*AB*) contains a focus of neutrophils (*NG inset* in *A*). Note the phagocytosed bacteria in one of the neutrophils that are further magnified in the large inset in **B**. The secondary abscess is formed by bacteria (*BA* in *oval inset*) from the apical root canal (*RC*) advancing into the chronic apical periodontitis lesion (*B*). Note the tissue necrosis immediately in front of the apical foramen and the bacterial front within the body of the lesion (*arrowhead in lower inset*). (*D*: dentin, *BV*: blood vessel.) (Magnifications: *A* × 130, *B* × 100, *oval inset* × 400, *inset* in *A* × 2' 680, *upper inset* in *B* × 4'900, *lower inset* in *B* × 250.) (From Nair PNR: Apical periodontitis: a dynamic encounter between root canal infection and host response, *Periodontology 2000* 13:121, 1997.)

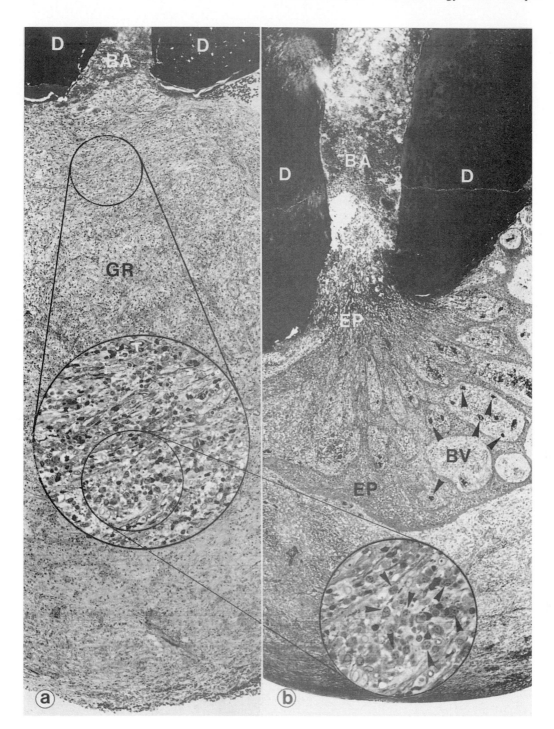

Fig. 12-11 Chronic asymptomatic apical periodontitis without (**A**) and with (**B**) epithelium (*EP*). The root canal contains bacteria (*BA*). Lesion *A* is without acute inflammatory cells (even at the mouth of the root canal) with visible bacteria at the apical foramen (*BA*). Note the collagen-rich maturing granulation tissue (*GR*) infiltrated with plasma cells and lymphocytes (*insets* in *A* and *B*). (*D*: dentin, *BV*: blood vessels.) (Magnifications: *A* × 80; *B* × 60, inset in *A* × 250, *inset* in *B* × 400.) (From Nair PNR: Apical periodontitis: a dynamic encounter between root canal infection and host response, *Periodontology 2000* 13:121, 1997.)

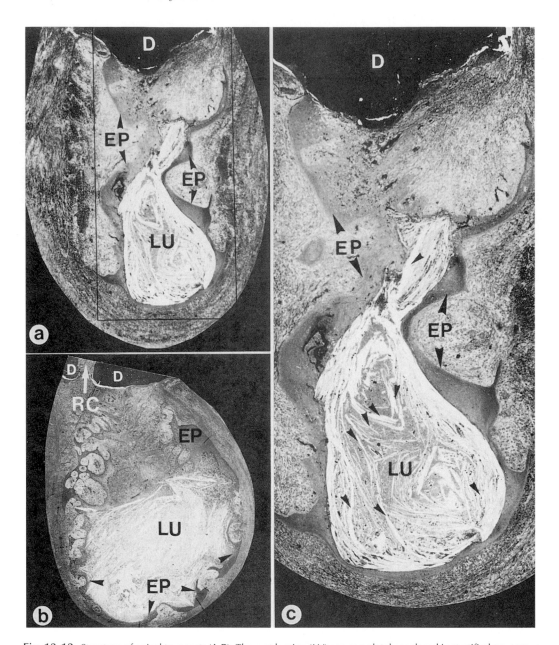

Fig. 12-12 Structure of apical true cysts (**A,B**). The cyst lumina (*LU*) are completely enclosed in stratified squamous epithelium (*EP*). Note the absence of any communication of the cyst lumen with the root canal (*RC* in *B*). The demarcated area in *A* is magnified in C. Arrowheads in c indicate cholesterol clefts. (Magnifications: *A* × 30, *B* × 17, *C* × 60.) (From Nair PNR, Pajarola G, Schroeder HE: Types and incidence of human periapical lesions obtained with extracted teeth, *Oral Surg Oral Med Oral Pathol* 81:93, 1996.)

There are two long-standing hypotheses regarding the formation of the cyst cavity:

1. The "nutritional deficiency theory" is based on the assumption that the central cells of the epithelial strands get removed from their source of nutrition and undergo necrosis and liquefactive degeneration. The accumulating products, in turn, attract neutrophilic granulocytes into the necrotic area. Such microcavities containing degenerating epithelial cells, infiltrating leukocytes, and tissue exudate coalesce to form the cyst cavity lined by stratified squamous epithelium.

2. The "abscess theory" postulates that the proliferating epithelium surrounds an abscess formed by tissue necrosis and lysis because of the inherent nature of epithelial cells to cover exposed connective tissue surfaces. During the third phase, the cyst grows, the exact mechanism of which has not yet been adequately clarified.

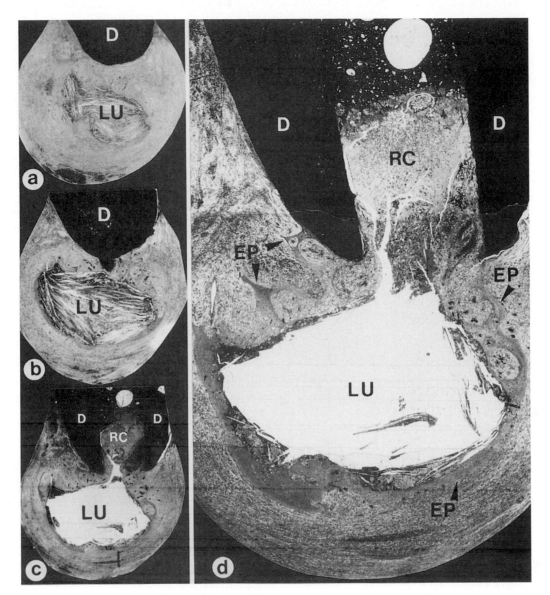

Fig 12-13 Structure of an apical pocket cyst. Axial sections passing peripheral to the root canal (**A,B**) give the false impression of the presence of a cyst lumen (*LU*) completely enclosed in epithelium. Sequential section (**C,D**) passing through axial plane of the root canal (*RC*) clearly reveals the continuity of the cystic lumen (*LU*) with the root canal (*RC*). Note the pouchlike lumen (*LU*) of the pocket cyst with the epithelium (*EP*) forming a collar at the root apex. (Magnifications: *A-C* × 15, *D* × 132.) (Adapted from Nair PNR: Eine neue Sicht der radikulären Zysten—Sind sie heilbar?, *Endodontie* 4:169, 1995.)

Theories based on osmotic pressure[119,299,300] have receded to the background in recent years as research attention has shifted in favor of finding a molecular basis for the cystogenesis.[29,40,96,97,293] The fact that apical pocket cyst (see Fig. 12-13) (with a lumen open to the necrotic root canal) can grow would eliminate osmotic pressure as a potential factor in the development of radicular cysts. Although no direct evidence is yet available, the tissue dynamics and the cellular components of radicular cysts suggest possible molecular pathways for cyst expansion. The neutrophils perishing in the cyst lumen provide a continuous source of prostaglandins,[81] which can diffuse through the porous epithelial wall[245] into the surrounding tissues. The cell population residing in the extraepithelial area contains numerous T-lymphocytes[306] and macrophages (Fig. 12-14, *A-B*) that are known to produce a battery of cytokines, particularly the IL-1β. The prostaglandins and the inflammatory cytokines can activate osteoclasts, culminating in bone resorption. The presence of

Table 12-2 THE INCIDENCE OF RADICULAR CYSTS AMONG PERIAPICAL LESIONS

Reference	Cysts %	Granuloma %	Others %	Total lesions n
Sommer & Kerr[258]	6	84	10	170
Block et al[33]	6	—	94	230
Sonnabend & Oh[259]	7	93	—	170
Winstock[326]	8	83	9	9804*
Linenberg et al[146]	9	80	11	110
Wais[318]	14	84	2	50
Patterson & Shafer[213]	14	84	2	510
Nair et al[192]	15	50	35	256
Simon[248]	17	54	23	35
Stockdale & Chandler[272]	17	77	6	1108
Lin et al[145]	19	—	81	150
Nobuhara & Del Rio[203]	22	59	19	150
Baumann & Rossman[17]	26	74	—	121
Mortensen et al[181]	41	59	—	396
Bhaskar[26]	42	48	10	2308
Spatafore et al[262]	42	52	6	1659
Lalonde & Luebke[137]	44	45	11	800
Seltzer et al[239]	51	45	4	87
Zain[336]	53	38	8	149
Priebe et al[218]	55	46	—	101

* Number of operations performed. The author does not explicitly say whether all the 9804 biopsies were subjected to histopathologic diagnosis.

effector molecules (i.e., MMP-1, MMP-2) have also been reported in human periapical cysts.[293]

Histopathologically there are four major components in an apical true cyst: (1) cyst cavity, (2) epithelial cyst wall, (3) extraepithelial tissue, and (4) collagenous capsule. The cavity, completely enclosed in an epithelial lining, generally reveals necrotic tissue and, on occasion, cholesterol clefts and erythrocytes (the presence of the latter is probably due to hemorrhage). The thickness of the stratified squamous epithelium can vary from a few to several cell layers. Scanning electron microscopy (SEM) (see Fig. 12-14, *A*) of the inner surface of the cyst wall reveals flat epithelial and globular cells (i.e., the surface of the epithelium and neutrophils protruding through the intercellular spaces). The basal cell side of the epithelium is irregular, so as to form ridges. Correlative studies using SEM, light microscopy (LM) and TEM of the specimens (see Fig. 12-14, *B*) show numerous intraepithelial neutrophils in the process of transmigration across the epithelium into the cyst lumen. The tissue existing between the epithelial lining and the fibrous capsule usually consists of numerous blood vessels and infiltrating cells, predominantly T-lymphocytes,[306] B-lymphocytes, plasma cells, and macrophages (see Fig. 12-14, *B*). Neutrophils, which are numerous in the epithelial lining, are rarely found in the extraepithelial area.

Periapical Pocket Cyst A periapical pocket cyst is probably initiated by the accumulation of neutrophils around the apical foramen in response to the bacterial presence in the apical root canal. The microabscess so formed can become enclosed by the proliferating epithelium that, on coming in contact with the root tip, forms an epithelial collar with "epithelial attachment."[195] The latter seals off the infected root canal and microabscess from the periapical milieu. When the externalized neutrophils die and disintegrate, the space occupied by them becomes a microcystic sac. The presence of microbes in the apical root canal, their products, and the necrosed cells in the cyst lumen attract more neutrophilic granulocytes by a chemotactic gradient. However, the pouchlike lumen, biologically outside the periapical milieu, acts as a "death trap" to the transmigrating neutrophils. As the necrotic cells accumulate, the saclike lumen enlarges to accommodate the debris and may form a voluminous diverticulum of the root canal space extending into the periapical area (see Fig. 12-13, *C* and *D*). Bone resorption and degradation of the matrices occurring in association with the enlargement of the pocket cyst may follow a similar molecular pathway, such as in the case of the periapical true cyst.[192] From the pathogenic, structural, tissue dynamic, and host benefit standpoint, the pouchlike extension of the root canal space has much in common with a marginal peri-

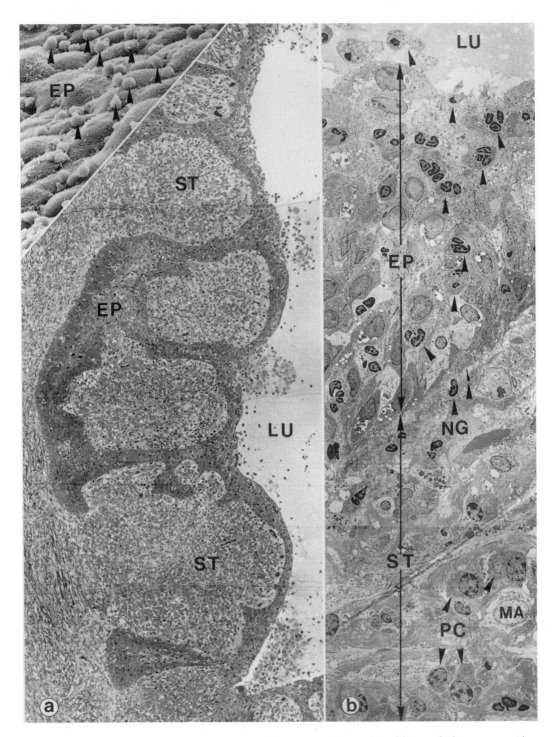

Fig. 12-14 Fine structure of an apical true cyst. **A**, A light microscopic overview of the stratified squamous epithelium (*EP*) that lines a true cyst lumen (*LU*). **B** is a transmission electron microscopic montage. The subepithelial tissue (*ST*) consists of plasma cells (*PC* in **B**), macrophages (*MA*), and lymphocytes. Neutrophils (*arrowheads* in B) transmigrate through the epithelium into the cyst lumen. The inset on the upper left-hand corner is a scanning electron microscopic view of the flat epithelial cells (*EP*) that line the inner wall of the lumen and globular neutrophilic granulocytes (*arrowheads*) emerging through the intercellular spaces into the lumen. (Magnifications: *A* × 83, *B* × 1400, *inset* × 700.) (From Nair PNR: Apical periodontitis: a dynamic encounter between root canal infection and host response, *Periodontology 2000* 13:121, 1997.)

odontal pocket; hence the name periapical pocket cyst.[192] Histologically the stratified squamous epithelial lining and the rest of the cyst wall are similar to those of a true cyst.

SPECIAL PATHOLOGIC MANIFESTATIONS

Transient Apical Periodontitis

Although no histologic evidence is yet available, "sterile" apical periodontitis of transient nature may develop as a result of moderate trauma of the periapical tissues. A periapical radiolucency developing after such injury to the apical periodontium that resolves without intervening treatment has been designated as transient apical breakdown.[9,34] In a radiographic analysis of 637 luxated teeth, such transient apical radiolucencies were found to occur in about 4% of the injured teeth.[9] The radiographic lesion appears sometime after the injury and is usually associated with discoloration of the tooth and loss of pulpal sensitivity. These changes are reversible, and the tooth will gradually return to normal. If a radiolucency is the principal criteria of diagnosis, the radiographic lesion may be incorrectly diagnosed as apical periodontitis developing as a consequence of endodontic infection, and invasive therapeutic procedures may follow. Therefore a diagnosis should be reached in association with the previous history of trauma and monitoring of the tooth for reversibility of the tooth discoloration, pulpal sensitivity, and apical radiolucency.

Condensing Apical Periodontitis

A special radiographic and histologic manifestation of chronic periradicular inflammation of pulpal origin has been known as condensing osteitis, or focal sclerosing osteomyelitis. The condition is more prevalent among young and middle-aged subjects, and diseased mandibular first molars are more commonly affected. The lesions appear as well-circumscribed radiopacities of periradicular bone[101] of teeth with necrotic pulps, which may or may not be sensitive to percussion stimuli. Histologically[172] such lesions reveal a dense mass of bony trabeculae, with limited marrow space. The osseous tissue is lined by osteoblasts, and the marrow space may be infiltrated with lymphocyte. Conventional root canal treatment usually results in a complete resolution of the condition.[101] However, it has to be differentially diagnosed from advanced stages of cemental dysplasia, which is a benign tumor of unknown cause that affects healthy teeth with vital pulps.

Cholesterol and Apical Periodontitis

Cholesterol[291] is a lipid of the steroid family that is present in almost all animal tissues. The name is derived from the Greek *Chole-stereos* (i.e., "bile solid"), because of its occurrence in gall stones. Cholesterol is a major structural component of animal plasma membranes and an important deter-minant of membrane properties. Therefore it is abundant in myelin and other "membrane-rich" tissues and cells. It is the precursor of bile acids, steroid hormones, and provitamin D_3.[332] Excess blood level of cholesterol is suspected to play a role in atherosclerosis as a result of its deposition in the vascular walls.[332,333] Local deposition of crystalline cholesterol also occurs in other tissues and organs, as in the case of otitis media and the "pearly tumor" of the cranium.[7] In the oral region, accumulation of cholesterol crystals occurs in apical periodontitis lesions,* with clinical significance in endodontics and oral surgery.[190,198]

Apical periodontitis lesions often contain deposits of cholesterol crystals (Fig. 12-15) that appear as narrow, elongated tissue clefts in histopathologic sections. The crystals dissolve in fat solvents used for the tissue processing and leave behind the spaces they occupied as clefts. The reported incidence of cholesterol clefts in apical periodontitis varies from 18% to 44% of such lesions.[38,63,244,313] The crystals are believed to be formed from cholesterol released by (1) disintegrating erythrocytes of stagnant blood vessels within the lesion[38]; (2) lymphocytes, plasma cells, and macrophages that die in great numbers and disintegrate in chronic periapical lesions[313]; and (3) the circulating plasma lipids.[244]

It is possible that all these sources may contribute to the concentration and crystallization of cholesterol in periapical area. Nevertheless, locally dying inflammatory cells may be the major source of cholesterol as a result of its release from disintegrating membranes of such cells in chronic, long-standing lesions.[198,238] The crystals are initially formed in the inflamed periapical connective tissue, where they act as foreign bodies and excite a giant-cell reaction.

In histologic sections it is common to observe numerous multinucleated giant cells around the cholesterol clefts (see Fig. 12-15). When a large number of crystals accumulate in the inflamed connective tissue, they passively move in the direction of least resistance. If the lesion happens to be a radicular cyst, the crystals move in the direction of the epithelium-lined cyst cavity, because moving through the outer collagenous capsule of the lesion is much more difficult. The slow, "glacierlike" movement of the crystal mass erodes the epithelial lining (see Fig. 12-15) and empties the crystals into the cyst lumen.

Periapical cysts[296] and apical granuloma[26] in which cholesterol clefts form a major component have been referred to as "cholesteatoma." This term is borrowed from general pathology, where it refers to a local accumulation of cholesterol crystals causing discomfort and dysfunction of the affected organs.[7] Therefore the term may be dropped altogether or used more specifically as "apical cholesteatoma," so as to distinguish the condition from cholesteatoma affecting other tissues and organs.[198]

Tissue reaction to cholesterol crystals is well understood in conjunction with the role of the crystals in cardiovascular diseases. Cholesterol crystals are intensely sclerogenic.[1,21]

---

*References 26,38,63,183,198,244,313.

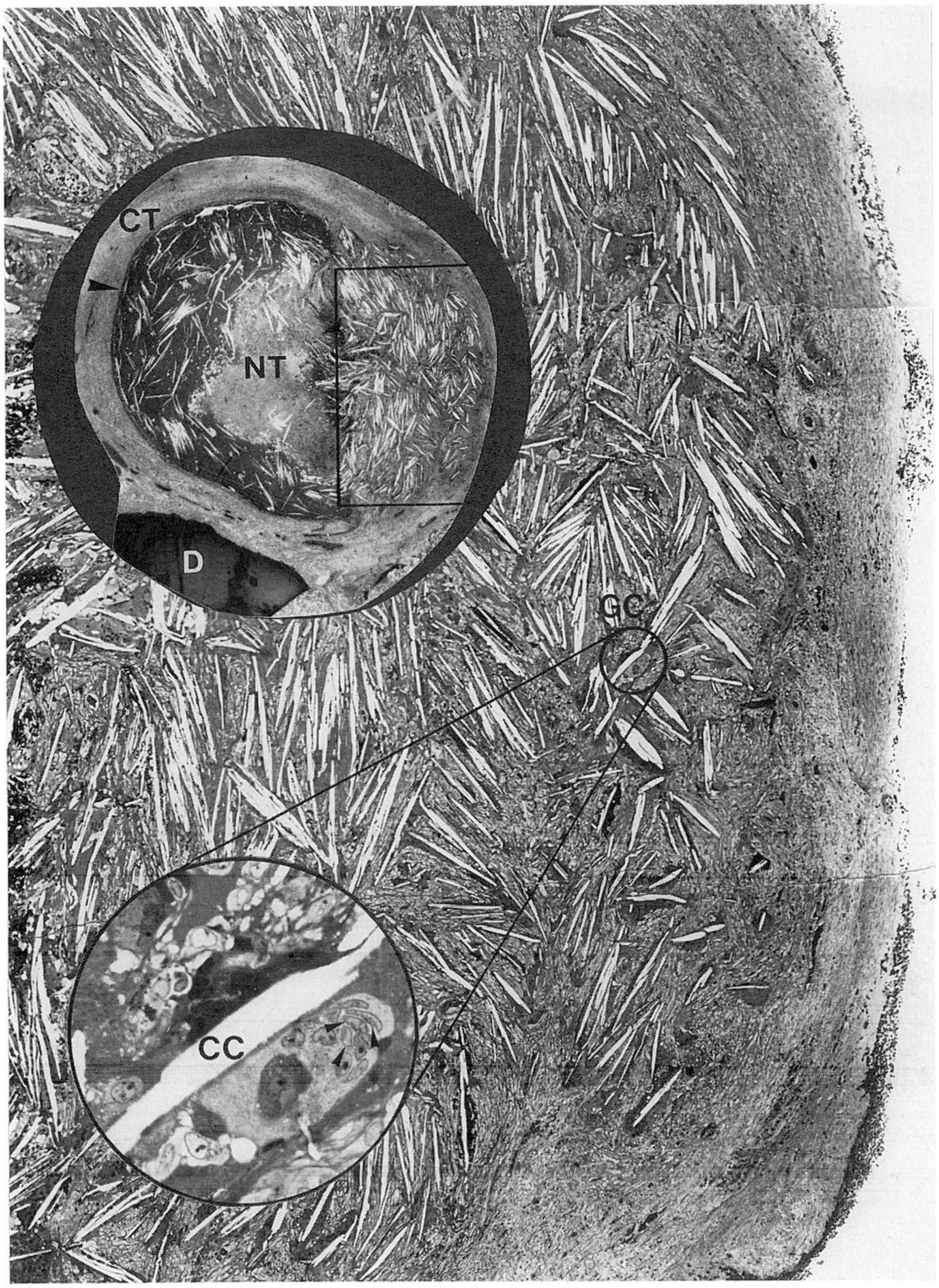

Fig. 12-15 Cholesterol in apical periodontitis: Overview of a histologic section (*upper inset*) of an asymptomatic apical periodontitis that persisted after conventional root canal treatment. Note the vast number of cholesterol clefts (*CC*) surrounded by giant cells (*GC*) of which a selected one with several nuclei (*arrowheads*) is magnified in the lower inset. (*D*: dentine, *CT*: connective tissue, *NT*: necrotic tissue.) (Magnifications: x 68, *upper inset* x 11, *lower inset* x 412.) (From Nair PNR: Cholesterol as an aetilogical agent in endodontic failures—a review, *Aus Endod J* 25:19, 1999.)

They have been shown to induce granulomatous lesions in dogs,[49] mice,[1,3,4,21,261] and rabbits.[106,260,261] These studies consistently showed that the cholesterol crystals were densely surrounded by macrophages and giant cells.

One experimental report specifically addressed the potential association of cholesterol crystals and nonresolving apical periodontitis lesions.[199] In this study on guinea pigs, the tissue reaction to cholesterol crystals was investigated by using a Teflon cage model[152] to answer the question as to whether aggregates of cholesterol crystals would induce and sustain a granulomatous tissue reaction in guinea pigs. Pure cholesterol crystals, prepared to a mushy form, were placed in Teflon cages that were implanted subcutaneously in guinea pigs. The cage contents were retrieved after 2, 4, and 32 weeks of implantation; they were then processed for LM and electron microscopy. The cages revealed delicate, soft connective tissue that grew in through perforations on the cage wall.

The crystals were densely surrounded by numerous macrophages and multinucleated giant cells, forming a well-circumscribed area of tissue reaction. The cells, however, were unable to eliminate the crystals during an observation period of 8 months. The tissue response to cholesterol crystals observed in the investigation was totally in agreement with the findings of previous morphologic investigations.* The congregation of macrophages and giant cells around cholesterol crystals suggests that the crystals induced a typical foreign-body reaction.[51,197,253]

In the context of periapical healing after root canal treatment, it is of interest to know to what extent the body cells are able to eliminate locally accumulated cholesterol crystals. Such degradation, if any, should happen via the phagocytic or biochemical pathways or both. To degrade tissue deposits of cholesterol crystals, the cells surrounding them should have the ability to attack the crystals chemically to disperse the crystals into the surrounding tissue fluid or to make them accessible to the cells themselves. Cholesterol crystals are highly hydrophobic, and their dispersal would necessitate making them hydrophilic and "soluble" in an aqueous medium.[1] The granulomatous and sclerogenic effects of cholesterol crystals can be prevented by the incorporation of phospholipids into subcutaneous implants of cholesterol.[3] This beneficial effect of phospholipids has been attributed to their "detergent" property and their role as donors of polyunsaturated fatty acids during esterification of the cholesterol.[1,4] The giant cells and macrophages are known to esterify and mobilize cholesterol in a lipid droplet form.[21] Macrophages can convert particulate cholesterol into a soluble form by incorporating it into a lipoprotein vehicle[66,302] so that the cholesterol can be readily esterified or added into the lipoprotein pool in circulation. These biologic findings, obviously in support of the possible ability of macrophages and giant cells to degrade particulate cholesterol, are not consistent with the histopathologic observation of spontaneous[26,198,295] and experimentally induced* cholesterol granuloma.

The characteristic feature of such lesions is the accumulation of macrophages and giant cells around the cholesterol clefts and their persistence for long periods of time. Therefore it is to be assumed that the macrophages and the multinucleate giant cells that congregate around cholesterol crystals are unable to destroy the crystals in a way beneficial to the host.[36]

Although the presence of cholesterol crystals in apical periodontitis lesions has long been observed to be a common histopathologic feature, its significance to failed root canal treatments has not yet been fully appreciated.[191] The tissue dynamics of apical periodontitis lesions containing cholesterol crystals are no longer dependent on the presence or absence of irritants in the root canal. The macrophages and giant cells that accumulate around cholesterol crystals are not only unable to degrade the crystalline cholesterol, they are major sources of apical inflammatory and bone-resorptive mediators.

Evidence shows that accumulation of cholesterol crystals in apical periodontitis lesions (see Fig. 12-15) can adversely affect posttherapeutic healing of the periapical tissues. This has been shown in a long-term, longitudinal follow up of a case in which the authors concluded that "the presence of vast numbers of cholesterol crystals . . . would be sufficient to sustain the lesion indefinitely."[198] The evidence presented from the general literature is clearly in support of that assumption. Therefore accumulation of cholesterol crystals in apical periodontitis lesions can prevent healing of periapical tissues after conventional root canal treatment. Endodontic retreatment is unlikely to resolve the problem of tissue-irritating cholesterol crystals[198] and other extraradicular agents* that sustain posttherapeutic periapical lesions, because they exist outside the root canal system. Apical surgery is indicated for successful outcome of such cases.

Periapical Actinomycosis

Actinomycosis is a chronic, granulomatous, infectious disease in man and animals that is caused by the genera *Actinomyces* and *Propionibacterium*.[164] The causative agent of bovine actinomycosis, *Actinomyces bovis*, was the first species to be identified.[99] The disease in cattle, known as "lumpy jaw" or "big head disease," is characterized by extensive bone rarefaction, swelling of the jaw suppuration, and fistulation. The causative agents were described as nonacidfast, nonmotile, gram-positive organisms, revealing characteristic branching filaments that end in clubs or hyphae. Because of the morphologic appearance, these organisms were considered fungi and the taxonomy of *Actinomyces* remained controversial for more than a century. The intertwining, filamentous colonies are often called "sulphur granules," because of their appearance as yellow specks in exudate. On careful crushing, the tiny clumps of branching microorganisms with radiating filaments in pus give a "starburst appearance" that prompted Harz[99] to coin the name

---

*References 1,3,21,49,260,261.

*References 131,133,194,197,198,252.

Actinomyces, or "ray fungus." Four years later *Actinomyces israelii* was isolated from humans in pure culture. Then it was characterized and its pathogenicity in animals demonstrated.[328] Many researchers, nevertheless, considered the human and bovine isolates as identical. However, *A. bovis* and *A. israelii* are now classified as two distinct bacterial species, and in natural infections the former is restricted to animals and the later to humans.

Human actinomycosis is clinically divided into cervicofacial, thoracic, and abdominal forms. About 60% of the cases occur in the cervicofacial region, 20% in the abdomen, and 15% in the thorax.[124,208] The most species isolated from humans is *A. israelii,* [328] which is followed by *Propionibacterium propionicum,*[41] *Actinomyces naeslundii,*[298] *Actinomyces viscosus,*[111] and *Actinomyces odontolyticus*[16] (in descending order).

Periapical actinomycosis (Fig. 12-16) is a cervicofacial form of actinomycosis. The endodontic infections are generally a sequel to caries. *A. israelii* is commensal of the oral cavity and can be isolated from tonsils, dental plaque, periodontal pockets, and carious lesions.[283] Most of the publications on periapical actinomycosis are case reports and have been reviewed.* Although periapical actinomycosis is considered to be rare,[194] it may not be so infrequent.[116,178,232] The data on the frequency of periapical actinomycosis among apical periodontitis lesions is scarce. A microbiologic control study revealed actinomycotic involvement in 2 of the 79 endodontically treated cases.[44] A histologic analysis showed the presence of characteristic actinomycotic colonies (see Fig. 12-16, *A*) in 2 of the 45 investigated lesions.[194] Identification of the species involved (and cause of infection) can be established only through laboratory culturing of the organisms[283] and by experimental induction of the lesion in susceptible animals.[79] However, the strict growth requirements of *A. israelii* make isolation in pure culture difficult. Therefore a laboratory diagnosis is generally reached on the basis of histologic demonstration of typical colonies[194] and by specific immunohistochemical staining of such colonies.[94,283] The characteristic light microscopic feature of an actinomycotic colony is the presence of an intensely dark staining, gram- and PAS-positive core, with radiating peripheral filaments (see Fig. 12-16, *A*) that gives the typical "star burst" or "ray fungus" appearance.

Ultrastructurally[79,194] the center of the colony consists of a dense aggregation of branching filamentous organisms held together by an extracellular matrix (see Fig. 12-16, *B*). Several layers of PMN usually surround an actinomycotic colony.

Because of the ability of certain actinomycotic organisms to establish extraradicularly (see Fig. 12-16) to perpetuate the inflammation at the periapex (even after proper root canal treatment), periapical actinomycosis is of special importance in endodontics.[93,94,194,252,283] *A. israelii* and *P. proprionicum* are the most consistently isolated and characterized microorganisms from the periapical tissue of teeth that did not respond to proper conventional endodontic treatment.[93,252] *A.*

israelii has been specifically implicated in periapical actinomycosis.[204,283] The biologic properties that enable these bacteria to establish in the periapical tissues are not fully understood, but they appear to involve the ability to build cohesive colonies (see Fig. 12-16) that enables them to escape the host defense system.[79]

Foreign-Body Reactions

There is general agreement that microorganisms are the main causative agents of apical periodontitis. Nevertheless, foreign materials trapped in periapical tissue[133,197] can initiate and perpetuate certain apical periodontitis lesions, particularly those persisting after root canal treatment. Endodontic clinical materials[133,197] and food particles[249] may reach the periapex and cause a foreign-body reaction that may appear radiolucent and remain asymptomatic for many years.[197]

Oral Pulse Granuloma   This lesion denotes a foreign-body reaction to particles of vegetable food materials, particularly leguminous seeds (i.e., pulses) that get lodged in the oral tissues. Oral pulse granuloma is a distinct histopathologic entity.[127] The lesions are also referred to as the giant cell hyalin angiopathy,[73,127] vegetable granuloma,[98] and food-induced granuloma.[36] Pulse granuloma have been reported in lungs,[100] stomach walls, and peritoneal cavities.[246] Experimental lesions have been induced in animals by intratracheal, intraperitonial, and submucous introduction of leguminous seeds.[129,288] Periapical pulse granuloma are associated with teeth grossly damaged by caries and with the history of endodontic therapy.[249,289] Pulse granuloma are characterized by the presence of intensely iodine- and PAS-positive hyaline rings or bodies, surrounded by giant cells and inflammatory cells.[171,249,288,289] The cellulose in plant materials has been suggested to be the granuloma-inducing agent.[129] However, leguminous seeds are the most frequently involved vegetable food material in such granulomatous lesions. This indicates that other components in pulses, such as antigenic proteins and mitogenic phytohaemaagglutinins, may also be involved in the pathologic tissue response.[129] The pulse granuloma are clinically significant because particles of vegetable food materials can get lodged under the mucous membrane by the pressure of dentures[289] or can reach the periapical tissue via root canals of teeth exposed to the oral cavity by trauma, carious damage, or endodontic procedures.[249]

Cellulose Granuloma   This term is more specifically used for pathologic-tissue reaction developing against particles of predominantly cellulose-containing materials that are used in endodontic practice.[131,132,236,323] Endodontic paper points are used for microbial sampling and drying of root canals. Medicated cotton wool has been used as an apical seal. Particles of these materials can dislodge or get pushed into the periapical tissue,[323] so as to induce a foreign-body reaction at the periapex. Such clinical situations can result in "prolonged, extremely troublesome and disconcerted course of events."[323]

---

*References 39,158,194,232,233,322.

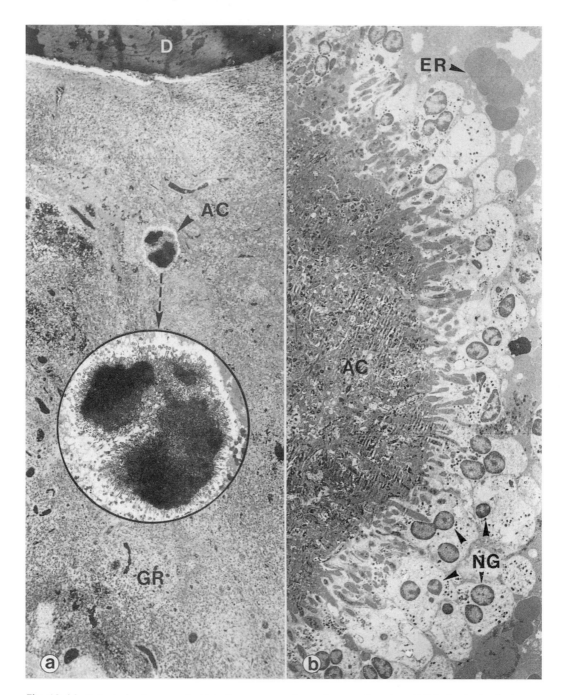

Fig. 12-16 Periapical actinomycosis. Note the presence of an actinomycotic colony (*AC*) in the body of a human apical periodontitis lesion (*GR*), revealing typical "starburst" appearance (*inset* in **A**). The transmission electron microscopic montage (**B**) shows the peripheral area of the colony with filamentous organisms surrounded by few layers of neutrophilic granulocytes (*NG*). (*D*: dentin, *ER*: erythrocytes.) (Magnifications: *A* × 70, *inset* × 250, *B* × 2' 200.) (Adapted from Nair PNR, Schroeder HE: Periapical actinomycosis, *J Endod* 10:567, 1984.)

Presence of cellulose fibers in periapical biopsies with a history of previous endodontic treatment has been reported.[131,132,236] The endodontic paper points and cotton wool consists of cellulose, which is neither digested by humans nor degraded by the body cells. They remain in tissues for long periods of time[236] and evoke a foreign-body reaction around them. The particles, when viewed in polarized light, reveal birefringence because of the regular struc-tural arrangement of the molecules within cellulose.[131] Infected paper points can project through the apical foramen into the periapical tissue (Fig. 12-17) and may allow bacterial plaque to grow around the paper point. This will sustain and intensify the apical periodontitis lesion.

Gutta-percha The major root canal sealant used in ortho-grade obturation of root canals is gutta-percha cone. It is

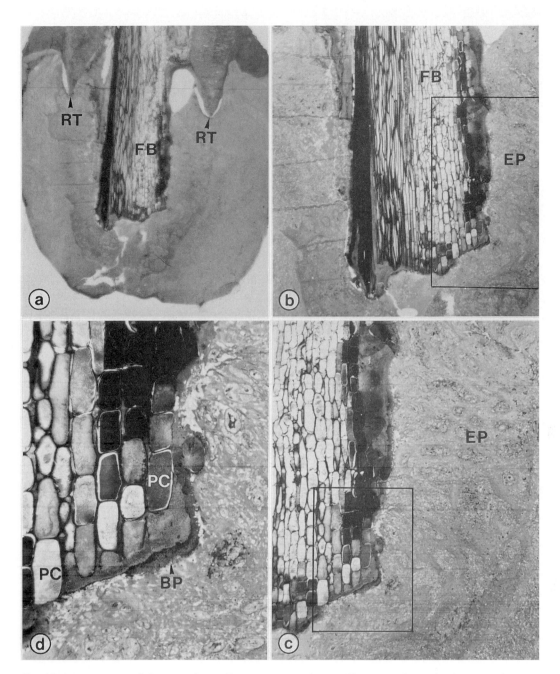

Fig. 12-17 A massive cellulose granuloma affecting a root canal–treated human tooth (**A**). The demarcated area in **B** is magnified in **C**, and it is further magnified in **D**. Note the tip of the foreign body (*FB*) projecting into the apical periodontitis lesion and the bacterial plaque (*BP*) adhering to the surface of the object. (*RT*: root tip, *EP*: epithelium, *PC*: plant cell.) (Magnifications: *A* × 20, *B* × 40, *C* × 60, *D* × 150.)

considered to be biocompatible and well tolerated by human tissues (a view inconsistent with the clinical observation that the presence of gutta-percha in excess is associated with interrupted or delayed healing of the periapex[125,197,240,251,274]). It has been convincingly shown in guinea pigs that large pieces of gutta-percha are well encapsulated in collagenous capsules, but fine particles of gutta-percha evoke an intense, localized tissue response (Fig. 12-18) characterized by the presence of macrophages and giant cells.[253] The accumulation of macrophages in conjunction with the fine particles of gutta-percha is significant for the clinically observed impairment in the healing of apical periodontitis when teeth are root filled with excess.

Gutta-percha cones may become contaminated with tissue-irritating substances that can initiate a foreign-body reaction at the periapex. In a follow-up study of nine asymp-

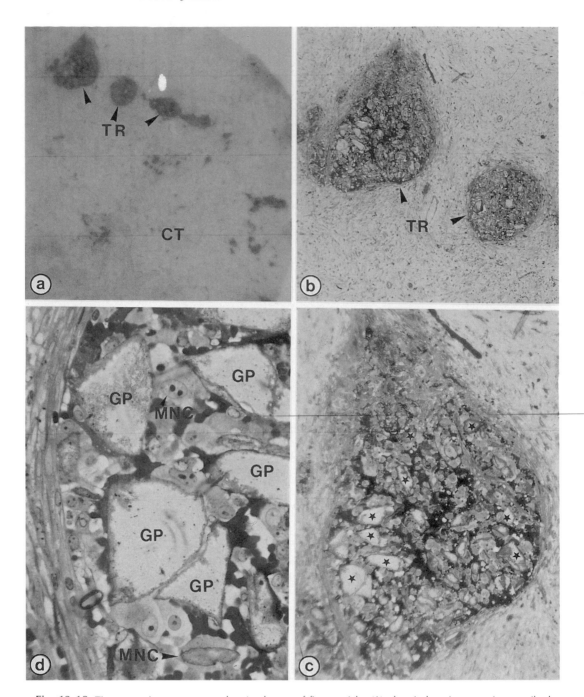

Fig. 12-18 Tissue reaction to gutta-percha. As clusters of fine particles (**A**), they induce intense, circumscribed tissue reaction (*TR*). Note that the fine particles of gutta-percha (* in **C**, *GP* in **D**) are surrounded by numerous mononuclear cells (*MNC*). (Magnifications: *A* × 30, *B* × 80, *C* × 200, *D* × 750.)

tomatic, persistent, apical periodontitis lesions that were removed as surgical block biopsies and analyzed by correlative LM and TEM, one biopsy (Fig. 12-19, *A-B*) revealed the involvement of contaminated gutta-percha.[197] The lesion persisted asymptomatically for a decade of postendodontic follow up. The most striking feature of the lesion was the presence of vast numbers of multinucleate giant cells, with characteristic birefringent inclusion bodies. In TEM the birefringent bodies were found to be highly electron dense.

Energy dispersive x-ray microanalysis of the inclusion bodies revealed the presence of magnesium and silicon. These elements are presumably the remnants of a talc-contaminated gutta-percha excess that protruded into the periapex and had been resorbed during the follow-up period.

Other Foreign Materials   Other foreign materials that commonly occur in periapical tissues include amalgam, endodontic sealants, and calcium salts derived from periapi-

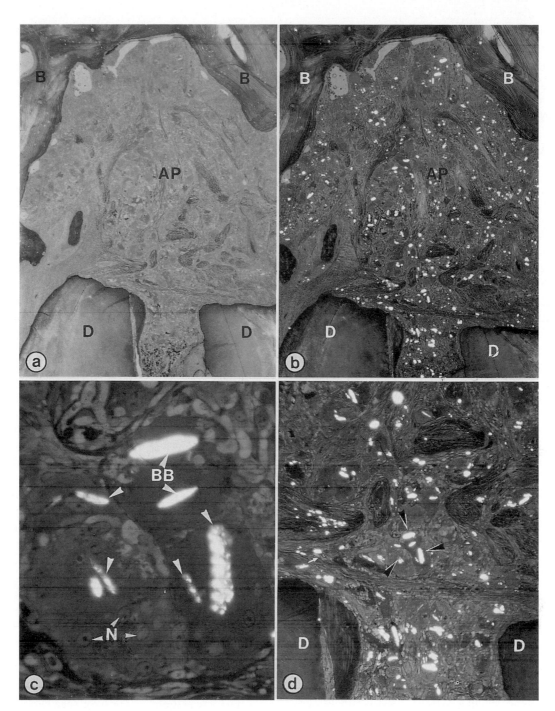

Fig. 12-19 Apical periodontitis (*AP*) characterized by foreign body–giant cell reaction to gutta-percha cones contaminated with talc (**A**). The same field when viewed in polarized lights (**B**). Note the birefringent bodies distributed throughout the lesion (**B**). The apical foramen is magnified in *D*, and the dark, arrow-headed cells in C are further enlarged in *C*. Note the birefringence (*BB*) emerging from slitlike inclusion bodies in multinucleated (*N*) giant cells. (*B*: bone, *D*: dentin.) (Magnifications: *A-B* × 25, *C* × 66, *D* × 300.) (From Nair PNR: Pathology of apical periodontitis. In Ørstavik D and Pitt-Ford TR, editors: *Essential endodontology*, Oxford, 1998, Blackwell.)

cally extruded $Ca(OH)_2$. In a histologic and x-ray microanalytic investigation of 29 apical biopsies, 31% of the specimens were found to contain materials compatible with amalgam and endodontic sealer components.[133]

CONTROVERSIES IN PERIAPICAL PATHOLOGY

Extraradicular Infections

Ever since Miller[169] demonstrated the presence of several distinct types of bacteria in diseased dental pulp, microorganisms have been suspected to play a causative role in the development of apical periodontitis. As a result, voluminous literature[325] exists that attempts to corroborate or disprove the presence of bacteria in apical periodontitis lesions. Samples of lesions gained after tooth extraction, recovered during endodontic treatment, or removed during apical surgery were bacteriologically and histopathologically studied. Many histobacteriologic studies were conducted on lesions removed *in toto,* with complete connective tissue encapsulation and firm attachment to the root apex. In a great majority of these lesions, it was not possible to demonstrate the presence of bacteria in the periapical tissue. However, bacteria could be found in abscessed lesions. Under these circumstances, Harndt[95] noted that solid granuloma are "sterile." These observations were largely supported by LM,[10,33,35,139] correlative LM, and TEM investigations.[187] As such, there has been a consensus of opinion that although "solid granuloma" may not harbor infectious agents within the inflamed periapical tissue, microorganisms are present in the periapical tissue of cases with clinical signs of exacerbation, abscesses formation, and draining sinuses.

However, in recent years there has been a resurgence of the idea of extraradicular microbes in apical periodontitis lesions,[2,118,311,312,321] with the implied, controversial suggestion that extraradicular infections are the cause of many failed endodontic treatments. Presence of several species of bacteria have been reported at extraradicular sites of lesions described as "asymptomatic periapical inflammatory lesions...refractory to endodontic treatment," with the declaration that "...our findings clearly end the era of sterile periapical granuloma."[312] It should be noted that in five out of the eight patients "long-standing fistulae to the vestibule were present."[312] The presence of sinus tracts is a clear sign of abscessed apical periodontitis having been drained by fistulation. Obviously the microbial samples of Tronstad et al[169] were obtained from periapical abscesses and erroneously presented as recovered from asymptomatic periapical lesions persisting after proper endodontic treatment.

Other independent investigations[118,321] also reveal serious materials and methodologic problems. Iwu et al[118] studied 16 periapical specimens that were collected "during normal periapical curettage, apectomy, or retrograde filling." A total of 58 specimens were investigated by Wayman et al,[321] of which "29 communicated with the oral cavity through vertical root fractures or fistulas." The specimens were obtained during routine surgery and were "submitted by seven practitioners." Obviously these researchers[118,312,321] failed to apply the knowledge gained more than 30 years ago in selecting appropriate cases in which to study the problem and in sampling cases with the utmost stringency needed to avoid bacterial contamination.[174]

The problem of microbial contamination of periapical samples appears to be inadequately understood. It is often thought of as something happening from the oral cavity and other extraneous sources only. Even if researchers succeed to avoid such microbial contamination, they cannot prevent contaminating the periapical specimens with microbes from the infected root canal. This is because microorganisms most often live at the apical foramen (Fig. 12-20) of teeth affected with apical periodontitis.[187,196,216,319] It is obvious that they can be easily scraped or dislodged during surgical manipulations of the lesion, resulting in contamination of the tissue sample with *intraradicular* microbes that, on cultivation, give false positive results that are interpreted as evidence for the presence of *extraradicular* infections. This may be the reason for the repeated reporting of bacteria in the periapical tissue of asymptomatic post-endodontic lesions in spite of having used "aseptic techniques."[2]

It has been convincingly shown by other investigators that most of the teeth with asymptomatic apical radiolucencies persisting after proper root canal treatment harbor microorganisms in the apical root canal system.[196] Correlative LM and TEM, using step serial sectioning technique of specimens removed as block biopsies during carefully planned, nonroutine, apical surgery, did not reveal any acute foci of PMN or microbes at extraradicular sites.[196] In experimentally induced apical periodontitis in monkeys,[319] and the development of such lesions in dogs after intentional microbial contamination of the root canals before obturation,[216] bacteria were consistently found in the apical root canal but not in the inflamed periapical tissue.

Extraradicular infections may, nevertheless, be found in the following situations:

1. Acute apical periodontitis lesions (see Figs. 12-9 and 12-10), as has been shown by TEM[187]
2. Periapical actinomycosis[93,94,194,252,283] (see Fig. 12-16)
3. In association with pieces of infected root dentine that may be displaced into the periapex during root canal instrumentation[109,335] or have been cut off from the rest of the root (Fig. 12-21) by massive apical resorption[141,314]
4. Infected periapical cysts (Fig. 12-22), particularly in periapical pocket cysts with cavities open to the root canal[187,192]

But for these exceptional situations, the long-standing idea[95,134] that solid granuloma generally do not harbor microorganisms is still valid.

Focal Infection, Bacteremia, and Systemic Effects

Centuries before the discovery of microorganisms and their role in infectious diseases, ancient cultures observed that the

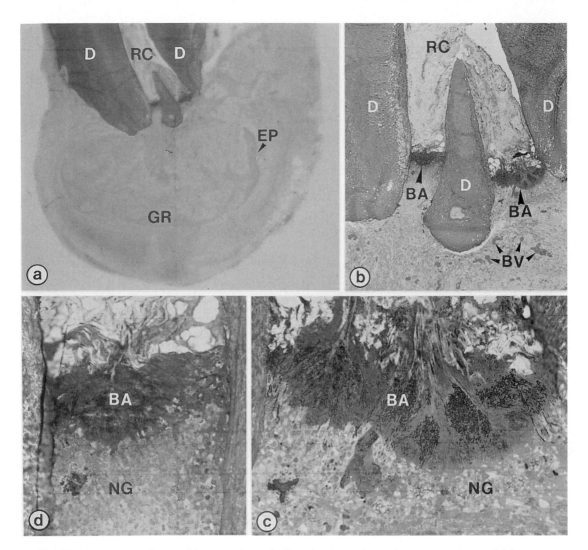

Fig. 12-20 Bacteria at the apical foramen of a tooth affected with apical periodontitis (*GR*). The apical delta in **A** is magnified in **B**. The canal ramifications on the right and left (**B**) are magnified in **C** and **D**, respectively. Note the strategic location of the bacterial clusters (*BA*) at the apical foramina. The bacterial mass appears to be held back by a distinct wall of neutrophilic granulocytes (*NG*). Obviously any surgical or microbial sampling procedures of the periapical tissue would contaminate the sample with the intraradicular flora. (*EP*: epithelium.) (Magnifications: *A* × 20, *B* × 65, *C-D* × 350.)

removal of a diseased tissue or organ could sometimes alleviate an ailment in a remote area of the body. Herein lay the roots of focal infection[27]: the controversial concept that microorganisms from a localized area of infection can be disseminated to other parts of the body and may cause metastatic local and systemic diseases. This concept had an enormous impact on the dental profession during the first half of the twentieth century. The years 1909 to 1937 came to be known as the era of focal infection.[23] For on October 3, 1910, William Hunter, a physician at Charring Cross Hospital, London, gave an address on "oral sepsis" and its relationship to systemic diseases at the McGill University in Montreal, Canada. This address was later published in the *Lancet*.[115]

Although focal infection theory has been attributed to Hunter,[115] he did not use the terminology in the lecture or in

his early writings.[114,115] Frank Billings[27] coined the term "focal infection," and his student, Edward Rosenow, defined "focus" as a circumscribed area of chronic infection.[227] The duo became foremost proponents of focal infection so that chronic diseases of unknown cause were referred to as Billings-Rosenow syndrome.[166] During the early years of the twentieth century when bacteriology was in its infancy, sepsis was the "modern subject" of discussion in many medical gatherings. The McGill lecture, later delivered in several other North American cities, received great media attention and created a furor. Hunter attacked conservative dentistry and blamed crown and bridgework as "a perfect gold trap of sepsis."[115] Nevertheless, public concern and criticism were directed against pulpless teeth and the practice of root canal treatment. This culminated in the "wholesale"[90] removal of both healthy and diseased teeth of people suffering from

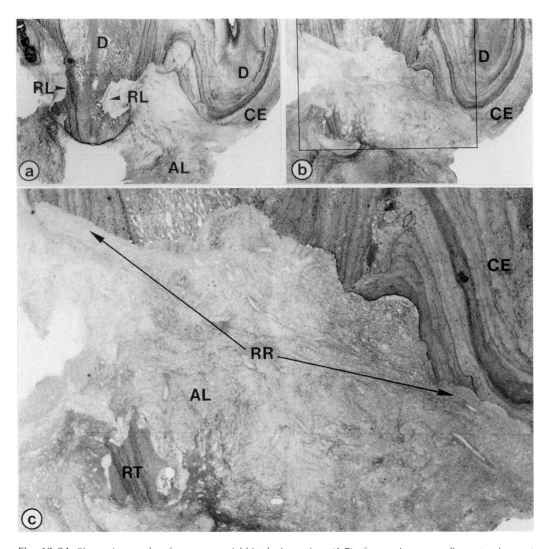

Fig. 12-21 Photomicrographs of two sequential histologic sections (**A,B**) of a specimen revealing extensive root resorption (*RR* in **C**). The demarcated area in **B** is magnified in **C**. Note the severe root resorption that resulted in shortening of the root length and detachment of a portion of the root tip (*RT*) into the body of the apical periodontitis lesion (*AL*). (*D*: dentine, *CE*: cementum, *RL*: resorption lacunae.) (Magnifications: *A-B* × 14, *C* × 40.) (From Laux M, Abbott P, Pajarola G, Nair PNR: Apical inflammatory root resorption: a correlative radiographic and histological assessment. *Int Endod J* 33:483, 2000.)

chronic diseases of unknown cause. Thus "Hunter, in 1910, gave dentistry in general, and root canal treatment in particular, a black eye from which it did not recover for about 30 years."[90]

By the middle of the twentieth century, the concept of focal infection fell into disrepute because of a combination of several factors. Many of the original claims of the link between a focus of infection and related systemic disease were anecdotal. Although the onus was on the proponents to bring forward scientific evidence to support their propositions, no such material was forthcoming and there has been no credible direct evidence of a cause-and-effect relationship. Observations that discredited focal infection theory include (1) patients with diseases presumed to be caused by foci of infection have not been relieved of their symptoms

after removal of the suspected foci, (2) patients suffering from the same ailment did not reveal any potential foci of infection, and (3) the supposed foci of infection are as common in healthy persons as with those with disease.

Despite the damaging legacy of Hunter,[115] there has been a resurgence of interest over the past several years in the relationships between systemic and oral health, with reports appearing in the general medical,[112] periodontal,* and endodontic[67-70] literature. A few animal experimental[103] and analytic epidemiologic investigations point to periodontal disease as a potential risk factor in several systemic conditions of immense social health importance, such as chronic cardiovascular diseases, acute myocardial and cerebral

---

*References 6,112,154,162,200,210,317.

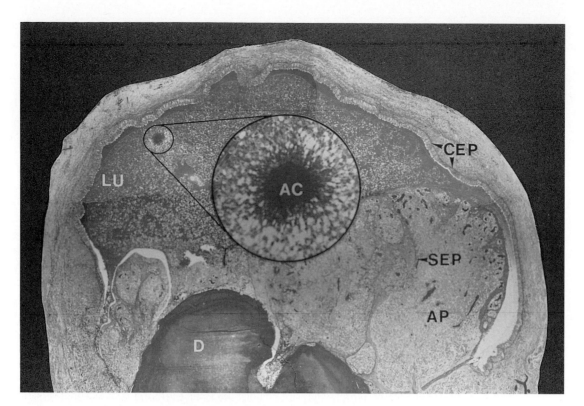

Fig. 12-22 Infected periapical cyst that affected a human maxillary premolar. The circular demarcated area is magnified in the inset. Note the distinct "ray-fungus" type of actinomycotic (*AC*) colony within the lumen. The cyst lumen is lined with ciliated columnar (*CEP*) and stratified squamous epithelia (*SEP*). (*D*: dentine.) (Magnifications: × 40, *inset* × 260.)

infarcts,[22] respiratory disorders, and adverse pregnancy outcomes.[64,65,104,205] However, it must be emphasized that a mere epidemiologic association does not imply a cause-and-effect relationship between certain oral infections and suspected systemic conditions. Further, a relationship between a suspected focus of oral infection and a disease manifestation attributed to it has not yet been substantiated by stringent scientific methods.

The reasons for the contemporary revival of interest in the once discredited concept of focal infection may not be based on scientific inquiry alone. Other factors, such as a highly competitive and grant-dependent dental research community and economic interests, may favor partnership between researchers and industry. Biomedic research–funding agencies have become "extremely supportive"[264] of such collaborative efforts. A certain eagerness to enhance the prestige of the dental profession by integrating it with general medicine is evidenced in statements such as, "This may lead to a time when we will be true oral physicians, less preoccupied with the commonest of human diseases..." confined to tooth structures.[200] The suspected association of oral infections and certain systemic conditions has been built around the pathologic effects of bacteremia, endotoxemia, and the possible entry of inflammatory mediators into blood circulation.[22,68,154,162,210] Apart from selected instances, such as infective endocarditis,

it is very unlikely that this is a significant phenomenon, because the normal function of the host defense is to quickly eliminate microbes from the circulation by phagocytic cells. Moreover, transient bacteremia is common in healthy persons after simple activities, such as chewing, tooth brushing, flossing, and various oral health procedures.[19,107] Yet diseases attributable to such bacteremia are rare.

What about the presence of apical periodontitis? Can it endanger the health of the patient? From pathogenic point of view there is a great similarity between periodontitis developing at the marginal and apical periodontal sites. Teeth with infected, necrotic pulps contain a predominantly anaerobic flora that has the potential to egress into the periapical tissue. As outlined earlier in this chapter, the body mounts an impressive defense consisting of several classes of cells, intercellular messengers, chemical weapons, and effector molecules. The clash between the microbes and the host defense results in the formation of an apical periodontitis, a lesion that is generally well barricaded in a tough, collagenous capsule. The periapical inflammatory response functions as a defense enclosure to prevent the spread of root canal infection into periradicular tissues and other parts of the body.

In spite of a formidable defense, the body's immune system cannot reach and eliminate the microbes living in the sanctuary of the necrotic root canal. There is a consensus of opinion that such diseased teeth should be treated promptly to achieve good oral health and general well being of the patient. The goal of endodontic treatment is to eliminate infection from the root canal and to prevent reinfection by obturation. When root canal treatment is done properly, a great majority of apical periodontitis heals by osseous regeneration* and any potential threat of inflammatory mediators emanating from the site is eliminated. In view of the close anatomic proximity of the endodontic flora and the blood capillaries of the inflamed periapical tissues (see Fig. 12-20), the clinician should aim to confine instrumentation to the root canal because, apart from the possibility of bacteremia, overinstrumentation can cause an increased risk of apical perforation, flare-up, and a higher endodontic failure rate.

Radicular Cysts and Periapical Healing

As stated before, the incidence of cysts among apical periodontitis lesions has been reported to vary from 6% to 55%. A correct histopathologic diagnosis of periapical cysts is possible only through serial sectioning or step serial sectioning of the lesions removed *in toto*. Most of the investigators (see Table 12-2) analyzed specimens obtained from wide sources for routine histopathologic reports. The statistically impressive 2,308 lesions analyzed in a study[26] were obtained from 314 contributors, and the 800 biopsies in another study[137] originated from 134 sources. Such diagnostic specimens, often derived through apical curettage, do not represent lesions *in toto*. In random sections from fragmented and epithelialized lesions, part of the specimens can give the appearance of epithelium-lined cavities that do not exist in reality. Seltzer et al[239] even defined a radicular cyst as one in which "a real or imagined lumen was lined with stratified squamous epithelium." Published photomicrographic illustrations[26,137] often represent only magnified views of selected small segments of epithelialized lesions that are not supported by overview pictures of lesser magnifications of sequential sections.

The vast discrepancy in the reported incidence of periapical cysts is probably due to the difference in the interpretation of the sections. Histopathologic diagnosis based on random or limited number of serial sections, usually leads to wrong categorization of epithelialized lesions as radicular cysts. This assumption is strongly supported by a recent study[192] in which an overall 52% of the lesions (n = 256) were found to be epithelialized, but only 15% were actually periapical cysts. In routine histopathologic diagnostic work, the structure of a radicular cyst in relation to the root canal of the affected tooth has not been taken into account. As apical

biopsies obtained by curettage do not include root tips of the diseased teeth, structural reference to the root canals of the affected teeth is not possible.

The low incidence of true cysts (<10%) among apical periodontitis lesions and the prevalence of two distinct histopathologic classes of periapical cysts have much clinical significance. Oral surgeons generally hold the view that cysts do not heal and have to be removed by surgery. It must be pointed out that apical periodontitis cannot be differentially diagnosed into cystic and noncystic lesions based on radiographs alone.* However, diagnostic laboratories and publications based on reviewing such histopathologic reports perpetuate the notion that nearly half of all apical periodontitis are cysts.

Consequently, a disproportionately large number of apical surgeries are performed to "enucleate" lesions that are clinically diagnosed as cysts. Studies based on meticulous serial sections show that the incidence of true radicular cysts is less than 10% of all periapical lesions. In fact, most of the cases in which apical surgery have been performed based on radiographic diagnosis of the presence of cysts might have resolved by conventional root canal treatment.

On the other hand, many endodontists are of opinion that majority of cysts heal after conventional root-filling therapy. A "success rate" of 85% to 90% has been recorded by many practitioners and endodontic investigators.[13,125,251,266] However, the histopathologic status of any apical radiolucent lesion at the time of treatment is unknown to the clinician who is also unaware of the differential diagnostic status of the "successful" and "failed" cases. Nevertheless, a great majority of the cystic lesions must heal to account for the "high success rate" after conventional endodontic treatment and the reported "high incidence" of radicular cysts.

The aim of conventional endodontic treatment has been the elimination of infectious agents from the root canal and the prevention of reinfection by obturation. A periapical pocket cyst is, therefore, likely to heal after conventional endodontic therapy.[192,198,248] However, the tissue dynamics of a true cyst is self-sustaining by virtue of its independence of the presence or absence of irritants in the root canal. Therefore, the true cysts, particularly the large ones containing cholesterol crystals, are less likely to be resolved by conventional endodontic therapy. This has been clearly shown in a longitudinal follow up of a case.[198]

ACKNOWLEDGEMENTS

The author is indebted to Mrs. Susy Münzel-Pedrazzoli for excellent technical assistance.

*References 87,125,176,177,240,250,251,273,274,281.

*References 17,26,136,146,181,218,318.

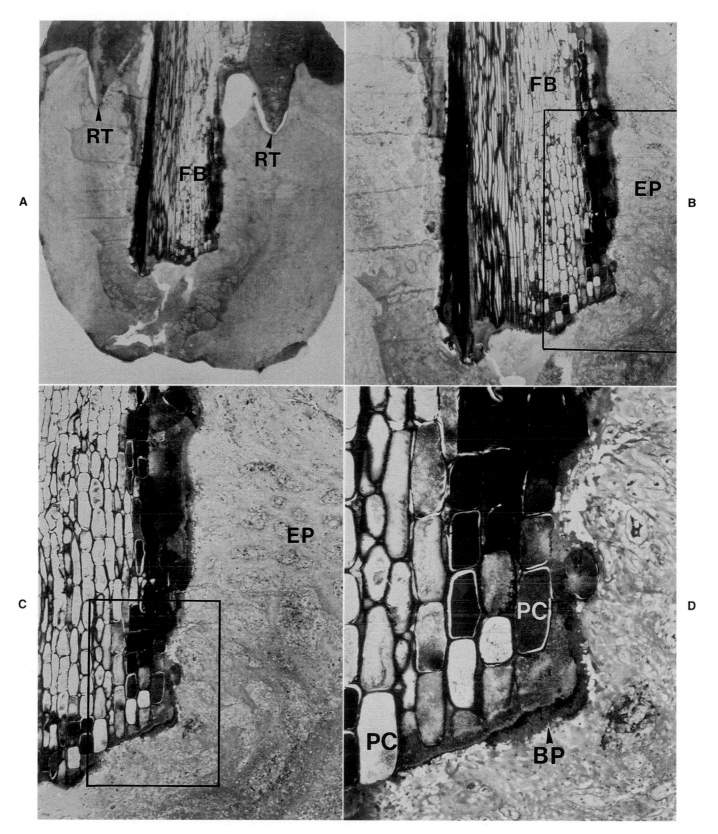

Plate 12-1 A massive paper point granuloma affecting a root canal–treated human tooth **(A).** The demarcated area in **B** is magnified in **C,** and it is further magnified in **D.** Note the tip of the paper point *(FB)* projecting into the apical periodontitis lesion and the bacterial plaque *(BP)* adhering to the surface of the paper point. *(RT,* Root tip; *EP,* epithelium; *PC,* plant cell.) (Magnifications: **A** × 20, **B** × 40, **C** × 60, **D** × 150.)

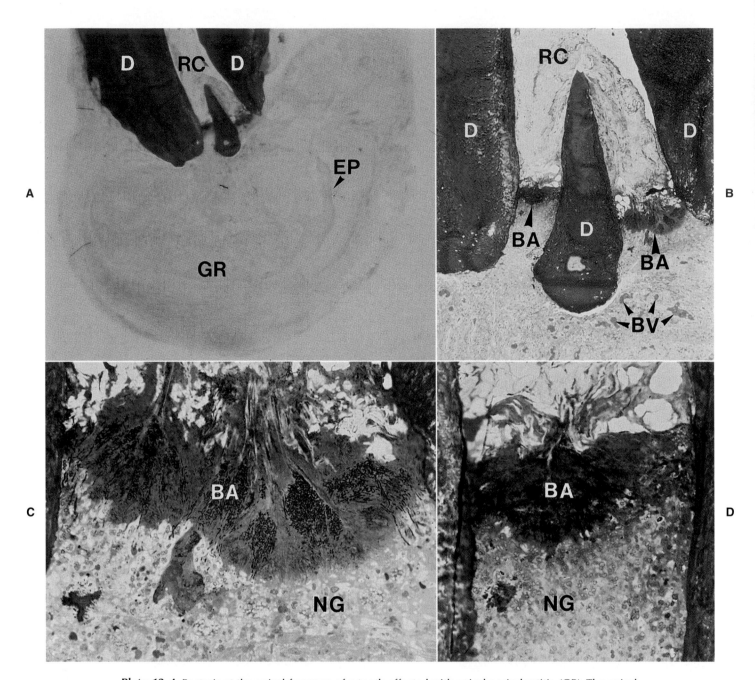

Plate 12-4 Bacteria at the apical foramen of a tooth affected with apical periodontitis *(GR)*. The apical delta in **A** is magnified in **B.** The canal ramifications on the right and left **(B)** are magnified in **C** and **D,** respectively. Note the strategic location of the bacterial clusters *(BA)* at the apical foramina. The bacterial mass appears to be held back by a distinct wall of neutrophilic granulocytes *(NG)*. Obviously any surgical or microbial sampling procedures of the periapical tissue would contaminate the sample with the intraradicular flora. *(EP,* Epithelium.) (Magnifications: **A** × 20, **B** × 65, **C-D** × 350.)

References

1. Abdulla YH, Adams CWM, Morgan RS: Connective tissue reactions to implantation of purified sterol, sterol esters, phosphoglycerides, glycerides and free fatty acids, *J Pathol Bacteriol* 94:63, 1967.
2. Abou-Rass M, Bogen G: Microorganisms in closed periapical lesions, *Int Endod J* 31:39, 1997.
3. Adams CWM, Bayliss OB, Ibrahim MZM, Webster MW Jr: Phospholipids in atherosclerosis: the modification of the cholesterol granuloma by phospholipid, *J Pathol Bacteriol* 86:431, 1963.
4. Adams CWM, Morgan RS: The effect of saturated and polyunsaturated lecithins on the resorption of 4-14C-cholesterol from subcutaneous implants, *J Pathol Bacteriol* 94:73, 1967.
5. Allard U, Nord CE, Sjöberg L, Strömberg T: Experimental infections with *Staphylococcus aureus, Streptococcus sanguis, Pseudomonas aeruginosa,* and *Bacteroides fragilis* in the jaws of dogs, *Oral Surg Oral Med Oral Pathol* 48:454, 1979.
6. American Academy of Periodontology: Position paper: periodontal disease as a potential risk factor for systemic diseases, *J Periodontol* 69:841, 1998.
7. Anderson WAD: *Pathology*, ed 5, St Louis, 1996, Mosby.
8. Ando N, Hoshino E: Predominant obligate anaerobes invading the deep layers of root canal dentine, *Int Endod J* 23:20, 1990.
9. Andreasen FM: Transient apical breakdown and its relation to color and sensibility changes after luxation injuries to teeth, *Endod Dent Traumatol* 2:9, 1985.
10. Andreasen JO, Rud J: A histobacteriologic study of dental and periapical structures after endodontic surgery, *Int J Oral Surg* 1:272, 1972.
11. Arden LA: Revised nomenclature for antigen non-specific T cell proliferation and helper factors, *J Immunol* 123:2928, 1979.
12. Artese L, Plattelli A, Quaranta M, Colasante A, Musiani P: Immunoreactivity for interleukin 1b and tumor necrosis factor-a and ultrastructural features of monocytes/macrophages in periapical granulomas, *J Endod* 17:483, 1991.
13. Barbakow FH, Cleaton-Jones PE, Friedman D: Endodontic treatment of teeth with periapical radiolucent areas in general dental practice, *Oral Surg Oral Med Oral Pathol* 51:552, 1981.
14. Barkhordar RA, Desouza YG: Human T-lymphocyte subpopulations in periapical lesions, *Oral Surg Oral Med Oral Pathol* 65:763, 1988.
15. Barkhordar RA, Hussain MZ, Hayashi C: Detection of Interleukin-1 beta in human periapical lesions, *Oral Surg Oral Med Oral Pathol* 73:334, 1992.
16. Batty I: *Actinomyces odontolyticus*, a new species of actinomycete regularly isolated from deep carious dentine, *J Pathol Bacteriol* 75:455, 1958.
17. Baumann L, Rossman SR: Clinical, roentgenologic, and histologic findings in teeth with apical radiolucent areas, *Oral Surg Oral Med Oral Pathol* 9:1330, 1956.
18. Baumgartner JC, Falkler WA: Bacteria in the apical 5 mm of infected root canals, *J Endod* 17:380, 1991.
19. Baumgartner JC, Heggers JP, Harrison JW: The incidence of bacteremias related to endodontic procedures. II. Surgical endodontics, *J Endod* 3:399, 1977.
20. Baumgartner JC, Watkins BJ, Bae K-S, Xia T: Association of black-pigmented bacteria with endodontic infections, *J Endod* 25:413, 1999.
21. Bayliss OB: The giant cell in cholesterol resorption, *Br J Exp Pathol* 57:610, 1976.
22. Beck JD, Offenbacher S, Williams R, Gibbs P, Garcia R: Periodontitis: A risk factor for coronary heart disease? *Ann Periodontol* 3:127, 1998.
23. Bellizzi R, Cruse WP: A historic review of endodontics, 1689-1963, part 3, *J Endod* 6:576, 1980.
24. Bergenholtz G: Micro-organisms from necrotic pulp of traumatized teeth, *Odont Revy* 25:347, 1974.
25. Bergenholtz G, Lekholm U, Liljenberg B, Lindhe J: Morphometric analysis of chronic inflammatory periapical lesions in root filled teeth, *Oral Surg Oral Med Oral Pathol* 55:295, 1983.
26. Bhaskar SN: Periapical lesion—types, incidence and clinical features, *Oral Surg Oral Med Oral Pathol* 21:657, 1966.
27. Billings F: *Focal infection: the Lane medical lectures*, New York, 1916, Appleton and Company.
28. Birch RH, Melville TH, Neubert EW: A comparison of root-canal and apical lesion flora, *Br Dent J* 116:350, 1964.
29. Birek C, Heersche D, Jez D, Brunette DM: Secretion of bone resorbing factor by epithelial cells cultured from porcine rests of Malassez, *J Periodontal Res* 18:75, 1983.
30. Birkedal-Hansen H: Role of matrix metalloproteinases in human periodontal diseases, *J Periodontol* 64:474, 1993.
31. Birkedal-Hansen H et al: Matrix metalloproteinases: a review, *Crit Rev Oral Biol Med* 4: 197, 1993.
32. Birkedal-Hansen H, Werb Z, Welgus HG, Van Wart HE: *Matrix metalloproteinases and inhibitors*, Stuttgart, 1992, Gustav Fischer Verlag.
33. Block RM, Bushell A, Rodrigues H, Langeland K: A histopathologic, histobacteriologic, and radiographic study of periapical endodontic surgical specimens, *Oral Surg Oral Med Oral Pathol* 42:656, 1976.
34. Boyd KS: Transient apical breakdown following subluxation injury: a case report, *Endod Dent Traumatol* 11:37, 1995.
35. Boyle PE: Intracellular bacteria in a dental granuloma, *J Dent Res* 14:297, 1934.
36. Brown AMS, Theaker JM: Food induced granuloma - an unusual cause of a submandibular mass with observations on the pathogenesis of hyalin bodies, *Br J Oral Maxillofac Surg* 25:433, 1987.
37. Brown LR Jr, Rudolph CE Jr: Isolation and identification of microorganisms from unexposed canals of pulp-involved teeth, *Oral Surg Oral Med Oral Pathol* 10:1094, 1957.
38. Browne RM: The origin of cholesterol in odontogenic cysts in man, *Arch Oral Biol* 16:107, 1971.
39. Browne RM, O'Riordan BC: Colony of Actinomyces-like organism in a periapical granuloma, *Br Dent J* 120:603, 1966.
40. Brunette DM, Heersche JNM, Purdon AD, Sodek J, Moe HK, Assuras JN: In vitro cultural parameters and protein and prostaglandin secretion of epithelial cells derived from porcine rests of Malassez, *Arch Oral Biol* 24:199, 1979.
41. Buchanan BB, Pine L: Characterization of a propionic acid producing actinomycete, *Actinomyces propionicus*, sp nov, *J Gen Microbiol* 28:305, 1962.

42. Burke GWJ, Knighton HT: The localization of microorganisms in inflamed dental pulps of rats following bacteremia, *J Dent Res* 39:205, 1960.

43. Byström A, Claeson R, Sundqvist G: The antibacterial effect of camphorated paramonochlrophenol, camphorated phenol, and calcium hydroxide in the treatment of infected root canals phenol, *Endod Dent Traumatol* 1:170, 1985.

44. Byström A, Happoneen RP, Sjögren U, Sundqvist G: Healing of periapical lesions of pulpless teeth after endodontic treatment with controlled asepsis, *Endod Dent Taumatol* 3:58, 1987.

45. Byström A, Sundqvist G: Bacteriological evaluation of the efficacy of mechanical root canal instrumentation in endodontic therapy, *Scand J Dent Res* 89:321, 1981.

46. Carlsson J: Microbiology of plaque associated periodontal disease. In Lindhe J, editor: *Textbook of clinical periodontology,* Copenhagen, 1990, Munksgaard.

47. Carlsson J, Frölander F, Sundqvist G: Oxygen tolerance of anaerobic bacteria isolated from necrotic dental pulps, *Acta Odontol Scand* 35:139, 1977.

48. Chirnside IM: A bacteriological and histological study of traumatised teeth, *N Z Dent J* 53:176, 1957.

49. Christianson OO: Observations on lesions produced in arteries of dogs by injection of lipids, *Arch Pathol* 27:1011, 1939.

50. Cohen S, Bigazzi PE, Yoshida T: Similarities of T cell function in cell-mediated immunity and antibody production, *Cell Immunol* 12:150, 1974.

51. Coleman DL, King RN, Andrade JD: The foreign body reaction: a chronic inflammatory response, *J Biomed Mater Res* 8:199, 1974.

52. Cotti E, Torabinejad M: Detection of leukotriene C4 in human periradicular lesions, *Int Endod J* 27:82, 1994.

53. Cymerman JJ, Cymerman DH, Walters J, Nevins AJ: Human T-lymphocyte subpopulations in chronic periapical lesions, *J Endod* 10:9, 1984.

54. Dahle UR, Tronstad L, Olsen I: Observation of an unusually large spirochete in endodontic infection, *Oral Microbiol Immunol* 8:251, 1993.

55. Dahle UR, Tronstad L, Olsen I: Characterization of new periodontal and endodontic isolates of spirochetes, *Eur J Oral Sci* 104:41, 1996.

56. Dahlén G: Studies on lipopolysaccharides from oral Gram-negative anaerobic bacteria in relation to apical periodontitis, doctoral thesis, Göteborg, Sweden, 1980, University of Göteborg.

57. Dahlén G, Bergenholtz G: Endotoxic activity in teeth with necrotic pulps, *J Dent Res* 59:1033, 1980.

58. Dahlén G, Fabricius L, Heyden G, Holm SE, Möller AJR: Apical periodontitis induced by selected bacterial strains in root canals of immunized and non-immunized monkeys, *Scand J Dent Res* 90:207, 1982.

59. Dahlén G, Fabricius L, Holm SE, Möller AJR: Circulating antibodies after experimental chronic infection in the root canal of teeth in monkeys, *Scand J Dent Res* 90:338, 1982.

60. Dahlén G, Haapasalo M: Microbiology of apical periodontitis. In Ørstavik D and Pitt-Ford TR, editors: *Essential Endodontology,* Oxford, 1998, Blackwell.

61. Dahlén G, Magnusson BC, Möller A: Histological and histochemical study of the influence of lipopolysaccharide extracted from *Fusobacterium nucleatum* on the periapical tissues in the monkey *Macaca fascicularis, Arch Oral Biol* 26:591,1981.

62. Damme JV: Interleukin-8 and related chemotactic cytokines. In Thomson AW, editor: *The cytokine handbook,* ed 2, London, 1994, Academic Press.

63. Darlington CG: "So called" tumors of special interest to the dentists, *Dental Cosmos* 75:310, 1933.

64. Dasnayake AP: Poor periodontal health of pregnant woman as a risk factor for low birth weight, *Ann Periodontol* 3:206, 1998.

65. Davenport ES et al: The east London study of maternal chronic peridontal disease and preterm low birth weight infants: study design and prevalence data, *Ann Periodontol* 3:213, 1998.

66. Day AJ: The macrophage system, lipid metabolism and atherosclerosis, *J Atheroscler Res* 4:117, 1964.

67. Debelian GJ: Bacteremia and fungemia in patients undergoing endodontic therapy, Dr. Odont. Thesis, Oslo, Norway, 1997, University of Oslo.

68. Debelian GJ, Olsen I, Tronstad L: Systemic diseases caused by oral microorganisms, *Endod Dent Traumatol* 10:57, 1994.

69. Debelian GJ, Olsen I, Tronstad L: Bacteremia in conjunction with endodontic therapy, *Endod Dent Taumatol* 11:142, 1995.

70. Debelian GJ, Olsen I, Tronstad L: Anaerobic bacteremia and fungimia in patients undergoing endodontic therapy: an overview, *Ann Periodontol* 3:281, 1998.

71. Delivanis PD, Fan VSC: The localization of blood-borne bacteria in instrumented unfilled and overinstrumented canals, *J Endod* 10:521, 1984.

72. Dubrow H: Silver points and gutta-percha and the role of root canal fillings, *J Am Dent Assoc* 93:976, 1976.

73. Dunlap CL, Barker BF: Giant cell hyalin angiopathy, *Oral Surg Oral Med Oral Pathol* 44:587, 1977.

74. Engström B, Frostell G: Bacteriological studies of the non-vital pulp in cases with intact pulp cavities, *Acta Odont Scand* 19:23, 1961.

75. Fabricius L: Oral bacteria and apical periodontitis. An experimental study in monkeys, doctoral thesis, Göteborg, Sweden, 1982, University of Göteborg.

76. Fabricius L, Dahlén G, Holm SC, Möller AJR: Influence of combinations of oral bacteria on periapical tissues of monkeys, *Scand J Dent Res* 90:200, 1982.

77. Fabricius L, Dahlén G, Öhman AE, Möller AJR: Predominant indigenous oral bacteria isolated from infected root canal after varied times of closure, *Scand J Dent Res* 90:134, 1982.

78. Fales WH, Warner JF, Teresa GW: Effects of *Fusobacterium necrophorum* leukotoxin on rabit peritoneal macrophages *in vitro, Am J Vet Res* 38:491, 1977.

79. Figdor D, Sjögren U, Sorlin S, Sundqvist G, Nair PNR: Pathogenicity of *Actinomyces israelii* and *Arachnia propionica*: experimental infection in guinea pigs and phagocytosis and intracellular killing by human polymorphonuclear leukocytes *in vitro, Oral Microbiol Immunol* 7:129, 1992.

80. Fish EW: Bone infection, *J Am Dent Assoc* 26:691, 1939.

81. Formigli L et al: Osteolytic processes in human radicular cysts: morphological and biochemical results, *J Oral Pathol* 24:216, 1995.

82. Freeman N: Histopathological investigation of dental granuloma, *J Dent Res* 11:176, 1931.

83. Fukushima H, Yamamoto K, Hirohata K, Sagawa H, Leung KP, Walker CB: Localization and identification of root canal bacteria in clinically asymptomatic periapical pathosis, *J Endod* 16:534, 1990.

84. Gardner AF: A survey of periapical pathology: part one, *Dent Dig* 68:162, 1962.

85. Gay CV: Osteoclast ultrastructure and enzyme histochemistry: functional implications. In Rifkin BR and Gay CV, editors: *Biology and physiology of the osteoclast*, Boca Raton, Fla, 1992, CRC Press.

86. Gier RE, Mitchel DF: Anachoretic effect of pulpitis, *J Dent Res* 47:564, 1968.

87. Grahnén H, Hansson L: The prognosis of pulp and root canal therapy: a clinical and radiographic follow-up examination, *Odontol Revy* 12:146, 1961.

88. Greening AB, Schonfeld SE: Apical lesions contain elevated immunoglobulin G levels, *J Endod* 12:867, 1980.

89. Grossman LI: Origin of microorganisms in traumatized, pulpless, sound teeth, *J Dent Res* 46:551, 1967.

90. Grossman LI: Endodontics 1776-1976: a bicentennial history against the background of general dentistry, *J Am Dent Assoc* 93:78, 1976.

91. Haapasalo M: *Bacteroides* sp in dental root canal infections, *Endod Dent Traumatol* 5:1, 1989.

92. Hampp EG: Isolation and identification of spirochetes obtained from unexposed canals of pulp-involved teeth, *Oral Surg Oral Med Oral Path* 10:1100, 1957.

93. Happonen RP: Periapical actinomycosis: a follow-up study of 16 surgically treated cases, *Endod Dent Traumatol* 2:205, 1986.

94. Happonen RP, Söderling E, Viander M, Linko-Kettungen L, Pelliniemi LJ: Immunocytochemical demonstration of *Actinomyces* species and *Arachnia propionica* in periapical infections, *J Oral Pathol* 14:405, 1985.

95. Harndt E: Histo-bakteriologische Studie bei Parodontitis chronika granulomatosa, *Korresp bl Zahnärzte,* 50:330, 1926.

96. Harris M, Goldhaber P: The production of a bone resorbing factor by dental cysts in vitro, *Br J Oral Surg* 10:334, 1973.

97. Harris M, Jenkins MV, Bennett A, Wills MR: Prostaglandin production and bone resorption by dental cysts, *Nature* 145:213, 1973.

98. Harrison JD, Martin IC: Oral vegetable granuloma: ultrastructural and histological study, *J Oral Pathol* 23:346, 1986.

99. Harz CO: *Actinomyces bovis,* ein neuer Schimmel in den Geweben des Rindes, *Dtsch Zschr Tiermed* 5 (suppl 2):125, 1879.

100. Head MA: Foreign body reaction to inhalation of lentil soup: giant cell pneumonia, *J Clin Pathol* 9:295, 1956.

101. Hedin M, Polhagen L: Follow-up study of periradicular bone condensation, *Scand J Dent Res* 79:436, 1971.

102. Heersche JN: Systemic factors regulating osteoclast function. In Rifkin BR and Gay CV, editors: *Biology and physiology of the osteoclast,* Boca Raton, FL, 1992, CRC Press.

103. Herzberg MC, Meyer MW: Dental plaque, platelets, and cardiovascular diseases, *Ann Periodontol* 3:151, 1998.

104. Hill GB: Preterm birth: Association with genital and possibly oral microflora, *Ann Periodontol* 3:222, 1998.

105. Hirano T: Interleukin-6. In Thomson AW, editor: *The cytokine handbook,* ed 2, London, 1994, Academic Press.

106. Hirsch EF: Experimental tissue lesions with mixtures of human fat, soaps and cholesterol, *Arch Pathol* 25:35, 1938.

107. Hockett RN, Loesche WJ, Sodeman TM: Bacteraemia in asymptomatic human subjects, *Arch Oral Biol* 22:91, 1977.

108. Holdeman LV, Cato EP, Moore WEC: Anaerobe laboratory manual, Blacksburg, VA, 1977, Virginia Polytechnic Institute and State University.

109. Holland R et al: Tissue reactions following apical plugging of the root canal with infected dentin chips, *Oral Surg Oral Med Oral Pathol* 49:366, 1980.

110. Horiba N, Maekawa Y, Matsumoto T, Nakamura H: A study of the detection of endotoxin in the dental wall of infected root canals, *J Endod* 16:331, 1990.

111. Howell A, Jordan HV, Georg LK, Pine L: *Odontomyces viscosus* gen nov spec nov. A filamentous microorganism isolated from periodontal plaque in hamsters, *Sabouraudia* 4:65, 1965.

112. Hughes RA: Focal infection revisited, *Br J Rheumatol* 33:370, 1994.

113. Hungate RE: The anaerobic mesophilic cellulolytic bacteria, *Bacteriol Rev* 14:1, 1950.

114. Hunter W: Oral sepsis as a cause of disease, *Br Med J* 2:215, 1900.

115. Hunter W: An address on the role of spesis and of antisepsis in medicine, *Lancet* 1:79, 1911.

116. Hylton RP, Samules HS, Oatis GW: Actinomycosis: is it really rare? *Oral Surg Oral Med Oral Pathol* 29:138, 1970.

117. Isaacs A, Lindenmann J: Virus interference. I. Interferon. *Proc R Soc Lond (Biol)* 147:258, 1957.

118. Iwu C, MacFarlane TW, MacKenzie D, Stenhouse D: The microbiology of periapical granulomas, *Oral Surg Oral Med Oral Pathol* 69:502, 1990.

119. James WW: Do epithelial odontomes increase in size by their own tension? *Proc R Soc Med* 19:73, 1926.

120. Jones OJ, Lally ET: Biosynthesis of immunoglobulin isotopes in human periapical lesions, *J Endod* 8:672, 1980.

121. Kakehashi S, Stanley HR, Fitzgerald RJ: The effects of surgical exposures of dental pulps in germ-free and conventional laboratory rats, *Oral Surg Oral Med Oral Pathol* 20:340, 1965.

122. Kamagata Y, Miyasaka N, Inoue H, Hashimoto J, Ida M: Cytokine production in inflamed human gingival tissues, Interleukin-6, *Nippon Shishubyo Gakkai Kaishi* 31:1081, 1989.

123. Kantz WE, Henry CA: Isolation and classification of anaerobic bacteria from intact pulp chambers of non vital teeth in man, *Arch Oral Biol* 19:91, 1974.

124. Kapsimalis P, Garrington GE: Actinomycosis of the periapical tissues, *Oral Surg Oral Med Oral Pathol* 26:374, 1968.

125. Kerekes K, Tronstad L: Long-term results of endodontic treatment performed with standardized technique, *J Endod* 5:83, 1979.

126. Killian M: Degradation of human immunoglobulins A1, A2 and G by suspected principal periodontal pathogens, *Infect Immun* 34:57, 1981.

127. King OH: "Giant cell hyaline angiopathy": Pulse granuloma by another name? Paper presented at the meeting of the American Academy of Oral Pathologists, Fort Lauderdale, Fla, April 23-29,1978.

128. Klevant FJH, Eggink CO: The effect of canal preparation on periapical disease, *Int Endod J* 16:68, 1983.

129. Knoblich R: Pulmonary granulomatosis caused by vegetable particles. So-called lentil pulse granuloma, *Am Rev Respir Dis* 99:380, 1969.
130. Kopp W, Schwarting R: Differentiation of T-lymphocyte subpopulations, macrophages, HLA-DR-restricted cells of apical granulation tissue, *J Endod* 15:72, 1989.
131. Koppang HS, Koppang R, Solheim T, Aarneals H, Stølen SØ: Cellulose fibers from endodontic paper points as an etiologic factor in postendodontic periapical granulomas and cysts, *J Endod* 15:369, 1989.
132. Koppang HS, Koppang R, Solheim T, Aarnes H, Stølen SØ: Identification of cellulose fibers in oral biopsis, *Scand J Dent Res* 95:165, 1987.
133. Koppang HS, Koppang R, Stølen SØ: Identification of common foreign material in postendodontic granulomas and cysts, *J Dent Assoc S Afr* 47:210, 1992.
134. Kronfeld R: *Histopathology of the teeth and their surrounding structures*, ed 2, Philadelphia, 1939, Lea & Febiger.
135. Kuntz DD, Genco RJ, Guttuso J, Natiella JR: Localization of immunoglobulins and the third component of complement in dental periapical lesions, *J Endod* 3:68, 1977.
136. Lalonde ER: A new rationale for the management of periapical granulomas and cysts. An evaluation of histopathological and radiographic findings, *J Am Dent Assoc* 80:1056, 1970.
137. Lalonde ER, Luebke RG: The frequency and distribution of periapical cysts and granulomas, *Oral Surg Oral Med Oral Pathol* 25:861, 1968.
138. Langeland K: Erkrankungen der Pulpa und des Periapex. In Guldener PHA, Langeland K, editors: *Endodontie,* ed 2, Stutgart, 1993, Georg Thieme.
139. Langeland MA, Block RM, Grossman LI: A histopathologic and histobacteriologic study of 35 periapical endodontic surgical specimens, *J Endod* 3:8, 1977.
140. Langworth BF: *Fusobacterium necrophorum*: its characteristics and role as an animal pathogen, *Bacteriol Rev* 41:373, 1977.
141. Laux M, Abbott P, Pajarola G, Nair PNR: Apical inflammatory root resorption: a correlative radiographic and histological assessement, *Int Endod J* 33:483, 2000.
142. Lerner UH: Regulation of bone metabolism by the kallikrein-kinin system, the coagulation cascade, and acute phase reactions, *Oral Surg Oral Med Oral Pathol* 78:481, 1994.
143. Lew M, Keudel KC, Milford AF: Succinate as a growth factor for Bacteroides melaninogenicus, *J Bacteriol* 108:175, 1971.
144. Lim CG, Torabinejad M, Kettering J, Linkhardt TA, Finkelman RD: Interleukin 1b in symptomatic and asymptomatic human periradicular lesions, *J Endod* 20:225, 1994.
145. Lin LM, Pascon EA, Skribner J, Gängler P, Langeland K: Clinical, radiographic, and histologic study of endodontic treatment failures, *Oral Surg Oral Med Oral Pathol* 71:603, 1991.
146. Linenberg WB, Waldron CA, DeLaune GF: A clinical roentgenographic and histopathologic evaluation of periapical lesions, *Oral Surg Oral Med Oral Pathol* 17:467, 1964.
147. Listgarten MA: Structure of the microflora associated with periodontal health and disease in man. A light and electron microscopic study, *J Periodontol* 47:1, 1976.
148. Listgarten MA, Lewis DW: The distribution of spirochetes in the lesion of acute necrotizing ulcerative gingivitis: an electron microscopical and statistical study, *J Periodontol* 38:379, 1967.
149. Loesche WJ, Gusberti F, Mettraux G, Higgins T, Syed S: Relationship between oxygen tension and subgingival bacterial flora in untreated human periodontal pockets, *Infect Immun* 42:659, 1983.
150. Love RM, McMillan MD, Jenkinson HF: Invasion of dentinal tubules by oral Streptococci is associated with collagen regeneration mediated by the antigen I/II family of polypeptides, *Infect Immun* 65:5157, 1997.
151. Lukic A, Arsenijevic N, Vujanic G, Ramic Z: Quantitative analysis of the immunocompetent cells in periapical granuloma: correlation with the histological characteristcs of the lesion, *J Endod* 16:119, 1990.
152. Lundgren D, Lindhe J: Exudation inflammatory cell migration and granulation tissue formation in preformed cavities, *Scand J Plast Reconstr Surg* 7:1, 1973.
153. Macdonald JB, Hare GC, Wood AWS: The bacteriologic status of the pulp chambers in intact teeth found to be nonvital following trauma, *Oral Surg Oral Med Oral Pathol* 10:318, 1957.
154. Maeley B: Influence of periodontal infection on systemic health, *Periodontol 2000* 21:197, 1999.
155. Main DMG: The enlargement of epithelial jaw cysts, *Odont Revy* 21:29, 1970.
156. Malassez ML: Sur l'existence de masses épithéliales dans le ligament alvéolodentaire chez l'homme adulte et à l'état normal, *Com Rend Soc Biol* 36: 241, 1884.
157. Malassez ML: Sur la role débris épithélaux paradentaris. In Mason G, editor: *Travaux de L'année 1885*, Paris, 1885, Librairie de l'Académie de Médicine.
158. Martin IC, Harrison JD: Periapical actinomycosis, *Br Dent J* 156:169, 1984.
159. Marton IJ, Kiss C: Characterization of inflammatory cell infiltrate in dental periapical lesions, *Int Endod J* 26:131, 1993.
160. Matsumoto Y: Monoclonal and oligoclonal immunoglobulins localized in human dental periapical lesion, *Microbiol Immunol* 29:751, 1985.
161. Matsuo T, Ebisu S, Nakanishi T, Yonemura K, Harada Y, Okada H: Interleukin-1a and interleukin-1b in periapical exudates of infected root canal: correlations with the clinical findings of the involved teeth, *J Endod* 20:432, 1994.
162. Mattila K: Systemic impact of periodontal infections. In Guggenheim B and Shapiro S, editors: *Oral biology at the turn of the century,* Basel, Switzerland, 1998, Karger.
163. McConnell G: The histo-pathology of dental granulomas, *Natl Dent Assoc J* 8:390, 1921.
164. McGhee JR, Michalek SM, Cassel GH: *Dental microbiology*, Philadelphia, 1982, Harper & Row.
165. McNicholas S, Torabinejad M, Blankenship J: The concentration of prostaglandin E2 in human periradicular lesions, *J Endod* 17:97, 1991.
166. Meinig GE: *Root-canal cover-up*, ed 2, Ojai, California, 1994, Bion Publishing.
167. Metchinkoff E: *Lectures on the comparative pathology of inflammation,* New York, 1968, Dover Publications.
168. Miller WD: *The micro-organisms of the human mouth*, Philadelphia, 1890, White Dental MFG Co.
169. Miller WD: An introduction to the study of bacterio-pathology of the dental pulp, *Dent Cosmos* 36:505, 1894.

170. Mims CA: *The pathogenesis of infectious disease*, ed 3, London, 1988, Academic Press.

171. Mincer HH, McCoy JM, Turner JE: Pulse granuloma of the alveolar ridge, *Oral Surg Oral Med Oral Pathol* 48:126, 1979.

172. Mixner D, Green TL, Walton R: Histologic examination of condensing osteitis (Abstract), *J Endod* 18:196, 1992.

173. Molander A, Reit C, Dahlén G, Kvist T: Microbiological status of root filled teeth with apical periodontitis, *Int Endod J* 31:1, 1998.

174. Möller ÅJR: Microbiological examination of root canals and periapical tissues of human teeth (thesis), Akademiförlaget, Göteborg, Sweden, 1966, University of Göteborg.

175. Möller ÅJR, Fabricius L, Dahlén G, Öhman AE, Heyden G: Influence on periapical tissues of indigenous oral bacteria and necrotic pulp tissue in monkeys, *Scand J Dent Res* 89:475, 1981.

176. Molven O: The frequency, technical standard and results of endodontic therapy, *Nor Tannlaegeforenings Tid* 86:142, 1976.

177. Molven O, Halse A: Success rates for gutta-percha and Klorperka N-Ø root fillings made by undergraduate students: radiographic findings after 10-17 years, *Int Endod J* 21:243, 1988.

178. Monteleone L: Actonomycosis, *J Oral Surg Anes Hosp Dent Serv* 21:313, 1963.

179. Moore WEC: Techniques for routine culture of fastidious anaerobes, *Int J Syst Bacteriol* 16:173, 1966.

180. Moore WEC: Microbiology of periodontal disease, *J Periodontol* 22:335, 1987.

181. Mortensen H, Winther JE, Birn H: Periapical granulomas and cysts, *Scand J Dent Res* 78:241, 1970.

182. Morton TH, Clagett JA, Yavorsky JD: Role of immune complexes in human periapical periodontitis, *J Endod* 3:261, 1977.

183. Nadal-Valldaura A: Fatty degeneration and the formation of fat-lipid needles in chronic granulomatous periodontitis, *Rev Esp Estomatol* 15:105, 1968.

184. Nagaoka S et al: Bacterial invasion into dentinal tubules in human vital and nonvital teeth, *J Endod* 21:70, 1995.

185. Nagase H, Barrett AJ, Woessner JF Jr: Nomenclature and glossary of the matrix metalloproteinases. In Birkedal-Hansen H et al, editors: *Matrix metalloproteinases and inhibitors,* Stuttgart, 1992, Gustav Fischer Verlag.

186. Naidorf IJ: Immunoglobulins in periapical granulomas: a preliminary report, *J Endod* 1:15, 1975.

187. Nair PNR: Light and electron microscopic studies of root canal flora and periapical lesions, *J Endod* 13:29, 1987.

188. Nair PNR: Apical periodontitis: a dynamic encounter between root canal infection and host response, *Periodontology 2000* 13:121, 1997.

189. Nair PNR: Pathology of apical periodontitis. In Ørstavik D, Pitt-Ford TR, editors: *Essential endodontology*, Oxford, 1998, Blackwell.

190. Nair PNR: New perspectives on radicular cysts: do they heal? *Int Endod J* 31:155, 1998.

191. Nair PNR: Cholesterol as an aetilogical agent in endodontic failures—a review, *Aus Endod J* 25:19, 1999.

192. Nair PNR, Pajarola G, Schroeder HE: Types and incidence of human periapical lesions obtained with extracted teeth, *Oral Surg Oral Med Oral Pathol* 81:93, 1996.

193. Nair PNR, Schmid-Meier E: An apical granuloma with epithelial integument, *Oral Surg Oral Med Oral Pathol* 62:698, 1986.

194. Nair PNR, Schroeder HE: Periapical actinomycosis, *J Endod* 10:567, 1984.

195. Nair PNR, Schroeder HE: Epithelial attachment at diseased human tooth-apex, *J Periodontal Res* 20:293, 1985.

196. Nair PNR, Sjögren U, Kahnberg KE, Krey G, Sundqvist G: Intraradicular bacteria and fungi in root-filled, asymptomatic human teeth with therapy-resistant periapical lesions: a long-term light and electron microscopic follow-up study, *J Endod* 16:580, 1990.

197. Nair PNR, Sjögren U, Krey G, Sundqvist G: Therapy-resistant foreign-body giant cell granuloma at the periapex of a root-filled human tooth, *J Endod* 16:589, 1990.

198. Nair PNR, Sjögren U, Schumacher E, Sundqvist G: Radicular cyst affecting a root-filled human tooth: A long-term post-treatment follow-up, *Int Endod J* 26:225, 1993.

199. Nair PNR, Sjögren U, Sundqvist G: Cholesterol crystals as an etiological factor in non-resolving chronic inflammation: an experimental study in guinea pigs, *Eur J Oral Sci* 106:644, 1998.

200. Newman HN: Focal infection, *J Dent Res* 75:1912, 1996.

201. Nijweide PJ, Grooth dR: Ontogeny of the osteoclast. In Rifkin BR and Gay CV, editors: *Biology and physiology of the osteoclast*, Boca Raton, FL, 1992, CRC Press.

202. Nilsen R, Johannessen A, Skaug N, Matre R: In situ characterization of mononuclear cells in human dental periapical lesions using monoclonal antibodies, *Oral Surg Oral Med Oral Pathol* 58:160, 1984.

203. Nobuhara WK, Del Rio CE: Incidence of periradicular pathoses in endodontic treatment failures, *J Endod* 19:315, 1993.

204. O'Grady JF, Reade PC: Periapical actinomycosis involving *Actinomyces israelii, J Endod* 14:147, 1988.

205. Offenbacher S et al: Potential pathogenic mechanisms of periodontitis-associated pregnancy complications, *Ann Periodontol* 3:233, 1998.

206. Okiji T, Morita I, Sunada I, Murota S: The role of leukotriene B4 in neutrophil infiltration in experimentally induced inflammation of rat tooth pulp, *J Dent Res* 70:34, 1991.

207. Oppenheim JJ: Forward. In Thomson AW, editor: *The cytokine handbook,* ed 2, London, 1994, Academic Press.

208. Oppenheimer S, Miller GS, Knopf K, Blechman H: Periapical actinomycosis, *Oral Surg Oral Med Oral Pathol* 46:101, 1978.

209. Ørstavik D, Pitt-Ford TR: Apical periodontitis: microbial infection and host response. In Ørstavik D and Pitt-Ford TR, editors: *Essential endodontology,* Oxford, 1998, Blackwell.

210. Page RC: The pathobiology of periodontal diseases may affect systemic diseases: inversion of a paradigm, *Ann Periodontol* 3:108, 1998.

211. Page RC, Schroeder HE: *Periodontitis in man and other animals,* Basel, Switzerland, 1982, Karger.

212. Papadimitriou JM, Ashman RB: Macrophages: current views on their differentiation, structure and function, *Ultrastruct Pathol* 13:343, 1989.

213. Patterson SS, Shafer WG, Healey HJ: Periapical lesions associated with endodontically treated teeth, *J Am Dent Assoc* 68:191, 1964.

214. Perez F, Calas P, de Falguerolles A, Maurette A: Migration of a *Streptococcus sanguis* through the root dentinal tubules, *J Endod* 19:297, 1993.

215. Piattelli A, Artese L, Rosini S, Quarenta M, Musiani P: Immune cells in periapical granuloma: morphological and immunohistochemical characterization, *J Endod* 17:26, 1991.

216. Pitt-Ford TR: The effects of the periapical tissues of bacterial contamination of the filled root canal, *Int Endod J* 15:16, 1982.

217. Poertzel E, Petschelt A: Bakterien in der Wurzelkanalwand bei Pulpagangrän, *Dtsch Zahnärztl Zschr* 41:772, 1986.

218. Priebe WA, Lazansky JP, Wuehrmann AH: The value of the roentgenographic film in the differential diagnosis of periapical lesions, *Oral Surg Oral Med Oral Pathol* 7:979, 1954.

219. Pulver WH, Taubman MA, Smith DJ: Immune components in human dental periapical lesions, *Arch Oral Biol* 23:435, 1978.

220. Puzas JE, Ishibe M: Osteoblast/osteoclast coupling. In Rifkin BR and Gay CV, editors: *Biology and physiology of the osteoclast,* Boca Raton, FL, 1992, CRC Press.

221. Rickert UG, Dixon CM: The controlling of root surgery. In *transactions of the eighth international dental congress*, Paris, 1931, The Congress.

222. Rietschel ET, Brude H: Bacterial endotoxins, *Sci Am* 267:54, 1992.

223. Robinson HBG, Boling LR: The anachoretic effect in pulpitis. Bacteriologic studies, *J Am Dent Assoc* 28:268, 1941.

224. Rohrer A: Die Aetiologie der Zahnwurzelzysten, *Dtsch Mschr Zahnhk* 45:282, 1927.

225. Roitt I: *Essential Immunology*, Oxford, 1994, Blackwell.

226. Rosebury T, Reynolds JB: Continuous anaerobiosis for cultivation of spirochetes, *Proc Soc Exp Biol Med* 117:813, 1964.

227. Rosenow EC: The relation of dental infection to systemic disease, *Dent Cosmos* 59:485, 1917.

228. Ruddle NH: Tumour necrosis factor-beta (Lymphotoxin-alpha). In Thomson AW, editor: *The cytokine handbook,* ed 2, London, 1994, Academic Press.

229. Ryan GB, Majno G: Acute inflammation, *Am J Pathol* 86:185, 1977.

230. Safavi KE, Rossomando ER: Tumor necrosis factor identified in periapical tissue exudates of teeth with apical periodontitis, *J Endod* 17:12, 1991.

231. Sahara N et al: Odontoclastic resorption of the superficial nonmineralized layer of predentine in the shedding of human deciduous teeth, *Cell Tissue Res* 277:19, 1994.

232. Sakellariou PL: Periapical actinomycosis: report of a case and review of the literature, *Endod Dent Traumatol* 12:151, 1996.

233. Samanta A, Malik CP, Aikat BW: Periapical actinomycosis, *Oral Surg Oral Med Oral Pathol* 39:458, 1975.

234. Samuelsson B: Leukotrienes: mediators of immediate hypersensitivity reactions and inflammation, *Science* 220:268, 1983.

235. Schein B, Schilder H: Endotoxin content in endodontically involved teeth, *J Endod* 1:19, 1975.

236. Sedgley CM, Messer H: Long-term retention of a paper-point in the periapical tissues: a case report, *Endod Dent Traumatol* 9:120, 1993.

237. Selle G: Zur Genese von Kieferzysten anhand vergleichender Untersuchungen von Zysteninhalt und Blutserum, *Dtsch Zahnärztl Z* 29:600, 1974.

238. Seltzer S: *Endodontology*, ed 2, Philadelphia, 1988, Lea & Febiger.

239. Seltzer S, Bender IB, Smith J, Freedman I, Nazimov H: Endodontic failures - an analysis based on clinical, roentgenographic, and histologic findings (Part I & II), *Oral Surg Oral Med Oral Pathol* 23:500, 1967.

240. Seltzer S, Bender IB, Turkenkopf S: Factors affecting successful repair after root canal treatment, *J Am Dent Assoc* 67:651, 1963.

241. Seltzer S, Soltanoff W, Bender IB: Epithelial proliferation in periapical lesions, *Oral Surg Oral Med Oral Pathol* 27:111, 1969.

242. Shah HN, Collins MD: Proposal for classification of *Bacteroides asaccharolyticus, Bacteroides gingivalis, and Bacteroides endodontalis* in a new genus, *Porphyromonas, Int J Syst Bacteriol* 38:128, 1988.

243. Shah HN, Collins MD: *Prevotella*, a new genus to include *Bacteroides melaninogenicus* and related species formerly classified in the genus *Bacteroides, Int J Syst Bacteriol* 40:205, 1990.

244. Shear M: The histogenesis of dental cysts, *Dent Pract* 13:238, 1963.

245. Shear M: *Cysts of the oral regions*, ed 3, Oxford:1992, Wright.

246. Sherman FE, Moran TJ: Granulomas of stomach. Response to injury of muscle and fibrous tissue of wall of human stomach, *Am J Cl Pathol* 24:415, 1954.

247. Shovelton DS: The presence and distribution of microorganisms within non-vital teeth, *Br Dent J* 117:101, 1964.

248. Simon JHS: Incidence of periapical cysts in relation to the root canal, *J Endod* 6:845, 1980.

249. Simon JHS, Chimenti Z, Mintz G: Clinical significance of the pulse granuloma, *J Endod* 8:116, 1982.

250. Sjögren U, Figdor D, Persson S, Sundqvist G: Influence of infection at the time of root filling on the outcome of endodontic treatment of teeth with apical periodontitis, *Int Endod J* 30:297, 1997.

251. Sjögren U, Hägglund B, Sundqvist G, Wing K: Factors affecting the long-term results of endodontic treatment, *J Endod* 16:498, 1990.

252. Sjögren U, Happonen RP, Kahnberg KE, Sundqvist G: Survival of *Arachnia propionica* in periapical tissue, *Int Endod J* 21:277, 1988.

253. Sjögren U, Sundqvist G, Nair PNR: Tissue reaction to guttapercha of various sizes when implanted subcutaneously in guinea pigs, *Eur J Oral Sci* 103:313, 1995.

254. Skaug N: Proteins in fluids from non-keratinizing jaw cysts: 4. Concentrations of immunoglobulins (IIgG, IgA and IgM) and some non-immunoglobulin proteins: relevance to concepts of cyst wall permeability and clearance of cyst proteins, *J Oral Pathol* 3:47, 1974.

255. Skaug N, Nilsen R, Matre R, Bernhoft C-H, Christine A: *In situ* characterization of cell infiltrates in human dental periapical granulomas 1. Demonstration of receptors for Fc region of IgG, *J Oral Pathol* 11:47, 1982.

256. Smith G, Matthews JB, Smith AJ, Browne RM: Immunoglobulin-producing cells in human odontogenic cysts, *J Oral Pathol* 16:45, 1987.

257. Socransky S, Macdonald JB, Sawyer S: The cultivation of *Treponema microdentium* as surface colonies, *Arch Oral Biol* 1:171, 1959.

258. Sommer RF, Kerr DA, Quoted in Sommer RF: *Clinical endodontics*, ed 3, Philadelphia, 1966, WB Saunders.

259. Sonnabend E, Oh C-S: Zur Frage des Epithels im apikalen Granulationsgewebe (Granulom) menschlicher Zähne, *Dtsch Zahnärztl Z* 21:627, 1966.

260. Spain D, Aristizabal N: Rabbit local tissue response to triglycerides, cholesterol and its ester, *Arch Pathol* 73:94, 1962.

261. Spain DM, Aristizabal N, Ores R: Effect of estrogen on resolution of local cholesterol implants, *Arch Pathol* 68:30, 1959.

262. Spatafore CM, Griffin JA, Keyes GG, Wearden S, Skidmore AE: Periapical biopsy report: an analysis over a 10-year period, *J Endod* 16:239, 1990.

263. Spinner JR: Vom Chemismus der Pulpagangrän. Ein akutes Problem der konservierenden Zahnheilkunde, *Zahnärztl Welt* 2:305, 1947.

264. Stamm JW: Periodontal sideases and human health: new directions in periodontal medicine, *Ann Periodontol* 3:1, 1998.

265. Stashenko P, Yu SM, Wang C-Y: Kinetics of immune cell and bone resorptive responses to endodontic infections, *J Endod* 18:422, 1992.

266. Staub HP: Röntgenologische Erfolgstatistik von Wurzelbehandlungen, doctoral thesis, Zurich, 1963, University of Zurich.

267. Stern MH, Dreizen S, Mackler BF, Levy BM: Antibody producing cells in human periapical granulomas and cysts, *J Endod* 7:447, 1981.

268. Stern MH, Dreizen S, Mackler BF, Levy BM: Isolation and characterization of inflammatory cells from the human periapical granuloma, *J Dent Res* 61:1408, 1982.

269. Stern MH, Dreizen S, Mackler BF, Selbst AG, Levy BM: Quantitative analysis of cellular composition of human periapical granuloma, *J Endod* 7:117, 1981.

270. Stern MH, Mackler BF, Dreizen S: A quantitative method for the analysis of human periapical inflammation, *J Endod* 7:70, 1981.

271. Stock CJR, Gulabivala K, Walker RT, Goodman JR: *Color atlas and text of endodontics*, ed 2, St Louis, 1995, Mosby.

272. Stockdale CR, Chandler NP: The nature of the periapical lesion—a review of 1108 cases, *J Dent* 16:123, 1988.

273. Storms JL: Factors that influence the success of endodontic treatment, *J Can Dent Assoc* 35:83, 1969.

274. Strindberg LZ: The dependence of the results of pulp therapy on certain factors. An analytic study based on radiographic and clinical follow-up examinations, *Acta Odontol Scand* 14 (suppl 21):1, 1956.

275. Sundqvist G: Bacteriological studies of necrotic dental pulps, doctoral thesis, Umeå, Sweden, 1976, University of Umeå.

276. Sundqvist G: Associations between microbial species in dental root canal infections, *Oral Microbiol Immunol* 7:267, 1992.

277. Sundqvist G: Ecology of the root canal flora, *J Endod* 18:427, 1992.

278. Sundqvist G: Taxonomy, ecology and pathogenicity of the root canal flora, *Oral Surg Oral Med Oral Pathol,* 78:522, 1994.

279. Sundqvist G, Carlsson J, Herrman B, Tärnvik A: Degradation of human immunoglobulins G and M and complement factor C3 and C5 by black pigmented *Bacteroides, J Med Microbiol* 19:85, 1985.

280. Sundqvist G, Figdor D: Endodontic treatment of apical periodontitis. In Ørstavik D and Pitt-Ford TR, editors: *Essential endodontology,* Oxford, 1998, Blackwell.

281. Sundqvist G, Figdor D, Persson S, Sjögren U: Microbiologic analysis of teeth with failed endodontic treatment and the outcome of conservative re-treatment, *Oral Surg Oral Med Oral Pathol* 85:86, 1998.

282. Sundqvist G, Johansson E, Sjögren U: Prevalence of black pigmented *Bacteroides* species in root canal infections, *J Endod* 15:13, 1989.

283. Sundqvist G, Reuterving CO: Isolation of *Actinomyces israelii* from periapical lesion, *J Endod* 6:602, 1980.

284. Sundqvist GK, Eckerbom MI, Larsson AP, Sjögren UT: Capacity of anaerobic bacteria from necrotic dental pulps to induce purulent infections, *Infect Immun* 25:685, 1979.

285. Szajkis S, Tagger M: Periapical healing in spite of incomplete root canal debridement and filling, *J Endod* 9:203, 1983.

286. Taichman NS, Dean RT, Sanderson CJ: Biochemical and morphological characterization of the killing of human monocytes by a leukotoxin derived from *Actinobacillus actinomycetemcomitans, Infect Immun* 28:259, 1980.

287. Taichman NS, Korchak H, Lally ET: Membranolytic activity of *Actinobacillus actinomycetemcomitans* leukotoxin, *J Periodontal Res* 26:258, 1991.

288. Talacko AA, Radden BG: The pathogenesis of oral pulse granuloma: an animal model, *J Oral Pathol* 17:99, 1988.

289. Talacko AA, Radden BG: Oral pulse granuloma: clinical and histopathological features, *Int J Oral Maxillofac Surg* 17: 343-346, 1988.

290. Tani-Ishii N, Wang C-Y, Stashenko P: Immunolocalization of bone-resorptive cytokines in rat pulp and periapical lesions following surgical pulp exposure, *Oral Microbiol Immunol* 10:213, 1995.

291. Taylor E: *Dorland's illustrated medical dictionary*, ed 29, Philadelphia, 2000, WB Saunders.

292. Ten Cate AR: Epithelial cell rests of Malassez and the genesis of the dental cyst, *Oral Surg Oral Med Oral Pathol* 34:956, 1972.

293. Teronen O, Salo T, Laitinen J, Törnwall J, Ylipaavainiemi P, Konttinen Y, Hietanen J, Sorosa T: Characterization of interstitial collagenases in jaw cyst wall, *Eur J Oral Sci* 103:141, 1995.

294. Thilo BE, Baehni P, Holz J: Dark-field observation of bacterial distribution in root canals following pulp necrosis, *J Endod* 12:202, 1986.

295. Thoma KH: A histo-pathological study of the dental granuloma and diseased root apex, *Natl Dent Assoc J* 4:1075, 1917.

296. Thoma KH, Goldman HM: *Oral pathology*, ed 5, St Louis, 1960, Mosby.

297. Thomas L: *The lives of a cell*, Toronto, 1974, Bantam Books.

298. Thompson L, Lovestedt SA: An actinomyces-like organism obtained from the human mouth, *Mayo Clin Proc* 26:169, 1951.

299. Toller PA: Experimental investigations into factors concerning the growth of cysts of the jaw, *Proc R Soc Med* 41:681, 1948.

300. Toller PA: The osmolarity of fluids from cysts of the jaws, *Br Dent J* 129:275, 1970.

301. Toller PA, Holborrow EJ: Immunoglobulin and immunoglobulin containing cells in cysts of the jaws, *Lancet* 2:178, 1969.

302. Tompkins DH: Reaction of the reticuloendothelial cells to subcutaneous injections of cholesterol, *Arch Pathol* 42:299, 1946.

303. Torabinejad M: The role of immunological reactions in apical cyst formation and the fate of the epithelial cells after root canal therapy: a theory, *Int J Oral Surg* 12:14, 1983.

304. Torabinejad M, Clagett J, Engel D: A cat model for evaluation of mechanism of bone resorption; induction of bone loss by simulated immune complexes and inhibition by indomethacin, *Calcif Tissue Int* 29:207, 1979.

305. Torabinejad M, Cotti E, Jung T: Concentration of leukotriene B4 in symptomatic and asymptomatic periapical lesions, *J Endod* 18:205, 1992.

306. Torabinejad M, Kettering J: Identification and relative concentration of B and T lymphocytes in human chronic periapical lesions, *J Endod* 11:122, 1985.

307. Torabinejad M, Kriger RD: Experimentally induced alterations in periapical tissues of the cat, *J Dent Res* 59:87, 1980.

308. Torneck CD: Reaction of rat connective tissue to polyethylene tube implants. I. *Oral Surg Oral Med Oral Pathol* 21: 379, 1966.

309. Torres JOC, Torabinejad M, Matiz RAR, Mantilla EG: Presence of secretory IgA in human periapical lesions, *J Endod* 20:87, 1994.

310. Tracey KJ: Tumour necrosis factor-alpha. In Thomson AW, editor: *The cytokine handbook,* ed 2, London, 1994, Academic Press.

311. Tronstad L, Barnett F, Cervone F: Periapical bacterial plaque in teeth refractory to endodontic treatment, *Endod Dent Traumatol* 6:73, 1990.

312. Tronstad L, Barnett F, Riso K, Slots J: Extraradicular endodontic infections, *Endod Dent Traumatol* 3:86, 1987.

313. Trott JR, Chebib F, Galindo Y: Factors related to cholesterol formation in cysts and granulomas, *J Can Dent Assoc* 38:76, 1973.

314. Valderhaug J: A histologic study of experimentally induced periapical inflammation in primary teeth in monkeys, *Int J Oral Surg* 3:111, 1974.

315. Van Dyke TE, Vaikuntam J: Neutrophil function and dysfunction in periodontal disease. In Williams RC, Yukna RA, Newman MG, editors: *Current opinion in periodontology,* ed 2, Philadelphia, 1994, Current Science.

316. Van Furth R et al: The mononuclear phagocyte system: a new classification of macrophages, monocytes and their precursors, *Bull World Health Organ* 46:845, 1972.

317. Van Velzen SKT, Abraham-Inpijn L, Moorer WR: Plaque and systemic disease: a reappraisal of the focal infection concept, *J Clin Periodontol* 11:209, 1984.

318. Wais FT: Significance of findings following biopsy and histologic study of 100 periapical lesions, *Oral Surg Oral Med Oral Pathol* 11:650, 1958.

319. Walton RE, Ardjmand K: Histological evaluation of the presence of bacteria in induced periapical lesions in monkeys, *J Endod* 18:216, 1992.

320. Wang CY, Stashenko P: The role of interleukin-1a in the pathogenesis of periapical bone destruction in a rat model system, *Oral Microbiol* 8:50, 1993.

321. Wayman BE, Murata M, Almeida RJ, Fowler CB: A bacteriological and histological evaluation of 58 periapical lesions, *J Endod* 18:152, 1992.

322. Weir JC, Buck WH: Periapical actinomycosis, *Oral Surg Oral med Oral Pathol* 54:336, 1982.

323. White EW: Paper point in mental foramen, *Oral Surg Oral Med Oral Pathol* 25:630, 1968.

324. World Health Organization: *Application of the international classification of diseases to dentistry and stomatology,* ed 3, Geneva, 1995, The Organization.

325. Winkler TF: Review of the literature: a histologic study of bacteria in periapical pathosis, *Pharmacol Ther Dent* 2:157, 1975.

326. Winstock D: Apical disease: an analysis of diagnosis and management with special reference to root lesion resection and pathology, *Ann R Coll Surg Engl* 62:171, 1980.

327. Wittgow WC Jr, Sabiston CB Jr: Microorganisms from pulpal chambers of intact teeth with necrotic pulps, *J Endod* 1:168, 1975.

328. Wolff M, Israel J: Ueber Reinkultur des Actinomyces und seine Ubertragbarkeit auf Thiere, *Virchows Arch Pathol Anat Physiol Klin Med* 126:11, 1891.

329. Yamasaki M, Nakane A, Kumazawa M, Hashioka K, Horiba N, Nakamura H: Endotoxin and Gram-negative bacteria in the rat periapical lesions, *J Endod* 18:501, 1992.

330. Yamazaki K, Nakajima T, Gemmeli E, Polak B, Seymour GJ, Hara K: IL-4 and IL-6-producing cells in human periodontal disease tissue, *J Oral Pathol Med* 23:347, 1994.

331. Yanagisawa W: Pathologic study of periapical lesions. I. Periapical granulomas: clinical, histologic and immunohistopathologic studies, *J Oral Pathol* 9:288, 1980.

332. Yeagle PL: *The biology of cholesterol*, Boca Raton, FL 1988, CRC Press.

333. Yeagle PL: *Understanding your cholesterol,* San Diego, 1991, Academic Press.

334. Ylipaavalniemi P: Cyst fluid concentrations of immunoglobulins a2-macroglobulin and a1-antitrypsin, *Proc Finn Dent Soc* 73:185, 1977.

335. Yusuf H: The significance of the presence of foreign material periapically as a cause of failure of root treatment, *Oral Surg Oral Med Oral Pathol* 54:566, 1982.

336. Zain RB: Radiographic evaluation of lesion sizes of histologically diagnosed periapical cysts and granulomas, *Ann Dent* 48:3, 1989.

Chapter 13

Endodontic Microbiology and Treatment of Infections

J. Craig Baumgartner, Jeffrey W. Hutter

Chapter Outline

There is no greater association between a basic science and the practice of endodontics than that of microbiology. The vast majority of diseases of the dental pulp and the periradicular tissues are associated with microorganisms. After microbial invasion of these tissues, the host responds with both nonspecific inflammatory responses and with specific immunologic responses. Both nonsurgical endodontic treatment and surgical endodontic treatment are essentially débridement procedures to disrupt and remove the microbial ecosystem that is associated with the disease process. It is important that clinicians understand the close relationship between the presence of microorganisms and endodontic disease processes to develop an effective rationale for treatment. Clinicians must also be constantly alert for avenues of cross contamination among patients and use "universal pre-cautions" to prevent passage of potential pathogens among patients and the dental staff. This chapter will focus on the role of microorganisms in the pathogenesis of endodontic infections and effective clinical treatment of the infections. In addition, the "Theory of Focal Infection" will be discussed because misinformation is being disseminated that recommends the extraction of teeth, rather than effective root canal treatment.

ASSOCIATION OF MICROBES IN PULPAL AND PERIRADICULAR DISEASES

All of the surfaces of the human body are colonized with microbes. Colonization is simply the establishment of microbes in a host if biochemical and physical conditions that are adequate for growth. It has been estimated that the average human body is colonized by ten times more bacteria (i.e., 10^{14} bacteria) than mammalian cells (i.e., 10^{13} cells).[68] Normal flora is the result of permanent colonization of microbes in a symbiotic relationship that produces beneficial results. However, given the proper conditions, normal oral flora may become "opportunistic pathogens." Opportunistic pathogens produce disease if they gain access to normally sterile areas of the body, such as the dental pulp or periradicular tissues. The degree of pathogenicity produced by microbes is referred to as *virulence*.

Pathogenic response also includes damage produced by the host in response to the microbes. The host's response includes both nonspecific inflammation and specific immunologic reactions. Pulpal injury produces pulpitis, with increased vascular permeability, vasodilation, pain, resorption of hard tissues, and, eventually, pulpal necrosis. Jontell et al[75-77] demonstrated the presence of dendritic cells in the pulp, which activate T-lymphocytes that, in turn, promote a local immune response. Hahn et al[64] showed production of specific IgG in the pulp specific for the bacteria in deep caries. If caries or infection of the root canal system is not treated, inflammation with accompanying bone resorption spreads to the contiguous periradicular tissues (Fig. 13-1).

501

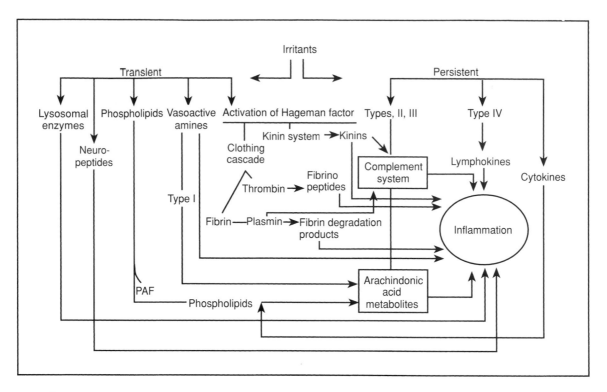

Fig. 13-1 Pathways of inflammation and bone resorption by nonspecific inflammatory mediators and specific immune reactions.

PATHWAYS OF PULPAL INFECTION

Dental caries is the most common pathway for microbes to the root canal system. When the tooth is intact, enamel and dentin provide protection against invasion of the pulp space. As caries approaches the pulp, reparative dentin is laid down to avert exposure, but it is rarely is able to prevent microbial entry without caries excavation.

Dentinal tubules range from 1 to 4 μm, whereas the majority of bacteria are less than 1 μm in diameter. Where the cementum is missing or after trauma, the dentinal tubules may be the pathway for microbial invasion of the pulp space. Bacterial movement is restricted by odontoblastic processes, mineralized crystals, and macromolecules, including immunoglobulins in the tubules.[64] Bacteria and their by-products may have an effect on the pulp before direct exposure.[27,85,140] If the caries is removed, the pulps can undergo healing.

When a healthy vital pulp is exposed as a result of trauma, the penetration of tissue is relatively slow. Bacterial penetration is less than 2 mm after 2 weeks.[35] If the pulp is necrotic, "dead tracts" of empty dentinal tubules are rapidly penetrated. Microbes rapidly reach the pulp space after direct exposure of the pulp from restorative procedures, a traumatic injury, or an anomalous tooth development. The breakdown products of the necrotic pulp, serous exudate, and bacterial by-products provide the nutrients for the invading organisms.

Controversy still exists as to whether periodontal disease directly causes pulpal disease.[37,86,89,130] Microbes and their by-products may reach the pulp space through the portals at the apex of a root and through other lateral, accessory, or furcation canals. Langeland et al[86] found that pulpal necrosis only occurred when the apical foramen was involved. For diagnostic purposes it has been shown that abscesses of periodontal origin contain 30% to 58% spirochetes, whereas abscesses of endodontic origin contain less than 10% spirochetes.[132]

Anachoresis may be defined as the transportation of microbes through the blood or lymph to an area of inflammation, such as a tooth with pulpitis. Anachoresis has been demonstrated in animals but is not believed to contribute to significant disease in humans.[6,53,104] It does seem possible that anachoresis may be the mechanism by which some traumatized teeth may become infected.[61] Anachoresis could not be demonstrated in instrumented but unfilled canals.[40,41]

MICROORGANISMS ASSOCIATED WITH ENDODONTIC DISEASE

In 1890 W.D. Miller, the father of oral microbiology, was the first investigator to associate the presence of bacteria with pulpal disease.[90] A classic study published in 1965 by Kakehashi et al proved the bacteria were the cause of pulpal and periradicular disease.[78] Exposure of the pulps in rats with normal microbial flora produced pulpal necrosis and periradicular lesion formation. No pathologic changes occurred

Table 13-1   BACTERIA FROM THE ROOT CANALS OF TEETH WITH APICAL RAREFACTIONS

Bacteria	Percentage of Incidence
Fusobacterium nucleatum	48
Streptococcus sp.	40
Bacteroides sp.*	35
Prevotella intermedia	34
Peptostreptococcus micros	34
Eubacterium alactolyticum	34
Peptostreptococcus anaerobius	31
Lactobacillus sp.	32
Eubacterium lentum	31
Fusobacterium sp.	29
Campylobacter sp.	25
Peptostreptococcus sp.	15
Actinomyces sp.	15
Eubacterium timidum	11
Capnocytophaga ochracea	11
Eubacterium brachy	9
Selenomonas sputigena	9
Veillonella parvula	9
Porphyromonas endodontalis	9
Prevotella buccae	9
Prevotella oralis	8
Proprionibacterium propionicum	8
Prevotella denticola	6
Prevotella loescheii	6
Eubacterium nodatum	6

*Nonpigmenting species
Other species isolated in low incidence included *Porphyromonas gingivalis, Bacteroides ureolyticus, Bacteroides gracilis, Lactobacillus minutus, Lactobacillus catenaforme, Enterococcus faecalis, Peptostreptococcus prevotii, Eienella corrodens,* and *Enterobacter agglomerans.*
(Adapted from Sundqvist: Taxonomy, ecology, and pathogenicity of the root canal, *Oral Surg* 78:522, 1994.)

the vast majority of bacteria isolated from an endodontic infection are anaerobic. Table 13-1 lists the organisms most often cultivated from endodontic infections. This is a relatively small, restricted group of organisms compared with normal oral flora, which contains over 500 species of cultivable bacteria. Strict anaerobes function at low oxidation–reduction potential and grow only in an absence of oxygen, but they vary in their sensitivity to oxygen. Most strictly anaerobic bacteria are missing the enzymes superoxide dismutase and catalase. Some species of bacteria are microaerophilic and can grow in the presence of oxygen but derive most of their energy from anaerobic energy pathways. Facultative anaerobic bacteria can grow in the presence or absence of oxygen. Obligate aerobes possess both superoxide dismutase and catalase enzymes, and they require oxygen for growth.

Kobayashi et al[82] have compared the bacteria isolated from root canals to those isolated from the sulcus of a periodontal pocket. Because similar species of bacteria were cultivated from the root canals as from the periodontal pockets, they believe that the sulcus is the source of bacteria in root canal infections.

The interrelationships of bacteria were studied in monkeys.[48,49,93] Root canals in the animals were infected with indigenous oral bacteria and then sealed in the teeth for intervals up to 1080 days. The results show that a selective process takes place over time that allows anaerobic bacteria to predominate.[48,49,93] After 1080 days, 98% of the bacteria that were cultured from the canals were strict anaerobes. Apparently tissue fluid, necrotic pulp tissue, low-oxygen tension, and bacterial by-products determine which bacteria will predominate. Some bacterial metabolites may be antagonistic to other bacteria. In addition, some species of bacteria produce bacteriocins which are proteins produced by one species that inhibit another species of bacteria.

When intact teeth with necrotic pulps are cultured, over 90% of the bacteria were strict anaerobes.[126] When the apical 5 mm of carious exposed teeth were cultured, 67% were strict anaerobes.[15] Therefore it seems that the polymicrobial ecosystem in an infected root canal system selects for anaerobes. Gomes et al[56,57] and Sundqvist et al[117,119] have used ratios to show how one species tends to associate with another species.

Some species of black-pigmented bacteria, peptostreptococci, peptococci, *Fusobacterium* sp., *Eubacterium* sp., and *Actinomyces* sp. have been implicated with certain clinical signs and symptoms.* However, no absolute correlation has been made between any species of bacteria and the severity of endodontic infections. This is probably related to the polymicrobial nature of endodontic infections and the synergistic relationship between bacteria or virulence factors that increase the overall pathogenic effect. Polymicrobial infections spread from the root canal to the contiguous periradicular tissues. Endodontic abscesses are mixed infections with

in germ-free rats when the pulps were exposed. The germ-free rats healed with dentinal bridging regardless of the severity of the pulpal exposure, showing that the presence or absence of bacteria was the determinant for pulpal and periapical disease.[78]

Endodontic infections are polymicrobial. As improved methods for culturing improved, the number of microorganisms detected in an endodontic infection increased to a range of 3 to 12 organisms per infected root canal associated with an apical lesion. The number of colony forming units (CFU) is usually between 10^2 and 10^8. A positive correlation exists between the number of bacteria in an infected root canal and the size of periradicular radiolucencies.[32,118]

Before 1970 only a few strains of anaerobic bacteria were isolated because of inadequate culturing methods. Currently,

*References 29,30,44,57-59,62,63,65-67,118,126,135,144

Box 13-1   RECENT TAXONOMIC CHANGES FOR PREVIOUS "BACTEROIDES" SPECIES

Porphyromonas: Black-pigmented (asaccharolytic *Bacteroides* species)
- Porphyromonas asaccharolyticus (usually nonoral)
- Porphyromonas gingivalis*
- Porphyromonas endodontalis*

Prevotella: Black-pigmented (saccharolytic *Bacteroides* species)
- Prevotella melaninogenica
- Prevotella denticola
- Prevotella loescheii
- Prevotella intermedia*
- Prevotella nigrescens†
- Prevotella corporis
- Prevotella tannerae

Prevotella: Nonpigmented (saccharolytic *Bacteroides* species)
- Prevotella buccae*
- Prevotella bivia
- Prevotella oralis
- Prevotella oris
- Prevotella oulorum
- Prevotella ruminicola

* Studies have associated species with clinical signs and symptoms.
† Most commonly isolated species of black-pigmented bacteria from endodontic infections.

several strains of bacteria cultured from each infection.* For example, it has been shown that strains of black-pigmented bacteria in pure culture produce only a mild infection in an animal model, but if mixed with another bacteria (e.g., *Fusobacterium nucleatum*), the combination produces abscesses and even death of the animals.†

In addition, our "state of the art" culturing techniques may be only detecting and identifying a portion of the total microbial population. Conventional identification of bacteria was based on gram-staining, colonial morphology, growth characteristics, and biochemical tests. Very often the best that could be done was a presumptive identification. Taxonomic revision based on DNA studies has left species identification in older studies in question. For example, using DNA methods, the black-pigmented bacteria previously in the genus *Bacteroides* have now been placed in the geneses *Porphyromonas* (asaccharolytic) and *Prevotella* (saccharolytic) (Box 13-1). Using DNA methods, the species *Prevotella nigrescens* was separated from *Prevotella intermedia*.[108] Based on this work it has been determined that

*References 29,30,44,57-59,62,63,65-67,118,126,135,144
†References 18,31,102,120,124,134

P. nigrescens is actually the black-pigmented bacteria most commonly cultivated from endodontic infections.[8,9,43,52]

More recently, molecular techniques were used to identify five strains of black-pigmented bacteria found to be *Prevotella tannerae*.[142] Using biochemical tests these five strains were originally identified as *P. intermedia*.[22] Using sodium dodecyl sulfate-polyacrylamide gel electrophoresis (SDS-PAGE), they were differentiated from *P. intermedia* and believed to be *P. nigrescens*.[9] However, using molecular methods and comparing gene sequences in a gene bank, they have been identified as *P. tannerae*.[142] When 118 samples from endodontic infections were examined using polymerase chain reaction (PCR) with specific primers for *P. tannerae*, 60% of the samples were positive for the presence of the organism.[142] This suggests that *P. tannerae* is commonly present in endodontic infections but not routinely cultivable. There may be many other species that are not cultivable, which include pathogenic organisms yet to be characterized.

It seems that the teleologic purpose of chronic periradicular lesions (i.e., periapical granulomas) is to prevent the spread of infection to surrounding tissues. Thus it has been stated that "a granuloma is not an area in which bacteria live, but in which they are destroyed."[83] Recently investigators have cultured bacteria from asymptomatic chronic periradicular lesions.[1,74,131,141] These studies have been criticized because of the probability of microbial contaminants, either from the surgical procedure, the presence of direct communication (e.g., from sinus tracts), or from the root apex during curettment of the sample. However, as evidenced by the presence of periapical abscesses, bacteria do invade periradicular tissues. Prior to formation of an abscess or cellulitis or both, there may be some point in time where microbial invasion takes place before a symptomatic inflammatory response is mounted against the invading organisms.

Nair[94] used both light and electron microscopy to observe microorganisms, both intracellular and extracellular, in four symptomatic granulomas and one asymptomatic cyst. With 25 other teeth that had asymptomatic, chronic inflammatory lesions, bacteria could not be identified beyond the root apex.[94] Species of *Actinomyces* and *Proprionibacteium* have been shown to be able to persist in inflammatory tissue.[65,99,127] *Actinomyces israelii* is a species of bacteria isolated from periapical tissues that does not always respond to conventional endodontic therapy.[65,99,127] However, both sodium hypochlorite and calcium hydroxide have been shown to be highly effective in killing *A. israelii*.[13] In addition, endodontic surgery apparently is an effective way to remove *A. israelii* from the periapex and seems to provide a high success rate without antibiotics.[13,65,127] However, when a periradicular infection with *A. israelii* is not resolved by surgery, antibiotic therapy is optimized by prescribing amoxicillin or cephalexin.[13] The need for this extended regimen of antibiotics is a relatively rare occurrence.

The presence of *A. israelii* should be confirmed with either a biopsy or a culture showing the presence of *Actinomyces* sp., without healing of the lesion after conventional treatment. Recent studies of endodontically treated teeth requiring retreatment have shown a prevalence of facultative bacteria, especially *Streptococcus faecalis,* instead of strict anaerobes that are predominant in the initial infections.[*] It has also been reported that complete periapical healing occurred in 94% that had negative cultures at the obturation appointment, whereas complete healing occurred in just 68% of cases with positive cultures at the time of obturation.[111] These results support previous studies showing that failure of healing is more likely when the canals are obturated in the presence of a persisting infection.[95,110]

Bacteria have long been associated with endodontic infections, but the role of other microbes, including viruses and fungi, has only recently been investigated.[54,55,95,106] Studies have identified the presence of fungi after therapy-resistant endodontic treatment.[95,125,138] A recent study by Waltimo et al showed that strains of *Candida albicans* required incubation with a saturated solution of calcium hydroxide for about 16 hours to kill 99.9% of the fungi.[137] Out of 692 samples of therapy-resistant, chronic apical periodontitis, Waltimo et al[138] identified 48 fungi in 47 (7%) samples. Sen et al[106] used scanning electron microscopy (SEM) to observe fungi in the dentinal tubules of 4 of 10 extracted human molars with infected root canals. In another recent study, the polymerase chain reaction was used to detect *Candida albicans* in 5 of 24 intact teeth with infected root canals (but not in 19 samples aspirated from periradicular abscesses or cellulitis[23]).

BACTERIAL VIRULENCE FACTORS

Although the initial injury may be associated with other causes (e.g., physical or chemical trauma), the majority of pathogenic responses are associated with microorganisms. Microbes have numerous virulence factors, which include bacterial capsules, fimbriae (pili), lipopolysaccharides (LPS), enzymes, extracellular vesicles, fatty acids, polyamines, ammonia, and hydrogen sulfides. Both gram-positive and gram-negative bacteria have capsules that may protect the bacteria from phagocytosis.[120]

Fimbriae and extracellular vesicles may participate in aggregation of bacteria or attachment to tissues.[80] Pili may extend form one bacterium to another during conjugation and exchange DNA for virulence factors, including resistance to antibiotics. When LPS is released from the outer membrane of gram-negative bacteria, it is called *endotoxin.* Endotoxin has several biologic effects, including the activation of complement and bone resorption.[46,72] It has been shown that the concentration of endotoxin in the canals of symptomatic teeth is higher than that in the canals of asymptomatic teeth.[71]

Enzymes are produced by bacteria and are detrimental to the host. It was recently shown that the gene for collagenase

could be detected in stains of *Porphyromonas gingivalis* but not *Porphyromonas endodontalis* isolated from endodontic infections.[97] Collagenase is a metalloprotease that seems to be associated with the spread of cellulitis.[11,128,129] Other enzymes produced by bacteria neutralize immunoglobulins and the components of complement.[121-123] In abscesses, neutrophils lyse and release their enzymes to the surrounding milieu to form purulent exudate. This enzyme-rich exudate has an adverse affect on the surrounding tissues.

Extracellular vesicles are formed from the outer membrane of gram-negative bacteria and have a trilaminar structure similar to the parent bacteria. Because they have the same surface antigens, they are capable of neutralizing antibodies against the parent organism. The vesicles may contain enzymes or other toxic agents. Extracellular vesicles are believed to be involved in hemagglutination, hemolysis, bacterial adhesion, and proteolytic action on host tissues.[80,107]

The short-chain fatty acids most commonly produced by bacteria in infected root canals are propionic, butyric, and isobutyric acids. Short-chain fatty acids affect neutrophil chemotaxis, degranulation, chemiluminescence, and phagocytosis. Butyric acid has the greatest inhibition of T-cell blastogenesis and stimulates the production of interleukin-1 (IL-1), which is associated with bone resorption.[47] Host cells and bacteria produce polyamines.

Polyamines are biologically active compounds involved in the regulation of growth, regeneration of tissues, and modulation of inflammation. They include spermine, spermidine, cadaverine, and putrescine. Polyamines, which are produced by both bacteria and host cells, are found in infected root canals. Teeth that are painful to percussion or have spontaneous pain have been shown to have a higher concentration of total polyamines (specifically putrescine) in necrotic pulps.[47]

PERIRADICULAR RESPONSE TO INFECTIONS

Numerous studies have analyzed the inflammatory cells in a chronic apical periodontitis.[*] The majority of cells associated with an untreated, infected root canal are T-lymphocytes. During the first 15 days of periapical lesion–development in a rat model, the Th (i.e., helper) cells outnumber the Ts (i.e., suppressor) cells.[114] However, after 15 days the Ts cells outnumber the Th cells.[114] The Th cells seem to be associated with bone resorption and lesion expansion. In another study, the cells associated with endodontically treated teeth had more B-lymphocytes than T-lymphocytes.[5] Thus the periradicular inflammatory tissue is capable of an immunologic response to bacteria and bacterial by-products.

Several studies using enzyme-linked immunosorbent assay (ELISA), radioimmunosorbent tests, and radial immunodiffusion assays have demonstrated the presence of IgG, IgA, IgM, or IgE.[†] In one study, IgG produced from peri-

---

[*]References 92,103,109,111,125

[*]References 5,7,12,26,36,88,96,101,115,130
[†]References 14,16,17,19,79

apical explants from humans was more often reactive with black-pigmented bacteria (e.g., *P. intermedia, P. endodontalis, P. gingivalis)* than the any of the other species of bacteria tested.[19] In addition, an increase in the level of serum IgG reactive with *P. intermedia* has been shown to be associated with patients having periodontal disease or combined endodontic and periodontal disease.[20]

Another investigation has shown that samples from root canals associated with symptomatic periapical lesions contain elevated amounts of ß-glucoronidase and interleukin-1ß.[84] Interleukin-1 and prostaglandins seem to be especially associated with bone resorption. However, other mediators, including prostanoids, kinins, and neuropeptides, are involved in the inflammatory response.[113] The antigens of bacteria and bacterial by-products stimulate both B-cells and T-cells. For example, LPS can produce both polyclonal stimulation of B-cells and induce macrophage activation.

Abscesses and cellulitis are the result of bacteria invading and infecting periradicular tissues. Chemotaxis of neutrophils is a nonspecific inflammatory response to the presence of bacteria in normally sterile tissues. With accumulation of neutrophils and the resulting purulent exudate, an acute apical inflammatory response develops. The seriousness of the infection is related to numbers and virulence of the bacteria, host resistance, and associated anatomic structures. By definition an *abscess* is an accumulation of purulent exudate, consisting of bacteria, bacterial by-products, inflammatory cells (mainly neutrophils), lysed inflammatory cells, and the contents of those cells (e.g., enzymes). A *cellulitis* is defined as a diffuse, erythemous, mucosal or cutaneous infection that may spread to deeper facial spaces and become life threatening. However, needle aspirates often reveal pockets of pus within a diffuse cellulitis. From a clinical viewpoint, a cellulitis and an abscess may be considered a continuum of the inflammatory process. It is just a matter of timing before purulence is visibly present in an area of cellulitis.

FASCIAL SPACE INFECTIONS

If bacteria from the infected pulp tissue gain entry into the periradicular tissue and the patient's immune system is not able to suppress the invasion, an otherwise healthy patient will eventually show signs and symptoms of an acute periradicular abscess, cellulitis, or both. Clinically, the patient experiences swelling and mild-to-severe pain. Depending on the relationship of the apices of the involved tooth to the muscular attachments, the swelling may be localized to the vestibule or extend into a fascial space. In addition, the patient may exhibit systemic manifestations, such as fever, chills, lymphadenopathy, headache, and nausea. Because the reaction to the infection may occur very quickly, the involved tooth may or may not show radiographic evidence of a widened periodontal ligament space. However, in most cases, the tooth will elicit a positive response to percussion, and the periradicular area will be tender to palpation. The tooth in

this case is indeed serving as a *focus of infection,* because it leads to periapical infection and secondary (i.e., metastatic) spread to the fascial spaces of the head and neck (resulting in cellulitis and systemic signs and symptoms of infection).

In most cases, treatment involves incision, for drainage, and root canal treatment of the involved tooth to remove the source of the infection. Antibiotic therapy may be indicated if the patient has a compromised host resistance, the presence of systemic symptoms, or fascial space involvement. Fascial space infections of odontogenic origin are infections that have spread into the fascial spaces from the periapical area of a tooth: the focus of infection. They are *not* examples of the *Theory of Focal Infection,* which describes the dissemination of bacteria or their toxic products from a distant focus of infection.

Fascial spaces are potential anatomic areas that exist between the fascia and underlying organs and other tissues. During an infection, these spaces are formed as a result of the spread of purulent exudate. The spread of infections of odontogenic origin into the fascial spaces of the head and neck is determined by the location of the root end of the involved tooth in relation to its overlying buccal or lingual cortical plate and the relationship of the apex with the attachment of a muscle. For example, if the source of the infection is a mandibular molar and the apices of the molar lie closer to the lingual cortical plate and above the attachment of the mylohyoid muscle of the floor of the mouth, the purulent exudate will break through the lingual cortical plate into the sublingual space (Fig. 13-2). If the apices, however, lie below the attachment of the mylohyoid muscle, the infection would spread into the submandibular space.

As described by Hohl et al,[70] the fascial spaces of the head and neck can be placed into four anatomic groups:
1. Mandible and below
2. Cheek and lateral face

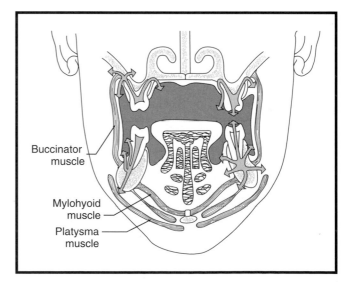

Fig. 13-2 Spread of odontogenic infections.

Buccinator muscle

Mylohyoid muscle

Platysma muscle

3. Pharyngeal and cervical
4. Midface

Swellings of and below the mandible include six anatomic areas or fascial spaces:

1. Buccal vestibule
2. Body of the mandible
3. Mental space
4. Submental space
5. Sublingual space
6. Submandibular space

The *mandibular buccal vestibule* is the anatomic area located between the buccal cortical plate, overlying alveolar mucosa and the buccinator muscle in the posterior (or mentalis) muscle in the anterior (Figs. 13-3 and 13-4). In this case the source of the infection is a mandibular posterior or ante-

rior tooth in which the purulent exudate breaks through the buccal cortical plate, and the apex or apices of the involved tooth lie above the attachment of the buccinator or mentalis muscle, respectively.

The *space of the body of the mandible* is that potential anatomic area that is located between the buccal or lingual cortical plate and its overlying periosteum. The source of infection is a mandibular tooth in which the purulent exudate has broken through the overlying cortical plate, but not yet perforated the overlying periosteum. Involvement of this space can also occur as a result of a postsurgical infection.

The *mental space* (Fig. 13-5) is the potential bilateral, anatomic area of the chin that lies between the mentalis muscle superiorly and the platysma muscle inferiorly. The source of the infection is an anterior tooth in which the purulent exudate breaks through the buccal cortical plate, and the apex of the tooth lies below the attachment of the mentalis muscle.

The *submental space* (Fig. 13-6) is that potential anatomic area that lies between the mylohyoid muscle superiorly and the platysma muscle inferiorly. The source of the infection is an anterior tooth in which the purulent exudate breaks through the lingual cortical plate, and the apex of the tooth lies below the attachment of the mylohyoid muscle.

The *sublingual space* (Fig. 13-7) is that potential anatomic area that lies between the oral mucosa of the floor of the mouth superiorly and the mylohyoid muscle inferiorly. The lateral boundaries of the space are the lingual surfaces of the mandible. The source of infection is any mandibular tooth in which the purulent exudate breaks through the lingual cortical plate and the apex or apices of the tooth lie above the attachment of the mylohyoid muscle.

The *submandibular space* (Fig. 13-8) is the potential space that lies between the mylohyoid muscle superiorly and the platysma muscle inferiorly. The source of infection is a posterior tooth, usually a molar, in which the purulent exudate breaks through the lingual cortical plate, and the apices of the tooth lie below the attachment of the mylohyoid mus-

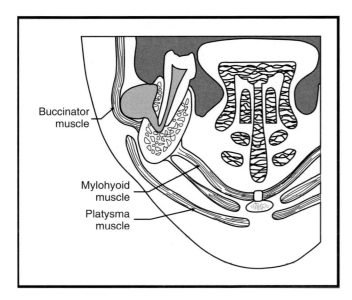

Fig. 13-3 Mandibular buccal vestibule (posterior tooth).

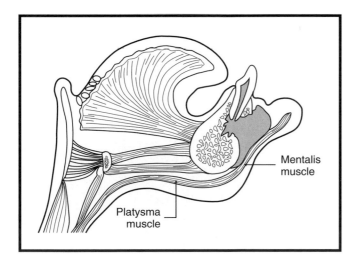

Fig. 13-4 Mandibular buccal vestibule (anterior tooth).

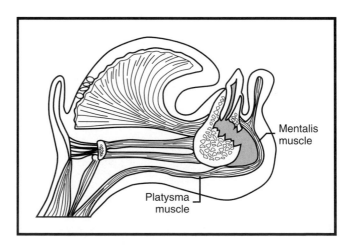

Fig. 13-5 Mental space.

cle. If the submental, sublingual, and submandibular spaces are involved at the same time, a diagnosis of *Ludwig's Angina* is made. This life-threatening cellulitis can advance into the pharyngeal and cervical spaces, resulting in airway obstruction.

Swellings of the lateral face and cheek include four anatomic areas or fascial spaces:

1. Buccal vestibule of the maxilla
2. Buccal space
3. Submasseteric space
4. Temporal space

Anatomically, the *buccal vestibular space* (Fig. 13-9) is located between the buccal cortical plate, the overlying mucosa, and the buccinator muscle. The superior extent of the space is the attachment of the buccinator muscle to the zygomatic process. The source of infection is a maxillary posterior tooth in which the purulent exudate breaks through the buccal cortical plate, and the apex of the tooth lies below the attachment of the buccinator muscle.

The *buccal space* (Fig. 13-10) is the potential space located between the lateral surface of the buccinator muscle and the medial surface of the skin of the cheek. The superior extent of the space is the attachment of the buccinator muscle to the zygomatic arch, whereas the inferior and posterior boundaries are the attachment of the buccinator to the inferior border of the mandible and the anterior margin of the masseter muscle, respectively. The source of the infection can be either a posterior mandibular or maxillary tooth in which the purulent exudate breaks through the buccal cortical plate, and the apex or apices of the tooth lie above the attachment of the buccinator muscle (i.e., maxilla) or below the attachment of the buccinator muscle (i.e., mandible).

As the name implies, the *submasseteric space* (Fig. 13-11) is the potential space that lies between the lateral surface of the ramus of the mandible and the medial surface of the masseter muscle. The source of the infection is usually an impacted third molar in which the purulent exudate breaks through the lingual cortical plate. The apices of the tooth lie very close to or within the space.

The *temporal space* (Fig. 13-12) is divided into two compartments by the temporalis muscle. The *deep temporal space* is the potential space that lies between the lateral sur-

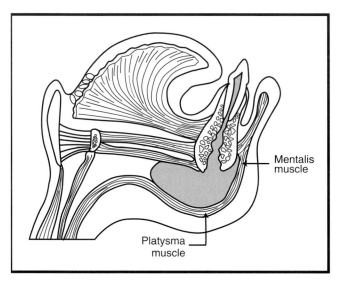

Fig. 13-6 Submental space.

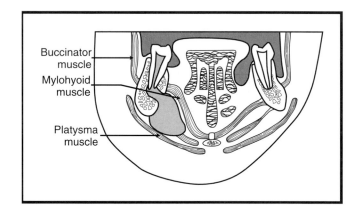

Fig. 13-8 Submandibular space.

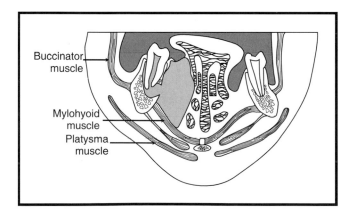

Fig. 13-7 Sublingual space.

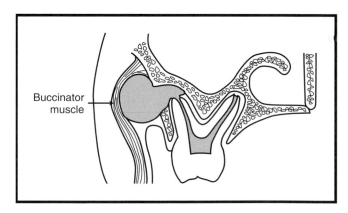

Fig. 13-9 Maxillary buccal vestibule.

face of the skull and medial surface of the temporalis muscle, whereas the *superficial temporal space* lies between the temporalis muscle and its overlying fascia. The deep and superficial temporal spaces are involved indirectly as a result of an infection spreading superiorly from the inferior pterygomandibular and submasseteric spaces, respectively.

Swellings of the pharyngeal and cervical areas include the following fascial spaces:

1. Pterygomandibular space
2. Parapharyngeal spaces
3. Cervical spaces

The *pterygomandibular space* (Fig. 13-13) is the potential space that lies between the lateral surface of the medial pterygoid muscle and the medial surface of the ramus of the mandible. The superior extent of the space is the lateral pterygoid muscle. The source of the infection is mandibular second or third molars in which the purulent exudate drains directly into the space. In addition, contaminated inferior alveolar nerve injections can lead to infection of the space.

The *parapharyngeal spaces* are comprised of the lateral pharyngeal and retropharyngeal spaces (Fig. 13-14). The *lateral pharyngeal space* is bilateral and lies between the lateral surface of the medial pterygoid muscle and the posterior surface of the superior constrictor muscle. The superior and inferior margins of the space are the base of the skull and the hyoid bone, respectively, whereas the posterior margin is the *carotid space,* or sheath, which contains the common carotid artery, internal jugular vein, and the vagus nerve. Anatomically, the *retropharyngeal space* lies between the anterior surface of the prevertebral fascia and the posterior surface of the superior constrictor muscle and extends inferiorly into the retroesophageal space, which extends into the posterior compartment of the mediastinum. The pharyngeal spaces usually become involved as a result of the secondary spread

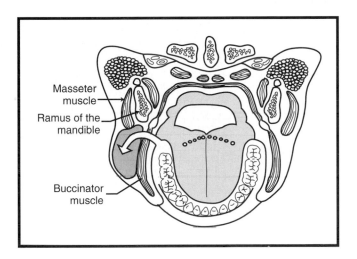

Fig. 13-10 Buccal space.

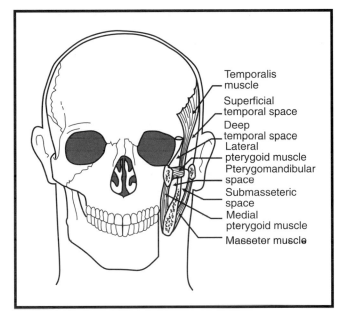

Fig. 13-12 Temporal spaces.

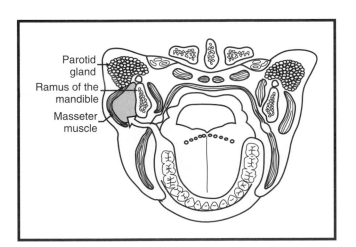

Fig. 13-11 Submasseteric space.

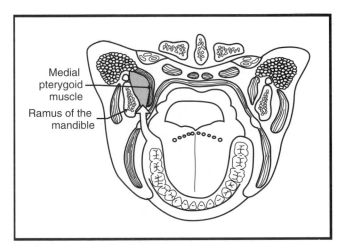

Fig. 13-13 Pterygomandibular space.

of infection from other fascial spaces or directly from a peritonsillar abscess.

The cervical spaces are comprised of the pretracheal, retrovisceral, danger, and prevertebral spaces (Fig. 13-15). The *pretracheal space* is the potential space surrounding the trachea. It extends from the thyroid cartilage *inferiorly* into the superior portion of the anterior compartment of the mediastinum to the level of the arch of the aorta. Because of its anatomic location, odontogenic infections do not spread to the pretracheal space. The *retrovisceral space* is comprised of the retropharyngeal space superiorly and the retroesophageal space inferiorly. The space extends from the base of the skull into the posterior compartment of the mediastinum to a level between vertebrae C-6 and T-4. The *danger space* (i.e., space 4), as originally described by Grodinsky and Holyoke,[60] is the potential space that lies between the alar and prevertebral fascia. Because this space is comprised of loose connective tissue, it is considered an actual anatomic space extending from the base of the skull into the posterior compartment of the mediastinum to a level corresponding to the diaphragm. The *prevertebral space* is the potential space surrounding the vertebral column. As such, it extends from vertebra C-1 to the coccyx. A retrospective study showed that 71% of the cases in which the mediastinum was involved resulted from the spread of infection from the retrovisceral space (21% from the carotid space and 8% from the pretracheal space[87]).

Swellings of the midface consist of four anatomic areas and spaces:
1. Palate
2. Base of the upper lip
3. Canine spaces
4. Periorbital spaces

Although not considered actual fascial spaces, odontogenic infections can spread into the area between the palate and its overlying periosteum and mucosa and the base of the upper lip, which lies superior to the orbicularis oris muscle.

The source of infection of the palate is any of the maxillary teeth in which the apex of the involved tooth lies close to the palate, whereas the source of infection of the base of the upper lip is a maxillary central incisor in which the apex lies close to the buccal cortical plate and above the attachment of the orbicularis oris muscle.

The *canine,* or *infraorbital space,* (Fig. 13-16) is the potential space that lies between the levator anguli oris muscle inferiorly and the levator labii superioris muscle superiorly. The source of infection is the maxillary canine or first premolar in which the purulent exudate breaks through the buccal cortical plate and the apex of the tooth lies above the attachment of the levator anguli oris muscle.

The *periorbital space* (see Fig. 13-16) is the potential space that lies deep to the orbicularis oculi muscle. The source of infection is the spread of infection from the canine or buccal spaces. Infections of the midface can be very dangerous because they can result in *cavernous sinus throm-*

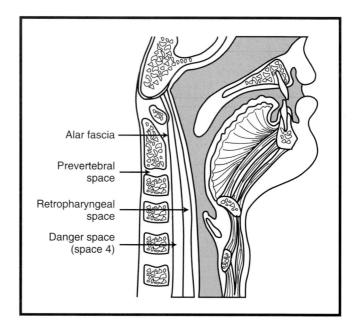

Fig. 13-15 Cervical spaces.

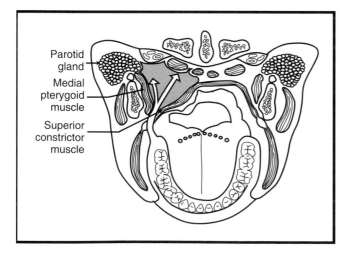

Fig. 13-14 Parapharyngeal spaces.

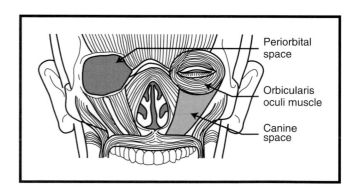

Fig. 13-16 Canine (infraorbital) and periorbital spaces.

bosis, a life-threatening infection in which a thrombus formed in the cavernous sinus breaks free, resulting in blockage of an artery or spread of infection. Under normal conditions, the angular and ophthalmic veins and the pterygoid plexus of veins flow into the facial and external jugular veins. If an infection has spread into the midfacial area, however, edema and resultant increased pressure from the inflammatory response causes the blood to back up into the cavernous sinus. Once in the sinus, the blood stagnates and clots. The resultant infected thrombi remain in the cavernous sinus or escape into the circulation.[100,145]

MANAGEMENT OF ABSCESSES AND CELLULITIS

Of most importance in effective patient management is the correct diagnosis and removal of the cause of an infection of endodontic origin. Chemomechanical débridement of the infected root canals and incision for drainage of periradicular swelling in an otherwise healthy patient will usually allow rapid improvement in the patient's clinical signs and symptoms. Most endodontic infections can be effectively treated without the use of adjunctive antibiotics. The appropriate treatment is removal of the cause of the inflammatory event.

The prescription of antibiotics (i.e., antimicrobials) is not recommended for irreversible pulpitis, acute apical periodontitis, a draining sinus tract, after endodontic surgery, or after incision for drainage of a localized swelling (without cellulitis, fever, or lymphadenopathy). In these situations, when ratio of risks to benefits are considered, an antibiotic may put the patient at risk for the side effects of the antimicrobial agent and select for resistant organisms.[51,139] Finally, analgesics (not antibiotics) are indicated for the treatment of pain.

The use of adjunctive antibiotics is recommended in conjunction with appropriate endodontic treatment for progressive or persistent infections or both, which have any of the following systemic signs and symptoms. These include fever (>100°F), malaise, cellulitis, unexplained trismus, and progressive or persistent swelling or both. With these signs and symptoms, the prescription of an antibiotic is indicated as adjunctive therapy to effective débridement of the root canal system, which is the reservoir of the organisms. In addition, aggressive incision for drainage is indicated for any infection with a cellulitis. Incision for drainage is indicated whether the cellulitis is indurated or fluctuant. It is important to provide a pathway of drainage to prevent further spread of the abscess and/or cellulitis. An incision for drainage allows decompression of the increased tissue pressure associated with edema and provides significant pain relief for the patient. The incision also provides a pathway for not only bacteria and bacterial by-products but also for the inflammatory mediators associated with the spread of cellulitis.

A minimum inhibitory concentration of antibiotic may not reach the source of the infection because of decreased blood flow and because the antibiotic must diffuse through the edematous fluid and pus. Drainage of edematous fluid and purulent exudate improves circulation to the tissues associated with an abscess or cellulitis, providing better delivery of the antibiotic to the area. Placement of a drain may not be indicated for localized fluctuant swellings if complete evacuation of the purulent exudate is believed to have occurred.

For effective drainage, a stab incision is made in the most dependent site of the swelling through the periosteum. The incision must be long enough to allow blunt dissection using a curved hemostat or periosteal elevator under the periosteum for drainage of pockets of inflammatory exudate. *A rubber dam drain (or preferably a penrose drain) is indicated for any patient having a progressive abscess or cellulitis to maintain an open pathway for drainage.* Patients should rapidly improve after the removal of the cause of the infection and drainage. Patients with cellulitis should be followed on a daily basis to ensure the infection is resolving.

Endodontic treatment should be completed as soon as possible after the incision for drainage to remove the cause of the infection. The drain can usually be removed in 1 or 2 days after improvement in clinical signs and symptoms. If there is not a significant improvement, then the diagnosis and treatment must be carefully reviewed. Consultation with a specialist and referral may be indicated for severe infections or with persistent infections. Likewise, patients requiring extraoral drainage should be referred to a clinician trained in the technique.

ANTIBIOTICS (ANTIMICROBIALS) FOR ENDODONTIC INFECTIONS

Ideally susceptibility testing would be done when antibiotics are indicated. However, because it may take from several days to weeks to do testing on strict anaerobes, empiric prescription of antibiotics is done. Empiric prescription of antibiotics is based on past knowledge of the organisms most likely associated with endodontic infections.

Clinicians should inform the patients of the benefits, risks, side effects, and problems if the proper dosing schedule is not followed. Although the antituberculosis drug rifampin seems to be the only antimicrobial proven to reduce the effectiveness of oral contraceptives, case reports have implicated other antibiotics.[69] Thus patients using oral contraception should be warned to use alternative methods of birth control.[69] The prudent use of antibiotics to treat endodontic infections is an integral part of appropriate treatment. In general an antibiotic should be taken for 2 to 3 days after resolution of the major clinical signs and symptoms. Thus the typical regimen to treat an endodontic infections is from 6 to 10 days on an around-the-clock schedule. Improvement should be seen in 24 to 48 hours after initial treatment and initiation of the prescription. A high-dose regimen for a short time is preferred to a low dose for a longer time. The latter is much more likely to select for resistant organisms. A loading dose is generally recommended to provide an initial effective serum level that is then followed by the maintenance dose.

Penicillin VK

Penicillin VK has a relatively narrow spectrum of microbial activity, which includes many of the bacteria most often identified from endodontic infections, including both facultative and anaerobic bacteria. Penicillin VK remains the antibiotic of choice for treatment of endodontic infections because of its efficacy and low toxicity.[10,103,136,143] However, all of the penicillins have up to a 10% allergy rate, which is a major concern. An oral loading dose of 1000 mg should be followed by 500 mg every 6 hours for 6 to 10 days. For severe infections the antibiotic may be prescribed every 4 hours to maintain a more level serum level.

Amoxicillin

Amoxicillin has a broader spectrum of activity than penicillin VK that includes bacteria usually not isolated from endodontic infections. It is absorbed more rapidly and gives a higher and more sustained serum level.[38] However, because of its wider spectrum, it will select for more resistant organisms, especially in the gastrointestinal tract. For patients that are immunocompromised or otherwise medically compromised, the prescription of a broader spectrum penicillin may be warranted. An oral loading dose of 1000 mg of amoxicillin should be followed by 500 mg every 8 hours for 6 to 10 days. The combination of amoxicillin with clavulanate (i.e., Augmentin) is not recommended for endodontic infections unless it is determined that ß lactamase–producing bacteria are causing the infection.

Clarithromycin and Azithromycin

Clarithromycin and azithromycin are macrolides (like erythromycin) but are effective against some of the anaerobic species of bacteria associated with endodontic infections (unlike erythromycin). They may be considered for mild infections in patients allergic to penicillin but do not have a long-term track record. They produce less gastrointestinal upset than erythromycin. Clarithromycin may be given with or without meals in a dose of 250 to 500 mg every 12 hours for 6 to 10 days. Aziththromycin should be taken 1 hour before meals or 2 hours after meals, with a loading dose of 500 mg on the first day, followed by 250 mg daily. These antimicrobials block the metabolism of a number of drugs, so care must be taken to check interaction with other drugs the patient may be taking. They block the metabolism of warfarin and anisindione, which can lead to serious bleeding in anticoagulated patients.[69]

Metronidazole

Metronidazole is an antimicrobial with excellent activity against strict anaerobes but ineffective against facultative bacteria. It can be used in conjunction with penicillin when the latter does not seem to be effective after 2 to 3 days of therapy without improvement of the patient's signs and symptoms. After reviewing the diagnosis and appropriate drainage, the addition of metronidazole to penicillin is indicated. Metronidazole is prescribed in a loading dose of 500 mg, followed by 250 to 500 mg every 6 hours. Penicillin should be continued because metronidazole is not effective against facultative bacteria. Patients taking metronidazole should not consume alcohol during therapy and for at least 3 days afterward because of a disulfiram type of reaction. Likewise, metronidazole should be avoided in patients taking lithium.

Clindamycin

Clindamycin is recommended for patients with a serious infection and an allergy to penicillin. It is effective against both facultative and strict anaerobes. Clindamycin is distributed throughout the body and concentrates in bone. Although antibiotic-associated colitis (i.e., pseudomembraneous colitis) has been linked to clindamycin, it only rarely occurs in the doses recommended for endodontic infections. In addition, antibiotic-associated colitis has been associated with numerous other antibiotics, with the exception of aminoglycosides. Clindamycin should be prescribed with a 300 mg loading dose and then 150 to 300 mg every 6 hours for 6-10 days.

ANTIBIOTICS FOR MEDICALLY COMPROMISED PATIENTS

The American Heart Association (AHA) has updated their guidelines for prophylactic antibiotic coverage for medically compromised patients.[38] The guidelines are not based on controlled clinical studies but on an analysis of relevant articles. The guidelines are published as an aid to clinicians and not intended as a standard of care or as a substitute for clinical judgment. If there is any doubt about the need for antibiotic prophylaxis, the clinician should request a consultation with the patient's physician.

The incidence of bacteremia is low for nonsurgical root canal therapy, but microorganisms can be extruded past the root apex.[21,25,39] A recent population-based study concluded that *dental treatments, in general, did not seem to be a risk factor for infective endocarditis.*[116] If more studies support these findings, future consideration should be given to downgrading antibiotic prophylaxis for most dental procedures, except for tooth extractions and gingival surgery.[45] The AHA recommends antibiotic endocarditis prophylaxis for root canal instrumentation or surgery beyond the root apex and for intraligamentary local anesthetic injections. Endocarditis prophylaxis in not recommended for non-intraligamentary local anesthetic injections, rubber dam placement, or the taking of radiographs.

For patients not allergic to penicillins, amoxicillin in a dose of 2 g, 1 hour before the dental procedure is recommended. Amoxicillin is recommended because it is better absorbed from the gastrointestinal tract and provides a higher

Table 13-2   **PROPHYLACTIC REGIMENS FOR DENTAL PROCEDURES**

Situation	Agent	Regimen*
Standard general prophylaxis	amoxicillin	Adults: 2.0 g Children: 50 mg/kg orally 1 hour before procedure
Unable to take oral medications	ampicillin	Adults: 2.0 g IM or IV Children: 50 mg/kg IM or IV within 30 min before procedure
Allergic to penicillin	clindamycin	Adults: 600 mg Children: 20 mg/kg orally 1 hr before procedure
	OR cephalexin†	Adults: 2.0 g Children: 50 mg/kg
	OR cefadroxil†	orally 1 hour before procedure
	OR azithromycin	Adults: 500 mg
	clarithromycin	Children: 15 mg/kg or orally 1 hour before procedure
Allergic to penicillin unable to take oral medications	clindamycin	Adults: 600 mg Children: 20 mg/kg and IV within 30 min before procedure
	OR cefazolin†	Adults: 1.0 g Children: 25 mg/kg IM or IV within 30 min before procedure

IM, Intramuscularly; *IV*, intravenously.
*Total children's dose should not exceed adult dose.
†Cephalosporins should not be used in individuals with immediate type of hypersensitivity reaction (i.e., urticaria, angioedema, or anaphylaxis) to penicillins.
(From: Dejani AD et al: Prevention of Bacterial endocarditis: recommendations by the American Heart Assocation, *JADA* 128:1142, August 1997.)

and longer sustained serum level than penicillin V. Table 13-2 gives alternative endocarditis prophylactic regimens.

Recent guidelines have also been updated for antibiotic prophylaxis for patients with total joint replacements.[3] Those considered to be at risk for prosthetic joint replacement include patients who are immunocompromised or immunosuppressed, patients who have insulin-dependent (i.e., Type I) diabetes, patients who have had joint replacement surgery less than two years prior to dental treatment, patients who have had previous prosthetic joint infections, patients with malnourishment, and patients with hemophilia.[3,4] The recommended regimen of antibiotics is 2 g of amoxicillin 1 hour before dental treatment. If patients are not able to take oral medication, then cefazolin (1 g) or ampicillin (2 g) intramuscularly or intravenously 1 hour before the dental procedure is recommended. If the patients are allergic to penicillin, clindamycin (600 mg) orally 1 hour before the dental treatment is recommended. Intravenous clindamycin (600 mg) may be used if the patient is not able to take oral medication.

MICROBIAL SAMPLES FOR LABORATORY SUPPORT

Most regimens of adjunctive antibiotics for treatment of endodontic infections are prescribed empirically; however, there are times when identification of the organisms or susceptibility tests may be valuable. For example, patients that are immunosuppressed after radiation or chemotherapy or at high risk of developing an infection (e.g., previous infective endocarditis) may need to have infective organisms better targeted by an antibiotic selected with laboratory support. Samples may be collected either from an infected root canal or from a periradicular abscess or cellulitis.

To obtain an aseptic sample from a root canal, the tooth must be isolated with a rubber dam. The surface of the tooth and surrounding field must be disinfected with NaOCl or other disinfectant. Access to the canal is made with sterile burs and instruments. If there is drainage the sample may be collected using a sterile needle and syringe or with the use of sterile paper points. Air should be vented from the syringe and the aspirate placed in anaerobic transport media provided by the laboratory. To sample a dry canal, the clinician should use a sterile syringe to place some sterile transport media into the canal. A sterile instrument is used to suspend microbes in the media, and the sample taken as described.

A sample from a mucosal swelling is best acquired by needle aspiration through the disinfected mucosal surface to avoid contamination with "normal oral flora." Once profound anesthesia is achieved, the patient is asked to rinse with chlorhexidine mouthwash and then the surface is scrubbed with an iodophor swab. The surface is then penetrated with a sterile 16-20 gauge needle and moved into the area of swelling, where a sample of the exudate is aspirated. A new sterile needle is then placed on the syringe and any air vented before the aspirate is injected into an anaerobic transport media recommended by the laboratory. After taking the specimen, an incision for drainage is made *and blunt dissec-*

tion with a periosteal elevator and curved hemostat is used to provide complete drainage from the tissues.

Good communication with the laboratory personnel is important so that they understand that "normal oral flora" may be "opportunistic pathogens." Although a gram stain may demonstrate the predominate morphologic type present, they must be identified or tested for susceptibility to alter the choice of antibiotic. Identification or susceptibility testing will establish which antibiotic is effective against the remaining resistant organisms. Unfortunately, it takes 1 to 2 weeks to identify many of the slow growing, strict anaerobes. In the near future, molecular techniques will be routinely available to give rapid results with 24 to 48 hours.

THEORY OF FOCAL INFECTION—DÉJÀ VU?

In 1952 an editorial in the *Journal of the American Medical Association* stated:

"After exerting a tremendous influence on the practice of medicine for a generation, the theory of focal infection in the past 10 or 15 years has fallen in part into disfavor. This has been due partly to the following observations that seem to discredit it: (1) Many patients with diseases presumably caused by foci of infection have not been relieved of their symptoms by removal of the foci. (2) Many patients with these same systemic diseases have no evident focus of infection. (3) Foci of infection are, according to some statistical studies, as common in apparently healthy persons as in those with disease."[112]

This editorial supposedly marked the end of the focal infection theory as it was known at that time. The focal infection theory as it applied to endodontics was the erroneous theory put forward in the early part of this century (1910 to 1940) stating that pulpless and endodontically treated teeth may leak bacteria or toxins or both into the body, causing arthritis and diseases of the kidneys and heart, as well as nervous, gastrointestinal, endocrine, and other systems. During this time most dentists and physicians accepted the theory. As a result, to cure a multitude of chronic illnesses, millions of teeth were needlessly extracted. In that era the term "pulpless tooth" was used to describe a tooth with a nonvital pulp associated with a periapical rarefaction. Currently, we define a pulpless tooth as a tooth from which the pulp has been removed.[2]

Numerous studies conducted by both medical and dental researchers during and after this dismal period in dental history thoroughly disproved the theory. In particular, epidemiologic and biologic studies showed that endodontic therapy was safe and it resulted in the saving of teeth. In addition, the investigations proved that teeth with a nonvital pulp or endodontically treated teeth were not the cause of chronic illnesses. Unfortunately, the theory (as it pertains to teeth with nonvital pulps or endodontically treated teeth) is still promulgated through anecdotal stories, *even though the concept is erroneous and has no scientific basis in fact.* There is

growing evidence that a correlation between systemic health and periodontal disease exists.

Historically, the origin of the focal infection theory dates back to 1888 when Dr. W.D. Miller proposed that necrotic pulps could act as centers of infection, resulting in alveolar abscesses.[91] Dr. Frank Billings, in 1904, reported for the first time a positive correlation between oral disease and endocarditis and defined a *focus of infection* as a "circumscribed area of tissue infected with pathogenic organisms."[28] In 1909 Dr. E.C. Rosenow, a student of Billing's, reported that organisms present in diseased organs could establish an infection in a distant organ. This "theory of elective localization" proposed that bacteria have a specific affinity for certain tissues and organs of the body. Rosenow went on to define *focal infection* as a "localized or generalized infection caused by the dissemination of bacteria or their toxic products from a distant focus of infection."[105]

In 1910 Dr. William Hunter, a British physician, presented a lecture entitled *The Role of Sepsis and Antisepsis in Medicine* to the faculty of McGill University in Montreal.[73] His presentation severely criticized dentistry in the United States and inadvertently affected the practice of root canal therapy for 40 years. In his address, Hunter stated the following:

"Gold fillings, gold caps, gold bridges, gold crowns, fixed dentures, built in, on, and around diseased teeth, form a veritable mausoleum of gold over a mass of sepsis to which there is no parallel in the whole realm of medicine or surgery. The medical ill effects of this septic surgery are to be seen every day in those who are the victims of this gilded dentistry—in their dirty gray, sallow, pale, waxlike complexions, and in the chronic dyspepsias, intestinal disorders, ill health, anemias, and nervous complaints from which they suffer."

Although the dental radiograph was not in use until 1913, the cause of the illnesses discussed in his address was misdirected to teeth with nonvital pulps and endodontically treated teeth. In reality, Hunter was actually referring to infections found around poorly fabricated restorations. His remarks, however, were used by some physicians as a means of explaining away those diseases for which they had no cure. Extraction of a tooth was much easier than actually finding an appropriate treatment. The dental community also supported the extraction of teeth if for no other reason than they feared reprisal from the medical profession or did not feel comfortable or efficient in performing technically demanding root canal therapy. As a result, the needless extraction of all teeth with nonvital pulps or with endodontic treatment by dentists, appropriately called "one hundred percenters," ensued.

During this period, case histories reporting cures after the extraction of teeth appeared in the dental literature. Although these reports were empirical and without appropriate follow up, they wrongfully justified the continued, unwarranted extraction of teeth for approximately 20 years. In time, however, the cures attributed to the extraction of the teeth proved to be short lived, psychologic, or a placebo effect. In nearly all cases the illness returned to the patient, who was now faced with the additional burden of dealing with a mutilated dentition.

Using Rosenow's theory of "Elective Localization of Bacteria," (i.e., Theory of Focal Infection) Dr. Westin Price, the chair of the ADA's research section, conducted research on the relationship of teeth with infected nonvital pulps or endodontically treated teeth with degenerative chronic illnesses. In 1923 his work was published in two books, *Dental Infections Oral and Systemic* and *Dental Infections and the Degenerative Diseases.*

In 1930 the following editorial rejecting the focal infection theory and the needless extraction of teeth appeared in *Dental Cosmos*:

> *"The policy of indiscriminate extraction of all teeth in which the pulps are involved has been practiced sufficiently long to convince the most rabid hundred percenter that it is irrational and does not meet the demands of either medical or dental requirements, and much less those of the patient. Now let us turn from the destructive policy, the path of least resistance, to the constructive, even though it be beset with more difficulties, it certainly offers more possibilities of making the masticatory apparatus a useful and helpful organ rather than a crippled and constant menace to the patient."[81]*

In 1938 physicians R.L. Cecil and D.M. Angevine reported in the *Annals of Internal Medicine* on a follow-up study of 156 patients with rheumatoid arthritis who had teeth or tonsils removed because they were considered foci of infection. Of the 52 patients who had teeth extracted, 47 did not get any better and three became more ill. This study was especially interesting because Cecil had been a strong advocate of the focal infection theory. Cecil suggested that the focal infection theory should be redressed and the further removal of foci of infection curtailed. In other words, subjective improvement of symptoms after extraction of a tooth did not mean that the tooth was the cause of the illness.[33,34]

Microbiologic studies also disputed the studies by Rosenow and Price. Fish and MacLean found that the root surfaces of extracted teeth and corresponding alveolar sockets were contaminated from the gingival sulcus during extraction.[50] In addition, Tunnicliff and Hammond reported that bacteriologic examination of the root surfaces of extracted teeth has no scientific standing unless the gingival tissue had been cauterized prior to extraction, and bacteria can be forced into the pulp tissue during extraction because of the pressure incurred during the rocking of the tooth.[133] In addition, it was determined that the scientific method of Rosenow and Price was flawed in three major areas:

1. Massive doses of bacteria were injected into the experimental animals
2. The experiments were not adequately controlled
3. The specificity of the bacteria involved was not proven

As a result of these clinical and scientific studies, both the medical and dental professions concluded that there was no relationship between teeth with nonvital pulps or endodontically treated teeth and any of the so-called degenerative diseases. Although the focal infection theory resulted in the needless extraction of millions of teeth, it definitely encouraged research that eventually led to the current scientific and biologic basis for root canal treatment.

It has been well established that bacteria play a definite role in the development of pulpitis and subsequent periradicular periodontitis. As a result a major goal of endodontic therapy is the elimination of bacteria and tissue substrate that supports bacterial growth from the root canal system. Working in an aseptic environment, this is accomplished by thorough cleansing, shaping, and obturation of the root canal system in three dimensions. Research has shown that the use of appropriate bactericidal irrigating solutions and inter-appointment medicaments, such as sodium hypochlorite and calcium hydroxide, during the cleaning and shaping phase of treatment will eliminate bacteria and bacterial substrate from the root canal and dentinal tubules. The use of modern obturating techniques (after appropriate cleaning and shaping) produces a predictably high success rate.

ASSOCIATION OF ORAL AND SYSTEMIC DISEASE

Practitioners are well aware of the relationship between bacteremias caused by various dental procedures and the resultant risk of infective endocarditis in those patients with damaged heart valves as a result of congenital or rheumatic heart disease. It must be pointed out that a bacteremia can also result from normal chewing and tooth brushing. Infective endocarditis is a classic example of a distant secondary infection that is not related to the focal infection theory proposed in 1910. The bacteremia occurs at the time of the dental procedure, not from bacteria leaking from a nonvital tooth or endodontically treated teeth. Because endocarditis is such a serious disease, susceptible patients are prescribed antibiotics, according to current AHA guidelines, to be taken prior to dental procedures known to cause bacteremia in an attempt to rid the circulation of the bacteria known to establish residence on the damaged heart valve (see Table 13-2).

Although the focal infection theory as it related to teeth with nonvital pulps and endodontically treated teeth has been disproved, there is growing evidence that a relationship does indeed exist between oral and systemic disease. Recent epidemiologic and case-based studies have shown a positive correlation between periodontitis and cardiovascular and cerebrovascular diseases and preterm low birth–weight babies. In 1993 DeStefano et al[42] reported that subjects with periodontitis had a 25% increased risk of coronary heart disease relative to those with minimal periodontal disease. Hypothesizing that periodontal disease, which is a chronic gram-negative infection, represents a previously unrecognized risk factor for atherosclerosis, Beck et al[24] conducted a cohort study of periodontal and cardiovascular disease. Subjects with a bone loss greater than 20% had approximately twice the incidence of fatal coronary heart disease; for every 20% increase in mean bone loss, the incidence of total coronary heart disease increased 40%. Periodontal disease results in a chronic systemic vascular challenge with endotoxin and host-derived inflammatory cytokines and prostaglandins that are capable of initiating and promoting the formation of atheromas. This is especially noteworthy in patients who possess a macrophage-positive phenotype, because they produce a threefold to tenfold increase in PGE2, IL-1B (i.e., interleukin 1B), and TNF-a (i.e., tumor necrosis factor-a) in response to endotoxin.

A case control study in which all known risk factors and covariates for preterm, low birth–weight were controlled found that periodontal disease increased the risk for preterm, low birth weight sixfold.[98] As with cardiovascular disease, periodontal disease serves as a chronic source of endotoxin. Local production of IL-1B and PGE2 in the periodontal tissues or the chorioamniotic and trophoblastic cells of the uterus elicited by the endotoxin results in premature parturition.[98]

Many questions remain to be answered regarding the exact role of oral bacteria in the onset and progression of systemic disorders. A cause-and-effect relationship between periodontal and systemic disease has to be studied, as well as the relevance of infections of endodontic origin to systemic disease. There is, however, *no scientific evidence that bacteria remaining in the dentinal tubules after properly performed endodontic treatment are a source of bacteria for chronic systemic diseases.*

References

1. Abou-Rass M, Bogen G: Microorganisms in closed periapical lesions, *Int Endod J* 31(31):39, 1998.
2. American Association of Endodontists: *Glossary - contemporary terminology for endodontics,* Chicago, 1998, The Association.
3. American Dental Association: Antibiotic prophylaxis for dental patients with total joint replacements, *JADA* 128:1004, 1997.
4. American Dental Association: Antibiotics use in dentistry, *J Am Dent Assoc* 128(5):648, 1997.
5. Alavi A, Gulabivala K, Speight P: Quantitative analysis of lymphocytes and their subsets in periapical lesions, *Int Endod J* 31:233, 1998.
6. Allard U, Nord CE, Sjoberg L, Stromberg T: Experimental infections with Staphylococcus aureus, Streptococcus sanguis, Pseudomonas aeruginosa, and *Bacteroides* fragilis in the jaws of dogs, *Oral Surg* 48(5):454, 1979.
7. Babál P et al: In situ characterization of cells in periapical granuloma by monoclonal antibodies, *Oral Surg* 64:348, 1987.
8. Bae K, Baumgartner J, Shearer T, David L: Occurrence of *Prevotella nigrescens* and *Prevotella intermedia* in infections of endodontic origin, *J Endod* 23(10):620, 1997.
9. Bae K et al: SDS-PAGE and PCR for differentiation of *Prevotella intermedia* and *P. nigrescens, J Endod* 25(5):324, 1997.
10. Baker PT, Evans RT, Slots J, Genco RJ: Antibiotic susceptibility of anaerobic bacteria from the human oral cavity, *J Dent Res* 64:1233, 1985.
11. Barkhordar RA: Determining the presence and origin of collagenase in human periapical lesions, *J Endod* 13(5):228, 1987.
12. Barkhordar RA, Desousa YG: Human T-lymphocyte subpopulations in periapical lesions, *Oral Surg* 65:763, 1988.
13. Barnard D, Davies J, Figdor D: Susceptibility of *Actinomyces israelii* to antibiotics, sodium hypochlorite and calcium hydroxide, *Int Endod J* 29:320, 1996.
14. Baumgartner JC: Microbiologic and pathologic aspects of endodontics, *Curr Opin Dent* 1(6):737, 1991.
15. Baumgartner JC, Falkler WA: Bacteria in the apical 5 mm of infected root canals, *J Endod* 17(8):380, 1991.
16. Baumgartner JC, Falkler WA: Biosynthesis of IgG in periapical lesion explant cultures, *J Endod* 17:143, 1991.
17. Baumgartner JC, Falkler WA: Detection of immunoglobulins from explant cultures of periapical lesions, *J Endod* 17(3):105, 1991.
18. Baumgartner JC, Falkler WA: Experimentally induced infection by oral anaerobic microorganisms in a mouse model, *Oral Microbiol Immunol* 7:253, 1992.
19. Baumgartner JC, Falkler WA: Reactivity of IgG from explant cultures of periapical lesions with implicated microorganisms, *J Endod* 17:207, 1991.
20. Baumgartner JC, Falkler WA: Serum IgG reactive with bacteria implicated in infections of endodontic origin, *Oral Microbiol Immunol* 7:106, 1992.
21. Baumgartner JC, Heggers J, Harrison J: The incidence of bacteremias related to endodontic procedures. I. Nonsurgical endodontics, *J Endod* 2:135, 1976.
22. Baumgartner JC, Watkins BJ: Prevalence of black-pigmented bacteria associated with root canal infections, *J Endod* 20(4):191, 1994.
23. Baumgartner JC, Watts CM, Xia T: Occurrence of *Candida albicans* infections of endodontic origin, *J Endod* 26(12):695, 2000.
24. Beck J et al: Periodontal disease and cardiovascular disease, *J Periodontol* 67:1123, 1996.
25. Bender IB, Seltzer S, Yermish M: The incidence of bacteremia in endodontic manipulation, *Oral Surg* 13(3):353, 1960.
26. Bergenholtz G, Lekholm U, Liljenberg B, Lindhe J: Morphometric analysis of chronic inflammatory periapical lesions in root-filled teeth, *Oral Surg* 55(3):295, 1983.
27. Bergenholtz G, Lindhe J: Effect of soluble plaque factors on inflammatory reactions in the dental pulp, *Scand J Dent Res* 83:153, 1975.
28. Billings F: Chronic infectious endocarditis, *Arch Int Med* 4:409, 1904.
29. Brook I, Frazier E: Clinical features and aerobic and anaerobic microbiological characteristics of cellulitis, *Arch Surg* 130:786, 1995.
30. Brook I, Frazier E, Gher MJ: Microbiology of periapical abscesses and associated maxillary sinusitis, *J Periodonol* 67(6):608, 1996.
31. Brook I, Walker RI: Infectivity of organisms recovered from polymicrobial abscesses, *Infect Immun* 42:986, 1983.
32. Byström A, Happonen RP, Sjögren U, Sundqvist G: Healing of periapical lesions of pulpless teeth after endodontic treat-

ment with controlled asepsis, *Endod Dent Traumatol* 3:58, 1987.

33. Cecil R, Angevine D: Clinical and experimental observations on focal infection with an analysis of 200 cases of rheumatoid arthritis, *Ann Intern Med* 12:577, 1938.
34. Cecil R, Archer B: Chronic infectious arthritis; analysis of 200 cases, *Am J Med Sci* 173:258, 1927.
35. Cvek M, Cleaton-Jones PE, Austin JC, Andreason JO: Pulp reactions to exposure after experimental crown fractures or grinding in adult monkeys, *J Endod* 8(9):391, 1982.
36. Cymerman JJ, Cymerman DH, Walters J, Nevins AJ: Human T-lymphocyte subpopulations in chronic periapical lesions, *J Endod* 10(1):9, 1984.
37. Czarnecki RT, Schilder H: A histological evaluation of the human pulp in teeth with varying degrees of periodontal disease, *J Endod* 5(8):242, 1979.
38. Dajani AD et al: Prevention of bacterial endocarditis: recommendations by the American Heart Association, *JAMA* 277(22):794, 1997.
39. Debelian GF, Olsen I, Tronstad L: Bacteremia in conjunction with endodontic therapy, *Endod Dent Traumatol* 11(3):142, 1995.
40. Delivanis PD, Fan VSC: The localization of blood-borne bacteria in instrumented unfilled and overinstrumented canals, *J Endod* 10(11):521, 1984.
41. Delivanis PD, Snowden RB, Doyle RJ: Localization of blood-borne bacteria in instrumented unfilled root canals, *Oral Surg* 52(4):430, 1981.
42. DeStefano F et al: Dental disease and risk of coronary heart disease and mortality, *Br Dent J* 306:688, 1993.
43. Dougherty W, Bae K, Watkins B, Baumgartner J: Black-pigmented bacteria in coronal and apical segments of infected root canals, *J Endod* 24(5):356, 1998.
44. Drucker D, Lilley J, Tucker D, Gibbs C: The endodontic microflora revisited, *Microbios* 71:225, 1992.
45. Durack D: Antibiotics for prevention of endocarditis during dentistry: time to scale back? *Ann Intern Med* 129(10):829, 1998.
46. Dwyer TG, Torabinejad M: Radiographic and histologic evaluation of the effect of endotoxin on the periapical tissues of the cat, *J Endod* 7(1):31, 1981.
47. Eftimiadi C et al: Divergent effect of the anaerobic bacteria by-product butyric acid on the immune response: suppression of T-lymphocyte proliferation and stimulation of interleukin-1 beta production, *Oral Microbiol Immunol* 6:17-23, 1991.
48. Fabricius L, Dahlén G, Holm SE, Möller ÅJR: Influence of combinations of oral bacteria on periapical tissues of monkeys, *Scand J Dent Res* 90:200, 1982.
49. Fabricius L, Dahlén G, Öhman AE, Möller ÅJR: Predominant indigenous oral bacteria isolated from infected root canals after varied times of closure, *Scand J Dent Res* 90:134, 1982.
50. Fish E, MacLean I: The distribution of oral streptococci in the tissues, *Br Dent J* 61:336, 1936.
51. Fouad A, Rivera E, Walton R: Pencillin as a supplement in resolving the localized acute apical abscess, *Oral Surg* 81(5):590, 1996.
52. Gharbia S et al: Characterization of *Prevotella intermedia* and *Prevotella nigrescens* isolates from periodontic and endodontic infections, *J Periodontol* 65(1):56, 1994.
53. Gier RE, Mitchell DF: Anachoretic effect of pulpitis, *J Dent Res* 47:564, 1968.
54. Glick M, Trope M, Pliskin M: Detection of HIV in the dental pulp of a patient with AIDS, *JADA* 119:649, 1989.
55. Glick M, Trope M, Pliskin E: Human immunodeficiency virus infection of fibroblasts of dental pulp in seropositive patients, *Oral Surg* 71:733, 1991.
56. Gomes B, Drucker D, Lilley J: Association of specific bacteria with some endodontic signs and symptoms, *Int Endod J* 27(6):291, 1994.
57. Gomes B, Drucker D, Lilley J: Positive and negative associations between bacterial species in dental root canals, *Microbios* 80(325):231, 1994.
58. Gomes B, Lilley J, Drucker D: Clinical significance of dental root canal microflora, *J Dent* 24(1-2):47, 1996.
59. Griffee MB et al: The relationship of *Bacteroides melaninogenicus* to symptoms associated with pulpal necrosis, *Oral Surg* 50:457, 1980.
60. Grodinsky M, Holyoke EA: The fasciae and fascial spaces of the head, neck, and adjacent regions, *Am J Anat* 63:367, 1938.
61. Grossman LI: Origin of microorganisms in traumatized pulpless sound teeth, *J Dent Res* 46:551, 1967.
62. Haapasalo M: *Bacteroides* spp. in dental root canal infections, *Endod Dent Traumatol* 5(1):1, 1989.
63. Haapasalo M, Ranta H, Ranta K, Shah H: Black-pigmented *Bacteroides* spp. in human apical periodontitis, *Infect Immun* 53:149, 1986.
64. Hahn CL, Overton B: The effects of immunoglobulins on the convective permeability of human dentine *in vitro*, *Arch Oral Biol* 42(12):835, 1997.
65. Happonen RP: Periapical actinomycosis: A follow-up study of 16 surgically treated cases, *Endod Dent Traumatol* 2(5):205, 1986.
66. Hashioka K et al: The relationship between clinical symptoms and anaerobic bacteria from infected root canals, *J Endod* 18(11):558, 1992.
67. Heimdahl A, Von Konow L, Satoh T, Nord CE: Clinical appearance of orofacial infections of odontogenic origin in relation to microbiological findings, *J Clin Microbiol* 22:299, 1985.
68. Henderson B, Wilson M: Commensal communism and the oral cavity, *J Dent Res* 77(9):1674, 1998.
69. Hersh EV: Adverse drug interactions in dental practice, *JADA* 130(2):236, 1999.
70. Hohl TH, Whitacre RJ, Hooley JR, Williams B: *A self-instructional guide: diagnosis and treatment of odontogenic infections*, Seattle, 1983, Stoma Press.
71. Horiba N et al: Correlations between endotoxin and clinical symptoms or radiolucent areas in infected root canals, *Oral Surg* 71:492, 1991.
72. Horiba N et al: Complement activation by lipopolysaccharides purified from gram-negative bacteria isolated from infected root canals, *Oral Surg* 74(5):648, 1992.
73. Hunter W: The role of sepsis and antisepsis in medicine and the importance of roal sepsis as its chief cause, *Dental Register* 65:579, 1911.
74. Iwu C, MacFarlane TW, MacKenzie D, Stenhouse D: The microbiology of periapical granulomas, *Oral Surg* 69:502, 1990.
75. Jontell M, Bergenholtz G, Scheynius A, Ambrose W: Dendritic cells and macrophages expressing Class II antigens in the normal rat incisor pulp, *J Dent Res* 67:1263, 1988.

76. Jontell M, Gunraj MN, Bergenholtz G: Immunocompetent cells in the normal dental pulp, *J Dent Res* 66(6):1149, 1987.

77. Jontell M, Okiji T, Dahlgren U, Bergenholtz G: Immune defense mechanisms of the dental pulp, *Crit Rev Oral Biol Med* 9(2):179, 1998.

78. Kakehashi S, Stanley HR, Fitzgerald RJ: The effects of surgical exposures of dental pulps in germ-free and conventional laboratory rats, *Oral Surg* 20:340, 1965.

79. Kettering JD, Torabinejad M, Jones SL: Specificity of antibodies present in human periapical lesions, *J Endod* 17(5): 213, 1991.

80. Kinder SA, Holt SC: Characterization of coaggregation between Bacteroides gingivalis T22 and Fusobacterium nucleatum T18, *Infect Immun* 57:3425, 1989.

81. Kirk EC: Focal infection, *Dental Cosmos* 72:408, 1930.

82. Kobayashi T et al: The microbial flora from root canals and periodontal pockets of non-vital teeth associated with advanced periodontitis, *Int Endod J* 23:100, 1990.

83. Kronfeld R: *Histopathology of the teeth and their surrounding structures*, Philadelphia, 1920, Lea & Febiger.

84. Kuo M, Lamster I, Hasselgren G: Host Mediators in endodontic exudates, *J Endod* 24(9):598, 1998.

85. Langeland K: Tissue changes in the dental pulp, *Odontol Tidskr* 65(239), 1957.

86. Langeland K, Rodrigues H, Dowden W: Periodontal disease, bacteria, and pulpal histopathology, *Oral Surg* 37(2):257, 1974.

87. Levitt GW: The surgical treatment of deep neck infections, *Laryngoscope* 81:403, 1970.

88. Lukic A, Arsenijevic N, Vujanic G, Ramic Z: Quantitative analysis of the immunocompetent cells in periapical granuloma: correlation with the histological characteristics of the lesions, *J Endod* 16(3):119, 1990.

89. Mazur B, Massler M: Influence of periodontal disease on the dental pulp, *Oral Surg* 17(5):592, 1964.

90. Miller W: An introduction in the study of the bacteriopathology of the dental pulp, *Dent Cosmos* 36:505, 1894.

91. Miller W: Gangrenous tooth pulps as centers of infection, *Dent Cosmos,* 30:213, 1888.

92. Molander A, Reit C, Dahlen G, Kvist T: Microbiological status of root-filled teeth with apical periodontitis, *Int Endod J* 31:1, 1998.

93. Moller AJR: Influence on periapical tissues of indigenous oral bacteria and necrotic pulp tissue in monkeys, *Scand J Dent Res* 89:475, 1981.

94. Nair PNR: Light and electron microscopic studies of root canal flora and periapical lesions, *J Endod* 13:29, 1987.

95. Nair PNR et al: Intraradicular bacteria and fungi in root-filled, asymptomatic human teeth with therapy-resistant periapical lesions: a long-term light and electron microscopic follow-up study, *J Endod* 16(12):580, 1990.

96. Nilson R, Johannessen AC, Skaug N, Matre R: In situ characterization of mononuclear cells in human dental periapical inflammatory lesions using monoclonal antibodies, *Oral Surg* 58:160, 1984.

97. Odell L, Baumgartner J, Xia T, David L: Detection of collagenase gene in *P. gingivalis* and *P. endodontalis* from endodontic infections, *J Endod* 25(8):555, 1999.

98. Offenbacher S et al: Periodontal infection as a possible risk factor for preterm low birth weight, *J Periodontol* 67:1103, 1996.

99. O'Grady JF, Reade PC: Periapical actinomycosis involving Actinomyces israelii, *J Endod* 14:147, 1988.

100. Ogundiya DA, Keith DA, Mirowski J: Cavernous sinus thrombosis and blindness as complications of an odontogenic infection, *Oral Maxillofac Surg* 47:1317, 1989.

101. Piattelli A et al: Immune cells in periapical granuloma: morphological and immunohistochemical characterization, *J Endod* 17(1):26, 1991.

102. Price SB, McCallum RE: Studies on bacterial synergism in mice infected with Bacteroides intermedius and Fusobacterium necrophorum, *J Basic Microbiol* 27:377, 1987.

103. Ranta H et al: Bacteriology of odontogenic apical periodontitis and effect of penicillin treatment, *Scan J Infect Dis* 20(2): 187, 1988.

104. Robinson HB, Boling LR: The anachoretic effect in pulpitis, *JADA* 28:268, 1941.

105. Rosenow E: Immunological and experimental studies on pneumococcus and staphylococcus endocarditis, *J Infect Dis* 6:245, 1909.

106. Sen B, Safavi K, Spangberg L: Growth patterns of candida albicans in relation to radicular dentin, *Oral Surg* 84(1):68, 1997.

107. Shah HH: *Biology of the species Porphyromonas gingivalis*, Ann Arbor, Mich, 1993, CRC Press.

108. Shah HN, Gharbia SE: Biochemical and chemical studies on strains designated *Prevotella intermedia* and proposal of a new pigmented species, *Prevotella nigrescens* sp. nov., *Int J Syst Bacteriol* 42(4):542, 1992.

109. Siren E et al: Microbiological findings and clinical treatment procedures in endodontic cases selected for microbiological investigation, *Int Endod J* 30(2):91, 1997.

110. Sjögren U: Success and failure in endodontics, thesis, Umea, Sweden, 1996, Umea University.

111. Sjögren U, Figdor D, Persson S, Sundqvist G: Influence of infection at the time of root filling on the outcome of endodontic treatment of teeth with apical periodontitis, *Int Endod J* 30:297, 1997.

112. Smith A: Focal infection, *JAMA* 150:490, 1952.

113. Stashenko P, Teles R, D'Souza R: Periapical inflammatory responses and their modulation, *Crit Rev Oral Bio Med* 9(4): 498, 1998.

114. Stashenko P, Wang SM: T helper and T suppressor cell reversal during the development of induced rat periapical lesions, *J Dent Res* 68:830, 1989.

115. Stern MH et al: Quantitative analysis of cellular composition of human periapical granuloma, *J Endod* 7:117, 1981.

116. Strom B et al: Dental and cardiac risk factors for infective endocarditis: a population-based, case-control study, *Ann Intern Med* 129(10):761, 1998.

117. Sundqvist GK: Associations between microbial species in dental root canal infections, *Oral Microbiol Immunol* 7:257, 1992.

118. Sundqvist GK: Bacteriological studies of necrotic dental pulps, doctoral dissertation, Umea, Sweden, 1976, University of Umea.

119. Sundqvist GK: Ecology of the root canal flora, *J Endod* 18(9): 427, 1992.

120. Sundqvist GK, Bloom GD, Enberg K, Johansson E: Phagocytosis of Bacteroides melaninogenicus and Bacteroides gingivalis in vitro by human neutrophils, *J Periodontal Res* 17:113, 1982.

121. Sundqvist GK, Carlsson J, Hänström L: Collagenolytic activity of black-pigmented Bacteroides species, *J Periodont Res* 22:300, 1987.

122. Sundqvist GK et al: Degradation in vivo of the C3 protein of guinea-pig complement by a pathogenic strain of Bacteroides gingivalis, *Scand J Dent Res* 92:14, 1984.

123. Sundqvist GK, Carlsson J, Herrmann BF, Tärnvik A: Degradation of human immunoglobulins G and M and complement factors C3 and C5 by black-pigmented Bacteroides, *J Med Microbiol* 19:85, 1985.

124. Sundqvist GK, Eckerbom MI, Larsson ÅP, Sjögren UT: Capacity of anaerobic bacteria from necrotic dental pulps to induce purulent infections, *Infect Immun* 25:685, 1979.

125. Sundqvist GK, Figdor D, Persson S, Sjögren U: Microbiologic analysis of teeth with failed endodontic treatment and the outcome of conservative re-treatment, *Oral Surg* 85(1): 86, 1998.

126. Sundqvist GK, Johansson E, Sjögren U: Prevalence of black-pigmented Bacteroides species in root canal infections, *J Endod* 15:13, 1989.

127. Sundqvist GK, Reuterving CO: Isolation of Actinomyces israelii from periapical lesion, *J Endod* 6:602, 1980.

128. Tamura M, Nagaoka S, Kawagoe M: Interleukin-1 stimulates interstitial collagenase gene expression in human dental pulp fibroblast, *J Endod* 22(5):240, 1996.

129. Topazian R, Goldberg M, Hupp JR: *Oral and maxillofacial infections*, ed 4, Philadelphia, WB Saunders (in press).

130. Torabinejad M, Kiger RD: A histologic evaluation of dental pulp tissue of a patient with periodontal disease, *Oral Surg Oral Med Oral Path* 59(2):198, 1985.

131. Tronstad L, Barnett F, Riso K, Slots J: Extraradicular endodontic infections, *Endod Dent Traumatol* 3(2):86, 1987.

132. Trope M, Rosenberg E, Tronstad L: Darkfield microscopic spirochete count in the differentiation of endodontic and periodontal abscesses, *J Endod* 18(2):82, 1992.

133. Tunnicliff R, Hammond C: Presence of bacteria in the pulps of intact teeth, *J Am Dent Assoc* 24:1663, 1937.

134. van Steenbergen TJ, Kastelein P, Touw JJ, de Graaff J: Virulence of black-pigmented Bacteroides strains from periodontal pockets and other sites in experimentally induced skin lesions in mice, *J Periodont Res* 17:41, 1982.

135. van Winkelhoff AJ, Carlee AW, de Graaff J: Bacteroides endodontalis and other black-pigmented Bacteroides species in odontogenic abscesses, *Infect Immun* 49:494, 1985.

136. Vigil GV et al: Identification and antibiotic sensitivity of bacteria isolated from periapical lesions, *J Endod* 23(2):110, 1997.

137. Waltimo TM, Siren EK, Orstavik D, Haapasalo M: Susceptibility of oral candida species to calcium hydroxide in vitro, *Int Endod J* 32(2):94, 1999.

138. Waltimo TM et al: Fungi in therapy-resistant apical periodontitis, *Int Endod J* 30:96, 1997.

139. Walton RE, Chiappinelli J: Prophylactic pencillin: effect on posttreatment symptoms following root canal treatment of asymptomatic periapical pathosis, *J Endod* 19(9):466, 1993.

140. Warfvinge J, Bergenholtz G: Healing capacity of human and monkey dental pulps following experimentally-induced pulpitis, *Endod Dent Traumatol* 2(6):256, 1986.

141. Wayman BE, Murata SM, Almeida RJ, Fowler CB: A bacteriological and histological evaluation of 58 peripical lesions, *J Endod* 18(4):152, 1992.

142. Xia T, Baumgartner JC, David LL: Isolation and identification of Prevotella tannerae from endodontic infections, *Oral Microbiol Immunol* (in press).

143. Yamamoto K, Fukushima H, Tsuchiya H, Sagawa H: Antimicrobial susceptibilities of Eubacterium, Peptostreptococcus, and Bacteroides isolated from root canals of teeth with periapical pathosis, *J Endod* 15(3):112, 1989.

144. Yoshida M et al: Correlation between clinical symptoms and microorganisms islolated from root canals of teeth with periapical pathosis, *J Endod* 13(1):24, 1987.

145. Yun MW, Hwang CF, Lui CC: Cavernous sinus thrombus following odontogenic and cervicofacial infection, *Eur Arch Othorhinolarygol* 248:422, 1991.

Chapter 14

 # Instruments, Materials, and Devices

Larz Spångberg

Chapter Outline

Many instruments, materials, and devices are required for adequate endodontic treatment. This chapter provides a broad orientation to these various groups and general instruction in their use during endodontic treatment. In recent years many new devices and instruments have been brought forward; therefore it is important that the clinician approaches these devices and instruments with some caution because few have yet been tried by time or scientific assessment. The outline of this chapter follows the natural progression of endodontic treatment.

DIAGNOSTIC MATERIALS AND DEVICES

Radiography is an essential part of endodontic diagnosis. Modern technology is rapidly shifting toward digital filmless imaging. It is important that the endodontist is well-informed in this diagnostic field, because modern technology has opened up new image-enhancing methods.*

Materials for Thermometric Evaluation

Pulp stimulation with heat or cold is the oldest method to evaluate pulpal health and ability to respond to external stimulation. This evaluation of pulpal response must not be confused with vitality testing, which requires the evaluation of pulpal circulation.

Heating of the pulp is commonly achieved by applying heated gutta-percha that may reach a temperature of 168.8° F (76° C) before burning. Special care should be taken not to damage the pulp with excessive heat. (Other methods for conducting a heat test are described in Chapter 1.)

A cold test is commonly done by applying ice, a liquid refrigerant, or dry ice. Ice (32° F, 0° C) is limited because it is normally only effective on intact teeth in the anterior part of the mouth. Ethyl chloride (Fig. 14-1) and liquid refrigerant, such as dichlorodifluoromethane (Endo Ice, Hygienic Corp., Akron, OH) (-21° F, -30° C), provide good sources for lowering the tooth temperature.[48] However, they are normally not sufficient for the stimulation of a tooth with very extensive restorations or full-crown coverage. In these cases dry ice (-108° F, 78° C) is an excellent stimulant (Figs. 14-2 and 14-3). A cold-water bath is the most effective method for testing because it is the only technique that immerses the tooth in chilled water. Therefore, regardless of the restoration, the cold test remains effective. See Chapter 1 for more details.

---

*References 27,103,132,149,168,174.

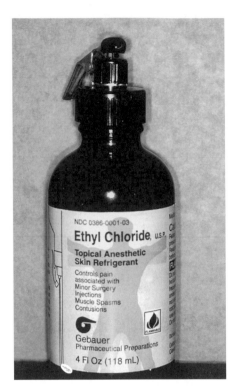

Fig. 14-1 Ethyl chloride.

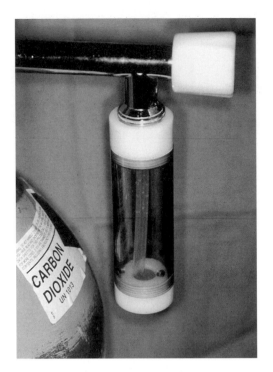

Fig. 14-2 Dry ice maker.

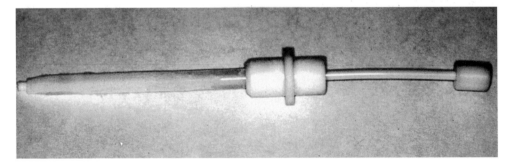

Fig. 14-3 Dry ice stick with holder and plunger.

Although both the levels of heat (168.8° F, 76° C) and cold (-108° F, -78° C) are extreme, it has been demonstrated that the effect on the pulp does not jeopardize the health of the pulp if used with care.[187] The understanding of pain responses to thermometric pulp testing has its basis in the hydrodynamic theory for the sensitivity of dentin because there are no thermosensing nerve endings in the pulp. Thus the pain sensation the patient experiences requires that some pulp tissue, including odontoblasts, is intact for the hydrodynamic mechanisms to function. In other words hot or cold sensation on stimulation is dependent on that a part of a morphologically intact pulp still exists.

Electrometric Pulp Testers

"The basic requirements are an adequate stimulus, an adequate technique of applying this to the teeth, and a careful interpretation of the result."[165] This exactly describes the problems and difficulties with electrical pulp testing, which is often overused and poorly understood.

Evaluation of responding nerve endings can be done with an electrical pulp tester (Figs. 14-4 and 14-5). Several such instruments are available on the commercial market. An electrical pulp tester, however, is only as good as the person interpreting the patient responses. The sensation the patient may feel when electrical current is passed through the tooth is the result of direct nerve stimulation. There is no reasonable assurance, however, that these nerves are located in an intact pulp. Necrotic and disintegrating pulp tissue often leaves an excellent electrolyte in the pulp space. This electrolyte can easily conduct the electrical current to nerves further down into the pulp space, simulating normal pulp response. This becomes even more complicated in a multirooted tooth, where the health status of the pulp may vary in each root.

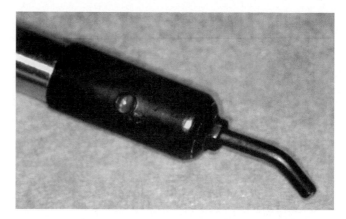

Fig. 14-5 Tooth electrode for electrical pulp tester (Analytic Technology, Redmond, WA).

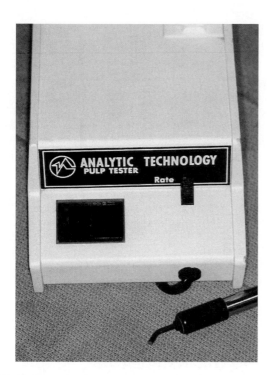

Fig. 14-4 Electrical pulp tester (Analytic Technology, Redmond, WA).

Positive response to electrometric recordings should not be used for differential diagnosis of pulpal disease.[128] Provided the examination was conducted properly, a lack of response suggests the lack of responding nerve endings. In most cases this means pulp necrosis. If the nerves to the pulp have been transected during surgery, the pulp could still be vital. Pulp tissue is much more sensitive to electrical stimulation than gingival and periapical tissues.[32] Most modern pulp testers cannot put out high enough energies to stimulate periradicular tissues.

Several pulp testers with different characteristics are commercially available. It has been shown that pulsating direct current with a duration of 5 to 15 ms provides the best nerve stimulation.[32,165] The optimal stimulation is achieved when the cathode is used for tooth stimulation. The faster the current is rising, the more effective is the stimulation, and the less compensation takes place in the nerves. Somewhat simplified, Ohm's law ($E = R \times I$) is applicable to electrical pulp testing, although the phenomenon most likely is a combination of impedance and resistance. This explains many phenomena occurring during electrometric pulp testing.

Pulp testers operate at a relatively high-potential difference (i.e., several hundred volts) but at a very low current (mA). Enamel and dentin constitute a very high resistance in the electrical circuit through the tooth. Of these, enamel has the highest resistance. In dentin the lowest resistance is parallel with the tubules. It is the product of E and I ($E \times I$) that results in nerve response. This energy can be "consumed" in the hard-tissue part of the tooth, leaving too low a level of stimulation for the pulpal nerves. Therefore to be able to compare recordings on the same tooth at different times, it is very important that the tooth electrode is applied at the same location and with the same conduction each time. This is practically impossible under clinical conditions. Electrometric recording is often used when monitoring traumatic injuries to the teeth. Under these conditions it must be understood that the need to increase stimulation from one observation time to another very often suggests increased hard-tissue formation in the pulp space (not real changes in the pulp's ability to respond).

It is also important that the tooth is kept very dry when performing electrometric recording. Due to the high electrical potential used, the current tends to creep along any wet external tooth surface to the gingiva, creating a short circuit and leaving too little energy for the pulp. This is also the reason why critical recordings must be done after the teeth are isolated from the saliva with a rubber dam and insulated from each other by inserting Mylar strips through the contact points.

Based on this relative shortcoming, the electrometric pulp tester should not be the primary instrument of choice when assessing pulpal health. A positive cold test provides a more accurate response that is easier to interpret. Neither of these tests ensures vitality of the pulp if the results are positive.

Pulp Vitality Testing

Vitality testing requires the measurement of pulpal blood flow. There are several devices regularly applied in medicine for the evaluation of circulatory changes. Several of these have been used for the experimental evaluation of pulpal health. Gazelius et al[80,81] reported the successful application of laser Doppler flowmetry for the study of human pulpal blood flow. The value of this method has been well documented, but its high cost and difficulty of use in clinical situations have slowed its application.[110,111,184,197]

Pulse oximeter is another nondestructive method for monitoring pulp vitality by recording the oxygenation of pulpal blood flow. It was evaluated as a clinical tool in a preliminary investigation and found to perform satisfactorily.[207] Special sensors were developed to study blood flow and blood oxygenation in vitro.[59,169] Further careful attempts to apply the technology to a clinically useful device have been disappointing.[115] Photoplethysmography of pulpal blood flow has also been evaluated for the assessment of pulp vitality.[60]

Although all these methods are successfully applied in medicine and in dental research, they have been less successfully applied to routine endodontic care. This is because the circulatory system of the pulp is encased in a rigid structure and is, therefore, difficult to study without tissue removal. Thus the need for an absolute rigid observation point when using the Doppler phenomenon and the interference of extra pulpal circulatory systems when using the pulse oximetry and photoplethysmography have limited the introduction of these interesting methods to endodontic practice.

Tooth Slooth

The Tooth Slooth (Fig. 14-6) has proven very useful for the differential diagnosis of various stages of incomplete crown fractures (cracks). It is designed in such way that chewing force can be applied selectively on one cusp at a time, thereby allowing the clinician to evaluate weaknesses in defined areas of a tooth. This device is much more effective than cotton rolls or wooden sticks, which are often suggested for this important examination to establish a differential diagnosis.

MATERIALS FOR ENDODONTIC FIELD ISOLATION

(The reader is referred to Chapter 5.)

ENDODONTIC INSTRUMENTS

Although most instruments used in general dentistry are applicable to endodontic work, some hand instruments are unique for endodontic procedures. In addition, there are many different instrument types for procedures performed inside the pulp space. They are hand-operated instruments for root canal preparation, engine-driven and energized instruments for root canal preparation, instruments for root canal obturation, and rotary instruments for post space preparation.

During the last 25 years extensive work has been done to standardize instruments to improve quality. For example, the

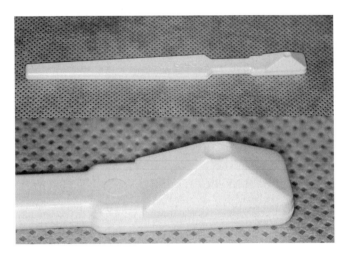

Fig. 14-6 Tooth Slooth.

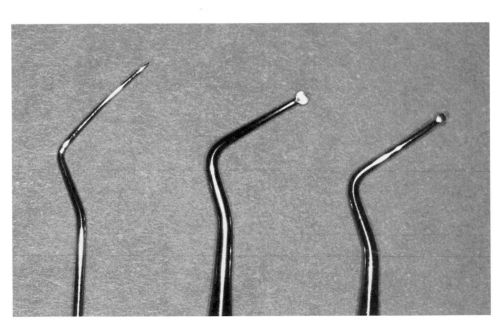

Fig. 14-7 Endodontic explorer (*left*) and endodontic spoons.

International Standards Organization (ISO) has been working with the Federation Dentaire Internationale (FDI) in the Technical Committee 106 Joint Working Group (TC-106 JWG-l). The American Dental Association (ADA) has also been involved in this development, together with the American National Standards Institute (ANSI).

There are two ISO and FDI standards pertaining to instruments. ISO and FDI no. 3630/1 deals with K-type files (ANSI and ADA no. 28), Hedström files (ANSI and ADA no. 58), and barbed broaches and rasps (ANSI and ADA no. 63). ISO and FDI no. 3630/3 deals with condensers, pluggers, and spreaders (ANSI and ADA no. 71).

Hand Instruments

Except for the mirror, all regular hand instruments used in endodontics are different from their regular dental counterparts. Thus the endodontic explorer has two straight and very sharp ends, angulated in two different directions from the long axis of the instrument (Fig. 14-7).

Several different types of endodontic spoons are available. They have a much longer offset (from the long axis of the instrument for better reach) than regular spoons. They are intended for pulp tissue excision and should, therefore, be kept well sharpened (see Fig. 14-7).

The locking pliers with grooves for holding paper and gutta-percha points are an important instrument for rapid-and-secure transfer during endodontic work with a chair side assistant (Fig. 14-8). This instrument is always superior to the College or Perry pliers for work with points. The latter,

however, is also needed for work within small pulp chambers, because the working ends of the "points pliers" often are too large.

Instruments for Pulp Space Preparation

The classification of endodontic instruments for root canal preparation is subdivided into three groups:

1. Group I includes hand- and finger-operated instruments, such as barbed broaches and K-type and H-type instruments.
2. Group II includes low-speed instruments where the latch type of attachment is in one piece with the working part. Typical instruments in this group are Gates-Glidden (GG) burs and Peeso reamers.
3. Group III includes engine-driven instruments of a similar type as Group I. However, the handles of the instruments in Group III are replaced with attachments for a latch type of hand piece. In the past, few instruments have been in this group because rotary root canal files were rarely used. In recent years, however, the nickel-titanium (NiTi) rotary instruments have become popular, and instruments like ProFile, LightSpeed, Quantec, POW-R, and Hero 624, although not standardized, could be included in this grouping.

Various, sometimes conflicting, techniques for using these instruments have been described; the dentist should take time to get acquainted with the different applications of the instrument for optimal use.

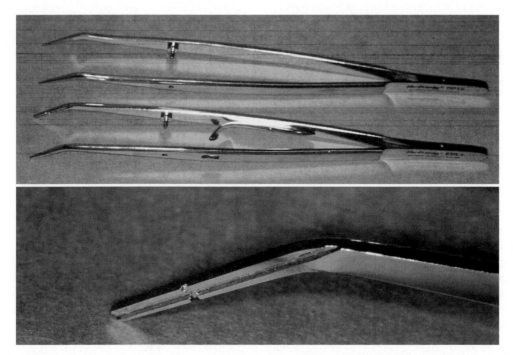

Fig. 14-8 Endodontic pliers. Nonlocking and locking pliers for gutta-percha and absorbent points. Note how the working part has grooves for holding of points.

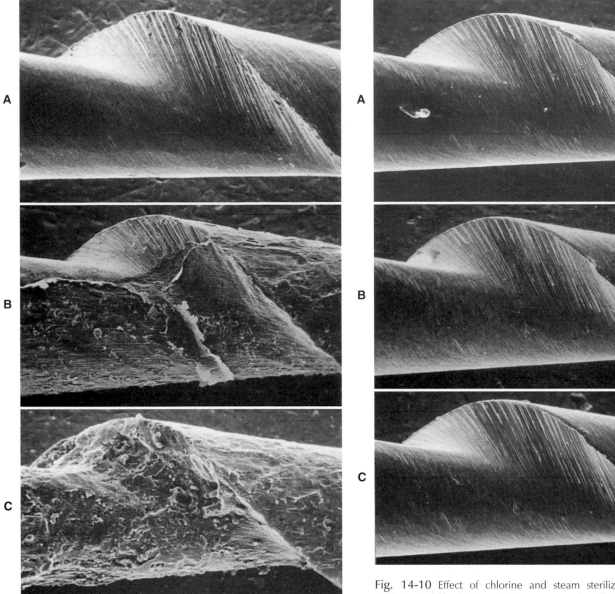

Fig. 14-9 Effect of chlorine and steam sterilization on carbon steel file. **A,** Untreated file. **B,** Five minutes exposure to 5% NaOCl followed by water rinse, drying, and autoclave sterilization. **C,** Same treatment as in **B** but repeated three times. Severe damage to the file. (Courtesy Dr. Evert Stenman.)

Fig. 14-10 Effect of chlorine and steam sterilization on SS file. **A,** Untreated file. **B,** Five minutes exposure to 5% NaOCl followed by water rinse, drying, and autoclave sterilization. **C,** Same treatment as in **B** but repeated three times. No damage to the file. (Courtesy Dr. Evert Stenman.)

Hand- and Finger-Operated Instruments

This group of instruments comprises all instruments that generally are included in the group of instruments called files. Barbed broach, rasps, and K-type and Hedström files are the old type of instruments in this category. Many new instrument designs have been brought to the market in recent years. These design changes affect the stiffness of the instrument, its efficiency, and the form of the cutting tip.

Traditionally, root canal instruments were manufactured from carbon steel. Its tendency to corrode because of the use of corrosive chemicals (e.g., iodine, chlorine) and during steam sterilization (Fig. 14-9) was a significant problem until stainless steel (SS) became the standard. SS has proven to be very valuable and has provided an improved quality of instruments (Fig. 14-10).[167,240]

New metal alloys have also been introduced as part of the attempt to improve the quality of endodontic files. The alloy with most promise at this time is nitinol, which is an equiatomic alloy of NiTi.[257] NiTi alloy has a low elastic modulus that provides very good elastic flexibility to instruments. This alloy is expensive and difficult to manufacture and mill. It belongs to a category of alloys called "shape memory alloys" that have some extraordinary qualities. The most

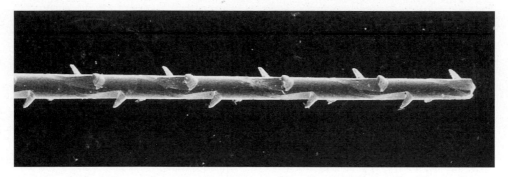

Fig. 14-11 Barbed broach (Union Broach, York, PA).

important characteristic of this alloy, applicable to its use in endodontic instruments, is its ability to recover from plastic strain when unloaded (i.e., pseudoelasticity). The alloy normally exists in an austenitic crystalline phase. On stressing at a constant temperature, the austenitic phase transforms to a martensitic structure. If the stress is released, the structure recovers to an austenitic phase and its original shape.

This phenomenon is not similar to conventional elastic deformation but totally related to a stress-induced thermoelastic transformation from austenitic phase to martensitic phase. In the martensitic phase only a light force is required for bending. There are, however, limits. When yield stress of the martensitic phase is reached, deformation occurs and fracture results. Thus this alloy differs from the traditionally used SS in that it may be strained much further than steel before it is permanently deformed. Resistance to fracture for K-files, however, measured as angular deflection before fracture, is higher for SS instruments than for NiTi instruments.[44] The alloy undergoes significant phase changes during stress. These can be slow thermoelastic or burst type of martensite. During these crystal changes the NiTi instrument is very prone to fracture. This is of special concern when used for rotary instruments. Attempts to improve the nitinol alloy are ongoing, and it was shown that the surface hardness could be greatly improved through the implantation of boron in the alloy.[134]

Barbed broach and rasps. The barbed broach and the rasp are the oldest endodontic intracanal instruments still being manufactured (Fig. 14-11). There are specifications for both the barbed broach and the rasp (ANSI no. 63, ISO no. 3630-1). Although similar in design, there are some significant differences in taper and barb size. Thus the broach has a taper of 0.007 to 0.010 mm/mm, and the rasp has a taper of 0.015 to 0.020 mm/mm. The barb height is much larger in the broach than in the rasp. As the barb comes out of the instrument core, the broach is a much weaker instrument than the rasp. The broaches and rasps were designed to extract pulp tissue from the root canal simply by attaching to the tissue remnants. This was especially useful when removing arsenic- or paraformaldehyde-devitalized pulps, which become very fibrous when coagulated. Vital pulps, low in collagen, are not easy to remove with a broach. Furthermore, it is impossible

with these instruments to sever the pulp in a calculated way. Therefore they have lost their usefulness in contemporary endodontics.

A barbed broach does not cut or machine dentin; however, it is an excellent tool for the removal of cotton or paper points that have accidentally been lodged in the root canal.

K-type instruments. The K-type file and reamer (originally produced by the Kerr Manufacturing Company in 1915) are the oldest useful instruments for cutting and machining of dentin (ANSI no. 28, ISO no. 3630/1) (Figs. 14-12 and 14-13). The instruments are made from a steel wire that is ground to a tapered square or triangular cross section. This wire is then twisted to generate a file or a reamer. During this process the steel is work hardened. The file has more flutes per length unit than the reamer. If the core is twisted more or the instrument is thicker, the work hardening increases. This changes the physical properties of the file, making the reamer, which is less twisted, more flexible than a comparable file.

The K-type instrument is useful for the penetration of root canals and increasing their size. The instrument primarily works by crushing the dentin when turned into a canal slightly smaller than the diameter of the instrument. Thus the apical enlargement with a K-type instrument is not an abrasive action but mainly a compression-and-release destruction of the dentin surrounding the canal.[215] Because of its dull flutes (i.e., rakes) and shallow concavities between the flutes, the K-type instrument does not easily thread itself deep into the dentin when used in rotary motion (compared with the H-type file). Although the reamer has fewer cutting rakes per length unit, it is as effective as a file in crushing and removing dentin, because there is more space between the flutes (allowing better transport of dentin debris).

The K-type instrument is poor in removing bulk dentin. Because of its working motion (i.e., rotation and pull) a K-type instrument used in a reaming motion causes little transport of the root canal, as the instrument tends to be self-centered in the canal. This is not true, however, if the K-type instrument is used in a filing motion.[255] The K-type file is strong and can easily be precurved to a desired form for filing. An advantage of the K-type design is that it is often obvious when a file has been stressed to permanent defor-

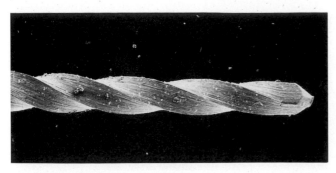

Fig. 14-12 K-type file (Kerr Manufacturing Co., Romulus, MI). Instrument fresh from a box displays significant amount of debris. This is not an uncommon observation in many brands of instruments. Therefore new instruments should be cleaned before being sterilized and used. Tip is blunted.

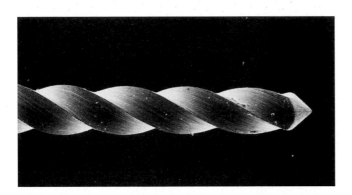

Fig. 14-13 K-type file no. 40 (Maillefer Instruments SA, Ballaiques, Switzerland). Note the clean surface and the well-rounded tip.

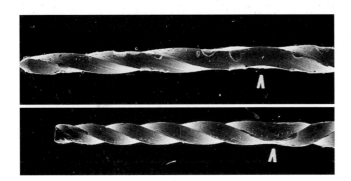

Fig. 14-14 K-type files stressed to deformation during clockwise and counterclockwise twisting. The deformed areas are marked with an arrow. These instruments are close to fracture.

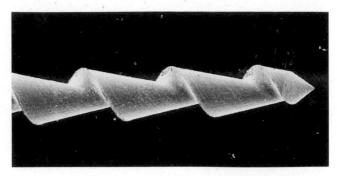

Fig. 14-15 Hedström file no. 45 (Maillefer Instruments SA, Ballaiques, Switzerland).

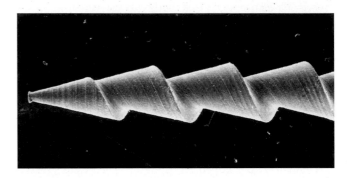

Fig. 14-16 Hedström file no. 50 (Antaeos, Vereinigte Dentalwerke, München, Germany). Steeper helical angle than file in Fig. 14-15. Note the blunted tip that is a common result of force used during attachment of handle.

mation. When this happens, the flutes on the working part of the file are wound tighter or opened up wider (Fig. 14-14). This sign is a clear indication that the file has been permanently deformed and must be discarded.

The K-type instrument and the hybrid files with the twisted K-type pattern fracture during clockwise motion after plastic deformation.[97] In counterclockwise motion little plastic deformation occurs before a brittle fracture occurs.[46]

These files have a similar torsional strength regardless if they are used in clockwise or counterclockwise motions. In counterclockwise rotation, breakage occurs in half (or less) of the rotations required for breakage in clockwise rotation.[46,127,131] Thus this type of instrument should be operated more carefully when forced in counterclockwise direction.

Hedström file. The H-type instrument (ANSI no. 58, ISO no. 3630/1) is a more aggressive instrument than the K-type instrument. The H-type file is ground from a round steel blank. Modern, computer-assisted machining technology has made it possible to develop H-type instruments with very complex forms. This technique makes it possible to adjust the rake angle and the helical angle. The edge that is facing the handle of the instrument can, therefore, be made rather sharp (Figs. 14-15 and 14-16).

The H-type file machines the root canal wall when the instrument is pulled but has no abrasive effect when pushed. The sharpness of these edges allows the file to self-thread into the root canal walls when turned clockwise. Combined with the compressibility of the dentin it is easy for the inexperienced user to enter into a situation where the file is so far into the dentin that it cannot be pulled or unscrewed but will fracture. This rarely happens with a K-type file or reamer. Because of these characteristics, an H-type file is less useful

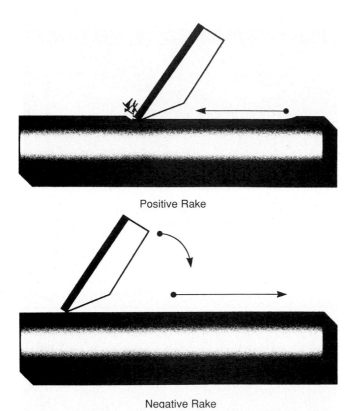

Positive Rake

Negative Rake

Fig. 14-17 Rake angle. **A,** Positive rake angle planes the substrate surface. **B,** Negative angle scrapes the surface.

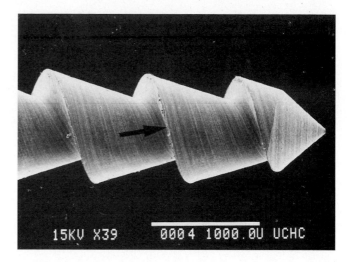

Fig. 14-18 Hedström file no. 100 (CC Cord, Roydent, Rochester Hills, MI). Rake angle close to neutral (*arrow*) makes this instrument very efficient during machining strokes.

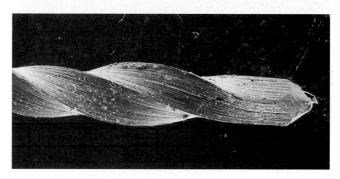

Fig. 14-19 K-Flex file no. 35 (Kerr Manufacturing Co., Romulus, MI). This file resembles a classic K-file with its twisted pattern (compare Fig. 14-16). The cross section of the blank is rhomboid, giving the instrument a small and a large diameter that can be seen clearly in this figure. Note the untwisted tip.

for reaming of a root canal but ideal for bulk removal of dentin.

In the design of an H-type file the rake angle and the distance between the flutes are important for the working of the file. The rake angle may be seen as the direction of the cutting edge if visualized as a surface (Figs. 14-17 and 14-18). If this surface is turned in the same direction as the force applied, the rake angle is positive. On the other hand, if the blade performs a scraping action faced away from the direction of the force, the rake angle is said to be negative. Most endodontic instruments have a slightly negative rake angle. If the rake angle is positive, the instrument actually works like a shaver on the dentin surface. Under such circumstances the instrument may dig itself into the dentin. Therefore the ideal instrument has a neutral or slightly positive rake for maximal effectiveness. The area between the flutes fills with dentin when the file is pulled over the root canal surface. The larger this groove, the longer the file is effective. When the groove is filled with dentin shavings, the instrument lifts off the surface and no longer planes effectively. Thus a file with a positive rake angle and a deep groove between the flutes is the most effective in removing dentin. This reduces the thickness of the core, however, making the instrument less stiff and more prone to fractures. The desire to have an aggressive instrument must, therefore, be balanced with the expectation of strength and must be considered seriously when choosing a brand.

Contrary to K-type instruments, the Hedström file is difficult to bend to the desired curvature without sharp nicks. The instrument may break through the development of cracks, followed by ductile failure.[97] Clinically, this happens without any physical external signs of stress, such as the flute changes observed on K-type instruments (see Fig. 14-14).

Hybrid instruments. Many new designs of files are simply modifications of the K-type and H-type files. These files are not made to any national or international standards, but their size designation often follows the specifications for K-type or H-type files. By changing the cross-sectional geometry of a K-type instrument from a square to rhomboid, it has been possible to create an instrument (using classic K-file manufacturing technique) that is more flexible because one cross section is smaller than the cross section determining the size. It also allows more space for dentin shavings between the root canal wall and the instrument. These types of files are known as "flex files" (Fig. 14-19).

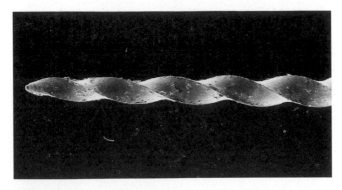

Fig. 14-20 Flex-R file (Union Broach, York, PA). This is a milled K-type instrument. The flutes are sharper with a less negative rake than a traditional twisted K-type file. The tip is well rounded.[178]

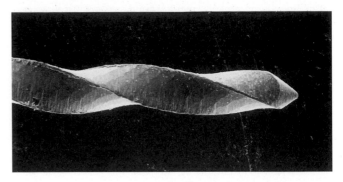

Fig. 14-22 Ultra Flex no. 30 (Texeed). Milled K-type NiTi file. Note the coarse surface, which is a typical result of milling in NiTi alloy. The flutes are less sharp than a steel counterpart and are often rolled over the edge.

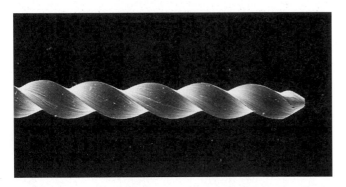

Fig. 14-21 FlexoFile (Maillefer Instruments SA, Ballaiques, Switzerland). Milled K-type instrument. Note the smooth surface and well-formed tip.

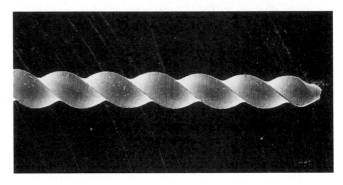

Fig. 14-23 Sureflex no. 30 (Caulk/Dentsply, Milford, DE). Milled K-type NiTi file with a higher helical angle than Ultra Flex (see Fig. 14-22). Compare design with the FlexoFile (see Fig. 14-21).

The use of modern computer-assisted grinding technology has also made it possible to fabricate (from a round blank) files similar to the K-type file. These files can be made with much sharper flutes to increase the machining qualities and with much deeper space between the flutes to allow for transport of more dentin shavings (Figs. 14-20 and 14-21). In regard to strength this type of instrument is more similar to H-type files than K-type files. Because of the sharper rake of ground K-type files, they also tend to become lodged in the root canal walls and break on unscrewing or removal.[214] These milled K-type instruments are also available in NiTi alloy (Figs. 14-22 and 14-23).

There are also many modifications of the H-type file. Thus several brands now supply H-type files with double-helix configuration (Figs. 14-24 and 14-25). Although this doubles the number of machining edges, the space between the edges is radically decreased; therefore overall effectiveness is not enhanced compared with conventional Hedström files.[120] Modified H-type files with continuously variable helical angle are also available. This variation reduces the chances that the instrument will thread itself into the dentin and then fracture on removal.

Tip design. It was observed by Weine et al[261] that the abrasive effect of the instrument tip had an important effect on the control of the root canal preparation. In a study of cutting efficiency of some endodontic files where the files were performing a quarter turn reciprocal drilling action in a Giromatic hand piece under 1000 g pressure, it was also found that the tip design had an effect on what was called "cutting efficiency."[157,158] These results are not surprising, because the instruments used in the study were larger than the predrilled hole they had to penetrate. Therefore the only way the instruments could advance is by using abrasive planes on the tip.

Abrasive tips may be helpful when penetrating canals smaller than the file. If steel files are used, however, the inherent stiffness of these files enhances the machining of dentin on the concave side of the curvature, resulting in some ledging. Much has been written about the importance of various sophisticated tip modifications to prevent such ledging, but there is no scientific proof that any one design is better than the other during clinical work.[121,180,181,188,192] The original K-type file had a tip that resembled a pyramid (Fig. 14-26). It was, therefore, very capable of lateral and apical machining. Practically all contemporary file designs have an acceptable nonaggressive tip design, and there should be little concern over tip geometry in the selection of files if they are within the ANSI and ISO guidelines (Fig. 14-27).

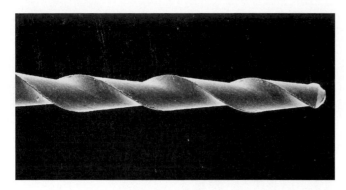

Fig. 14-24 Hyflex X-file (Hygenic Corp., Akron, OH). Hedström type NiTi file with double helix.

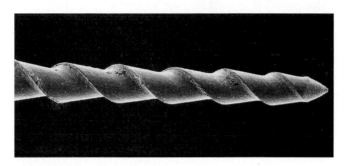

Fig. 14-25 Mity Turbo (JS Dental, Ridgefield, CT). Hedström type NiTi file with tighter double helix than the Hyflex X-file. This file is much less efficient in machining a substrate than the Hyflex X-file seen in Fig. 14-24.[113]

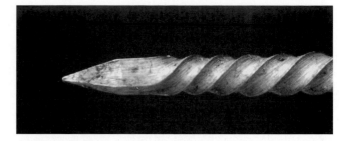

Fig. 14-26 K-type instrument with aggressive pyramid type of tip.

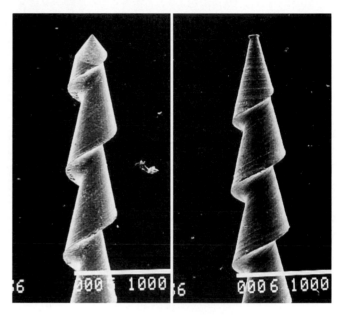

Fig. 14-27 Hedström files with different tip designs. Although sold as standardized files, these files (of the same size) display very different tips.

Rotary Instruments—Low Speed   Many types of rotary instruments are used during endodontic treatment procedures. In addition to regular burs adapted for endodontics, there are various types of root canal reamers for preparation of the root canal or for the removal of root canal–filling materials and preparation for post space.

Burs.   In addition to conventional burs, burs with extended shanks are useful for preparation in the pulp space. Many burs are available in surgical length (i.e., 26 mm) and some in extralong shank (i.e., 34 mm) for low-speed contraangle hand pieces (Fig. 14-28). The extralong shank model (e.g., Brasseler, Shank 25) is exceptionally helpful in deep preparation in the pulp chamber and root canals, because it allows good visibility and control.

After access has been achieved, there is little need for high-speed preparation in the pulp chamber. Low-speed preparation with sharp burs is as effective as high-speed preparation and allows a better tactile control during this critical phase of preparation.

GG burs and Peeso reamers are examples of common rotary reamers. The GG bur is commonly used during initial root canal preparation for opening of orifices and coronal root canal preparation. This reamer is available both in a 32-mm length and a shorter 28-mm length for posterior teeth (Fig. 14-29).

The risk for perforation with GG burs is less than with other types of burs, because the short head is less self-guiding (Fig. 14-30). It is self-centering in the root canal, however. This may result in unexpected thinning of the furcation wall of root canals when larger sizes are used. This is especially pronounced on the furcation sides of mesial roots of molars. GG instruments are also available in NiTi (Fig. 14-31).

The Peeso reamer is an instrument mostly used for post space preparation (Fig. 14-32). It is a stiff instrument and, therefore, does not follow the root canal if there is a slight curvature. This reamer easily cuts laterally, causing perforations, despite the "safety tip." The inexperienced user should be especially careful when using Peeso reamers.

Rotary Instruments—Engine Driven   With the advent of NiTi for endodontic files, the idea of a safe rotary file was born. Attempts to use conventional steel files for instrumentation of root canals have been ongoing for many years with

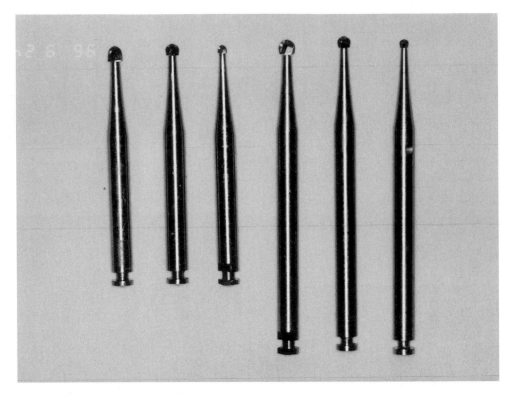

Fig. 14-28 Round burs for endodontic use. The burs to the left have a length of 26 mm (Brasseler, Shank 24), whereas the burs to the right are 32 mm long (Brasseler, Shank 25). This extra length allows direct view around the head of the hand piece during pulp chamber preparation.

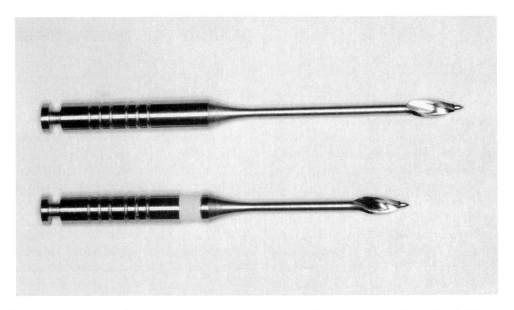

Fig. 14-29 GG burs made of SS (Union Broach, York, PA). Normal length (32 mm) and short length (28 mm).

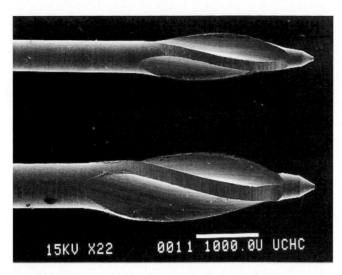

Fig. 14-30 Working part of GG bur made of SS. Note the rounded safety tip and the lack of sharp cutting edges. The instrument has a marginal land to center the drill in the canal and more safely machine the canal walls.

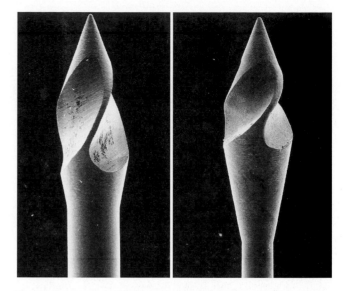

Fig. 14-31 Working part of NiTi GG bur (Tulsa Dental Products, Tulsa, OK). Small size to the left and a large instrument to the right. Compare design with the LightSpeed rotary instrument in Figure 14-38.

little success. The steel file does not have the flexibility to be used for rotary movements in a curved root canal without significantly altering the canal configuration and perforating the canal wall. In addition, the design of the instruments was such that they easily became overstressed and fractured. The rotary instrument device that best survived through many years was the Giromatic hand piece. This provided a quarter turn reciprocal movement of the instruments used. Most common for Giromatic hand pieces were the rasps and barbed broaches, but K-type and H-type instruments were also used. The Giromatic hand piece was an ineffective instrument that never became an important addition to the endodontic armamentarium. With NiTi it became practical to develop a file type of instrument that could be effectively used as a rotary root canal instrument in moderately curved root canals. Presently there are at least five major instruments available that provide useful alternatives:

1. ProFile and ProFile GT (Tulsa Dental Products, Tulsa, OK)
2. LightSpeed (Light Speed Technology, Inc., San Antonio, TX)
3. Quantec (Analytic, Orange, CA)
4. POW-R (Union Broach, York, PA)
5. Hero 642 (MicroMega, Geneva, Switzerland)

The ProFile, LightSpeed, and Quantec are somewhat similar in design in that they feature U-grooves and radial lands that prevent the instrument from cutting into the root canal walls in an uncontrolled fashion, causing premature fractures, perforations, and transportation. The land also contributes significantly to the strength of the instrument by the relatively large peripheral mass. This peripheral strengthening has been further accentuated in the Quantec instrument. The POW-R is designed with a triangular passive flute. The newest instru-

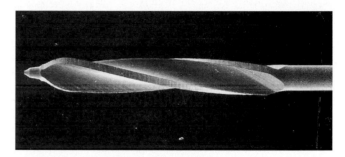

Fig. 14-32 Peeso reamer (Union Broach, York, PA). Note safety tip and guiding marginal lands on machining surfaces.

ment is Hero 642 (MicroMega), which has a different design from earlier successful rotary instruments. The Hero 642 has a trihelical Hedström design with rather sharp flutes. Because of a progressively changing helical angle for the flutes, there is a reduced risk for binding in the root canal. The Hero 642 is designed to operate at 500 to 600 RPM.

Only LightSpeed provides instruments of such size that proper apical preparation can be done in slightly curved root canals. Quantec provides 0.02 mm/mm taper instruments to a size no. 60 and Hero 642 to a size no. 45. A high frequency of root canals have apical canal sizes that exceed these instrument sizes.[79,123] *Therefore most root canals need final hand instrumentation with conventional files to complete the apical preparation.* Rotary NiTi instruments require constant speed to prevent stress fractures. Although it may sometimes be possible to operate these NiTi instruments with an air-driven hand piece, it is highly recommended that an electric hand piece (Fig. 14-33) be used, because the speed can

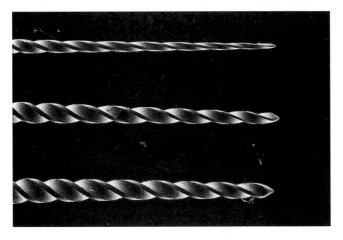

Fig. 14-33 Electrical hand piece with different gear reductions and motor controller (Aseptico, Kirkland, WA).

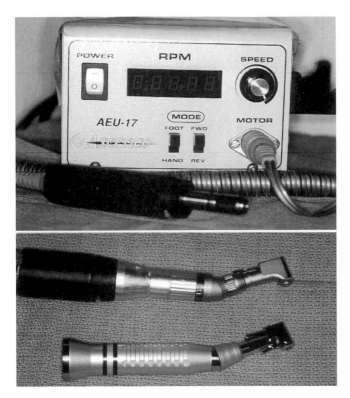

Fig. 14-34 Rotary ProFile NiTi instruments (Tulsa Dental Products, Tulsa, OK). Sizes no. 3, no. 5, and no. 6. The instruments have marginal lands that guide the instrument in the center of the canals and around curvatures.

be maintained more evenly and at the right RPM. Torque control motors (Dentsply, Tulsa Dental, Tulsa, OK) are now available, but their utility is still unknown.

ProFile and ProFile GT. ProFile was the original NiTi rotary instrument made by Tulsa Dental (Tulsa, OK). The standard taper is 0.04 mm/mm. In addition, some of the instrument sizes are available in 0.06 mm/mm and 0.08

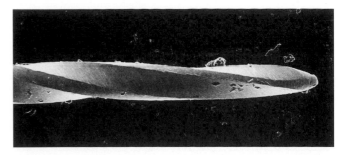

Fig. 14-35 Rotary ProFile NiTi instruments (Tulsa Dental Products, Tulsa, OK). Size no. 3..

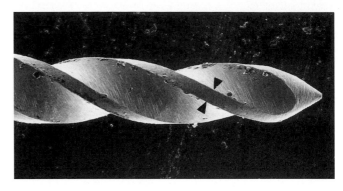

Fig. 14-36 Rotary ProFile NiTi instruments (Tulsa Dental Products, Tulsa, OK). Size no. 5. Note the wide marginal land of the instrument (*arrows*).

mm/mm taper (Fig. 14-34). The instrument is sized in the ISO and ANSI standard. Because of the large taper the instrument becomes rather stiff before the apical preparation has been sufficiently enlarged.[79,123] This places some limitations on its use in narrow, curved root canals. The instrument is well manufactured and true to design at all sizes (Figs. 14-35 and 14-36). ProFile GT is an addition to the original instrument sequence. The standard ProFile GT set consists of four instruments, size no. 20, with taper 0.06, 0.08, 0.10, and 0.12 mm/mm. The largest taper is also available in sizes no. 35, no. 50, and no. 70. The instrument has well-developed lands in a trihelical arrangement (Fig. 14-37). The rotational speed used for ProFile is in the range of 150 to 300 RPM.

LightSpeed. LightSpeed resembles the GG reamer, with a long shaft and a short flame-formed cutting head (Fig. 14-38). It comes in sizes no. 020 to no. 140 (according to ISO and ANSI). It also includes "half" sizes (e.g., 022.5, 027.5) up to no. 060. In the smaller sizes the head is less well defined (Fig. 14-39). The design has been shown to vary with the instrument size.[144] With careful use this instrument is not more prone to fracture than other NiTi rotary instruments. It is of essence, however, that the manufacturers' instructions are followed to the letter and that no sizes are skipped during preparation when increasing the canal size. The instrument works very well and prepares ideal canals with little or no

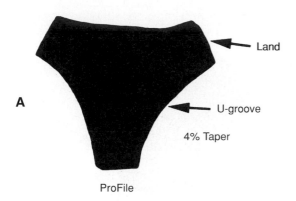

A

Land

U-groove

4% Taper

ProFile

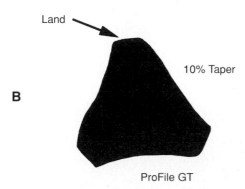

Land

B

10% Taper

ProFile GT

Fig. 14-37 Microphoto of ground cross section of ProFile/ProFile GT instruments showing the triple helical configuration. **A**, ProFile no. 45 with 0.04 mm/mm taper. Note the symmetrical U grooves and the three lands. **B**, ProFile GT no. 20 with 0.10 mm/mm taper. The cross section is similar to ProFile but with less clear U grooves. (Tulsa Dental Products, Tulsa, OK).

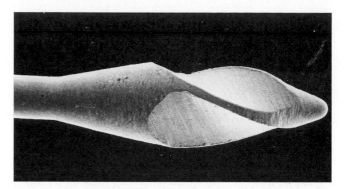

Fig. 14-38 LightSpeed rotary NiTi instruments (LightSpeed Technologies, San Antonio, TX). Size no. 90. Well-outlined instrument head with radial lands.

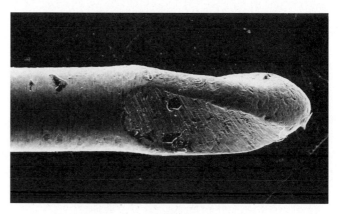

Fig. 14-39 LightSpeed rotary NiTi instruments (LightSpeed Technologies, San Antonio, TX). Size no. 20. Working head is slightly larger than the shaft. Radial lands are poorly defined.

transportations. The excessive number of instruments for a complete instrumentation is a strain, however. The rotational speed used for LightSpeed is in the range of 1000 to 2000 RPM. Under no circumstances should the speed be below 750 RPM.

Quantec. In many aspects, the design of the Quantec and ProFile instruments are similar. The lands of the Quantec instrument are much wider, however, with a modification that provides enhanced strength to the instrument (Fig. 14-40). The Quantec file is available with two types of tip design, a noncutting tip and a safe-cutting tip (Fig. 14-41). Quantec has recently reformulated its sortiment of instruments to a formula similar to ProFile and ProFile GT. Thus the manufacturer advocates a crown-down technique with large taper instruments and an apical size instrumentation of no more than size no. 25. All instrument sizes are standardized (ISO and ANSI). Instruments come in 0.02, 0.03, 0.04, 0.05, 0.06, 0.08, 0.10, and 0.12 mm/mm taper. The old sortiment of 0.02 mm/mm taper instruments in sizes no. 15 to no. 60 is also available. The rotational speed used for Quantec is in the range of 150 to 300 RPM. Quantec has a double helical flute design and extensive peripheral mass (Fig. l4-42).

During milling of nitinol there is always a certain degree of rollover at sharp edges (Fig. 14-43).

Hero 642. The Hero 642 has a trihelical Hedström design with rather sharp flutes (Fig. 14-44). Due to a progressively increasing distance between the flutes, there is a reduced risk for binding in the root canal when used. The Hero 642 is designed to operate at 500 to 600 RPM. This instrument is available in ISO sizes no. 20 to no. 45. All sizes are available in 0.02 mm/mm taper, and no. 20, no. 25, and no. 30 also are available in 0.04 and 0.06 mm/mm taper. A crown-down technique is recommended with an apical preparation of at least size no. 30. The Hero 642 has a large central core that provides extra strength (Fig. 14-45). Despite its aggressive design the instrument is easy to operate, with no higher apparent fracture risk than other rotary instruments.

Sonic and Ultrasonic Instruments   A radically different way of instrumenting root canals was introduced when files were activated with electromagnetic ultrasonic energy.[186] Currently, piezoelectrical ultrasonic units are also available for this purpose. These units activate an oscillating sinusoidal wave in the file with a frequency around 30 kHz.

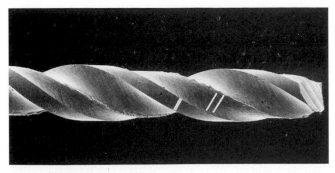

Fig. 14-40 Quantec rotary NiTi instrument (Analytic, Orange, CA). Size no. 10. Taper 0.02 mm/mm. Note the typical double land that characterizes the Quantec instrument. Higher marginal land performs the machining (*wide white bar*) of the root canal, whereas the lower reduced peripheral surface (*double white bars*) contributes to peripheral strength. Note the sharp and blunt tip.

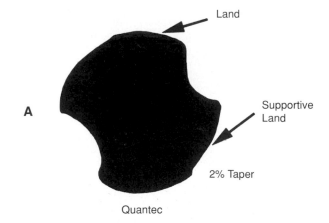

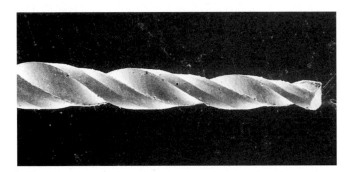

Fig. 14-41 Quantec rotary NiTi instrument (Analytic, Orange, CA). Orifice opener no. 1. Taper 0.06 mm/mm. Note the blunt and sharp tip of the instrument.

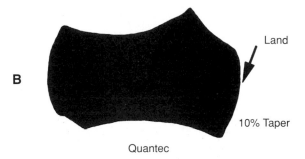

Fig. 14-43 Quantec NiTi Rotary instrument (Analytic, Orange, CA). Microphoto of ground cross section showing the double helix configuration. **A**, Quantec no. 45 with 0.02 mm/mm taper. The metal core of the instrument is big, with the land and supportive land occupying major portions of the periphery. The supportive land is slightly lower than the land. **B**, Quantec no. 25 with 0.10 mm/mm taper. The land and the small supportive lands occupy only a small part of the periphery.

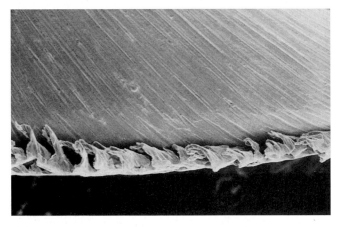

Fig. 14-42 Quantec rotary NiTi instrument (Analytic, Orange, CA). High magnification of edge between the reduced peripheral surface and the U groove. Because of the difficulties in milling NiTi alloys, edges are often "rolled over" like this. Similar rollover can be seen when NiTi instruments wear (see Fig. 14-22).

There are principally two different types of devices: (1) the ultrasonic device, at 25 to 30 kHz (e.g., CaviEndo [magnetostrictive] [Fig. 14-46], ENAC, EMS Piezon Master 400, Piezo-Ultrasonic [piezoelectrical] [Fig. 14-47]) and (2) the sonic device, at 2 to 3 kHz (e.g., Sonic Air MM 1500, Megasonic 1400, Endostar). The ultrasonic devices use regular type of instruments (e.g., K-type files), whereas the sonic devices use special instruments known as Rispi Sonic, Shaper Sonic, Trio Sonic, and Heli Sonic files.

Although similar in function, the piezoelectrical design has advantages over the magnetostrictive systems (Caulk/Dentsply, Milford, DE). For example, little heat is generated by piezoelectrical devices; therefore no cooling is needed for the electrical hand piece. In addition, the piezoelectrical transducer transfers more energy to the file than the magnetostrictive system, making it more powerful.[10] The magnetostrictive system generates a large amount of heat, and a special cooling system is needed in addition to the irrigation system for the root canal (see Fig. 14-46).

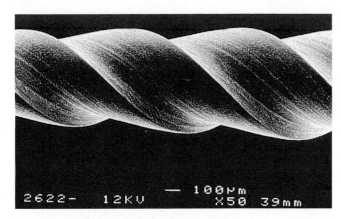

Fig. 14-44 SEM photo of Hero 642 (MicroMega, Geneva, Switzerland). Note the positive rake and the similarity to a trihelical Hedström file (Courtesy MicroMega, Geneva, Switzerland).

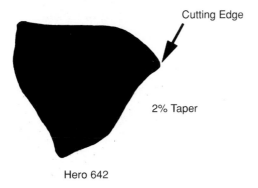

Fig. 14-45 Hero 642 (MicroMega, Geneva, Switzerland). Microphoto of ground cross section (no. 45 with 0.02 mm/mm taper) showing the triple helical Hedström configuration. This instrument has a strong core with cutting edges of a slightly positive rake angle.

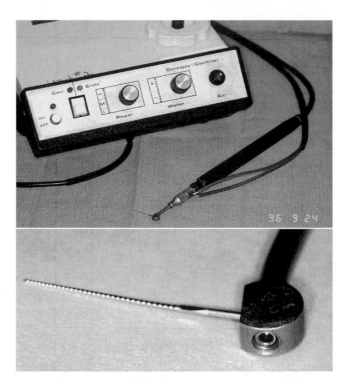

Fig. 14-46 Cavi-Endo ultrasonic device (Caulk/Dentsply, Milford, DE). The unit allows setting for endodontic work or periodontal scaling. The top lid covers a container for irrigation solution. Power and irrigation rate can be adjusted. The irrigation and cooling drain are attached close to the working head. Files are attached with a hexscrew.

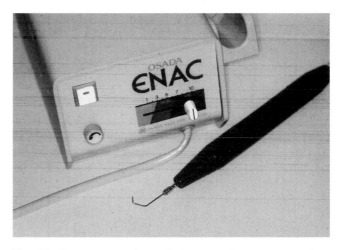

Fig. 14-47 ENAC piezoelectrical ultrasonic device (Osada, Tokyo, Japan). The hand piece has adapters for periodontal scaling or endodontic work. Power and water flow can be adjusted.

The file in an ultrasonic device vibrates in a sinus wave-like fashion. In a standing wave there are areas with maximal displacement (i.e., antinodes) and areas with no displacement (i.e., nodes). The tip of the instrument exhibits an antinode. If powered too high, the instrument may break because of the intense vibration. Therefore files must be used only a short time and with careful setting of power. The frequency of breakage in files used for more than 10 minutes may be as high as 10% and normally occurs at the nodes of vibrations.[3]

Ultrasonic devices have a very efficient system for irrigation into the pulp space during operation. During free ultrasonic vibration in a fluid, two significant physical effects are observed: (1) cavitation and (2) acoustic streaming. During the oscillation in a fluid a positive pressure is followed by a negative pressure in the fluid. If the tensile strength of the fluid is exceeded during this oscillation of pressure gradients, a cavity is formed in the fluid in the negative phase. During the next positive pressure phase the cavity implodes with great force. This is *cavitation*. The power of dental ultrasonic units is too low during normal clinical conditions to create significant cavitation effects on the dentin walls.[7,8] *Acoustic streaming* creates small, intense, circular fluid movement (i.e., eddy flow) around the instruments. The eddying occurs closer to the tip than in the coronal end of the file, with an apically directed flow at the tip. Acoustic streaming increases the cleaning effect of the irrigant in the pulp space through hydrodynamic shear stress. Increased amplitude occurring at smaller file sizes enhances the acoustic streaming.[6] This has proven to be of great value in the cleaning of root canals, because conventional irrigation solutions do not penetrate small spaces well.[155,196,213]

Acoustic streaming has little direct antimicrobial effect.[4,9] Both cavitation and acoustic streaming are dependent on the free vibration of the file. The limits of the space in a root canal significantly inhibit the practical utility of ultrasonic devices for root canal cleaning. Depending on size and power the file tip may have an amplitude of 20 to 140 mm, requiring a canal size of at least a no. 30 file through a no. 40 file for free oscillation. Any contact with the root canal walls dampens oscillation. As the contact with the canal wall increases, the oscillation is dampened and too weak to maintain acoustic streaming. Small file size, with minimal contact to the root canal wall, provides optimal cleaning conditions.[11]

Ultrasonic devices are disappointing as instruments to enhance the removal of dentin from the root canal walls.[156,178] These devices enhance the ability to clean the pulp space and difficult-to-debride areas through acoustic streaming.[16,52,53,263] It is unclear, however, if this can be achieved during regular preparation when the file is actively dampened and little acoustic streaming takes place.[239,258,259] Cleaning is further enhanced by the excellent irrigation systems provided in some of the devices. Applying a freely oscillating file with sodium hypochlorite (NaOCl) irrigation for a couple of minutes to aid in the pulp space disinfection is, therefore, believed to be useful after good biomechanic instrumentation of the pulp space.[218]

Sonic devices are more useful for true hard-tissue removal during root canal preparation.[156,271] Because the files operate like a conventional hand piece, the file vibrations are less likely to be dampened by contact with the root canal walls. Therefore the special files used in these systems are true bulk dentin removers. The Rispi Sonic file is less aggressive than the Shaper Sonic file. The instruments come in lengths from 17 to 29 mm and in various sizes from no. 010 and up. Because of the rasplike design of the instruments, they tend to leave a rougher canal surface than many other devices.

The working length and the apical part of the root canal are normally prepared with conventional files, after which the sonic files are used. Both sonic and ultrasonic instruments are prone to cause canal transport if used carelessly.[5,124,142] Various, often conflicting, techniques for using these instruments have been described, and the individual user should take time to be acquainted with the instrument for optimal use.

National and International Standards for Instruments

As a result of concerns nearly 40 years ago, efforts were made to standardize endodontic files and root-filling materials. This resulted in an international standard for endodontic files known in the United States as the ANSI no.

Table 14-1 DIMENSIONS OF STANDARDIZED K-TYPE FILE, H-TYPE FILE, AND GUTTA-PERCHA CONES (ANSI NOS. 28, 58, AND 78)*

Size	D_0	D_{16}	Color
006	*0.06*	*0.38*	*No color assigned*
008	*0.08*	*0.40*	*No color assigned*
010	0.10	0.42	Purple
015	0.15	0.47	White
020	0.20	0.52	Yellow
025	0.25	0.57	Red
030	0.30	0.62	Blue
035	0.35	0.67	Green
040	0.40	0.72	Black
045	0.45	0.77	White
050	0.50	0.82	Yellow
055	0.55	0.87	Red
060	0.60	0.92	Blue
070	0.70	1.02	Green
080	0.80	1.12	Black
090	0.90	1.22	White
100	1.00	1.32	Yellow
110	1.10	1.42	Red
120	1.20	1.52	Blue
130	1.30	1.62	Green
140	1.40	1.72	Black

*Sizes denoted in italics are only for files, commercially available but not part of ANSI No. 28 or No. 58. Colors on instrument handles or gutta-percha cones are not mandatory. The size must be printed on the handles. The tolerance for files is ± 0.02 mm and for gutta-percha cones is ± 0.05 mm. Length for the gutta-percha cones is ≥ 30 mm ± 2 mm.

58 for Hedström files and ANSI no. 28 for K-type files (Table 14-1). There are several similarities in these standards, but there are also some important differences. Fig. 14-48 illustrates the important measurements dictated by the standard. The size designation is derived from the projected diameter at the tip of the instrument. This is an imaginary measurement and is not reflected in the real size of the working part of the instrument. The taper of the instruments are prescribed to be 0.02 mm/mm of length, starting at the tip. Thus the working diameter is the product of taper and the length of the tip. Three standard lengths are available at 21 mm, 25 mm, and 31 mm. The working part of the instrument must be at least 16 mm.

This system of numbering files with at least 15 different sizes replaced the old, somewhat imperfect system that numbered the sizes from no. 0 through no. 6. Although the new standard includes many sizes, rational clinicians may compose the proper collection of fewer instrument sizes for their special work habit.

In recent years suggestions to change the numbering system for files with different sizes have been implemented by several manufacturers. One system has introduced "half"

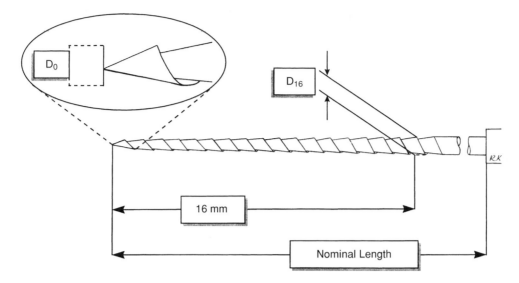

Fig. 14-48 Measuring points for ANSI and ADA no. 28 and no. 58 for K-type and H-type instruments. The measuring point for the diameter of the instrument (*size*) is imaginary (D_o) and projects the taper of the instrument at the tip. Thus an instrument with a short tip is more true to its size than instruments with long tip. D_{16} represents the diameter at the end of the working part that must be at least 16 mm long.

sizes in the range of no. 15 through no. 60. Thus there are instruments in sizes no. 15, no. 17.5, no. 20, no. 22.5, etc. Considering the fact that most manufacturers already are unable to size their instruments within accepted range (Fig. 14-49),[244] the introduction of "half" sizes makes no rational sense. It is reasonable, however, if standards are strictly adhered to, to use "half" sizes for instrument systems like the LightSpeed, where the strength of the instrument is so low that full-size increments may generate stresses beyond the tolerance of the instrument.

Effectiveness and Wear of Instruments   Although the advertising literature is rich in claims of various forms of superiority of file designs, few claims can be verified in objective endodontic literature. There are no standards for the cutting or machining effectiveness of endodontic files, neither are there clear requirements regarding resistance to wear.

When studying the effectiveness of instruments, there are two measurements to investigate: (1) the instrument's effectiveness in cutting or breaking loose dentin and (2) the effectiveness in machining dentin. These two measurements are radically different. There are methods to quantitate machining, but as of now there is no good method that measures cutting. Some studies have attempted evaluation of cutting, but the methodologies have involved the drilling motion with K-type instruments and at high speed compared with clinical use.[71,256] There are studies of machining, however, that evaluate the effectiveness of an instrument when used in a linear movement.[119,120,166,241-243,260] They show that instruments are very different when comparing brands and types but also within one brand and type. For K-type files the effectiveness varies 2 to 12 times between files of the same brand. The

variation for Hedström files is larger and varies between 2.5 to more than 50 times.[154,242] The greater variation among Hedström files is easy to understand because the H-type file is the result of more individual grinding during manufacturing than the conventional K-type file, which is difficult to alter much during manufacturing. During the grinding of a Hedström file, it is possible to modify the rake angle to neutral or even slightly positive. This is impossible to achieve with a K-type file. The Hedström file is, therefore, approximately 10 times more effective in removing dentin than the K-type file (Fig. 14-50).

In the machining process the rake edge shaves off dentin that accumulates in the grooves between the rake edges. The deeper and larger this space is, the longer the stroke can be before the instrument is riding on its own debris, making it ineffective. These design variations and the rake angle of the edges determine the effectiveness of a Hedström file. Of the hybrid files the K-Flex file, which is a modified K-type file, shows variables similar to K-type files. The Flex-R file, which is a ground instrument, is more similar to H-type files in its variation in effectiveness. It is also much more effective in substrate removal than the K-type files but cannot measure up to the H-type files' ability to machine.

NiTi alloy instruments are as effective or better than comparable SS instruments in machining dentin. Steel files wear significantly when used on dentin.[119] After 300 pull strokes on dentin, the instruments may lose up to 55% of their original effectiveness. NiTi files also wear noticeably, but they are much more resistant to wear than the steel files (Figs. 14-51 and 14-52).[120] The NiTi file is significantly more expensive than the steel file, and it is important from a cost-effective point of view to decide what instruments to use.

Text continued on p. 542

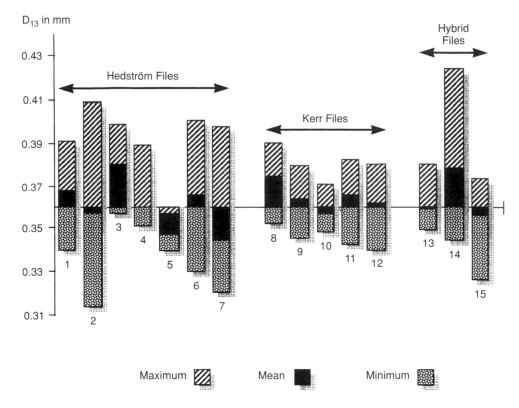

Fig. 14-49 Results from a study of the size of standardized root canal instrument (no. 030). Measurements made 3 mm from the tip where a conforming instrument should measure 0.36 ± 0.02 mm. Mean marked in black. Shaded areas indicate maximal and minimal values. Few instruments conform to the standard. For details see Stenman and Spångberg.[234] *1*, Antaeos; *2*, Hygenic; *3*, Miltex; *4*, Maillefer; *5*, J.S. Dental; *6*, Union Broach; *7*, Brasseler; *8*, Antaeos; *9*, Miltex, *10*, Maillefer; *11*, J.S. Dental; *12*, Brasseler; *13*, S-File; *14*, K-Flex; *15*, Flex-R.

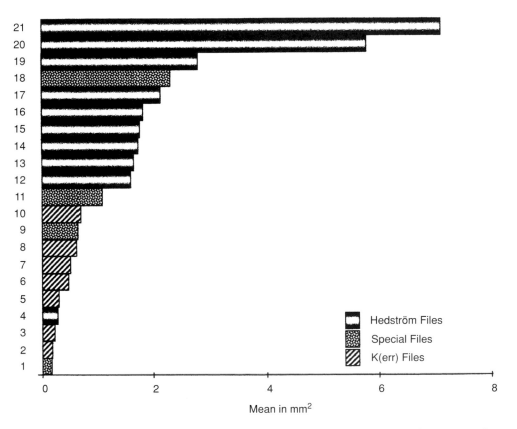

Fig. 14-50 Comparison of effectiveness of various endodontic instruments in machining. Substrate removal measured in mm². Hedström files are, in general, much more efficient than K-type instruments. For details see Stenman and Spångberg.[243] *1*, Trio-Cut; *2*, Miltex; *3*, Brasseler; *4*, Brasseler; *5*, Healthco Delux; *6*, J.S. Dental; *7*, Aristocrat; *8*, Antaeos; *9*, K-Flex; *10*, Maillefer; *11*, Flex-R; *12*, Union Broach; *13*, Maillefer; *14*, Miltex; *15*, J.S. Dental; *16*, Healthco Delux; *17*, Hygenic; *18*, S. File; *19*, Aristocrat; *20*, Zipperer; *21*, Antaeos.

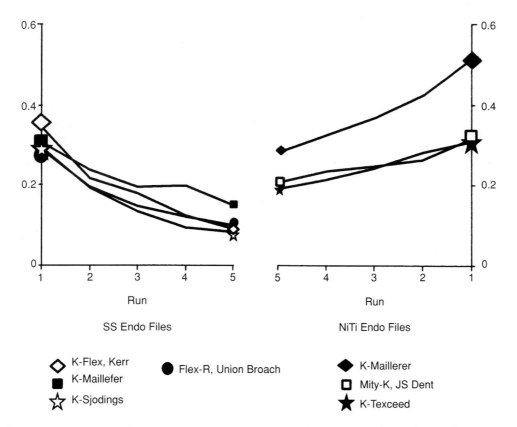

Fig. 14-51 Wear of endodontic K-type instruments manufactured in SS or NiTi. The machining efficiency measured in mm². The efficiency measured after one, two, three, four, and five runs in dentin. The files lose their efficiency as they wear after contact with dentin. NiTi instruments maintain their abrasive efficiency better than SS files.

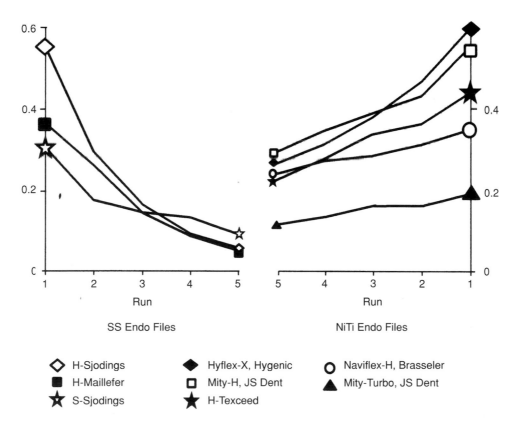

Fig. 14-52 Wear of endodontic H-type instruments manufactured in SS or NiTi. The machining efficiency measured in mm². The efficiency measured after one, two, three, four, and five runs in dentin. The files lose their efficiency as they wear after contact with dentin. NiTi instruments maintain their abrasive efficiency better than SS files.

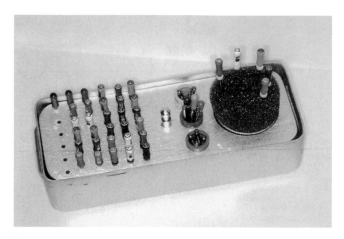

Fig. 14-53 Simple file box for organization of endodontic files and extended round burs. GG burs, finger spreaders, and pluggers (Union Broach).

Modern endodontic SS instruments are fabricated from excellent metal alloys, and their resistance to fracture is great. With careful application of force and a strict program to discard instruments after use, few instrument fractures should occur. SS files are so inexpensive that adequate cleaning and sterilization for reuse of files in sizes up to no. 60 may not be cost effective. Therefore *files in the range up to no. 60 should be considered disposable instruments*. Fig. 14-53 suggests a file setup that provides efficient overview of the instruments. In a disposable file system the sponge used to hold treatment instruments will be disposed of along with the files.

Devices for Root Canal Length Measurements

Traditionally, measurements during root canal instrumentation have been made by exposing radiographs with a root canal file in place in the canal. Based on this information the working length has normally been determined.

Sundada[244] suggested that the apical foramen could be localized with the use of an electrical current. This early, often imperfect, technique has undergone significant and successful modifications. Currently, the apex locator is an accurate tool for the determination of working length.[73,75,76,77] Apex locators are still sensitive to individual interpretation, however, and the user must carefully train with the instrument to be proficient. In addition, many instruments are very sensitive to the type of tissue or fluid content of the root canal.

Two of the best modern apex locators are Endex Plus, or Apit, (Osada Inc., Los Angeles, CA) and the Root ZX (J. Morita Co., Kyoto, Japan).[76,130] These devices, which are easy to use and less sensitive to the root canal content, measure the electrical impedance between the file and the mucosa. Normally two electrical currents at different frequency are emitted, and the apex is related to the place of

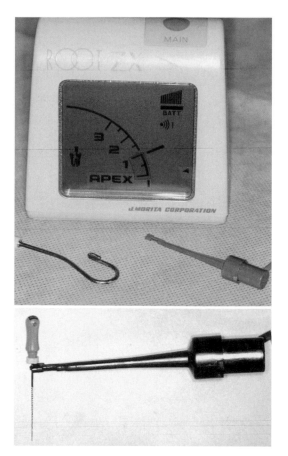

Fig. 14-54 Root ZX apex locator with lip clip and file holder (J. Morita, Kyoto, Japan).

maximal difference calculated by subtraction or division. The Endex device uses 1 and 5 kHz and provides apex location based on subtraction. The Root ZX emits currents at frequencies of 8 and 0.4 kHz and provides apex location based on the resulting quotient. When the file tip reaches the apical foramen area, the instrument gives some type of signal. There are typically three parts to an apex locator: (1) the lip clip, (2) the file clip, and (3) the instrument itself, which has a display indicating the advancement of the file toward the apex (Fig. 14-54).

On average the best of these instruments provides accurate measurements to within 0.5 mm of the apex.[76,130] Therefore to achieve a "safe" measurement, 1 mm should be subtracted from the instruments' measurements. The final measurement can then be established with a radiograph. Electronic measurements provide more accurate estimates of working length than the normal subtraction of 2 mm from a preoperative radiograph. In a recent study comparing the radiographic method of apex location with the Endex apex locator, it was found that the electronic device was slightly more reliable.[182] However, clinicians must keep in mind that Electrical devices, such as apex locators, should not be used on patients with pacemakers without careful consultation with the patient's cardiologist.[23,74]

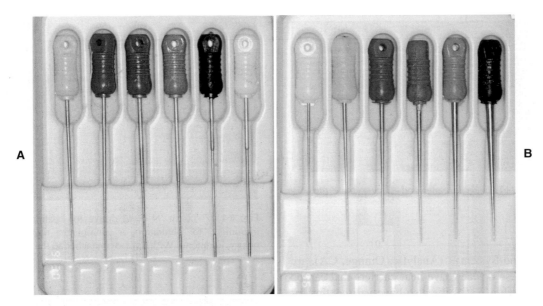

Fig. 14-55 Sets of finger spreaders and pluggers made of NiTi alloy (HyFlex; Hygenic, Akron, OH). **A,** Spreaders in sizes extra fine, fine-fine, medium-fine, fine, and medium. **B,** Pluggers in sizes no. 20, no. 25, no. 30, no. 35, no. 40, and no. 45.

Instruments for Root Canal Obturation

When the root canal has been properly cleaned and enlarged, the space is obturated with a manufactured material. A number of obturation methods are practiced, but the lateral and vertical condensations are the two most common.

There are a great number of specialized instruments for each method practiced. Gutta-percha cones are best handled with a grooved endodontic pliers, allowing a firm-and-controlled grip of the cones (see Fig. 14-8). The pliers are also available with a lock to accommodate various working preferences. Other significant instruments for obturation are spreaders and pluggers. The spreader is a tapered-and-pointed instrument intended to laterally displace gutta-percha for insertion of additional accessory gutta-percha cones. The plugger is a similar instrument, but it has a blunt end. In smaller sizes the spreader and the plugger are often used interchangeably. These instruments are available as a handled instrument or as a finger-held instrument (Fig. 14-55). The handled instruments are potentially dangerous, because the tips of the working ends are offset from the long axes of the handles. This arrangement results in strong lateral wedging forces on the working ends if the instruments are not firmly operated.

The risk of inducing vertical damage to the root is greatly reduced with finger spreaders and pluggers. Each clinician must choose the appropriate spreader and plugger according to personal working preferences. There are standardized instruments with the same taper as the files (e.g., 0.02 mm/mm). Considering the greater taper of standardized accessory gutta-percha cones (Table 14-2), it may sometimes be better to use nonstandardized spreaders with a larger taper to better accommodate the gutta-percha.

Table 14-2   SIZE DESIGNATION FOR AUXILIARY GUTTA-PERCHA CONES*

Designation	D_3	D_{16}	Taper
XF†	0.20	0.45	0.019
FF	0.24	0.56	0.025
MF‡	0.27	0.68	0.032
F	0.31	0.80	0.038
FM	0.35	0.88	0.041
M	0.40	1.10	0.054
ML§	0.43	1.25	0.063
L	0.49	1.55	0.082
XL	0.52	1.60	0.083

*The cones are pointed. The diameters 3 mm (D_3) and 16 mm (D_{16}) from the tip are prescribed. Tolerance is ± 0.05 mm. Length is ≥ 30 mm ± 2 mm.
†X, Extra; F, fine.
‡M, Medium
§L, Large.

In recent years spreaders and pluggers have become available in NiTi. In curved canals these instruments are superior, because they easily follow canal curvatures and are less likely to be deformed during use (Fig. 14-56).

Heat carriers are used for vertical condensation obturation techniques. Traditionally, heat carriers are handled instruments similar to pluggers. They are used to transfer heat to the gutta-percha in the root canal, allowing apical and lateral displacement of the gutta-percha. Electrical heat carriers, such as Endotec (Caulk/Dentsply, Milford, DE) and

NaOCl.[98,101,102] This proves little, because there are poor correlations between tissue damage and clinical symptoms.

Commercial NaOCl is buffered to a pH of approximately 12 to 13. This adds another toxic component to that of NaOCl to make the solution even more caustic. Therefore if commercial bleach is used as a base for preparing a 1% irrigation solution, it is better to use sterile 1% sodium bicarbonate as a dilutent instead of water. This helps in adjusting the pH to a less caustic level. Diluted and buffered NaOCl has a limited shelf life and should be stored in a dark, cool place no longer than 1 to 2 weeks.

There are few clinical complications to the use of NaOCl. The most common complication is accidental injection of NaOCl into periradicular tissue.[24,191] This results in excruciating pain, periapical tissue bleeding, and extensive swelling. The pain normally subsides within 2 to 3 days. The swelling increases for the first day, after which healing occurs. The prognosis is good.

Detergents   Detergents are often used as irrigation solutions, because they are very effective in removing fatty tissue residues that are by-products of tissue necrosis. The more common materials used are in the family of quaternary ammonium compounds. These compounds were once considered optimal for antimicrobial therapy and effective in very low concentrations. This has proven wrong, and the preparations have a toxicity comparable with other irrigation solutions and a rather narrow bactericidal spectrum.[26,191] Quaternary ammonium antiseptics are normally used in water solution at 0.1% to 1%. Zephiran Chloride is a compound that has been commonly used as an endodontic irrigation solution. Considering its toxicity and low antimicrobial effectiveness, there are no reasons to use this detergent rather than a mild (i.e., 1% or less) NaOCl solution.

Another group of antimicrobial agents with detergent effects are the iodophors. Wescodyne and Iodopax are common products in this line of antiseptics. These organic iodine products are not allergenic and are effective at low concentrations. They are antimicrobially effective at an iodine concentration of 0.05% (volume/volume). Detergents have also been mixed with calcium hydroxide for irrigation.[21]

Decalcifying Materials   During preparation of the root canal a smear layer is formed. There is no clear scientifically based understanding if this smear layer must be removed or can be left. There are, however, a multitude of opinions on both sides of this question. In addition to weak acids, solutions for the removal of the smear layer include carbamide peroxide, aminoquinaldinium diacetate (i.e., Salvizol), and EDTA. In objective studies, carbamide peroxide and Salvizol appear to have little effect on the smear layer buildup.[28,189] A 25% citric acid solution also failed to provide reliable smear layer removal.[272]

EDTA is often suggested as an irrigation solution, because it has the capability to chelate and remove the min-

eralized portion of smear layers.[83,84,147,148,170] It also can decalcify up to a 50-mm thin layer of the root canal wall if used liberally.[254,262] EDTA is normally used in a concentration of 17%. It removes smear layers in less than 1 minute if the fluid is able to reach the root canal wall surface. Under clinical conditions, reports suggest that the fluid should be kept in the root canal for at least 15 minutes to obtain optimal results. The decalcifying process is self-limiting, because the chelator is used up. To achieve continuous effect the EDTA must be replaced through frequent irrigation.[84] For root canal preparation, EDTA has limited value as an irrigation fluid. It may open up a hair-fine canal if given the time to soften the 50 mm it is capable of decalcifying. This amount, at two opposite canal walls, results in 100 mm. This is equivalent to the tip of a no. 010 file.

The smear layer consists of both an organic and an inorganic component. To remove this smear layer effectively, it is normally insufficient to use EDTA only. A proteolytic component (e.g., NaOCl) must also be added for removal of the organic components of the smear layer.[86]

A commercially available product, EndoDilator N-Ø (Union Broach, York, PA), is a combination of EDTA and a quaternary ammonium compound. Such irrigation fluid has a slight detergent effect mixed with the chelating effect.

Intracanal Disinfection Materials

Biomechanic instrumentation and irrigation with an antimicrobial solution is essential for the disinfection of the pulp space, but some suggest it may not be sufficient for the complete elimination of microorganisms in a necrotic pulp space.[39,40,92] Therefore further disinfection with an effective antimicrobial agent may be necessary (see Fig. 14-59). The most commonly used intracanal disinfectants belong to the family of phenol or phenol derivatives. Antiseptics on a chlorine or iodine base are also common. In recent years more attention has been given to the use of calcium hydroxide as intracanal dressing for the treatment of infected pulp necrosis. Conventional antiseptics are generally toxic, and care must be taken not to induce undue tissue damage (Table 14-3).

Phenolic Preparations   Phenol (C_6H_5OH) or carbolic acid is one of the oldest antimicrobial agents used in medicine. Despite its severe toxicity, derivatives of phenol, such as paramonochlorphenol (C_6H_4OHCl), thymol ($C_6H_3OHCH_3C_3H_7$), and cresol ($C_6H_4OHCH_3$), are still in common use for endodontic treatment. Phenol is a nonspecific protoplasm poison, having optimal antibacterial effect at 1% to 2%. Many dental preparations use much too high concentration of phenol (i.e., in the range of 30%). At such concentration the antimicrobial effect in vivo is lower than optimal and of very short duration.[153] Derivatives of phenol are stronger antiseptics and toxins than phenol alone. The phenolic compounds are often available as camphorated solutions. Camphoration results in a less toxic phenolic compound because of a slower release of toxins to the surrounding tissues.

Studies in vitro have shown that phenol and phenol derivatives are highly toxic to mammalian cells and that the antimicrobial effectiveness of phenol and phenol derivatives does not correspond favorably to their toxicity.[233,234] Experimentation in vivo also demonstrated that phenol and phenol derivatives induce inflammatory changes at much lower concentrations than many other antimicrobial agents.[236]

Phenols are ineffective antiseptics under clinical conditions. Two weeks of intracanal dressing, where the canals were filled with camphorated phenol or camphorated parachlorophenol, failed to eliminate intracanal bacteria in a third of the cases studied[38] (see Fig. 14-56). Phenolic compounds are also unable to release an effective antimicrobial vapor and are, therefore, ineffective when placed on a cotton pellet in the pulp space.[62,236]

Formaldehyde Formaldehyde has been extensively used in endodontic therapy and still enjoys great popularity despite its high toxicity and mutagenic potential.[138] The compound of interest when discussing pulp space disinfection is formocresol. The formaldehyde component of formocresol may vary substantially between 19% formaldehyde to 37% formaldehyde. Tricresol formalin is another formaldehyde preparation containing 10% tricresol and 90% formaldehyde. Thus all these preparations contain formaldehyde well above the 10% normally used for fixation of pathologic specimens.

Formaldehyde is volatile and, therefore, releases antimicrobial vapors if applied on a cotton pellet for pulp chamber disinfection. All these formaldehyde preparations are potent toxins with an antimicrobial effectiveness much lower than their toxicity.[67,234,236] The formaldehyde in contact with tissue in the pulp and periapical tissues is transported to all parts of the body.[15,34] Considering the outright toxic and tissue-destructive effects and the mutagenic and carcinogenic potential, *there is no clinical reason to use formocresol as an antimicrobial agent for endodontic treatment.* The alternatives are better antiseptics with significantly lower toxicity.

Halogens Chlorine has been used for many years for irrigation of root canals. It is also sometimes used as intracanal dressing in the form of Chloramine-T.[65,67]

Iodine, in the form of iodine potassium iodide, is a very effective antiseptic solution[175,233] with a low tissue toxicity.[65,67,234,236] It was shown in vitro that iodine potassium iodide (i.e., IKI 2%) penetrated more than 1000 μm of dentin in 5 minutes.[175] It is an effective disinfectant for infected dentin, and it is capable of killing bacteria in infected dentin in 5 minutes in vitro.[195] Iodine potassium iodide releases vapors that have a strong antimicrobial effect.[62,236] This solution can be prepared by mixing 2 g of iodine in 4 g of potassium iodide. This mixture is then dissolved in 94 ml of distilled water. Tincture of iodine (5%) has also proven to be one of the few reliable agents for the disinfection of rubber dam and tooth surfaces during the preparation of an aseptic endodontic working field.[160]

Calcium Hydroxide The use of calcium hydroxide ($Ca[OH]_2$) in endodontics was introduced by Hermann in 1920.[104] Although well documented for its time, the clinical applications during the following 25 years were not well-known.[105] Calcium hydroxide cannot be categorized as a conventional antiseptic, but it does kill bacteria in the root canal space. It has been routinely used by many endodontists during the last 40 years. The value of calcium hydroxide in endodontic treatment of necrotic infected teeth is now well documented.[38,217] Calcium hydroxide is normally used as a

Table 14-3   **TISSUE IRRITATION OF ANTISEPTICS USED FOR INTRACANAL DRESSINGS***

Dilution	IKI 2%	CP	FC	Cresatin	CPC
1:16	26.9 ± 3.0	—	—	—	—
1:32	2.9 ± 0.3	—	—	—	—
1:64	3.3 ± 0.4	33.8 ± 3.1	21.6 ± 0.8	—	—
1:128	1.6 ± 0.2	16.1 ± 1.4	15.7 ± 1.0	29.7 ± 2.2	33.4 ± 2.7
1:256	1.6 ± 0.1	2.1 ± 0.1	17.0 ± 3.5	19.9 ± 2.2	28.2 ± 2.4
1:512	1.1 ± 0.1	1.1 ± 0.1	11.1 ± 1.7	12.2 ± 0.8	23.0 ± 1.8
1:1024	—	—	4.5 ± 0.9	0.5 ± 0.2	1.9 ± 0.5
1:2048	—	—	1.6 ± 0.4	—	—

IKI, Iodine potassium iodide; *CP*, camphorated phenol; *FC*, formocresol; *CPC*, camphorated parachlorophenol.
*Measurement of enhanced vascular permeability after intradermal injection of 0.1 ml of the diluted antiseptic. Figures indicate leaked albumine measured after 3 hr as μg of Evans blue. Normal values <3 μg. Formocresol causes inflammation when diluted 1000 times; formocresol, cresatin, and camphorated parachlorophenol when diluted 500 times; and camphorated phenol at a dilution of 128 times. Iodine potassium iodide is the least irritating antiseptic. M ± SD. See Spångberg et al.[235] for details.

slurry of calcium hydroxide in a water base. At body temperature, less than 0.2% of the calcium hydroxide is dissolved into Ca^{++} and OH^- ions. Calcium hydroxide needs water to dissolve. Therefore it is most advantageous to use water as the vehicle for the calcium hydroxide paste. In contact with air, calcium hydroxide forms calcium carbonate ($CaCO_3$). This is an extremely slow process, however, and of little clinical significance.

Calcium hydroxide paste with a significant amount of calcium carbonate feels granular, because the carbonate has a very low solubility. It has been suggested to use Cresatin or camphorated parachlorophenol as the mixing vehicle. Mixing with Cresatin results in the formation of calcium cresylate and acetic acid, whereas mixing with camphorated parachlorophenol results in calcium parachlorphenolate. In both instances the hydrolysis is inhibited, and the advantageous high pH is not reached.[14, 216]

Calcium hydroxide is a slowly working antiseptic. Direct contact experiments in vitro require a 24-hour contact period for complete kill of enterococci.[195] In clinical experimentation, one week of intracanal dressing has been shown to safely disinfect a root canal system.[217] In addition to killing the bacteria, calcium hydroxide has an extraordinary quality in its ability to hydrolyze the lipid moiety of bacterial lipopolysaccharides, thereby inactivating the biologic activity of the lipopolysaccharide.[193,194] This is a very desirable effect because dead cell wall material remains after killing of the bacteria that causes the root canal infection. Calcium hydroxide not only kills the bacteria, but it also reduces the effect of the remaining cell wall material lipopolysaccharide (LPS).

Calcium hydroxide may be mixed with sterile water or saline, but this formula is also available commercially from a number of manufacturers in sterile single-dose packages (Calasept, J.S. Dental, Ridgefield, CT; Centrix Inc., Shelton, CT; DT Temporary Dressing, Global Dental Products, North Bellmore, NY) (Fig. 14-60). It should be mixed to a thick mixture to carry as much calcium hydroxide particles as possible. This slurry is best applied with a lentulo spiral. For maximal effectiveness it is important that the root canal is filled homogeneously to the working length. Saturated calcium hydroxide solution mixed with a detergent is an effective antimicrobial agent suitable for irrigation.[21]

ROOT CANAL–FILLING MATERIALS

After the pulp space has been appropriately prepared, it must be obturated with a material that is capable of completely preventing communication between the oral cavity and the periapical tissue wound. The prepared apical connective tissue wound area cannot heal with epithelium. Therefore the root filling placed against this wound serves as an alloplastic implant. These expectations regarding physical and biologic properties make the selection of a good obturation material critical. The materials commonly used for root canal fillings

can normally be divided into a solid phase and a cementing medium (i.e., a sealer).

Solid Materials

Gutta-Percha   Gutta-percha is the most commonly used material. Gutta-percha is the dried juice of the Taban tree (i.e., *Isonandra percha*). It was first introduced to the Royal Asiatic Society of England in 1843 by Sir Jose d'Almeida and was introduced into dentistry in the late 1800s. It occurs naturally as 1, 4-polyisoprene and is harder, more brittle, and less elastic than natural rubber. A linear crystalline polymer like gutta-percha melts at a set temperature, and a random but distinct change in structure results.

The crystalline phase appears in two forms: (1) the alpha phase and (2) the beta phase. The forms differ only in the molecular repeat distance and single-bond form. The alpha form is the material that comes from the natural tree product. The processed form, called beta form, is used in gutta-percha for root fillings.[203] When heated, gutta-percha undergoes phase transitions. Thus when the temperature increases, there is a transition from beta phase to alpha phase at around 115° F (46° C). This then changes to an amorphous phase at around 130° to 140° F (54° to 60° C). When cooled very slowly (i.e., 1° F per hour), it crystallizes to the alpha phase. Normal cooling returns the gutta-percha to the beta phase. Gutta-percha cones soften at a temperature above 147° F (64°

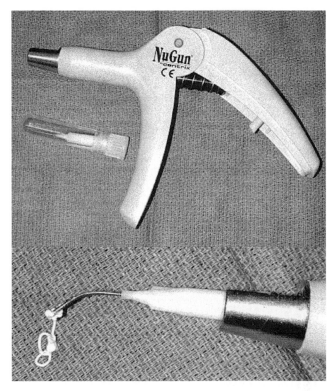

Fig. 14-60 SteriCal (Centrix Inc., Shelton, CT). Single dose calcium hydroxide paste in sterile saline. "Centrix" syringe used for dispensing of paste directly into root canal.

C).[88,203] It can easily be dissolved in chloroform and halothane.

Modern gutta-percha cones for root fillings contain only about 20% gutta-percha (Table 14-4). The major content is zinc oxide, which constitutes 60% to 75% of the material. The zinc oxide content provides a major part of the radiopacity of endodontic gutta-percha. The remaining 5% to 10% consists of various resins, waxes, and metal sulfates. The specific content is normally a manufacturing secret. Antiseptic gutta-percha with various antimicrobial agents has been suggested, but no credible information is available concerning the effect of these additives. Gutta-percha cone material that is 1-mm thick has a radiopacity corresponding to 6.44 mm aluminum.[31]

Because gutta-percha cannot be heat sterilized, other methods for decontamination must be used. The most practical method is to *disinfect the gutta-percha in NaOCl before use.* This can be done in 1 minute if submerged in a 5% solution of NaOCl.[212] It is imperative, however, after this disinfection that the gutta-percha is rinsed in ethyl alcohol to remove crystallized NaOCl before obturation; crystals of NaOCl on the gutta-percha cones impair the obturation seal.

Gutta-percha is normally applied using some form of condensation pressure. It has been shown, however, that real compression of gutta-percha is practically impossible.[204] Thus compression during root canal–filling procedures cannot be expected to compress gutta-percha but dislodge gutta-percha points to a more complete fill of the root canal. Gutta-percha may also be plasticized with a solvent or through heating to better fit the pulp space for the obturation. Both methods result in a slight shrinkage of approximately 1% to 2% when the gutta-percha has solidified.[150,268] It has been suggested that shrinkage in warmed gutta-percha may be prevented if not heated above 113° F (45° C). This is, however, practically impossible when performing vertical warm condensation.[87,94,95,205] It is important, however, to carefully control the temperature during warm condensation to prevent focal areas of unnecessary high temperatures. The first line of defense would be to use devices that can provide better temperature control than an open flame.[113] Several such electricalally controlled heating devices are available. The Touch 'N Heat and System B (Analytic, Orange, CA) are the more commonly used devices for this purpose (Fig. 14-61). Gutta-percha oxidizes in air and exposure to light and becomes brittle.[172] Therefore it should be stored in a cool, dry place for better shelf life. Methods to rejuvenate aged gutta-percha have been suggested.[224]

Gutta-percha cannot be used as the sole filling material because it lacks the adhering quality that is necessary to seal the root canal space. Several techniques have been described to use heat or solvents to adapt the gutta-percha to the canal space better, but a sealer and cement is always needed for the final seal. Gutta-percha cannot seal, because it lacks adhesive properties.

Endodontic gutta-percha is sold as cones in a variety of shapes and tapers (Fig. 14-62). There are two types: (1) "core" points used as master cones and (2) "auxiliary" points used for lateral condensation. There is an accepted international standard for gutta-percha points. Thus the sizing of gutta-percha core points (i.e., master cones) is based on similar size and taper standards as the endodontic files (ANSI and ADA no. 78) (see Table 14-1). It is very important to realize, however, that the tolerance is much less stringent for gutta-percha. An endodontic file must be manufactured with a tolerance of ± 0.02 mm, but the gutta-percha must only measure up to ± 0.05 mm. The consequence is that at the same size of instrument and gutta-percha point, there could

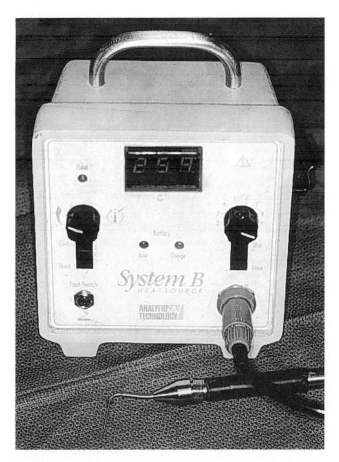

Fig. 14-61 System B (Analytic Technology, Redmond, WA) heating device for vertical compaction and removal of gutta-percha.[267]

Table 14-4 **COMPOSITION OF GUTTA-PERCHA FOR ENDODONTIC USE**

Gutta-Percha Cones	
Gutta-percha	19-22%
Zinc oxide	59–79%
Heavy metal salts	1–17%
Wax or resin	1–4%

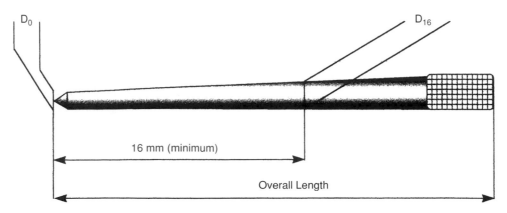

Fig. 14-62 Gutta-percha cone measurement points according to ADA and ANSI no. 78.

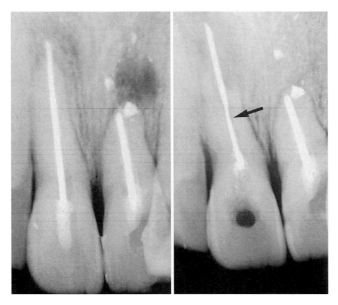

Fig. 14-63 Silver cone root filling. Poorly performed silver cone obturation shows extensive corrosion (*arrow*) 2 years after placement.

be a 0.07 mm difference (greater than one file size) in diameter. This discrepancy could be even larger in the cases when the standards are not strictly followed by the manufacturer.[244]

The auxiliary points have a larger taper and a pointed tip. They are also standardized but in a very different system (see Table 14-2). They are normally supplied in sizes such as *fine, fine-medium, medium-fine, medium,* and *medium-large.* These gutta-percha cones are usually used as accessory points during lateral condensation. Although core points often are used as master cones for obturation, there are also applications where the auxiliary cone is more suited.

Silver Cones   Pure silver molded in a conical shape has also been used for root canal fillings since the 1930s.[112,252] The use of silver cones is becoming increasingly rare. It was often used for the obturation of very narrow canals. Because

of the stiffness of silver, this technique was easier than using gutta-percha. In recent years, SS files have been used for root canal obturation in clinical situations with heavily calcified, dilacerated, narrow canals.

Obtaining good obturation with silver is difficult, because it cannot be made to conform with the pulp space like gutta-percha. Most silver cones contain small amounts of other trace metals (e.g., 0.1% to 0.2%), such as copper and nickel. This adds to the corrosion of silver cones (a very common complication in clinical cases [36,100,122,276]) (Fig. 14-63). Other reasons for the corrosion of silver in situ are the presence of metal restorations and posts that may have been used in teeth in the area. The silver corrosion products are highly toxic and may in themselves cause severe tissue injury.[82,211] Corrosion has been suggested as a reason for the failure of many silver cone root fillings, but despite numerous reports of silver corrosion in situ, it is not clear if the high failure rate of silver root fillings is associated with the corrosion or simply is the result of poor obturation with such rigid material.

Like all solid materials currently available, silver cones or SS files also have the drawback that they cannot independently seal the root canal (because these materials do not stick to the dentin walls). Therefore the metal core material must always be used with a cementing material and endodontic sealer.

Sealers and Cements

Endodontic Sealers   In the root canal filling the sealer plays an important role. The sealer fills all the space the gutta-percha is unable to fill because of gutta-percha's physical limitations. A good sealer must have adhesive strength to the dentin and to the core material, which usually is gutta-percha. In addition, the sealer must have cohesive strength to hold the obturation together. The sealers are usually a mixture that hardens through a chemical reaction. Such reaction normally includes the release of toxic material, making the sealer less biocompatible. In general the sealer is the critical part when assessing the toxicity of materials used.

Several sealer and cements, such as AH26, AH Plus, Ketac-Endo, and Diaket, may be used as the sole filling material because they have sufficient volume stability to maintain a seal. Under such use preventing excess is often difficult, because the sealer is applied with a lentulo spiral.

The sealer is expected to have some degree of radiopacity to be clearly visible on adequately exposed radiographs. Additives used to enhance radiopacity are silver, lead, iodine, barium, and bismuth. Compared with gutta-percha cones most sealers have a slightly lower radiopacity. There are a variety of sealers from among which to choose, and the clinician must be careful to evaluate all characteristics of a sealer before selecting.

Zinc Oxide–Eugenol Cements
Many endodontic sealers are simply zinc oxide–eugenol cements that have been modified for endodontic use. The mixing vehicle for these materials is mostly eugenol. The powder contains zinc oxide that is finely sifted to enhance the flow of the cement. Setting time is adjusted to allow for adequate working time. One millimeter of zinc oxide–eugenol cement has a radiopacity corresponding to 4 to 5 mm of aluminum, which is slightly lower than gutta-percha.[31] These cements easily lend themselves to the addition of chemicals, and paraformaldehyde is often added for antimicrobial and mummifying effects, germicides for antiseptic action, rosin or Canada balsam for greater dentin adhesion, and corticosteroids for suppression of inflammatory reactions.

Zinc oxide is a valuable component in the sealer (Table 14-5). It is effective as an antimicrobial agent[247] and has been shown to provide cytoprotection to tissue cells. The incorporation of rosins in sealers may initially have been for the adhesive properties.[93] Rosins (i.e., colophony), which are derived from a variety of conifers, are composed of approximately 90% resin acid. The remaining parts are volatile and nonvolatile compounds, such as terpene alcohol, aldehydes, and hydrocarbons. Resin acids are monobasic carboxylic acids with the basic molecular formula $C_{20}H_{30}O_2$. Resin acids are amphiphilic, with the carbon group being lipophilic, affecting the lipids in the cell membranes. This way the resin acids have a strong antimicrobial effect that, on mammalian cells, is expressed as cytotoxicity. The resin acids work in a similar way to quaternary ammonium compounds by increasing the cell membrane permeability of the affected cell. Although toxic, the combination of zinc oxide and resin acids may be overall beneficial. The antimicrobial effect of zinc oxide in both gutta-percha cones and in many sealers brings a low level of long-lasting antimicrobial effect. The resin acids are both antimicrobial and cytotoxic, but the combination with zinc oxide exerts a significant level of cytoprotection.[222, 246, 247]

Resin acids may under certain conditions, react with zinc, forming resin acid salt (i.e., resinate). This matrix-stabilized zincresinate is only slightly soluble in water.[146,223] Therefore zinc oxide–eugenol cements with resin components are less soluble than regular zinc oxide–eugenol cements.

The setting of zinc oxide–eugenol cements is a chemical process combined with physical embedding of zinc oxide in a matrix of zinc eugenolate. Particle size of zinc oxide, pH, and the presence of water regulate the setting and other additives that might be included in special formulas. The formation of eugenolate constitutes the hardening of the cement. Free eugenol always remains in the mass and acts as an irritant. Some more common zinc oxide–eugenol cements are Rickert's sealer (Kerr, Romulus, MI), Proco-Sol (Star Dental, Conshohocken, PA), U/P-Grossman's sealer (Sultan Chemists, Englewood, NJ), Wach's sealer (Sultan Chemists), Tubli-Seal (Kerr), Endomethasone (Septodont, Saint-Maur, France), and N2 (Agsa, Locarno, Switzerland). Zinc oxide–eugenol cements lose some volume with time because of dissolution in tissues with the release of eugenol and zinc oxide. This volume loss was measured in pure zinc oxide–eugenol cements over a 180-day period and found to be over 11%.[118] It can be expected that the addition of resin acids to the zinc oxide–eugenol cement significantly reduces this dissolution.[146]

For a long time it has been common to mix formaldehyde into endodontic sealers. The most common combinations have been zinc oxide–eugenol cements mixed with formaldehyde (Table 14-6). This is an undesirable additive to any sealer, because it only adds to the already toxic effect of eugenol and prevents or delays healing. The use of endodontic materials with formaldehyde content has been popular because formaldehyde necrotizes the nerve endings in the tissue area and, therefore, masks the inflammatory processes. Thus despite the necrotic effect of formaldehyde, the patients have few immediate symptoms and the damage is only clinically noticeable years later.

Chloropercha
Chloropercha (Moyco, Union Broach, York, PA) is another type of sealer that has been in use for many years. It is made by mixing white gutta-percha (i.e., alba) with chloroform. This will allow a gutta-percha root filling to fit better in the canal. It is important to recognize, however, that chloropercha has no adhesive properties. Another commercial form of chloropercha, called Kloroperka N-Ø (N-Ø Therapeutics, Oslo, Norway), contains resins and Canada balsam, thereby providing better adhesive properties (Table 14-7). Various forms of chloropercha have a radiodensity (1 mm thick) corresponding to only 1.2 to 2.7 mm of aluminum, which is much less than 1 mm of gutta-percha at 6.4 mm of aluminum.[31] These sealers appear vague on a radiograph. The general problem with most chloropercha products is their shrinkage during the evaporation or disappearance of the chloroform. Some brands, such as Kloroperka N-Ø, contain filler particles (e.g., zinc oxide) to reduce the shrinkage. Zinc oxide also increases radiopacity.

Another variation on the chloropercha technique is to use a mixture of 5% to 8% of rosins in chloroform.[41] A rosin chloroform wash of the root canal leaves a very adhesive residue. This residue in combination with dipping of the

Table 14-5   **COMPOSITION OF SOME COMMON ZINC OXIDE–EUGENOL ENDODONTIC CEMENTS**

	Kerr Sealer (Rickert's)	Proco-Sol	Proco-Sol (Nonstaining)	Grossman's Sealer	Wach's Paste	Tubli-Seal
Powder						
Zinc oxide	34.0–41.2	45.0	40.0	42.0	61.3	57.4–59.0
Silver (molecular/precipitated)	25.0–30.0	17.0				
Oleoresins	16.0–30.0					18.5–21.3
Resin (hydrogenated)		36.0				
Staybelite resin			30.0	27.0		
Dithymoliodide	11.0–12.8					
Magnesium oxide U.S.P.		2.0				
Calcium phosphate					12.3	
Bismuth subcarbonate			15.0	15.0		
Bismuth subnitrate					21.5	
Bismuth subiodide					1.8	
Bismuth trioxide						7.5
Barium sulfate			15.0	15.0		
Sodium borate (anhydrous)				1.0		
Heavy magnesium oxide					3.1	
Thymol iodide						3.8–5.0
Oils and waxes						10.0–10.1
Liquid						
Oil of cloves	78.0–80.0				22.2	
Eugenol		90.0	83.3	100.0		*
Canada balsam	20.0–22.0	10.0			74.2	
Sweet oil of almond			16.7			
Eucalyptol					1.8	
Beechwood creosote					1.8	
Polymerized resin						*
Annidalin						*

*Proportions of components not disclosed.

gutta-percha cone in resin chloroform provides the sealer in this technique. This is a difficult technique, because there is no sealer to fill areas where there are voids between the gutta-percha cones. Chloroform technique for obturation requires that the operator has good basic skills with various obturation techniques, because the technique is very sensitive to proper manipulations (Fig. 14-64). When the chloroform technique is correctly used, the shrinkage is not greater than when gutta-percha is plasticized by heat.[269] The use of chloroform has been sharply curtailed in recent years because of its projected toxicity. In endodontics, however, the amounts used are normally insignificant and cause no health hazard. One must, however, take prudent steps to reduce the vaporization during use, because chloroform is highly volatile. Thus when used for softening of gutta-percha during revision of old root fillings, the chloroform should be dispensed through a syringe and hypodermic needle. For other uses the *exposure time, amounts used,* and *chloroform surface exposed* should all be kept to a minimum.

There are some chloroform substitutes in use, such as halothane and turpentine. Halothane is less effective in softening gutta-percha than chloroform, is hepatotoxic like chloroform, and has a higher local toxicity than chloroform (Table 14-8). Therefore halothane is not a good substitute. Turpentine is not carcinogenic but is reported to easily cause allergic reactions. It has a high local toxicity and dissolves gutta-percha poorly. Therefore there are presently no good substitutes to the use of chloroform in endodontic treatment procedures. With careful workplace hygiene there is little risk associated with the occasional use of minuscule amounts of chloroform in endodontics.[19,143]

Calcium Hydroxide Sealers   Recently several calcium hydroxide (Ca[OH]$_2$)–based sealers have been brought to the market. Examples of such sealers are Sealapex (Kerr), CRCS (Hygenic Corp., Akron, OH), and Apexit (Vivadent, Schaan, Liechtenstein). These sealers are promoted as having therapeutic effect because of the calcium hydroxide content (Box 14-1). However, no such convincing results from scientific

Table 14-6　COMPOSITION OF TWO ZINC OXIDE–EUGENOL ENDODONTIC CEMENTS WITH FORMALDEHYDE

	Endomethasone*			
	Type A	Type B	Type C	N2 and RC-2B
Powder				
Zinc oxide	+	+	+	62.0–69.0
Bismuth subcarbonate				5.0–9.0
Bismuth subnitrate	+	+	+	2.0–4.0
Barium sulfate				2.0–3.0
Dexamethasone	+	+	+	
Hydrocortisone acetate			+	
Hydrocortisone				1.2
Prednisolone				0.2
Tetraiodothymol	+	+	+	
Paraformaldehyde	+	+	+	6.5
Titanium dioxide				2.0–3.0
Phenylmercuric borate				0.16
Lead tetroxide				11.0–12.0
Liquid				
Eugenol	+	+	+	92.0–100.0
Geraniol				8.0

*Amounts are not disclosed by the manufacturer; + indicates part of formula.

Table 14-7　COMPOSITION OF GUTTA-PERCHA SEALERS*

	Kloroperka N-Ø	Chloropercha
Powder		
Canada balsam	19.6	
Resin	11.8	
Gutta-percha	19.6	9.0
Zinc oxide	49.0	
Liquid		
Chloroform	100.0	91.0

*Chloropercha is a premixed sealer. Kloroperka N-Ø is a powder/liquid mixture.

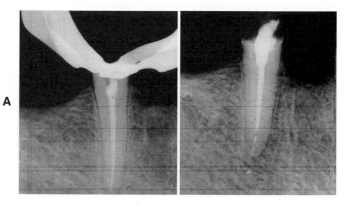

A　　　　**B**

Fig. 14-64　Root filling performed with a resin chloroform dip method. Too much chloroform has been used. Obturation seems good at time of filling (**A**), but at a follow-up 2 weeks later (**B**), when the chloroform had evaporated, the gutta-percha mass has lost significant volume and "dropped" into the periapical tissue.

trials have been shown. To be therapeutically effective calcium hydroxide must be dissociated into Ca^{++} and OH^-. Therefore to be effective, an endodontic sealer based on calcium hydroxide must dissolve and the solid consequently lose content. Thus one major concern is that the calcium hydroxide content may dissolve, leaving obturation voids. This would ruin the function of the sealer, because it would disintegrate in the tissue. These sealers also have poor cohesive strength.[265] There is no objective proof that a calcium hydroxide sealer provides any advantage for root canal obturations or has any of the desirable biologic effects of calcium hydroxide paste. In a study of diffusion of hydroxyl ions into surrounding dentin after root filling with Sealapex and Apexit, no traces were found in teeth filled with Apexit. Some hydroxyl ions could be detected in the dentin close to the root filling with Sealapex.[238] In a similar study of calcium and hydroxyl ion release from Sealapex and CRCS negligible release was noted from CRCS. Sealapex released more ions but disintegrated in the process.[252] Studies in vivo of Sealapex and CRCS have demonstrated that Sealapex and CRCS easily disintegrate in the tissue.[221] They both cause chronic inflammation.[222,253] Considering the alternatives, calcium-containing sealers are not a practical choice of material.

Polymers　New sealers are mostly polymers (Table 14-9). The more common brands are Endofill (Lee Pharmaceuticals, South El Monte, CA), AH26, AH Plus (Caulk/Dentsply, Milford, DE), and Diaket (ESPE, Seefeld, Germany). AH26 is an epoxy resin that initially was developed to serve as a single-filler material.[209,210] Because of its good handling characteristics it has been extensively used as a sealer. It has a good flow, seals well to dentin walls, and allows for a sufficient working time.[141,210] One millimeter of AH26 has a radiopacity corresponding to 6.66 mm of aluminum; thus it is very similar to gutta-percha.[31] Like most sealers, AH26 is very toxic when freshly prepared.[176,225-229] This toxicity decreases rapidly during the setting, and after 24 hours the cement has one of the lowest toxicities of endodontic sealers. The reason for the toxicity of the AH26 sealer is the release of a very small amount of formaldehyde as a result of the chemical setting process. This amount of brief release of formaldehyde, however, is thousands of times lower than the long-term release from conventional formaldehyde-containing sealers, such as N2.[232] After the initial setting, AH26 exerts little toxic effect in vitro or in vivo.[29,176,208,264] A new formulation of AH26 is now available called AH Plus. This is a paste and paste-mixing system that assures a better mixture. It has an increased radiopacity, shorter setting time (approximately 8 hours), lower solubility, and a better flow compared with AH26.

Diaket is a polyketone compound containing vinyl polymers that, mixed with zinc oxide and bismuth phosphate, forms an adhesive sealer.[206] Small amounts of camphor and phenol interact negatively with the setting process and must be carefully removed before obturation. The material sets quickly in the root canal at body temperature but remains soft longer at room temperature. The volume stability is good and the solubility low.[91,106,107] It is highly toxic in vitro and causes extensive tissue necrosis. The irritation is long lasting.[176,225-229]

Table 14-8   TOXIC EFFECT OF GUTTA-PERCHA SOLVENTS ON L929 CELLS IN VITRO*

Time	Control	Chloroform	Halothane	Turpentine
Air Evaporation				
Fresh mix	7.2 ± 0.7	94.4 ± 3.0	102.5 ± 7.5	87.3 ± 2.2
1 day	10.1 ± 0.4	11.3 ± 1.8	12.6 ± 0.9	66.6 ± 5.3
7 days	9.5 ± 0.4	11.6 ± 0.9	14.8 ± 1.0	12.5 ± 2.8
Liquid Evaporation				
Fresh mix	7.2 ± 0.7	102.1 ± 6.4	98.4 ± 6.6	87.0 ± 2.1
1 day	10.1 ± 0.4	89.1 ± 6.7	103.9 ± 9.0	71.8 ± 4.7
7 days	9.5 ± 0.4	11.6 ± 5.8	10.1 ± 2.8	64.2 ± 3.9

From Barbosa SV et al: *J Endod* 20:6, 1994.
*Gutta-percha (2.5 g) was dissolved in either chloroform, halothane, or turpentine (5 ml). The cell response was measured as radiochromium release at various times after mixing. The solvents were allowed to evaporate in air or through a liquid layer. The higher the release, the higher is the toxicity. M ± SD.

Box 14-1   CONTENT OF CALCIUM HYDROXIDE SEALERS: SEALAPEX, CRCS, AND APEXIT*

Sealapex			**Apexit**	
Base			*Base*	
Calcium hydroxide	25.0%		Calcium hydroxide	31.9%
Zinc oxide	6.5%		Zinc oxide	5.5%
Catalyst			Calcium oxide	5.6%
Barium sulfate	18.6%		Silicon dioxide	8.1%
Titanium dioxide	5.1%		Zinc stearate	2.3%
Zinc stearate	1.0%		Hydrogenized colophony	31.5%
			Tricalcium phosphate	4.1%
CRCS			Polydimethylsiloxane	2.5%
Powder			*Activator*	
Calcium hydroxide			Trimethyl hexanedioldisalicylate	25.0%
Zinc oxide			Bismuth carbonate basic	18.2%
Bismuth dioxide			Bismuth oxide	18.2%
Barium sulfate			Silicon dioxide	15.0%
Liquid			1.3-Butanedioldisalicylate	11.4
Eugenol			Hydrogenized colophony	5.4%
Eucalyptol			Tricalcium phosphate	5.0%
			Zinc stearate	1.4%

*Proportions are unavailable for CRCS and incomplete for Sealapex.

Glass Ionomer Cement   Recently glass ionomer cements have been introduced as endodontic sealers (Ketac-Endo, ESPE). Glass ionomer cements are known to cause little tissue irritation.[275] It also has a low toxicity in vitro.[179] Little biologic data are available relative to its use as an endodontic sealer, so safety and efficacy of glass ionomer cements have not been established. There are questions about the quality of the seal with Ketac-Endo because of observed dentin and sealer adhesive failures.[58,220]

Formaldehyde-Containing Sealers   A large group of endodontic sealers and cements have substantial additives of paraformaldehyde. Some of the more common are Endomethasone, Kri paste, Riebler's paste, and N2. Although not much different in content as far as toxicity is concerned, N2 has been the material most commonly focused on when discussing this phenomenon. This material is also known as RC 2B or the "Sargenti technique." Throughout the years it has been heavily commercialized. It is difficult to understand that anyone can subscribe to the idea that treating the apical pulp wound with a strong tissue-coagulating toxic material may enhance healing.

N2 is basically a zinc oxide–eugenol sealer. Its composition has been varied extensively throughout the years. The significant content of lead oxide[64,266] and smaller amount of organic mercury (Fig. 14-65) that formerly were major toxic components of N2 are often missing in recent formulas. However, this material still contains large amounts of formaldehyde. It seals well in combination with a core.[37,90] Because it contains 6% to 8% paraformaldehyde (and sometimes hydrocortisone and prednisolone), it loses substantial volume when exposed to fluid.[91] It also absorbs more than 2% of fluid during the first week in situ.[106]

Table 14-9   **COMPOSITION OF RESIN-TYPE ENDODONTIC SEALERS**

	Resins		
	AH26	Diaket	Riebler's Paste
Powder			
Silver powder	10%		
Zinc oxide		98.0%	*
Bismuth oxide	60%		
Bismuth phosphate		2.0%	
Hexamethylenetetramine	25%		
Titanium oxide	5%		
Fromaldehyde (polymerized)			*
Barium sulfate			*
Phenol			*
Liquid			
Bisphenoldiglycidyl ether	100%		
2.2'-Dihydroxy 5.5'-dichlorodiphenylmethane		*	
Propionylacetophenone		*	
Triethanolamine		*	
Caproic acid		*	
Copolymers of vinyl acetate, vinyl chloride, and vinyl isobutylether		*	
Formaldehyde			*
Sulfuric acid			*
Ammonia			*
Glycerin			*

*Proportions not available.

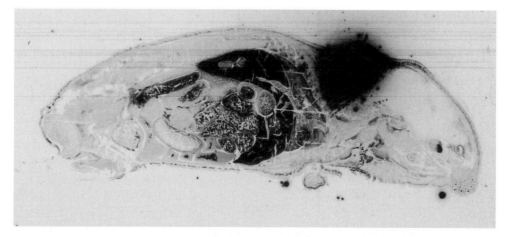

Fig. 14-65 Freshly mixed paste of N2 was injected in the neck skin of newborn mouse. Mercury in the powder had been made radioactive. Twenty-four hours after injection the mouse was instantly frozen and sectioned. This figure shows the autoradiogram resulting from such section. Neck area where the injection was done is highly radioactive, but practically all parts of the body are radioactive (*black*) to some degree. This shows that any zinc oxide–eugenol cement introduced into the tissue allows leakage of components that are transported to all parts of the body.

N2 is very toxic in experiments in vitro[235] and in animal experiments.[96,129,225-230] The tissue reaction normally observed is a coagulation necrosis within a very short time, reaching its maximum in less than 3 days. The coagulated tissue is altered to such an extent that it cannot undergo any repair for months because it is formaldehyde impregnated. With time the formaldehyde is washed out of the necrotic tissue,[15,35] allowing either bacteria to be established in the necrosis or, if the blood supply is adequate, repair to take place.[225-230] In clinical applications this untoward tissue reaction can be seen as localized inflammatory reactions in the periapical tissues.[66]

Standards and Properties

Physical Properties   ADA and ANSI document no. 57 outlines various test methods for the evaluation of physical properties of endodontic sealer-filling materials. Sealers are classified into two categories (i.e., types), depending on the intended use: Type I materials are intended to be used with core material, and Type II materials are intended for use with or without core material or sealer. Type I materials are divided into three classes. Class I includes materials in the form of powder and liquid that set through a nonpolymerizing process. Class 2 includes materials in the form of two pastes that set through a nonpolymerizing process. Finally, Class 3 includes polymer and resin systems that set through polymerization. The subclasses for Type II materials are the same as for Type I materials, except that metal amalgams are also included. Document no. 57 describes testing methods for working time, setting time, flow, film thickness, solubility, and disintegration. There is also a specific requirement for radiodensity.[31]

Despite these often detailed requirements there are still significant disagreements on ideal properties. Therefore most of these expectations are guidelines that have not significantly affected the industry.

Biologic Properties   ADA and ANSI document no. 41 recommends various protocols for the biologic evaluation of dental materials. This document outlines recommended test protocols for various dental materials, including certain guidelines for endodontic filling materials. These methods include general toxicity assessments (LD_{50}), cytotoxicity assessments in vitro, sensitization assays, mutagenicity assays, implantation tests, and usage tests. For each of these items there are several test methods to choose from depending on type of material.

Root canal–filling materials are generally toxic, and none fulfills the expectations that document no. 41 requires. However, in an attempt to select more biologically acceptable materials it is possible to use methods described in document no. 41 to distinguish more toxic materials from less toxic materials. This results in a less intensive or long-lasting chemical insult to the remaining apical pulp or apical peri-odontium. If the wound area is free from bacteria when the initial chemical necrosis occurs, there is no reason to believe that tissue repair would not take place as the initial irritant decreases in intensity. There may be some tissue irritation because of phagocytosis of particles of the material, but the result would not be an expanding lesion.[219]

Discounting paraformaldehyde-containing endodontic materials, endodontic sealers should not be implicated as the cause for the development of a periradicular bone lesion. When the tissue in the apical root area is not sterile, however, a chemical pulp or periapical necrosis is a good area for microbial expansion. Thus materials that cause extensive tissue necrosis (either inside the root canal or when extruded as an excess of filling material) are, in fact, vehicles for the development of a failing endodontic treatment (Fig. 14-66). This supports the idea that treatment should focus on the proper application of asepsis and antisepsis and use materials that cause as few tissue injuries as possible.

Gutta-percha as a root canal–filling material has been extensively investigated and found to be biocompatible. In comparison with sealers used for root canal obturations it clearly has the lowest tissue toxicity (Fig. 14-67). In implantation studies ranging up to 6 months in length, gutta-percha has been shown to heal in well, with minimal irritation.* Similar findings were reported from implantation in humans. After implantation the gutta-percha is normally surrounded by a defined capsule rich in cells but without significant presence of inflammatory cells. However, there is some presence of macrophages (Fig. 14-68). Results from more sensitive assays in vitro support the in vivo results suggesting that gutta-percha for root canal fillings have a low toxicity.[176,225-228,235] Gutta-percha in the form of small particles induces an intensive foreign-body reaction with massive accumulation of mononucleated and multinucleated macrophages.[219] This is not surprising, however, because material normally considered inert, such as Teflon, causes similar reactions when presented to the tissues as an irregular surface or particles.[43]

Sealers and cements are the very toxic component of a gutta-percha root filling (Fig. 14-69). Therefore great care must be given to the selection of materials and the understanding of what each material may contribute to a disease process. Zinc oxide–eugenol cements have a significant drawback in their release of free eugenol and loss of volume during the hydrolysis that takes place after setting. Several of the polymer materials have a high toxicity during the polymerization phase (AH26, Diaket, Endofill) but may become practically inert when polymerized (AH26, Endofill) (Fig. 14-70). AH Plus has a lower cytotoxicity and is less genotoxic than AH26.[139] Sealers with inclusions of dissolvable components, such as calcium hydroxide, lose these components in the tissue with a compromise of the integrity of the fill.

---

*References 29,30,69,70,109,159,219,225-229,231.

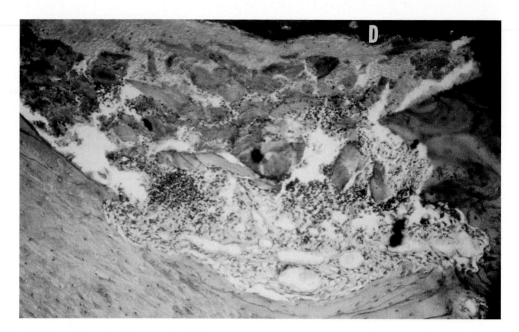

Fig. 14-66 Implant of Diaket (ESPE, Seefeld, Germany) in mandible of guinea pig. Material has necrotized the surrounding bone that contains sequestered bone and severe accumulation of all forms of inflammatory cells. Diaket at *D*.

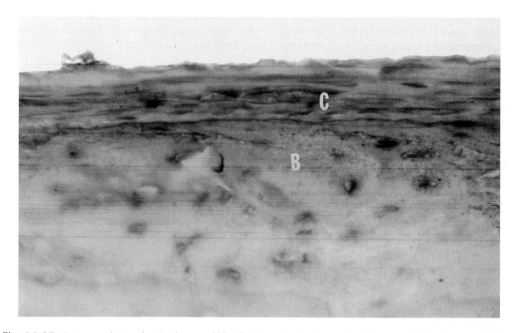

Fig. 14-67 Gutta-percha implant in the mandible of guinea pig. Twelve weeks. Gutta-percha implant (*on top*) has healed in well with a thin connective tissue interface (*C*) between the healed bone (*B*) and the implant that was lost during histologic preparation. Compare tissue reaction with Fig. 14-66.

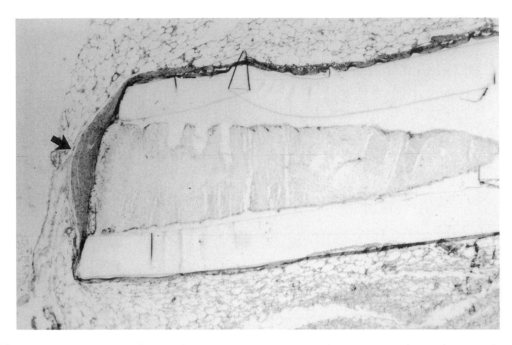

Fig. 14-68 Gutta-percha implant in subcutaneous connective tissue of guinea pig. Twelve weeks. Material was implanted in a Teflon tube. The tissue has responded with a connective tissue capsule (*arrow*) that is thicker than tissue surrounding the tube. No sign of inflammatory cells.

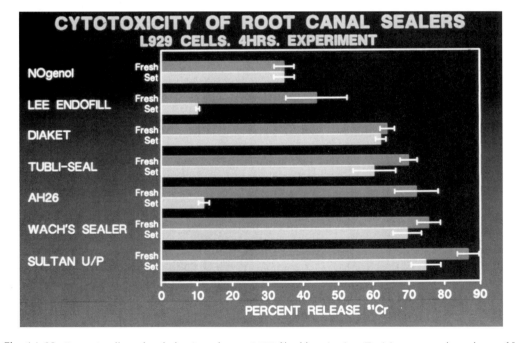

Fig. 14-69 Cytotoxic effect of endodontic sealers on L929 fibroblasts in vitro. Toxicity measured as release of [51] Cr. The more release the more cytotoxic is the material. Freshly prepared sealers are always more toxic than set sealers. Many sealers stay toxic even after setting.

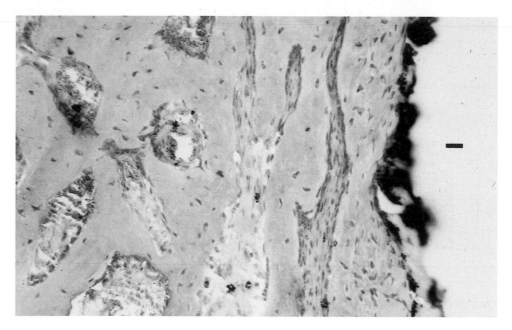

Fig. 14-70　Implant of AH26 in the mandible of the guinea pig at 12 weeks. Bone has grown up and integrated with the implant. Remnants of the AH26 implant, which was lost during histologic preparation, can be seen as a black area at the top. Complete healing observed without signs of inflammation.

DELIVERY SYSTEMS FOR ROOT CANAL–FILLING MATERIALS

The search for simplification and increased proficiency has led to the development of many new hybrid materials. All hybrids currently available are based on gutta-percha. The differences focus on alternative methods to introduce the gutta-percha into the root canal system with maintained control. The methods presently in use are either injection techniques or gutta-percha cones attached to a more rigid skeleton.

Most hybrid obturation methods require modification in the outline of the root canal preparation. Therefore for optimal results the clinician should consider technique variations before attempting hybrid obturation method.[268]

A comparison of the more commonly practiced obturation methods with an objective and sensitive dye penetration method failed to show any major difference in the quality of the obturation (Fig. l4-71).[57]

Rigid Systems

ThermaFil Plus (Tulsa Dental Products, Tulsa, OK; Densfil, Caulk/Dentsply, Milford, DE) is an obturation system where the gutta-percha is preapplied to a core skeleton that resembles an endodontic file (Fig. 14-72). The gutta-percha obturator is heated in a special heater (Fig. 14-73) (ThermaPrep Plus Oven, Tulsa Dental Products, Tulsa, OK) to the appropriate softness and the obturation is done with the complete device (i.e., gutta-percha + core). A sealer must be used for complete obturation. These devices are available with a plastic, SS, or titanium core. The plastic core material can, if needed, be softened with chloroform or heated (System B)[267] for easy removal. These obturators offer an alternative method for obturation with gutta-percha.

Injection Techniques

Several techniques have been described for introducing gutta-percha into the root canal system after the gutta-percha has been plasticized with heat. Obtura II (Fig. 14-74) (Obtura Spartan, Fenton, MO),[273] is presently the most common delivery system for gutta-percha. It dispenses a heavy form of gutta-percha heated to a high temperature (302° to 338° F, 150° to 170° C).

Although the temperature of the gutta-percha in the Obtura II injection gun is as high as 302° to 338° F (150° to 170° C), the temperature of the extruded material may vary between 140° to 176° F (60° to 80° C)[94,95] and 280° F (138° C).[61] The intracanal temperatures after delivery have been measured, with intracanal thermocouples, to be 107.6° to 192.2° F (42° to 89° C) with the Obtura system. With the high temperatures resulting from injection of gutta-percha with the Obtura system, periodontal injuries have been reported after endodontic treatment of teeth in the ferret and the dog.[161,199,200]

Shrinkage of gutta-percha in these injectable gutta-percha systems does not appear to be different from the shrinkage of normal gutta-percha. When plasticized by heat, gutta-percha has a volume loss of approximately 2% when cooling.[89]

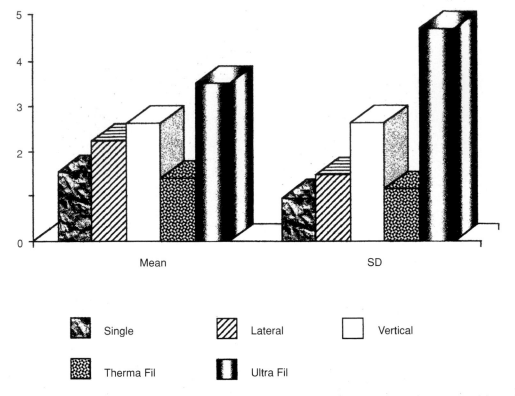

Fig. 14-71 Comparison of dye penetration after various obturation methods using AH26 sealer. Dye was delivered with a vacuum method. Measured as millimeters of leakage. Single cone technique and ThermaFil resulted in the least leakage followed by lateral condensation, vertical condensation, and UltraFil. Standard deviation is high, as is common for leakage studies, reflecting the variability in the obturation method. The less complicated the obturation method, the lower is the standard deviation.[57]

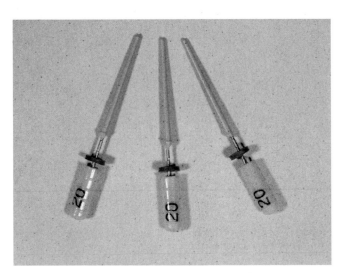

Fig. 14-72 ThermaFil obturators (Tulsa Dental Products, Tulsa, OK).

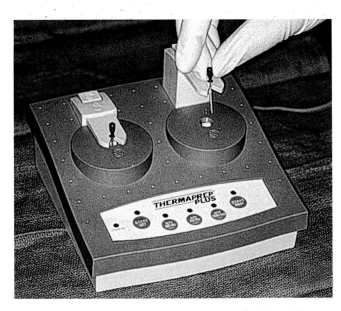

Fig. 14-73 ThermaPrep Plus heating oven for ThermaFil.

Rotary Techniques

Heat softening of gutta-percha can be achieved using frictional heat. This was first suggested with the introduction of the McSpadden compactor instrument. This technique has seen many variations[198,249] and the development of several compaction instruments. The generated heat may exceed safe levels for other heat compaction techniques.[199,200] One device called Quickfil (J.S. Dental, Ridgefield, CT) is commercially available. The ability to obturate root canals with this device and friction heating was found to be as good as lateral condensation.[201] Volumetric changes in the gutta-

percha after friction heat compaction are similar to other types of gutta-percha condensations using heat.[47]

TEMPORARY CEMENTS

If endodontic therapy cannot be completed in one visit, the pulp space must be closed with a sealing temporary cement. This cement must be capable of providing a satisfactory seal to prevent bacteria and fluid products from the oral cavity from contaminating the pulp space. This cement must have enough structural strength to withstand the masticatory forces and retain the seal. The most common materials are IRM (L.D. Caulk, Milford, DE), TERM (L.D. Caulk. Milford, DE), and Cavit (ESPE, Seefeld, Germany). IRM is a reinforced zinc oxide cement available as a powder or liquid in single-dose mixing capsules. Cavit is a premixed material composed of zinc oxide, calcium sulfate, glycol and polyvinyl acetate, polyvinyl chloride, and triethanolamine. It sets on contact with water. TERM is a filled composite resin that is light activated. Of these, TERM and Cavit provide better seal than IRM at any thickness of the restorations.[12,99,117] IRM has extensive marginal leakage of fluid, whereas Cavit seems to absorb fluid into the entire body of the restoration. These findings are surprising; however, IRM may, because of its eugenol content, provide a bacterial barrier but allow leakage of other liquid substances (Figs. 14-75 and 14-76). Therefore if Cavit or other types of relatively soft temporary cements are used, they must be placed at a thickness of at least 4 to 5 mm. If a more robust temporary restoration is required for a longer than 1 week, the soft cement must be covered with a harder cement, such as IRM or glass ionomer cement.

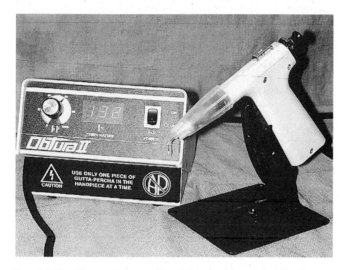

Fig. 14-74 Obtura II system for delivery of heat plasticized gutta-percha (Obtura Spartan, Fenton, MO).

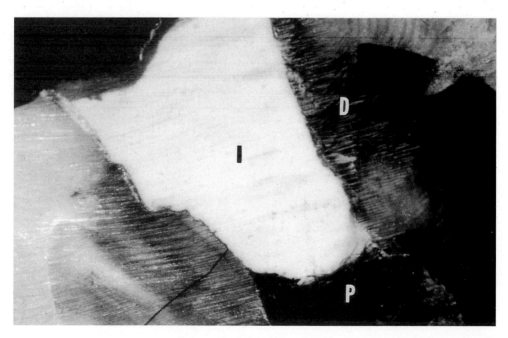

Fig. 14-75   Temporary filling of IRM (white at *I*). Dye has penetrated the margins and dyed the content of the pulp chamber (*P*). Dentin (*D*) has been stained by the dye penetrating the margins.

RETROGRADE ENDODONTIC TREATMENT

Root End Preparation

Root end preparation has classically been done with rotary instruments. Because of the restriction in available space in the periapical area, special hand pieces have been developed (Fig. 14-77). In recent years there has been extensive use of ultrasonic and sonic preparation of the root end. Such preparation can be done more conservatively than preparation with a bur and still be made deeper into the root canal. It also requires less angulated resection of the root apex. Because of their higher strength the piezoelectrical units have a clear advantage (because this type of preparation requires power) (Figs. 14-78 and 14-79). A serious concern was raised, however, over reports of a high frequency of apical cracks of the dentin in the resected area.[133,202] This cracking was especially pronounced at higher power settings. Other studies, however, have been unable to find any connection between root end cracks and ultrasonic preparation.[25,162] This phenomenon requires further careful assessment, because initial crack lines may propagate a more extensive fracture years later.

Root End–Filling Materials

The choice of root end–filling materials is a subject of great controversy among endodontic surgeons. The classic material in the past was silver amalgam, but it was suggested that the zinc normally found in the alloy may cause tissue damage.[173] This would be because of the precipitation of toxic zinc carbonate in the tissue associated with such root end amalgam filling. Despite the lack of more solid information regarding zinc in amalgam and its consequences, it has become a standard to use zinc-free alloys for root end fillings. More recent studies of the possible formation of zinc carbonate in the tissue has been unsuccessful. Thus there is no solid evidence that zinc-containing amalgams would be less suitable for retrograde obturations[125,126,140,145] (Figs. 14-80 and 14-81). Zinc is toxic in excess, however, and the tissue tolerance is rather low. Thus in evaluations in vitro, amalgams containing zinc are slightly more toxic than zinc-free amalgams (Table 14-10).

Because of various concerns about the use of silver amalgam other materials, such as zinc oxide–eugenol cements (e.g., IRM, Super EBA), glass ionomer cements, composite resins, and Cavit, have been used. The attempt to use Cavit as a retrograde obturation material was unsuccessful.[72]

Glass ionomer cements have generally been evaluated and compared with amalgam and gutta-percha with some success.[42,56,116,274,275] Silver glass ionomer cement (i.e., Ketac-Silver) was evaluated and compared with zinc oxide–eugenol cements and amalgam, and it was found to be superior in *in vitro* and *in vivo* applications.[33,179]

Mineral trioxide aggregate (MTA) is presently a root end repair material in great vogue. It is commercially available under the name ProRoot MTA (Dentsply/Tulsa Dental, Tulsa, OK). The material has been suggested to be used for a variety of endodontic procedures from pulp capping to perforation repair. Because of its high surface pH it supports tissue repairs similar to repairs seen with calcium hydroxide.[108] Contrary to calcium hydroxide, however, MTA pro-

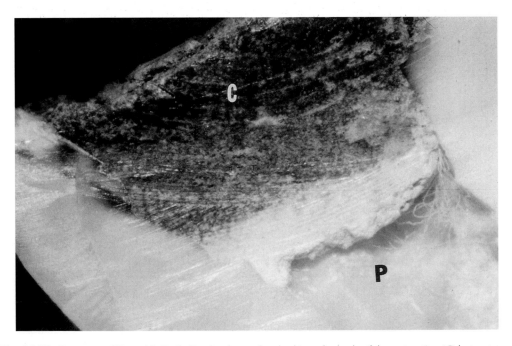

Fig. 14-76 Temporary filling with Cavit. Dye has been absorbed into the body of the restoration (*C*) but not penetrated to the pulp chamber (*P*) that is filled with white cotton. Inner part of the Cavit has no stain.

vides a hard setting nonresorbable surface with cavity adaptation comparable to Super-EBA.[22] From available literature, MTA appears to be an excellent material for root end fillings and perforation repairs.

All these materials have been used as alternatives to silver amalgam, but no clear-and-objective preferential material can be found. Results are highly variable after root end surgery and retrograde obturation, and it is possible to find data in the literature to support most of these materials, including silver amalgam. Therefore it is reasonable to believe that, within the scope of the reviewed materials, the material may be just one of several factors that determine success or failure after root end surgery.

LASERS

Laser applications in endodontics are still in their infancy. It remains unclear if the use of laser technology will ever have a practical application in this field of dentistry. Numerous papers have been written on the subject but mostly with inadequate documentation. Presently there is little support for the unbounded enthusiasm found in many commercial brochures and professional publications.

The lasers most commonly applied in endodontic research are the carbon dioxide laser (10,600 nm wavelength), the Nd:YAG laser (1064 nm), the argon laser (418 to 515 nm), and the xenon chloride excimer laser (308 nm). There are many factors affecting laser and tissue interaction.

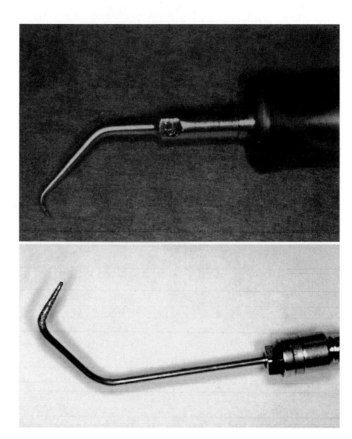

Fig. 14-79 Working tips for root end preparation. *Top,* a Spartan steel tip. *Bottom,* a diamond-coated tip for an Enac unit.

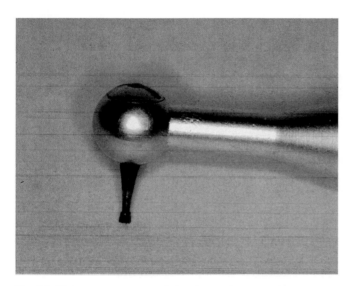

Fig. 14-77 Miniature contraangle hand piece for root end preparation.

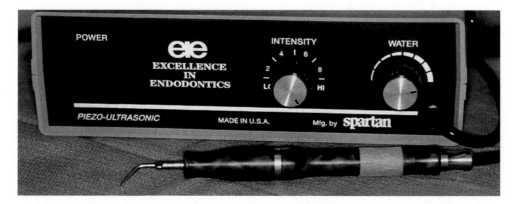

Fig. 14-78 Spartan piezoelectrical ultrasonic device with sterilizable hand piece. Power and irrigation flow can be adjusted (Obtura Spartan, Fenton, MO.)

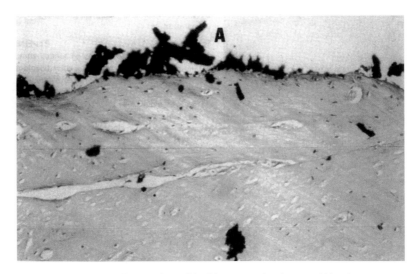

Fig. 14-80 Silver amalgam (Dispersalloy) implanted freshly prepared in the mandible of guinea pig. Twelve weeks. Remnants of the amalgam (A), which were removed during the histologic preparation, are black. Bone has healed and integrated with the amalgam without any layer of soft connective tissue.

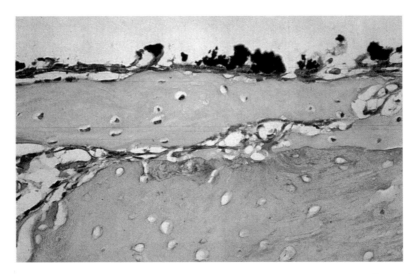

Fig. 14-81 Zinc-free amalgam implanted freshly prepared in the mandible of guinea pig. Twelve weeks. Remnants of the amalgam, which were removed during the histologic preparation, are black. Bone has healed and integrated with the amalgam without any layer of soft connective tissue.

One significant factor is the relationship between wavelength and tissue absorption of the energy. Thus the wavelength of a carbon dioxide laser is highly absorbed by water in the tissues. The Nd:YAG laser is almost transparent to water but absorbed in pigmented tissue and hemoglobin. Therefore it may cause deeper damage to tissue than a carbon dioxide laser. Refraction and diffuse scattering of radiation is another serious concern when operating in crystalline structures, such as teeth. Some of the attempted applications in endodontics have been related to lowering dentin permeability, instrumenting, cleaning and disinfecting root canals, and root end surgery.

Various attempts have been made to decrease dentin permeability by fusing the dentin surface with carbon dioxide and Nd:YAG lasers. Lowered permeability after treatment with carbon dioxide and Nd:YAG lasers has been reported,[155,251] but increased permeability has also been reported.[177] The xenon chloride excimer laser has been shown to occlude dentin tubules.[237]

The use of lasers for root canal preparation has not been successful. Levy[137] suggested that it was possible to clean root canals effectively with an air-and-water-cooled Nd:YAG laser. The illustrations in the publication, however, did not support the claims because they did not demonstrate root

Table 14-10   TOXICITY OF TWO AMALGAMS FOR ROOT END FILLING*

| | Cell Material Contact Time | | | |
| | 4 hr | | 24 hr | |
	Experiment	Control	Experiment	Control
Kerr Zinc-Free Amalgam				
In vitro				
Fresh mix	12.1 ± 0.9	7.7 ± 0.4	34.9 ± 1.2	25.7 ± 0.8
Set 1 day	7.7 ± 0.4	7.7 ± 0.4	28.7 ± 1.9	24.7 ± 1.8
Set 7 days	—	—	31.9 ± 1.8	25.7 ± 0.8
Implanted				
Retrieved	9.0 ± 0.3	9.4 ± 0.5	25.1 ± 1.0	25.4 ± 1.2
Corroded	—	—	45.6 ± 10.2	26.7 ± 0.8
Repolished	6.9 ± 0.6	7.5 ± 0.5	30.7 ± 1.9	25.7 ± 0.8
Dispersalloy				
In vitro				
Fresh	37.1 ± 1.0	6.0 ± 0.8	—	—
Set 1 day	9.8 ± 0.2	7.4 ± 0.1	67.9 ± 0.8	24.5 ± 0.8
Set 7 days	7.4 ± 0.5	6.0 ± 0.8	61.8 ± 3.0	28.9 ± 0.6
Implanted				
Retrieved	9.7 ± 1.8	9.4 ± 0.5	49.0 ± 7.6	25.4 ± 1.2
Corroded	—	—	44.8 ± 7.0	26.7 ± 0.8
Repolished	7.3 ± 0.4	7.5 ± 0.5	31.5 ± 1.3	25.7 ± 0.8

*Cytotoxicity measured as release of radiochromium from L929 cells in vitro. The amalgams were prepared and tested immediately, after 1 day and after 1 week. Amalgam samples were also prepared and implanted subcutaneously in guinea pigs for 3 months, retrieved, and tested for cytotoxicity. Samples were also corroded in saline for 3 months and tested for cytotoxicity. The samples were then polished and once again tested for cytotoxicity. The zinc-free amalgam showed a slightly lower cytotoxicity than the amalgam containing zinc. M ± SD.

canal walls but dentin cut parallel to the dentin tubules. Another study using an Nd:YAG laser showed that the heat generation during laser treatment of the root canals in the teeth of dogs resulted in necrosis of periodontal tissue and subsequent ankylosis.[17] Some Nd:YAG lasers have air-and-water cooling to decrease the heat buildup. It is highly questionable, however, if it is advisable to force water at a pressure of 2 psi and air at 10 psi down the pulp space to control temperature increases.[155]

The argon laser (as an adjunct to regular instrumentation and irrigation) was shown to improve the cleanliness of the root canal walls.[163] Root canal disinfection with Nd:YAG laser has been attempted with poor results.[164] Superficially infected root canals were lased in attempts to disinfect the canals, and the laser was found to reduce the number of bacteria in the root canal. The laser treatment was much less effective, however, than a 2-minute dressing with 1% NaOCl, which killed all bacteria. In similar studies, NaOCl was found superior to CO_2 and Er:YAG lasers.[135,152]

Argon, Nd:YAG, and carbon dioxide lasers have been tried for the softening of gutta-percha during root canal obturation.[13] During these procedures significant temperature increases were found on the external root surfaces. Depending on the type of laser and procedure the increases were recorded between 50.54° to 57.92° F (10.3° and 14.4° C). In an in vivo situation this would correspond to 117.14° to 124.52° F (47.3° to 51.4° C) in the periodontal tissues. This is uncomfortably close to a temperature of 127.4° F (53° C) that has been reported as dangerous for bone tissues.[68] Furthermore, these recordings were in vitro without the tissue absorption that occurs because of pigments and scattered radiation.

Lasers have also been used for root end surgery but with poor results.[78,185,270]

Another potential problem with significant consequences is the observation that smoke generated by laser treatment may carry infectious agents present in the burned area.[151]

SUMMARY

The reader is urged to use only instruments, materials, and devices that are deemed safe and effective by long-term, independent studies.

References

1. Abou-Rass M, Patonai FJ: The effects of decreasing surface tension on the flow of irrigating solutions in narrow root canals, *Oral Surg Oral Med Oral Pathol* 53:524, 1982.

2. Abou-Rass M, Piccinino MV: The effectiveness of four clinical irrigation methods on the removal of root canal debris, *Oral Surg Oral Med Oral Pathol* 54:323, 1982.

3. Ahmad M: An analysis of breakage of ultrasonic files during root canal instrumentation, *Endod Dent Traumatol* 5:78, 1989.

4. Ahmad M: Effect of ultrasonic instrumentation on Bacteroides intermedius, *Endod Dent Traumatol* 5:83, 1989.

5. Ahmad M, Pitt-Ford TR: A comparison using macroradiography of canal shapes in teeth instrumented ultrasonically and by hand, *J Endod* 15:339, 1989.

6. Ahmad M, Pitt-Ford TR, Crum LA: Ultrasonic débridement of root canals: acoustic streaming and its possible role, *J Endod* 13:490, 1987.

7. Ahmad M, Pitt-Ford TR, Crum LA: Ultrasonic débridement of root canals: an insight into the mechanisms involved, *J Endod* 13:93, 1987.

8. Ahmad M, Pitt-Ford TR, Crum LA, Walton AJ: Ultrasonic débridement of root canals: acoustic cavitation and its relevance, *J Endod* 14:486, 1988.

9. Ahmad M, Pitt-Ford TR, Crum LA, Wilson RF: Effectiveness of ultrasonic files in the disruption of root canal bacteria, *Oral Surg Oral Med Oral Pathol* 70:328, 1990.

10. Ahmad M, Roy RA, Ghanikamarudin AG: Observations of acoustic streaming fields around an oscillating ultrasonic file, *Endod Dent Traumatol* 8:189, 1992.

11. Ahmad M, Roy RA, Ghanikamarudin A, Safar M: The vibratory pattern of ultrasonic files driven piezoelectrically, *Int Endod J* 26:120, 1992.

12. Anderson RW, Powell BJ, Pashley DH: Microleakage of three temporary endodontic restorations, *J Endod* 14:497, 1988.

13. Anić I, Matsumoto K: Dentinal heat transmission induced by a laser-softened gutta-percha obturation technique, *J Endod* 21:470, 1995.

14. Anthony DR, Gordon TM, del Rio CE: The effect of three vehicles on the pH of calcium hydroxide, *Oral Surg Oral Med Oral Pathol* 54:560, 1982.

15. Araki K, Isaka H, Ishii T, Suda H: Excretion of ^{14}C-formaldehyde distributed systematically through root canal following pulpectomy, *Endod Dent Traumatol* 9:196, 1993.

16. Archer R, Reader A, Nist R, Beck M, Meyers WJ: An in vivo evaluation of the efficacy of ultrasound after step-back preparation in mandibular molars, *J Endod* 18:549, 1992.

17. Bahcall J, Howard P, Miserendino L, Walia H: Preliminary investigation of the histological effects of laser endodontic treatment on the periradicular tissues in dogs, *J Endod* 18:47, 1992.

18. Baker NA, Eleazer PD, Averbach RE, Seltzer S: Scanning electron microscopic study of the efficacy of various irrigating solutions, *J Endod* 1:127, 1975.

19. Barbosa SV, Burkard DH, Spångberg LSW: Cytotoxic effect of gutta-percha solvents, *J Endod* 20:6, 1994.

20. Barbosa SV, Safavi KE, Spångberg LSW: Influence of sodium hypochlorite on the permeability and structure of cervical human dentine, *Int Endod J* 27:309, 1994.

21. Barbosa SV, Spångberg LSW, Almeida D: Low surface tension calcium hydroxide solution is an effective antiseptic, *Int Endod J* 27:6, 1994.

22. Bates CF, Carnes DL, del Rio CE: Longitudinal sealing ability of mineral trioxide aggregate as a root end filling material, *J Endod* 22:575, 1996.

23. Beach CW, Bramwell JD, Hutter JW: Use of an electronic apex locator on a cardiac pacemaker patient, *J Endod* 22:182, 1996.

24. Becker GL, Cohen S, Borer R: The sequelae of accidentally injecting sodium hypochlorite beyond the root apex, *Oral Surg Oral Med Oral Pathol* 38:633, 1974.

25. Beling KL, Marshall JG, Morgan LA, Baumgartner JC: Evaluation for cracks associated with ultrasonic root end preparation of gutta-percha filled canals, *J Endod* 23:323, 1997.

26. Bengmark S, Rydberg B: Cytotoxic action of cationic detergents on tissue growth in vitro, *Acta Chir Scand* 134:1, 1968.

27. Benz C, Mouyen F: Evaluation of the new RadioVisioGraphy system image quality, *Oral Surg Oral Med Oral Pathol* 72:627, 1991.

28. Berg MS, Jacobsen EL, BeGole EA, Remeikis NA: A comparison of five irrigating solutions: a scanning electron microscopic study, *J Endod* 12:192, 1986.

29. Bergdahl M, Wennberg A, Spångberg L: Biologic effect of polyisobutylene on bony tissue in guinea pigs, *Scand J Dent Res* 82:618, 1974.

30. Bernhardt H, Eulig HG: Die reaktion des knochengewebe auf in die Markhöhle bei meerschweinchen implantierte gutta-percha, *Dtsch Zahnärztl Z* 7:295, 1953.

31. Beyer-Olsen EM, Ørstavik D: Radiopacity of root canal sealers, *Oral Surg Oral Med Oral Pathol* 51:320, 1981.

32. Björn H: Electrical excitation of teeth, *Svensk Tandläk Tidskr* 39:(suppl.), 1946.

33. Blackman R, Gross M, Seltzer S: An evaluation of the biocompatibility of a glass ionomer-silver cement in rat connective tissue, *J Endod* 15:76, 1989.

34. Block RM et al: Systemic distribution of ^{14}C-labeled paraformaldehyde Incorporated within formocresol following pulpotomies in dogs, *J Endod* 9:175, 1983.

35. Block RM et al: Systematic distribution of N2 paste containing ^{14}C paraformaldehyde following root canal therapy in dogs, *Oral Surg Oral Med Oral Pathol* 50:350, 1980.

36. Brady JM, del Rio CE: Corrosion of endodontic silver cones in humans: a scanning electron microscope and x-ray microprobe study, *J Endod* 1:205, 1975.

37. Brown BDK, Kafrawy AH, Patterson SS: Studies of Sargenti technique of endodontics - autoradiographic and scanning electron microscope studies, *J Endod* 5:14, 1979.

38. Byström A, Claesson R, Sundqvist G: The antimicrobial effect of camphorated paramonochlorphenol, camphorated phenol, and calcium hydroxide in the treatment of infected root canals, *Endod Dent Traumatol* 1:170, 1985.

39. Byström A, Sundqvist G: The antibacterial action of sodium hypochlorite and EDTA in 60 cases of endodontic therapy, *Int Endod J* 18:35, 1985.

40. Byström A, Sundqvist G: Bacteriological evaluation of the effect of 0.5 percent sodium hypochlorite in endodontic therapy, *Oral Surg Oral Med Oral Pathol* 55:307, 1983.

41. Callahan JR: Rosin solution for the sealing of the dentinal tubuli and as an adjuvant in the filling of root canals, *J Allied Dent Society* 9:53, 1914.

42. Callis PD, Santini A: Tissue response to retrograde root fillings in the ferret canine: a comparison of a glass ionomer cement and gutta-percha with sealer, *Oral Surg Oral Med Oral Pathol* 64:475, 1987.

43. Calnan J: The use of inert plastic material in reconstructive surgery, *Br J Plast Surg* 16:1, 1963.

44. Canalda-Sahli C, Brau-Aguadé E, Berástegui-Jimeno E: A comparison of bending and torsional properties of K-files manufactured with different metallic alloys, *Int Endod J* 29: 185, 1996.

45. Carrel A: Abortive treatment of wound infection, *Br Med J* 2:609, 1915.

46. Chernick LB, Jacobs JJ, Lautenschlager EP, Heuer MA: Torsional failure of endodontic files, *J Endod* 2:94, 1976.

47. Cohen BD, Combe EC, Lilley JD: Effect of thermal placement techniques on some physical properties of gutta-percha, *Int Endod J* 25:292, 1992.

48. Cohen HP, Cha BY, Spångberg LSW: Endodontic anesthesia in mandibular molars: a clinical study, *J Endod* 19:370, 1993.

49. Cunningham WT, Balekjian AY: Effect of temperature on collagen-dissolving ability of sodium hypochlorite endodontic irrigant, *Oral Surg Oral Med Oral Pathol* 49:175, 1980.

50. Cunningham WT, Cole JS, Balekjian AY: Effect of alcohol on the spreading ability of sodium hypochlorite endodontic irrigant, *Oral Surg Oral Med Oral Pathol* 53:333, 1982.

51. Cunningham WT, Joseph SW: Effect of temperature on the bactericidal action of sodium hypochlorite endodontic irrigant, *Oral Surg Oral Med Oral Pathol* 50:569, 1980.

52. Cunningham WT, Martin H: A scanning electron microscope evaluation of root canal débridement with the endosonic ultrasonic synergistic system, *Oral Surg Oral Med Oral Pathol* 53:527, 1982.

53. Cunningham WT, Martin H, Forrest WR: Evaluation of root canal débridement by the endosonic synergistic system, *Oral Surg Oral Med Oral Pathol* 53:401, 1982.

54. Dakin HD: The antiseptic action of hypochlorite: the ancient history of the new antiseptic, *Br Med J* 2:809, 1915.

55. Dakin HD: On the use of certain antiseptic substances in treatment of infected wounds, *Br Med J* 2:318,1915.

56. Dalal MB, Cohil KS: Comparison of silver amalgam, glass ionomer cement and gutta percha as retrofilling materials, and in vivo and an in vitro study, *J Indian Dent Assoc* 55:153, 1983.

57. Dalat DM, Spångberg LSW: Comparison of apical leakage in root canals obturated with various gutta-percha techniques using a dye vacuum tracing method, *J Endod* 20:315, 1994.

58. DeGee AJ, Wu MK, Wesselink PR: Sealing properties of a Ketac-Endo glass ionomer cement and AH26 root canal sealer, *Int Endodont J* 27:239, 1994.

59. Diaz-Arnold AM, Arnold MA, Wilcox LR: Optical detection of hemoglobin in pulpal blood, *J Endod* 22:19, 1996.

60. Diaz-Arnold AM, Wilcox LR, Arnold MA: Optical detection of pulpal blood, *J Endod* 20:164, 1994.

61. Donley DL, Weller RN, Kulild JC, Jurcak JJ: In vitro intracanal temperatures produced by low- and high-temperature thermoplasticized injectable gutta-percha, *J Endod* 17:307, 1991.

62. Ellerbruch ES, Murphy RA: Antimicrobial activity of root canal medicament vapors, *J Endod* 3:189, 1977.

63. Engfelt NO: Die wirkung der dakinschon hypochloritlösong auf gewisse organische substansen, *Hoppe Seylers Z Physiol Chem* 121:18, 1922.

64. England MC, West NM, Safavi K, Green DB: Tissue lead levels in dogs with RC-2B root canal fillings, *J Endod* 6:728, 1980.

65. Engström B, Spångberg L: Effect of root canal filling material N2 when used for filling after partial pulpectomy, *Svensk Tandläk Tidskr* 62:815, 1969.

66. Engström B, Spångberg L: Studies on root canal medicaments. I. Cytotoxic effect of root canal antiseptics, *Acta Odontol Scand* 25:77, 1967.

67. Engström B, Spångberg L: Toxic and antimicrobial effects of antiseptics *in vitro*, *Svensk Tandläk Tidskr* 62:543, 1969.

68. Eriksson AR, Albrektsson T: Temperature threshold levels for heat-induced bone tissue injury: a vital-microscopic study in the rabbit, *J Prosth Dent* 50:101, 1983.

69. Eulig HG, Bernhardt H: Die reaktion verschiedener gewebe auf implantiertes palavit, paladon und gutta-percha, *Dtsch Zahnärztebl Z* 7:227, 1953.

70. Feldmann G, Nyborg H: Tissue reaction to root filling materials. I. Comparison between gutta-percha and silver amalgam implanted in rabbit, *Odontol Revy* 13:1, 1962.

71. Felt RA, Moser JB, Heuer MA: Flute design of endodontic instruments: its influence on cutting efficiency, *J Endod* 8:253, 1982.

72. Finne K, Nord PG, Persson G, Lennartsson B: Retrograde root filling with amalgam and cavit, *Oral Surg Oral Med Oral Pathol* 43:621, 1977.

73. Fouad AF: The use of electronic apex locators in endodontic therapy, *Int Endod J* 26:13, 1993.

74. Fouad AF et al: The effects of selected electronic dental instruments on patients with cardiac pacemakers, *J Endod* 16: 188, 1990.

75. Fouad AF, Krell KV: An in vitro comparison of five root canal length measuring instruments, *J Endod* 15:573, 1989.

76. Fouad AF et al: A clinical evaluation of five electronic root canal length measuring instruments, *J Endod* 16:446, 1990.

77. Fouad AF, Rivera EM, Krell KV: Accuracy of the endex with variations in canal irrigants and foramen size, *J Endod* 19:63, 1993.

78. Friedman S, Rotstein I, Mahamid A: *In vivo* efficacy of various retrofills and of CO₂ laser in apical surgery, *Endod Dent Traumatol* 7:19, 1991.

79. Gani O, Visvisian C: Apical canal diameter in the first upper molar at various ages, *J Endod* 25:689, 1999.

80. Gazelius B, Olgart L, Edwall B: Restored vitality in luxated teeth assessed by laser Doppler flowmetry, *Endod Dent Traumatol* 4:265, 1988.

81. Gazelius B, Olgart L, Edwall B, Edwall L: Noninvasive recording of blood flow in human dental pulp, *Endod Dent Traumatol* 2:219, 1986.

82. Goldberg F: Relation between corroded silver points and endodontic failures, *J Endod* 7:224, 1981.

83. Goldberg F, Abramovich A: Analysis of the effect of EDTAC on the dentinal walls of the root canal, *J Endod* 3:101, 1977.

84. Goldberg F, Spielberg C: The effect of EDTAC on the variation of its working time analyzed with scanning electron microscopy, *Oral Surg Oral Med Oral Pathol* 53:74, 1982.

85. Goldman M et al: The efficacy of several endodontic irrigation solutions: a scanning electron microscopic study: part 2, *J Endod* 8:487, 1982.

86. Goldman M et al: New method of irrigation during endodontic treatment, *J Endod* 2:257, 1976.

87. Goodman A, Schilder H, Aldrich W: The thermomechanical properties of gutta-percha. II. The history and molecular chemistry of gutta-percha, *Oral Surg Oral Med Oral Pathol* 37:954, 1974.

88. Goodman A, Schilder H, Aldrich W: The thermomechanical properties of gutta-percha. Part IV. A thermal profile of the warm gutta-percha packing procedure, *Oral Surg Oral Med Oral Pathol* 51:544, 1981.

89. Grassi MD, Plazek DJ, Michanowicz AE, Chay I-C: Changes in the physical properties of the ultrafill low-temperature (70° C) thermoplasticized gutta-percha system, *J Endod* 15:517, 1989.

90. Grieve AR, Parkholm JDD: The sealing properties of root filling cements, further studies, *Br Dent J* 135:327, 1973.

91. Grossman LI: The effect of pH of rosin on setting time of root canal cements, *J Endod* 8:326, 1982.

92. Grossman LI: Irrigation of root canals, *JADA* 30:1915, 1943.

93. Grossman LI: Solubility of root canal cements, *J Dent Res* 57:927, 1978.

94. Gutmann JL, Creel DC, Bowles WH: Evaluation of heat transfer during root canal obturation with thermoplasticized gutta-percha. Part I. In vitro heat levels during extrusion, *J Endod* 13:378, 1987.

95. Gutmann JL, Rakusin H, Powe R, Bowles WH: Evaluation of heat transfer during root canal obturation with thermoplasticized gutta-percha. Part II. In vivo response to heat levels generated, *J Endod* 13:441, 1987.

96. Guttuso J: A histopathological study of rat connective tissue responses to endodontic materials, *Oral Surg Oral Med Oral Pathol* 16:713, 1962.

97. Haikel Y, Gasser P, Allemann C: Dynamic fracture of hybrid endodontic hand instruments compared with traditional files, *J Endod* 17:217, 1991.

98. Hand RE, Smith ML, Harrison JW: Analysis of the effect of dilution on the necrotic dissolution property of sodium hypochlorite, *J Endod* 4:60, 1978.

99. Hansen-Bayless J, Davis R: Sealing ability of two intermediate restorative materials in bleached teeth, *Am J Dent* 5:151, 1992.

100. Harris WE: Disintegration of two silver cones, *J Endod* 7:426, 1981.

101. Harrison JW, Baumgartner JC, Zielke DR: Analysis of interappointment pain associated with the combined use of endodontic irrigants and medicaments, *J Endod* 7:272, 1981.

102. Harrison JW, Svec TA, Baumgartner JC: Analysis of clinical toxicity of endodontic irrigants, *J Endod* 4:6, 1978.

103. Hedrick RT, Dove SB, Peters DD, McDavid WD: Radiographic determination of canal length: direct digital radiography versus conventional radiography, *J Endod* 20:320, 1994.

104. Hermann BW: Calciumhydroxyd als mittel zum behandel und füllen von zahnwurzelkanälen, Würzburg, *Med.Diss.V.* German dissertation, 1920.

105. Hermann BW: Dentin obliteration der wurzelkanäle nach behandlung mit calcium, *Zahnärtzl Rundschau* 39:888, 1930.

106. Hertwig G: Wandständigkeit und durchlässigkeit von wurzelfüllmitteln, *Zahnärztl Praxis* 9:1, 1958.

107. Higginbotham TL: A comparative study of the physical properties of five commonly used root canal sealers, *Oral Surg Oral Med Oral Pathol* 24:89, 1967.

108. Holland R et al: Reaction of dog's teeth to root canal filling with mineral trioxide aggregate or a glass ionomer sealer, *J Endod* 25:728, 1999.

109. Hunter HA: The effect of gutta-percha, silver points and Rickert's root sealer on bone healing, *J Can Dent Assoc* 23: 385, 1957.

110. Ingólfsson ÆR, Tronstad L, Hersh E, Riva CE: Effect of probe design on the suitability of laser Doppler flowmetry in vitality testing of human teeth, *Endod Dent Traumatol* 9:65, 1993.

111. Ingólfsson ÆR, Tronstad L, Riva CE: Reliability of laser Doppler flowmetry in testing vitality of human teeth, *Endod Dent Traumatol* 10:185, 1994.

112. Jasper EA: Root canal therapy in modern dentistry, *Dent Cosmos* 75:823, 1933.

113. Jerome CE: Warm vertical gutta-percha obturation: a technique update, *J Endod* 20:97, 1994.

114. Jung S, Safavi K, Spångberg L: The effectiveness of chlorhexidine in the prevention or root canal reinfection, *J Endod* 25:288, 1999.

115. Kahan RS, Gulabivala K, Snook M, Setchell DJ: Evaluation of a pulse oximeter and customized probe for pulp vitality testing, *J Endod* 22:105, 1996.

116. Kawahara H, Imanishi Y, Oshima H: Biologic evaluation on glass ionomer cement, *J Dent Res* 58:1080, 1979.

117. Kazemi RB, Safavi KE, Spångberg LSW: Assessment of marginal stability and permeability of an interim restorative endodontic material, *Oral Surg Oral Med Oral Pathol* 78: 788, 1994.

118. Kazemi RB, Safavi KE, Spångberg LSW: Dimensional changes of endodontic sealers, *Oral Surg Oral Med Oral Pathol* 76:766, 1993.

119. Kazemi RB, Stenman E, Spångberg LSW: The endodontic file is a disposable instrument, *J Endod* 21:451, 1995.

120. Kazemi RB, Stenman E, Spångberg LSW: Machining efficiency and wear resistance of NiTi endodontic files, *Oral Surg Oral Med Oral Pathol Oral Radiol Endod* 81:596, 1996.

121. Keate KC, Wong M: A comparison of endodontic file tip quality, *J Endod* 16:486, 1990.

122. Kehoe JC: Intracanal corrosion of a silver cone producing a localized argyria: scanning electron microscope and energy dispersive x-ray analyzer analyses, *J Endod* 10:199, 1984.

123. Kerekes K, Tronstad L: Morphometric observations on the root canals of human molars, *J Endod* 3:114, 1977.

124. Kielt LW, Montgomery S: The effect of endosonic instrumentation in simulated curved root canals, *J Endod* 13:215, 1987.

125. Kimura JT: A comparative analysis of zinc and nonzinc alloys used in retrograde endodontic surgery. Part 1: apical seal and tissue reaction, *J Endod* 8:359, 1982.

126. Kimura JT: A comparative analysis of zinc and nonzinc alloys used in retrograde endodontic surgery. Part 2: optical emission spectrographic analysis for zinc precipitation, *J Endod* 8:407, 1982.

127. Krupp JD, Brantley WA, Gerstein H: An investigation of the torsional and bending properties of seven brands of endodontic files, *J Endod* 10:372, 1984.

128. Lado EA, Richmond AF, Marks RG: Reliability and validity of a digital pulp tester as a test standard for measuring sensory perception, *J Endod* 14:352, 1988.

129. Langeland K, Guttuso J, Langeland L, Tobon G: Methods in the study of biologic responses to endodontic materials, *Oral Surg Oral Med Oral Pathol* 27:522, 1969.

130. Lauper R, Lutz F, Barbakow F: An in vivo comparison of gradient and absolute impedance electronic apex locators, *J Endod* 22:260, 1996.

131. Lautenschlager EP, Jacobs JJ, Marshall GW, Heuer MA: Brittle and ductile torsional failures of endodontic instruments, *J Endod* 3:175, 1977.

132. Lavelle CLB, Wu CJ: Digital radiographic images will benefit endodontic services, *Endod Dent Traumatol* 11:253, 1995.

133. Layton CA, Marshall JG, Morgan LA, Baumgartner JC: Evaluation of cracks associated with ultrasonic root-end preparation, *J Endod* 22:157, 1996.

134. Lee DH, Park B, Saxena A, Serene TP: Enhanced surface hardness by boron implantation in nitinol alloy, *J Endod* 22:543, 1996.

135. LeGoff A et al: An Evaluation of the CO_2 laser for endodontic disinfection, *J Endod* 25:105, 1999.

136. Levine M, Rudolph AS: Factors affecting the germicidal efficiency of hypochlorite solutions, *Bull 150 Iowa Exp Sta*, 1941.

137. Levy G: Cleaning and shaping the root canal with a Nd:YAG laser beam: a comparative study, *J Endod* 18:123, 1992.

138. Lewis BB, Chester SB: Formaldehyde in dentistry: a review of mutagenic and carcinogenic potential, *J Am Dent Assoc* 103:429, 1981.

139. Leyhausen G et al: Genotoxicity and cytotoxicity of the epoxy resin-based root canal sealer AH Plus, *J Endod* 25:109, 1999.

140. Liggett WR, Brady JM, Tsaknis PJ, del Rio CE: Light microscopy, scanning electron microscopy, and microprobe analysis of bone response to zinc and nonzinc amalgam implants, *Oral Surg Oral Med Oral Pathol* 49:254, 1980.

141. Limkangwalmongkol S et al: A comparative study of the apical leakage of four root canal sealers and laterally condensed gutta-percha, *J Endod* 17:495, 1991.

142. Loushine RJ, Weller RN, Hartwell GR: Stereomicroscopic evaluation of canal shape following hand, sonic, and ultrasonic instrumentation, *J Endod* 15:417, 1989.

143. Margelos J, Verdelis K, Eliades G: Chloroform uptake by gutta-percha and assessment of its concentration in air during the chloroform-dip technique, *J Endod* 22.547, 1996.

144. Marsicovetere ES, Clement DJ, del Rio CE: Morphometric video analysis of the engine-driven NiTi lightspeed instrument system, *J Endod* 22:231, 1996.

145. Martin LR et al: Histologic response of rat connective tissue to zinc-containing amalgam, *J Endod* 2:25, 1976.

146. Matsuya Y, Matsuya S: Effect of abietic acid and polymethyl methacrylate on the dissolution process of zinc oxide–eugenol cement, *Biomaterials* 15:307, 1994.

147. McComb D, Smith DC: A preliminary scanning electron microscopic study of root canals after endodontic procedures, *J Endod* 1:238, 1975.

148. McComb D, Smith DC, Beagrie GS: The results of in vivo endodontic chemomechanical instrumentation—a scanning electron microscopic study, *Br Endod Soc* 9:11, 1976.

149. McDonnell D, Price C: An evaluation of the Sens-A-Ray digital dental imaging system, *Dentomaxillofac Radiol* 22:121, 1993.

150. McElroy DL: Physical properties of root canal filling materials, *J Am Dent Assoc* 50:433, 1955.

151. McKinley IB, Lublow MO: Hazards of laser smoke during endodontic therapy, *J Endod* 20:558, 1994.

152. Mehl A, Folwaczny M, Haffner C, Hickel R: Bactericidal effects of 2.94 mm Er:YAG laser radiation in dental root canals, *J Endod* 25:490, 1999.

153. Messer HH, Feigal RJ: A comparison of the antibacterial and cytotoxic effects of parachlorphenol, *J Dent Res* 64:818, 1985.

154. Miserendino LJ, Brantley WA, Walia HD, Gerstein H: Cutting efficiency of endodontic hand instruments. IV. Comparison of hybrid and traditional instrument designs, *J Endod* 14:451, 1988.

155. Miserendino LJ, Levy GC, Rizoiu IM: Effects of Nd:YAG laser on the permeability of root canal wall dentin, *J Endod* 21:83, 1995.

156. Miserendino LJ et al: Cutting efficiency of endodontic instruments. III. Comparison of sonic and ultrasonic instrument systems, *J Endod* 14:24, 1988.

157. Miserendino LJ, Moser JB, Heuer MA, Osetek EM: Cutting efficiency of endodontic instruments. I. A quantitative comparison of the tip and fluted region, *J Endod* 11:435, 1985.

158. Miserendino LJ, Moser JB, Heuer MA, Osetek EM: Cutting efficiency of endodontic instruments. II. An analysis of the design of the tip, *J Endod* 12:8, 1986.

159. Mitchell DF: The irritational qualities of dental materials, *J Am Dent Assoc* 59:954, 1959.

160. Möller ÅJR: Microbiological examination of root canals and periapical tissues of human teeth, *Odontol Tidskr* 74:1, 1966 (special issue).

161. Molyvdas I, Zervas P, Lambrianidis T, Veis A: Periodontal tissue reaction following root canal obturation with an injection-thermoplasticized gutta-percha technique, *Endod Dent Traumatol* 5:32, 1989.

162. Morgan LA, Marshall JG: A scanning electron microscopic study of in vivo ultrasonic root-end preparations, *J Endod* 25:567, 1999.

163. Moshonov J et al: Nd:YAG laser irradiation in root canal disinfection, *Endod Dent Traumatol* 11:220, 1995.

164. Moshonov J et al: Efficacy of argon laser irradiation in removing intracanal debris, *Oral Surg Oral Med Oral Pathol Oral Radiol Endod* 79:221, 1995.

165. Mumford JM, Björn H: Problems in electrical pulp-testing and dental algesimetry, *Int Dent J* 12:161, 1962.

166. Neal RG, Craig RG, Powers JM: Cutting ability of K type endodontic files, *J Endod* 9:52, 1983.

167. Neal RG, Craig RG, Powers JM: Effect of sterilization and irrigants on the cutting ability of stainless steel files, *J Endod* 9:93, 1983.

168. Nelvig P, Wing K, Welander U: Sens-A Ray: a new system for direct digital intraoral radiography, *Oral Surg Oral Med Oral Pathol* 74:818, 1992.

169. Noblett WC et al: Detection of pulpal circulation in vitro by pulse oximetry, *J Endod* 22:1, 1996.

170. Nygaard-Østby B: Chelation in root canal therapy, *Odont T* 65:3, 1957.

171. Ohara PK, Torabinejad M, Kettering JD: Antibacterial effects of various endodontic irrigants on selected anaerobic bacteria, *Endod Dent Tramatol* 9:95, 1993.

172. Oliet S, Sorin SM: Effect of aging on the mechanical properties of hand-rolled gutta-percha endodontic cones, *Oral Surg Oral Med Oral Pathol* 43:954, 1977.

173. Omnell K: Electrolytic precipitation of zinc carbonate in the jaw, *Oral Surg Oral Med Oral Pathol* 12:846, 1959.

174. Ørstavik D, Farrants G, Wahl T, Kerekes K: Image analysis of endodontic radiographs: digital subtraction and quantitative densitometry, *Endod Dent Traumatol* 6:6, 1990.

175. Ørstavik D, Haapasalo M: Disinfection by endodontic irrigants and dressings of experimentally infected dentinal tubules, *Endod Dent Traumatol* 6:142, 1990.

176. Pascon E, Spångberg LSW: In vitro cytotoxicity of root canal filling materials: 1. gutta-percha, *J Endod* 16:429, 1990.

177. Pashley EL, Horner JA, Liu M, Pashley DH: Effects of CO_2 laser energy on dentin permeability, *J Endod* 18:257, 1992.

178. Pedicore D, El Deeb ME, Messer HH: Hand versus ultrasonic instrumentation: its effect on canal shape and instrumentation time, *J Endod* 12:375, 1986.

179. Pissiotis E, Sapounas G, Spångberg LSW: Silver glass ionomer cement as a retrograde filling material: a study in vitro, *J Endod* 17:225, 1991.

180. Powell SE, Simon JHS, Maze B: A comparison of the effect of modified and nonmodified instrument tips on apical canal configuration, *J Endod* 12:293, 1986.

181. Powell SE, Wong PD, Simon JHS: A comparison of the effect of modified and nonmodified instrument tips on apical canal configuration. Part II, *J Endod* 14:224, 1988.

182. Pratten DH, McDonald NJ: Comparison of radiographic and electronic working lengths, *J Endod* 22:173, 1996.

183. Ram Z: Effectiveness of root canal Irrigation, *Oral Surg Oral Med Oral Pathol* 44:306, 1977.

184. Ramsay DS, Årtun J, Martinen SS: Reliability of pulpal blood-flow measurements utilizing laser Doppler flowmetry, *J Dent Res* 70:1427, 1991.

185. Read RP, Baumgartner JC, Clark SM: Effects of a carbon dioxide laser on human root dentin, *J Endod* 21:4, 1995.

186. Richman MJ: The use of ultrasonic in root canal therapy and root resection, *J Dent Med* 12:12, 1957.

187. Rickoff B et al: Effects of thermal vitality tests on human dental pulp, *J Endod* 14:482, 1988.

188. Roane JB, Sabala CL, Duncanson MG: The "balanced force" concept for instrumentation of curved canals, *J Endod* 11: 203, 1985.

189. Rome WJ, Doran JE, Walker WA: The effectiveness of glyoxide and sodium hypochlorite in preventing smear layer formation, *J Endod* 11:281, 1985.

190. Rutberg M, Spångberg E, Spångberg L: Evaluation of enhanced vascular permeability of endodontic medicaments in vivo, *J Endod* 3:347, 1977.

191. Sabala CL, Powell SE: Sodium hypochlorite injection into periapical tissues, *J Endod* 15:490, 1989.

192. Sabala CL, Roane JB, Southard LZ: Instrumentation of curved canals using a modified tipped instrument: a comparison study, *J Endod* 14:59, 1988.

193. Safavi KE, Nichols FC: Alteration of biological properties of bacterial lipopolysaccharide by calcium hydroxide treatment, *J Endod* 20:127, 1994.

194. Safavi KE, Nichols FC: Effect of calcium hydroxide on bacterial lipopolysaccharide, *J Endod* 19:76, 1993.

195. Safavi KE, Spångberg L, Langeland K: Root canal dentinal tubule disinfection, *J Endod* 16:207, 1990.

196. Salzgeber RM, Brilliant JD: An in vivo evaluation of the penetration of an irrigating solution in root canals, *J Endod* 3:394, 1977.

197. Sasano T, Kuriwada S, Sanjo D: Arterial blood pressure regulation of blood flow as determined by laser Doppler, *J Dent Res* 68:791, 1989.

198. Saunders EM: The effect of variation in the thermomechanical compaction techniques upon the quality of the apical seal, *Int Endod J* 22:163, 1989.

199. Saunders EM: *In vivo* findings associated with heat generation during thermomechanical compaction of gutta-percha. Part 1. Temperature levels at the external surface of the root, *Int Endod J* 23:263, 1990.

200. Saunders EM: *In vivo* findings associated with heat generation during thermomechanical compaction of gutta-percha. Part II. Histological response to temperature elevation on the external surface of the root, *Int Endod J* 23:268, 1990.

201. Saunders EM, Saunders WP: Long-term coronal leakage of JS Quickfill root filling with Sealapex and Apexit sealers, *Endod Dent Traumatol* 11:181, 1995.

202. Saunders WP, Saunders EM, Gutmann JL: Ultrasonic root-end preparation. Part 2. Microleakage of EBA root-end fillings, *Int Endodon J* 27:325, 1994.

203. Schilder H, Goodman A, Aldrich W: The thermomechanical properties of gutta-percha. I. The compressibility of gutta-percha, *Oral Surg Oral Med Oral Pathol* 37:946, 1974.

204. Schilder H, Goodman A, Aldrich W: The thermomechanical properties of gutta-percha. III. Determination of phase transition temperatures for gutta-percha, *Oral Surg Oral Med Oral Pathol* 38:109, 1974.

205. Schilder H, Goodman A, Aldrich W: The thermomechanical properties of gutta-percha. Part V. Volume changes in bulk gutta-percha as a function of temperature and its relationship to molecular phase transformation, *Oral Surg Oral Med Oral Pathol* 59:285, 1985.

206. Schmitt W: Die chemischen grundlagen der erhartenden wurtzelfüllungen, *Zahnärztl Welt* 5:560, 1951.

207. Schnettler JM, Wallace JA: Pulse oximetry as a diagnostic tool of pulp vitality, *J Endod* 17:488, 1991.

208. Schroeder A: Gewebsverträglichkeit des Wurzelfüllmittels AH 26, *Histologische und klinische Prüfung*, 58:563, 1957.

209. Schroeder A: Mitteilungen über die abschlussdichtigkeit von wurzelfüllmaterialien und erster hinweis auf ein neuartiges wurzelfüllmittel, *Schweiz Monatsschr Zahnmed* 64:921, 1954.

210. Schroeder A: Zum problem der bacteriendichten Wurzelkanalversorgung, *Zahnärztl Welt Zahnärztl Reform* 58:531, 1957.

211. Seltzer S, Green DB, Weiner N, De Renzis F: A scanning electron microscope examination of silver cones removed from endodontically treated teeth, *Oral Surg Oral Med Oral Pathol* 33:589, 1972.

212. Senia ES, Marraro RV, Mitchell JL, Lewis AG, Thomas L: Rapid sterilization of gutta-percha cones with 5.25% sodium hypochlorite, *J Endod* 1:136, 1975.

213. Senia ES, Marshall FJ, Rosen S: The solvent action of sodium hypochlorite on pulp tissue of extracted teeth, *Oral Surg Oral Med Oral Pathol,* 31:96, 1971.

214. Seto BG, Nicholls JI, Harrington GW: Torsional properties of twisted and machined endodontic files, *J Endod* 16:355, 1990.

215. Shoji Y: Study on the mechanism of the mechanical enlargement of root canals, *J Nihon Univ School Dent* 7:71, 1965.

216. Siqueira JF Jr, Lopes HP: Mechanisms of antimicrobial activity of calcium hydroxide: a critical review, *Int Endod J* 32:361, 1999.

217. Sjögren U, Figdor D, Spångberg L, Sundqvist G: The antimicrobial effect of calcium hydroxide as a short-term intracanal dressing, *Int Endod J* 24:119, 1991.

218. Sjögren U, Sundqvist G: Bacteriologic evaluation of ultrasonic root canal instrumentation, *Oral Surg Oral Med Oral Pathol* 63:366, 1987.

219. Sjögren U, Sundqvist G, Nair PNR: Tissue reaction to gutta-percha particles of various sizes when implanted subcutaneously in guinea pigs, *Eur J Oral Sci* 103:313, 1995.

220. Smith MA, Steinman HR: An in vitro evaluation of microleakage of two new and two old root canal sealers, *J Endod* 20:18, 1994.

221. Soares I, Goldberg F, Massone EJ, Soares IM: Periapical tissue response to two calcium hydroxide-containing endodontic sealers, *J Endod* 16:166, 1990.

222. Söderberg TA: Effects of zinc oxide, rosin and resin acids and their combinations on bacterial growth and inflammatory cells, doctoral dissertation, Umeå, Sweden, 1990, Umeå University.

223. Soltes EDJ, Zinkel DF: Chemistry of rosin. In Zinkel DF and Russell J, editors: *Naval stores production, chemistry, utilization,* New York, 1989, Pulp Chemical Association.

224. Sorin SM, Oliet S, Pearlstein F: Rejuvination of aged (brittle) endodontic gutta-perch cones, *J Endod* 5:233, 1979.

225. Spångberg L: Biological effects of root canal filling materials. II. Effect in vitro of water-soluble components of root canal filling materials on HeLa cells, *Odontol Revy* 20:133, 1969.

226. Spångberg L: Biological effects of root canal filling materials. IV. Effect in vitro of solubilized root canal filling materials on HeLa cells, *Odontol Revy* 20:289, 1969.

227. Spångberg L: Biological effects of root canal filling materials. V. Toxic effect in vitro of root filling materials on HeLa cells and human skin fibroblasts, *Odontol Revy* 20:427, 1969.

228. Spångberg L: Biological effects of root canal filling materials. VI. The inhibitory effect of solubilized root canal filling materials on respiration of HeLa cells, *Odont Tidskr* 77:1, 1969.

229. Spångberg L: Biological effects of root canal filling materials. VII. Reaction of bony tissue to implanted root canal filling material in guinea pigs, *Odont Tidskr* 77;133, 1969.

230. Spångberg L: Biological effects of root canal filling materials: the effect on bone tissue of two formaldehyde-containing root canal filling pastes; N2 and Rieblers paste, *Oral Surg Oral Med Oral Pathol* 38:934, 1974.

231. Spångberg L, Engström B: Studies on root canal medicaments. IV. Antimicrobial effect of root canal medicaments, *Odontol Revy* 19:187, 1968.

232. Spångberg L, Engström B, Langeland K: Biologic effect of dental materials. III. Toxicity and antimicrobial effects of endodontic antiseptics in vitro, *Oral Surg Oral Med Oral Pathol* 36:856, 1973.

233. Spångberg L, Langeland K: Biologic effect of dental materials. I. Toxicity of root canal filling materials on HeLa cells in vitro, *Oral Surg Oral Med Oral Pathol* 35:402, 1973.

234. Spångberg L, Rutberg M, Rydinge E: Biological effects of endodontic antimicrobial agents, *J Endod* 5:166, 1979.

235. Spångberg LSW, Barbosa SV, Lavigne GD: AH26 releases rormaldehyde, *J Endod* 19:596, 1993.

236. Stabholz A et al: Sealing of human dentinal tubules by XeCl 308-nm excimer laser, *J Endod* 19:267, 1993.

237. Staehle HJ, Spiess V, Heinecke A, Müller H-P: Effect of root canal filling materials containing calcium hydroxide and the alkalinity of root dentin, *Endod Dent Traumatol* 11:163, 1995.

238. Stamos DE, Sadeghi EM, Haasch GC, Gerstein H: An in vitro comparison study to quantitate the débridement ability of hand, sonic, and ultrasonic instrumentation, *J Endod* 13:434, 1987.

239. Stenman E: Effects of sterilization and endodontic medicaments on mechanical properties of root canal instruments, doctoral dissertation, Umeå, Sweden, 1977, Umeå University.

240. Stenman E, Spångberg LSW: Machining efficiency of endodontic files: a new methodology, *J Endod* 16:151, 1990.

241. Stenman E, Spångberg LSW: Machining efficiency of endodontic K files and Hedstrom files, *J Endod* 16:375, 1990.

242. Stenman E, Spångberg LSW: Machining efficiency of Flex-R, K-Flex, Trio-Cut, and S Files, *J Endod* 16:575, 1990.

243. Stenman E, Spångberg L: Root canal instruments are poorly standardized, *J Endod* 19:327, 1993.

244. Sundada I: New method for measuring the length of the root canal, *J Dent Res* 41:375, 1962.

245. Sunzel B: Interactive effects of zinc, rosin and resin acids on polymorphonuclear leukocytes, gingival fibroblasts and bacteria, doctoral dissertation, Umeå, Sweden, 1995, Umeå University.

246. Sunzel B et al: The effect of zinc oxide *on Staphylococcus aureus* and polymorphonuclear cells in a tissue cage model, *Scand J Plast Reconstr Surg* 24:31, 1990.

247. Svec TA, Harrison JW: The effect of effervescence on débridement of the apical regions of root canals in single-rooted teeth, *J Endod* 7:335, 1981.

248. Tagger M: Use of thermo-mechanical compactors as an adjunct to lateral condensation, *Quintessence Int* 15:27, 1984.

249. Tagger M, Tagger E, Kfir A: Release of calcium and hydroxyl ions from set endodontic sealers containing calcium hydroxide, *J Endod* 14:588, 1988.

250. Tani Y, Kawada H: Effects of laser irradiation on dentin. I. Effect on smear layer, *J Dent Mater* 6:127, 1987.

251. Trebitsch H: Über die Verwertung der heilkraft des Silbers, *Zahnäztl Rdsch* 38:1009, 1929.

252. Tronstad L, Barnett F, Flax M: Solubility and biocompatibility of calcium hydroxide-containing root canal sealers, *Endod Dent Traumatol* 4:152, 1988.

253. van der Fehr FR, Nygaard-Østby B: Effect of EDTAC and sulfuric acid on root canal dentine, *Oral Surg Oral Med Oral Pathol* 16:199, 1963.

254. Vessey RA: The effect of filing versus reaming on the shape of the prepared root canal, *Oral Surg Oral Med Oral Pathol* 27:543, 1969.

255. Villalobos RL, Moser JB, Heuer MA: A method to determine the cutting efficiency of root canal instruments in rotary motion, *J Endod* 6:667, 1980

256. Walia H, Brantley WA, Gerstein H: An initial investigation of the bending and torsional properties of nitinol root canal files, *J Endod* 14:246, 1988.

257. Walker TL, del Rio CE: Histological evaluation of ultrasonic and sonic instrumentation of curved root canals, *J Endod* 15: 49, 1989.

258. Walker TL, del Rio CE: Histological evaluation of ultrasonic débridement comparing sodium hypochlorite and water, *J Endod* 17:66, 1991.

259. Webber J, Moser JB, Heuer MA: A method to determine the cutting efficiency of root canal instruments in linear motion, *J Endod* 6:829, 1980.

260. Weine FS, Kelly RF, Lio PS: The effect of preparation procedures on original canal shape and apical foramen shape, *J Endod* 1:255, 1975.

261. Weinreb MM, Meier E: The relative efficiency of EDTA, sulfuric acid, and mechanical instrumentation in the enlargement of root canals, *Oral Surg Oral Med Oral Pathol* 19:247, 1965.

262. Weller RN, Brady JM, Bernier WE: Efficacy of ultrasonic cleaning, *J Endod* 6:740, 1980.

263. Wennberg A, Bergdahl M, Spångberg L: Biologic effect of polyisobutylene on HeLa cells and on subcutaneous tissue in guinea pigs, *Scand J Dent Res* 82:613, 1974.

264. Wennberg A, Ørstavik D: Adhesion of root canal sealers to bovine dentine and gutta-percha, *Int Endod J* 23:13, 1990.

265. West NM, England MC, Safavi K, Green DB: Levels of lead in blood of dogs with RC-2B root canal fillings, *J Endod* 6:598, 1980.

266. Wolcott JF, Himel VT, Hicks ML: Thermafil retreatment using a new system B technique or a solvent, *J Endod* 25:761, 1999.

267. Wong M, Peters DD, Lorton L: Comparison of gutta-percha filling techniques, compaction (mechanical), vertical (warm), and lateral condensation techniques, part 1, *J Endod* 7:551, 1981.

268. Wong M, Peters DD, Lorton L, Bernier WE: Comparison of gutta-percha filling techniques: three chloroform-gutta-percha filling techniques, part 2, *J Endod* 8:4, 1982.

269. Wong WS, Rosenberg PA, Boylan RJ, Schulman A: A comparison of the apical seals achieved using retrograde amalgam fillings and the Nd:YAG laser, *J Endod* 20:595, 1994.

270. Yahya AS, ElDeeb ME: Effect of sonic versus ultrasonic instrumentation on canal preparation, *J Endod* 15:235, 1989.

271. Yamada RS, Armas A, Goldman M, Sun Lin P: A scanning electron microscopic comparison of a high volume final flush with several irrigating solutions: part 3, *J Endod* 9:137, 1983.

272. Yee FS, Krakow A, Gron P: Three-dimensional obturation of the root canal using injection-molded thermoplasticized dental gutta-percha, *J Endod* 3:168, 1977.

273. Zetterqvist L, Anneroth G, Danin J, Roding K: Microleakage of retrograde filling - a comparative investigation between amalgam and glass ionomer cement in vitro, *Int Endod J* 21:1, 1988.

274. Zetterqvist L, Anneroth G, Nordenram A: Glass ionomer cement as retrograde filling material - an experimental investigation in monkeys, *Int J Oral Maxillofac Surg* 16:459, 1987.

275. Zmener O, Dominquez FV: Corrosion of silver cones in the subcutaneous connective tissue of the rat: a preliminary scanning electron microscope, electron microprobe, and histology study, *J Endod* 11:55, 1985.

276. Zmener O, Dominquez FV: Tissue response to a glass ionomer used as an endodontic cement, *Oral Surg Oral Med Oral Pathol* 56:198, 1983.

Chapter 15

 Pulpal Reaction to Caries and Dental Procedures

Syngcuk Kim, Henry Trowbridge, Hideaki Suda

Chapter Outline

One of the most important contributions to dental health in the last 50 years was the identification of fluoride as an agent that reduces or prevents caries. Through water fluoridation and addition of fluoride to toothpaste, there has been a significant reduction in caries (especially caries in caries-prone children). Theoretically, caries can be eliminated. However, dentistry is far from this goal: caries is still a significant health problem. This chapter will examine new research findings on caries, with emphasis on the defensive mechanisms of the dental pulp in response to invading caries.

Of the various forms of dental treatment, operative procedures are the most frequent cause of pulpal injury. It is accepted that trauma to the pulp cannot always be avoided, particularly when the tooth requires extensive restoration. Nonetheless, the competent clinician, by recognizing the hazards associated with each step of the restorative process, can often minimize (if not prevent) trauma to preserve the vitality of the tooth. In recent years laser systems have been added to the armamentarium of the dentist and the manufacturers claim that these lasers provide advantages over the use of traditional tools for tooth preparation and the management of hypersensitive teeth. Some of these claims are examined critically, especially whether lasers can be used for operative dentistry without harming the pulp.

In the past, pulpal responses to various dental procedures and materials have been discussed almost exclusively from a histologic perspective. Fortunately, active physiologic investigations in the last decade have shed new light on the dynamic changes in the pulp in response to dental procedures and materials. It is the purpose of this chapter to help the clinician understand pulpal responses to caries and to various restorative procedures and materials.

DENTAL CARIES

Dental caries is a localized, progressive destruction of tooth structure. If neglected, it is the most common cause of pulp disease. It is now generally accepted that for caries to develop, specific bacteria must exist on the tooth surface. Products of bacterial metabolism, notably organic acids and proteolytic enzymes, cause the destruction of enamel and dentin. Bacterial metabolites are also capable of eliciting an inflammatory reaction. Eventually extensive invasion of the dentin results in bacterial infection of the pulp. Three basic reactions tend to protect the pulp against caries: (1) a decrease in the permeability of the dentin, (2) the formation of new dentin, and (3) inflammatory and immune reactions.

Inward diffusion of toxic substances from carious lesions occurs mainly through the dentinal tubules. Therefore the extent to which toxins permeate the tubules and reach the pulp is of critical importance in determining the extent of pulpal injury. *The most common response to caries is dentin sclerosis.* In this reaction the dentinal tubules become partially or completely filled with mineral deposits consisting of apatite and whitlockite crystals. Researchers[72] reported finding dentin sclerosis at the periphery of carious lesions in 95.4% of 154 teeth examined. Studies using dyes, solvents, and radioactive ions have shown that dentin sclerosis has the effect of decreasing the permeability of dentin, thus shielding the pulp from irritation.[4] Evidence suggests that for sclerosis to occur, vital odontoblast processes must be present within the tubules.[30]

The ability of the pulp to produce reparative dentin beneath a carious lesion is another mechanism for limiting the diffusion of toxic substances to the pulp (see Fig. 11-48). Researchers[72] reported the presence of reparative dentin in 63.6% of teeth with carious lesions and found that it often occurred in combination with dentinal sclerosis. The characteristics of reparative dentin have already been discussed (see Chapter 11). In general, the amount of reparative dentin formed is proportional to the amount of primary dentin destroyed. The rate of carious attack also seems to be an influencing factor, because more dentin is formed in response to slowly progressing chronic caries than to rapidly advancing acute caries. For this reason, carious exposure of the pulp is likely to occur earlier in acute caries than in chronic caries.

Research has shown that along the border zone between primary and reparative dentin, the walls of dentinal tubules are thickened and the tubules are frequently occluded with material resembling peritubular dentin.[64] Thus the border zone appears to be considerably less permeable than ordinary dentin and may serve as a barrier to the ingress of bacteria and their products.

The formation of a dead tract in dentin is yet another reaction that may occur in response to caries. Unlike dentinal sclerosis and the formation of reparative dentin, this response is not considered to be a defense reaction. A dead tract is an area in dentin within which the dentinal tubules are devoid of odontoblast processes. The origin of these tracts in dental caries is uncertain, but most authorities are of the opinion that they are formed as a result of the early death of odontoblasts. Dead tracts are most often observed in young teeth affected by rapidly progressing lesions. Because dentinal tubules of dead tracts are patent, they are highly permeable. Therefore they are a potential threat to the integrity of the pulp. Fortunately, the healthy pulp responds to the presence of a dead tract by depositing a layer of reparative dentin over its surface, thus sealing it off.

Dentin is demineralized by organic acids (principally lactic acid) that are products of bacterial fermentation. These acids also play a role in degrading the organic matrix of enamel and dentin. Although very few oral bacteria possess collagenases, the collagenous matrix of dentin can be degraded by bacterial proteases if the collagen is first denatured by acid.

There is some controversy as to when caries first elicits an inflammatory response in the underlying pulp. One study observed an accumulation of chronic inflammatory cells in the pulp beneath enamel caries that had not yet invaded dentin.[13] Another study,[43] however, did not observe pulpal inflammation until the caries had penetrated beyond the enamel. There is general agreement that by the time caries has invaded the dentin, some changes are occurring in the pulp. These changes represent a response to the diffusion of soluble irritants and inflammatory stimuli into the pulp. Such substances include bacterial toxins, bacterial enzymes, antigens, chemotoxins, organic acids, and products of tissue destruction. Substances also pass outward from the pulp to the carious lesion. Researchers reported finding plasma proteins, immunoglobulins, and complement proteins in carious dentin.[50] It is conceivable that some of these factors are capable of inhibiting bacterial activity in the lesion.

Unfortunately, diagnosis of the extent of pulpal inflammation beneath a carious lesion is difficult. Many factors play a role in determining the nature of the caries process, so the individuality of each carious lesion should be recognized. The response of the pulp may vary depending on whether the caries process is progressing rapidly or slowly or is completely inactive (i.e., arrested caries). Moreover, caries tends to be an intermittent process, with periods of rapid activity alternating with periods of quiescence.[43] The rate of attack may be influenced by any or all of the following:

- Age of the host
- Composition of the tooth
- Nature of the bacterial flora of the lesion
- Salivary flow
- Buffering capacity of the saliva
- Antibacterial substances in the saliva
- Oral hygiene
- Cariogenicity of the diet and frequency with which acidogenic food is ingested
- Caries-inhibiting factors in the diet

Early morphologic evidence of a pulpal reaction to caries is found in the underlying odontoblast layer. Even before the appearance of inflammatory changes in the pulp, there is an overall reduction in the number and size of odontoblast cell bodies.[79] Although odontoblasts are normally tall, columnar

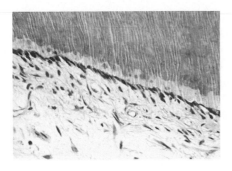

Fig. 15-1 Low cuboidal odontoblasts beneath a carious lesion.

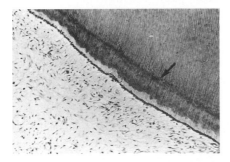

Fig. 15-2 Hyperchromatic line *(arrow)* in dentin beneath a carious lesion. (From Trowbridge H: Pathogenesis of pulpitis resulting from dental caries, *J Endod* 7:52, 1981.)

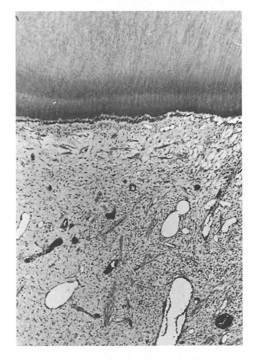

Fig. 15-3 Chronic inflammatory response evoked by a carious lesion in the overlying dentin.

cells, odontoblasts affected by caries appear flat to cuboidal in shape (Fig. 15-1). Electron microscopic examination of odontoblasts beneath carious lesions has revealed signs of cellular injury in the form of vacuolization, ballooning degeneration of mitochondria, and reduction in the number and size of other cytoplasmic organelles, particularly the endoplasmic reticulum.[42] These findings are in accord with biochemical studies[35] in which a reduction in the metabolic activity of odontoblasts was noted.

Concomitant with changes in the odontoblastic layer, a hyperchromatic line (i.e., calciotraumatic response) may develop along the pulpal margin of the dentin (Fig. 15-2). Formation of this line is thought to represent a disturbance in the normal equilibrium of the odontoblasts. It may also delineate the point at which the primary odontoblasts succumbed to the caries process and were replaced by odontoprogenitor cells arising from the cell-rich zone. In either event as new dentin is formed, the hyperchromatic line persists and becomes permanently embedded in the dentin.

The relationship between external caries environments and pulp and dentin complex reactions has been examined in several studies, which included the following:

1. Cytoplasm (nucleus ratio of primary odontoblast cells)
2. Cell-to-dentin tubule ratio
3. Adjacent predentin area
4. Nucleus ratio of nonodontoblastic cells and secondary odontoblast-like cells in the cytoplasm[7,8]

The results of these studies suggested a strong relationship between caries and the dentin and pulp complex. For instance, tertiary dentin appeared more atubular in the closed, active lesions with dentin exposure than in the open, slow-progressing lesions with dentin exposure. Furthermore, stimuli from the cariogenic biomasses in the enamel and enamel and dentin border caused an alteration in odontoblast cell population and the odontoblast and predentin region. Previous thoughts that enamel caries have little or no effect on the pulp have been challenged by this finding. The clinical significance is that any symptomatic pulp in the presence of incipient and shallow caries must be considered at risk, considering the possible implications of pulpal inflammation.

Dental caries is a protracted process, and lesions progress over a period of months or years. One investigator found that the average time from the stage of incipient caries to clinically detectable caries in children is 18 ± 6 months. Consequently, it is not surprising that pulpal inflammation evoked by carious lesions begins insidiously as a low-grade, chronic response rather than an acute reaction (Fig. 15-3). The initial inflammatory cell infiltrate consists principally of lymphocytes, plasma cells, and macrophages.[15]

Within this infiltrate are immunologically competent cells responding to antigenic substances diffusing into the pulp from the carious lesion.[72] Additionally, there is a proliferation of small blood vessels and fibroblasts and the deposition of collagen fibers. This pattern of inflammation is regarded as an inflammatory, reparative process. It is wise to remember that not all injuries result in permanent damage. Should the carious lesion be eliminated or become arrested, connective tissue repair would ensue.

The extent of pulpal inflammation beneath a carious lesion depends on the depth of bacterial invasion and the degree to which dentin permeability has been reduced by dentinal sclerosis and reparative dentin formation. In a study involving 46 carious teeth, investigators found that if the distance between the invading bacteria and the pulp (including the thickness of reparative dentin) averaged 1.1 mm or more; the inflammatory response was negligible.[62] When the lesions reached to within 0.5 mm of the pulp, there was a significant increase in the extent of inflammation, but it was not until the reparative dentin that had formed beneath the lesion was invaded by bacteria that the pulp became acutely inflamed.

As bacteria converge on the pulp, the characteristic features of acute inflammation become manifest. These include vascular and cellular responses in the form of vasodilation, increased vascular permeability, and the accumulation of leukocytes. Neutrophils migrate from blood vessels to the site of injury in response to certain split products of complement that are strongly chemotactic. These products are formed when complement is activated in the presence of antigen and antibody complexes.

Defense of the Dentin and Pulp Complex to Caries and the Role of Dentin Permeability

Similar to other biologic systems the pulp also defends itself against invasion. It is widely accepted that the dentin and pulp complex responds to cariogenic stimuli as a biologic continuum and exhibits a variety of interrelated defensive reactions, such as reparative-dentin formation and pulpal

inflammation. As discussed previously, the permeability of carious dentin plays an important role in determining the extent of the defensive response.[3] Many factors potentially influence the permeability of the carious dentin. These include the presence or absence of sclerotic dentin, the amount and quality of reparative dentin, the depth of the carious lesion, and the integrity of the odontoblastic layer. The critical element of the defense is dentinal fluid.

When microorganism lipopolysaccharide (LPS) invades the dentin, the first line of defense seems to be mobilization of immunosurveillance components from the pulp. These antigen-expressing cells are identified as the pulpal Ia antigen-expressing cells and macrophage-associated antigen-expressing cells.[34] Initial pulpal response to experimentally induced superficial caries in rats was characterized by a localized accumulation of Ia antigen-expressing cells beneath the corresponding dentin tubules (Fig. 15-4). As the caries extended deeper into the dentin there was a corresponding increase in Ia antigen-expressing cells and macrophages in the coronal pulp (Fig. 15-5). Because there was an intense accumulation of these cells under the dentin of the reparative dentin, the intensity of the defensive reaction may be correlated with the permeability of carious dentin (Fig. 15-6).[3,79]

Immunodefense of the Dentin and Pulp Complex to Caries

In addition to active participation of antigen-expressing cells in the dentin and pulp complex in response to caries, there is

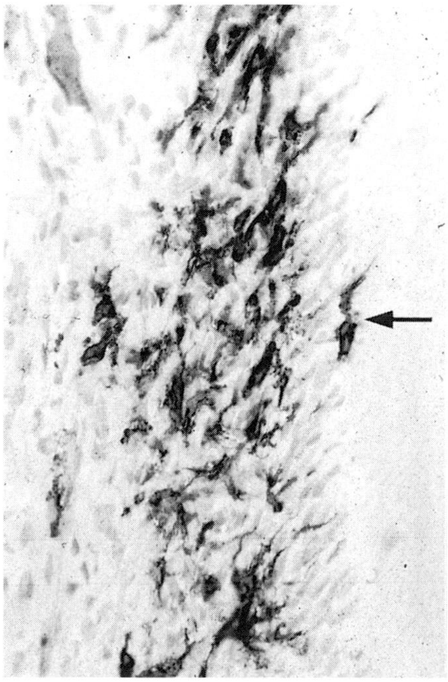

Fig. 15-4 OX6+ (anti–Ia antigen) cells accumulated near the pulp (*arrow*) of infected dental tubules from an 8-week-old superficial caries of a rat tooth.

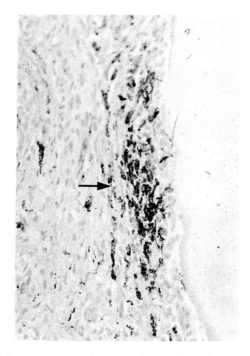

Fig. 15-5 Immunoperoxidase stained section from the caries-induced response in Fig. 15-4, showing accumulation of ED1+ (antimacrophase and dendritic cell marker) (*arrow*) at the pulpal end of the infected dental tubules (520 × magnification).

a delicate neuroimmune interaction that plays a modulatory role in the immunodefense. In a human caries study simultaneous immunohistochemical observation of neural elements were made.[63] The elements were labeled with anti–low-affinity nerve growth factor receptor microorganism (NFRG) and pulpal dendritic cells (PDC) were labeled with anti–HLA-DR or anticoagulation factor XIIIa (Fig. 15-7). The results showed the localized accumulation of both PDC and neural elements in the paraodontoblastic region corresponding to the pulpal end of carious dental tubules (Fig. 15-8). Even in the same tooth, factor-XIIA representing PDCs and NFRG imunoreactivities were significantly higher in the carious regions than those in the noncarious regions.

PDCs are considered to be a major constituent of the pulpal immune system, because of their putative potential of acting as antigen-presenting cells, which can uptake, process, and present foreign antigens to CD4+ T-lymphocytes. Investigators[51] suggested that neuropeptides may have some modulatory (i.e., stimulatory and inhibitory) role in the interaction of PDCs+ with T-lymphocytes. This interaction is supposed to facilitate immune-cellular infiltration by the generation of cytokines that can up regulate the expression of adhesion molecules on vascular endothelial cells.[32] Such a mechanism might have some implications in the initial immunodefense of the dental pulp against caries antigens. This finding also challenges the accepted notion that shallow caries have little or no effect on the pulp. Therefore clinicians may conclude that endodontic treatment is indicated. However, as pointed out by many researchers, the pulp has effective protective and healing mechanisms. Thus clinicians should not condemn these pulps too prematurely. A discussion of how the immunodefense system works in response to mechanical trauma, such as tooth preparation appears later in the chapter.

Pulpal Abscesses

When all the pulp's defense systems are overwhelmed, often the result of long-standing neglected caries, a pulpal abscess develops. Carious exposure of the pulp results in progressive mobilization of neutrophils and eventually to suppuration, which may be diffuse or localized in the form of an abscess.

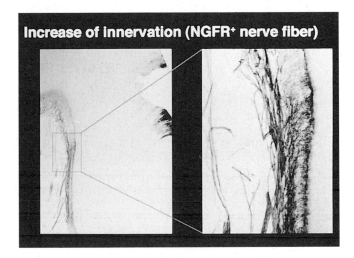

Fig. 15-7 NGFR-immunoreactive neural elements (i.e., dendritic cells) under the caries affected area (*left*). The larger magnification (*right*) shows an increased density of immunopositive staining in the region where the accumulation of HLA-DR–positive cells is observed. The top right corner of the left diagram shows the caries lesion.

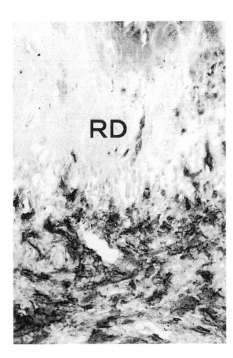

Fig. 15-6 A section from the 16-week-old group showing dense accumulation of OX6+ cells under the caries-affected reparative dentin (*RD*) (210 × magnification).

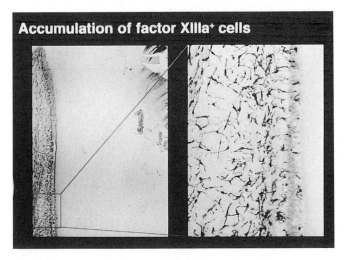

Fig. 15-8 Factor XIIIa ± immunoreactive neural elements (i.e., dendritic cells) under the caries-affected area (*left*). An enlarged view of the box, showing a dense accumulation of factor XIIIa ± immunoreactive cells. The top right corner of the left diagram shows the caries lesion.

The exudate associated with this reaction is called *pus*. Pus is formed when neutrophils release their lysosomal enzymes and the surrounding tissue is digested (a process known as liquefaction necrosis). The digested tissue has a greater osmotic pressure than the surrounding tissue, and this pressure differential is one of the reasons that abscesses are often painful and why drainage provides relief.

Few bacteria are found in an abscess, because bacteria entering the lesion are promptly destroyed by the antibacterial products of neutrophils. In addition, many bacteria cannot tolerate the low pH resulting from the release of lactic acid from neutrophils. However, as the size of the exposure enlarges and an ever-increasing number of bacteria enter the pulp, the defending forces are overwhelmed. It must be remembered that the pulp has a finite blood supply. Therefore when the demand for inflammatory elements exceeds the ability of the blood to transport them to the site of bacterial penetration, the bacteria become too numerous for the defenders and are able to proliferate without constraint. This ultimately leads to pulp necrosis.

Chronic Ulcerative Pulpitis

In some cases an accumulation of neutrophils may produce surface destruction (ulceration) of the pulp rather than an abscess. This is apt to occur when drainage is established through a pathway of decomposed dentin. The ulcer represents a local excavation of the surface of the pulp resulting from liquefaction necrosis of tissue. Because drainage prevents the buildup of pressure, the lesion tends to remain localized and asymptomatic. The base of the ulcer consists of necrotic debris and a dense accumulation of neutrophils. Granulation tissue infiltrated with chronic inflammatory cells is found within the deeper layers of the lesion. Eventually a space is created between the area of suppuration and the wall of the pulp chamber, giving the lesion the appearance of an ulcer (Fig. 15-9).

Hyperplastic Pulpitis

Hyperplastic pulpitis occurs almost exclusively in primary and immature permanent teeth with open apices. It develops in response to carious exposure of the pulp when the exposure enlarges to form a gaping cavity in the roof of the pulp chamber. This opening provides a pathway for drainage of the inflammatory exudate. Once drainage is established, acute inflammation subsides and chronic inflammatory tissue proliferates through the opening created by the exposure from a "pulp polyp" (Fig. 15-10). Presumably the young pulp does not become necrotic after exposure because its natural defenses and rich supply of blood allow it to resist bacterial infection. Clinically, the lesion has the appearance of a fleshy mass that may cover most of what remains of the crown of the tooth.

EFFECTS OF LOCAL ANESTHETICS ON THE PULP

The purpose of adding a vasoconstrictor to local anesthetics is to potentiate and prolong the anesthetic effect by reducing blood flow in the area in which the anesthetic is adminis-

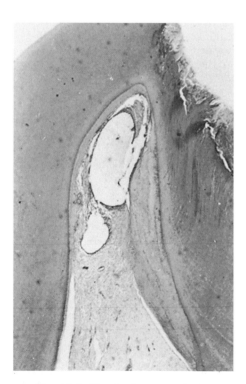

Fig. 15-9 Chronic ulcerative pulpitis.

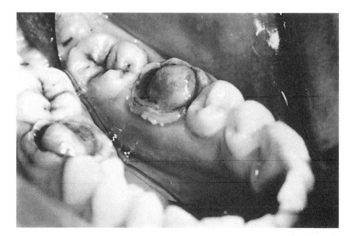

Fig. 15-10 Hyperplastic pulpitis (i.e., pulp polyp) in a lower first permanent molar. (Courtesy Dr. A. Stabholz, Hebrew University School of Dental Medicine, Jerusalem, Israel.)

tered. Although this enhances anesthesia, a recent study has shown that an anesthetic such as 2% lidocaine with 1:100,000 epinephrine is capable of significantly decreasing pulpal blood flow.[40] This reduction in blood flow may place the pulp in jeopardy for reasons explained later. Both infiltration and mandibular block injections cause a significant decrease in pulpal blood flow, although the flow reduction lasts a relatively short time (Fig. 15-11). With the ligamental injection, pulpal blood flow ceases completely for about 30 minutes when 2% lidocaine with 1:100,000 epinephrine is used (Fig. 15-12). With a higher concentration of epinephrine the cessation of pulp flow lasts even longer.

There is a direct relationship between the length of the flow cessation and the concentration of the vasoconstrictor used.[39] Because the rate of oxygen consumption in the pulp is relatively low, the healthy pulp can probably withstand a period of reduced blood flow. Researchers reported that pulpal blood flow and sensory nerve activity returned to normal levels after 3 hours of total cessation of blood flow.[52] However, a prolonged reduction in oxygen transport could interfere with cellular metabolism and alter the response of the pulp to injury. Irreversible pulpal injury is particularly apt to occur when dental procedures, such as full-crown preparations, are performed immediately after a ligamental injection. At least four documented cases have occurred in which the mandibular anterior teeth were devitalized as a result of crown preparation after ligamental injection.[39] Presumably irreversible pulp damage resulting from tooth preparation is caused by the release of substantial amounts of vasoactive agents, such as substance P, into the extracellular

compartment of the underlying pulp.[50] Under normal circumstances these vasoactive substances are quickly removed from the pulp by the bloodstream. However, when blood flow is drastically decreased or completely arrested, the removal of vasoactive substance from the pulp is greatly delayed; accumulation of these substances and other metabolic waste products may result in permanent damage to the pulp. One investigator has shown that the concentration of substances diffusing across the dentin into the pulp depends in part on the rate of removal via the pulpal circulation.[54] Thus a significant reduction in blood flow during a restorative procedure could lead to an increase in the concentration of irritants accumulating within the pulp. *Therefore, whenever possible, it is advisable to use vasoconstrictor-free local anesthetics for restorative procedures on vital teeth.* Because the addition of epinephrine at a concentration of 1:100,000 to local anesthetics appears to provide adequate vasoconstriction, stronger concentrations should be avoided during routine restorative procedures.

For dental treatments where clinicians need not be concerned about the vitality of the pulp, such as endodontic therapy and extractions, the use of a vasoconstrictor-containing local anesthetic is recommended. When used with an epinephrine-containing anesthetic, the ligamental injection is effective in obtaining anesthesia (Fig. 15-13). Over 80% of the problem teeth were successfully anesthetized with 1:100,000 epinephrine-containing anesthetic. Endodontists have found the ligamental injection to be an important tool to obtain profound anesthesia when treating "hot" mandibular molars.

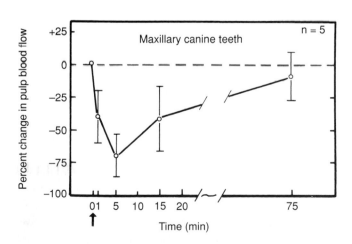

Fig. 15-11 Effects of infiltration anesthesia (i.e., 2% lidocaine with 1:100,000 epinephrine) on pulpal blood flow in the maxillary canine teeth of dogs. There is a drastic decrease in pulpal blood flow soon after the injection. Arrow indicates the time of injection. Bars depict standard deviation. (From Kim S: Effects of local anesthetics on pulpal blood flow in dogs, *J Dent Res* 63[5]:650, 1984.)

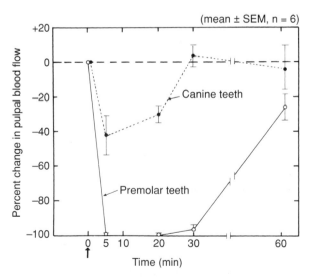

Fig. 15-12 Effects of ligamental injection (i.e., 2% lidocaine with 1:100,000 epinephrine) on pulpal blood flow in the mandibular canine and premolar teeth of dogs. Injection was given at the mesiodistal sulcus of the premolar teeth. Injection caused total cessation of pulpal blood flow, which lasted about 30 minutes in the premolar teeth. Arrow indicates the time of injection. (From Kim S: Ligamental injection: a physiological explanation of its efficacy; *J Endod* 12[10]:486, 1986.)

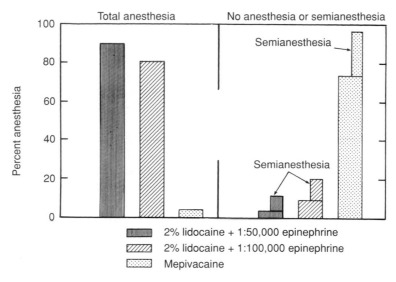

Fig. 15-13 Ligamental injection was effective in obtaining anesthesia in about 90% of cases with 2% lidocaine with 1:50,000 epinephrine and in about 80% of cases with 2% lidocaine with 1:100,000 epinephrine. Injection with mepivacaine (i.e., Carbocaine) practically failed to achieve anesthesia. Criterion for total anesthesia is no pain to pulp extirpation and canal instrumentation; semianesthesia is characterized by discomfort as a file approaches the apex.

Neurophysiologic Basis of Intraligamental Injection and Effects of Epinephrine

Electrical stimulation of the inferior alveolar nerve of cats revealed the significantly faster onset of intraligamental anesthesia than conventional infiltration anesthesia.[73] The onset time of 0.2 ml of lidocaine was 46 seconds in the intraligamental injection group, and 13 minutes and 24 seconds in the infiltration anesthesia group (Fig. 15-14). No significant difference was found in the effective and recovery times between the two injection groups. These experimental results confirmed the empirical clinical findings in humans that the intraligamental injection resulted in anesthesia much faster than the infiltration injection.

Epinephrine is an integral component of local anesthetic. The purpose of incorporating epinephrine in local anesthetics was to prolong the anesthetic effect by effecting vasoconstriction of the surrounding tissues. Recent studies showed that in addition to vasoconstriction, epinephrine also causes anesthesia. Simultaneous recording of antidromic responses and intradental nerve activity after intraligamental injection of 1:80,000 epinephrine showed cessation of nerve activity in both recordings, suggesting that epinephrine alone can cause an anesthetic effect.[73]

CAVITY AND CROWN PREPARATION

"Cooking the pulp in its own juice" is how Bodecker described tooth preparation without proper coolant. As shown in Fig. 15-15, pulpal responses to cavity and crown preparation depend on many factors. These include thermal injury, especially frictional heat, transaction of the odontoblastic processes, crown preparation, vibration, desiccation of dentin, pulp exposure, smear layer, remaining dentin thickness, and acid etching.

Thermal Injury

Cutting of dentin with a rotating bur or stone produces a considerable amount of frictional heat. The amount of heat produced is determined by speed of rotation, size and shape of the cutting instrument, length of time the instrument is in contact with the dentin, and amount of pressure exerted on the handpiece. If high temperatures are produced in deep cavities by continuous cutting without proper cooling, the underlying pulp may be severely damaged. According to one investigator,[87] the production of heat within the pulp is the most severe stress that restorative procedures impart to the pulp. If damage is extensive and the cell-rich zone of the pulp is destroyed, reparative dentin may not form.[48]

The thermal conductivity of dentin is relatively low. Therefore heat generated during the cutting of a shallow cavity preparation is much less likely to injure the pulp than a deep cavity preparation. One study found that temperatures and stresses developed during dry cutting of dentin were sufficiently high to be detrimental to tooth structure.[17] These investigators found that the greatest potential for damage was within a 1- to 2-mm radius of the dentin being cut.

The importance of the use of water and air spray during cavity preparation has been well established.[74,75] For example, more than 15 years ago it was reported that high-speed cutting with an adequate coolant caused cooling of the

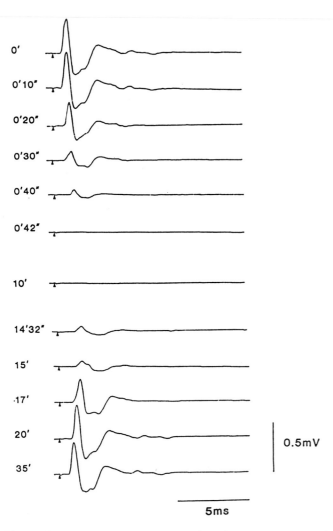

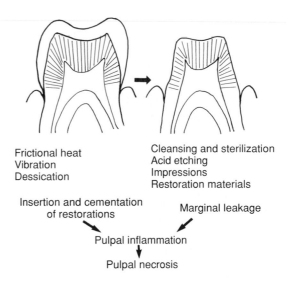

Fig. 15-15 Schematic illustration of factors that might cause pulpal reaction.

Fig. 15-14 An example of the changes of antidromic action potential in the intraligamental injection group with 0.2 ml of 2% lidocaine Note that the anesthesia was achieved immediately (i.e., 42 seconds) after the intraligamental injection (From: Suda H, Sunakawa M, Ikeda H, Yamamoto H: A neurophysiological evaluation of intraligamentary anesthesla, *Den Jpn [Tokyo]* 31:46, 1994.)

pulp to a subambient level.[87] Without a coolant the pulpal temperature rose to a critical level, 11° F (-11.6° C) above the ambient temperature. The same is true in the case of slow-speed cutting (i.e., 11,000 RPM). The reaction of the pulp to cavity preparation with and without a water spray has been studied histologically (Figs. 15-16 and 15-17).[70] When water and air spray were used, there was a negligible response, providing the remaining dentin thickness was greater than 1 mm (see Fig. 15-16). However, when the same procedure was performed without using a water spray, severe damage was found underneath the cutting site (Fig. 15-18). The flow was further reduced 1 hour after the completion of the crown preparation, suggesting irreversible damage. In a similar experiment using a water and air spray, only minor changes in pulpal blood flow were observed (Fig. 15-19).

Other researchers[48] investigated the effects of heat on the pulps of anesthetized young premolar teeth scheduled for orthodontic extraction. Class V cavities were prepared in the teeth, leaving an average of 0.5 mm remaining dentin thickness. Subsequently, a constant heat of 302° F (150° C) was applied to the surface of the exposed dentin for 30 seconds. After this procedure the teeth remained asymptomatic for a month, after which the teeth were extracted. Histologic examination of the pulps revealed varying degrees of pathosis, which included development of a homogenized collagenous zone along the dentin wall, disappearance of the "cell-rich" zone, and generalized cellular degeneration. Localized abscesses were observed in some of the teeth.

"Blushing" of teeth during or after cavity or crown preparation has been attributed to frictional heat. Characteristically the coronal dentin develops a pinkish hue very soon after the dentin is cut. This pinkish hue represents vascular stasis in the subodontoblastic capillary plexus blood flow. Under favorable conditions this reaction is reversible and the pulp will survive. However, a dark purplish color indicates thrombosis, and this is associated with a poorer prognosis. Histologically, the pulp tissue adjacent to the blushed dentinal surface is engorged with extravasated red blood cells, presumably as a result of the rupture of capillaries in the subodontoblastic plexus.[45] The incidence of dentinal blushing is greatest beneath full-crown preparations in teeth that were anesthetized by ligamental injection using 2% lidocaine plus 1:100,000 epinephrine.[39] In such cases the cessation of pulpal blood flow after ligamental injection may be a contributing factor. Tooth preparation may lead to the release of various vasoactive substances, such as substance P, and accumulation of such agents as a result of cessation of pulpal blood flow after ligamental injection may cause the tooth to blush.

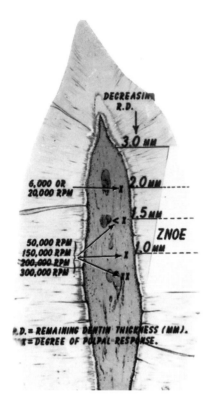

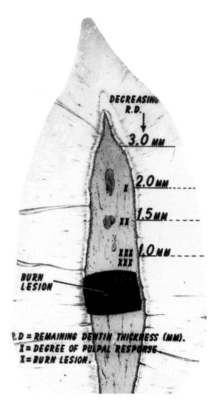

Fig. 15-16 With adequate water and air spray coolant, the same cutting tools, and a comparable remaining dentin thickness, the intensity of the pulpal response with high-speed techniques (i.e., decreasing force) is considerably less traumatic than with lower speed techniques (i.e., increasing force). (From Stanley HR, Swerdlow H: An approach to biologic variation in human pulpal studies, *J Prosthet Dent* 14:365, 1964.)

Fig. 15-17 Without adequate water coolant, larger cutting tools (e.g., no. 37 diamond point) create typical burn lesions within the pulp when the remaining dentin thickness becomes less than 1.5 mm. (From Stanley HR, Swerdlow H: An approach to biologic variation in human pulpal studies, *J Prosthet Dent* 14:365, 1964.)

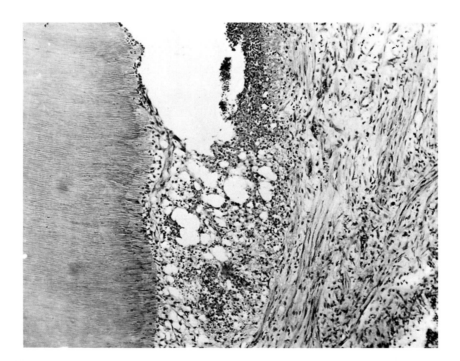

Fig. 15-18 Burn lesion with necrosis and expanding abscess formation in a 10-day specimen. Cavity prepared dry at 20,000 RPM, with remaining dentin thickness is 0.23 mm. (From Swerdlow H, Stanley HR: Reaction of human dental pulp to cavity preparation, *J Am Dent Assoc* 56:317, 1958.)

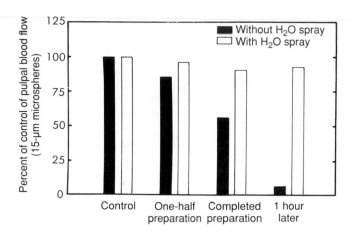

Fig. 15-19 Effects of crown preparation in dogs, with and without water and air spray (at 350,000 RPM) on pulpal blood flow. Tooth preparation without water and air spray caused a substantial decrease in pulpal blood flow, whereas that with water and air spray caused insignificant changes in the flow.

Transection of the Odontoblastic Processes and Its Implication in the Dentin and Pulp Complex

The length of the odontoblast process in fully formed teeth is still a matter of controversy. For many years it was believed that the process is confined to the inner third of the dentin. However, recent scanning electron microscopy (SEM) studies have provided evidence suggesting that many of the processes extend all the way from the odontoblast layer to the dentinoenamel junction.[37] In any event, amputation of the distal segment of odontoblast processes is often a consequence of cavity or crown preparation. Histologic investigation would indicate that amputation of a portion of the process does not invariably lead to death of the odontoblast. We know from numerous cytologic studies involving microsurgery that amputation of a cellular process is quickly followed by repair of the cell membrane. However, it would appear that amputation of the odontoblast process close to the cell body results in irreversible injury.

It is not always possible to determine the exact cause of death when odontoblasts disappear after a restorative procedure, because these cells may be subjected to a variety of insults. Frictional heat, vibration, amputation of processes, displacement as a result of desiccation, exposure to bacterial toxins, and other chemical irritants may each play a role in the demise of odontoblasts.

Investigators[19] studied the effects of class V cavity preparation on rat molar odontoblasts and observed a significant decrease in the amount of rough endoplasmic reticulum and number of mitochondria. There was also a loss of tight junctions between adjacent odontoblasts. Under the conditions of this experiment, these changes were reversible. Tight junctions provide a semipermeable barrier that prevents the passage of macromolecules from the pulp into the predentin. It has been shown that cavity preparation disturbs this barrier, thus increasing the permeability of the odontoblast layer.[83] The disruption of tight junctional complexes in the odontoblast layer could increase the potential for entry of toxic substances into the subjacent pulp tissue.

Taylor et al[76] observed an extensive increase in calcitonin gene-related peptide (CGRP) immunoreactive nerve fibers in the odontoblast layer beneath superficial dentinal cavities in rat molars. It was postulated that this increase represented nerve sprouting. The greatest number of nerve endings was observed at a postoperative interval of 4 days, but within 21 days these fibers had disappeared. The function of nerve sprouting in tissue injury is still unclear. Investigators[49] reported that pulpal dendritic cells showed a marked accumulation along the pulp and dentin border of the corresponding dentinal tubules after cavity preparation in rat molars. These findings, together with Taylor's, support the concept that pulpal dendritic cells and nerve sproutings play a critical role in the initial defense of the pulp against transdentinal antigenic stimuli.

Crown Preparation

Researchers[22] studied the long-term effects of crown preparation on pulp vitality and found a higher incidence of pulp necrosis associated with full-crown preparation (13.3%) as compared with partial veneer restorations (5.1%) and unrestored control teeth (0.5%). The placement of foundations for full-crown restorations was associated with an even greater incidence of pulp morbidity (17.7%).

Vibratory Phenomenon

Surprisingly little is known about the vibratory agitation that may be produced by high-speed cutting procedures. One study[28] demonstrated violent disturbances in the pulp chambers of teeth beneath the point of application of the bur and at other points remote from the cavity preparation. According to the observations the shock waves produced by vibration were particularly pronounced when the cutting speed was reduced; therefore stalling of the bur by increased digital pressure on the handpiece should be avoided. Obviously this problem deserves further study.

Desiccation of Dentin

When the surface of freshly cut dentin is dried with a jet of air there is a rapid outward movement of fluid through the dentinal tubules as a result of the activation of capillary forces within it.[11] According to the hydrodynamic theory of dentin sensitivity, this movement of fluid results in stimulation of the sensory nerve of the pulp. Fluid movement is also capable of drawing odontoblasts up into the tubules. These "displaced" odontoblasts soon die and disappear as they undergo autolysis. However, desiccation of dentin by cutting procedures or with a blast of air does not injure the pulp.[11] Although the clinician might expect that death of odontoblasts would evoke an inflammatory response, it is likely that too few cells are involved to evoke a significant reaction. Moreover, because death occurs within the dentinal tubules, dentinal fluid would dilute the products of cellular degeneration that might otherwise initiate an inflammatory response. Ultimately, odontoblasts that have been destroyed as a result of desiccation are replaced by new odontoblasts that arise from the cell-rich zone of the pulp, and in 1 to 3 months reparative dentin is formed.

Pulp Exposure

Exposure of the pulp during cavity preparation occurs most often in the process of removing carious dentin. Accidental mechanical exposure may result during the placement of pins or retention points in dentin. In both types of exposure, injury to the pulp primarily appears to be because of bacterial contamination. Investigators demonstrated that surgical exposure of the pulps of germ-free rats was followed by complete healing with no appreciable inflammatory reaction.[33] Another investigator has shown that pulps exposed during the removal of carious dentin become infected by bacteria that are carried into the pulp by dentin chips harboring microorganisms. It is safe to state that carious exposure results in much more bacterial contamination than does mechanical exposure.

Smear Layer

The smear layer is an amorphous, relatively smooth layer of microcrystalline debris with a featureless surface that cannot be seen with the unaided eye.[55] Although the smear layer may interfere with the adaptation of restorative materials to dentin, it may not be desirable to remove the entire layer because its removal greatly increases dentin permeability. By removing most of the layer but leaving plugs of grinding debris in the apertures of the dentinal tubules, dentin permeability is not increased, yet the walls of the cavity are relatively clean. Whether or not the smear layer should be removed is a matter of controversy. One view is that microorganisms present in the smear layer may irritate the pulp. Initially few bacteria are present in the smear layer; however, if conditions for growth are favorable, these will multiply, particularly if a gap between the restorative material and the dentinal wall permits the ingress of saliva.[12] Brännström believes that most restorative materials do not adhere to the dentinal wall.[12] Consequently, contraction gaps form between such materials and the adjacent tooth structure, and these gaps are invaded by bacteria either from the smear layer or from the oral cavity. As a result, bacterial metabolites diffuse through the dentinal tubules and injure the pulp.

Remaining Dentin Thickness

Dentin permeability increases almost logarithmically with increasing cavity depth because of the difference in size and number of dentinal tubules (see Chapter 11). In short, permeability of the dentin is of great importance in determining the degree of pulpal injury resulting from restorative procedures and materials. Stanley[70] found that the distance between the floor of the cavity preparation and the pulp (i.e., the remaining dentin thickness) greatly influences the pulpal response to restorative procedures and materials. He suggested that a remaining dentin thickness of 2 mm would protect the pulp from the effects of most restorative procedures, provided that all other operative precautions are observed.

Acid Etching

Although acid etching of cavity walls is cleansing, acid etching is specifically designed to enhance the adhesion of restorative materials. In the case of dentin, however, the ability of acid etching to improve long-term adhesion has been questioned. Acid cleansers applied to dentin have been shown to widen the openings of the dentinal tubules, increase dentin permeability, and enhance bacterial penetration of the dentin. One study showed that in deep cavities, pretreatment of the dentin with 50% citric or 50% phosphoric acid for 60 seconds is capable of significantly increasing the response of the pulp to restorative materials.[71] Results of one physiologic investigation have shown that acid etching a small class V cavity having a remaining dentin thickness of 1.5 mm has little effect on pulpal blood flow.[69] Thus direct effect of the acid on the pulpal microvascular vessels appears to be negligible, possibly because of a rapid buffering of the acid by the dentinal fluid. However, it is possible that in very deep cavities acid etching may contribute to pulpal injury.

Immunodefense of the Pulp to Tooth Preparation

As discussed earlier in the section on caries, the pulp undergoes significant cellular alterations in response to tooth preparation. The degree of cellular change is proportional to the tooth preparation. For instance, a shallow preparation with copious water coolant would cause minor odontoblast aspirations. A deeper preparation impacts the pulp more severely, with a concomitantly stronger pulpal cell reaction. In response to tooth preparation the sensory nerve cells release a number of neuropeptides, especially substance P.[16] In addition, pulp blood flow initially increases and then decreases severely because of the low-compliance environment of the pulp. Finally, immunodefense cells of the same type that appeared in response to caries accumulate underneath the area of tooth preparation. Simultaneous immunohistochemical observation of neural elements labeled with anti–low-affinity NFRG and PDC (labeled with anti–HLA-DR or anti-coagulation factor XIIIa) after tooth preparation showed the localized accumulation of both PDC and neural elements in the corresponding paraodontoblastic region.[63] Sensory nerve sprouting is also reported, suggesting that the tooth pulp would mobilize all the cellular elements to defend if it senses that mechanical trauma is inflammatory.

Comparison of Cavity Preparation by High-Speed Handpiece and Bur and Er:YAG Laser

For details of the physical properties of the Er:YAG laser system, please see the subsequent section on lasers. This section will compare the histopathologic reactions of the pulp to a cavity preparation by Er:YAG lasing versus with a high-speed bur.[65] Class V cavities were prepared on dog teeth by either Er:YAG laser with output energy ranging from 100 to 200 mj at 10 pulses per second (pps) or by conventional, high-speed cutting method with water-cooling equipment.

Test cavities were filled with glass ionomer cement after preparation. All samples were divided into two groups according to the remaining dentin thickness (RDT). A histopathologic comparison of the pulps was made between the high-speed handpiece group and the Er:YAG laser group postoperatively at 1, 2, 4, 7, and 28 days. Fig. 15-20 is a SEM display of the high-speed cutting and laser cutting. The high-speed cutting shows a smooth surface, with a smear layer covering the surface. The laser-cutting surface is granulated and rough, with exposed dentin tubules with a sparse smear layer.

One day postoperatively, all preparations (regardless of depth and preparation method) showed varying degree of histopathologic reactions: there were displacement and aspiration of odontoblasts, infiltration of inflammatory cells, and hemorrhage below the prepared cavities. These histopathologic changes were more severe in teeth treated by the Er:YAG laser (Fig. 15-21, *A* and *B*). In the 7-day postoperative specimen, pulpal reactions were generally mild under the shallow cavities, compared with the deep-cavity preparations group. Histopathologic changes were limited to the area of the pulp below the cavities both in the laser and the high-speed handpiece groups. The 28-day postoperative specimen showed repair of the odontoblastic layers in both laser and high-speed handpiece groups. Especially in the shallow RDT groups the pulp was almost normal with no noticeable histopathologic differences between the laser and high-speed handpiece groups (Fig. 15-22, *A* and *B*). In general, there were little or no noticeable pulpal reactions in both groups, suggesting that complete healing took place and that the cavity preparation by Er:YAG lasing is safe to the pulp. With the safety of the Er:YAG laser for cavity preparation confirmed, the question to be asked now is whether the laser is more efficient than the high-speed handpiece for this purpose.

RESTORATIVE MATERIALS

How do restorative materials evoke a response in the underlying pulp? For many years it was believed that toxic ingredients in the materials were responsible for pulpal injury. However, pulpal injury associated with the use of these materials could not be correlated with their cytotoxic properties. Thus irritating materials such as zinc oxide–eugenol (ZOE) produced a very mild pulpal response when placed in cavities, whereas less toxic materials, such as composite resins and amalgam, produced a much stronger pulp response. In addition to chemical toxicity, some of the properties of materials that might be capable of producing injury include the following:

1. Acidity (hydrogen ion concentration)
2. Absorption of water during setting
3. Heat generated during setting
4. Poor marginal adaptation resulting in bacterial contamination

Investigators[58] found that the pulpal response beneath a material is not associated with the material's hydrogen ion concentration. The acid content in restorative materials is probably neutralized by the dentin and dentinal fluid.[15] As the superficial dentin is demineralized, phosphate ions are liberated, thus producing a buffering effect. However, placement of an acidic material, such as zinc phosphate, at luting consistency in a deep cavity may have a toxic effect on the pulp, because the diffusion barrier is extremely thin. One study showed that zinc phosphate cement of luting consistency placed on a deep (i.e., 0.5 mm remaining dentin layer) and large class V cavity on canine tooth caused a moderate decrease in pulpal blood flow as measured with the 15 mm microsphere method. After the cement had hardened for about 30 minutes, blood flow had again increased, suggesting that the cement had a temporary and transitory effect on the pulpal circulation (Fig. 15-23). The changes in pulpal blood flow may have been caused by chemical or exothermal effects of the cement. One study[58] found that of all the materials studied, zinc phosphate cement was associated with the greatest temperature rise: an increase of 35.85° F (2.14° C).[58]

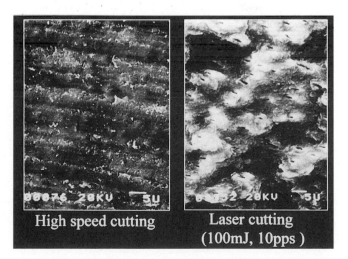

High speed cutting   **Laser cutting (100mJ, 10pps)**

Fig. 15-20 Scanning electron microscopic picture of high speed cutting (*left*) and ER:YAG lase cutting on a dentin surface. The high-speed cutting shows a smear layer, however, the laser cutting shows an irregular surface with open tubules.

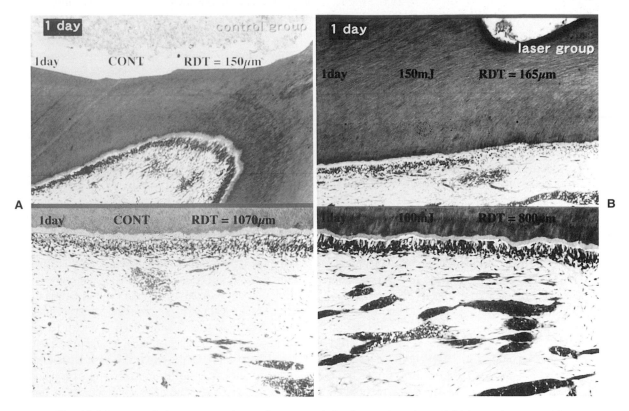

Fig. 15-21 Histopathologic picture of control group (**A**) defined as tooth cutting with high-speed motor and bur and ER:YAG laser cutting (**B**) after 1 day postpreparation in dog teeth. The top picture represents deep cutting (around 150 mm remaining dentin thickness [RD]), and the bottom picture represents shallow cutting (around 1000 mm RD). Varying reaction of cellular changes are observed regardless of the methods of preparations.

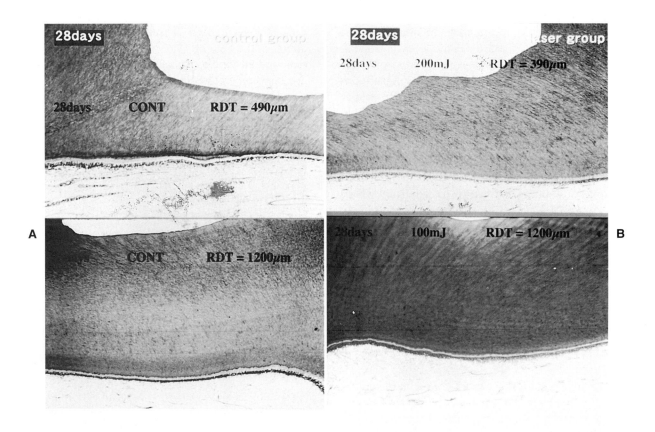

Fig. 15-22 **A** and **B**, The same condition as Fig. 15-21. This is 28 days postpreparation. Regardless of the cutting methods the pulps show little or no histopathologic changes, suggesting that repair has taken place.

This amount of temperature increase, however, is not sufficient to produce tissue injury.[87]

In a microcirculatory study using hamster cheek pouch, a drop of zinc phosphate liquid caused stasis, followed by hemolysis, resulting in total cessation of blood flow in the vessels that were in contact with the liquid. Thus there seems to be a real possibility of pulpal damage if the pulp is in close contact with the liquid portion of the cement. Absorption of water during the setting of a material can also be ruled out as a cause of pulpal injury. Compared with the removal of fluid from dentin by an airstream during cavity preparation (which produces no inflammatory response in the pulp), absorption of water by a material is insignificant. Researchers[58] found no relationship between the hydrophilic properties of materials and their effect on the pulp.

This brings us to bacterial contamination. It has long been recognized that, in general, dental materials do not adapt to tooth structure well enough to provide a hermetic seal. Thus it has been acknowledged that bacteria may penetrate the gap between the restored material and the cavity wall. Presumably bacteria growing beneath restorations create toxic products that can diffuse through the dentinal tubules and evoke an inflammatory reaction in the underlying pulp. Converging evidence suggests that *products of bacterial metabolism are the major cause of pulpal injury resulting from the insertion of restorations.*

One investigator showed that material such as composite resins, zinc phosphate, and silicate cements produced only a localized tissue reaction when placed directly on exposed pulps in germ-free animals.[71] The same procedure in conventional animals resulted in total pulp necrosis. Employing bacterial staining methods, researchers[15] demonstrated that the growth of bacteria under restorations was correlated with the degree of inflammation of the adjacent pulp tissue. They also found that bacteria did not grow when the outer portions of restorations were replaced with ZOE, thus producing a surface seal (Fig. 15-24). When bacterial growth was thus inhibited, pulpal inflammation was negligible. Similar studies[4] showed that colonies of bacteria become established under restorative materials that do not provide an adequate marginal seal. Of the materials tested (Dispersalloy amalgam [Johnson & Johnson Products Co., East Windsor, NJ], Concise composite resin [3M Co., St. Paul, MN], Hygienic guttapercha [Hygienic Corp., Akron, OH], MQ silicate cements [S.S. White Dental Products, Philadelphia, PA], and ZOE) only ZOE consistently prevented bacteria from becoming established beneath the restoration. Using ZOE as a surface seal, Cox et al[20] found that materials such as amalgam, composites, silicate cement, zinc phosphate cement, and ZOE produced only a thin zone of contact necrosis and no inflammation when placed directly on primate pulps (Fig. 15-25).

In vitro and in vivo studies on marginal adaptation of restorative materials have often yielded conflicting results. Obviously it is difficult to duplicate clinical conditions in the laboratory. Two important factors affecting marginal adaptation are temperature changes and masticatory forces. Nelson

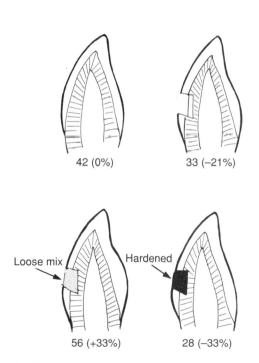

Fig. 15-23 Effects of zinc phosphate cement on pulpal blood flow (ml/min/100 g). Cement of luting consistency was placed in a deep and large class V cavity in the canine teeth of dogs, and pulpal blood flow was measured. A 33% increase was observed initially, but the hardened cement caused a decrease in pulpal blood flow.

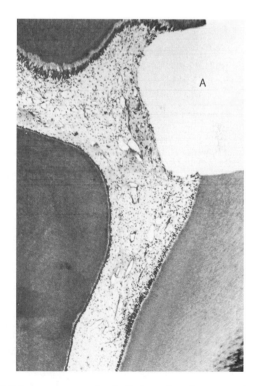

Fig. 15-24 Appearance of pulp 7 days after placement of amalgam restoration (**A**) directly against pulp tissue. Note absence of inflammatory response. (From Cox CF et al: Biocompatibility of various surface-sealed dental materials against exposed pulps, *J Prosthet Dent* 57:1, 1987.)

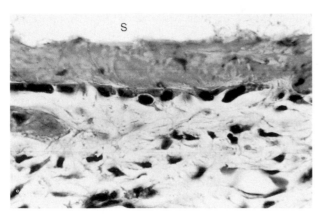

Fig. 15-25 Pulpal response 21 days after placement of silicate cement (S) directly against the pulp. Silicate was surface sealed with ZOE. Note formation of hard tissue and new odontoblasts. (From Cox CF et al: Biocompatibility of various surface-sealed dental materials against exposed pulps, *J Prosthet Dent* 57:1, 1987.)

et al[46] were the first to study the opening and closing of the margin of restorations that were subjected to temperature changes. If a material has a different coefficient of thermal expansion than tooth structure, temperature change is likely to produce gaps between the material and the cavity wall. Another investigator[61] demonstrated a marked effect of functional mastication on marginal adaptation of composite restorations. He found gap formation along 71% of the restorations in teeth that were in functional occlusion, whereas leakage occurred in only 28% of teeth with no antagonist.

As yet no permanent filling material has been shown to consistently provide a perfect marginal seal, so leakage and bacterial contamination are always a threat to the integrity of the pulp. Consequently, an adequate cavity liner or cement base should be employed to seal the dentinal tubules before inserting restorative materials. Despite these findings, it must be acknowledged that pulps frequently remain healthy under restorations that leak. Factors that determine whether bacterial growth beneath a restoration will injure the pulp probably include pathogenicity of the microorganisms, permeability of the underlying dentin (i.e., degree of sclerosis, number of tubules, thickness of dentin), and the ability of the irritated pulp to produce reparative dentin.

Because there is convincing evidence that bacterial growth beneath restorations is the primary cause of pulpal injury, the antibacterial properties of filling materials may be of considerable importance. Not all materials have been studied, but there is evidence that ZOE, calcium hydroxide, and polycarboxylate cement has some ability to inhibit bacterial growth. Zinc phosphate cement, the restorative resins, and silicate cements lack antibacterial ingredients, and these materials are most often associated with injury to the pulp.

Zinc Oxide and Eugenol

ZOE is used for a variety of purposes in dentistry. In addition to being a popular temporary filling material, it is used for provisional and permanent cementation of inlays, crowns, and bridges and as a pulp-capping agent and a cement base. Eugenol, a phenol derivative, is known to be toxic, and it is capable of producing thrombosis of blood vessels when applied directly to pulp tissue.[60] It also has anesthetic properties, and is used as an anodyne in relieving the symptoms of painful pulpitis. This presumably results from its ability to block the transmission of action potentials in nerve fibers.[82] Experimentally, ZOE has been shown to suppress nerve excitability in the pulp when applied to the base of a deep cavity.[80] This effect is obtained only when a fairly thin mix of ZOE (e.g., powder to liquid ratio 2:1 wt/wt) is used. Presumably it is the free eugenol in the cement that is responsible for the anesthetic effect. ZOE has two important properties that explain why it is such an effective base material: (1) it adapts very closely to dentin, thus providing a good marginal seal, and (2) its antibacterial properties inhibit bacterial growth on cavity walls. However, because eugenol injures cells, some authorities question whether ZOE should be used in very deep cavity preparations where there is a risk of pulp exposure.

Zinc Phosphate Cement

One study[29] found that when a liner was omitted, severe pulpal reactions (principally abscess formation) occurred in all teeth in which deep class V cavities were restored with zinc phosphate cement. The pulpal response was attributed to the phosphoric acid contained in the cement. In retrospect, however, it is likely that irritation to the pulp was due primarily to marginal leakage rather than to acidity. Because of its high modulus of elasticity, zinc phosphate is the cement base of choice for amalgam restorations. This results from the fact that it is better able to resist the stresses of mastication than other cements.

Zinc Polycarboxylate Cements

Polycarboxylate cement is well tolerated by the pulp, being roughly equivalent to ZOE cements in this respect.[29] This may be due to its ability to adapt well to dentin. It also has been reported that this cement has bactericidal qualities.[6]

Restorative Resins

The original unfilled resins were associated with severe marginal leakage, caused by dimensional changes that resulted from a high coefficient of thermal expansion. This, in turn, resulted in marked pulpal injury. The development of sulfuric acid catalyst systems and the nonpressure insertion techniques have improved the performance of resins considerably. The epoxide resins with a benzoyl peroxide catalyst that are 75% filled with glass or quartz (the so-called composite resins) represent another group of resins. These have much more favorable polymerization characteristics and a lower coefficient of thermal expansion than the original unfilled resins. The marginal seal has been further improved by acid etching of beveled enamel and the use of a bonding agent or primer. This reduces the risk of microbial invasion but does not eliminate bacteria that may be present on cavity walls. However, it has been shown that the initial marginal seal tends to deteriorate as the etched composite restoration ages. Furthermore, one study showed that functional mastication is capable of producing gaps that result in increased leakage.[61] Many investigators[15] have shown that unlined composite resins are harmful to the pulp, primarily because of bacterial contamination beneath the restoration. Thus the use of a cavity liner is strongly recommended. Because copal varnish is not compatible with the restorative resins, the use of a polystyrene liner has been advocated.[11] Bases containing calcium hydroxide have also been shown to provide good protection against bacteria.

Glass Ionomer Cement Restorations

Studies on glass ionomer cements indicate that they are well tolerated by the pulp.[36] However, researchers[1] have shown that leakage may occur around such fillings, so this material should be used in conjunction with a liner or base. There have been reports of postcementation tooth sensitivity after the use of glass ionomer cements to cement gold castings, but the cause of this sensitivity has not been determined. It appears that sensitivity is not the result of marginal leakage, because the results of an in vitro leakage study demonstrated that glass ionomer–luting cements provide a good marginal seal.[26]

Dental Amalgam

Dental amalgam, first used for the restoration of carious teeth in the sixteenth century, is still the most popular restorative material in dentistry. Unvarnished amalgam restorations leak severely when they are first inserted, but within a period of 12 weeks a marginal seal develops that resists dye penetration beyond the dentinoenamel junction. Investigators[27] found that pulp responses to unlined amalgams (Sybraloy [Kerr Manufacturing Co., Romulus, MI], Dispersalloy [Johnson & Johnson, East Windsor, NJ], Tytin [S.S. White Dental Products, Philadelphia, PA], and Spheraloy [Kerr Manufacturing Co., Romulus, MI]) consisted of slight-to-moderate inflammation. The inflammation tended to diminish with time, and within a few weeks reparative dentin was deposited. Other investigators[60] theorized that the high mercury content of amalgam may exert a cytotoxic effect on the pulp; they found that mercury penetrates into the dentin and pulp beneath an amalgam restoration. They have also reported that rubbing the bottom of the cavity with a calcium hydroxide and water mixture protects the pulp from the irritating effects of amalgam. Bacteria were found beneath unlined amalgams, whereas the pulps of teeth in which a ZOE liner was used exhibited a milder response and no bacteria were present. In vitro bacterial tests indicated that amalgam has no inhibitory effect on bacterial growth.

It is well known that insertion of amalgam restorations may result in postoperative thermal sensitivity, even when amalgam is placed in a shallow cavity. Brännström[10] is of the opinion that such sensitivity results from expansion or contraction of fluid that occupies the gap between the amalgam and the cavity wall. This fluid is in communication with fluid in the subjacent dentinal tubules, so variations in temperature would cause axial movement of fluid in the tubules. According to the hydrodynamic theory of dentin sensitivity, this fluid movement would stimulate nerve fibers in the underlying pulp, thus evoking pain.[80] The use of a cavity varnish or base is recommended to seal the dentinal tubules and prevent this form of postoperative discomfort.

Cavity Varnish

The effectiveness of cavity varnish in providing protection for the pulp is highly controversial. One study[23] has called attention to the fact that in vivo surfaces are wet and, therefore, the application of liners or varnishes may not result in an impervious coating. Even the application of two or three coats of varnish may not prevent gaps from occurring in the lining. Furthermore, other investigators[14] have reported that a double layer of Copalite did not prevent bacterial leakage and growth of bacteria on the cavity walls. Nonetheless, several reports indicate that varnish can act as a barrier to the toxic effects of restorations.[68] One study[47] assessed the ability of several commercial varnishes to decrease microleakage beneath a high copper–spherical alloy restorative material and found Copalite to be the most effective.

EFFECTS OF LASING ON THE PULP AND DENTIN COMPLEX

The successful use of various laser systems in medicine has stimulated its application in dentistry. Manufacturers of laser systems make the following claims: lasers can remove caries, modify the dentin surface for stronger bonding, eliminate pits and fissures, and anesthetize and treat hypersensitive teeth. These claims are made for several laser systems with differing wavelengths and energy outputs.[21,59] Two laser systems, the carbon dioxide and Nd:YAG, have demonstrated significant possibilities in clinical dentistry, such as those mentioned previously. Such results, however, are not the only criteria for evaluating the usefulness and value of lasers in clinical dentistry. Two other requirements are critical for the effectiveness of lasers and the health of the tooth: lasing must provide superior results over traditional procedures, and it must not damage the vital pulp in the process. Recently, Er:YAG laser has been shown to ablate dental hard tissue with minimal damage to the pulp at specific energy settings; thus it can theoretically replace the conventional drill for cavity preparation. We discussed this issue in the previous sections.

Transmissivity of Lasers Through Dentin

The interaction between laser light and substrate is expressed in terms of reflection, absorption and transmission, which

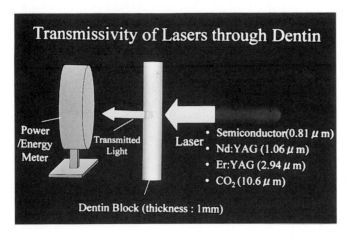

Fig. 15-26 A schematic diagram illustrating a model system to test transmissivity of various laser systems through dentin.

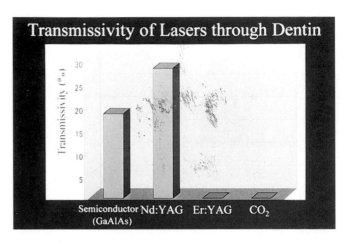

Fig. 15-27 Diode and Nd:YAG lasers have the more transmissivity through the 1 mm dentin than ER:YAG and CO_2 lasers, indicating that the former laser systems may be more harmful to the pulp when lased on the dentin surface.

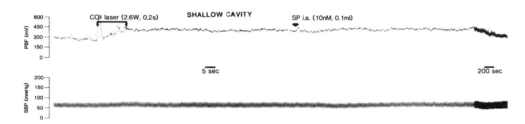

Fig. 15-28 Effect of carbon dioxide lasing on a cat canine pulp blood flow measured with laser Doppler flowmetry. Lasing at 2.6 W/0.2 ms/15 sec caused a 50% flow increase. There was no change in systemic blood pressure or flow response to intraarterial substance P injection, which was used to test vascular reactivity.

are wavelength-dependent.[41,88] In clinical dentistry, the three key elements are very important because use of any laser system on dentin and enamel must preserve the integrity of the pulp. A simple experiment using a 1 mm dentin block, power energy meter and varying laser beams can measure the degree of the transmissivity of lasers through dentin (Fig. 15-26). As shown in Fig. 15-27, 17% of diode laser (semiconductor) and 27% of Nd:YAG laser transmit through 1 mm thick dentin. In contrast, there is almost no transmitted light detected in ER:YAG and CO_2 lasers, suggesting that these laser beams are either absorbed or reflected. Clinically Er:YAG and CO_2 laser systems will do less harm to the pulp than the Nd:YAG and diode laser systems. Our animal experiment results support these claims.

Carbon Dioxide Laser

The carbon dioxide laser is well known for cutting soft tissue without bleeding; thus its use in soft tissue management in periodontal and oral surgery procedures has been well established. However, its utility in hard tissue management can be contested. Lasing effects on the pulp and dentin complex had

not been considered by evaluations of the system, and it has been subsequently shown in several studies that the dentin and the pulp are detrimentally affected by most lasing procedures. For instance, a cat's tooth with a remaining dentin thickness of 1 mm lased at a low-energy setting of 2.6 W showed a 50% increase in pulpal blood flow when measured with laser Doppler flowmetry (Fig. 15-28). This indicates a dilation of the blood vessels in response to noxious thermal stimulus. The moderately higher energy of 5 W caused an irreversible flow reduction, indicating damage to the pulp. The most likely cause of the blood flow reduction is an excessive thermal effect.[24] Dentin permeability measured by Pashley's in vitro dentin disk technique also revealed that permeability increased significantly after lasing. Thus the utility and safety of carbon dioxide laser systems for hard tissues is questionable with the systems currently available.

Nd:YAG Laser

A pulsed Nd:YAG laser with 1.06 mm wavelength has been the most widely tested and used laser system in dentistry with mixed results. White et al[86] reported that dentin modifi-

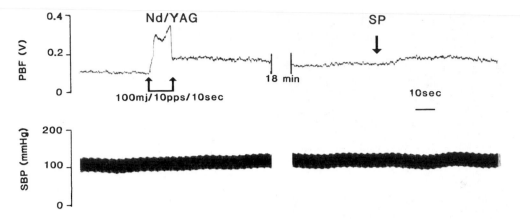

Fig. 15-29 Effect of Nd:YAG lasing on cat canine pulp blood flow measured with laser Doppler flowmetry. Lasing at 100 mj/10 pps/10 sec caused a moderate increase in flow, whereas intraarterial substance P injection caused a slight increase, indicating vascular reactivity after lasing.

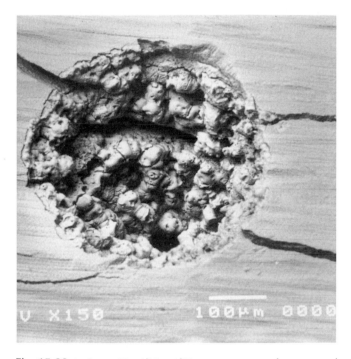

Fig. 15-30 Lasing at 30 mj/10 pps/10 sec at one spot of an extracted human tooth dental surface by Nd:YAG laser. Ablation and melting of the dentin at the irradiated area are found.

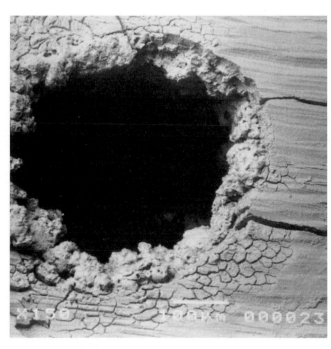

Fig. 15-31 Same tooth as in Fig. 15-30 at the same energy level but at a different site for 30 seconds. Complete removal of the dentin is causing a hole connecting to the pulp.

cation by laser increased dentin microhardness, making it more resistant to acid demineralization (i.e., caries). As far as pulp safety is concerned, White et al also reported that a histologic examination indicated this laser to be safe for the human pulp when used within limited parameters. However, other studies[66] show that the effect of Nd:YAG laser system on the pulp varies greatly, depending on the remaining dentin thickness. For instance, using 100 mj/10 pps/10 second, pulpal blood flow did not change significantly with lasing of

the intact enamel. Blood flow increased moderately after lasing of a shallow cavity with a remaining dentin thickness of 1 mm and was irreversibly altered at high energy levels (Fig. 15-29). The pulse per second rate also seems to play an important role. Similarly, when the laser is applied to one area for more than 10 seconds, significant structural damage is caused (Fig. 15-30). When lasing an area just longer than 15 seconds, a crater resulted (almost exposing the pulp) (Fig. 15-31).

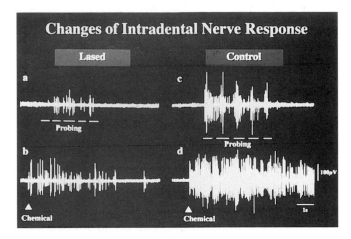

Fig. 15-32 Intradental recording of feline teeth subject to Nd:YAG lasing. Lased group with probing (*a*) and chemical application (*b*) are compared with the control group. There is a significant reduction in sensory nerve activities with laser group.

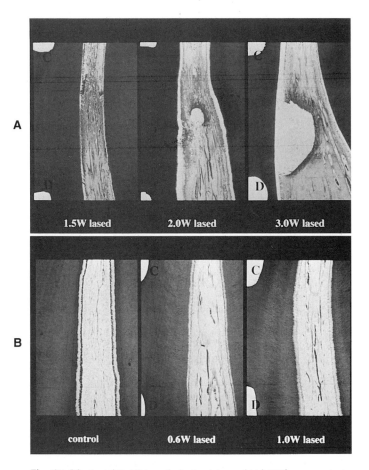

Fig. 15-33 **A** and **B,** Histopathologic picture of Nd:AG laser specimen with an increasing power. There is direct relationship between the degree of pathologic changes and the increasing power of the laser. In fact, 1.5 W and the greater power cause permanent damage to the pulp.

Recent studies examining pulpal nerve responses and corresponding histopathologic manifestations after spot lasing of cat teeth with an Nd:YAG laser also revealed interesting and important findings. First, the number of impulses evoked by various stimuli, such as chemical and mechanical stimuli, in the scanning lased group was significantly lower than in the control (i.e., nonscanned) group (Fig. 15-32). Second, single-fiber recordings of A-d and C-fiber after the scanning laser irradiation showed there is significant alteration and reduction of nerve activity.[18] Third, antidromic compound action potentials in the intradental nerves was diminished from the coronal tip to the cervix of the canine after the lasing. Furthermore, the coronal antidromic compound action potentials disappeared in all tested teeth during the lasing, and the time required to stop them was significantly shortened with increases in lasing power. These physiologic findings suggest that it may be dangerous to apply pulsed Nd:YAG laser on the vital pulp with the intention to reduce pulpal pain. Histologic investigation showed that spot irradiation produced severe damage in the pulp tissue in a dose-dependent manner (Fig. 15-33, *A* and *B*).[77]

These findings, together with previous investigations, clearly suggest that Nd:YAG laser may have certain beneficial effects on the dentin but not on the pulp. The pulp damage includes nerve injury and hemorrhage leading to irreversible damage. Identifying an energy level at a given dentin thickness that provides the desired effects on the dentin for operative dentistry without harming the pulp would be an important step in laser research.

Er:YAG Laser

Numerous studies have shown that the Er:YAG laser can ablate dental hard tissue with minimal damage to the dental pulp. In clinical studies little or no pain response to cavity preparation by this laser system has been reported. Researchers investigated the responses of intradental nerves to Er:YAG laser and compared the results with those obtained with the conventional drill (i.e., micromotor) during tooth cutting.[18] The nerve-firing rate during the lasing was significantly higher than during the micromotor cutting irrespective of the distance from the pulp. There was also no selective nerve firing. All of the nerve fibers (i.e., A-d, A-b) that responded to mechanical stimuli responded vigorously.

The mechanism of tooth cutting by Er:YAG laser is based on its high absorption into the water component of the hard tissue. This may cause a quick temperature increase within a small volume of the tissue. Thus both enamel and dentin are removed partly by a continuous vaporization process and partly by microexplosion. SEM studies also showed the opening of dentinal tubules after the lasing (see Fig. 15-20). These physiologic and structural findings indicate that there might be rapid fluid movement in dentinal tubules during laser cutting, causing intradental nerve firing based on the hydrodynamic theory.

Lasers for Hypersensitive Teeth

In view of such a damaging effects of the Nd:YAG laser on the pulp, it is difficult to see how the lasing can be used to manage hypersensitive teeth. Because lasing alters the dentin surface, including blocking of dentin tubules by melted and glazing dentin, some clinicians advocate lasing of the hypersensitive dentin as the means of curing the disorder. Pashley's dentin permeability study showed that lasing the dentin surface using carbon dioxide and Nd:YAG systems did not provide sufficient blocking of the dentin tubules. However, other research[77] shows that the Nd:YAG system provides transient anesthesia in cat teeth up to 5 hours as measured with a sensory nerve recording technique. Thus successful results obtained in managing hypersensitive teeth using the various laser systems may be because of permanently damaged sensory nerves or transient anesthesia. These studies also indicate that lasing the hypersensitive dentin does not cause pain but desensitizes the tooth only temporarily (with a more severe return of the sensitivity after a short period). Thus at present the use of lasers for hypersensitive teeth has no biologic basis or benefit.

POSTOPERATIVE SENSITIVITY

Although postoperative discomfort is usually transient, it indicates that the restorative procedure has inflicted trauma on the tooth or the supporting structures. Severe, persistent pain almost certainly signifies that pulpal inflammation has resulted in hyperalgesia. Researchers[67] examined 40 patients who had received dental treatment involving insertion of amalgam and composite restorations. They found that 78% of the patients experienced some degree of postoperative discomfort. Sensitivity to cold was the most frequent complaint, whereas sensitivity to heat occurred much less often. Another study[31] found there was a positive correlation between heat sensitivity and pulpal inflammation. The significance of sensitivity to cold has not been fully established. Because the response occurs very soon after stimuli such as ice, cold water, and cold air come into contact with the tooth, it is believed that pain is caused by the stimulation of sensory nerve fibers of the pulp by hydrodynamic forces.[81] Because these fibers have a relatively low excitability threshold, they respond to low-level stimuli that do not necessarily produce tissue injury. However, the presence of hyperalgesia associated with inflammation produces an exaggerated response to cold. Sensitivity that develops soon after a restoration is placed may also be due to poor marginal adaptation, resulting in leakage of saliva under the filling.

Mechanisms of Hypersensitive Teeth

Tooth sensitivity to various stimuli is a persisting problem that affects as many as one of seven adult dental patients.[25] Although the clinical features of tooth hypersensitivity are well described, the exact causes and their physiologic mechanisms are only beginning to be understood.

Mechanisms   The enamel and cementum covering the dentin, and thus the dentinal nerves, are protective layers. When these protective layers are removed and the dentin tubules are exposed by various means (e.g., scaling, caries, fracture, restorative procedures), the teeth often become hypersensitive. Dentin sensitivity is the result of activation of Ad-type nerve fibers located in the dentinal tubules. Hypersensitivity is characterized as sharp, transient, and well localized. Two mechanisms account for the pain: (1) stimulation of the dentinal *nerves* and (2) dynamics of *exposed dentin.* These two mechanisms are interrelated.

According to the hydrodynamic theory, dentin sensitivity should be proportional to the hydraulic conductance of dentin. According to Pashley[53] the most important variable related to hydraulic conductance in dentin is the condition of the tubule aperture. Anything, or any agent, that makes the dentin hypoconducting by blocking the aperture alleviates the hypersensitive teeth syndrome.

Another mechanism involves the intradental nerves. Although the nerves themselves are unaffected, the environment surrounding them might be changed so that the normal stimuli, which under normal conditions do not evoke sensation, now evoke the sensation. The causes in the environment may be because of changes in ionic concentration (e.g., excessive sodium or potassium around the nerve terminals in the tubules as the result of pulpal inflammation or exposed dentin).

Hypersensitive teeth and inflamed pulps in many ways present the same symptoms, such as sensitivity to cold, air, and heat. Hypersensitivity because of inflammation of the pulp is the result of excitation of C fibers, which release neuropeptides (e.g., CGRP, substance P) in the pulp. These neuropeptides play a key role in neurogenic inflammation by increasing blood flow and capillary permeability. In the dental pulp in its low-compliance environment the increase in flow and permeability causes a dramatic increase in tissue pressure, which can lower the excitatory threshold level of the intradental nerves, resulting in hypersensitivity.

Management of Hypersensitive Dentin

Agents That Block Exposed Dentinal Tubules   As previously discussed, one of the two possible causes of hypersensitive teeth is exposed dentin. To block the exposed tubules would be a simple solution, but finding agents or instruments to do just that has turned out to be not that simple. After many years of experimentation clinicians still do not have an agent or agents that completely block the tubules. Nevertheless, there has been substantial progress in discovering an agent that blocks dentinal tubules sufficiently to reduce hypersensitivity. Using dentin permeability techniques and SEM examination of the dentin surface, Pashley[53] discovered that oxalate salts are effective agents to block dentinal tubules. Fig. 15-34 shows a dentin surface that was treated with oxalate salts for 2 minutes. When applied to the exposed dentin, potassium oxalate solution forms a microcrystal consisting of calcium oxalate. The calcium oxalate crystals are small enough to block the tubules and thus reduce hydraulic conductance. According to Pashley,[53] the oxalate salts reduced dentin permeability by more than 95%.

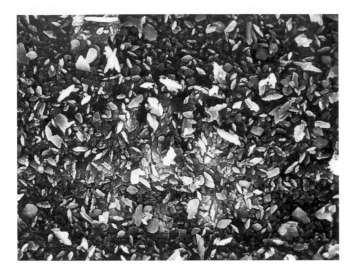

Fig. 15-34 Smear layer treated with 30% dipotassium oxalate for 2 minutes plus 3% monopotassium and monohydrogen oxalate for 2 minutes. Dentin surface is completely covered with calcium oxalate crystals (original magnification × 1900). (From Pashley DH, Galloway SE: The effects of oxalate treatment on the smear layer of ground surfaces of human dentins, *Arch Oral Biol* 30:731, 1985.)

Results of the clinical studies also agree with experimental results.

Agents That Reduce Intradental Nerve Excitability

The electrophysiologic method has been used to assess the function of the sensory nerves in response to various potentially useful chemical agents.[38] Sodium, lithium, and aluminum compounds have insignificant effects on reducing sensory nerve activity. Potassium compounds, however, were most effective ingredients for sensory nerve activity reduction. Important potassium compounds were potassium oxalate, potassium nitrate, and potassium bicarbonate. This finding lends credence to the hypothesis that reduction in sensory nerve activity is caused by the increase in potassium concentration around the nerve terminals in the dentinal tubules.

Fig. 15-35 provides the summary diagram illustrating the mechanisms and solutions to these problems. The far left-hand slice represents the sensitive dentin with open tubules. The second slice represents a smear layer covering the exposed dentin surface and occluding the dentinal tubules. However, this smear layer is extremely acid fibril and is easily removed; therefore it cannot be considered an effective way of managing the problem. The third slice represents other ways of occluding the dentinal tubules. Calcium oxalate is the crystallized product of the chemical reaction between potassium oxalate and dentinal calcium, and it is very effective in occluding the tubules. Calcium fluoride and silver nitrate are other agents that showed reasonable effectiveness. Tubular occlusion can also occur from the pulp side, mainly by plasma protein, especially fibrinogen, which is released from blood vessels.[56] The right-hand slice represents desensitization by altering nerve excitability by potassium and possibly by eugenol.

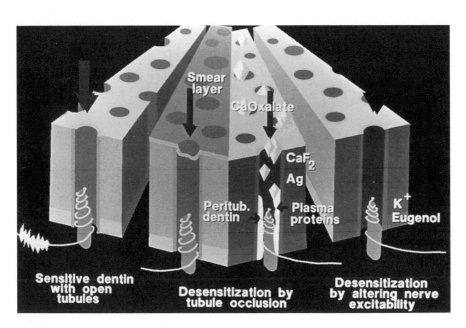

Fig. 15-35 Summary diagram illustrates the mechanisms and solutions to hypersensitivity problems. (Courtesy Dr. D.H. Pashley, Medical College of Georgia, Augusta, GA.)

CURRENT THINKING ON THE CAUSE OF PULPAL REACTION TO RESTORATION

In the past, pulp reactions to dental procedures were thought to be because of mechanical insults, such as frictional heat; generally this is true. The reaction to dental materials, on the other hand, has been attributed to chemical effects, such as acidity of the restorative materials. Although the chemical effects cannot be entirely discounted, especially in a deep cavity where only a very thin layer of dentin remains, in current thinking *pulpal injury is primarily due to microleakage through gaps between the filling material and the walls of the cavity.* It is believed that bacteria growing in these gaps elaborate products that diffuse through the dentinal tubules and irritate the pulp. It must be recognized that *all* permanent filling materials may allow these gaps to form. It is a miracle that all restored teeth do not show some degree of pulpal inflammation. On the other hand, it is not surprising that many teeth that have been restored require endodontic therapy. One study[5] reported that the quantity of bacterial toxins filtered from the base of a class V cavity depends on the type of restorative material used. The greatest amount of leakage occurred with silicate cements, followed by composite resins and amalgam fillings. Little or no leakage occurred when ZOE was used. Even full-crown restorations have been found to leak.

It is impossible to examine pulpal reactions without understanding structural and functional properties of the dentin. Pulp reactions begin when irritants make contact with the surface of the dentin. As the dentin's thickness decreases, the danger of pulpal reaction increases dramatically. A simple physiologic law of diffusion states that the rate of diffusion of substances depends on two factors: (1) the concentration gradient of the substances and (2) the surface area available for diffusion. Of importance in determining the extent of pulp reactions is the surface area of dentin available for diffusion. Because the dentinal tubules vary in diameter and density across the thickness of the dentin, the surface area (i.e., product of tubular area and density) available for diffusion varies from one region of the dentin to the other. Table 15-1 demonstrates the available dentin surface for diffusion at various distances from the pulp. For example, the diffusible surface area is 1% of the total dentin surface area at the dentin and enamel junction (DEJ), whereas it is 22% at the pulp. Thus the harmful effects of an insult increase significantly as the thickness of dentin over the pulp decreases.

The natural defense mechanisms of the tooth should be recognized. In some situations the dentinal tubules may become blocked by hydroxyapatite and other crystals, a condition known as dentinal sclerosis. Another reaction resulting in a decrease in dentin permeability is reparative dentin formation.

The smear layer also influences the permeability of dentin and thus protects the pulp by hindering the diffusion of toxic substances through the tubules.[57] According to one investigation, the smear layer accounts for 86% of the total resistance to flow fluid.[55] Thus acid etching, which removes the smear layer, greatly increases permeability by increasing the diffusible surface area (Fig. 15-36). The question arises of what to do with the smear layer. Should it be removed or left alone? Some authorities are of the opinion that it should be removed, because the smear layer may harbor bacteria. Yet the presence of a smear layer constitutes a physical barrier to bacterial penetration of the dentinal tubules.[44] However, another investigator demonstrated that the presence of the smear layer cannot prevent diffusion of bacterial products, although it effectively blocks actual bacterial invasion.[2] It has been shown that bacterial products reaching the pulp are capable of evoking an inflammatory response.[2] It follows that the best way to solve the problem is to remove the smear layer and replace it with a "sterile, nontoxic," artificial smear

Table 15-1   **SURFACE AREA OF DENTIN AVAILABLE FOR DIFFUSION AT VARIOUS DISTANCES FROM THE PULP**

Distance from Pulp (mm)	Number of Tubules (million/cm²) Mean	Range	Tubular Radius (cm × 10⁴) Mean	Range	Area of Surface (Ap) (%)* Mean	Range
	4.5	3.0-5.2	1.25	2.0-3.2	22.1	9-42
0.1-0.5	4.3	2.2-5.9	0.95	1.0-2.3	12.2	2-25
0.6-1.0	3.8	1.6-4.7	0.80	1.0-1.6	7.6	1-9.0
1.1-1.5	3.5	2.1-4.7	0.60	0.9-1.5	4.0	1-8.0
1.6-2.0	3.0	1.2-4.7	0.55	0.8-1.6	2.9	1-9.0
2.1-2.5	2.3	1.1-3.6	0.45	0.6-1.3	1.5	0.3-6
2.6-3.0	2.0	0.7-4.0	0.40	0.5-1.4	1.1	0.1-6
3.1-3.5	1.9	1.0-2.5	0.40	0.5-1.2	1.0	0.2-3

*$Ap = nr^2$, where n is the number of tubules/cm²; Ap represents the percentage of the total area of the physical surface available for diffusion. (Modified from: Garberoglio and Brännström [1976]; from Pashley DH: Smear layer: physiological consideration, *Oper Dent* 3:13, 1984.)

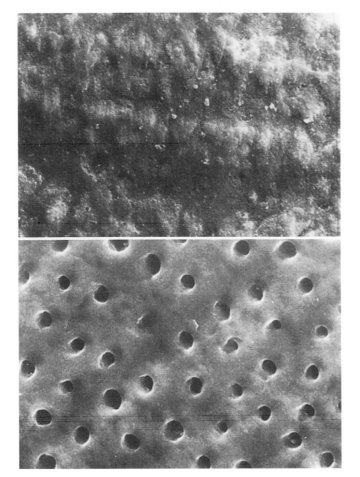

Fig. 15-36 Scanning electron microscopic photomicrographs of smear layer intact and smear layer removed. Notice the patent dentinal tubules. (Courtesy Dr. D.H. Pashley, Medical College of Georgia, Augusta, GA.)

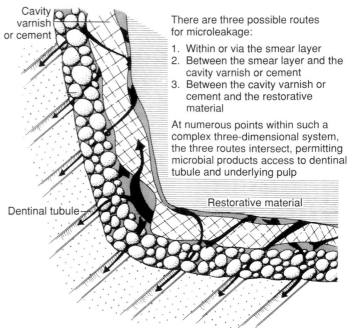

Fig. 15-37 Schematic representation of the interface of dentin and restorative material in a typical cavity. Granular constituents of the smear layer have been exaggerated out of their normal proportion for emphasis. Three theoretical routes for microleakage are indicated by arrows. (From Pashley DH et al: Effect of molecular size on permeability coefficients in human dentin, *Arch Oral Biol* 23:391, 1978.

layer. Research in the field has yielded some agents that look promising, two of which are potassium oxalate and 5% ferric oxalate.[9]

Because at the present time there is no material that can bond chemically to dentin and thus prevent leakage, the use of a cavity liner to seal dentin is highly recommended. According to one investigator, there are three possible routes for microleakage: (1) within or via the smear layer, (2) between the smear layer and the cavity varnish or cement, and (3) between the cavity varnish or cement and the restorative material (Fig. 15-37).[55]

COMPENSATORY PULPAL REACTION TO OUTSIDE INSULTS

Mechanisms exist by which the pulp is able to ward off insults. The ability of the pulp to deposit reparative dentin beneath a restoration is an excellent example. In addition, the vascular system is able to respond to mechanical insults. For example, it has been shown that deep drilling without proper water coolant causes a profound decrease in pulpal blood

flow in the area of injury. Blood is shunted away from the area by an abrupt increase in the flow of blood through arteriovenous anastomoses (AVA) or U-turn loops located in the dental pulp (Fig. 15-38). It is possible that opening of the previously closed AVA occurs as pulpal tissue pressure increases to critical levels. The opening of the AVA is a compensatory mechanism of the pulp to maintain blood flow within physiologically normal limits (see Fig. 15-38).

It should be remembered that the pulp is a very resilient tissue and that is has a great potential for healing. It is only when all compensatory mechanisms fail that the pulp becomes necrotic. Fig. 15-39 depicts the current thinking on the pathophysiologic mechanisms involved in pulp necrosis. Because the pulp is rigidly encased in mineralized tissues, it is protected from most forms of trauma to which the tooth is exposed. Nevertheless, insults (e.g., dental caries, restorative procedures) are capable of producing localized inflammatory lesions in the pulp. The tissue adjacent to the inflammatory lesion may show no sign of inflammation, and physiologic analysis may reveal no abnormalities. Thus investigators found that pulpal tissue pressure near a site of localized inflammation was almost normal.[78] This indicates that tissue pressure changes do not spread rapidly. Similar findings have been reported by another researcher.[84]

Local insults cause inflammation by triggering the release of various inflammatory mediators and reducing vascular reactivity. These mediators produce vasodilation and decrease the flow resistance in the resistance vessels. Vasodi-

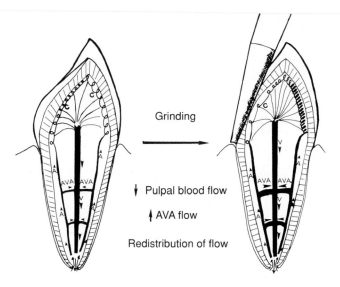

Grinding

↓ Pulpal blood flow

↕ AVA flow

Redistribution of flow

Fig. 15-38 Schematic representation of the changes in pulpal blood flow distribution in response to dry preparation. Notice there is an increase in flow through the arteriovenous anastomoses.

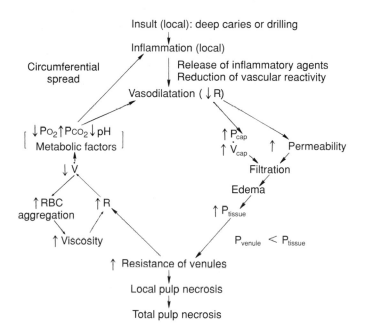

Insult (local): deep caries or drilling

Inflammation (local)

Circumferential spread

Release of inflammatory agents
Reduction of vascular reactivity

Vasodilatation (↓ R)

[↓Po₂ ↑Pco₂ ↓pH]
Metabolic factors

↓ V

↑RBC aggregation   ↑R

↑ Viscosity

↑ Resistance of venules

Local pulp necrosis

Total pulp necrosis

↑P_{cap}
↑$\dot{V}_{cap}$ ↑ Permeability

Filtration

Edema

↑ P_{tissue}

$P_{venule} < P_{tissue}$

Fig. 15-39 Pathophysiologic mechanism of pulp inflammation and necrosis. This hypothetical mechanism is constructed from the results of many structural and functional investigations.

lation and decreased flow resistance cause an increase in both intravascular pressure and blood flow in the capillaries, which in turn precipitate an increase in vascular permeability, favoring filtration of serum proteins and fluid from the vessels. As a result, the tissue becomes edematous. This results in an increase in the tissue pressure. Because the pulp is encased in mineralized tissue, it is in a low-compliance environment. As the tissue pressure increases it may exceed that of the venules, in which case the venules are compressed (producing an increase in flow resistance). This, in turn,

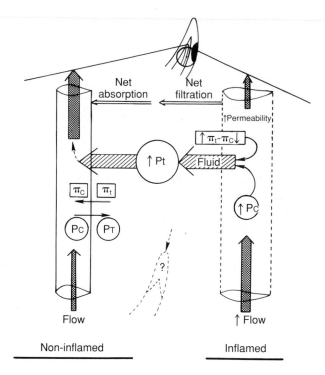

Net absorption   Net filtration

↑Permeability

↑π_t-π_C↓

Fluid

↑ Pt

π_C π_t

↑Pc

Pc   PT

Flow   ↑ Flow

Non-inflamed   Inflamed

Fig. 15-40 Schematic representation of the compensatory mechanism of the pulp during inflammation. *PC* and *PT*, hydrostatic pressure of capillary and tissue, respectively; pc and pt, osmotic pressure of capillary and tissue, respectively.

results in a decrease in blood flow, because the venous drainage is impeded. The sluggish blood flow causes the red blood cells to aggregate, resulting in an elevation of blood viscosity. This vicious cycle leads to even greater problems by producing hypoxia; thus suppressing cellular metabolism in the affected area of the pulp. The stagnation of blood flow not only causes rheologic changes (i.e., red blood cell aggregation, increased blood viscosity), it also causes an increase in carbon dioxide and a decrease in pH levels in the blood. The increase in PCO₂ results from impaired removal of waste products from the tissue. These changes in local metabolism lead to vasodilation in the adjacent area and the gradual spread of inflammation. The spread of inflammation is circumferential as was demonstrated in an elegant experiment by Van Hassel.[84] Thus total pulp necrosis is the gradual accumulation of local necroses.

It has been shown that the pulp has tremendous healing potential. This raises the question as to how the pulp recovers from the adverse effects of localized inflammation. Although the exact physiologic mechanisms are not yet known, recent research findings suggest the following. First, as the tissue pressure increases as a result of an increase in blood flow, the AVA or the U-turn loop vessels open and shunt the blood before it reaches the inflamed region of the coronal pulp. This prevents a further increase in blood flow and tissue pressure. Also the increase in tissue pressure pushes macromolecules back into the bloodstream via the venules in the adjacent healthy region (Fig. 15-40). Once the macromolecules and accompanying fluid leave the extracellular tissue space through the venule, the tissue pressure decreases and normal blood flow is restored.

Prevention

To preserve the integrity of the pulp, the dentist should observe certain precautions while rendering treatment. The following is a list of dos and don'ts that should prevent or minimize injury to the pulp:

- Cutting procedures: Use light, intermittent cutting, an efficient cooling system, and high speeds of rotation.
- Avoid desiccating the dentin: Do not overdry the cavity preparation.
- Do not apply irritating chemicals to freshly cut dentin.
- Choose restorative materials carefully, considering the physical and biologic properties of the material.
- Do not use caustic cavity sterilizing agents.
- Assume that all restorative materials will leak: Use a cavity liner or base to seal the openings of exposed dentinal tubules.
- Do not use excessive force when inserting a restoration.
- Employ polishing procedures that do not subject the pulp to excessive heat.
- Establish a patient recall system that ensures periodic evaluation of the status of pulps that have been exposed to injury.

(Supported in part by NIDR grants DEO-5605 and DEO-0121.)

References

1. Alperstein KS, Graver HT, Herold RCB: Marginal leakage of glass-ionomer cement restorations, *J Prosthet Dent* 50:803, 1983.
2. Bergenholtz G: Effect of bacterial products on inflammatory reactions in the dental pulp, *Scand J Dent Res* 85:122, 1977.
3. Bergenholtz G: Pathogenic mechanisms in pulpal disease. *J Endod* 16:98, 1990.
4. Bergenholtz G, Cox CF, Loesche WJ, Syed SA: Bacterial leakage around dental restorations: its effect on the dental pulp, *J Oral Pathol* 11:439, 1982.
5. Bergenholtz G, Reit C: Reactions of the dental pulp to microbial provocation of calcium hydroxide treated dentin, *Scand J Dent Res* 88:187, 1980.
6. Berggren H: The reaction of the translucent zone to dyes and radioisotopes, *Acta Odontol Scand* 23:197, 1965.
7. Bjorndal L, Darvann T: A light microscopic study of odontoblastic and non-odontoblastic cells involved in tertiary dentinogenesis in well-defined cavitated carious lesions, *Caries Res* 33:50, 1998.
8. Bjorndal L, Darvann T, Thylstrup A: A Quantitative light microscopic study of the odontoblast and subodontoblastic reactions to active and arrested enamel caries without cavitation, *Caries Res* 32:59, 1998.
9. Bowen RL, Cobb EN, Rapson JE: Adhesive bonding of various materials to hard tooth tissues: improvement in bond strength to dentin, *J Dent Res* 61:1070, 1982.
10. Brännström M: A new approach to insulation, *Dent Pract* 19:417, 1969.
11. Brännström M: Communication between the oral cavity and the dental pulp associated with restorative treatment, *Oper Dent* 9:57, 1984.
12. Brännström M: *Dentin and pulp in restorative dentistry,* London, 1982, Wolfe Medical Publications Ltd.
13. Brännström M, Lind PO: Pulpal response to early dental caries, *J Dent Res* 44:1045, 1965.
14. Brännström M et al: Protective effect of polystyrene liners for composite resin restorations, *J Prosthet Dent* 49:331, 1983.
15. Brännström M, Vojinovic O, Nordenvall KJ: Bacterial and pulpal reactions under silicate cement restorations, *J Prosthet Dent* 41:290, 1979.
16. Brodin E et al: Tissue concentration and release of substance P-like immunoreactivity in the dental pulp, *Acta Physiol Scand* 111:141, 1981.
17. Brown WS, Christensen DO, Lloyd BA: Numerical and experimental evaluation of energy inputs, temperature gradients, and thermal stresses during restorative procedures, *J Am Dent Assoc* 96:451, 1978.
18. Chaiyavej S et al: Intradental nerve response to tooth cutting by Er:YAG laser, *J Dent Res* 79(special issue):175, 2000.
19. Chiego DJ Jr, Wang RF, Avery JK: Ultrastructural changes in odontoblasts and nerve terminals after cavity preparations, *J Dent Res* 68(special issue):1023, 1989 (abstract 1251).
20. Cox CF et al: Biocompatibility of various surface-sealed dental materials against exposed pulps, *J Prosthet Dent* 57:1, 1987.
21. Featherstone J, Nelson D: Laser effects on dental hard tissue, *Adv Dent Res* 1:21, 1987.
22. Felton D: Long term effects of crown preparation on pulp vitality, *J Dent Res* 68(special issue):1009, 1989 (abstract 1139).
23. Frank RM: Reactions of dentin and pulp to drugs and restorative materials, *J Dent Res* 54:176, 1975.
24. Friedman S, Liu M, Dörscher-Kim J, Kim S: In-situ testing of CO2 laser on dental pulp function: the effects on microcirculation, *Lasers Surg Med* 11:325, 1991.
25. Graf H, Galasse R: Mobidity, prevalence and intraoral distribution of hypersensitive teeth, *J Dent Res* 162(special issue A): 2, 1977.
26. Graver T, Trowbridge H, Alperstein K: Microleakage of castings cemented with glass ionomer cements, *Oper Dent* 15(1):2, 1990.
27. Heys DR et al: Histologic and bacterial evaluation of conventional and new copper amalgams, *J Oral Pathol* 8:65, 1979.
28. Holden GP: Some observations on the vibratory phenomena associated with high-speed air turbines and their transmission to living tissue, *Br Dent J* 113:265, 1962.
29. Jendresen M, Trowbridge H: Biologic and physical properties of a zinc polycarboxylate cement, *J Prosthet Dent* 28:264, 1972.
30. Johnson NW, Taylor BR, Berman DS: The response of deciduous dentine to caries studied by correlated light and electron microscopy, *Caries Res* 3:348, 1969.
31. Johnson RH, Daichi SF, Haley JV: Pulpal hyperemia: a correlation of clinical and histological data from 706 teeth, *J Am Dent Assoc* 81:108, 1970.
32. Jontell M, Okiji T, Dahlgren U, Bergenholtz G: Immune defense mechanisms of the dental pulp, *Crit Rev Oral Biol Med* 9(2):179, 1998.

33. Kakehashi S, Stanley HR, Fitzgerald RJ: The effects of surgical exposures of pulps in germ-free and conventional rats, *Oral Surg* 20:340, 1965.

34. Kamal A, Okiji T, Kawashima N, Suda H: Defense responses of dentin/pulp complex to experimentally induced caries in rat molars: an immunohistochemical study on kinetics of pulpal Ia antigen-expressing cells and macrophages, *J Endod* 23:115, 1997.

35. Karkalainen S, LeBell Y: Odontoblast response to caries. In Thylstrup A, Leach SA, Qvist V, editors: *Dentine and dentine reactions in the oral cavity,* Oxford, 1987, IRL Press.

36. Kawahara H, Imanishi Y, Oshima H: Biological evaluation of glass ionomer cement, *J Dent Res* 58:1080, 1979.

37. Kelley KW, Bergenholtz G, Cox CF: The extent of the odontoblast process in rhesus monkeys *(Macaca mulatta)* as observed by scanning electron microscopy, *Arch Oral Biol* 26:893, 1981.

38. Kim S: Hypersensitive teeth: desensitization of pulpal sensory nerves, *J Endod* 12:482, 1986.

39. Kim S: Ligamental injection: a physiological explanation of its efficacy, *J Endod* 12:486, 1986.

40. Kim S, Edwall L, Trowbridge H, Chien S: Effects of local anesthetics on pulpal blood flow in dogs, *J Dent Res* 63:650, 1984.

41. Kumazaki M, Toyoda K: Removal of hard tissue (cavity preparation) with Er:YAG laser, *J Jpn Soc Laser Dent* 6:16, 1995.

42. Magloire H et al: Ultrastructural alterations of human odontoblasts and collagen fibers in the pulpal border zone beneath early caries lesions, *Cell Molec Biol* 27:437, 1981.

43. Massler M: Pulpal reaction to dentinal caries, *J Dent Res* 17:441, 1967.

44. Michelich VJ, Schuster GS, Pashley DH: Bacterial penetration of human dentin in vitro, *J Dent Res* 59:1398, 1980.

45. Mullaney TP, Laswell HR: Iatrogenic blushing of dentin following full crown preparation, *J Prosthet Dent* 22:354, 1969.

46. Nelson RJ, Wolcott RB, Paffenbarger GC: Fluid exchange at the margins of dental restorations, *J Am Dent Assoc* 44:288, 1952.

47. Newman SM: Microleakage of a copal rosin cavity varnish, *J Prosthet Dent* 51:499, 1984.

48. Nyborg H, Brännström M: Pulp reaction to heat, *J Prosthet Dent* 19:605, 1968.

49. Ohshima H et al: Responses of immunocompetent cells to cavity preparation in rat molars: an immunohistochemical study using OX6-monoclonal antibody, *Connect Tissue Res* 32:303, 1995.

50. Okamura K et al: Dentinal response against carious invasion: localization of antibodies in odontoblastic body and process, *J Dent Res* 59:1368, 1980.

51. Okiji T et al: Structural and functional association between substance-P and calcitonin gene-related peptide-immunoreactive nerves and accessory cells in the rat dental pulp, *J Dent Res* 76:1818, 1997.

52. Olgart L, Gazalius B: Effects of adrenaline and felypressin (Octapressin) on blood flow and sensory nerve activity on the tooth, *Acta Odontol Scand* 35:69, 1977.

53. Pashley DH: Dentin permeability, dentin sensitivity and treatment through tubule occlusion, *J Endod* 12:465, 1986.

54. Pashley DH: The influence of dentin permeability and pulpal blood flow on pulpal solute concentrations, *J Endod* 5:355, 1979.

55. Pashley DH: Smear layer: physiological consideration, *Oper Dent* 3:13, 1984.

56. Pashley DH, Galloway SE, Stewart F: Effects of fibrinogen in vivo on dentin permeability in the dog, *Arch Oral Biol* 29:725, 1984.

57. Pashley DH, Michelich V, Kehl T: Dentin permeability: effects of smear layer removal, *J Prosthet Dent* 46:531, 1981.

58. Plant CG, Jones DW: The damaging effects of restorative materials. I. Physical and chemical properties, *Br Dent J* 140:373, 1976.

59. Pogrel M, Muff D, Marshall G: Structural changes in dental enamel induced by high energy continuous wave carbon dioxide laser, *Lasers Surg Med* 13:89, 1993.

60. Pohto M, Scheinin A: Microscopic observations on living dental pulp. IV. The effects of oil of clove and eugenol on the circulation of the pulp in the rat's lower incisor, *Dent Abstr* 5:405, 1960.

61. Qvist V: The effect of mastication on marginal adaptation of composite restorations in vivo, *J Dent Res* 62:904, 1983.

62. Reeves R, Stanley HR: The relationship of bacterial penetration and pulpal pathosis in carious teeth, *Oral Surg* 22:59, 1966.

63. Sakurai K, Okiji T, Suda H: Co-increase of nerve fibers and HLA-DR-and/or Factor-XIIIa-expressing dendritic cells in dentinal caries-affected regions of the human dental pulp: an immunohistochemcial study, *J Dent Res* 78(10):1596, 1999.

64. Scott JN, Weber DF: Microscopy of the junctional region between human coronal primary and secondary dentin, *J Morphol* 154:133, 1977.

65. Sekine Y et al: Histopathologic study of Er:YAG laser application to cavity preparation, *Japan J Conserv Dent* 38:211, 1995.

66. Shamul J: *Effects of pulsed Nd:YAG laser on pulpal blood flow in cat teeth,* master's thesis, New York, 1992, Columbia University.

67. Silvestri AR, Cohen SN, Wetz JH: Character and frequency of discomfort immediately following restorative procedures, *J Am Dent Assoc* 95:85, 1977.

68. Sneed WD, Hembree JH, Welsh EL: Effectiveness of three varnishes in reducing leakage of a high-copper amalgam, *Oper Dent* 9:32, 1984.

69. Son HG, Kim S, Kim SB: Pulpal blood flow and bonding, *J Dent Res* 65 (special issue):726, 1986.

70. Stanley HR: Pulpal response. In Cohen S and Burns R, editors: *Pathways of the pulp,* ed 3, St Louis, 1984, Mosby.

71. Stanley HR, Going RE, Chauncey HH: Human pulp response to acid pretreatment of dentin and to composite restoration, *J Am Dent Assoc* 91:817, 1975.

72. Stanley HR et al: The detection and prevalence of reactive and physiologic sclerotic dentin, reparative dentin and dead tracts beneath various types of dental lesions according to tooth surface and age, *J Pathol* 12:257, 1983.

73. Suda H, Sunakawa M, Ikeda H, Yamamoto H: A neurophysiological evaluation of intraligamentary anesthesia, *Dent Jpn (Tokyo)* 31:46, 1994.

74. Swerdlow H, Stanley HR: Reaction of human dental pulp to cavity preparation. I. Effect of water spray at 20,000 RPM, *J Am Dent Assoc* 56:317, 1958.

75. Swerdlow H, Stanley HR: Reaction of human dental pulp to cavity preparation, *J Prosthet Dent* 9:121, 1959.

76. Taylor PE, Byers MR, Redd PE: Sprouting of CGRP nerve fibers in response to dentin injury in rat molars, *Brain Res* 461: 371, 1988.
77. Tokita Y, Sunakawa M, Suda H: Pulsed Nd:YAG laser irradiation of the tooth pulp in the cat: I. Effect of spot lasing. *Lasers Surg Med* 26(4):398, 2000.
78. Tönder K, Kvinnsland I: Micropuncture measurement of interstitial tissue pressure in normal and inflamed dental pulp in cats, *J Endod* 9:105, 1983.
79. Trowbridge HO: Pathogenesis of pulpitis resulting from dental caries, *J Endod* 7:52, 1981.
80. Trowbridge HO, Edwall L, Panopoulos P: Effect of zinc oxide and eugenol and calcium hydroxide on intradental nerve activity, *J Endod* 8:403, 1982.
81. Trowbridge HO, Franks M, Korostoff E, Emling R: Sensory response to thermal stimulation in human teeth, *J Endod* 6(1): 405, 1980.
82. Trowbridge HO, Scott D, Singer J: Effects of eugenol on nerve excitability, *J Dent Res* 56:115, 1977.
83. Turner DF, Marfurt CF, Sattleberg C: Demonstration of physiological barrier between pulpal odontoblasts and its perturbation following routine restorative procedures: horseradish peroxidase tracing study in the rat, *J Dent Res* 68:1261, 1989.
84. Van Hassel HJ: Physiology of the human dental pulp. In Siskin M, editor: *The biology of the human dental pulp,* St Louis, 1973, Mosby.
85. Watts A: Bacterial contamination and toxicity of silicate and zinc phosphate cements, *Br Dent J* 146:7, 1979.
86. White J, Goodis H, Daniel T: Effects of Nd:YAG cases on pulps of extracted teeth, *Lasers Life Sci* 4:191, 1991.
87. Zach L: Pulp liability and repair: effect of restorative procedures, *Oral Surg* 33:111, 1972.
88. Zennyu K et al: Transmission of Nd:YAG laser through human dentin *J Japan Soc Laser Dent* 7:37, 1996.

PART THREE

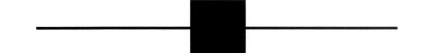

Related Clinical Topics

Chapter 16

 # Traumatic Injuries

Martin Trope, Noah Chivian, Asgeir Sigurdsson, William F. Vann, Jr.

Chapter Outline

INCIDENCE

Dental injuries can occur at any age; however, they are most common between the ages of 8 and 12, when children are most active. Childhood dental injuries as a result of bicycle, skateboard, playground, or sports accidents can affect the permanent teeth.[121,131] By the time students complete high school it is estimated that as many as one out of three boys and one out of four girls will have suffered a dental injury.[131] This seemingly high incidence of injuries to the permanent teeth is the result of the collective activities of young people throughout their school years. One fourth of dental injuries in public schools have been observed to be because of fighting and pushing.[47,59,110]

During high school the increased participation of boys and girls in sports increases the risk of dental injury. Before the 1960s, boys had three times as many injuries as girls.

603

However, the increase in women's athletics has reduced this ratio: today boys have just one and one half as many injuries as girls.[85,178]

The tooth that is most vulnerable to injury is the maxillary central incisor, which sustains approximately 80% of dental injuries. This is followed by the maxillary lateral and the mandibular central and lateral incisors.[85,176]

HISTORY AND CLINICAL EXAMINATION

Dental injuries are never convenient for the patient or the clinician. Consequently, one of the challenges facing clinicians is to control the situation in the dental office by calming the patient or parents or both and taking the necessary time to conduct a qualitative evaluation of the patient's injuries. Without such control by the clinician, significant injuries are easily missed in the haste of the moment.

The medical history (see Fig. 1-2) is fundamental to all evaluation and treatment of the patient. Even local anesthesia cannot be administered safely without the completion of a standard medical questionnaire.

History of the Accident

The *when, how,* and *where* of the accident are significant.[14] *When* the accident occurred is most important. With the passage of time, blood clots begin to form, periodontal ligaments of teeth dry out, and saliva contaminates the wound; these conditions influence the decisions that need to be made concerning the sequence of treatment.

Understanding *how* the accident occurred will assist the clinician in locating specific injuries. A blow to the lips and anterior teeth could possibly cause crown, root, or bone fractures to the anterior region and is therefore less likely to injure the posterior regions. A blow under the chin or jaw could cause fractures to any tooth in the mouth. A padded blow (e.g., a fall against a covered chair arm) could cause a root fracture or tooth displacement, whereas a hard blow (e.g., a fall on a concrete walk) would tend to cause coronal fractures.

Where the trauma occurred becomes significant for prognosis. The necessity for prophylactic tetanus toxoid is influenced by the location of the accident. Where the trauma occurred may also be significant for insurance and litigation purposes.

Another important question to ask is whether treatment of any kind has been given for the injury by a parent, coach, physician, school nurse, teacher, or ambulance attendant. A normal-appearing tooth may have been replanted or repositioned previously by any of these individuals or by the patient, and this will influence the prognosis for treatment and sequence of treatment.

Clinical Examination

Chief Complaint   Aside from pain and bleeding, there may be a specific complaint that will assist in the diagnosis. If the complaint is that the teeth "Don't fit together now!" the clinician must consider possible displacements or a bone fracture. Pain that occurs *only* when the patient closes the teeth together could indicate crown, root, or bone fractures or displacement.

Neurologic Examination   While the clinician is obtaining the history of the accident and chief complaint, the patient should be observed for neurologic or other medical complications[35] (Box 16-1). Dental injuries may occur

---

Box 16-1   **OUTLINE OF INITIAL NEUROLOGIC ASSESSMENT FOR THE PATIENT WITH TRAUMATIC DENTAL INJURIES**

Notice unusual communication or motor functions.
Look for normal respiration without obstruction of the airway or danger of aspiration.
Replant avulsed teeth as indicated.
Obtain a medical history and information on the accident.
Determine blood pressure and pulse.
Examine for rhinorrhea or otorrhea.
Evaluate function of the eyes—Is diplopia or nystagmus apparent? Are pupillary activity and movement of the eyes normal?
Evaluate movement of the neck—Is there pain or limitation?
Examine the sensitivity of the surface of the facial skin—Is paresthesia or anesthesia apparent?
Confirm that there is normal vocal function.
Confirm patient's ability to protrude the tongue.
Confirm hearing—Is tinnitus or vertigo apparent?
Evaluate the sense of smell.
Ensure follow-up evaluation.

From Croll TP et al: *J Am Dent Assoc* 100:530, 1980.

simultaneously with other head and neck injuries. A note should be made of whether the patient is communicating coherently. Does the patient have difficulty focusing or rotating the eyes or breathing? Can the patient turn the head from side to side? Is there any paresthesia of the lips or tongue? Does the patient complain of ringing in the ears? Has the patient experienced persistent headaches, dizziness, drowsiness, or vomiting since the accident? Airway obstruction by dental appliances must also be considered.

Before analgesics are prescribed or sedation by inhalation of nitrous oxide and oxygen is used, the clinician must be satisfied that there are no neurologic injuries.[35,90] If there is any question about this, the patient should be referred immediately for appropriate medical treatment.

External Examination   Before having the patient open the mouth for an intraoral examination, the clinician should first look for external signs of injury. Lacerations of the head and neck are easily detected. However, deviations of normal bone contours must be closely investigated. The temporomandibular joint (TMJ) should be palpated externally while the patient opens and closes. Does the patient's opening and closing pattern deviate to either side? If so, this could indicate a unilateral mandibular fracture. Similarly, the zygomatic arch, angle, and lower border of the mandible should be bilaterally palpated and note made of any areas of tenderness, swelling, or bruising of the face, cheek, neck, or lips. They could be clues to possible bone fractures.

Intraoral Soft-Tissue Examination   Next the clinician should look for lacerations of the lips, tongue, cheek, palate, and floor of the mouth. The facial and lingual gingivae and oral mucosa are palpated, with note made of areas of tenderness, swelling, or bruising. The anterior border of the ramus of the mandible is palpated. Any abnormal findings suggest possible tooth or bone injuries, and further radiographic examination of the area is indicated. Lacerations of the lips and tongue must be felt and radiographed for embedded foreign objects.[29,76]

Hard-Tissue Examination   One of the best examinations for evidence of traumatic injuries is simply to look carefully. Each tooth and its supporting structures must be examined with an explorer and periodontal probe. Basic questions (e.g., Is the occlusal plane disturbed? Are there any missing teeth?) must be answered before any thermal or electric tests are begun.

Initially, the examiner looks for gross evidence of injury. If several teeth are out of alignment, a bone fracture is the most reasonable explanation. The mandible should be examined for fractures by placing the forefinger on the occlusal plane of the posterior teeth with the thumbs under the mandible. Then the clinician should rock the mandible from side to side and from anterior to posterior. A mandibular fracture will cause discomfort with these motions, and the grating sound of broken fragments may be heard.[29] Gentle-

but-firm pressure should be used to prevent possible additional trauma to the inferior alveolar nerve and blood vessels.

The clinician can also try to move the individual teeth with finger pressure. Any looseness is indicative of displacement from the alveolar socket; movement of several teeth together is evidence of an alveolar fracture. Mobility of the crown must be differentiated from the mobility of the tooth. In instances of coronal fractures the crown will be mobile but the tooth will remain in position. Occasionally root fractures can be felt by placing a finger on the mucosa over the tooth and moving the crown.

Any freshly fractured cusps or incisal edge fractures should be recorded. Incomplete cusp fractures can be noted by using the tip of a dental explorer as a wedge in the occlusal grooves of the posterior teeth to elicit movement of any cusps. The patient may be asked to bite on a rubber-polishing wheel with each tooth (in succession) to locate tenderness that could indicate an incomplete cusp fracture or displaced tooth.

Each incisal edge and cusp can be gently percussed with the mirror handle to locate incomplete fractures or teeth that have been slightly displaced from the alveolar socket. Accumulation of extravasated fluid and tearing of periodontal fibers around a minimally displaced tooth will make the tooth tender to percussion.

Hemorrhage in the gingival sulcus may indicate a displaced tooth or tooth segment. Any discoloration of the teeth should be noted; viewing from the lingual surface of anterior teeth with a reflected light will help.

Obvious pulp exposures should be noted. Crown fractures with minute pulp exposures can be detected with a cotton pellet soaked in saline and pressed against the area of the suspected exposure.[14] The mechanical pressure of the cotton against an exposure will elicit a response. A dry cotton pellet can confuse the diagnosis by dehydrating dentinal tubules in a near exposure, causing pain sensation. Therefore it should not be used.

When the visual examination is complete and all abnormal findings are noted, radiographs of the injured areas should be taken. These can be processed while additional tests are being conducted.

Thermal and Electric Tests   A few general statements in regard to pulp tests on traumatized teeth may be helpful in trying to interpret the results. (See Chapter 1 for specific descriptions of pulp tests.)

For decades, controversy has surrounded the validity of thermal and electric tests on traumatized teeth. Only generalized impressions may be gained from these tests subsequent to a traumatic injury. They are, in reality, sensitivity tests for nerve function and do *not* indicate the presence or absence of blood circulation within the pulp. It is assumed that, subsequent to traumatic injury, the conduction capability of the nerve endings or sensory receptors or both is sufficiently deranged to inhibit the nerve impulse from an electric or thermal stimulus. This makes the traumatized tooth vulnerable to false negative readings from these tests.

The clinician should not assume that teeth that give a positive response at the initial examination are healthy or that they will continue to give a positive response. Teeth that yield a negative response (or no response) cannot be assumed to have necrotic pulps, because they may give a positive response later. It has been demonstrated that it may take as long as 9 months for normal blood flow to return to the coronal pulp of a traumatized, fully formed tooth. As circulation is restored, the responsiveness to pulp tests returns.[60]

The transition from a negative to a positive response at a subsequent test may be considered a sign of a healthy pulp. The repetitious finding of positive responses may be taken as a sign of a healthy pulp, and the transition from a positive to a negative response may be taken as an indication that the pulp is probably undergoing degeneration. The persistence of a negative response would suggest that the pulp has been irreversibly damaged, but even this is not absolute.[23]

In testing teeth for response to cold, the dry ice pencil (i.e., carbon dioxide stick) is the most effective test. It gives more accurate responses than does a water ice pencil, because the intense cold ($-78°$ C) seems to penetrate the tooth and covering splints or restorations and reach the deeper areas of the tooth. In addition, dry ice does not form ice water, which could disperse over adjacent teeth or gingiva to give a false-positive response. Thermal and electric pulp tests of all teeth in the traumatized area should be performed at the time of the initial examination and carefully recorded to establish a baseline for comparison with subsequent repeated tests in later months. These tests should be repeated at 3 weeks; 3, 6, and 12 months; and at yearly intervals after the accident. The purpose of the tests is to establish a trend as to the physiologic status of the pulps of these teeth (see Chapter 1).

Radiographic Examinations   Radiographs are essential to the thorough examination of traumatized hard tissue. They may reveal root fractures, subgingival crown fractures, tooth displacements, bone fractures, or foreign objects.

However, the fracture line may run in a mesiodistal direction in the tooth and not be evident on the radiograph. Also the fracture line may be diagonal in a facial lingual direction and not obvious on the film. Similarly, a hairline fracture may not be evident on the radiograph at the initial examination but may later become obvious as tissue fluids and mobility spread the broken parts.

In instances of soft-tissue laceration it is advisable to radiograph the injured area before suturing to be sure that no foreign objects have been embedded. A soft-tissue radiograph with a normal-sized film that is briefly exposed at a reduced kilo-voltage should reveal the presence of many foreign substances, including tooth fragments.

In reviewing the films of traumatized teeth, special attention should be directed to the dimension of the root canal space, the degree of apical closure of the root, the proximity of fractures to the pulp, and the relationship of root fractures to the alveolar crest. Whereas conventional periapical films are generally useful, an occlusal or Panorex film can supplement them when the examiner is looking for bone fractures or the presence of foreign objects.

In summary, the examination of traumatic injuries must be thorough and meticulously recorded. Some type of insurance covers most injuries, and many will eventually be involved in litigation. When asked to describe the condition of the patient at the time of the initial examination, months or years after the accident, the dentist will find a completely documented patient record, including quality radiographs, to be of immense assistance. These records form the basis for the justification of subsequent treatment and the associated professional fees. In addition, the rapid increase in professional liability claims against dentists further emphasizes the need for complete-and-accurate patient records (described in greater detail in Chapter 10).

PREVENTION OF DENTAL INJURIES

Wearing a face guard or mouth guard or both is the best way to effectively prevent (or significantly reduce) dental injuries when participating in sports in which there is a risk of falling or being hit by an object. It has been reported that before the mandate of wearing face and mouth guards in U.S. high school football, facial and oral injuries constituted up to 50% of all reported football injuries.[31] Subsequent to that mandate a significant drop was noted in reported injuries.[89]

Face Guards

Face guards are usually prefabricated, cage-type guards that are attached to helmets or helmet straps. Recently, face guards (either prefabricated or custom-made) of clear polycarbonate plastic have become available. All of these face guards provide good protection to the face and the teeth, but they are not applicable to all activities and do not protect the teeth if the individual is hit under the chin.

Mouth Guards

Several studies have shown that a good mouth guard is very effective in reducing the severity and number of dental injuries.[89,120] In a recent in vitro study using sheep mandibles it was shown that it required fourteenfold more force to cause an injury to a tooth that was covered with a custom-made mouth guard compared with an unprotected tooth.[83] It has been speculated that in addition to tooth protection, mouth guards could also reduce the likelihood of brain concussion, cerebral hemorrhage, and brain stem damage[83] by absorbing some of the forces when an athlete is hit under the chin.

There are three types of mouth guards on the market: (1) the stock mouth guard; (2) the mouth-formed, or boil-and-bite, mouth guard; and (3) the custom-made mouth guard.

The stock mouth guard is the preformed rubber or polyvinyl-type polymer guard. The main benefit of this type of mouth guard is that it is inexpensive and ready to use without modifications. It is also usable for children with mixed dentition and patients with orthodontic brackets. All studies have proven[48,61,134] that this type of mouth guard provides the least protection of all available types because of its poor fit. Additionally it is rather uncomfortable for the wearer because it tends to obstruct speech and breathing (because the wearer is required to keep it in place by either clenching the teeth together or supporting the mouth guard with the lips or tongue or both).

The second main type is often referred to as the mouth-formed, or boil-and-bite, mouth guard. There are two basic types of these mouth guards. The first type of mouth-formed mouth guard is a preformed shell of semirigid polyvinyl with an inner lining of silicone or plasticized acrylic gel. The gel is mixed and allowed to set in the mouth, covering the maxillary teeth (resulting in increased retention of the mouth guard). Initially many of these types of mouth guards fit fairly well and have some retention, but over time the inner lining has the tendency to creep or spread, causing decreased retention. The second type of mouth-formed mouth guard is a preformed thermoplastic copolymer of polyvinyl acetate and polyethylene. This prefabricated mouth guard is softened for a few seconds in hot or boiling water and then placed in the athlete's mouth and adapted to the dentition. These mouth guards tend to be bulky, especially those lined with silicone. Mouth guards that are heated and then adapted to the teeth can be a good alternative to a custom-made mouth guard, especially if formed by a dental professional. They are especially valuable for those athletes that have fixed orthodontic appliances.

The third main type of mouth guard is the custom-made version. These mouth guards are fabricated on a plaster cast, usually of the upper dentition and surrounding tissues, and are made of polyvinyl acetate and polyethylene or other rubber materials that are heated and then either vacuumed down on the cast or pressured down with positive pressure. This mouth guard is by far the best available protection and offers the most comfort for the wearer.[48,109] However, they are the most expensive to make. Recently several modifications have been offered, including multilaminated stock sheets that have harder inserts to further support the palatal side of the incisors (Fig. 16-1).

To gain maximal benefit from this type of mouth guard, several steps must be properly performed (if not, the benefits could be severely compromised):

1. The impression that is taken must include the gum area all the way to the vestibule, and the cast must reflect this extension (Fig. 16-2). If this is not done, significant reduction of retention and potential loss of protection may occur because of reduced strength.
2. The heated polyvinyl must be allowed to adapt well to the cast and cool in place. If this is not done there will be poor adaptation and poor retention.
3. The polyvinyl must be properly trimmed with scissors or a special heated knife after the guard has completely cooled. The mouth guard should extend as far up in the vestibule as tolerated by the athlete, with appropriate clearance of the buccal and labial frenum. In addition, it should extend as far back on the palate as reasonable to both increase anterior strength and retention. It is advisable to replace the mouth guard on the cast after all the trimming is done, flame the edges with an alcohol torch, and then smooth them with wet fingers or a small spatula. To improve comfort further it is possible to heat the occlusal surface gently and have the athlete bite down with the guard in place. This will even the occlusal contact throughout the dentition, thereby increasing

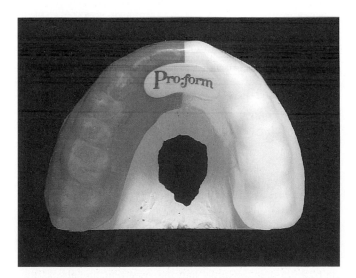

Fig. 16-1 Multilaminated custom-made mouthguard. The kidney shaped area on the palatal side of the incisor area is a harder plastic insert that increases the strength of the mouth guard in that area. Note the extension of the mouthguard in the palatal area.

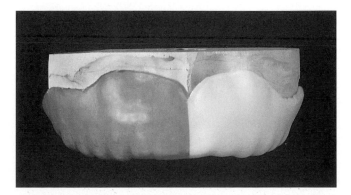

Fig. 16-2 Anterior view of a two-colored mouth guard on the plaster cast. The mouthguard is trimmed as high in the vestibule as the cast allows (within 2 mm of the vestibular reflection). When the mouthguard is fitted in the athlete's mouth, this extension should be trimmed as needed for comfort.

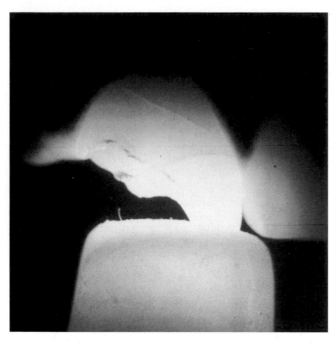

Fig. 16-3 Photograph of traumatized tooth illuminated with a resin-curing light. Enamel craze lines are clearly visible.

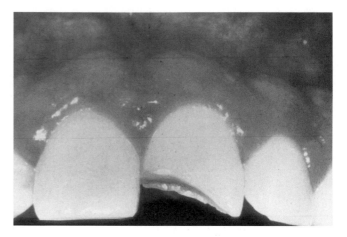

Fig. 16-4 Maxillary right central incisor with an uncomplicated crown fracture involving the enamel and dentin.

comfort and ensuring maximum force absorption in the event of a blow to the chin.[109]

CROWN INFRACTION

A crown infraction is an incomplete fracture of enamel without loss of tooth structure.[14]

Biologic Consequences

Theoretically these fractures are "weak points" through which bacteria and their by-products can travel to challenge the pulp. However, in the vast majority of cases, the pulp, if vital after the initial injury, will overcome the challenge.

Crown infraction rarely occurs alone and can be a sign of a concomitant attachment injury (see section on "Luxation Injuries"). The force taken up by the attachment injury leaves only sufficient force to crack (not completely fracture) the enamel.

Diagnosis and Clinical Presentation

Crack or craze lines can occasionally be observed during routine examination. However, indirect light or transillumination is of great value for their diagnosis.[14] A fiber-optic or resin-curing light is particularly useful (Fig. 16-3). In fact, indirect light and transillumination should be used routinely when examining all traumatic injuries because these injuries often occur in teeth adjacent to those that have sustained more serious injuries.

Treatment

Treatment involves establishing a baseline pulp status with routine sensitivity testing.

Follow-Up

The clinician should schedule follow-up examinations at 3, 6, and 12 months and annually thereafter.

Prognosis

Pulpal complications are extremely rare (i.e., 0.1%).[139]

UNCOMPLICATED CROWN FRACTURE

An uncomplicated crown fracture is a fracture of the enamel or the enamel and dentin without pulp exposure.[14]

Incidence

This type of injury is very common, accounting for approximately one third of all dental injuries.[151]

Biologic Consequences

If the fracture involves the enamel only, the consequences are minimal and any complications may be because of a concomitant injury to the attachment apparatus.

However, if dentin is exposed a direct pathway exists for noxious stimuli to pass through the dentinal tubules to the pulp. Although the pulp has the potential to successfully defend itself with partial closure of the dentinal tubules and reparative dentin,[28] chronic pulpal inflammation (or even necrosis) may still occur.[179] The reaction of the pulp depends on a number of factors, including time of treatment, distance

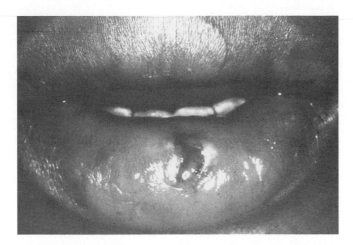

Fig. 16-5 Lip laceration as a result of an injury to the maxillary incisors.

of the fracture from the pulp, and size of the dentinal tubules.[46,135,179]

Diagnosis and Clinical Presentation

Enamel fracture includes a superficial, rough edge that may cause irritation to the tongue or lip. Sensitivity to air or liquids (hot or cold) is not a complaint. Although an enamel and dentin fracture also includes a rough edge on the tooth (Fig. 16-4), sensitivity to air and hot and cold liquids may be a chief complaint. Commonly a lip bruise or laceration is present because pursing of the lips is automatic when the injury occurs (Fig. 16-5).

Treatment

Enamel Fracture Only   Smooth the sharp edges and leave, if esthetically acceptable. Placing bonded composite resins may be necessary for esthetics.

Enamel and Dentin Fracture   Treatment should take place as soon as possible.[135] A hard-setting calcium hydroxide base is placed[39] over exposed dentinal tubules to disinfect the fractured dentinal surface and stimulate closure of the tubules, making them less permeable to noxious stimuli.[22,113,169] This is followed by restoration with a bonded-resin technique. Controversy exists as to whether dentin bonding can be carried out without an intermediate calcium hydroxide base. Some authors think that the modern bonding systems seal the cavity sufficiently to protect the pulp. However, although research is abundant as to the increased bond strength with modern dentin bonding systems,[75,87] information is scarce as to whether these bonding systems create a tight enough seal to protect the pulp.[98] It is the author's opinion that direct dentinal bonding (without an intermediate base) should be used on uncomplicated crown fractures that

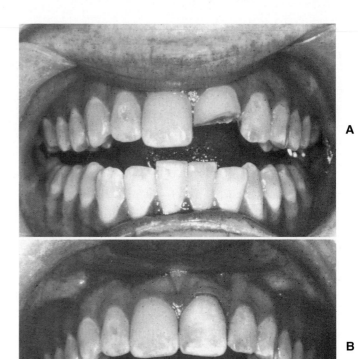

Fig. 16-6 **A**, Uncomplicated crown fracture of the maxillary central incisor. **B**, The fractured segment is bonded to tooth after placement of a calcium hydroxide base.

are superficial. Direct dentinal bonding without a base should be avoided on deep fractures or in young teeth with wide dentinal tubules.

It is essential to account for the fractured tooth fragment. If it can be located and is found intact, it is possible to bond this fragment to the crown with excellent esthetic results and an acceptable strength[115] (Fig. 16-6, *A* and *B*). If the tooth fragment is not located, a lip radiograph should be taken to ensure the fragment has not lodged in the lip. If a lip laceration is present, it must be thoroughly cleansed and sutured. In some cases a consultation with a plastic surgeon may be prudent. Sensitivity testing should be carried out to establish a baseline pulpal status.

Follow-Up

The clinician should schedule follow-up examinations at 3, 6, and 12 months and annually thereafter.

Prognosis

The prognosis for this type of injury is extremely good, with pulpal complications minimal.[14]

COMPLICATED CROWN FRACTURE

A complicated crown fracture involves the enamel, dentin, and pulp.[14]

Incidence

Complicated crown fractures occur in 2% to 13% of all dental injuries.[101,151]

Biologic Consequences

A crown fracture involving the pulp, if left untreated, will always result in pulp necrosis.[86] However, the manner and time sequence in which the pulp becomes necrotic allows a great deal of potential for successful intervention to maintain pulp vitality. The first reaction after the injury is hemorrhage and local inflammation.[99,146] Subsequent inflammatory changes are usually proliferative but can be destructive. A proliferative reaction is favored in traumatic injuries because the fractured surface is usually flat, allowing salivary rinsing with little chance of impaction of contaminated debris. Therefore unless impaction of contaminated debris is obvious, it is expected that in the first 24 hours after the injury a proliferative response (with inflammation extending not more than 2 mm into the pulp) will be present[37,41,72] (Fig. 16-7). In

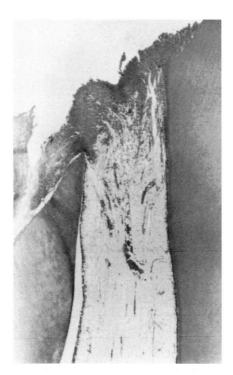

Fig. 16-7 Histologic appearance of the superficial pulp 24 hours after exposure. A proliferative response with inflammation extending 1 to 2 mm into the pulp is seen.

time the bacterial challenge will result in local pulpal necrosis and a slow apical spread of the pulpal inflammation.

Treatment

There are two treatment options: (1) vital pulp therapy comprising pulp capping, partial pulpotomy, and cervical pulpotomy or (2) pulpectomy. Choice of treatment depends on the stage of development of the tooth, time between the accident and treatment, concomitant periodontal injury, and restorative treatment plan.

Stage of Development of the Tooth
Loss of vitality in an immature tooth can have catastrophic consequences. Root canal treatment on a tooth with a blunderbuss canal is time consuming and difficult. Perhaps of more importance is the fact that necrosis of the pulp of an immature tooth leaves the tooth with thin dentinal walls that are susceptible to fracture during and after the apexification procedure.[87] Therefore every effort must be made to keep the tooth vital (at least until the apex and cervical root have completed their development).

Removal of the pulp in a mature tooth is not as significant as in an immature tooth because a pulpectomy has an extremely high success rate.[64,155] However, it has been shown that vital pulp therapy on a mature tooth performed under optimal conditions can be carried out successfully.[106,173] Therefore this form of therapy can be an option under certain circumstances even though a pulpectomy is the treatment that affords the most predictable success. In an immature tooth, vital pulp therapy should always be attempted if at all feasible, because of the tremendous advantages of maintaining the vital pulp.

Time Between the Accident and Treatment
For 24 hours after a traumatic injury, the initial reaction of the pulp is proliferative, with no more than 2-mm depth of pulpal inflammation (see Fig. 16-7). After 24 hours, chances of direct bacterial contamination from the pulp increase with resultant progression of the zone of inflammation in an apical direction.[41] Thus as time progresses the chance of successfully maintaining a healthy pulp decreases.

Concomitant Attachment Damage
A periodontal injury will compromise the nutritional supply of the pulp. This fact is particularly important in mature teeth where the chance of pulp survival is not as good as for immature teeth.[10,50]

Restorative Treatment Plan
Unlike an immature tooth where the benefits of maintaining vitality of the pulp are so great, a mature tooth pulpectomy is a viable treatment option. However, if performed under optimal conditions, vital pulp therapy after traumatic exposures can be successful. Thus if the restorative treatment plan is simple and a

composite resin restoration will suffice as the permanent restoration, this treatment option should be given serious consideration. If, on the other hand, a more complex restoration is to be placed (e.g., a crown or bridge abutment), pulpectomy may be the more predictable treatment method.

Vital Pulp Therapy

Requirements for Success   Vital pulp therapy has an extremely high success rate if the clinician strictly adheres to the following requirements.

Treatment of a Noninflamed Pulp   Treatment of a healthy pulp has been shown to be an essential requirement for successful therapy.[162] Vital pulp therapy of the inflamed pulp, however, affords an inferior success rate.[162] Therefore the optimal time for treatment is in the first 24 hours when pulp inflammation is superficial. As time increases between the injury and therapy, pulp removal must be extended in an apical direction to ensure that inflamed pulp has been removed and noninflamed pulp has been reached.

Bacteria-tight seal.   A bacteria-tight seal protecting the healing pulp is the most critical factor for successful treatment, because challenge by bacteria during the healing phase will cause failure.[34] On the other hand, if the exposed pulp is effectively sealed from bacterial leakage, successful healing of the pulp with a hard-tissue barrier will occur independent of the dressing placed on the pulp.[34]

Pulp dressing.   Presently, calcium hydroxide is the most common dressing used for vital pulp therapy. Its advantages are that it is antibacterial[32,145] and will disinfect the superficial pulp. Pure calcium hydroxide necroses about 1.5 mm of pulp tissue,[111] removing superficial layers of inflamed pulp if present (Fig. 16-8). The high pH of 12.5 of calcium hydroxide causes a liquefaction necrosis in the most superficial layers,[140] and the toxicity of the calcium hydroxide appears to be quickly neutralized as deeper layers of pulp are affected (causing coagulative necrosis at this level). The coagulative necrotic tissue causes a mild irritation to the adjacent vital pulp tissue.[140] This mild irritation will initiate an inflammatory response and, in the absence of bacteria (because of the bacteria-tight seal), will heal with a hard-tissue barrier.[139,140] Hard-setting calcium hydroxide will not necrose the superficial layers of pulp, but it has been shown to initiate healing with a hard-tissue barrier as with pure calcium hydroxide.[153,159]

A major disadvantage of calcium hydroxide is that it does not seal the fractured surface. Therefore an additional material must be used as a base to ensure that bacteria do not challenge the pulp, particularly during the critical healing phase. Zinc oxide–eugenol or glass ionomer base materials have been commonly used for this purpose.

Many materials such as zinc oxide–eugenol,[162] tricalcium phosphate,[73] and composite resin[34] have been proposed as medicaments for vital pulp therapy. However, none have

afforded the predictability of calcium hydroxide used in conjunction with a maximally sealed coronal restoration. Mineral trioxide aggregate (MTA), a new material, has been reported to show promise as a pulp-capping agent,[128] but the reproducibility of these results and its long-term success has not been tested.

Treatment Methods

Pulp Capping   Pulp capping implies placing the dressing directly onto the pulp exposure.

Indications   This technique is used on immature, permanent teeth; on a very recent exposure (< 24 hours); and possibly on a mature, permanent tooth with a simple restorative plan.

Technique   After adequate anesthesia, a rubber dam is placed and the crown and exposed dentinal surface is thoroughly rinsed with saline followed by disinfection with 0.12% chlorhexidine or betadine. Pure calcium hydroxide mixed with sterile saline (anesthetic solution can also be used) is carefully placed over the exposed pulp and dentinal surface. The surrounding enamel is acid etched and bonded with composite resin.

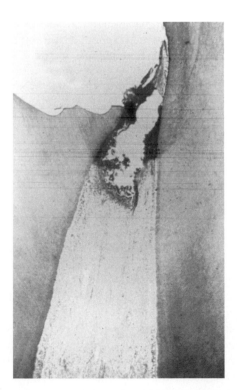

Fig. 16-8 Histologic appearance of the pulp 7 days after capping with pure calcium hydroxide. The calcium hydroxide has necrosed about 1 to 2 mm of the superficial pulp.

Follow-up   Advantages of pulp capping are that the final restorative treatment can be completed at the emergency visit and that pulp tissue remains coronal to the gingival margin, allowing periodic sensitivity testing to be performed. Electric pulp testing, thermal testing, palpation tests, and percussion tests should be carried out at 3 weeks; 3, 6, and 12 months; and yearly thereafter. A radiographic examination is extremely important in these cases. A hard-tissue barrier can sometimes be visualized as early as 6 weeks posttreatment. Signs of apical periodontitis, an indirect sign of an unhealthy pulp, can also be seen as an apical radiolucency. Most importantly, continued root development of the immature root, which was the primary reason for performing the procedure, is checked with this periodic radiographic examination.

Prognosis   The success of the pulp-capping procedure relies on the ability of the calcium hydroxide to disinfect the superficial pulp and dentin and to necrose the zone of superficially inflamed pulp. Also the quality of the bacteria-tight seal provided by the enamel-bonded resin restoration is an important factor in successful pulp capping. Reported prognosis is in the range of 80%.[55,91,132]

Partial Pulpotomy

Partial pulpotomy implies the removal of coronal pulp tissue to the level of healthy pulp. This procedure is commonly called the "Cvek Pulpotomy."

Indications   As with pulp capping, the zone of inflammation in the pulp has extended more than 2 mm in an apical direction but has not reached the root pulp (e.g., a traumatic exposure a few days postinjury in a large, young pulp). For reasons to be discussed, this treatment method is superior to pulp capping and affords a better prognosis.

Technique   Anesthesia is administered, a rubber dam is placed, and superficial disinfection is performed as described with pulp capping.

A 1- to 2-mm deep cavity is prepared into the pulp using a sterile diamond bur of appropriate size with copious water coolant[65] (Fig. 16-9). Use of a slow-speed bur or spoon excavator should be avoided unless cooling of the high-speed bur is not possible. If bleeding is excessive, the pulp is amputated deeper until only moderate hemorrhage is seen. Excess blood is carefully removed by rinsing with sterile saline or anesthetic solution and dried with a sterile cotton pellet. Care must be taken not to allow a blood clot to develop, because this will compromise the prognosis.[37,139] If the pulp is of sufficient size to allow 1 to 2 mm additional pulp necrosis, a thin layer of pure calcium hydroxide is mixed with sterile saline or anesthetic solution and carefully placed. If the pulp size does not permit additional loss of pulp tissue, a commercial hard-setting calcium hydroxide can be used.[153] The prepared cavity is filled with a material with the best chance of a bacteria-tight seal (i.e., zinc oxide–eugenol, glass ionomer

cement) to a level that is flush with the fractured surface. The material in the pulpal cavity and all exposed dentinal tubules are covered with hard-setting calcium hydroxide and the enamel is etched and restored with bonded composite resin as in pulp capping.

Follow-up   As with pulp capping, the emphasis is placed on maintenance of positive sensitivity tests and radiographic evidence of continued root development (Fig. 16-10).

Prognosis   This method affords many advantages over pulp capping. Superficial inflamed pulp is removed in the preparation of the pulpal cavity. Calcium hydroxide disinfects dentin and pulp, removing additional pulpal inflammation. Most importantly, space is provided for a material that will provide a bacteria-tight seal, allowing pulpal healing with hard tissue under optimal conditions. Additionally, coronal pulp remains, which allows sensitivity testing to be carried out at the follow-up visits. Prognosis is extremely good (94% to 96%).[37,56]

Full (Cervical) Pulpotomy

Full, or cervical, pulpotomy involves removal of the entire coronal pulp to the level of the root orifices. This level of pulp amputation is chosen arbitrarily because of its anatomic convenience. Therefore because the inflamed pulp sometimes extends past the canal orifices into the root pulp, many "mistakes" are made resulting in treatment of an inflamed rather than noninflamed pulp.

Indications   When the prediction is that the pulp is inflamed to the deeper levels of the coronal pulp, full pulpotomy is indicated. This treatment may also be indicated for carious exposure and traumatic exposure (after 72 hours). Because of the reasonably good chance that the dressing will be placed on inflamed pulp, full pulpotomy is contraindicated in mature teeth. However, benefits outweigh risks for this treatment in the immature tooth with incompletely formed apices and thin dentinal walls.

Technique   After anesthesia, a rubber dam is placed and superficial disinfection is instituted (as in pulp capping and partial pulpotomy). The coronal pulp is removed as in a partial pulpotomy, but only to the level of the root orifices. Calcium hydroxide dressing, bacteria-tight seal, and coronal restoration are carried out as in partial pulpotomy.

Follow-up   The clinician should schedule follow-up as would be done for pulp capping and partial pulpotomy. A major disadvantage of this treatment method is the fact that sensitivity testing is not possible because of the loss of coronal pulp. Therefore radiographic follow up is extremely important with this form of treatment to assess for signs of apical periodontitis and to ensure the continuation of root formation.

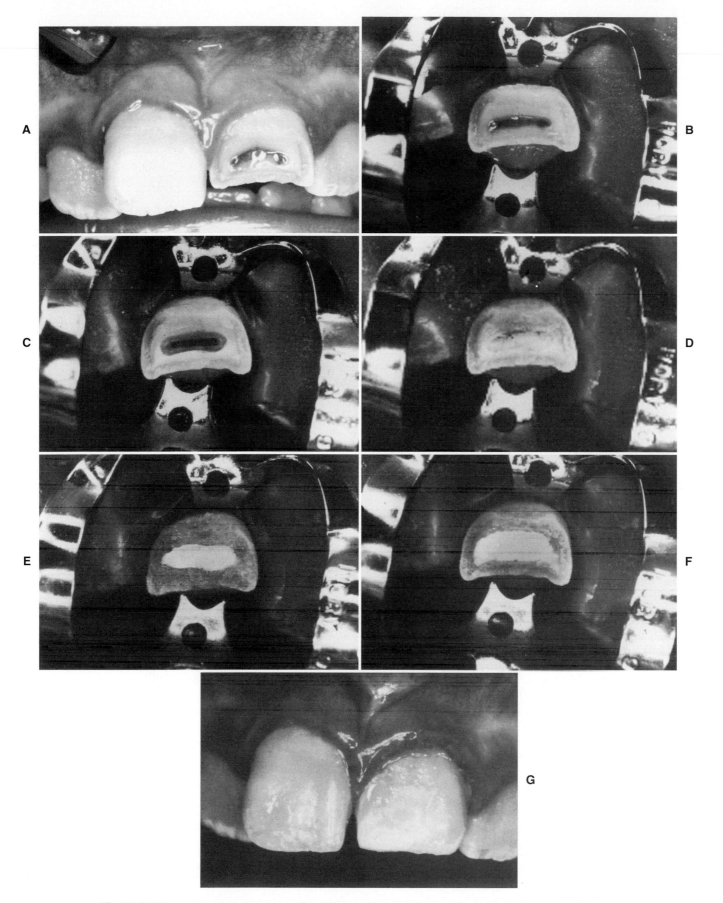

Fig. 16-9 Pulp-capping procedure on maxillary left central incisor with a complicated crown fracture. **A,** Tooth on presentation to the dentist. **B,** Anesthesia is administered, a rubber dam is placed, and superficial disinfection is performed. **C,** A cavity is prepared 1 to 2 mm into the pulp with a high-speed diamond bur with copious water spray. **D,** A thin layer of calcium hydroxide is placed on the pulp tissue. **E,** A bacteria-tight seal is created by the placement of a ZOE temporary restoration into the cavity to the level flush with the fractured dentinal surface. **F,** A calcium hydroxide base is placed to cover the ZOE and protect the exposed dentin. **G,** The restoration is completed with bonded composite resin.

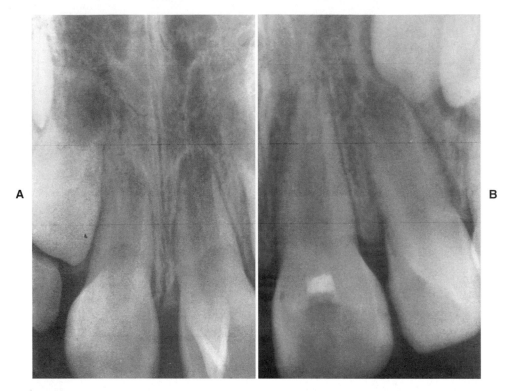

Fig. 16-10 Radiographic follow-up after pulp capping procedure. **A**, Preoperative radiograph before the procedure. **B**, Follow-up radiograph 1 year later showing continued root development.

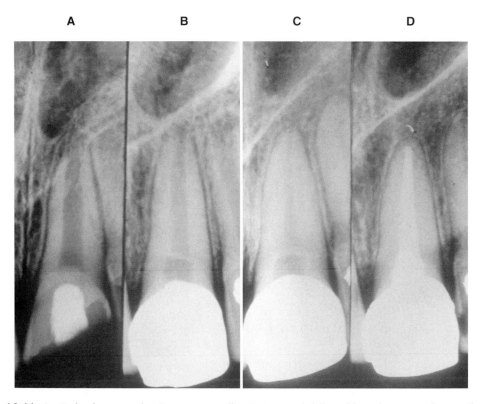

Fig. 16-11 Cervical pulpotomy of an immature maxillary incisor tooth followed by pulpectomy after root formation. **A**, Pulpotomy is initiated. **B**, Six months later a hard-tissue barrier has formed and the root continues to develop. **C**, One year later root development is complete. **D**, A pulpectomy followed by a permanent root canal therapy is performed.

Prognosis   Because the full pulpotomy is performed on pulps that are expected to have deep inflammation and the site of pulp amputation is arbitrary, many more "errors" are made leading to treatment of the inflamed pulp. Consequently, the prognosis in the range of 75% is poorer than for partial pulpotomy.[60,66] Because of the inability to evaluate pulp status after full pulpotomy, some authors have recommended pulpectomy after the roots have fully formed (Fig. 16-11). This philosophy is based on the fact that the pulpectomy procedure has a success rate in the range of 95%, whereas the prognosis of root canal treatment drops significantly to about 80% if apical periodontitis develops.[64,142]

Pulpectomy

Pulpectomy implies removal of the entire pulp to the level of the apical foramen.

Indications   This treatment is indicated for complicated crown fracture of mature teeth (if conditions are not ideal for vital pulp therapy).

Technique   (See Chapters 8 and 9.)

Follow-up   (See Chapter 22.)

Prognosis   Reported prognosis for pulpectomy under optimal conditions is above 90%.[64,155] However, no pulpectomy prognosis study has been limited to teeth that have undergone a traumatic injury. It is not known if the attachment injury and possible disruption of the apical blood supply that occur in most traumatic injuries affects the prognosis of pulpectomy in these teeth.

Treatment of the Nonvital Pulp

Mature Tooth   (See Chapters 8 and 9.)

Immature Tooth—Apexification
Indications.   This technique is indicated for teeth with open apices in which standard instrumentation techniques cannot create an apical stop to facilitate effective obturation of the canal.

Biologic Consequences   A nonvital, immature tooth presents a number of difficulties for adequate endodontic therapy. The canal is wider apically than coronally, necessitating the use of a soft gutta-percha technique to mold the gutta-percha to the shape of the apex. Because the apex is extremely wide, no barrier exists to stop this softened gutta-percha from moving into and traumatizing the apical periodontal tissues. Also, the lack of an apical stop and subsequent extrusion of material through the canal may result in a canal that is underfilled and susceptible to leakage. An additional problem in immature teeth with thin dentinal walls is their susceptibility to fracture both during and after treatment.[38,154]

These problems are overcome by creating an environment that will allow the formation of a hard-tissue barrier so that obturation of the canal can take place under the most ideal circumstances. In addition, the weakened root is reinforced against fracture both during and after apexification.[87]

Technique
Disinfection of the canal.   Because in the vast majority of cases nonvital teeth are infected,[21,156] the first phase of treatment is to disinfect the root canal system to ensure periapical healing.[32,42,86] The canal length is estimated with a parallel preoperative radiograph. After access to the canals is achieved, a file is placed to this length. When the length has been confirmed radiographically, *light* filing (because of the thin dentinal walls) is performed with *copious* irrigation, with 0.5% sodium hypochlorite* (NaOCl).[42,150] An irrigation needle that can passively reach close to the apical length is useful in disinfecting the canals of these immature teeth. The canal is dried with paper points and a soft mix of calcium hydroxide spun into the canal with a lentulo spiral instrument.

The addition of calcium hydroxide is effective in further disinfecting the canal; research indicates that it should be left in place for at least 1 week.[145] Further treatment should not be delayed more than 1 month, because the calcium hydroxide can be washed out by tissue fluids (through the open apex), leaving the canal susceptible to reinfection.

Stimulation of a hard-tissue barrier.   The formation of the hard-tissue barrier at the apex requires a similar environment to that required for hard-tissue formation in vital pulp therapy (i.e., a mild inflammatory stimulus to initiate healing and a bacteria-free environment to ensure that the inflammation is not progressive). As with vital pulp therapy, calcium hydroxide is presently the medicament of choice for this procedure.[38,71,74]

Pure calcium hydroxide powder is mixed with sterile saline (or anesthetic solution) to a thick (powdery) consistency (Fig. 16-12). Premixed commercial calcium hydroxide can also be used. The calcium hydroxide is packed against the apical soft tissue with a plugger or thick gutta-percha point to initiate hard-tissue formation. This step is followed by backfilling with calcium hydroxide to completely obturate the canal, thus ensuring a bacteria-free canal with little chance of reinfection during the 6 to 18 months required for hard-tissue formation at the apex. The calcium hydroxide is meticulously removed from the access cavity to the level of the root orifices, and a well-sealing temporary filling is placed in the access cavity. A radiograph is taken, and the canal should appear to have become calcified (indicating that the entire canal has been filled with the calcium hydroxide). Because calcium hydroxide washout is evaluated by its rela-

---

*Note: Many knowledgeable clinicians may use higher concentrations of NaOCl.

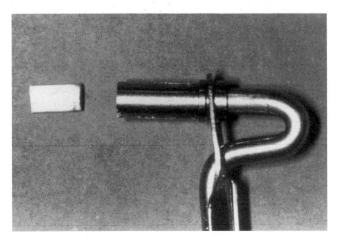

Fig. 16-12 Calcium hydroxide mixed to a thick, powdery consistency that allows it to be deposited in the access cavity with an amalgam carrier.

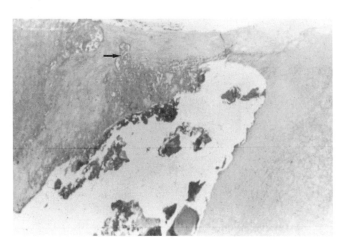

Fig. 16-13 Histologic appearance of hard-tissue barrier at the apex of a tooth. It consists of irregularly arranged layers of coagulated soft tissue, calcified tissue, and cementum-like tissue. Included are islands of soft tissue (*arrow*).

tive radiodensity in the canal, it is prudent to use a calcium hydroxide mixture without the addition of a radiopaquer, such as barium sulphate. These additives do not wash out as readily as calcium hydroxide so that (if present in the canal) evaluation of washout is not possible.

A radiograph is taken at 3-month intervals to evaluate whether a hard-tissue barrier has formed and if the calcium hydroxide has washed out of the canal. If calcium hydroxide washout is seen the calcium hydroxide is replaced. If no washout is evident it can be left intact for another 3 months. Excessive calcium hydroxide dressing changes should be avoided if at all possible because the initial toxicity of the material is thought to delay healing.[93]

When completion of a hard-tissue barrier is suspected, the calcium hydroxide should be washed out of the canal with NaOCl and a radiograph made to evaluate the radiodensity of the apical stop. A file of a size that can easily reach the apex can be used to gently probe for a stop at the apex. When a hard-tissue barrier is indicated radiographically and can be probed with an instrument, the canal is ready for obturation.

Obturation of the root canal. Because the apical diameter is larger than the coronal diameter of most of these canals, a softened gutta-percha technique is indicated in these teeth (see Chapter 9). Care must be taken to avoid excessive lateral force during obturation because of the thin walls of the root. The hard-tissue barrier consists of irregularly arranged layers of coagulated soft tissue, calcified tissue, and cementum-like tissue (Fig. 16-13). Also included are islands of soft connective tissue, giving the barrier a "Swiss cheese" consistency.[24,44] Because of the irregular nature of the barrier, it is not unusual for cement or softened gutta-percha to be pushed through it into the apical tissues during obturation. Formation of the hard-tissue barrier may be some distance short of the radiographic apex, because the

barrier forms wherever the calcium hydroxide contacts vital tissue. In teeth with wide-open apices vital tissue can survive and proliferate from the periodontal ligament a few millimeters into the root canal. Obturation should be completed to the level of the hard-tissue barrier and not forced toward the radiographic apex.

Reinforcement of the thin dentinal walls. The apexification procedure with long-term calcium hydroxide has become a predictably successful procedure (see Prognosis).[39,52] However, the thin dentinal walls still present a clinical problem. Should secondary injuries occur, teeth with thin dentinal walls are more susceptible to fractures, rendering them unrestorable.[49,157] It has been reported that approximately 30% of these teeth will fracture during or after endodontic treatment.[88] Consequently, some clinicians have questioned the advisability of the apexification procedure and have opted for more radical treatment procedures, including extraction[154] followed by extensive restorative procedures (e.g., dental implants). Recent studies have shown that intracoronal, acid-etched, bonded resins can internally strengthen endodontically treated teeth and increase their resistance to fracture.[130,164]

A new technique has been described to internally strengthen nonvital, immature teeth using the Luminex post system. A clear post is used to assist in curing the resin in the deeper layers of the canal. After curing of the resin, the post is removed to allow a channel for calcium hydroxide replenishment and obturation of the canal (Fig. 16-14). In vitro studies have shown the technique to be effective in strengthening these teeth.[87]

Follow-up Routine recall evaluation should be performed to determine the success in the prevention or treatment of apical periodontitis. Restorative procedures should be assessed to ensure that they never promote root fractures.

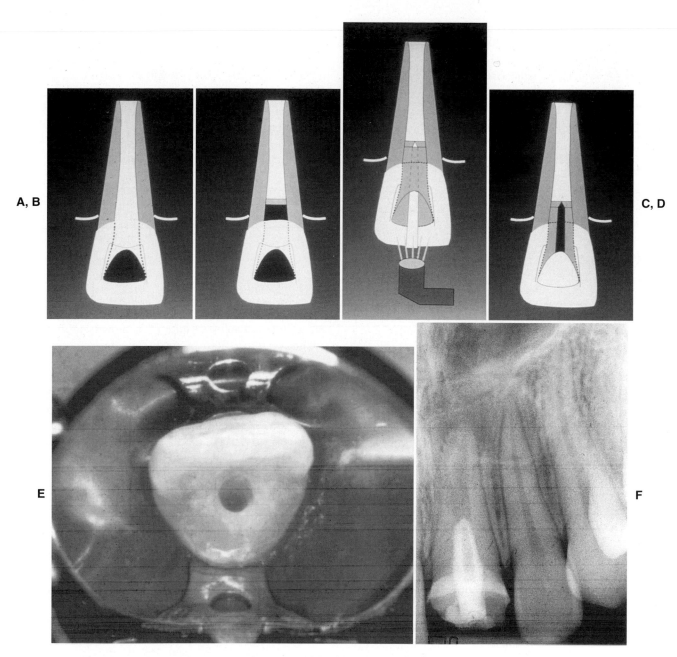

Fig. 16-14 Method for strengthening the root against fracture during the apexification procedure. **A,** The canal is filled with a thick mixture of calcium hydroxide. **B,** The calcium hydroxide is removed to below the level of the bone, a thin layer of glass ionomer cement is placed over it, and a clear Luminex post is seated into the glass ionomer cement parallel to the long axis of the tooth. **C,** Composite resin is packed into the access cavity, the post is pushed through it to seat into the glass ionomer cement, and it is cured in the same manner as the glass ionomer cement. **D,** After the resin is cured the post is removed, leaving a reinforced root and a channel through which medicament changes and obturation can take place. **E,** Clinical picture of the channel that is sealed with a temporary stopping between medicament changes and is filled with composite resin after obturation. The channel can be widened with a fissure bur to facilitate medicament changes and obturation, after which it is repaired with resin using the same method of curing. **F,** Radiograph of composite resin reinforcement of the root with channel.

Prognosis Periapical healing and the formation of a hard-tissue barrier can occur predictably (i.e., 79% to 96%) with long-term calcium hydroxide treatment.[38,88] However, long-term survival can be jeopardized by the fracture potential of the thin dentinal walls of these teeth. It is expected that the newer techniques of internal strengthening will increase long-term survivability.

CROWN AND ROOT FRACTURE

A crown and root fracture is a fracture involving enamel, dentin, and cementum. The pulp may or may not be involved.

Incidence

The incidence of crown and root fractures as a direct result of traumatic injuries has been reported to be 5% of all dental injuries.[11]

Biologic Consequences

The biologic consequences of a crown root fracture are identical to an uncomplicated (if the pulp is not exposed) or complicated (if the crown is exposed) crown fracture. In addition, periodontal complications are present because the fracture may encroach on the attachment apparatus. The seriousness of the complication is dependent on the apical extent of the attachment injury.

Diagnosis and Clinical Presentation

In most cases, crown root fractures are the result of direct trauma that produces a chisel type of fracture, with a fragment or fragments below the lingual gingiva[14] (Fig. 16-15). The fragments may be firm, loose, and attached only by the periodontal ligament, or they may be lost. The periodontal injury causes pain on pressure and biting, and exposed dentin or pulp causes pain to air and hot or cold liquids. Indirect light and transillumination is an effective way of diagnosing these fractures.

The "cracked tooth syndrome" in a posterior tooth is also an example of a crown root fracture. However, because this syndrome is not always the result of an acute traumatic injury, it will not be discussed in this chapter (see Chapter 1).

Treatment

These injuries are treated in the same manner as uncomplicated or complicated crown fractures, with additional treatment for any attachment injury. If a crown and root fracture cannot be turned into a crown fracture by periodontal or orthodontic therapy or both, the tooth should be extracted.

After adequate anesthesia, all loose fragments are removed. A periodontal assessment is made as to whether the tooth can be treated periodontally to allow it to be adequately restored. Periodontal therapy could involve a simple removal of tissue with a scalpel, electro-surgical or a laser procedure to allow for adequate sealing of the restoration, or forced eruption to extrude the fractured area above the attachment level to allow for adequate restoration.

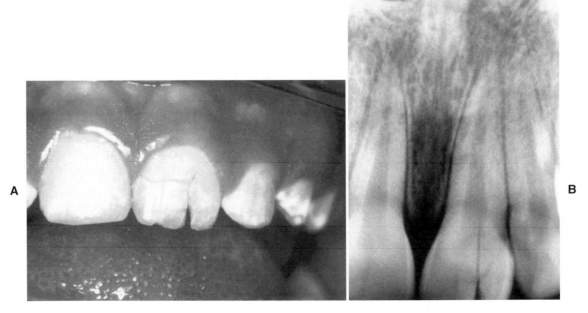

Fig. 16-15 Crown and root fracture of maxillary left central incisor. **A,** Chisel type of fracture has resulted in multiple fragments, one of which extends below the attachment level. **B,** Radiograph of the same tooth.

Follow-Up and Prognosis

The clinician should schedule follow-up as would be done for uncomplicated and complicated crown fractures. Because long-term success is dependent on the quality of the coronal restoration, success (particularly at the gingival sulcus) should be reassessed at each visit.[103] Prognosis is similar to that described for uncomplicated or complicated crown fractures.

ROOT FRACTURE

A root fracture is a fracture of the cementum and dentin involving the pulp.

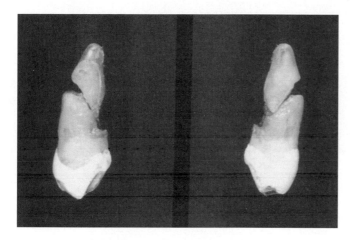

Fig. 16-16 Extracted tooth with an oblique (facial to palatal) root fracture.

Incidence

These injuries are relatively infrequent, occurring in less than 3% of all dental injuries.[177] Incompletely formed roots with vital pulps rarely fracture horizontally.[4]

Biologic Consequences

When a root fractures horizontally, the coronal segment is displaced to a varying degree; generally the apical segment is not displaced. Because the apical pulpal circulation is not disrupted, pulp necrosis in the apical segment is extremely rare. Pulp necrosis of the coronal segment results because of its displacement and occurs in about 25% of cases.[6,7,81]

Rigid stabilization of the segments (for 2 to 4 months) will allow healing and "reattachment" of the fractured segments. The speed at which the emergency treatment is rendered will probably determine the proximity to which the root segments can be repositioned, which may be the most important determinant of favorable healing results.

Diagnosis and Clinical Presentation

Clinical presentation is similar to that of luxation injuries. The extent of displacement of the coronal segment is usually indicative of the location of the fracture and can vary from simulating a concussion injury (i.e., apical fracture) to simulating an extrusive luxation (i.e., cervical fracture).

Radiographic examination for root fractures is extremely important. Because a root fracture is usually oblique (facial to palatal) (Fig. 16-16), one periapical radiograph may easily miss its presence. It is imperative to take at least three angled radiographs (45, 90, and 110 degrees) so that at least at one angulation the x-ray beam will pass directly through the fracture line to make it visible on the radiograph (Fig. 16-17).

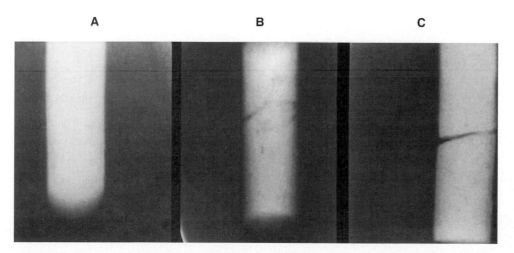

Fig. 16-17 Chalk cut horizontally and radiographed at different angles, illustrating the different radiographic pictures that can be obtained. **A**, At this angle, no "fracture" is seen. **B**, The "fracture" appears complicated in nature. **C**, Only at this angle, the true nature of the fracture can be seen. (Courtesy Dr. I.B. Bender.)

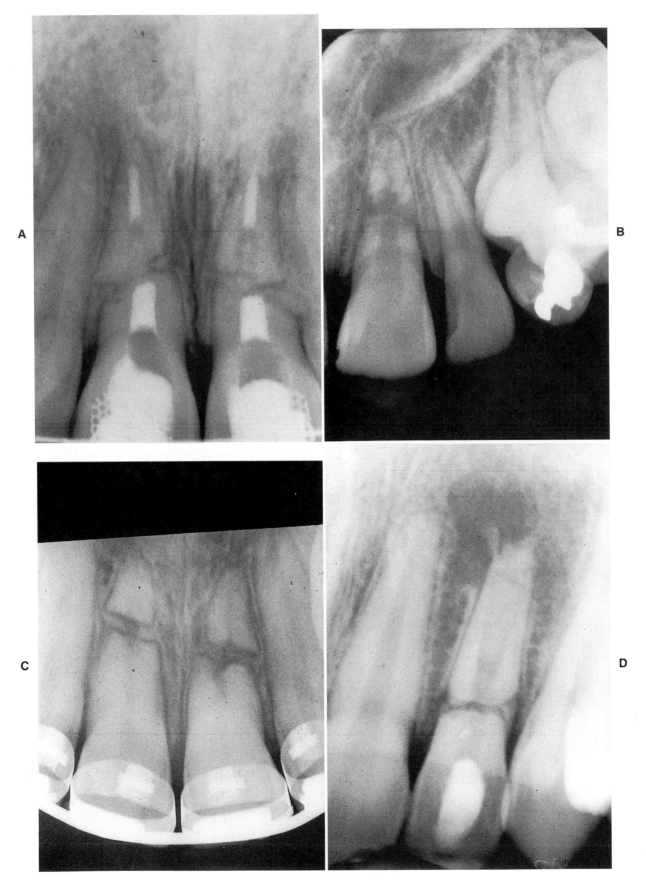

Fig. 16-18 Healing patterns after horizontal root fractures. **A**, Healing with calcified tissue. **B**, Healing with interproximal connective tissue. **C**, Healing with bone and connective tissue. **D**, Interproximal connective tissue without healing.

Treatment

Emergency treatment involves repositioning of the segments in as close proximity as possible and rigidly splinting to adjacent teeth for 2 to 4 months.[129] If a long period has elapsed between the injury and treatment, it will likely not be possible to reposition the segments close to their original position, compromising the long-term prognosis of the tooth.

Healing Patterns

Andreasen and Hjorting-Hansen[16] have described four types of healing of root fractures:

1. Healing with calcified tissue—Radiographically, the fracture line is discernible, but the fragments are in close contact.
2. Healing with interproximal connective tissue—Radiographically, the fragments appear separated by a narrow radiolucent line, and the fractured edges appear rounded.
3. Healing with interproximal bone and connective tissue—Radiographically, a distinct bony ridge separates the fragments (Fig. 16-18, *A*).
4. Interproximal inflammatory tissue without healing—Radiographically, a widening of the fracture line, a developing radiolucency corresponding to the fracture line, or both become apparent (Fig. 16-18, *B*).

The first three types of healing patterns are considered successful. The teeth are usually asymptomatic and respond positively to sensitivity testing. Coronal yellowing is possible because calcification of the coronal segment is not unusual.[82,177]

The fourth type of healing pattern is typical when the coronal segment loses its vitality. The infective products in the coronal pulp cause an inflammatory response and typical radiolucencies at the fracture line[17] (Fig. 16-19).

Treatment of Complications

Coronal Root Fractures   Historically it had been thought that fractures in the coronal segment had a poor prognosis, and extraction of the coronal segment was recommended. Research does not support this treatment; in fact, if these coronal segments are rigidly splinted, chances of healing do not differ from midroot or apical fracture.[177] However, if the fracture occurs at the level of or coronal to the crest of the alveolar bone, the prognosis is extremely poor.

If reattachment of the fractured segments is not possible, extraction of the coronal segment is indicated. The level of fracture and length of the remaining root are evaluated for restorability. If the apical root segment is long enough, forced eruption of this segment can be carried out to enable a restoration to be fabricated (Fig. 16-20).

Mid-root, Apical Root Fracture   Pulp necrosis occurs in 25% of root fractures. In almost all cases the necrosis occurs in the coronal segment only, with the apical segment remaining vital. Therefore endodontic treatment is indicated in the coronal root segment only, unless periapical pathology is seen in the apical segment. In most cases the pulpal lumen is wide at the apical extent of the coronal segment so that long-term calcium hydroxide treatment is indicated (see "Apexification"). The coronal segment is obturated after a hard-tissue barrier has formed apically in the coronal segment and periradicular healing has taken place.

In rare cases when both the coronal and apical pulp are necrotic, treatment is more complicated. Endodontic treatment through the fracture is extremely difficult. Endodontic manipulations, medicaments, and filling materials all have a detrimental effect on healing of the fracture site (Fig. 16-21). If healing of the fracture has been completed, followed by necrosis of the apical segment, the prognosis is much improved.

In more apical root fractures, necrotic apical segments can be surgically removed. This is a viable treatment if the remaining root is long enough to provide adequate periodontal support. Removal of the apical segment in midroot fractures leaves the coronal segment with a compromised attachment; often endodontic implants are used to provide additional support to the tooth.

Follow-Up

After the splinting period is completed, the clinician should schedule follow-up examinations at 3, 6, and 12 months and yearly thereafter.

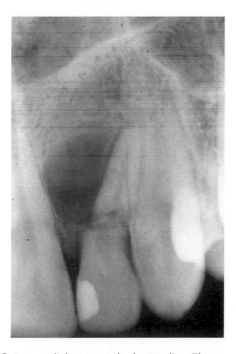

Fig. 16-19 Large radiolucency at the fracture line. The coronal pulp is nonvital, resulting in an inflammatory response at the fracture line.

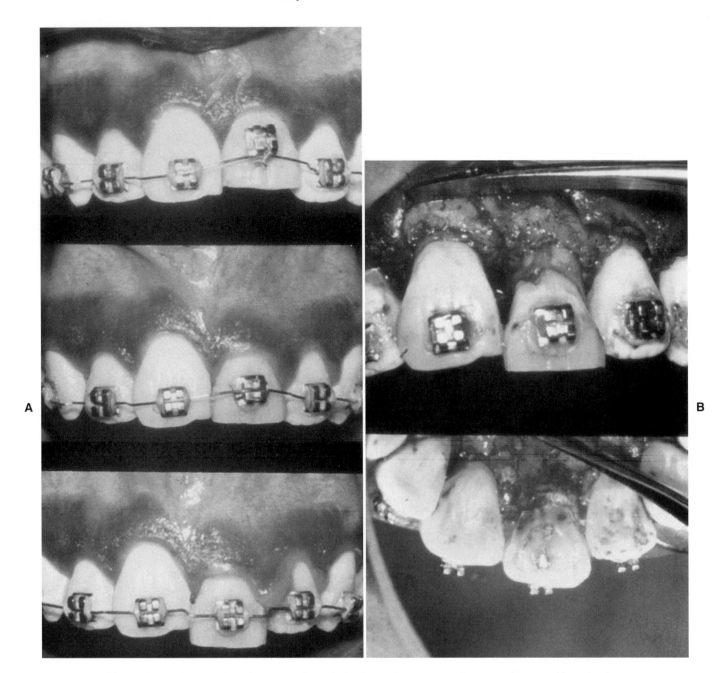

Fig. 16-20 Orthodontic forced eruption of a tooth that has undergone a root fracture at the cervical bone level. **A,** Endodontic treatment is performed. A temporary post is cemented through the crown into the root. The root is erupted approximately 2 mm over a 4-week period. **B,** A flap procedure is performed to ensure that enough tooth structure remains to construct the restoration and to adjust the gingival and bone levels to be compatible with the adjacent teeth.

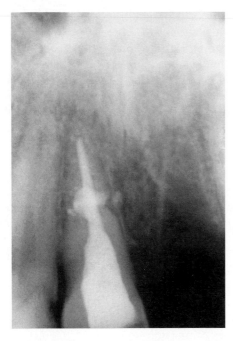

Fig. 16-21   Conservative root canal treatment of the coronal and apical segments. Note the filling material in the fracture line that compromises the healing response.

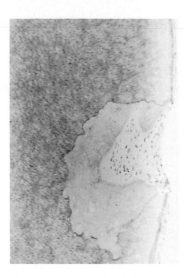

Fig. 16-22   Histologic appearance of surface resorption. Repair of the resorption lacuna with cementum-like tissue is evident (stain: H&E). (Courtesy Dr. Leif Tronstad.)

Prognosis

There are three factors that influence repair success:

1. The degree of dislocation and mobility of the coronal fragment are extremely important.[4,82,151,177] Increased dislocation and coronal fragment mobility result in a decreased prognosis.
2. Immature teeth are seldom involved in root fractures; when they are the prognosis is good.[78]
3. Prognosis increases with quick treatment, close reduction of the root segments, and rigid splinting for 2 to 4 months.[82,129,151] Therefore the quality of treatment is also important.

There are two complications to repair success:

1. Pulp necrosis, which can be treated successfully[36,81] by treating the coronal segment with long-term calcium hydroxide and obturation when a hard-tissue barrier has formed.
2. Root canal obliteration is not uncommon if the root segment (coronal or apical) remains vital.

LUXATION INJURIES

There are five kinds of luxation injury:

1. Concussion—An injury involving no displacement, mobility, or sensitivity to percussion.
2. Subluxation—An injury involving sensitivity to percussion, increased mobility, and no displacement.
3. Lateral luxation—An injury involving displacement labially, lingually, distally, or incisally.
4. Extrusive luxation—An injury involving displacement in a coronal direction.
5. Intrusive luxation—An injury involving displacement in an apical direction into the alveolus.

Note: The previous definitions describe injuries of increasing magnitude in terms of intensity of the injury and subsequent sequelae.

Incidence

Luxation injuries are the most common of all dental injuries, with reported incidences ranging from 30% to 44%.[91,157]

Biologic Consequences

Luxation injuries result in damage to the attachment apparatus (i.e., periodontal ligament, cemental layer), the severity of which is dependent on the type of injury sustained (concussion least, intrusion most). The apical neurovascular supply to the pulp is also affected to varying degrees, resulting in an unreliable response to electric pulp testing, and thus an altered or complete loss of vitality to the tooth.

Sequelae of Attachment Damage

Surface resorption. During a luxation injury mechanical damage to the cementum surface occurs and a local inflammatory response and localized area of root resorption results. If no further inflammatory stimulus is present, periodontal healing and root surface repair will occur within 14 days.[67] These small resorptive lacunae have been termed *surface resorption* (Fig. 16-22). It is symptomless and, in most cases, cannot be visualized on routine radiographs.

Dentoalveolar ankylosis and replacement resorption. If the trauma is extensive (e.g., intrusive luxation) with a large area of damage involving more than 20% of the root surface,[94,97] an abnormal attachment can occur after healing. After the initial inflammatory response to remove debris resulting from the injury, a root surface devoid of cementum results.[67,97] Cells in the vicinity of the denuded root now compete to repopulate it.[18] Often cells that are precursors of bone (rather than the slower moving periodontal ligament cells) will move across from the socket wall and populate the damaged root, and bone comes into direct contact with the root without an intermediate attachment apparatus. This phenomenon is termed *dentoalveolar ankylosis*.[68]

Bone resorbs and reforms physiologically throughout life. The osteoclasts in contact with the root resorb the dentin as though it was bone; in the reforming phase, osteoblasts lay down new bone in the area that was previously root, eventually replacing it. This progressive replacement of the root by bone is termed *replacement resorption*.[68] It is characterized histologically by direct contact between bone and dentin without a separating periodontal ligament and cemental layer[14] (Fig 16-23). Radiographically, the distinction between the root and surrounding bone (a traceable lamina dura) is lost and a "moth eaten" appearance results[14,160] (Fig. 16-24). Clinically, lack of mobility of the tooth and a metallic sound to percussion is pathognomonic,[12] as is infraocclusion in the developing dentition (see Fig. 16-24). Ultimately the tooth is lost because of loss of root support.

Consequences of Apical Neurovascular Supply Damage

Pulp canal obliteration. Pulp canal obliteration is common after luxation injuries. The frequency of pulp canal obliteration appears inversely proportional to that of pulp necrosis. The exact mechanism of pulp canal obliteration is not known. It has been theorized that the sympathetic and parasympathetic control of blood flow to the odontoblasts is altered, resulting in uncontrolled reparative dentin.[4] Another theory is that hemorrhage and blood clot formation in the pulp after injury is a nidus for subsequent calcification if the pulp remains vital.[4] Pulp canal obliteration can usually be diagnosed within the first year after injury.[9] Pulp canal obliteration was found to be more frequent in teeth with open apices (> 0.7 mm radiographically), in teeth with extrusive and lateral luxation injuries, and in teeth that have been rigidly splinted.[9]

Pulp necrosis. The factors most important for the development of pulp necrosis are the type of injury (concussion least, intrusion most) and the stage of root development (mature apex > immature apex).[8]

Pulp necrosis can lead to infection of the root canal system with the following consequences:

Apical periodontitis with apical root resorption Practically all teeth exhibiting apical periodontitis exhibit apical

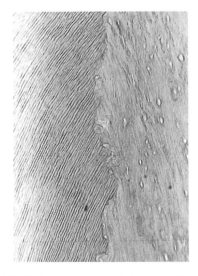

Fig. 16-23 Histologic appearance of dentoalveolar ankylosis with replacement resorption. Note the absence of the periodontal ligament and cemental layer and the direct union of the bone and root.

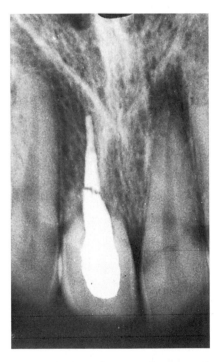

Fig. 16-24 Radiograph of maxillary central incisor with replacement resorption. Note the lack of the lamina dura and the moth-eaten appearance of the roots. Infraocclusion of the tooth relative to the surrounding teeth is also apparent.

resorption (Fig. 16-25). The resorption can be minor and practically invisible radiographically, or it can be so extensive that a significant amount of root tip is lost (Fig. 16-26). The cemental layer is a physical barrier that separates the root canal system from the surrounding periodontal attachment. If the cemental layer stays intact after the traumatic injury, it will not allow the passage of toxins through it. Therefore the only communication between the root canal system and periodontal ligament remains the apical foramen, causing an apical periodontitis with apical root resorption. It appears that the intense and progressive inflammation confined at the apex overcomes the resistance of the cemental layer to resorption.

Apical root resorption is asymptomatic; symptoms that may lead to its diagnosis would be associated with the periapical inflammation. Radiographically, the diagnosis is made by radiolucencies at the root tip and adjacent bone. (Pathognomonic of root resorption at all root locations is concomitant resorption of the adjacent bone.) Treatment is conventional root canal treatment (as described in Chapters 8 and 9) (Fig. 16-27) that has a reasonably good success rate.[108,116,125] Apical closure techniques with long-term calcium hydroxide treatment can also be used to ensure a better prognosis for future nonsurgical endodontic therapy.[88]

Periradicular periodontitis with root resorption   After a more serious injury, portions of the cemental covering of the root are damaged and the protective (i.e., insulating) quality is lost. If the pulp is necrotic and infected, the bacterial toxins may now pass through the dentinal tubules, stimulating an inflammatory response in the corresponding periodontal ligament. The result will be resorption of the root and bone. This process is termed *inflammatory root resorption*.[12,14] The periodontal infiltrate consists of granulation tissue with lymphocytes, plasma cells, and polymorphonuclear leukocytes. Multinucleated giant cells resorb the denuded root surface and will continue until the stimulus (i.e., pulp space bacteria) is removed[67] (Fig. 16-28).

Radiographically, inflammatory root resorption is observed as progressively forming radiolucent areas of the root and adjacent bone (Fig. 16-29). When inflammatory root resorption is treated by root canal disinfection, a large area denuded of attachment can result when the inflammation subsides. The competition between cells for the denuded root surface (previously described) occurs under these circumstances as well, possibly resulting in replacement resorption.

It is important to diagnose these resorptive complications because periradicular inflammatory root resorption can be reversed. If ankylosis is present long-term treatment alternatives must be planned. To diagnose these complications it is important to have knowledge of and be able to differentiate it from other types of root resorption.

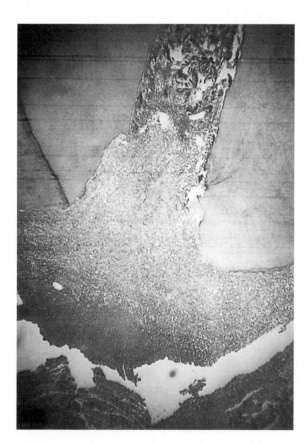

Fig. 16-25 Histologic appearance of apical resorption because of an infected root canal. Chronic inflammation is present apically. Resorption of the external and internal aspect of the root can be seen (stain: H&E). (Courtesy Dr. S. Seltzer.)

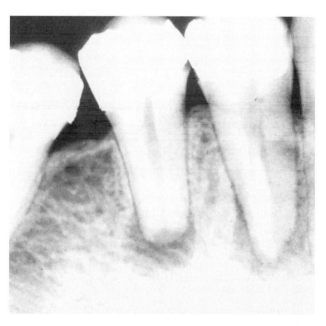

Fig. 16-26 Mandibular premolar with external apical resorption because of apical periodontitis. Pulp of the tooth is necrotic and infected.

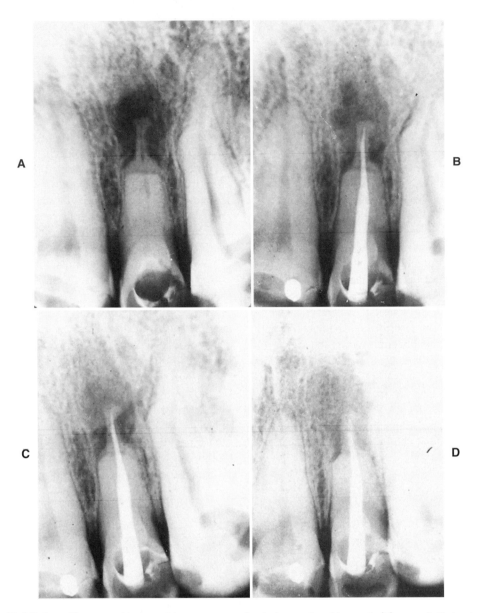

Fig. 16-27 A maxillary central incisor with severe external apical resorption. Nonsurgical therapy. **A**, Pretreatment. Extensive resorption in the apical third, but the canal is intact. **B**, After instrumentation and disinfection, obturation with lateral condensation. **C**, Follow-up 6 months after treatment. There is some evidence of bone repair. **D**, Follow-up 5 years after treatment. Continued bone remineralization.

ROOT RESORPTION DEFECTS MIMICKING PERIRADICULAR INFLAMMATORY ROOT RESORPTION OF PULPAL ORIGIN

Cervical Root Resorption

Cervical root resorption is a progressive root resorption of inflammatory origin usually occurring immediately below the epithelial attachment of the tooth (but not exclusively in that area).[14,160,176] It appears to be a delayed reaction after an injury; however, its exact pathogenesis is not fully understood. The name *cervical root resorption* implies that the resorption must occur at the cervical area of the tooth. However, the periodontal attachment of teeth is not always located at the cervical margin and may occur more apically on the root surface. The anatomic connotation of its name has led to confusion and misdiagnosis of this condition. Because of this confusion many attempts have been made to rename this type of external resorption.[20,53,62]

Cause   Because its histologic appearance and progressive nature is identical to other forms of progressive inflammatory root resorption, it appears logical that the pathogenesis would be the same (i.e., an unprotected or altered root sur-

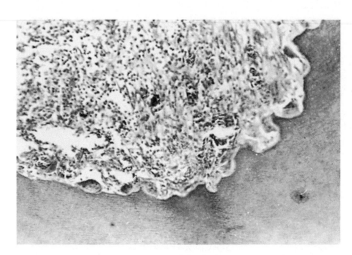

Fig. 16-28 Histologic appearance of inflammatory resorption. Granulomatous tissue in relation to the resorbed root surface. Multinucleated giant cells are present in the areas of active resorption on the root surface (stain: H&E). (Courtesy Dr. Leif Tronstad.)

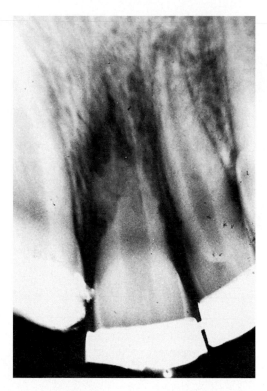

Fig. 16-29 Maxillary left incisor with inflammatory resorption 3 months after replantation without appropriate endodontic treatment. Resorption of the root and bone is apparent. Original root canal can still be traced radiographically.

face attracting resorbing cells and an inflammatory response maintained by infection). Cervical root resorption can occur long after orthodontic treatment (Fig. 16-30), orthognathic surgery, periodontal treatment, nonvital bleaching, or trauma (Fig. 16-31).[69,160] It is assumed that these procedures are the cause of removal of the protective layer or alteration of the root surface immediately below the epithelial attachment. *The pulp plays no role in cervical root resorption and is usually normal in these cases.*

Because the source of stimulation (i.e., infection) is not the pulp, it has been postulated that it is bacteria found in the sulcus of the tooth that stimulate and sustain an inflammatory response in the periodontium at the attachment level of the root.[62,160] The delayed nature (sometimes by many years) of this type of resorption is difficult to explain. It is possible that the inflammatory process does not reach the damaged root surface initially, and that only after years, with eruption of the tooth or periodontal recession, are the chemotactic factors of inflammation close enough to attract resorbing cells to the appropriate root surface. However, it would seem logical that if a stimulus were not present immediately after the injury to the root surface, repair would take place and the root surface would no longer be susceptible to resorption.

An alternate theory is that the procedures mentioned previously cause alteration in the ratio of organic and inorganic cementum,[136] making it relatively more inorganic and less resistant to resorption when challenged by inflammation. It has also been speculated that the altered root surface registers in the immune system as a different tissue and is attacked as a foreign body.[92] Thus these root surfaces do not possess their original antiresorptive properties on healing and would be susceptible to resorption at all times.

When, owing to periodontal recession or tooth eruption, the inflammation in the sulcular gingival area reaches the

altered root surface, resorption takes place. Obviously, the *pathogenesis of cervical root resorption is not yet fully understood,* and further research is required in this area.

Clinical Manifestations   Cervical resorption presents no symptoms; often it is detected only through routine radiographs. As mentioned previously, the pulp is not involved in this type of resorption, and sensitivity test results would be within normal limits. On occasion, if the pulp is exposed by an extensive resorptive defect, abnormal sensitivity to thermal stimuli may be experienced; however, pain to percussion and palpation is not to be expected. The resorption starts on the root surface. However, when the predentin is reached the resorptive process is resisted and the resorption proceeds laterally and in an apical and coronal direction, enveloping the root canal (Fig. 16-32).

When cervical root resorption is long standing, the granulation tissue can be seen undermining the enamel of the crown of the tooth, giving it a pinkish appearance (Fig. 16-33). This "pink spot" has traditionally been used to describe the pathognomonic clinical picture of internal root resorption, resulting in many cervical root resorption cases being misdiagnosed and treated as internal root resorption.

Because (as with other types of inflammatory resorption) adjacent bone and root are resorbed and, in this type of

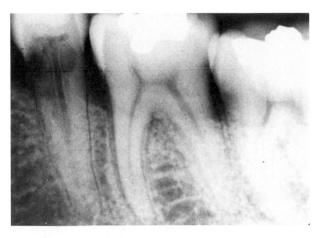

Fig. 16-30 Cervical root resorption on mandibular bicuspid 6 years after completion of orthodontic treatment. Note the mottled appearance of the resorptive defect and the outline of the root canal within the defect.

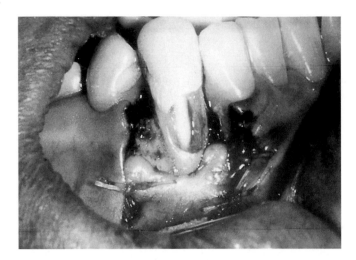

Fig. 16-32 Mandibular canine after removal of granulation tissue of a cervical resorption defect. Note the extensive nature of the defect in the dentin, although the root remains intact. (Courtesy Dr. Henry Rankow.)

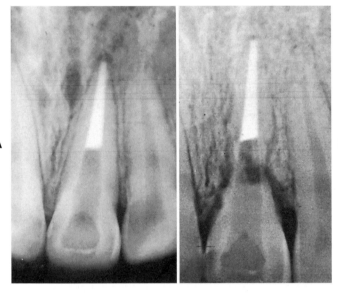

A   **B**

Fig. 16-31 **A,** Maxillary incisor after completion of root canal therapy and immediate bleaching procedure. **B,** Sixteen-month follow-up showing severe cervical root resorption. (Courtesy Dr. William Goon and Dr. Stephen Cohen.}

resorption, the bone loss is below the epithelial attachment, this condition is commonly misdiagnosed as an infrabony pocket of periodontal origin. However, when the "pocket" is probed copious bleeding and a spongelike feeling are observed when the granulation tissue of the resorptive defect is disturbed.

Radiographic Appearance   The radiographic appearance of cervical root resorption can vary. If the resorptive process occurs mesially or distally on the root surface, it is common to see a small, radiolucent opening into the root. The radiolucency may expand coronally and apically in the dentin, and it may reach but not perforate the root canal (Fig. 16-34). If the resorptive process is buccal or palatal-lingual, the radiographic picture is dependent on the extent to which the resorptive process has spread in the dentin. Initially, radiolucency near the attachment level (i.e., cervical margin) would be seen. However, if the process is long standing and extensive, the radiolucent area can extend a considerable way in a coronal and apical direction. The resorption site may have a mottled appearance, owing to deposition of calcified reparative tissue within the resorptive lesion.[144] Because the pulp in the root canal is not involved in this type of resorption, it is usually possible to clearly distinguish the outline of the canal through the radiolucency of the external resorptive defect (see Figs. 16-30 and 16-33).

Histologic appearance   The histologic appearance of cervical root resorption is similar to that of other types of inflammatory root resorption (i.e., chronic inflammation, multinucleated resorbing cells). It is also common to see histologic evidence of attempts at repair by cementum-like and bonelike material. Union of bone and dentin (i.e., replacement resorption) sometimes occurs.

Internal Root Resorption

Internal root resorption is *rare* in permanent teeth. Internal resorption is characterized by an oval-shaped enlargement of the root canal space.[14] External resorption, which is much more common, is often misdiagnosed as internal resorption.

Cause   Internal root resorption is characterized by resorption of the internal aspect of the root by multinucleated giant cells adjacent to granulation tissue in the pulp (Fig. 16-35).

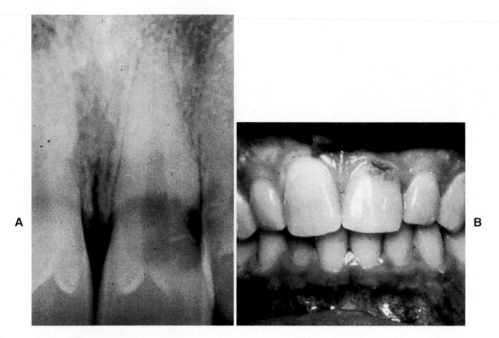

Fig. 16-33 **A,** Maxillary incisor with cervical root resorption extending coronally. **B,** Clinical appearance shows a pink spot on the labial surface of the tooth, close to the gingival margin.

Chronic inflammatory tissue is common in the pulp, but only rarely does it result in resorption. There are different theories on the origin of the pulpal granulation tissue involved in internal resorption. The most logical explanation is that it is pulp tissue that is inflamed because of an infected coronal pulp space. Communication between the coronal necrotic tissue and the vital pulp is through appropriately oriented dentinal tubules[158,171] (Fig. 16-36).

One investigator reports[152] that resorption of the dentin is frequently associated with deposition of hard tissue resembling bone or cementum but not dentin. He postulates that the resorbing tissue is not of pulpal origin but is "metaplastic" tissue derived from the pulpal invasion of macrophage-like cells.[67] Others[172] concluded that the pulp tissue was replaced by periodontium-like connective tissue when internal resorption was present. In addition to the requirement of the presence of granulation tissue, root resorption takes place only if the odontoblastic layer and predentin are lost or altered.[160,172] Reasons for the loss of predentin adjacent to the granulation tissue are not obvious. Trauma frequently has been suggested as a cause.[45,141]

Some researchers[171] report that trauma may be recognized as an initiating factor in internal resorption. These resorptions are divided into transient-type resorption and progressive-type resorption, the latter requiring continuous stimulation by infection. Another reason for the loss of predentin may be extreme heat produced when cutting on dentin without adequate water spray. The heat presumably would destroy the predentin layer, and if later the coronal aspect of the pulp became infected the bacterial products could initiate the typical inflammation in conjunction with resorbing giant cells in

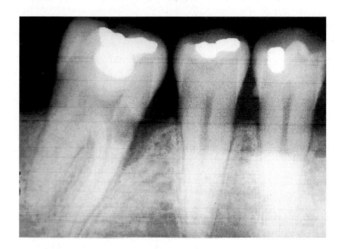

Fig. 16-34 Mandibular molar with cervical resorption on its mesial aspect. Note the small opening into the root and the extensive resorption in the dentin; however, the pulp is not exposed. Also notice that a resorptive defect is present in the adjacent bone, appearing radiographically similar to an infrabony pocket.

the vital pulp adjacent to the denuded root surface. Internal root resorption has been produced experimentally by the application of diathermy.[63]

Clinical Manifestations   Internal root resorption is usually asymptomatic and is first recognized clinically through routine radiographs. Pain may be a presenting symptom if perforation of the crown occurs and the metaplastic tissue is

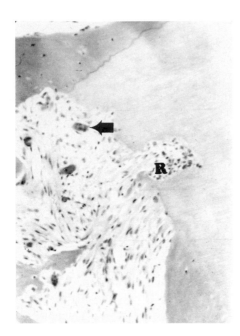

Fig. 16-35 Histologic appearance of internal resorption. Granulation tissue, including multinucleated giant cells (*arrow*) is present. Resorptive lacunae (*R*) in dentin (stain: H&E) (original magnification: × 100). (Courtesy Dr. Harold Stanley.)

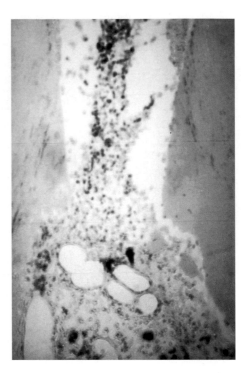

Fig. 16-36 Histologic section of internal resorption stained with Brown and Brenn. Bacteria are seen (in the dentinal tubules) communicating between the necrotic coronal segment and the apical granulation tissue and resorbing cells. (Courtesy Dr. Leif Tronstad.)

exposed to oral fluids. For internal resorption to be active, at least part of the pulp must be vital so that a positive response to pulp sensitivity testing is possible. The clinician should remember that the coronal portion of the pulp is often necrotic, whereas the apical pulp, which includes the internal resorptive defect, can remain vital. Therefore a negative sensitivity test result does not rule out active internal resorption. It is also possible that the pulp becomes nonvital after a period of active resorption, giving a negative sensitivity test, radiographic signs of internal resorption, and radiographic signs of apical inflammation (Fig. 16-37). Traditionally, the pink tooth has been thought pathognomonic of internal root resorption. The pink color is caused by granulation tissue in the coronal dentin undermining the crown enamel. The pink tooth can also be a feature of cervical root resorption, which must be ruled out before a diagnosis of internal root resorption is made.

Radiographic Appearance   The usual radiographic presentation of internal root resorption is a fairly uniform, radiolucent enlargement of the pulp canal (Fig. 16-38). Because the resorption is initiated in the root canal, the resorptive defect includes some part of the root canal space. Therefore the original outline of the root canal is distorted. Only on rare occasions when the internal resorptive defect penetrates the root and impacts the periodontal ligament does the adjacent bone show radiographic changes.

Histologic Appearance   Like that of other inflammatory resorptive defects, the histologic picture of internal resorption is granulation tissue with multinucleated giant cells (see Fig. 16-35). An area of necrotic pulp is found coronal to the granulation tissue. Dentinal tubules containing microorganisms and communicating between the necrotic zone and the granulation tissue can sometimes be seen[*] (see Fig. 16-36). Unlike external root resorption, resorption of the adjacent bone does not occur with internal root resorption.

Diagnostic Features of External Versus Internal Root Resorption

It is often very difficult to distinguish external from internal root resorption, so misdiagnosis and incorrect treatment result. What follows is a list of typical diagnostic features of each resorptive type.

Radiographic Features   A change of angulation of radiographs should provide a fairly good indication of whether a resorptive defect is internal or external. A lesion of internal origin appears close to the canal regardless of the angle of the radiograph exposure (Fig. 16-39). On the other hand, a defect on the external aspect of the root moves away from the canal as the angulation changes (Fig. 16-40). In addition, by using

[*]References 160,161,163,165,170,171

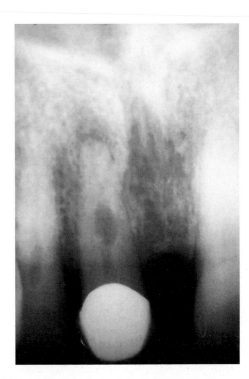

Fig. 16-37 Maxillary incisor with midroot radiolucency typical of internal resorption. Apical radiolucency is also present. Internal resorption must have occurred before the pulp became nonvital.

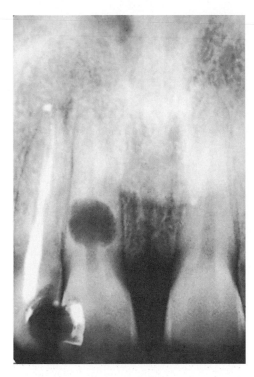

Fig. 16-38 A maxillary incisor with internal root resorption. Uniform enlargement of the pulp space is apparent. Outline of the canal cannot be seen in the resorptive defect.

the buccal-object rule it is usually possible to distinguish if the external root defect is buccal or palatal-lingual.

In internal resorption, the outline of the root canal is usually distorted and the root canal and the radiolucent resorptive defect appear contiguous (see Figs. 16-37 and 16-38). When the defect is external, the root canal outline appears normal and can usually be seen "running through" the radiolucent defect (see Fig. 16-33).

External inflammatory root resorption is always accompanied by resorption of the bone (see Figs. 16-31 and 16-34). Therefore radiolucencies are apparent in both the root and the adjacent bone. Internal root resorption does not involve the bone, and as a rule the radiolucency is confined to the root (see Figs. 16-37 through 16-39). On rare occasions if the internal defect perforates the root, the bone adjacent to it is resorbed and appears radiolucent on the radiograph.

Vitality Testing   External inflammatory resorption of the apical and lateral aspects of the root involves an infected pulp space, so a negative response to sensitivity tests is required to support the diagnosis. On the other hand, because cervical root resorption does not involve the pulp (the bacteria are thought to originate in the sulcus of the tooth), a normal response to sensitivity testing is usually associated with this type of resorption. Internal root resorption usually occurs in teeth with vital pulps and gives a positive response to sensitivity testing. However, it is not uncommon to register

a negative response to sensitivity testing in teeth that exhibit internal root resorption, because often the coronal pulp has been removed or is necrotic and the active resorbing cells are more apical in the canal. In addition, the pulp may have become necrotic after active resorption has taken place.

Pink Spot   With apical and lateral external root resorption the pulp is nonvital; therefore the granulation tissue that produces the pink spot is not present in these cases. For cervical and internal root resorption the pink spot caused by granulation tissue undermining the enamel is a possible sign.

Summary of Possible Diagnostic Features

Inflammatory Root Resorption

Apical.   These teeth (with or without a history of trauma) often produce negative pulp sensitivity tests.

Lateral.   These teeth often have a history of trauma, negative pulp sensitivity tests, lesions that move on angled radiographs, root canals that are visualized radiographically overlying the defect, and bony radiolucencies that are apparent to the clinician.

Cervical.   These teeth have a history of trauma (often forgotten or not identified by the patient), positive pulp sensitivity tests, lesions located at the attachment level of the teeth, lesions that move on angled radiographs, root canal outlines that are undistorted and can be visualized radio-

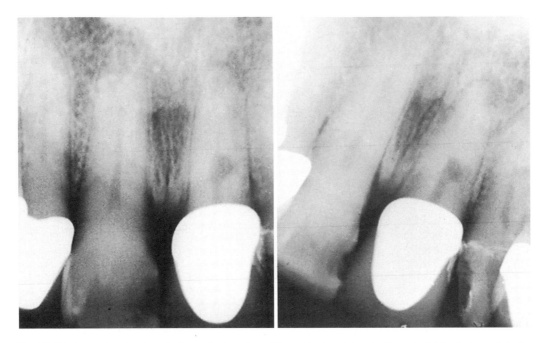

Fig. 16-39 Internal resorption. Radiographs from two different horizontal projections depict the lesion within the confines of the root canal on both views.

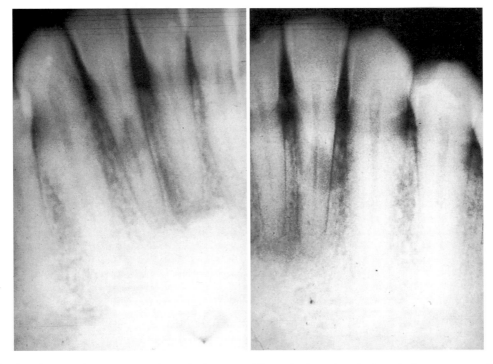

Fig. 16-40 External resorption. Radiographs from two different horizontal projections depict movement of the lesion to outside the confines of the root canal.

graphically, and crestal bony defects associated with the lesions. Pink spots are also possible.

Internal.   These teeth have a history of trauma, crown preparation, or pulpotomy. In addition, positive pulp sensitivity tests are likely, and they may occur at any location along the root canal (not only at the attachment level). Lesions remain associated with the root canal on angled radiographs, and radiolucencies are contained in the root without an adjacent bony defect. Pink spots are also possible.

The majority of misdiagnoses of resorptive defects are made between cervical and internal root resorptions. The diagnosis should always be confirmed while treatment is proceeding. If root canal therapy is the treatment of choice for an apparent internal root resorption, the bleeding within the canal should cease quickly after pulp extirpation because the blood supply of the granulation tissue is the apical blood vessels. If bleeding continues during treatment (particularly if it is still present at the second visit) the source of the blood supply is external and treatment for external resorption should be completed. On obturation it should be possible to fill the entire canal from within in internal resorption. Failure to achieve dense, homogeneous obturation should make the clinician suspicious of an external lesion. Finally, if the blood supply of an internal resorption defect is removed on pulp extirpation, any continuation of the resorptive process on recall radiographs should alert the dentist to the possibility that an external resorptive defect was misdiagnosed.

DIAGNOSIS OF LUXATION INJURIES AT THE EMERGENCY VISIT

Evaluation

Patients will report a history of a recent traumatic injury, a varying degree of displacement of the tooth, and pain to percussion. A thorough history (medical and dental) must be taken and clinical assessment of the teeth made, with particular emphasis on pain to percussion and mobility. Radiographic assessment (see "Root Fractures") is extremely important to assess the extent of displacement (if present) and to assess the presence or absence of a root fracture.

Diagnosis and Emergency Treatment

Concussion

Diagnosis and clinical presentation.   Concussion injuries include no displacement or mobility of the tooth. Pain to percussion is the only feature of this type of injury. A history of the recent traumatic injury, in addition to the pain to percussion, makes the diagnosis possible.

Treatment.   Baseline sensitivity tests should be performed. A possible root fracture must be ruled out with angled radiographs (see "Root Fractures"). The occlusion must be checked and adjusted if necessary. With concussion injuries (as with other luxation injuries) it is possible to have

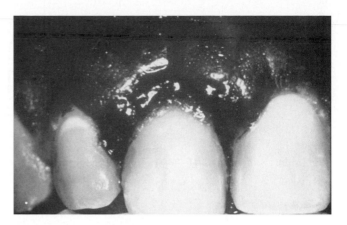

Fig. 16-41 Maxillary central incisor after luxation injury. Sulcular bleeding is an indication that the tooth was displaced in the socket.

a negative response to sensitivity testing and also discoloration of the crown. Endodontic treatment should not be carried out at this visit because both the negative sensitivity testing and crown discoloration can be reversible.[4]

Follow-up.   The clinician should schedule follow-up examinations at 3 weeks; 3, 6, 12 months; and yearly thereafter. The major concern in follow-up examinations is the development of pulp necrosis. Sensitivity tests are performed as are tests for periapical inflammation (i.e., percussion, palpation, radiographic signs of apical periodontitis). Pulp necrosis has been reported to be discernable within 3 months.[4] Because concussion injuries are relatively minimal injuries in terms of attachment damage, a conservative approach is feasible if sensitivity tests are negative but no signs of apical periodontitis are present.

Subluxation

Diagnosis and clinical presentation   Clinical presentation of subluxation is similar to concussion. In addition, the tooth is slightly mobile and typically has clinical signs of sulcular bleeding (Fig. 16-41).

Treatment   The clinician should provide treatment as would be done with concussion.

Follow-up   The clinician should schedule follow-up examinations as would be done with concussion.

Lateral Luxation

Diagnosis and clinical presentation.   History of a recent traumatic injury. The tooth is displaced laterally (usually the crown toward the palatal) and sulcular bleeding is usually present. The tooth is usually extremely sensitive to touch or percussion.

Treatment.   In most cases of lateral luxation the crown of the tooth is moved palatally and the apex facially (Fig. 16-42, *A*). Often the apical root is forced through the labial cortical plate and the tooth is then frequently locked into its new position and difficult to dislodge. The tooth must be dislodged from the labial cortical plate by moving it coronal and then apical. This is performed as gently as possible by placing coronal and palatal pressure on the apical root with the index finger and labial pressure on the crown with the thumb (Fig. 16-42, *B*). Thus the tooth is moved first coronally out of the buccal plate of bone and "snaps back" into its original position. Local anesthetic is usually required for repositioning. If the tooth is mobile after repositioning, it should be splinted with an acid etched technique (see "Avulsion"). Sensitivity testing is of little value at this visit.

Follow-up

Mature tooth   Although pulp survival is possible in a small number of cases,[4] if sensitivity testing indicates pulp necrosis at the 3-week follow-up visit, endodontic treatment should be performed. Root canal treatment of a noninfected pulp space has an extremely high success rate in a mature tooth[64,155] and should be performed rather than risk external root resorption complications.

Immature tooth   Immature teeth present a dilemma. Chances of pulpal vitality (i.e., maintenance or revascularization) are fairly good. However, if necrosis and infection do occur, teeth that have undergone cemental damage because of traumatic injury are susceptible to inflammatory root resorption and could be lost in a short period of time. Careful follow-up is very important. At the first sign (clinical or

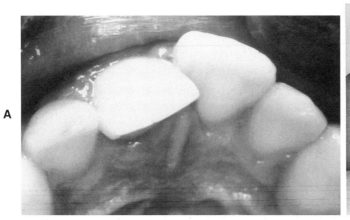
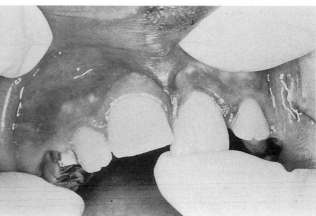

A   B

Fig. 16-42 Lateral luxation of maxillary central incisor. **A**, Crown is moved palatally and the root apex facially. **B**, The tooth is moved coronally out of the buccal plate with the index finger and facially with the thumb.

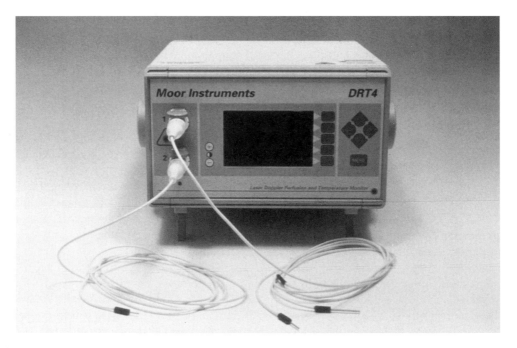

Fig. 16-43 Laser Doppler flowmeter used in the diagnosis of revascularization in luxated and avulsed immature teeth. (From Mesaros S, Trope M: Revascularization of traumatized teeth assessed by laser Doppler flowmetry: case report, *Endod Dent Traumatol* 13[1]:24,1997.)

radiographic) of apical or periradicular root resorption, endodontic treatment should be initiated (see "Avulsion"). The laser Doppler flowmeter is a promising tool in the diagnosis of revascularization in these young teeth (Fig. 16-43).[112]

Extrusive Luxation   Diagnosis and clinical presentation, treatment, and follow-up are essentially the same as with lateral luxations.

Intrusive Luxations

Diagnosis and clinical presentation   The tooth may be pushed into its socket, sometimes giving the appearance that it may have been avulsed (Fig. 16-44). The tooth presents with the clinical presentation of ankylosis because the tooth is firm in the socket, gives a metallic sound to the percussion test, and after the injury is in infraocclusion. The obvious difference is the recent traumatic injury. Radiographic evaluation is essential to evaluate the extent and the position of the intruded tooth.

Treatment.   Intrusive luxation is probably the most damaging injury that a tooth can sustain. The movement of the tooth into the socket results in extensive attachment damage, with resultant dentoalveolar ankylosis and replacement resorption almost a certainty. In addition, pulp necrosis is extremely common so that inflammatory root resorption will result if timely and adequate endodontic treatment is not performed.

Initial treatment depends on the stage of development of the tooth. Immature teeth usually will reerupt spontaneously and establish their original position within a few weeks or months.[79] If reeruption stops before normal occlusion is attained, orthodontic movement should be initiated quickly before the tooth is ankylosed in position (Fig. 16-45). Intruded mature teeth must be repositioned immediately as not to ankylose in the intruded position.[14] If an orthodontic appliance can be attached to the tooth, orthodontic repositioning is favored. If the tooth is severely intruded, surgical access can be made to attach an orthodontic appliance or the tooth can be repositioned by loosening it surgically and immediately repositioning it into alignment with the adjacent teeth. Endodontic treatment protocols are similar to those of an avulsed tooth (see "Avulsion").

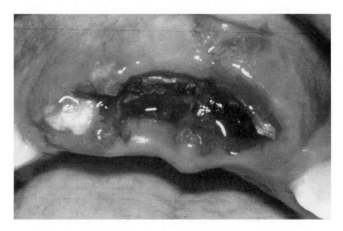

Fig. 16-44 Severely intruded maxillary incisor teeth mistaken as having been avulsed.

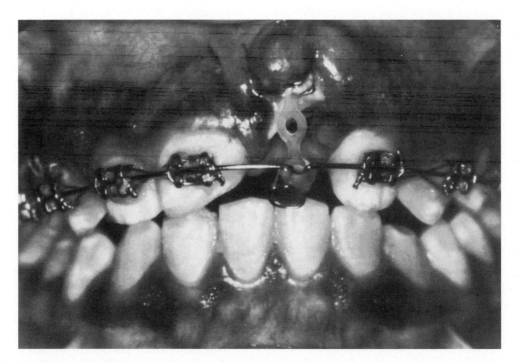

Fig. 16-45 Intruded maxillary incisor is to be orthodontically moved into position soon after the injury. If treatment is delayed, the tooth will be ankylosed in the intruded position.

Prognosis of Luxation Injuries

Pulp Necrosis   Pulp necrosis is common after luxation injuries. Even a subluxation injury that appears to be minimal results in pulp necrosis in the range of 12% to 20% of cases.[102,151] For lateral or extrusive luxations over half of the pulps will eventually become necrotic.[10,80,135,151] Intrusive injuries result in an extremely high incidence of necrosis. Infection of the necrotic pulp will take place after a variable amount of time. Therefore signs of apical periodontitis, including pain to percussion, can take months or even years to appear.[80]

Pulp Canal Obliteration   Pulp canal obliteration is a fairly common occurrence in luxated teeth.[10,102,138] Endodontic treatment is *not* routinely indicated (see "Biologic Consequences").

Root Resorption   Root resorption occurs in 5% to 15% of luxation injuries.[102,119,151] Inflammatory root resorption can be treated with a high degree of success with adequate endodontic therapy.[38] However, ankylosis is irreversible, and when it occurs a long-term treatment plan for the ultimate loss of the tooth must be made.

AVULSION

Avulsion, or exarticulation, implies complete displacement of the tooth from the alveolus.

Incidence

The reported incidence of tooth avulsion ranges from 1% to 16% of all traumatic injuries to the permanent dentition.[51] Like most dental trauma, maxillary central incisors are the most frequently avulsed in the permanent dentition.[51] Sports and automobile accidents are the most frequent cause,[70] and the most frequently involved age group is children 7 to 10 years old.[16]

Biologic Consequences

The biologic consequences of tooth avulsion are the same as described for tooth luxation. In addition, the drying damage that occurs to the periodontal ligament when the tooth is out of the mouth has extremely detrimental effects on healing. Pulpal necrosis always occurs after an avulsion injury, but revascularization is possible in teeth with immature apices. Therefore complications after avulsion injuries are common, but treatment must be carried out in a timely and correct fashion to prevent or limit these complications.

Treatment Objectives

Treatment is directed at avoiding or minimizing the effects of the two main complications of the avulsed tooth, namely attachment damage and pulpal infection. Attachment damage as a direct result of the avulsion injury cannot be avoided. However, considerable additional damage can occur to the periodontal membrane in the time that the tooth is out of the mouth (primarily because of drying). Treatment is directed at minimizing this damage so that the fewest possible complications result. When extreme damage has occurred and replacement resorption is considered certain, steps must be taken to slow the resorptive process to maintain the tooth in the mouth for as long as possible. In the open-apex tooth, all efforts must be made to promote revitalization of the pulp. In the closed-apex tooth or in the open-apex tooth in which revitalization is unsuccessful, all treatment efforts must be made to eliminate potential toxins from the root canal space.

Clinical Management

Management Outside of the Dental Office   The damage to the attachment apparatus that occurs during an initial injury is unavoidable. However, all efforts are made to minimize necrosis of the remaining periodontal ligament while the tooth is out of the mouth. Pulpal sequelae are not an initial concern but will be dealt with at a later phase of treatment.

The single most important factor in the success of replantation is the *speed* with which the tooth is replanted.[13,14] Of utmost importance is the prevention of drying, which causes loss of normal physiologic metabolism and morphology of the periodontal ligament cells.[18,148] Every effort should be made to replant the tooth within the first 15 to 20 minutes.[13,16] This usually requires emergency personnel with experience in this type of injury. The dentist should give careful instructions to the person at the scene of the accident over the phone. A clean tooth with an undamaged root should be replanted with as little force as possible. The person should be instructed to hold the tooth by the crown, wash the root gently (but not excessively) in running water or saline, and gently place it back in the socket. The patient should be brought to the office immediately.

If doubt exists that the tooth can be replanted adequately, the tooth should quickly be stored in an appropriate medium until the patient can arrive at the dental office for replantation. Suggested storage media include the vestibule of the mouth, physiologic saline, milk, and cell culture media in specialized transport containers.[77] Water is the least desirable storage medium because the hypotonic environment causes rapid cell lysis.[26] Storage in the vestibule of the mouth keeps the tooth moist but is not ideal because of incompatible osmolality, pH, and the presence of bacteria.[95] Saliva, however, allows storage for up to 2 hours.[27] Milk is considered the best storage medium for uncomplicated avulsion because it is usually readily available at or near an accident site, it has a pH and osmolality compatible to vital cells, and it is relatively free of bacteria. Milk effectively maintains the vitality of periodontal ligament cells for 3 hours, which usually allows adequate time for the patient to reach the dentist for replantation.[26] Cell culture media have also been tested as storage media for avulsed teeth and have great potential.[14] However, culture media are seldom available near the site of an accident, rendering their use impractical and of academic interest only.

Recently, an avulsed-tooth preserving system (Save-A-Tooth) that contains Hank's Balanced Salt Solution (HBSS) (Biologic Rescue Products, Conshohocken, PA), a pH-preserving fluid and trauma-reducing suspension apparatus, has become available and has many potential advantages. This system should be available at schools and contact sport events, in ambulances and hospital emergency rooms, or even in the home. The system makes the use of a variety of storage media practical and enhances the possibility of maintaining the viability of the periodontal ligament cells for an extended time after avulsion. Thus teeth avulsed in serious accidents (when replantation is not immediately possible) may be stored in these devices and replanted after the crisis is over. Media storage extends the storage period significantly as compared with milk.[77,165]

Management in the Dental Office

Emergency visit. Recognizing that the dental injury may be secondary to a more serious injury is essential. If on examination a serious injury is suspected, immediate referral to the appropriate expert is the first priority. The focus of the emergency visit is the attachment apparatus. The aim is to replant the tooth with the maximal number of periodontal ligament cells that have the potential to regenerate and repair the damaged root surface. Necrotic and irreversibly damaged cells should be removed before replantation if possible. If maintaining the periodontal ligament in a viable state is not possible, steps must be taken to alter the root so as to slow the inevitable resorption. The necrotic pulp is not of immediate concern because toxins are usually not present initially in a great enough concentration to elicit an inflammatory response. Endodontics is not initiated at the emergency visit and is not performed extraorally if any hope exists of maintaining vital periodontal fibers on the root surface.

A medical history is extremely important and cannot be overlooked. The possible presence of a more serious trauma than the avulsion must be assessed; therefore obtaining a full history of the accident is essential. Reconstruction of the events of the accident gives the practitioner a good idea of the extent of injury to the attachment apparatus and the likelihood of damage to other teeth or structures. Information about where the tooth was recovered, dry time, storage media, and mode of transportation of the patient and tooth is essential for formation of the correct treatment choices.

Local anesthesia is usually recommended for conductance of a thorough clinical examination. If the tooth was replanted at the accident site, its positioning in the socket is assessed and a radiograph is made. If unacceptable, the tooth is gently removed and replanted. Once the tooth is positioned correctly, splinting, soft-tissue management, and adjunctive

therapy are the next steps. The following clinical steps minimize root resorption when the tooth is not replanted at the accident site:

Diagnosis and treatment planning   The tooth should immediately be placed in an appropriate storage medium while a history of the accident is obtained and the clinical examination is conducted. As previously mentioned, HBSS is presently considered the best medium for this purpose. It is commercially available and has a shelf life of 2 years or more. Milk or physiologic saline is also appropriate for storage purposes.

The clinical examination should include an examination of the socket to ascertain if it is intact and suitable for replantation. This is accomplished by palpation facially and palatally. The socket is gently rinsed with saline and (when cleared of any clot and debris) its walls are examined directly for the presence, absence, or collapse of the socket wall. Using palpation of the socket and surrounding apical areas and applying pressure on surrounding teeth are used to ascertain if an alveolar fracture is present in addition to the avulsion. Movement of a segment of bone and multiple teeth is suggestive of an alveolar fracture. The socket and surrounding areas, including the soft tissues, should be radiographed.[14] Three vertical angulations are required for diagnosis of the presence of a horizontal root fracture in adjacent teeth or foreign objects. The remaining teeth in both jaws should be examined for crown damage. Any soft-tissue lacerations should be noted. *Sensitivity testing at the emergency visit is always inconclusive and, therefore, of limited value; it should be delayed until the next visit.*

Preparation of the root

Extraoral dry time less than 20 minutes, closed apex.   If the tooth has a closed apex, revitalization is not possible. However, if the tooth was dry for less than 20 minutes (i.e., replanted or placed in appropriate medium) the chance for periodontal healing is excellent. The root should be rinsed of debris with water or saline and replanted in as gentle a fashion as possible.[14]

Extraoral dry time less than 20 minutes, open apex.   In an open-apex tooth, revascularization of the pulp and continued root development is possible (Fig. 16-46). One study[41] revealed that soaking the tooth in doxycycline (i.e., 1 mg in approximately 10 ml of physiologic saline) for 5 minutes before replantation significantly enhanced revascularization. The doxycycline inhibits bacteria in the pulpal lumen, thus removing the major obstacle to revascularization.[41] As with the tooth with the closed apex, the open-apex tooth is then rinsed with water or saline and gently replanted.

Extraoral time 20 to 60 minutes, closed and open apices. For drying periods of 20 to 60 minutes most authors suggest rinsing the tooth gently and replanting it as soon as possible, accepting that complications are inevitable. Previously mentioned was an attempt was made to soak the tooth is saline for approximately 30 minutes before replantation with limited success.[107] The theory behind soaking is that dead periodontal ligament cells will wash off the root surface, thus remov-

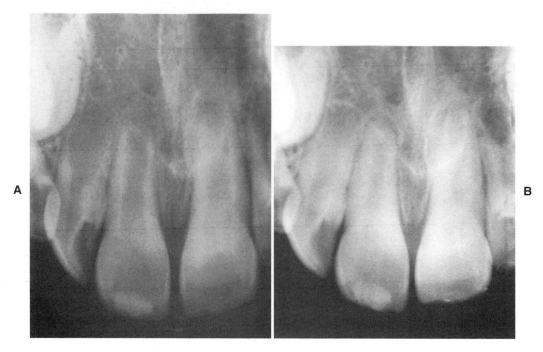

Fig. 16-46 Maxillary incisor with open apex that maintained vitality and continued root development after tooth replantation. **A,** Taken at the time of replantation. **B,** At the 2-year follow-up the pulp is still vital and the root is fully formed. (Courtesy Dr. Joe H. Camp.)

ing a stimulus for inflammation on replantation. In addition, it was believed that the soaking medium may revitalize cells affected by the extended drying time. A recent study tested newer storage media for soaking of teeth left dry for between 20 and 60 minutes.[124] Although HBSS was not beneficial for healing after soaking, ViaSpan, a liver transplant medium, did decrease the incidence of complications after replantation.[124] Although the results of this study do not yet justify the recommendation to soak such teeth, the newer media shows promise that this may be a recommendation in the future.

Extraoral dry time greater than 60 minutes, open and closed apices.   When the root has been dry for 60 minutes or more all periodontal cells have died,[96,141,148] soaking is ineffective.[107] In these cases the root should be prepared to be as resistant to resorption as possible (attempting to slow the process). These teeth should be soaked in citric acid for 5 minutes to remove all remaining periodontal ligament cells, in 2% stannous fluoride for 5 minutes, then replanted.[25,143] If the tooth has been dry for more than 60 minutes and no consideration has been given to preserving the periodontal ligament, the endodontics could be performed extraorally.

In the case of a tooth with a closed apex, no advantage exists to this additional step at the emergency visit. However, in a tooth with an open apex the endodontic treatment, if performed after replantation, involves a long-term apexification procedure. In these cases completing the root canal treatment extraorally, where a seal in the blunderbus apex is easier to achieve, may be advantageous. When endodontic treatment is performed extraorally, it must be performed aseptically

with the utmost care to achieve a root canal system that is free of bacteria.

Preparation of the socket   The socket should be left undisturbed before replantation.[68] Emphasis is placed on removal of obstacles within the socket to facilitate replacement of the tooth.[165] New evidence suggests that the environment in the socket may change with time, contributing to the prognosis of the replantation.[165,167] These changes have yet to be defined and no procedures for preparation of the socket can yet be suggested. The socket should be lightly aspirated if a blood clot is present. If the alveolar bone has collapsed and may prevent replantation or cause it to be traumatic, a blunt instrument should be inserted carefully into the socket in an attempt to reposition the wall.

Splinting.   A splinting technique that allows physiologic movement of the tooth during healing and that is in place for a minimal time period results in a decreased incidence of ankylosis.[3,14] Semirigid (i.e., physiologic) fixation for 7 to 10 days is recommended.[3,14] The splint should allow movement of the tooth, should have no memory (so the tooth is not moved during healing), and should not impinge on the gingiva or prevent maintenance of oral hygiene in the area. Many types of splints fulfill these requirements (Fig. 16-47, *A-C*). The acid-etch resin and arch wire splint is probably the most commonly used splint for traumatic injuries. A passive wire (size 0.015 to 0.030) is shaped to conform to the facial aspect of the avulsed tooth and one or two teeth on either side. The middle third of the facial surface of the teeth is acid etched and light-cured composite resin is used to attach the wire to the teeth on either side of the affected tooth. When the wire is satisfactorily in place the patient is asked to bite lightly into a bite block (softened pink wax is useful) and gently force the avulsed tooth as far into the socket as possible. The avulsed tooth is then added to the splint with light-cured composite resin (Fig. 16-48). After the splint is in place, a radiograph should be taken to verify the positioning of the tooth and as a preoperative reference for further treatment and follow-up. When the tooth is in the best possible position, adjusting the bite to ensure that it has not been splinted in a position causing traumatic occlusion is important. One week is sufficient for creating periodontal support to maintain the avulsed tooth in position.[14] Therefore the splint should be removed after 7 to 10 days. The only exception is with avulsion in conjunction with alveolar fractures, for which 4 to 8 weeks is the suggested time of splinting.[14]

Management of soft tissues.   Soft-tissue lacerations of the socket gingiva should be tightly sutured. Lacerations of the lip are fairly common with these types of injuries. The dentist should approach lip lacerations with some caution and a consultation with a plastic surgeon may be prudent. If these lacerations are sutured, care must be taken to clean the wound thoroughly beforehand, because dirt or even minute tooth fragments left in the wound can affect healing and the esthetic result.

Adjunctive therapy.   Systemic antibiotics given at the time of replantation and before endodontic treatment are effective in preventing bacterial invasion of the necrotic pulp and, therefore, subsequent inflammatory resorption.[68] In addition, the use of tetracycline antibiotics have antiresorptive properties in addition to their antibacterial properties.[137] The administration of systemic antibiotics is recommended beginning at the emergency visit and continuing until the splint is removed (in 7 to 10 days). The bacterial content of the sulcus also should be controlled during the healing phase by stressing the need for adequate oral hygiene to the patient, including the use of chlorhexidine rinses for 7 to 10 days. The chlorhexidine rinses assist the patient in maintaining good oral hygiene in the initial stages when the tooth is still painful because of the trauma and also when the splint is in place, making adequate brushing and flossing difficult. The need for analgesics should be assessed on an individual case basis. The use of pain medication stronger than nonprescription, nonsteroidal, antiinflammatory drugs is unusual. *The patient should be sent to a physician for consultation regarding a tetanus booster within 48 hours of the initial visit.*

Second visit.   This visit should take place 7 to 10 days after the emergency visit. At the emergency visit, emphasis is placed on the preservation and healing of the attachment apparatus. The focus of the second visit is the prevention or elimination of potential irritants from the root canal space. These irritants, if present, provide the stimulus for the progression of the inflammatory response and bone and root resorption. The course of systemic antibiotics is also completed at the second visit; the chlorhexidine rinses can be stopped, and the splint can be removed.

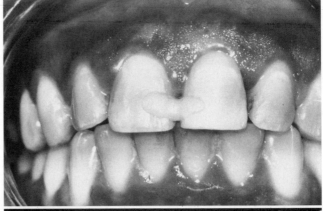

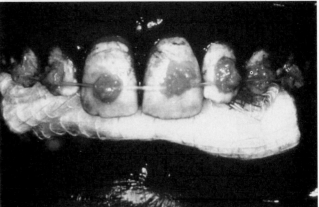

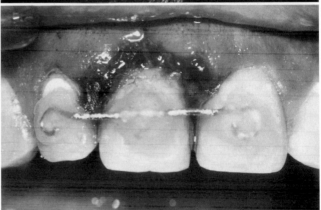

Fig. 16-47   Semirigid splints acceptable for the avulsed tooth. **A,** Acid-etched resin splint between the avulsed tooth and an adjacent tooth. The splint is constructed with resin only and should not extend further than two teeth without wire reinforcement. **B,** Long-span splint constructed with nylon fishing line bonded to the teeth with acid-etched resin. **C,** Wire-reinforced resin splint spanning three teeth.

Endodontic treatment

Tooth with an open apex and less than 60 minutes extraoral dry time   Teeth with open apices have the potential to revascularize and continue root development. Therefore initial treatment is directed toward reestablishment of the blood supply (see Fig. 16-55).[147] Even when a traumatic injury has not occurred, the assessment of a necrotic pulp in young teeth is difficult with the sensitivity methods currently

available.[57,58] The addition of traumatic injury in these immature teeth is an especially difficult diagnostic problem.[118]
After trauma, diagnosis of a necrotic pulp is particularly
desirable because infection in these teeth is potentially more
harmful because of cemental damage accompanying the
traumatic injury. Inflammatory root resorption can be
extremely rapid in these young teeth because the tubules are
wide and allow the irritants to move freely to the external
surface of the root.[14]

Patients are recalled every 3 to 4 weeks for sensitivity
testing. Recent reports indicate that thermal tests with carbon dioxide snow ($-78°$ C) or difluordichlormethane
($-50°$ C) placed at the incisal edge or pulp horn are the best
methods of sensitivity testing, particularly in young permanent teeth (Fig. 16-49).[57] One of these two tests must be
included in the sensitivity testing of these traumatized teeth.
Radiographic signs (i.e., apical breakdown, lateral root
resorption) and clinical symptoms (i.e., pain to percussion

and palpation) of pathosis are carefully assessed. At the first
sign of pathosis, endodontic treatment should be initiated.
After disinfection of the root canal space an apexification
procedure should be performed.

*Tooth with an open apex and extraoral dry time of
more than 60 minutes*   In these teeth the chance of revascularization is extremely poor.[13,163] Therefore no attempt is
made to revitalize them. An apexification procedure is initiated at the second visit if root canal treatment was not performed at the emergency visit. If endodontics was performed
at the emergency visit, the second visit is used to assess initial healing only.

Tooth with a closed apex   No chance exists for revitalization of these teeth, and endodontic treatment should be
initiated at the second visit at 7 to 10 days.[14,41] If therapy is
initiated at this optimum time, the pulp should be ischemi-
cally necrosed without infection (or with only minimal infection[9,163,166]).Therefore endodontic therapy with an effective

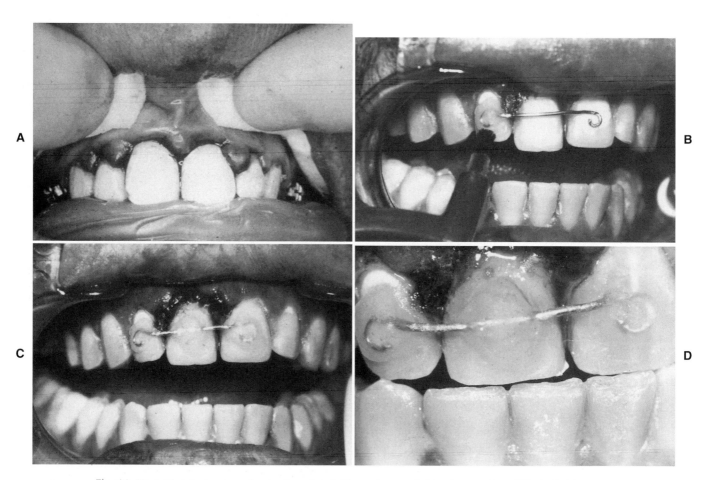

Fig. 16-48 Acid-etched resin and arch wire splint. **A,** The patient gently bites into a softened block of pink wax to
assure that the avulsed tooth can be replaced close to its original position. **B,** A passive wire is shaped to conform to
the facial aspect of the avulsed tooth and to a tooth on either side of it. The middle third of the tooth crown is acid-
etched, and light-cured composite resin attaches the wire to the adjacent teeth. **C,** After the avulsed tooth is correctly positioned by again biting into the pink wax, it is added to the splint with light-cured composite resin. **D,** The
position of the avulsed tooth and the occlusal adjustment is carefully checked to eliminate the possibility of additional trauma to the tooth during function.

interappointment antibacterial agent[32] over a relatively short period (i.e., 7 to 10 days) is sufficient to ensure effective disinfection of the canal.[145]

If the dentist is confident of complete patient cooperation, long-term therapy with calcium hydroxide remains an excellent treatment method.[160,166] The advantage of its use is that it allows the dentist to have a temporary obturating material in place until an intact periodontal ligament space is confirmed. Long-term calcium hydroxide treatment should always be used when the injury occurred more than 2 weeks before initiation of the endodontic treatment or if radiographic evidence of resorption is present.[166]

The root canal should be thoroughly instrumented, irrigated, and then filled with a thick (powdery) mix of calcium hydroxide and sterile saline (anesthetic solution is also an acceptable vehicle). The calcium hydroxide should be changed every 3 months for 6 to 24 months. The canal is obturated when a radiographically intact periodontal membrane can be demonstrated around the root (Fig. 16-50). Calcium hydroxide is an effective antibacterial agent,[32,145] and favorably influences the local environment at the resorption site, theoretically promoting healing.[161] It also changes the environment in the dentin to a more alkaline pH, which may slow the action of the resorptive cells and promote hard-tissue formation.[161] However, the changing of the calcium hydroxide should be kept to a minimum (i.e., not more than every 3 months) because it has a necrotizing effect on the cells attempting to repopulate the damaged root surface.[93]

Although calcium hydroxide is considered the drug of choice in the prevention and treatment of inflammatory root resorption, it is not the only medicament recommended in these cases. Some attempts have been made not only to remove the stimulus for the resorbing cells but also to affect them directly. The antibiotic corticosteroid paste Ledermix is effective in treating inflammatory root resorption by inhibiting the spread of dentinoclasts[125,127] without damaging the

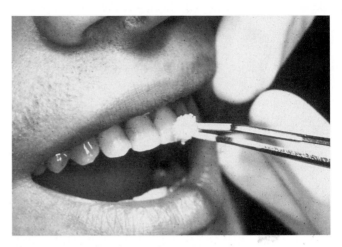

Fig. 16-49 Sensitivity test of previously avulsed tooth. Cotton pellet that was sprayed with dichlorodifluoromethane (−58° F, −50° C) was placed on the incisal edge of maxillary incisor tooth.

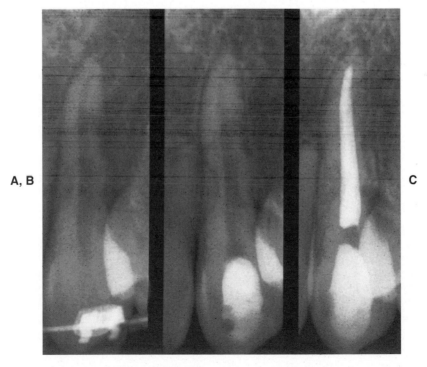

Fig. 16-50 **A**, Active resorption is seen soon after the tooth was replanted. **B**, After long-term Ca(OH)$_2$ treatment, the resorptive defects have healed and an intact lamina dura can be traced around the root. **C**, The tooth is obturated.

periodontal ligament. Its ability to diffuse through human tooth roots has been demonstrated.[1] Its release and diffusion is enhanced when used in combination with calcium hydroxide paste.[2] Calcitonin, a hormone that inhibits osteoclastic bone resorption, also is an effective medication in the treatment of inflammatory root resorption.[126]

Temporary restoration Effectively sealing the coronal access is essential to prevent infection of the canal between visits. Recommended temporary restorations are reinforced zinc oxide–eugenol cement, acid-etch composite resin, or glass-ionomer cement.[174] The depth of the temporary restoration is critical to its sealability. A depth of at least 4 mm is recommended so that a cotton pellet sometimes cannot be placed; the temporary restoration is placed directly onto the calcium hydroxide in the access cavity.[114] Calcium hydroxide should first be removed from the walls of the access cavity because it is soluble and will wash out when it comes into contact with saliva, leaving a defective temporary restoration.

After initiation of the root canal treatment, the splint is removed. If time does not permit complete removal of the splint at this visit, the resin tacks are smoothed so as not to irritate the soft tissues and the residual resin is removed at a later appointment.

At this appointment, healing is usually sufficient to perform a detailed clinical examination on the teeth surrounding the avulsed tooth. The sensitivity tests, reaction to percussion and palpation, and periodontal probing measurements should be carefully recorded for reference at follow-up visits.

Obturation visit. Obturation should take place 7 to 14 days after the second visit or, in the case of long-term calcium hydroxide therapy, when an intact lamina dura is traced (see Fig. 16-50).

If the endodontic treatment was initiated 7 to 10 days after the avulsion and clinical and radiographic examinations do not indicate pathosis, obturation of the root canal at this visit is acceptable,[163,166] although the use of long-term calcium hydroxide is a proven option for these cases.[160,166] The canal is reinstrumented and irrigated under strict asepsis. After completion of the instrumentation the canal can be obturated by any acceptable technique with special attention to an aseptic technique and the best possible seal of the obturating material.

Permanent restoration. Much evidence exists that coronal leakage caused by defective temporary and permanent restoration results in a clinically relevant amount of bacterial contamination of the root canal after obturation.[104,133] Therefore the tooth should receive a permanent restoration at or soon after the time of obturation of the root canal. As with the temporary restoration, the depth of restoration is important for its seal; therefore the deepest restoration possible should be made. A post should be avoided, if possible. Because most avulsions occur in the anterior region of the mouth where esthetics is important, composite resins with the addition of dentin-bonding agents are usually recommended in these cases. They have the additional advantage of

internally strengthening the tooth against fracture, should another trauma occur.[75]

Follow-up care. Follow-up care should transpire every 6 months for 5 years and yearly for as long as possible. Follow-up of avulsion cases (after completion of the obturation of the canal) is extremely important. If replacement resorption is identified (see Fig. 16-24), timely revision of the long-term treatment plan is indicated. In the case of inflammatory root resorption (Fig. 16-51), a new attempt at disinfection of the root canal space by standard retreatment can reverse the process. Teeth adjacent to and surrounding the avulsed tooth or teeth may show pathologic changes long after the initial accident. Therefore these teeth should be tested at recall and the results compared with those collected soon after the accident.

TRAUMATIC INJURIES TO THE PRIMARY DENTITION

The pulpal and periodontal consequences of traumatic injuries to the primary dentition are similar to those of the permanent dentition with one important difference: the risk of subsequent injury to the developing permanent teeth that may occur when the primary tooth is damaged. Therefore all evaluations and treatment decisions are made not so much in terms of the short-term maintenance of the primary tooth but on the long-term health of the permanent successor.

There are three treatment goals for traumatic injuries to the primary dentition:
1. To protect the patient's health
2. To protect the developing tooth bud (if any)
3. To maintain the integrity of the injured tooth

Epidemiology

The reported frequency of trauma to the primary dentition varies widely, depending on the study setting, design, and country of origin. One comprehensive review of the literature[175] reported frequency of injuries ranging from 4% to 33% of all children. The frequency of injuries among genders varies from study to study and country to country, but most experts report slightly more injuries among males. Maxillary central incisors are involved as much as 70% of the time.[59]

Causes of primary tooth injuries generally include falls, bike accidents, sports play, auto accidents, child abuse, and iatrogenic injuries (e.g., trauma during intubation).[149] There is good consensus among experts that the typical primary tooth injury is caused by falls inside the home during the time children are learning to walk.[175] The combination of newly discovered mobility and limited coordination causes children to fall against hard objects and traumatize their maxillary central incisors. Knowing this, epidemiologic information gives clinicians great insights into counseling parents of toddlers on prevention: a safe home environment

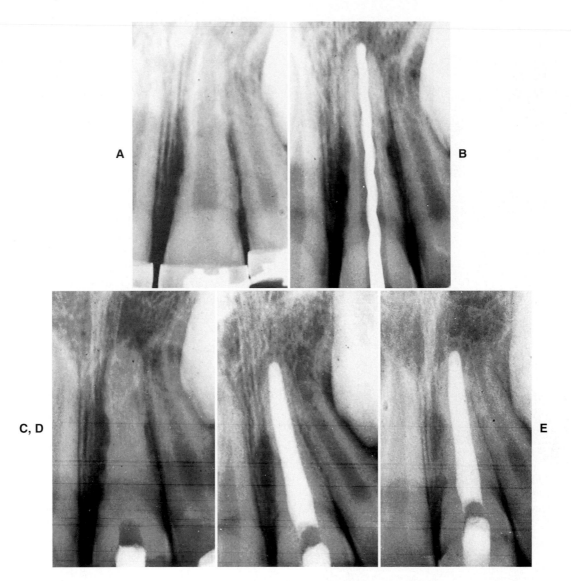

Fig. 16-51 Long-term calcium hydroxide therapy of lateral inflammatory root resorption. **A**, Maxillary central incisor shows radiographic signs of root resorption 1 month after a severe luxation injury. Sensitivity test result is negative. **B**, Root canal therapy is initiated. **C**, Thick mixture of calcium hydroxide and anesthetic solution is packed into the canal. **D**, Nine-month recall. Resorption has been abated, and there is evidence of bone regeneration. Canal is obturated. **E**, One-year recall. Continued healing is apparent.

would be one free of coffee tables or other similar hard objects that may be encountered by young who are learning to walk.

Classification

Injuries to primary teeth only are classified as crown infraction, crown fracture (with and without pulp exposure), crown and root fracture, and root fracture.[28] Injuries to the periodontal attachment are classified as concussion, subluxation, extrusion, lateral luxation, intrusion, and avulsion.[28] Although tooth-only and periodontal attachment injuries occur in primary teeth, by far the most prominent injury involves the attachment. One study reports tooth-only frac-

ture 16% of the time of the time in children in the primary dentition years.[28]

Treatment of Primary Tooth Trauma

These treatment options are described on the assumption that all the initial evaluations and tests have been performed as described for the permanent dentition.

Tooth Injuries[54]

Crown infraction and crown fractures that do not involve the pulp.   Treatment options include no treatment, smoothing rough edges, or placement of bonded-resin restorations.

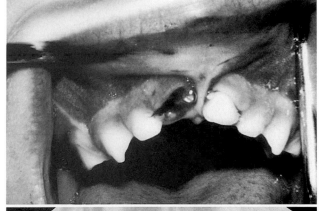

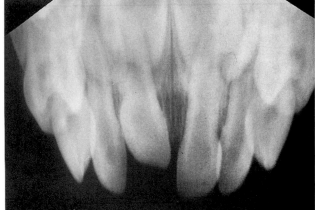

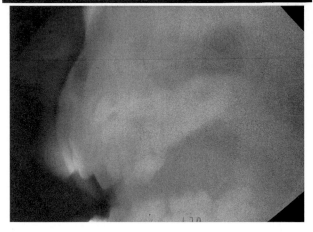

Fig. 16-52 Intruded tooth. **A**, Clinical picture of a 3-year-old child after the intrusion of the upper right maxillary primary incisor. **B**, Periapical radiograph to verify the intrusion. **C**, A lateral anterior view to verify that the apex of the primary tooth is facial to the developing permanent tooth bud.

Crown fractures involving the pulp. Treatment options include pulp therapy and resin restorations or full-coverage, stainless steel (SS) or tooth-colored crowns.

Crown and root fractures. These teeth are usually extracted, but pulp therapy and full coverage is an option in some instances.

Root fractures. Treatment options include no treatment, splinting mobile teeth, or extraction.

Periodontal Treatment of Attachment Injuries

Concussion and subluxation. Treatment options should focus on an occlusal evaluation and alignment as needed.

Lateral luxation and extrusion. Treatment options include no treatment, alignment, realignment, and splinting and extraction.

Intrusion. Treatment options include no treatment and extraction. This is potentially the most damaging of the traumatic injuries because of the potential for the primary tooth root to be forced into the developing permanent tooth follicle. When this occurs, the primary tooth should be extracted.[14]

In most instances of intrusion, the apex of the primary tooth root will be forced facial to the developing follicle and even through the facial plate of bone. This results because of the more facial developmental location of the follicle and the fact that the maxillary incisor roots have a slightly labial curvature in their apical one third.

When treating intruded maxillary primary incisors, palpation or radiographs should verify the juxtaposition of the apex to the developing tooth follicle. If the apex is clear of the follicle, the intruded tooth should be monitored for reeruption[14] (Fig. 16-52).

Avulsion. Although there are occasional case reports of replanted avulsed primary teeth, all experts are in agreement that this should not be attempted because of the possible untoward sequelae for the developing permanent tooth.[15]

Reaction of Primary Incisors to Trauma
Various authors have reported on the complications after primary tooth trauma and many such complications can be listed. Because of the inconsistency of trauma classification systems used and the fact that most studies are cross-sectional in nature, there is little evidence-based data on sequelae of primary teeth after trauma. The best data available emerged from an extensive clinical trial in Copenhagen[28] that carefully tracked 545 traumatized maxillary central incisors over 15 years.

The reported frequencies of complications are as follows:

1. Color change (Fig. 16-53)	62%
2. Pulp necrosis (Fig. 16-54)	28%
3. Pulp canal obliteration	42%
4. Gingival retraction	7%
5. Permanent displacement	3%
6. Surface resorption	1%
7. Inflammatory resorption	13%
8. Ankylosis	1%
9. Disturbed physiologic resorption	5%
10. No complications	12%

It should be noted that the complications are often related to the type of periodontal attachment, and their associations are reported in more detail in this investigation.[28]

Damage to the Developing Permanent Tooth Bud
The most frequently reported defect to permanent teeth after primary tooth trauma include enamel hypoplasia, crown

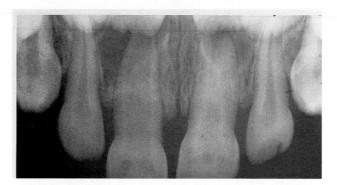

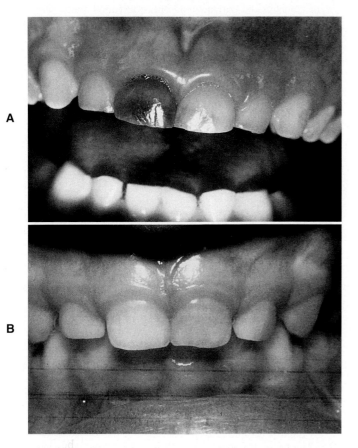

Fig. 16-54 Periapical radiograph of necrotic primary central incisors. Periapical inflammation could potentially be harmful to the permanent tooth bud.

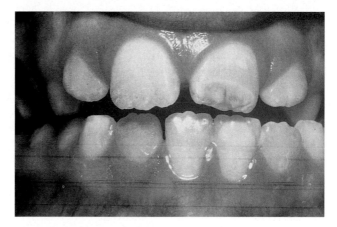

Fig. 16-53 Discoloration of traumatized primary teeth. **A**, Dark gray-and-black discoloration suggestive of pulp necrosis. **B**, Yellow discoloration suggestive of canal space obliteration.

Fig. 16-55 Enamel hypoplasia of left central incisor as a result of damage from a traumatized primary tooth.

dilaceration, root formation, and dome-shaped teeth.[168] The extent of damage depends on the age of the patient at the time of trauma and the nature of the traumatic injury.

The most damage to the permanent tooth bud follows intrusive luxation of primary central incisors. The younger the child, the greater the extent of damage to the permanent tooth bud.[15] The most common defect is enamel hypoplasia. (Fig. 16-55) The defect has been reported as frequently as 69% after intrusive luxation, with corresponding percentages of 52%, 34%, and 27% for avulsions, luxations, and subluxations.[15]

References

1. Abbott PV, Heithersay GS, Hume WR: Release and diffusion through human tooth roots in vitro of corticosteroid and tetracycline trace molecules from Ledermix paste, *Endod Dent Traumatol* 4:55, 1988.

2. Abbott PV, Hume WR, Heithersay GS: Effects of combining Ledermix and calcium hydroxide pastes on the diffusion of corticosteroid and tetracycline through human roots in vitro, *Endod Dent Traumatol* 5:188, 1989.

3. Andersson L, Friskopp J, Blomlof L: Fiber-glass splinting of traumatized teeth, *J Dent Child* 3:21, 1983.

4. Andreasen FM: Pulpal healing after tooth luxation and root fractures in the permanent dentition, thesis, Copenhagen, Denmark, 1995, University of Copenhagen.

5. Andreasen FM: Transient apical breakdown and its relation to color and sensibility changes after luxation injuries to teeth, *Endod Dent Traumatol* 2:9, 1986.

6. Andreasen FM, Andreasen JO: Resorption and mineralization processes following root fracture of permanent incisors, *Endod Dent Traumatol* 4:202, 1988.

7. Andreasen FM, Andreasen JO, Bayer T: Prognosis of root-fractured permanent incisors—prediction of healing modalities, *Endod Dent Traumatol* 5:11, 1989.

8. Andreasen FM, Pedersen BV: Prognosis of luxated permanent teeth and the development of pulp necrosis, *Endod Dent Traumatol* 1:207, 1985.

9. Andreasen FM, Zhijie Y, Thomsen BL, Andersen PK: The occurrence of pulp canal obliteration after luxation injuries in the permanent dentition, *Endod Dent Traumatol* 3:103, 1987.

10. Andreasen JO: Luxation of permanent teeth due to trauma. A clinical and radiographic follow-up study of 189 injured teeth, *Scand J Dent Res* 78:273, 1970.

11. Andreasen JO: Etiology and pathogenesis of traumatic dental injuries, *Scand J Dent Res* 78:329,1970.

12. Andreasen JO: Periodontal healing after replantation of traumatically avulsed human teeth: assessment by mobility testing and radiography, *Acta Odontol Scand* 33: 325, 1975.

13. Andreasen JO: The effect of extra-alveolar period and storage media upon periodontal and pulpal healing after replantation of mature permanent incisors in monkeys, *Int J Oral Surg* 10: 43, 1981.

14. Andreasen JO, Andreasen FM: *Textbook and color atlas of traumatic injuries to the teeth,* ed 3, St Louis, 1994, Mosby.

15. Andreasen JO, Andreasen FM: *Essentials of traumatic injuries of the teeth,* ed 2, Copenhagen, Denmark, 2000, Munksgaard International Publishers.

16. Andreasen JO, Hjorting-Hansen E: Replantation of teeth. I. Radiographic and clinical study of 110 human teeth replanted after accidental loss, *Acta Odontol Scand* 24:263, 1966.

17. Andreasen JO, Hjorting-Hansen E: Intra-alveolar root fractures: radiographic and histologic study of 50 cases, *J Oral Surg* 25:414, 1967.

18. Andreasen JO, Kristersson L: The effect of limited drying or removal of the periodontal ligament: periodontal healing after replantation of mature permanent incisors in monkeys, *Acta Odontol Scand* 39:1, 1981.

19. Andreasen JO, Ravn JJ: Epidemiology of traumatic dental injuries to primary and permanent teeth in a Danish population sample, *Int J Oral Surg* 1:235, 1972.

20. Antrim DD, Hicks ML, Altaras DE: Treatment of subosseous resorption: a case report, *J Endod* 8:567, 1982.

21. Bergenholtz G: Microorganisms from necrotic pulp of traumatized teeth, *Odont Revy* 25:247, 1974.

22. Bergenholtz G, Reit C: Pulp reactions on microbial provocation of calcium hydroxide treated dentin, *Scand J Dent Res* 88:187, 1980.

23. Bhaskar SN, Rappaport HM: Dental vitality tests and pulp status, *J Am Dent Assoc* 86:409, 1973.

24. Binnie WH, Rowe AHR: A histological study of the periapical tissues of incompletely formed pulpless teeth filled with calcium hydroxide, *J Dent Res* 52:1110, 1973.

25. Bjorvatn K, Selvig KA, Klinge B: Effect of tetracycline and SnF_2 on root resorption in replanted incisors in dogs, *Scand J Dent Res* 97:477, 1989.

26. Blomlof L: Milk and saliva as possible storage media for traumatically exarticulated teeth prior to replantation, *Swed Dent J* 8(suppl):1, 1981.

27. Blomlof L et al: Storage of experimentally avulsed teeth in milk prior to replantation, *J Dent Res* 62:912, 1983.

28. Borum MK, Andreasen JO: Sequelae of trauma to primary maxillary incisors. I. Complications to the primary dentition. *Endod Dent Traumatol* 14:33, 1998.

29. Braham RL, Roberts MW, Morris ME: Management of dental trauma in children and adolescents, *J Trauma* 17:857, 1977.

30. Brannstrom M: Observations on exposed dentine and corresponding pulp tissue. A preliminary study with replica and routine histology, *Odont Revy* 13:253, 1952.

31. Bureau of Dental Health Education: Mouth protectors: 11 years later, *J Am Dent Assoc* 86:1365, 1973.

32. Bystrom A, Claesson R, Sundqvist G: The antibacterial effect of camphorated paramonochlorphenol, camphorated phenol and calcium hydroxide in the treatment of infected root canals, *Endod Dent Traumatol* 1:170, 1985.

33. Cameron CE: The cracked tooth syndrome: additional findings, *J Am Dent Assoc* 93:971, 1976.

34. Cox CF, Keall HJ, Ostro E, Bergenholtz G: Biocompatibility of surface-sealed dental materials against exposed pulps, *Prosthet Dent* 57:1, 1987.

35. Croll TO et al: Rapid neurologic assessment and initial management for the patient with traumatic dental injuries, *J Am Dent Assoc* 100:530, 1980.

36. Cvek M: Treatment of non-vital permanent incisors with calcium hydroxide. IV. Periodontal healing and closure of the root canal in the coronal fragment of teeth with intra-alveolar fracture and vital apical fragment, *Odont Revy* 25:239, 1974.

37. Cvek M: A clinical report on partial pulpotomy and capping with calcium hydroxide in permanent incisors with complicated crown fracture, *J Endod* 4:232, 1978.

38. Cvek M: Prognosis of luxated non-vital maxillary incisors treated with calcium hydroxide and filled with gutta-percha, a retrospective clinical study, *Endod Dent Traumatol* 8:45, 1992.

39. Cvek M: Endodontic treatment of traumatized teeth. In Andreasen JO, Andreasen FM, editors: *Textbook and color atlas of traumatic injuries to the teeth*, ed 3, St Louis, 1994, Mosby.

40. Cvek M, Cleaton-Jones, P, Austin J: Effect of topical application of doxycycline on pulp revascularization and periodontal healing in reimplanted monkey incisors, *Endod Dent Traumatol* 6:170,1990.

41. Cvek M et al: Pulp reactions to exposure after experimental crown fractures or grinding in adult monkeys, *J Endod* 8:391,1982.

42. Cvek M, Hollender L, Nord C-E: Treatment of non-vital permanent incisors with calcium hydroxide. VI. A clinical, microbiological and radiological evaluation of treatment on one sitting of teeth with mature and immature roots, *Odont Revy* 27:93, 1976.

43. Cvek M, Nord C-E, Hollender L: Antimicrobial effect of root canal débridement in teeth with immature root, *Odont Revy* 27:1, 1976.

44. Cvek M, Sundstrom B: Treatment of non-vital permanent incisors with calcium hydroxide. V. Histological appearance of roentgenologically demonstrable apical closure of immature roots, *Odont Revy* 25:379, 1974.

45. Dargent P: A study of root resorption, *Acta Odontostomatol* 117:47, 1977.

46. Darling AI: Response of pulpodential complex to injury. In Gorlin RJ, Goldman H, editors: *Thoma's oral pathology*, ed 6, St Louis, 1970, Mosby.

47. Davis GT, Knott SC: Dental trauma in Australia, *Aust Dent J* 29:217, 1984.

48. Deyoung AK, Robinson E, Godwin WC: Comparing comfort and wearability: custom-made vs. self-adapted mouthguards, *J Am Dent Assoc* 125:1112, 1994.

49. Deutsch AS et al: Root fracture during insertion of prefabricated posts related to root size, *J Prosthet Dent* 53:786, 1985.

50. Eklund G, Stalhane I, Hedegard B: A study of traumatized permanent teeth in children aged 7-15. III. A multivariate analysis of post-traumatic complications of subluxated and luxated teeth, *Sven Tandläk Tidskr* 69:179, 1976.

51. Fountain SB, Camp JH: Traumatic injuries. In Cohen S, Burns RC, editors: *Pathways of the pulp*, ed 6, St Louis, 1994, Mosby.

52. Frank AL: Therapy for the divergent pulpless tooth by continued apical formation, *J Am Dent Assoc* 72:87, 1966.

53. Frank AL, Bakland LK: Nonendodontic therapy for supraosseous extracanal invasive resorption, *J Endod* 13:348, 1987.

54. Fried I, Erickson P: Anterior tooth trauma in the primary dentition: incidence, classification, treatment methods and sequelae, *J Dent Child* 2:256, 1956.

55. Fuks AB, Bielak S, Chosak A: Clinical and radiographic assessments of direct pulp capping and pulpotomy in young permanent teeth, *Pediatr Dent* 24:240, 1982.

56. Fuks A, Chosak A, Eidelman E: Partial pulpotomy as an alternative treatment for exposed pulps in crown-fractured permanent incisors, *Endod Dent Traumatol* 3:100, 1987.

57. Fulling HJ, Andreasen JO: Influence of maturation status and tooth type of permanent teeth upon electrometric and thermal pulp testing procedures, *Scand J Dent Res* 84:266, 1976.

58. Fuss Z et al: Assessment of reliability of electrical and thermal pulp testing agents, *J Endod* 12:301, 1986.

59. Galea H: An investigation of dental injuries treated in an acute care general hospital, *J Am Dent Assoc* 109:434, 1984.

60. Gazelius B, Olgart L, Edwall B: Restored vitality in luxated teeth assessed by laser Doppler flowmeter, *Endod Dent Traumatol* 4:265, 1988.

61. Gelbier MJ, Winter GB: Traumatized incisors treated by vital pulpotomy: a retrospective study, *Br Dent J* 164:319, 1988.

62. Going RE, Loehaman RD, Chan MS: Mouthguard materials: their physical and mechanical properties, *J Am Dent Assoc* 89:132, 1974.

63. Gold SI, Hasselgren G: Peripheral inflammatory root resorption, *J Periodontol* 19:523, 1992.

64. Gottlieb B, Orban B: Veranderunngen in Periodontium nach chirurgischer Diathermie, *ZJ Stomatol* 28:1208, 1930.

65. Grahnen H, Hansson L: The prognosis of pulp and root canal therapy. A clinical and radiographic follow-up examination, *Odont Revy* 12:146, 1961.

66. Granath LE, Hagman G: Experimental pulpotomy in human bicuspids with reference to cutting technique, *Acta Odontol Scand* 29:155, 1971.

67. Hallet GE, Porteous JR: Fractured incisors treated by vital pulpotomy. A report on 100 consecutive cases, *Br Dent J* 115:279, 1963.

68. Hammarstrom L, Lindskog S: General morphologic aspects of resorption of teeth and alveolar bone, *Int Endod J* 18:93, 1985.

69. Hammarstrom L et al: Tooth avulsion and replantation: a review, *Endod Dent Traumatol* 2:1, 1986.

70. Harrington GW, Natkin E: External resorption associated with bleaching of pulpless teeth, *J Endod* 5:344, 1979.

71. Hedegard B, Stalhone I: A study of traumatized permanent teeth in children aged 7-15 years, part I, *Swed Dent J* 66:431, 1973.

72. Heithersay GS: Calcium hydroxide in the treatment of pulpless teeth with associated pathology, *J Br Endod Soc* 8:74, 1962.

73. Heide S, Mjor IA: Pulp reactions to experimental exposures in young permanent teeth, *Int Endod J* 16:11, 1983.

74. Heller AL et al: Direct pulp capping of permanent teeth in primates using resorbable form of tricalcium phosphate ceramics, *J Endod* 1:95, 1975.

75. Herforth A, Strassburg M: Zur Therapie der chronischapikalen paradontitis bei traumatisch beschadigten frontzahnen mit nicht abgeschlossenen wurzelwachstrum, *Dtsch Zahnärzt Z* 32:453, 1977.

76. Hernandez R, Bader S, Boston D, and Trope M: Resistance to fracture of endodontically treated premolars restored with new generation dentin bonding systems, *Int Endod J* 27:281, 1994.

77. Hill FJ, Picton JF: Fractured incisor fragment in the tongue: a case report, *Pediatr Dent* 3:337, 1981.

78. Hiltz J, Trope M: Vitality of human lip fibroblasts in milk, Hanks Balanced Salt Solution and Viaspan storage media, *Endod Dent Traumatol* 7:69, 1991.

79. Jacobsen I: Root fractures in permanent anterior teeth with incomplete root formation, *Scand J Dent Res* 84:210, 1976.

80. Jacobsen I: Clinical follow-up study of permanent incisors with intrusive luxation after acute trauma, *J Dent Res* 62:4, 1983.

81. Jacobsen I, Kerekes K: Long-term prognosis of traumatized permanent anterior teeth showing calcific processes in the pulp cavity, *Scand J Dent Res* 85:588, 1977.

82. Jacobsen I, Kerekes K: Diagnosis and treatment of pulp necrosis in permanent anterior teeth with root fracture, *Scand J Dent Res* 88:370, 1980.

83. Jacobsen I, Zachrisson BU: Repair characteristics of root fractures in permanent anterior teeth, *Scand J Dent Res* 83:355, 1975.

84. Johnston T, Messer LB: An in vitro study of the efficacy of mouthguard protection for dentoalveolar injuries in deciduous and mixed dentitions, *Endod Dent Traumatol* 12:277, 1996.

85. Jarvinen S: Incisal overject and traumatic injuries to upper permanent incisors: a retrospective study, *Acta Odontol Scand* 36:359, 1978.

86. Jarvinen S: Fractured and avulsed permanent incisors in Finnish children: a retrospective study, *Acta Odontol Scand* 37:47, 1979.

87. Kakehashi S, Stanley HR, Fitzgerald RJ: The effect of surgical exposures on dental pulps in germ-free and conventional laboratory rats, *Oral Surg* 20:340, 1965.

88. Katebzadeh N, Dalton C, Trope M: Strengthening immature teeth during and after apexification, *J Endod* 11:256, 1998.

89. Kerekes K, Heide S, Jacobsen I: Follow-up examination of endodontic treatment in traumatized juvenile incisors, *J Endod* 6:744, 1980.

90. Kerr LI: Mouth guards of the prevention of injuries in contact sports, *Sports Med* 3:415, 1986.

91. Kopel HM, Johnson R: Examination and neurologic assessment of children with oro-facial trauma, *Endod Dent Traumatol* 1:155, 1985.

92. Kozlowska I: Pokrycie bezposrednie miazgi preparatem krajowej produccji, *Czas Stomatol* 13:375, 1960.

93. Lado EA, Stanley HR, Weissman MI: Cervical resorption in bleached teeth, *Oral Surg* 55:78, 1983.

94. Lengheden A, Blomlof L, Lindskog S: Effect of delayed calcium hydroxide treatment on periodontal healing in contaminated replanted teeth, *Scand J Dent Res* 99:147, 1991.

95. Lindskog A et al: The role of the necrotic periodontal membrane in cementum resorption and ankylosis, *Endod Dent Traumatol* 1:96, 1985.

96. Lindskog S, Blomlof L: Influence of osmolality and composition of some storage media on human periodontal ligament cells, *Acta Odontol Scand* 40:435, 1982.

97. Lindskog S, Blomlof L, Hammarstrom L: Repair of periodontal tissues in vivo and in vitro, *J Clin Periodontol* 10: 188, 1983.

98. Loe H, Waerhaug J: Experimental replantation of teeth in dogs and monkeys, *Arch Oral Biol* 3:176, 1961.

99. Lundin S-A, Noren JG, Warfvinge J: Marginal bacterial leakage and pulp reactions in Class II composite resin restorations in vivo, *Swed Dent J* 14:185, 1990.

100. Luostarinen V, Pohto M, Sheinin A: Dynamics of repair in the pulp, *J Dent Res* 45: 519, 1966.

101. Mackie IC, Bentley EM, Worthington HV: The closure of open apices in non-vital immature incisor teeth, *Br Dent J* 165:169, 1988.

102. Macko DJ et al: A study of fractured anterior teeth in a school population, *J Dent Child* 46:130, 1979.

103. Magnusson B, Holm A: Traumatized permanent teeth in children—a follow-up. I. Pulpal complications and root resorption, *Swed Dent J* 62:61, 1969.

104. Magnusson B, Holm A, Berg H: Traumatized permanent teeth in children—a follow-up. II. The crown fractures, *Swed Dent J* 62:71, 1969.

105. Magura M et al: Human saliva coronal microleakage in obturated canals: an in vitro study, *J Endod* 17:324, 1991.

106. Makkes PG, Thoden van Velzen SK: Cervical external root resorption, *J Dent Res* 3:217, 1975.

107. Masterton JB: The healing of wounds of the dental pulp of man. A clinical and histological study, *Br Dent J* 120:213, 1966.

108. Matsson L et al: Ankylosis of experimentally reimplanted teeth related to extra-alveolar period and storage environment, *Pediatr Dent* 4:327, 1982.

109. Maurice CG: Selection of teeth for root canal treatment, *Dent Clin North Am* 761, 1957.

110. McClelland C, Kinirons M, Geary L: A preliminary study of patient comfort associated with customized mouthguards, *Br J Sports Med* 33:186, 1999.

111. Meadow D, Needleman H, Lindner G: Oral trauma in children, *Pediatr Dent* 6:248, 1984.

112. Mejare I, Hasselgren G, Hammarstrom LE: Effect of formaldehyde-containing drugs on human dental pulp evaluated by enzyme histochemical technique, *Scand J Dent Res* 84:29, 1976.

113. Mesaros SV, Trope M: Revascularization of traumatized teeth assessed by laser Doppler flowmetry: case report, *Endod Dent Traumatol* 1:24, 1997.

114. Mjor IA, and Tronstad L: The healing of experimentally induced pulpitis, *Oral Surg* 38:115, 1974.

115. Moller AJR: Microbiologic examination of root canals and periapical tissues of human teeth, thesis, Goteborg, Sweden, 1966, University of Goteborg.

116. Munksgaard EC et al: Enamel-dentin crown fractures bonded with various bonding agents, *Endod Dent Traumatol* 7:73, 1991.

117. Nichols E: An investigation into the factors which may influence the prognosis of root canal therapy, master's thesis, London, 1960, University of London.

118. Nicholls E: Endodontic treatment during root formation, *Int Dent J* 31:49, 1981.

119. Ohman A: Healing and sensitivity to pain in young replanted human teeth: an experimental and histologic study, *Odontol Tidskr* 73:166, 1965.

120. Oikarinen K, Gundlach KKH, Pfeifer G: Late complications of luxation injuries to teeth, *Endod Dent Traumatol* 3:296, 1987.

121. Oikarinen KD, Salonen MAM: Introduction of four custom made protectors constructed of single and double layers for activists in contact sports, *Endod Dent Traumatol* 9:19, 1993.

122. O'Mullane DM: Injured permanent incisor teeth: an epidemiological study, *J Ir Dent Assoc* 18:160, 1972.

123. Olgart L, Brannstrom M, Johnsson G: Invasion of bacteria into dentinal tubules. Experiments in vivo and in vitro, *Acta Odontol Scand* 32:61, 1974.

124. Penick EC. The endodontic management of root resorption, *Oral Surg* 16:344, 1963.

125. Pettiette M et al: Periodontal healing of extracted dog teeth air dried for extended periods and soaked in various media, *Endod Dent Traumatol* 13:113, 1997.

126. Pierce A, Lindskog S: The effect of an antibiotic corticosteroid combination on inflammatory root resorption, *J Endod* 14:459, 1988.

127. Pierce A, Berg JO, Lindskog S: Calcitonin as an alternative therapy in the treatment of root resorption, *J Endod* 14:459, 1988.

128. Pierce A, Heithersay G, Lindskog S: Evidence for direct inhibition of dentinoclasts by a corticosteroid/antibiotic endodontic paste, *Endod Dent Traumatol* 4:44, 1988.

129. Pitt-Ford TR et al: Using mineral trioxide aggregate as a pulp-capping material, *J Am Dent Assoc* 127:1491, 1996.

130. Rabie G, Barnett F, Tronstad L: Long-term splinting of maxillary incisor with intra-alveolar root fracture, *Endod Dent Traumatol* 4:99, 1988.

131. Rabie G et al: Strengthening and restoration of immature teeth with an acid-etch resin technique, *Endod Dent Traumatol* 1:246, 1985.

132. Ravn JJ: Dental injuries in Copenhagen school children, school years 1967-1972, *J Ir Dent Assoc* 2:231, 1974.

133. Ravn JJ: Follow-up study of permanent incisors with complicated crown fractures after acute trauma, *Scand J Dent Res* 90:363, 1982.

134. Ray H, Trope M: Periapical status of endodontically treated teeth in relation to the technical quality of the root filling and the coronal restoration, *Int Endod J* 28(1):12, 1995.

135. American Dental Association: Report of the joint commission on mouth protectors of the American Dental Association for health, physical education and recreation, Chicago, 1960, The Association.

136. Rock WP et al: The relationship between trauma and pulp death in incisor teeth, *Br Dent J* 136:236, 1974.

137. Rotstein I, Lehr Z, Gedalia I: Effect of bleaching agents on inorganic components of human dentin and cementum, *J Endod* 18:290, 1992.

138. Sae-Lim V, Wang CY, Choi GW, Trope M: The effect of systemic tetracycline on resorption of dried replanted dogs' teeth, *Endod Dent Traumatol* 14:127, 1998.

139. Schindler WG, Gullickson DC: Rationale for the management of calcific metamorphosis secondary to traumatic injuries, *J Endod* 14:408, 1988.

140. Schroder U: Reaction of human dental pulp to experimental pulpotomy and capping with calcium hydroxide (thesis), *Odont Revy* 24: (suppl 25)97, 1973.

141. Schroder U, Granath LE: Early reaction of intact human teeth to calcium hydroxide following experimental pulpotomy and its significance to the development of hard tissue barrier, *Odont Revy* 22:379, 1971.

142. Seltzer S: *Endodontology*, Philadelphia, 1988, Lea & Febiger.

143. Seltzer S, Bender IB, Turkenkopf S: Factors affecting successful repair after root canal therapy, *J Am Dent Assoc* 52: 651, 1963.

144. Selvig KA, Zander HA: Chemical analysis and microradiography of cementum and dentin from periodontally diseased human teeth, *J Periodontol* 33:303, 1962.

145. Seward GR: Periodontal disease and resorption of teeth, *Br Dent J* 34:443, 1963.

146. Sjogren U, Figdor D, Spangberg L, Sundqvist G: The antimicrobial effect of calcium hydroxide as a short-term intracanal dressing, *Int Endod J* 24:119, 1991.

147. Sheinin A, Pohto M, Luostarinen V: Defense mechanisms of the pulp with special reference to circulation. An experimental study in rats, *Int Dent J* 17: 461, 1967.

148. Skoglund A, Tronstad L: Pulpal changes in replanted and autotransplanted immature teeth of dogs, *J Endod* 7:309, 1981.

149. Soder PO et al: Effect of drying on viability of periodontal membrane, *Scand J Dent Res* 85:167, 1977.

150. Soporowski NJ, Allred EN, Needleman HL: Luxation injuries of primary anterior teeth – prognosis and related correlates, *Pediatr Dent* 16:23, 1994.

151. Spangberg L, Rutberg M, Rydinge E: Biologic effects of endodontic antimicrobial agents, *J Endod* 5:166, 1979.

152. Stalhane I, Hedegard B: Traumatized permanent teeth in children aged 7-15 years. Part II, *Swed Dent J* 68:157, 1975.

153. Stanley HR: Diseases of the dental pulp. In Tieck RW, editor: *Oral Pathology*, New York, 1965, McGraw-Hill.

154. Stanley HR, Lundi T: Dycal therapy for pulp exposures, *Oral Surg* 34:818, 1972.

155. Stormer K, Jacobsen I: Hvor funksjonsdyktige blir rotfylte unge permanente incisiver? Nordisk forening for pedodonti Arsmote, Bergen, Norway, 1988.

156. Strinberg LZ: The dependence of the results of pulp therapy on certain factors. An analytic study based on radiographic and clinical follow-up examinations, *Acta Odont Scand* 14 (Suppl 21), 1956.

157. Sundqvist G: Ecology of the root canal flora, *J Endod* 18:427, 1992.

158. Trabert KC, Caput AA, Abou-Rass M: Tooth fracture, a comparison of endodontic and restorative treatments, *J Endod* 4:341, 1978.

159. Tronstad L: Pulp reactions in traumatized teeth. In Gutman JL, Harrison JW, editors: *Proceedings of the international conference on oral trauma,* Chicago, 1984, American Association of Endodontists Endowment and Memorial Foundation.

160. Tronstad L: Reaction of the exposed pulp to Dycal treatment, *Oral Surg* 34:477, 1974.

161. Tronstad L: Root resorptionæetiology, terminology and clinical manifestations, *Endod Dent Traumatol* 4:241, 1988.

162. Tronstad L et al: pH changes in dental tissues following root canal filling with calcium hydroxide, *J Endod* 7:17, 1981.

163. Tronstad L, Mjor IA: Capping of the inflamed pulp, *Oral Surg* 34:477, 1972.

164. Trope M et al: Effect of different endodontic treatment protocols on periodontal repair and root resorption of replanted dog teeth, *J Endod* 18:492, 1992.

165. Trope M, Maltz DO, Tronstad L: Resistance to fracture of restored endodontically treated teeth, *Endod Dent Traumatol* 1:108, 1985.

166. Trope M, Friedman S: Periodontal healing of replanted dog teeth stored in Viaspan, milk and Hanks Balanced Salt Solution, *Endod Dent Traumatol* 8:183, 1992.

167. Trope M et al: Short versus long term $Ca(OH)_2$ treatment of established inflammatory root resorption in replanted dog teeth, *Endod Dent Traumatol* 11:124, 1995.

168. Trope M, Hupp JG, Mesaros SV: The role of the socket in the periodontal healing of replanted dog teeth stored in ViaSpan for extended periods, *Endod Dent Traumatol* 13:171, 1997.

169. Von Arx T: Developmental disturbances of permanent teeth following trauma to the primary dentition, *Aust Dent J* 38:1, 1993.

170. Warfvinge J, Rozell B, Hedstrom KG: Effect of calcium hydroxide treated dentin on pulpal responses, *Int Endod J* 20:183, 1987.

171. Wedenberg C: Evidence for a dentin-derived inhibitor of macrophage spreading, *Scand J Dent Res* 95:381, 1987.

172. Wedenberg C, Lindskog S: Experimental internal resorption in monkey teeth, *Endod Dent Traumatol* 1:221, 1985.

173. Wedenberg C, Zetterqvist L: Internal resorption in human teeth—a histological, scanning electron microscope and enzyme histo-chemical study, *J Endod* 13:255, 1987.

174. Weiss M: Pulp capping in older patients, *N Y State Dent J* 32:451, 1966.

175. Wilcox LR, and Diaz-Arnold A: Coronal microleakage of permanent lingual access restorations in endodontically treated anterior teeth, *Int Endod J* 23:321, 1990

176. Wilson CFG: Management of trauma to primary and developing teeth, *Dent Clin North Am* 39:133, 1995.

177. York AH et al: Dental injuries to 11-13 year old children, *N Z Dent J* 74:218, 1978.

178. Zachrisson BU, Jacobsen I: Long-term prognosis of 66 permanent anterior teeth with root fracture, *Scand J Dent Res* 83: 345, 1975.

179. Zadik D, Chosack A, Eidelman E: A survey of traumatized incisors in Jerusalem school children, *J Dent Child* 39:185, 1972.

180. Zadik D et al: The prognosis of traumatized permanent teeth with fracture of enamel and dentin, *Oral Surg* 47:173, 1979.

Chapter 17

Endodontic and Periodontic Interrelationships

Hom-Lay Wang, Gerald N. Glickman

Chapter Outline

The interrelationships between pulpal and periodontal disease primarily occur via the intimate anatomic and vascular connections between the pulp and the periodontium; these interrelationships have been traditionally demonstrated using radiographic, histologic, and clinical criteria. Pulpal and periodontal problems are responsible for more than 50% of tooth mortality.[12] Diagnosis is often challenging because these diseases have been primarily studied as separate entities, and each primary disease may mimic clinical characteristics of the other disease. Pulp tissue succumbs to degeneration via a multitude of insults, such as caries, restorative procedures, chemical and thermal insults, trauma, and periodontal disease. When products from pulp degeneration reach the supporting periodontium, rapid inflammatory responses can ensue that are characterized by bone loss, tooth mobility, and sometimes sinus tract formation. If this occurs in the apical region a periradicular lesion forms. If this occurs with crestal extension of the inflammation a ret-

rograde periodontitis or reverse pocket is formed. However, the lesion formed has little anatomic similarity to a periodontally induced defect.

Periodontal disease, on the contrary, is a slow progressing disease that may have a gradually atrophic effect on the dental pulp. Therefore, periodontal lesion is used to denote an inflammatory process in the periodontal tissues resulting from dental plaque accumulation on the external tooth surfaces. Research has shown the presence of localized inflammation and/or tissue infarction, a decrease in cells, resorption, fibrosis, and coagulation necrosis.* Dystrophic calcification may cause some degeneration in the pulp and further influence periodontal disease. In addition, periodontal treatments such as deep root planing and/or curettage, usage of localized medicaments, and gum injury or wounding may accelerate further pulpal inflammation and provoke the interrelated disease process.[58,65,66]

In recent years periodontal disease has been shown to be related to (and even the cause of) pulpal disease, and pulpal disease may cause periodontal lesions that behave differently from chronic destructive periodontitis. The effects of periodontal disease on the pulp and the potential for healing of certain periodontal lesions after endodontic therapy have been documented extensively.† In this chapter the intercommunications between pulpal and periodontal tissues, the effects of pulpal disease on the periodontium, periodontal disease and its effects on the pulp, as well as the classification, differential diagnosis, and management and prognosis of endodontic and periodontic problems will be discussed.

INTERCOMMUNICATION BETWEEN PULPAL AND PERIODONTAL TISSUE

Several possible channels between the pulp and periodontium that lead to the interaction of the disease process in both tissues have been suggested. These include neural (i.e.,

---

*References 38, 42, 53, 58, 63, 65.
†References 5, 14, 36, 41, 55, 66.

Table 17-1   **INCIDENCE OF FURCATION CANALS**

Investigators	Techniques	% Incidence
Rubach & Mitchell (1965)[53]	Sectioned teeth	45%
Lowman et al (1973)[41]	Dissecting microscope	59% maxillary molars 55% mandibular molars
Burch & Hulen (1974)[10]	Radiopaque dye	76% accessory furca canals
Vertucci & Williams (1974)[70]	Hematoxylin dye	46%
Kirkham (1975)[34]	Radiopaque dye	23%
Gutmann (1978)[27]	Safranin dye	28.4% maxillary molars 27.4% mandibular molars

reflex) pathways, lateral canals, dentinal tubules, palato-gingival grooves, periodontal ligament, alveolar bone, apical foramina, and common vasculolymphatic drainage pathways. The most interconnected and evidenced relationship between the two tissues is via the vascular system as illustrated anatomically by the presence of the apical foramen, lateral (i.e., accessory) canals, and dentinal tubules.* These communications, when they exist, may serve as potential paths for inflammatory reciprocity.[10,27,36,41,53]

The apical foramen is the most direct route of communication to the periodontium, but by no means is it the only location where pulpal and periodontal tissues communicate with each other. Lateral and accessory canals, mainly in the apical area and in the furcation of molars, also connect the dental pulp with the periodontal ligament. Table 17-1 lists the incidence of furcation canals. These have been suggested as a direct pathway between pulp and periodontium and typically contain connective tissue and vessels that connect the circulatory system of the pulp with that of the periodontium. Research has demonstrated that inflammation in the interradicular periodontal tissues will develop by induction of pulpal inflammation.[57,58] Serial sectioning of 74 teeth has revealed 45% of accessory canals are present primarily in the apical region.[53] More significantly, lateral accessory canals in eight teeth were located more coronally on the roots. Among them, connection of the accessory canals with periodontal pockets was microscopically demonstrable in five of the specimens. Gutmann introduced safranin dye into 102 molar teeth that were placed in a vacuum chamber and found 28.4% of the teeth had furcation canals, although only 10.2% of the total group exhibited canals on the lateral root surface.[27]

In addition to the apical foramen and lateral accessory canals, dentinal tubules have also been suggested as another common pathway between periodontium and pulpal tissue. Dentinal tubules contain cytoplasmic extensions or odontoblastic processes that extend from the odontoblasts at the pulp and dentin border to the dentin and enamel junction (DEJ) or dentin and cementum junction (CDJ). It has been reported that the pulp chamber can communicate with the external root surface via dentinal tubules, especially when the cementum is denuded.[27,74]

Palatogingival grooves are developmental anomalies of the maxillary incisor teeth, with lateral incisors more often affected than central incisors (4.4% versus 0.28%, respectively).[73] These usually begin in the central fossa, cross the cingulum, and extend apically with varying distances. Generally the incidence of palatogingival grooves ranges from 1.9% to 8.5%.[20,73] Everett and Kramer reported that 0.5% of the teeth examined had a palatogingival groove extension to the root apex, thus contributing to an endodontic pathologic condition.[20]

Perforation of the root creates a communication between the root canal system and the periodontal ligament. This may occur as a result of overinstrumentation during endodontic procedures, internal or external root resorption, or caries invading through the floor of the pulp chamber. The prognosis for teeth with root perforation is usually determined by the location of the perforation, the time left unsealed, the ability to seal the perforation, the chance of building new attachments, and the accessibility of the remaining root canals. Teeth that have perforations in the middle or apical third of the root have the greatest chance of healing. The closer the perforation is to the gingival sulcus, particularly into the coronal third of the root or the furcation region, the greater the likelihood of apical migration of the gingival epithelium in initiation of a periodontal lesion.

A vertical root fracture can produce a "halo" effect around the tooth radiographically.[51] Deep periodontal pocketing and localized destruction of alveolar bone are often related to long-standing root fractures. The fractured root can mimic a radiographic profile of occlusal trauma, with localized loss of lamina dura, altered trabecular pattern, and a widened periodontal ligament. The fractured site provides a portal of entry for irritants from the root canal system to the surrounding periodontal ligament. Vertical root fractures have contributed to the progression of periodontal destruction in the presence of apparently successful endodontic tooth therapy and overall periodontal site stability.[52]

*References 5, 14, 37, 41, 55, 66.

INFLUENCE OF PULPAL PATHOLOGIC CONDITION ON THE PERIODONTIUM

Pulpal pathology as a cause of periodontal disease has received much attention during the last decade. Pulpal degeneration results in necrotic debris, bacterial byproducts, and other toxic irritants that can move toward the apical foramen, causing periodontal tissue destruction apically and potentially migrating toward the gingival margin. Simring and Goldberg termed this "retrograde periodontitis" to differentiate the process from "marginal periodontitis" in which the disease proceeds physically from the gingival margin toward the root apex. When pulpal disease progresses beyond the confines of the tooth, inflammation extends and affects the adjacent periodontal attachment apparatus.[62] This inflammatory process often results in dysfunction of the periodontal ligament, as well as resorption of alveolar bone, cementum, and even dentin. The endodontic infection has been regarded as a local modifying risk factor for periodontitis progression if left untreated.[18] It is believed that an unresolved periapical infection could sustain endodontic pathogen growth, and infectious products would egress into the periodontium via the apex and lateral or accessory canals, as well as encourage osteoclastic activity. These may aggravate periodontal pocket formation, bone loss, and impair wound healing to further accelerate periodontal disease development and progression. In addition, the medicaments (e.g., high concentrations of calcium hydroxide, corticosteroids, antibiotics) used for root canal therapy can also irritate the periodontal attachment apparatus.[7,8] However, the nature and extent of periodontal destruction is dependent on several factors, including virulence of the irritating stimuli present in the root canal system (e.g., microbiota, medications, foreign-body reactions), duration of the disease, and host defense mechanisms.[12]

The ability of the periodontium to regenerate lost attachment apparatus on pulpless teeth has been questioned, especially if these teeth contain a root canal filling and have been denuded of cementum. Sanders suggested that endodontically treated teeth may not respond as well as untreated teeth to periodontal procedures. He found 60% osseous regeneration of periodontal defects in nonendodontically treated teeth, compared with 33% defect fill in endodontically treated teeth.[54] However, in a monkey study, Diem et al reported that all tissue of the periodontium had a potential for regeneration after periodontal surgery, regardless of the status of the pulp (vital, filled, medicated, or open).[16] Perlmutter et al also failed to prove the hypothesis that pulp has an influence on initial cementogenesis and that substances leaching from certain root canal–filling materials may prevent deposition of new cementum.[49]

Although endodontic infections have been highly correlated with deeper periodontal pockets and furcation involvement in mandibular molars, the causal relationship between the two tissues has not yet been established.[31] It has been suggested that endodontic treatment should occur before treatment of furcation lesions (i.e., bone regeneration) to ensure successful results. Thus extensive evidence is lacking to prove this hypothesis. However, there is general agreement that with the proper endodontic treatment, periodontal disease of pulpal origin should heal. Hence the question of whether endodontic infections play a significant role in affecting the health of the periodontium remains to be further elucidated.[45]

INFLUENCE OF PERIODONTAL INFLAMMATION ON THE PULP

Clinically, it is not uncommon to observe an advanced periodontitis spreading to the apical foramen and causing pulp necrosis. It is also recognized that infection from a periodontal pocket may spread to the pulp through accessory canals, which occur most often in the furcation and closer to the apex of teeth. Rubach et al proved that pulpitis and pulp necrosis can occur as a result of periodontal inflammation involving accessory and apical canals.[53] In addition, bacterial products and toxins may also gain access to the pulp via exposed dentinal tubules. The pulpal reaction is not only influenced by the stages of periodontal disease but also by the type of periodontal treatment such as scaling, root planing, and administration of medication.[26] Inflammatory lesions of varying severity and necrotic pulp tissue are usually found in teeth with large canals or in cases where periodontal breakdown has extended to the apex.[26] Moreover, Whyman stated that during periodontal therapy the blood vessels supplying the pulp via accessory canals may be damaged.[74] Bergenholtz and Lindhe, in an animal study, found that 70% of root specimens examined showed no pathologic changes, despite the fact that 30% to 40% of the periodontal attachment was lost.[6] The remaining 30% of roots displayed only small inflammatory cell infiltrates or formation of reparative dentin or both in areas where pulp was adjacent to root exposed through periodontal destruction. These tissue changes were frequently associated with root surface resorption, suggesting that dentinal tubules must be uncovered before irritation can be transmitted.

These observations suggest that the presence of an intact cementum layer is important for the protection of the pulp from toxic elements produced by the plaque microbiota. Hence, periodontal disease and periodontal treatments should be regarded as potential causes of pulpitis and pulpal necrosis. It has also been reported that the pulps of teeth with long-standing periodontal disease develop fibrosis and various forms of mineralization. Canals associated with periodontally involved teeth were reported to be narrower than canals of nonperiodontally involved teeth. This result is thought to be a reparative process rather than an inflammatory response.[5,39]

Although consensus supports the influence that a degenerating or inflamed pulp can have on the periodontium, not all researchers are in agreement about the effect of periodontal disease upon the pulp. Specifically, inflammatory alterations and localized pulp necrosis have been observed

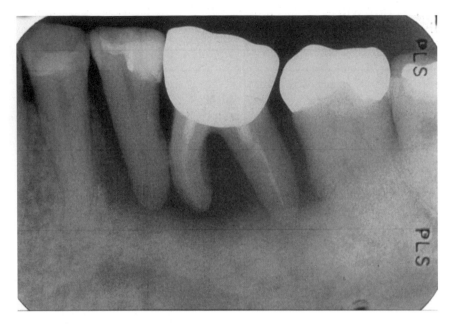

Fig. 17-6 True combined pulpal and periodontal lesions on mandibular second premolar and first molar. Periodontal probing depths were to the apices in both teeth.

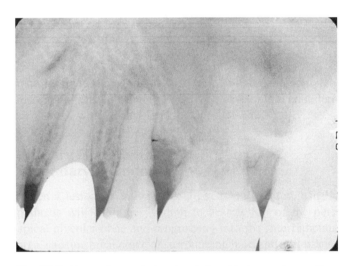

Fig. 17-7 Concomitant pulpal and periodontal lesion on the maxillary second premolar. An endodontic lesion was noted at the apex with a noncommunicating periodontal pocket on the distal side.

must resist the temptation to label everything a "combined lesion." Table 17-2 summarizes the differential diagnosis between pulpal and periodontal lesions and highlights a number of common characteristics between these lesions.

Root fractures, especially vertical root fractures, present particular problems in diagnosis (Fig. 17-8). Symptoms and signs associated with vertical root fractures show a varying character and are frequently difficult to distinguish from those associated with periodontal and endodontic lesions. Breakdown can manifest itself radiographically in a number

of different ways. It is imperative for the clinician to take more than one radiograph at different angles, especially when no clear diagnosis emerges. In these cases, a minor alteration in the angulation may reveal a tooth fracture or periodontal furcation involvement. The diagnosis of vertical root fractures is often difficult because the fracture is usually not detectable by clinical inspection and radiographic examination, unless there is a clear separation of the root fragments.

Often the definitive diagnosis of vertical root fractures has to be confirmed by exploratory surgical exposure of the root for direct visual examination.[71] Vertical root fractures have been associated with root-filled teeth where excessive lateral forces were applied during condensation, or possibly with stress induced by a post placement in root-filled teeth.[46] Clinical survey of fractured teeth also reveals fractures are more common in teeth with extensive restorations, in older patients, and in mandibular posterior teeth.[24] Vertical root fractures that involve the gingival sulcus and periodontal pocket area usually have a hopeless prognosis because of continuous bacterial invasion of the fracture space from the oral environment. Single-rooted teeth are generally extracted. In multirooted teeth, a treatment alternative is hemisection or resection of the fractured root.

Developmental grooves, primarily found in maxillary central and lateral incisors, are also capable of initiating localized periodontal destruction along the root surface.[20,40] It is thought that they may be a genetic attempt to form an accessory root. However, once plaque and calculus invade the epithelial attachment, the groove becomes a cove for microbia and food debris, heading to create a a self-supporting periodontal destruction pathway. The bone deso-

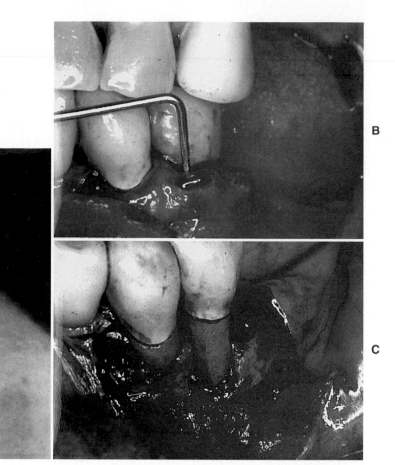

Fig. 17-8 Vertical root fracture. **A,** Radiograph revealed widened periodontal ligament with J-shaped radiolucency around the apex. **B,** Periodontal probe indicated more than 12 mm of probing depth. **C,** Exploratory surgery confirmed vertical root fracture.

Table 17-2   DIFFERENTIAL DIAGNOSIS BETWEEN PULPAL AND PERIODONTAL DISEASE

	Pulpal	Periodontal
Clinical		
Cause	Pulp infection	Periodontal infection
Vitality	Nonvital	Vital
Restorative	Deep or extensive	Not related
Plaque/Calculus	Not related	Primary cause
Inflammation	Acute	Chronic
Pockets	Single, narrow	Multiple, wide coronally
pH value	Often acid	Usually alkaline
Trauma	Primary or secondary	Contributing factor
Microbial	Few	Complex
Radiographic		
Pattern	Localized	Generalized
Bone loss	Wider apically	Wider coronally
Periapical	Radiolucent	Not often related
Vertical bone loss	No	Yes
Histopathology		
Junctional epithelium	No apical migration	Apical migration
Granulation tissues	Apical (minimal)	Coronal (larger)
Gingival	Normal	Some recession
Therapy		
Treatment	Root canal therapy	Periodontal treatment

lation follows the path of the groove. Palatogingival grooves are often associated with poor periodontal health due to their inability to keep these areas clean; therefore, a poor prognosis is usually assigned regardless of proper conventional therapy.[24,73] It is easy to identify these grooves if one is aware of their existence. Clinically, these grooves may be asymptomatic, or symptomatic periodontal problems (either acute or chronic). It is also thought that the pulp of these teeth may become secondarily involved and demonstrate symptoms of pulpal disease (Fig. 17-9). These lesions are often confused with the enamel projections in the furcation area of mandibular molars.[43] The prevalence of cervical enamel projections (Fig. 17-10) ranges from 18% to 45%.[30,43] Depending on the apical extent of these cervical grooves, these authors also find a high association with pathologic furcation involvement (up to 82.5%[30]).

There are cases that either do not fit a characteristic endodontic or periodontal lesion or do not respond to treatment as expected. A biopsy and histologic analysis is often recommended. Systemic diseases such as scleroderma, metastatic carcinoma, and osteosarcoma can mimic endodontic and periodontal disease visible on a radiograph. The conscientious clinician must always be alert for lesions of nonendodontic or nonperiodontal origin and look for other causes.

TREATMENT ALTERNATIVES

When traditional endodontic and periodontal treatments prove insufficient to stabilize an affected tooth, the clinician must consider treatment alternatives. Generally, a localized periodontal defect associated with an endodontically untreatable tooth or an iatrogenic tooth problem are reasons to explore other treatment options. Alternate treatments often consist of resective or regenerative approaches. Resec-

tive techniques focus on eliminating the diseased roots or teeth; regenerative efforts are aimed at restoring lost biologic structures. Resective methods involve removal of affected roots or extraction of involved teeth. When a tooth requires extraction, the option for restoring occlusal function should include placement of dental implants with hybrid prostheses. Bone replacement grafts using guided tissue and bone regeneration techniques are ways to reestablish biologic structures that were lost during this disease process.

Root resection is the removal of a root with accompanying odontoplasty, before or after endodontic treatment.[21] Formerly, it was used when root canal therapy was considered too difficult, but now its indications are restricted to multirooted teeth where one or more roots cannot be saved. The indications for root resection often include (but are not limited to) root fracture, perforation, root caries, dehiscence, fenestration, external-root resorption involving one root, impaired endodontic treatment of a particular root, severe periodontitis affecting only one root, and severe Grade II or III furcation involvement. Root resection is a technique-sensitive procedure (Fig. 17-11) requiring a careful diagnostic process for selection of those teeth that would likely be successful candidates, followed by meticulous interdisciplinary treatment. Factors such as occlusal forces, tooth restorability, and the value of the remaining roots must be examined before treatment. A carefully constructed treatment plan is crucial to the success of this resection procedure.[25] Proper reshaping of the occlusal table and restoration of the clinical crown are essential, and the root surface must be recontoured to remove the root stump, thus avoiding formation of a potential food trap.[33]

The effectiveness of this approach remains controversial based on the disparity of results reported in several long-term studies.[3,7,9,11,19,21,35] Retrospective longitudinal studies

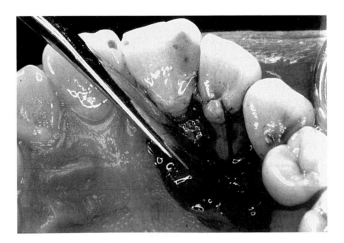

Fig. 17-9 Palato-gingival groove on maxillary lateral incisor with periodontal defect.

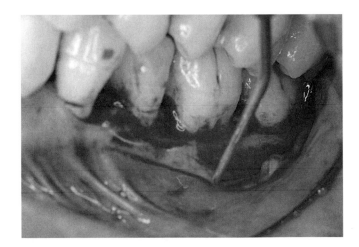

Fig. 17-10 Cervical enamel projection on mandibular molar.

have followed the fate of sectioned teeth for time frames ranging from 3 to 12 years and have reported success rates ranging from 62% to 100%, with a low incidence (i.e., 10%) of periodontal breakdown. However, as most long-term studies will point out, the major cause of failure of resection procedures resides in failure of the endodontic and restorative components. Unique anatomic features, such as root length, curvature, shape, size, position of adjacent teeth, and bone density, may influence the end result. For example, root fusion makes resection all but impossible. The removal of roots purely to eliminate a resorptive or traumatic perforation defect, fractured root, or endodontically inoperable root usually results in definitive treatment. If, however, localized or generalized periodontal disease is present, conditions favorable for healing must be created, and concomitant periodontal therapeutic procedures can be implemented to restore the health of the periodontium.[25] The final restoration of root-resected teeth will depend significantly on the nature of the resection, the amount of remaining tooth structure, periodontal status, and the patient's occlusion. The prosthetic aspects of tooth restoration must be carefully assessed and integrated into the anticipated surgical procedure to ensure proper positioning of tooth margins relative to the osseous crest and also to manage the anticipated changes in occlusal relationships and masticatory forces.[72]

Controversy has also existed regarding the benefits and need for endodontic therapy before root resection. Instances develop, however, where exploratory surgery is necessary, and should the periodontal problem be more extensive than that determined presurgically, the removal of a root should be carried out at that time. In these instances, removal of the involved root without endodontic treatment would be acceptable, but root canal therapy should be performed as soon as possible after root removal.[23,64] After resection of a vital root, the pulpal opening in the crown may be sealed and restored with a permanent amalgam restoration or sedative base material (e.g., Dycal) as a temporary solution. Filipowicz et al evaluated vital-root resection in maxillary molar teeth for 9 years.[21] Amputated pulps were covered with Dycal base and amalgam. At 1 year, 38% of molar teeth remained vital; however, at 5 years only 13% maintained vitality. These findings imply that the long-term prognosis for vital-root resection is poor, hence it is advised to have endodontic therapy done before or immediately after resection. Contrary to this study, Haskell reported that vitality of resected teeth can be maintained even after 16 years.[29] Nonetheless, it is generally agreed that whenever possible, endodontics should be performed in advance (before root resection). If this is not possible the endodontic treatment should be performed within 2 to 3 weeks after vital-root amputation. Otherwise, pulpal complications, such as internal resorption, pulpal inflammation, and necrosis, may occur.[2,67]

Recently the concepts of guided tissue regeneration (GTR) or guided bone regeneration (GBR) have been used to promote bone healing after endodontic surgery.[47] Fig. 17-12 illustrates an endodontic defect successfully treated with this approach. Theoretically, the GTR barrier prevents contact of connective tissue with the osseous walls of the defect, protecting the underlying blood clot and stabilizing the wound.[28] Pecora treated large periradicular lesions with GTR barrier membranes and demonstrated that periradicular healing occurred more rapidly at membrane sites than at control sites.[47,48] The quality and quantity of the regenerated bone was superior with adjunctive use of the membrane than without such use. Similar findings were published in a case report with histologic examination of biopsy material obtained at barrier removal.[50] In addition, when examining clinical cases, the closer the lesion is to the gingival margin, the greater the fluid-and-bacterial contamination from the sulcus (and also a greater risk of mechanic trauma). Thus the combined endodontic and periodontal lesion probably has the least favorable prognosis when GTR is used.[47]

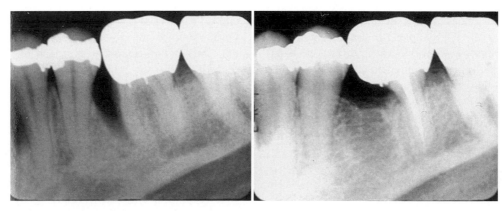

Fig. 17-11   Root resection to correct endodontic and periodontic defect. Preop radiograph depicts severe periodontal involvement on the mesial (*left*). Endodontic treatment was performed before surgical removal of the mesial root. Five year follow-up shows the remaining tooth well maintained (*right*).

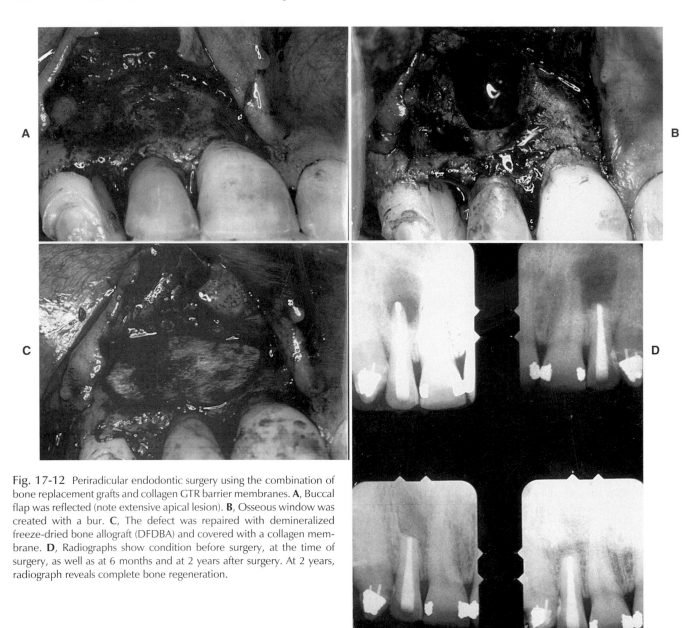

Fig. 17-12 Periradicular endodontic surgery using the combination of bone replacement grafts and collagen GTR barrier membranes. **A,** Buccal flap was reflected (note extensive apical lesion). **B,** Osseous window was created with a bur. **C,** The defect was repaired with demineralized freeze-dried bone allograft (DFDBA) and covered with a collagen membrane. **D,** Radiographs show condition before surgery, at the time of surgery, as well as at 6 months and at 2 years after surgery. At 2 years, radiograph reveals complete bone regeneration.

There are many varieties of GTR membranes available for clinical use. However, it is logical to use bioresorbable collagen-and-polymer membranes because there is no need for a second surgery to retrieve the membrane. In addition, studies reveal similar results achieved with nonresorbable and resorbable membranes.[13] It should be noted, though, that long-term studies are still needed to critically evaluate the effect of this newly developed approach.

For more than 40 years bone grafts have been used to treat osseous defects associated with periodontal disease.[56] Because the "apicoectomy" (i.e., root-end resection) defect has a surrounding bony wall, it is questionable as to the need for adjunctive bone grafting during this procedure (unless it is exceptionally large in diameter). With the introduction of the GTR concept a combination of bone replacement graft

and GTR membrane has shown promising results.[1,17,32,50,69] Further studies are required to explore the true benefit of this combination treatment approach in root-end resection procedures.

SUMMARY

Endodontic and periodontal lesions result from the close interrelationship of pulp tissue and the periodontium. The major pathways of communication between the two types of tissue are the apical foramina, lateral and accessory canals, and dentinal tubules. The differential diagnosis of endodontic and periodontal lesions is not always straightforward and requires clinical data accumulation from a number of diagnostic tests to obtain a correct diagnosis. When examining and treating the combined or individual lesion in endodontics and periodontics, the clinician must bear in mind that successful treatment depends on a correct diagnosis. Lesions with combined cause will require both endodontic and periodontal therapy, and endodontic therapy should usually be completed first. In addition, root resective and regenerative techniques offer alternative approaches, thus enhancing the clinician's ability to deal with these complex clinical problems.

References

1. Abramowitz PN, Rankow H, Trope M: Multidisciplinary approach to apical surgery in conjunction with the loss of buccal cortical plate, *Oral Surg Oral Med Oral Pathol Oral Radiol Endod* 77:502, 1994.

2. Allen AL, Gutmann JL: Internal root resorption after vital root resection, *J Endod* 3:438, 1977.

3. Basten CH-J, Ammons WF Jr, Persson R: Long-term evaluation of root resected molars: a retrospective study, *Int J Periodontics Restorative Dent* 16:207, 1996.

4. Belk CE, Gutmann JL: Perspectives, controversies, and directives on pulpal-periodontal relationship, *J Can Dent Assoc* 56:1013, 1990.

5. Bender IB, Seltzer S: The effect of periodontal disease on the pulp, *Oral Surg Oral Med Oral Pathol Oral Radiol Endod* 33:458, 1972.

6. Bergenholtz G, Lindhe J: Effect of experimentally induced marginal periodontitis and periodontal scaling on the dental pulp, *J Clin Periodontol* 5:59, 1978.

7. Blomlof L, Jansson L, Applegren R, Ehnevid H, Lindskog S: Prognosis and mortality of root-resected molars, *Int J Periodon Rest Dent* 17:191, 1997.

8. Blomlof L, Lengheden A, Linskog S: Endodontic infection and calcium hydroxide treatment effects on periodontal healing in mature and immature replanted monkey teeth, *J Clin Periodontol* 29:652, 1992.

9. Buhler H: Evaluation of root resected teeth. Results after 10 years, *J Periodontol* 59:805, 1988.

10. Burch JG, Hulen S: A study of the presence of accessory foramina and the topography of molar furcations, *Oral Surg Oral Med Oral Pathol* 38:451, 1974.

11. Carnevale G, DiFebo G, Tonelli MP, Marin C, Fuzzi MA: Retrospective analysis of the periodontal-prosthetic treatment of molars and interradicular lesions, *Int J Periodontics Restorative Dent* 11:189, 1991.

12. Chen SY, Wang HL, Glickman GN: The influence of endodontic treatment upon periodontal wound healing, *J Clin Periodontol* 24:449, 1997.

13. Christgau M, Schmalz G, Reich E, Wenzel A: Clinical and radiographical split-mouth study on resorbable versus nonresorbable GTR-membranes, *J Clin Periodontol* 22:306, 1995.

14. Cutright DE, Bhaskar SN: Pulpal vasculature as demonstrated by a new method, *Oral Surg Oral Med Oral Pathol* 27:678, 1969.

15. Czarnecki RT, Schilder H: A histological evaluation of human pulp in teeth with varying degrees of periodontal disease, *J Endod* 5:242, 1979.

16. Diem CR, Bower GM, Ferrigno PD, Fedi PF Jr: Regeneration of the attachment apparatus on pulpless teeth denuded of cementum in Rhesus money, *J Periodontol* 45:18, 1974.

17. Duggins I, Clay J, Himel V, Dean J: A combined endodontic retrofill and periodontal guided tissue regeneration for the repair of molar endodontic furcation perforations: Report of a case, *Quintessence Int* 25:109, 1994.

18. Ehnevid H, Jansson L, Lindskog S, Blomlof L: Endodontic pathogens: propagation of infection through patent dentinal tubules in traumatized monkey teeth, *Endod Dent Traumatol* 11:229, 1995.

19. Erpenstein H: A three year study of hemisections molars, *J Clin Periodontol* 10:1, 1983.

20. Everett FG, Kramer GM: The disto-lingual groove in the maxillary lateral incisor: a periodontal hazard, *J Periodontol* 443:352, 1972.

21. Filipowicz F, Umstott P, England M: Vital root resection in maxillary molar teeth: a longitudinal study, *J Endod* 10:264, 1984.

22. Garrett S: Periodontal regeneration around natural teeth, *Ann Periodontol* 1:621, 1996.

23. Gerstein K: The role of vital root resection in periodontics, *J Periodontol* 48,478, 1977.

24. Gher ME, Dunlap RM, Anderson MH, Kuhl LV: Clinical survey of fractured teeth, *J Am Dent Assoc* 114:174, 1987.

25. Green EN: Hemisection and root amputation, *J Am Dent Assoc* 112:511, 1986.

26. Guldener PH: The relationship between periodontal and pulpal disease, *Int Endod J* 18:41, 1985.

27. Gutmann JL: Prevalence, location and patency of accessory canals in the furcation region of permanent molars, *J Periodontol* 49:21, 1978.

28. Hany JM, Nilveus RE, McMillan PJ, Wikesjo UME: Periodontal repair in dogs: expanded polytetrafluoroethylene barrier membranes support would stabilization and enhance bone regeneration, *J Periodontol* 64:883, 1993.

29. Haskell E: Vital root resection: a case report of long-term follow-up, *Int J Periodontics Restorative Dent* 4(6):57, 1984.

30. Hou GL, Tsai C: Relationship between periodontal furcation involvement and molar cervical enamel projections, *J Periodontol* 58:715, 1987.

31. Jansson LE, Ehnevid H: The influence of endodontic infection on periodontal status in mandibular molars, *J Periodontol* 69:1392, 1998.

32. Kellert M, Chalfin H, Solomon C: Guided tissue regeneration: an adjunct to endodontic surgery, *J Am Dent Assoc* 125:1229, 1994.

33. Kirchoff DA, Gerstein H: Presurgical occlusal contouring for root amputation procedures, *Oral Surg* 27:379, 1969.

34. Kirkham DB: The location and incidence of accessory pulpal canals in periodontal pockets, *J Am Dent Assoc* 91:353, 1975.

35. Klavan B: Clinical observation following root amputation in maxillary molar teeth, *J Periodontol* 46:105, 1975.

36. Koenigs JF, Brilliant JD, Foreman DW: Preliminary scanning electron microscope investigations of accessory foramina in the furcation areas of human molar teeth, *Oral Surg Oral Med Oral Pathol* 38:773, 1974.

37. Kramer IRH: The vascular architecture of the human dental pulp, *Arch Oral Biol* 2:177, 1960.

38. Langeland K, Rodrigues H, Dowden W: Periodontal disease, bacteria and pulpal histopathology, *Oral Surg Oral Med Oral Pathol Oral Radiol Endod* 37:257, 1974.

39. Lantelme RL, Handelman SL, Herbison RJ: Dentin formation in periodontally diseased teeth, *J Dent Res* 55:48, 1976.

40. Lee KW, Lee EC, Poon KY: Palato-gingival grooves in maxillary incisors, *Br Dent J* 124:14, 1968.

41. Lowman JV, Burke RS, Pelleu GB: Patent accessory canals: incidence in molar furcation region, *Oral Surg Oral Med Oral Pathol* 36:580, 1973.

42. Mandi FA: Histological study of the pulp changes caused by periodontal disease, *J Br Endod Soc* 6:80, 1972.

43. Masters DH, Hoskins SW: Projection of cervical enamel into molar furcations, *J Periodontol* 35:49, 1964.

44. Mazur B, Massler M: Influence of periodontal disease on the dental pulp, *Oral Surg Oral Med Oral Pathol Oral Radiol Endod* 17:592, 1964.

45. Miyashita H, Bergenholtz G, Grondahl K, Wennstrom JL: Impact of endodontic conditions on marginal bone loss, *J Periodontol* 69:158, 1998.

46. Obermayr G, Walton RE, Leary JM, Krell KV: Vertical root fracture and relative deformation during obturation and post cementation, *J Prosthet Dent* 66:181, 1991.

47. Pecora G, Baek SH, Rethnam S, Kim S: Barrier membrane techniques in endodontic microsurgery, *Dent Clin North Amer* 41:585, 1997.

48. Pecora G, Kim S, Celleti R, Davarpanah M: The guided tissue regeneration principle in endodontic surgery: one year postoperative results of large periapical lesions, *Int Endod J* 7:76, 1995.

49. Perlmutter S, Tagger M, Tagger E, Abram M: Effect of the endodontic status of the tooth on experimental periodontal reattachment in baboons: a preliminary investigation, *Oral Surg Oral Med Oral Pathol* 63:232, 1987.

50. Pinto VS, Zuolo ML, Mellonig JT: Guided bone regeneration in the treatment of a large periapical lesion: a case report, *Pract Periodontics Aesthet Dent* 7:76, 1995.

51. Pitts DL, Natkin E: Diagnosis and treatment of vertical root fractures, *J Endod* 9:338,1983.

52. Polson AM: Periodontal destruction associated with vertical root fracture: report of four cases, *J Periodontol* 48:27, 1977.

53. Rubach WC, Mitchell DF: Periodontal disease, accessory canals and pulp pathosis, *J Periodontol* 36:34, 1965.

54. Sanders J et al: Clinical evaluation of freeze-dried bone allograft in periodontal osseous defects. III. Composite freeze-dried bone allografts with and without autogenous bone grafts, *J Periodontol* 54:1, 1983.

55. Saunders RL, de CH: X-Ray microscopy of the periodontal and dental pulp vessels in the monkey and in man, *Oral Surg Oral Med Oral Pathol* 22:503, 1966.

56. Schallhorn RG: Long-term evaluation of osseous grafts in periodontal therapy, *Int Dent J* 30:101, 1980.

57. Seltzer S, Bender IB, Nazimov H, Sinai I: Pulpitis induced interradicular periodontal change in experimental animals, *J Periodontol* 38:124, 1967.

58. Seltzer S, Bender IB, Ziontz M: The interrelationship of pulp and periodontal disease, *Oral Surg Oral Med Oral Pathol Oral Radiol Endod* 16:1474, 1963.

59. Silverstein L, Shatz PC, Amato AL, Kurtzman D: A guide to diagnosing and treating endodontic and periodontal lesions, *Dent Today* 17(4):112, 1998.

60. Simon JHS, Glick DH, Frank AL: The relationship of endodontic-periodontic lesions, *J Periodontol* 43:202, 1972.

61. Simon JH, Werksman LA: Endodontic-periodontal relations. In Cohen S, Burns RC, editors: *Pathways of the Pulp*, ed 6, St Louis, 1994, Mosby.

62. Simring M, Goldberg M: The pulpal pocket approach. Retrograde periodontitis, *J Periodontol* 35:22, 1964.

63. Sinai I, Soltanoff W: The transmission of pathologic changes between the pulp and the periodontal structures, *Oral Surg Oral Med Oral Pathol* 36:558, 1973.

64. Smukler H, Tagger M: Vital root amputation. A clinical and histologic study, *J Periodontol* 47:324, 1976.

65. Stahl SS: Pathogenesis of inflammatory lesions in pulp and periodontal tissues, *Periodontics* 4:190, 1966.

66. Stallard RE: Periodontic-endodontic relationships, *Oral Surg Oral Med Oral Pathol* 34:314, 1972.

67. Tagger M, Perlmutter S, Tagger E, Abrams M: Histological study of untreated pulps in hemisected teeth in baboons, *J Endod* 14:288, 1988.

68. Torabinejad M, Kiger RD: A histologic evaluation of dental pulp tissue of a patient with periodontal disease, *Oral Surg Oral Med Oral Pathol Oral Radiol Endod* 59:198, 1985.

69. Tseng CC, Chen YH, Huang CC, Bowers GM: Correction of a large periradicular lesion and mucosal defect using combined endodontic and periodontal therapy: a case report, *Int J Periodontics Restorative Dent* 15:377, 1995.

70. Vertucci FJ, Williams RG: Furcation canals in the human mandibular first molar, *Oral Sug Oral Med Oral Pathol* 38: 308, 1974.

71. Walton RE, Michelich RJ, Smith GN: The histopathogenesis of vertical root fractures, *J Endod* 10:48, 1984.

72. Ward HE: Preparation of furcally involved teeth, *J Prosthet Dent* 48:261, 1982.

73. Withers J, Brunsvold M, Killoy W, Rahe A: The relationship of Palato-gingival grooves to localized periodontal disease, *J Periodontol* 52:41, 1981.

74. Whyman RA: Endodontic-periodontic lesion. I. Prevalence, etiology, and diagnosis, *NZ Dent J* 84:74, 1988.

Chapter 18

Endodontic Pharmacology

Kenneth M. Hargreaves, Jeffrey W. Hutter

Chapter Outline

The effective management of pain is a hallmark of clinical excellence. Pain management is an integral part of endodontics, and the practice of endodontics requires a thorough understanding of pain mechanisms and management.[5] To treat pain effectively and efficiently, the skilled clinician should understand mechanisms of pain and analgesics and strategies for the management of pain, including the use of analgesic drugs. Accordingly, this chapter reviews mechanisms of hyperalgesia and the management of odontogenic pain, with an emphasis on endodontic pharmacology. A comprehensive review of pain will also include diagnosis of odontogenic pain (see Chapters 1 and 2), nonodontogenic pain (see Chapter 3), neuroanatomy of pulp (see Chapter 11), mechanisms of dentinal hypersensitivity (see Chapter 11), mediators activated in inflamed pulpal and periapical tissue (see Chapters 12 and 13), and the pharmacology of local anesthetics and anxiolytics (see Chapter 20). Fortunately, all of these topics are reviewed in this text.

MECHANISMS OF PAIN

Odontogenic pain is usually caused by either noxious physical stimuli or the release of inflammatory mediators that stimulate receptors located on terminal endings of nociceptive (i.e., "pain detecting") afferent nerve fibers.* Nociceptive fibers are distributed throughout the body and are prevalent in trigeminal nerves innervating tooth pulp and periapical tissue. As described in other chapters there are two major classes of nociceptors: (1) C fibers and (2) A-delta fibers (Fig. 18-1). In tooth pulp there are at least three to eight times more unmyelinated C fibers as compared with A-delta fibers.[21,22,84,159] Activation of dental pulp nerves by thermal, mechanical, chemical, or electrical (e.g., electrical pulp tester) stimuli results in a nearly pure sensation of pain.[17] Pulpal C fibers are thought to have a predominant role for encoding inflammatory pain arising from dental pulp and periradicular tissue. This hypothesis is supported by the distribution of C fibers in dental pulp, their responsiveness to inflammatory mediators,[100,120,121] and the strikingly similar perceptual qualities (e.g., dull, aching) of pain associated with C fiber activation and with pulpitis.

After activation the C and A-delta fibers from the orofacial region transmit nociceptive signals primarily via trigeminal nerves to the trigeminal nucleus caudalis (N. caudalis) located in the medulla.[67,97,119,144] The N. caudalis is an important, but not exclusive, site for processing orofacial nociceptive input.[41,101,145] Blockade of input from C and A-delta fibers by the use of long-acting local anesthetics evokes profound postoperative analgesia.[32,63,83,110]

The N. caudalis has been termed the "medullary dorsal horn," because its anatomical organization is similar to that seen in the spinal dorsal horn. The medullary dorsal horn is not simply a relay station where nociceptive signals are passively transferred to higher brain regions; rather the N. caudalis plays an important role in processing nociceptive signals, and the output to higher brain regions can be increased (e.g., hyperalgesia), decreased (e.g., analgesia), or misinterpreted (e.g., referred pain) as compared with incoming activity from the relevant C and A-delta fibers. For example,

---

*References 67,72,97,168,172

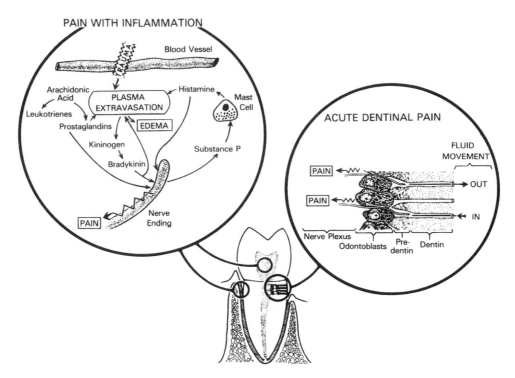

Fig. 18-1 Schematic diagram of two mechanisms for the peripheral stimulation of nociceptive nerve fibers in tooth pulp. Acute dentinal pain (*insert*). According to the hydrodynamic theory, stimuli that cause fluid movement in exposed dentinal tubules results in the stimulation of nociceptive nerve fibers. Pain with inflammation (*insert*). Inflammation is associated with the synthesis or release of mediators, including prostaglandins, bradykinin, substance P, and histamine (and other mediators not shown). The interrelationships of these inflammatory mediators form a positive feedback loop, allowing inflammation to persist far beyond cessation of the dental procedure. (From Hargreaves KM, Troullos E, Dionne R: Pharmacologic rationale for the treatment of acute pain, *Dent Clin North Am* 31:675, 1987.)

during tissue inflammation or after pulpal extirpation there is a dramatic change in the responsiveness or receptor field size of neurons in the medullary dorsal horn; these and other changes are called dorsal horn plasticity to denote the dramatic alteration in neuronal activity produced by peripheral inflammation.*

MEDULLARY DORSAL HORN

The medullary dorsal horn contains at least four major components related to the processing of nociceptive signals: (1) central terminals of afferent fibers, (2) local-circuit neurons, (3) projection neurons, and (4) descending neurons. In the first component, primary nociceptive afferents (e.g., C and A-delta fibers) enter the medullary dorsal horn via the trigeminal tract (Fig. 18-2). The central terminals of these C and A-delta fibers end primarily in the outer layers of the medullary dorsal horn. These sensory fibers transmit information by releasing excitatory amino acids, such as glutamate or neuropeptides (e.g., substance P or calcitonin gene–

related peptide [CGRP]). In animal studies the administration of receptor antagonists to glutamate (in particular) and antagonists to SP and CGRP (to a lesser extent) has been shown to block hyperalgesia.[24,40,134,171] Evidence gathered in animal studies strongly implicates antagonists to the glutamate N-methyl D-aspartate (NMDA) receptor as being particularly effective in reducing hyperalgesia. These compounds are likely to serve as prototypes for future classes of analgesic drugs.[172]

Local-circuit neurons are a second component of the dorsal horn, and they regulate transmission of nociceptive signals from the primary afferent fibers to projection neurons.[41,97,168] The third component of the dorsal horn is the projection neurons; the cell bodies of these neurons are within the medullary dorsal horn and their axons make up the output system for sending orofacial pain information to more rostral brain regions. A major projection pathway for these axons is the trigeminothalamic tract. This tract crosses to the contralateral side of the medulla and ascends to the thalamus (see Fig. 18-2). From the thalamus, additional neurons relay this information to the cerebral cortex via a thalamocortical tract.

Evidence exists that referred pain is caused by the convergence of afferent input from cutaneous and visceral noci-

*References 24,40,146,147,177

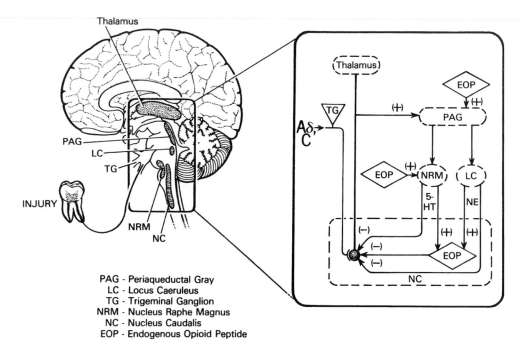

PAG - Periaqueductal Gray
LC - Locus Caeruleus
TG - Trigeminal Ganglion
NRM - Nucleus Raphe Magnus
NC - Nucleus Caudalis
EOP - Endogenous Opioid Peptide

Fig. 18-2 Schematic diagram of the perception and modulation of orofacial pain. Activation of A-delta or C-nociceptive fibers leads to the entry of a nociceptive signal that is conveyed across a synapse in the nucleus caudalis of the trigeminal system. The second order neuron projects to the thalamus; the information is then relayed to the cortex. Endogenous pain suppression system (*insert*). This insert depicts the functional relationship of several neurotransmitters for the modulation of nociceptive information at the nucleus caudalis (the actual anatomical relationships are more complex). As in the large figure, peripheral activation of A-delta or C fibers stimulates the projection neuron in the N. caudalis (filled cell body), which relays to the thalamus. This signal is also transmitted to the periaqueductal gray (*PAG*), which receives additional input from other areas not shown. The PAG, in turn, activates the nucleus raphe magnus (*NRM*) and the locus coerulius (*LC*). The NRM sends fibers to the first synapse in the N. caudalis, where it inhibits the transmission of nociceptive information by the secretion of serotonin (*5-HT*) and other neurotransmitters. In a similar fashion the LC sends fibers to the first synapse, where norepinephrine (*NE*) is released to inhibit transmission. Note that neurons secreting endogenous opioid peptides (*EOP*) are present at all three levels of this system. The "+" sign indicates an excitatory action, whereas the "−" sign denotes an inhibitory action. (From Hargreaves KM, Troullos E, Dionne R: Pharmacologic rationale for the treatment of acute pain, *Dent Clin North Am* 31:675, 1987.)

ceptors onto the same projection neurons. For example, nociceptors in the maxillary sinus and maxillary molars may stimulate the same neuron located in the N. caudalis. This convergence of sensory input probably mediates referred pain.[145] Indeed, about 50% of neurons in the N. caudalis exhibit convergence of sensory input from cutaneous and visceral structures.[147] In one example a single neuron in the N. caudalis received input from sensory neurons innervating the maxillary skin, cornea, mandibular canine, mandibular premolar, and maxillary premolar.[145]

The theory of convergence has been used to explain the clinical observation of a patient complaining of pain originating from an inflamed mandibular molar and radiating to the preauricular region (or of pain originating in inflamed maxillary sinuses and radiating to the maxillary posterior teeth). Moreover, the convergence theory forms the basis for the diagnostic use of local anesthetics to establish the origin of difficult to locate pain. For example, Okeson describes the selective injection of local anesthetics as a clinical test to dis-

tinguish the site of pain origin from the area of pain referral.[126]

The fourth component of the medullary dorsal horn consists of the terminal endings of descending neurons (see Fig. 18-2). These terminals act to inhibit the transmission of nociceptive information.[12] Important components of this endogenous analgesic system are the endogenous opioid peptides (EOP). The EOPs are a family of peptides that possess many of the properties of exogenous opioids, such as morphine and codeine. The EOP family includes the enkephalins, dynorphins, and beta-endorphin–related peptides. Importantly, EOPs are found at several levels of the pain suppression system. This fact underlies the analgesic efficacy of endogenous and exogenous opioids, because their administration conceivably activates opioid receptors located at all levels of the neuraxis.

The EOPs are probably released during dental procedures because blockade of the actions of endogenous opioids by administration of the antagonist naloxone can significantly

Table 18-1 **SIGNS OF HYPERALGESIA AND ENDODONTIC DIAGNOSTIC TESTS**

Sign of Hyperalgesia	Related Diagnostic Test or Symptom
Spontaneous pain	Spontaneous pain
Reduced pain threshold	Percussion test, Palpation test, Throbbing pain
Increased response to painful stimuli	Increased response to pulp test (EPT or thermal test)

(From Hargreaves et al: Pharmacology of peripheral neuropeptide and inflammatory mediator release, *Oral Surg Oral Med Oral Pathol* 78: 503,1994.)
EPT, Electric pulp test.

Box 18-1 **PERIPHERAL MECHANISMS CONTRIBUTING TO HYPERALGESIA**

Mechanism
- Composition and concentration of inflammatory mediators[69]
- Changes in afferent fiber: activation and sensitization[90,106,142]
- Changes in afferent fiber: sprouting[20]
- Changes in afferent fiber: proteins[20,62,172]
- Tissue pressure[120,121]
- Tissue temperature[108]
- Sympathetic primary afferent fiber interactions[82,94,130]
- A-beta fiber plasticity[122]

(Modified from Hargreaves et al: Pharmacology of peripheral neuropeptide and inflammatory mediator release, *Oral Surg Oral Med Oral Pathol* 78:503,1994.)

increase the perception of dental pain.[63,66,92] Another example is the endogenous cannabinoid system that inhibits central terminals of C fibers; hypoactivity of this system may mediate some forms of chronic pain.[135,136] Cannabinoids may have profound effects for modulating pain because there are about 10 times more cannabinoid receptors in the central nervous system (CNS) as compared with the opioid receptors. Additional studies have demonstrated cannabinoid receptors on sensory neurons and dental pulp, where they may act to inhibit peripheral terminals of unmyelinated nociceptors.[78,137,174]

MECHANISMS OF HYPERALGESIA

The pain system can undergo dramatic changes in response to peripheral inflammation, leading to the development of hyperalgesia.[40,42,167,172] Hyperalgesia can be characterized as spontaneous pain, reduced pain threshold (i.e., allodynia), and increased pain perception to noxious stimuli.[69,167] Most of us have experienced hyperalgesia; common examples include a sunburn or a thermal injury. Sunburn will often induce spontaneous pain, a reduced pain threshold (e.g., wearing a shirt is painful), and increased pain responsiveness (e.g., increased pain perception occurs when someone slaps sunburned skin). Thus a peripheral injury evokes fundamental changes in the response properties of the pain system.

Hyperalgesia also occurs during inflammation of pulpal or periradicular tissue. Indeed, the outcome of endodontic diagnostic tests and patient symptoms can be used to determine the presence of hyperalgesia (Table 18-1). For example, percussion of a tooth with a mirror handle (see Chapter 1) tests for one aspect of hyperalgesia, called *allodynia*: a reduction in the mechanical nociceptive thresholds of neurons innervating the periodontal ligament. Under normal conditions, this innocuous stimulation does not elicit pain.

However, under conditions of hyperalgesia the mechanical pain threshold is reduced to the point where tapping with a mirror handle is now perceived as tender or painful. Similarly, studies in cats have shown that pulpal inflammation lowers the mechanical threshold of pulpal fibers to the level where increases in systolic blood pressure can activate pulpal neurons. The synchrony of firing of pulpal fibers in response to the heartbeat is thought to mediate the "throbbing" pain of pulpitis.[22,121] Additional studies have shown that the thermal threshold of nociceptors can be reduced to the point where normal physiologic temperature (i.e., 37° C) can activate these peripheral neurons. This may explain the clinical observation of patients using ice water to relieve pain caused by severe, irreversible pulpitis, because the neurons would be expected to stop firing when the tissue is cooled. Accordingly, the study of mechanisms and management of hyperalgesia are important issues in the field of endodontics.[69]

Hyperalgesia is caused by both peripheral and central mechanisms.* Several mechanisms appear to contribute to peripheral hyperalgesia (Box 18-1). It is important to note that dental procedures, such as the incision and drainage of an abscess or a pulpectomy, may reduce pain by reducing concentrations of mediators and lowering tissue pressure. Many inflammatory mediators found in inflamed pulp or periradicular tissue (see Chapters 12 and 13) can either activate or sensitize nociceptors and evoke pain when administered to human volunteers (Table 18-2).

Activation of a nociceptor is caused by a membrane depolarization sufficient to elicit an action potential that is then propagated along the neuron to central terminals located in the brainstem trigeminal nuclei. Sensitization of a nociceptor is caused by receptor-mediated events leading to spontaneous activity, a decreased threshold for depolarization, and prolonged responses (i.e., after discharges) to suprathreshold

*References 40,42,167,170,171,172

Table 18-2   EFFECT OF INFLAMMATORY MEDIATORS ON NOCICEPTIVE AFFERENT FIBERS

Mediator	Effect on Nociceptors	Effect on Human Volunteers
Potassium[86]	Activate	++
Protons[98,150]	Activate	++
Serotonin[14,86]	Activate	++
Bradykinin[14,86,93]	Activate	+++
Histamine[86]	Activate	+
Tumor Necrosis Factor α[160,176]	Activate	?
Prostaglandins[15]	Sensitize	±
Leukotrienes[15,100]	Sensitize	±
Nerve Growth Factor[95,131]	Sensitize	++
Substance P[65]	Sensitize	±
Interleukin-1[49]	Sensitize (?)	?

+ Positive, ++; very positive; +++, extremely positive; ±, equivalent; ?, unknown. (Modified from Fields H: *Pain*, New York, 1987, McGraw-Hill.)

Box 18-2   CENTRAL MECHANISMS CONTRIBUTING TO HYPERALGESIA

- Mechanism
- Increased neurotransmitter release from primary afferent fibers[55]
- Changes in postsynaptic receptors[54]
- Changes in second messenger systems[56,107]
- Changes in protooncogenes[38,177]
- Changes in endogenous opioids[38,64,66,92]
- Central sensitization[79,161,170]
- Wind up[171]
- Dark Neurons[151]

(Modified from Hargreaves et al: Neuroendocrine and immune responses to injury, degeneration, and repair. In Sessle BJ, Dionne RA, Bryant P, editors: *Temporomandibular disorders and related pain conditions*, Seattle, 1995, IASP Press.)

stimuli. The action of peripheral analgesics is based, in part, upon the ability of these drugs to reduce nociceptor activation or sensitization by reducing tissue levels of inflammatory mediators. Predictably, drugs that inhibit the actions of these mediators exhibit analgesic activity in models of hyperalgesia.[28,139] Considerable research is being directed to understanding the mechanisms of sensitization of nociceptors in the hope of developing new classes of analgesic drugs.[43,133,172]

In addition to activation and sensitization, the peripheral afferent fiber responds to mediators (e.g., nerve growth factor [NGF]) by increasing protein synthesis of substance P and CGRP and by undergoing sprouting of terminal fibers in the inflamed tissue.[18,20,88] Sprouting increases the density of innervation in inflamed tissue and may contribute to increased pain sensitivity in chronic pulpal or periradicular inflammation.[20] Certain afferent fibers also respond to inflammatory mediators by synthesizing other proteins, such as TTX-resistant sodium channels.[3,43,165] These ion channels are synthesized by a major class of nociceptors and undergo activation by inflammatory mediators.[7,61,62] Unlike the typical class of TTX-sensitive sodium channels found on sensory neurons, local anesthetics poorly block the TTX-resistant class of sodium channels. Indeed, it takes about four times more lidocaine to block TTX-resistant channels as it takes to block the typical class of TTX-sensitive ion channels.[140] Given this disparity in lidocaine potency, the synthesis of new types of ion channels on sensory neurons may well contribute to the clinical finding of difficulty in obtaining local anesthesia in certain endodontic pain cases. Indeed,

interventions that block the expression of one member of the class of TTX-resistant sodium channels (the PN3 channel), have a significant effect in reducing nociception in rat models of inflammatory and neuropathic pain.[132]

In addition to these peripheral mechanisms, several central mechanisms of hyperalgesia have also been proposed (Box 18-2).* For example, pulpectomy can evoke a central sensitization as measured both by an expansion of receptive field sizes and an increase in spontaneous activity.[147] In addition, central terminals of afferent fibers continue to exhibit increased release of CGRP even after removal from the animal.[55] Thus even in the absence of peripheral input, central mechanisms of hyperalgesia can persist for some time. Because at least some components of hyperalgesia can persist even without continued sensory input from inflamed tissue, it is not surprising that up to 80% of endodontic patients experiencing pain before treatment continue to report pain after treatment.[104,105] Drugs that block mechanisms of hyperalgesia may well offer new advances in the control of endodontic pain.[40,56,107] Taken together, it is apparent that the mechanisms of hyperalgesia are clinically significant factors in understanding strategies for diagnosing and managing the patient with endodontic pain.

PREDICTORS OF POSTOPERATIVE ENDODONTIC PAIN

Although present day endodontic treatment can be virtually pain free during the actual procedure itself, patients may still experience some pain after their appointments. Early studies investigating postoperative endodontic pain have reported an incidence of moderate-to-severe pain in the range of 15% to 25%.[25,75,125] In a prospective clinical study, 57% of patients

*References 40,42,70,167,172

TABLE 18-3 FACTORS RELATED TO POSTENDODONTIC PAIN

Author/Year	N	Preop Hyperalgesia	Preop Swelling	Necrotic Pulp	Apical Periodontitis	Re-Tx	Tooth Type	Sex	Age	Hx of Allergy	Intracanal Medicament	Apical Patency	One-Step vs. Multiappt
Seltzer et al, 1968[143]	698	+							+		=		
Frank et al, 1968[52]	585				AP < Pain						=		
Fox et al, 1970[51]	291	+		=	AP < Pain		=	+	=			+	
Clem, 1970[25]	318			+			+	=					
O'Keefe, 1976[125]	147	+		=	=		+	=	+		=		=
Maddox et al, 1977[99]	252			=				=	=		=		
Soltantoff, 1978[148]	281						+						Multi is <
Harrison et al, 1979[73]	195			=	=		+						
Rowe et al., 1980[141]	150	+	+	=	=								
Harrison et al, 1981[74]	245			=	=		=				=		
Pekruhn, 1981[128]	102												=
Mulhern et al, 1982[117]	60	+			=		=	+	=				=
Oliet, 1983[127]	387			=			=	=	+				=
Harrison et al, 1983[75]	229			=			=						
Harrison et al, 1983[76]	229			=	AP > Pain		=				+		1-Step is <
Roane et al, 1983[138]	359			=			=						
Balaban et al, 1984[10]	157						+	+					
Creech and Walton, 1984[29]	49	+											
Jostes and Holland, 1984[85]	58	+											
Marshall and Walton, 1984[104]	50	+		=	=		=	=	=				=
Georgopoulou et al, 1986[59]	245			=	=		=		=				
Morse et al, 1987[112]	106	+		=	AP > Pain		+	+	+			=	
Flath et al, 1987[48]	116	+		=	=							=	
Genet et al, 1987[58]	443	+		+	AP > Pain		+	+	=			=	
Torabinejad et al, 1988[153]	2000	+			AP < Pain	+	+	+	+	+	=	=	=
Fava, 1989[46]	60												
Trope, 1990[156]	474				AP > Pain	+					=		
Trope, 1991[157]	226				AP > Pain	+							
Mor, 1992[111]	334			+	AP < Pain		=	=					=
Walton and Fouad, 1992[163]	946	+	+	+	AP > Pain	=	=	=	=				
Marshall and Liesinger, 1993[103]	106			=	AP < Pain		=		=				
Torabinejad et al, 1994[154]	588	+											
Abbott, 1994[2]	100										+		
Imura and Suolo, 1995[80]	1012	+		=	AP > Pain	+	=	=	=				1-Step is <
Eleazor and Eleazor, 1998[45]	402												1-Step is <
Albashaireh, 1998[4]	300												1-Step is <
Total	12300												

Note: A "+" sign indicates that a positive correlation was found between this factor and the presence of pain. A "=" sign indicates that no correlation was found between this factor and the presence of pain. The absence of either sign indicates that the study did not address this factor. "AP > Pain" indicates that the presence of apical periodontitis was associated with more postoperative pain.

reported no pain after débridement and shaping of the root canal system, although 21% had slight pain, 15% had moderate pain, and 7% had severe pain.[59] Although some patients may experience moderate-to-severe pain after endodontic treatment, very few experience what is now commonly referred to as a flare-up or a postoperative problem requiring an unscheduled visit with unplanned treatment intervention to manage the patient's symptoms. Patients with a flare-up will usually describe severe pain, swelling, or the sensation of pressure within their mandible or maxilla. The incidence of flare-up varies across studies and ranges from about 2% to about 20% of patients.[11,114,156,157]

To better predict when postoperative endodontic pain or a flare-up is more likely to occur, numerous studies have evaluated factors related to their occurrence. Table 18-3 summarizes the results of studies evaluating more than 12,000 patients for predictors of postoperative pain. Although a direct comparison between studies is confounded because of differences in experimental design, it is interesting to note that the presence of *preoperative* hyperalgesia (defined as preoperative pain or percussion sensitivity) was a positive predictor of postoperative pain in 14 studies out of 14 involving more than 6600 patients (see Table 18-3).

Other factors were more variable in their predictive value of postoperative pain. For example, in a retrospective study the dental records of 1000 patients who had received nonsurgical root canal treatment and experienced no flare-ups (i.e., unscheduled patient return visits) were compared with the records of 1000 patients who experienced flare-ups after the cleansing and shaping of their necrotic root canals. The results showed that factors, such as presence of preoperative pain, tooth type, sex, age, history of allergy, and retreatment, were significantly predictive for the incidence of flare-up, although intracanal medicaments, systemic disease, and establishment of patency of the apical foramen had no significant relation to the incidence of flare-ups.[153]

Specifically, the highest incidences of flare-ups were associated with mandibular teeth, retreatments, females over the age of 40, and patients with a history of allergies.[153] In another retrospective study, Mor et al. determined the flare-up rate in patients treated in multiple visits by undergraduate dental students.[111] The flare-up incidence was 4.2%, and there was a positive correlation between flare-ups and teeth with necrotic pulp. There was, however, no correlation between the occurrence of a flare-up and the presence or absence of a periradicular radiolucency.

In a prospective study of one-visit treatments, the overall flare-up rate was only 1.8%.[157] However, this same study determined that one-visit endodontic retreatment cases involving teeth with apical periodontitis had almost a tenfold higher incidence of flare-ups (13.6%), with the recommendation that retreatment of teeth with apical periodontitis should not be completed in one visit. Another prospective clinical study reported an overall flare-up rate of 3.17% of 946 endodontic cases.[163] Patients with severe preoperative pain had a flare-up rate of 19%, although the presence of localized or diffuse swelling related to an incidence of 15%.

In this study pulpal status predicted the flare-up rate, with necrotic teeth having a significantly greater incidence of flare-ups compared with vital teeth (6.5% versus 1.3%). Periradicular status also predicted flare-up rates, with differences noted between chronic apical periodontitis (3.4%), acute apical periodontitis (4.8%), and acute apical abscess (13.1%). There was no significant difference between single and multiple visits. Finally, there was no significant increase in flare-ups for teeth undergoing retreatment of a failed root canal, although a subset analysis of retreatment with or without apical periodontitis was not performed.

In summary, the most consistent factor that predicts post-endodontic pain is the presence of preoperative hyperalgesia. Although no single factor completely predicts the occurrence and magnitude of postoperative pain, the astute clinician often interprets the presence of preoperative hyperalgesia as a warning sign in selecting the pain control regimen for each patient.

NON-NARCOTIC ANALGESICS

Management of endodontic pain is multifactorial and is directed at reducing the peripheral and central components of hyperalgesia (see Boxes 18-1 and 18-2) through combined endodontic procedures and pharmacotherapy. One major class of drugs for managing endodontic pain is nonnarcotic analgesics, which include both the nonsteroidal antiinflammatory drugs (NSAIDs) and acetaminophen. NSAIDs have been shown to be very effective for managing pain of inflammatory origin and, by virtue of their binding to plasma proteins, actually exhibit increased delivery to inflamed tissue.[19,36,71] Although these drugs are classically thought to produce analgesia through peripheral mechanisms, it should be pointed out that the CNS is now believed to be an additional site of action.[102]

Numerous NSAIDs are available for management of pain and inflammation (Table 18-4). Unfortunately, comparatively few studies (particularly for endodontic pain) directly compare one NSAID to one another for analgesia and side effect liability. The lack of comprehensive comparative studies in endodontic models means that only general recommendations can be made, and the clinician is encouraged to be familiar with several of these drugs. Ibuprofen is generally considered the prototype of NSAIDs and has a well-documented efficacy and safety profile.[31] Other NSAIDs may offer certain advantages over ibuprofen. For example, etodolac (i.e., Lodine) has minimal gastrointestinal (GI) irritation,[8] and ketoprofen (i.e., Orudis) has been shown in some studies to be somewhat more analgesic than ibuprofen.[26] The advantages of NSAIDs include their well-established analgesic efficacy for inflammatory pain. Indeed, many of the NSAIDs listed in Table 18-4 have been shown to be more effective than traditional acetaminophen and opioid combinations, such as Tylenol with codeine no. 3.[28,32,158]

The introduction in 1999 of selective inhibitors of cyclooxygenase-2 (COX-2) offers the potential for both

Table 18-4 **SUMMARY OF SELECTED NON-NARCOTIC ANALGESICS**

Analgesic Drug	Maximum Trade Name	Dose Range (mg)	Dose/Day (mg)
Acetaminophen	Tylenol et al	325-1000	4000
Aspirin	Many	325-1000	4000
Diflunisal	Dolobid	250-1000	1500
Diclofenac potassium	Cataflam	50-100	150-200
Etodolac	Lodine	200-400	1200
Fenoprofen	Nalfon	200	1200
Flurbiprofen	Ansaid	50-100	200-300
Ibuprofen	Motrin et al	200-400	2400 (Rx)
Ketorolac*	Toradol	10 (oral)	40
Naproxen Na	Anaprox et al	220-550	1650 (Rx)
Naproxen	Naprosyn	250-500	1500
Ketoprofen	Orudis	25-75	300 (Rx)
Rofecoxib	Vioxx	12.5-50	50

*A new package insert for ketorolac tablets contains the instructions that the drug should be used only as a transition from injectable ketorolac and for no more than 5 days.
Rx: Prescription strength.
(Modified from Cooper SA: Treating acute dental pain, *Postgrad Dentistry* 2:7, 1995.)

analgesic and antiinflammatory benefits and reduced GI irritation.[33] Oral surgery pain studies evaluating COX-2 inhibitors have indicated that rofecoxib (i.e., Vioxx) has significant analgesic efficacy in this model.[44] In one study, rofecoxib at a 50 mg dose produced equivalent analgesia compared with ibuprofen 400 mg, with both drugs displaying similar times for onset of analgesia.[44] Another COX-2 inhibitor, celecoxib (i.e., Celebrex), appears to have less conclusive analgesic efficacy and did not receive Food and Drug Administration (FDA) approval for treatment of acute pain. Recently concern has been raised that the COX-2 inhibitors may also display at least some GI irritation in cases with preexisting disease, suggesting some caution with use of these drugs.[162] However, when indicated, these drugs may have utility for endodontic pain because recent COX-2 levels are increased in inflamed human dental pulp, compared with levels in control dental pulp.[118]

LIMITATIONS AND DRUG INTERACTIONS

In addition to their analgesic efficacy, the clinician should be aware of limitations and drug interactions when considering the use of nonnarcotic analgesics for managing endodontic pain. For example, NSAIDs exhibit an analgesic ceiling that limits the maximal level of analgesia and induces side effects, including those affecting the GI (i.e., 3% to 11% incidence) and CNS (i.e., a 1% to 9% incidence of dizziness and headache) systems. They are contraindicated in patients with ulcers and aspirin hypersensitivity.[27,28,39,53,175] Indeed, NSAIDs are associated with severe GI complications and the risk of adverse effects increases with increasing lifetime-

accumulated dose of these drugs.[35,169] Moreover, the NSAIDs have been reported to interact with a number of other drugs (Table 18-5). Acetaminophen and opioid combination drugs represent an alternative to those patients unable to take NSAIDs.[27] Further information is available on the pharmacology and adverse effects of this important class of drugs.[35,39,53,175] Other venues (e.g., internet drug search engines, such as *www.rxlist.com*, *www.pharminfo.com*, *www. Epocrates.com*, *www.Endodontics.UTHSCSA.edu*) are also available for evaluating drug interactions.

OPIOID ANALGESICS

Opioids are potent analgesics and are often used in dentistry in combination with acetaminophen, aspirin, or ibuprofen. Most clinically available opioids activate the mu opioid receptor. This opioid receptor is located at several important sites in the brain (see Fig. 18-2) and its activation inhibits the transmission of nociceptive signals from the trigeminal nucleus to higher brain regions. However, recent studies indicate that opioids also activate peripheral opioid receptors, and intraligamentary injection of morphine has been shown to significantly reduce pain in endodontic patients and other inflammatory pain states.[36,68] Moreover, there appears to be gender-dependent differences in responsiveness to at least the kappa opioid agonists. For example, women have a greater analgesic response to pentazocine compared with men.[57]

Although opioids are effective as analgesics for moderate-to-severe pain, their use is generally limited by their adverse side effect profile. Opioids induce numerous side effects, including nausea, emesis, dizziness, drowsiness, and the

Table 18-5   A SUMMARY OF SELECTED NSAID DRUG INTERACTIONS

Drug	Possible Effect
Anticoagulants	Increase in prothrombin time or bleeding with anticoagulants (e.g., coumarins)
ACE inhibitors	Reduced antihypertensive effectiveness of captopril (especially indomethacin)
Beta blockers	Reduced antihypertensive effects of beta blockers (e.g., propranolol, atenolol, pindolol)
Cyclosporine	Increased risk of nephrotoxicity
Digoxin	Increase in serum digoxin levels (especially ibuprofen, indomethacin)
Dipyridamole	Increased water retention (especially indomethacin)
Hydantoins	Increased serum levels of phenytoin
Lithium	Increased serum levels of lithium
Loop diuretics	Reduced effectiveness of loop diuretics (e.g., furosemide, bumetanide)
Methotrexate	Increased risk of toxicity (e.g., stomatitis, bone marrow suppression)
Penillamine	Increased bioavailability (especially indomethacin)
Sympathomimetics	Increased blood pressure (especially indomethacin with phenylpropanolamine)
Thiazide diuretics	Reduced antihypertensive effectiveness

Data from *Drug facts and comparisons,* ed 54, St Louis, 2000, Facts and Comparisons; Gage T, Pickett F: *Mosby's dental drug reference,* ed 5, St Louis, 2000, Mosby; Wynn R, Meiller T, Crossley H: *Drug information handbook for dentistry,* Hudson, Ohio, 2000, Lexi-Comp.

potential for respiratory depression and constipation. Chronic use is associated with tolerance and dependence. Because the dose of opioids is limited by their side effect profile, opioids are almost always used in combination drugs for management of dental pain. A combination formulation is preferred, because it permits a lower dose of the opioid to reduce patient side effects (Table 18-6).

Codeine is often considered the prototype opioid for orally available combination drugs. Most studies have found that the 60 mg dose of codeine (the amount in two tablets of Tylenol with codeine no. 3) produces significantly more analgesia than placebo, although it often produces less analgesia than either aspirin 650 mg or acetaminophen 600 mg.[27,28,71] In general, patients taking only 30 mg of codeine report about as much analgesia as those taking a placebo.[13,158] Accordingly, Table 18-7 provides doses of other opioids equivalent to the 60 mg dose of codeine.

Table 18-6   ANALGESIC DOSES OF REPRESENTATIVE OPIOIDS

Drug	Dose Equivalent to Codeine 60 mg
Codeine	60
Oxycodone	5-6
Hydrocodone	10
Dihydrocodeine	60
Propoxyphene HCl	102
Proxyphene N	146
Meperidine	90
Tramadol	50

Modified from Troullos E, Freeman R, Dionne RA: The scientific basis for analgesic use in dentistry, *Anesth Prog* 33:123, 1986.

Table 18-7   SELECTED OPIOID COMBINATION ANALGESIC DRUGS

Formulation	Trade name*	Possible Rx
APAP 300 mg & codeine 30 mg	Tylenol with codeine no. 3	2 tabs q4h
APAP 500 mg & hydrocodone 5 mg	Vicodin, Lortab 5/500	1-2 tabs q6h
APAP 325 mg & oxycodone 5 mg	Percocet	1 tab q6h
APAP 500 mg & oxycodone 5 mg	Tylox	1 tab q6h
ASA 325 mg & codeine 30 mg	Empirin with codeine no. 3	2 tabs q4h
ASA 325 mg & oxycodone 5 mg	Percodan	1 tab q6h

APAP, Acetaminophen; *ASA,* aspirin; *Rx,* prescription.
*Several generics are available for most formulations.

ROLE OF CORTICOSTEROIDS IN THE PREVENTION OF POSTTREATMENT ENDODONTIC PAIN AND FLARE-UP

The cause of postoperative pain or flare-up after endodontic treatment can be attributed to inflammation or infection or both occurring in the periradicular tissues. The act of establishing patency and subsequently débriding and shaping the root canal system directly irritates the periradicular tissues and inadvertently introduces bacteria, bacterial products, necrotic pulp tissue, or caustic irrigating solution through the apical foramen.

In response to this irritation, inflammatory mediators, such as prostaglandins, leukotrienes, bradykinin, platelet-activating factor, substance P, vasoactive intestinal peptide, and other neuropeptides, are released into the tissues surrounding the apical area of the tooth. As a result, pain fibers are directly stimulated or sensitized. In addition, the increase in vascular dilation and permeability results in edema and increased interstitial tissue pressure.

Glucocorticosteroids are known to reduce the acute inflammatory response by suppressing vasodilation, PMN migration, and phagocytosis, and by inhibiting the formation of arachidonic acid from neutrophil and macrophage cell membrane phospholipids, thus blocking the cyclooxygenase and lipoxygenase pathways and respective synthesis of prostaglandins and leukotrienes. Therefore it is not surprising that a number of investigations have evaluated the efficacy of corticosteroids (administered either via intracanal or systemically) on the prevention or control of postoperative endodontic pain or flare-ups.

Intracanal Administration

Several studies have evaluated intracanal administration of steroids. In 50 consecutive patients requiring nonsurgical root canal treatment of vital teeth, Moskow et al alternately placed a dexamethasone solution or saline placebo as intracanal medicaments after the root canals were cleansed and shaped.[116] Pain ratings were collected preoperatively and at 24, 48, and 72 hours after treatment. Results indicated a significant reduction in pain at 24 hours, but no significant difference at 48 and 72 hours. In a similar double blind clinical trial, the intracanal placement of a 2.5% steroid solution or saline placebo upon completion of instrumentation resulted in a significant reduction of the incidence of postoperative pain in teeth in which the pulp was vital.[23] When the pulp was necrotic, however, there was no significant difference between the steroid and placebo in reducing postoperative discomfort.

In another study, Trope found no significant difference in the flare-up rate when formocresol (the corticosteroid antibiotic paste), Ledermix, or calcium hydroxide was placed as an intracanal medicament in strict sequence, irrespective of the presence or absence of symptoms or radiographic signs of apical periodontitis.[156] Thus intracanal steroids appear to have most consistent effects for reducing postoperative pain

when used for vital cases. The reduced efficacy in necrotic cases may be caused by poor efficacy for this route of administration, to diffusion of inadequate amounts of the drug into the periradicular tissue, or to other factors (e.g., experimental design, statistical power).

Systemic Administration

Other studies have evaluated the systemic route of administration of corticosteroids on postoperative pain or flare-ups. In one double blind, randomized, placebo-controlled study, dexamethasone (4 mg/ml) or saline was injected intramuscularly at the conclusion of a single-visit, endodontic appointment or at the first visit of a multivisit procedure.[104] The results indicated that the steroid significantly reduced the incidence and severity of pain at 4 hours when compared with the placebo. Pain was reduced at 24 hours, but it was not statistically significant, and there was no difference in incidence or severity at 48 hours between the two groups.

In a similar study, 106 patients with irreversible pulpitis and acute periradicular periodontitis were administered either an intraoral, intramuscular injection of dexamethasone at different doses upon completion of a single-visit, endodontic treatment or after the first visit of a multivisit procedure.[96] Systemic administration of dexamethasone was shown to significantly reduce the severity of pain at 4 and 8 hours, with an optimum dose between 0.07 and 0.09 mg/kg. There was, however, no significant reduction in the severity of pain at 24, 48, and 72 hours, and no overall effect on the incidence of pain. Another study compared the effect an intraligamentary injection of methylprednisolone, mepivacaine, or placebo in preventing posttreatment endodontic pain.[87] The results showed that methylprednisolone significantly reduced postoperative pain within a 24-hour follow-up period.

Animal studies have histologically evaluated the antiinflammatory effects that corticosteroids have on inflamed periradicular tissues.[124] After inducing an acute inflammatory reaction in the molar teeth of rats by overextending endodontic instruments, sterile saline or dexamethasone was infiltrated supraperiosteally into the buccal vestibule adjacent to the treated teeth. The results demonstrated that dexamethasone significantly reduced the number of neutrophils present and, thus, had an antiinflammatory effect on the periradicular tissues of the teeth in which endodontic treatment had been performed.

Other systemic administration studies have evaluated the efficacy of oral administration of corticosteroids on the incidence and severity of posttreatment endodontic pain. In a double blind, controlled, clinical trial, 50 patients randomly received either a 0.75 mg dexamethasone or placebo tablet orally after their initial endodontic treatment.[89] Administration of oral dexamethasone significantly reduced postoperative pain after 8 and 24 hours, when compared with the subjects who received a placebo. A follow-up study evaluated the effect a larger oral dose of dexamethasone (i.e., 12 mg dexamethasone given every 4 hours) on the severity of posttreatment endodontic pain.[60] Results showed that the dexamethasone as prescribed was effective in reducing posttreatment endodontic pain up to 8 hours after the treatment was completed. There appeared to be no affect on the severity of pain at 24 and 48 hours after treatment. Collectively, these studies on systemic steroid administration indicate that corticosteroids reduce the severity of posttreatment endodontic pain as compared with placebo treatment, but with a time course of approximately 8 to 24 hours.

ROLE OF ANTIBIOTICS IN THE PREVENTION OF POSTTREATMENT ENDODONTIC PAIN AND FLARE-UP

Because bacteria are involved in endodontic cases with apical periodontitis, the incidence of a posttreatment infection or flare-up is of concern to practitioners providing endodontic treatment. As such, it might make sense that patients be prescribed an antibiotic prophylactically to prevent such an occurrence. This use of antibiotics, however, is controversial for several reasons. First, the overprescribing of antibiotics, especially when not indicated, has led to increased bacterial resistance and patient sensitization. Second, antibiotics have been mistakenly prescribed in patients with severe pain, but having a vital tooth (i.e., when bacteria are not likely to be a causative factor in periradicular pain). Third, even in cases where bacteria are likely to be present, data from controlled clinical trials provide little to no support for the hypothesis that antibiotics reduce pain.

A series of clinical studies have evaluated the efficacy of prophylactically administered systemic antibiotics for preventing posttreatment endodontic flare-ups.* Working on the premise that the incidence of infectious flare-ups after endodontic treatment is 15%, Morse et al. randomly prescribed a prophylactic dose of either penicillin or erythromycin to patients after their endodontic treatment of teeth with a diagnosis of necrotic pulp and chronic periradicular periodontitis (i.e., no placebo was used).[114] The results showed that the overall incidence of flare-ups was 2.2%, with no difference between penicillin or erythromycin. Similar results were obtained in a similar study in which dental students (instead of private practitioners) provided the endodontic treatment.[2] In this follow-up study, a 2.6% flare-up incidence was found, with no statistically significant differences between penicillin or erythromycin.

To ascertain whether the timing of the administration of an antibiotic alters the occurrence of flare-ups and nonflare-up–associated swelling and pain, analysis of components of two separate prospective studies of patients undergoing endodontic treatment for teeth with a diagnosis of necrotic pulp and chronic periradicular periodontitis was done. In the first study, prophylactic penicillin was provided, while in the second study the patients were instructed to take penicillin or

erythromycin if allergic to penicillin at the first sign of swelling.[112,114] When the results were compared, the authors concluded that the use of prophylactic antibiotics is preferable to the patient taking the antibiotics at the first sign of an infection.

Another study of similar design compared the incidence of flare-up when a cephalosporin or erythromycin was given prophylactically.[115] When the data from previous studies were pooled and retrospectively compared, the authors concluded that prophylactically administered antibiotics, including cephalosporins, significantly reduced the incidence of flare-ups in those endodontic cases with a diagnosis of necrotic pulp and chronic periradicular periodontitis. However, these studies have been questioned because of the lack of concurrent placebo-treated groups and the use of historic controls.

In a multicenter, two-part clinical study, 588 consecutive patients received one of nine medications or placebos and were monitored for 72 hours after treatment.[154,155] The results showed that ibuprofen, ketoprofen, erythromycin, penicillin, and penicillin plus methylprednisolone significantly reduced the severity of pain within the first 48 hours after treatment.[154] The second part of the study then evaluated the incidence of posttreatment pain after obturation of the same teeth in the first phase of the study.[155] Although only 411 of the original 588 patients participated in this phase, they were randomly given the same medications or placebo after completion of the obturation appointment. The results showed that the incidence of posttreatment pain is less after obturation (i.e., 5.83%) than after cleansing and shaping (i.e., 21.76%) of the root canal system, and there was no significant difference between the effectiveness of the various medications and placebo in controlling posttreatment pain after obturation.

Walton and Chiappinelli[164] were concerned that previous studies were uncontrolled, retrospective, or carried out on different patient groups at different times and with different treatment modalities. They conducted a randomized prospective double-blind clinical trial to test the hypothesis that an antibiotic (e.g., penicillin) can prevent a posttreatment endodontic flare-up.[164] Eighty patients with a diagnosis of necrotic pulp and chronic periradicular periodontitis were randomly divided into three groups. The first two groups were administered either penicillin or a placebo 1 hour before and 6 hours after their individual appointments on a double-blind basis. Upon completion of their individual endodontic appointments, which included débridement, shaping, and possibly obturation of the root canal system, the patients completed questionnaires at 4, 8, 12, 24, and 48 hours. The results indicated that there was no significant difference among the three groups in the incidence of flare-ups, pain or swelling. The authors concluded that the use of prophylactic penicillin offers no benefit for postoperative pain or flare-up and is not indicated for routine administration in patients undergoing endodontic treatment of necrotic teeth and chronic periradicular periodontitis.

In another randomized, prospective, placebo-controlled clinical study, Fouad et al. examined whether supplemental

*References 2,112-115

penicillin reduced the symptoms or course of recovery of emergency patients with a diagnosis of necrotic pulp and acute apical abscess.[50] Patients were randomly given penicillin, a placebo, or no medication. Using a visual analog scale, the subjects then evaluated their postoperative pain and swelling for up to 72 hours. The results showed that there was no significant difference between the three groups. Recovery occurred as a result of endodontic treatment alone.

It is well recognized that antibiotics may be indicated when managing infections of endodontic origin. However, a review of the available literature indicates that their prophylactic use is contraindicated in immunocompetent patients in which there are no systemic signs of infection present and swelling is localized to the vestibule. Under these conditions, controlled clinical studies indicate that antibiotics offer little to no benefit for pain reduction. However, antibiotics may be indicated for immunocompromised patients and those cases in which the patient has systemic signs and symptoms of an infection or the infection has spread into the fascial spaces of the head and neck.

PAIN MANAGEMENT STRATEGIES

When managing pain in an individual patient, the skilled clinician must customize the treatment plan, balancing the general principles of endodontics, mechanisms of hyperalgesia, and pain management strategies with the particular factors of the individual patient (e.g., medical history, concurrent medications). The following discussion reviews general considerations for pain management strategies.

Effective management of the endodontic pain patient starts with the "three Ds": *diagnosis, definitive* dental treatment, and *drugs* (Box 18-3). Comprehensive reviews on *diagnosis* and *definitive* dental treatment (e.g., incision and drainage, pulpectomy) are provided elsewhere in this text (see Chapters 1, 2, 3, 8, and 9). As described earlier in this chapter, the management of endodontic pain should focus on removal of peripheral mechanisms of hyperalgesia (see Box 18-1). This generally requires treatment that removes and reduces causative factors (e.g., bacterial and immunologic factors). For example, both pulpotomy and pulpectomy have been associated with substantial reduction in patient reports of pain as compared with their pretreatment pain levels.[37,77,129] However, pharmacotherapy is often required to reduce continued nociceptor input (e.g., NSAIDs, local anesthetics) and suppress central hyperalgesia (e.g., opioids).

Pretreatment

Pretreatment with an NSAID before a procedure has been demonstrated to produce a significant benefit in many[32,81] but not all studies.[123] The rationale for pretreatment is to block the development of hyperalgesia by reducing the input from peripheral nociceptors. Interestingly, patients who cannot take NSAIDs may still benefit because pretreatment with

acetaminophen also has been shown to reduce postoperative pain.[109] Patients can be pretreated 30 minutes before the procedure with either an NSAID (e.g., ibuprofen 400 mg or flurbiprofen 100 mg) or with acetaminophen 1000 mg.[37,81,109]

Long-Acting Local Anesthetics

A second pharmacologic approach for pain management is the use of long-acting, local anesthetics. Bupivacaine and etidocaine are two long-acting local anesthetics available for use (see Chapter 20). Clinical trials indicate that the local-acting, local anesthetics not only provide anesthesia during the procedure but also significantly delay the onset of post-treatment pain as compared with lidocaine-containing local anesthetics.[30,32,63,83] Indeed, the use of long-acting, local anesthetics by block injection have been shown to reduce postoperative pain for to 2 to 7 days after the oral procedure[63,83] because an afferent barrage of nociceptors can induce central hyperalgesia.[170,171,172] The analgesic benefit of long-acting, local anesthetics is observed to a greater extent when administered by block injections as compared with infiltration injections. However, the clinician should also be aware of adverse effects attributed to the long-acting, local anesthetics.[9,110]

Flexible Plan

A third pharmacologic approach is the use of a flexible plan for prescribing analgesics (Fig. 18-3).[6,28,71,158] A flexible prescription plan serves to minimize both postoperative pain and side effects. With this goal in mind, the strategy is to first achieve a maximally effective dose of the nonnarcotic analgesic (either an NSAID or acetaminophen for patients who cannot take NSAIDs). Second, in those rare cases where the patient is still experiencing moderate-to-severe pain, the clinician should consider adding drugs that increase NSAID analgesia. Because of its predictive value, the presence of preoperative hyperalgesia may serve as an indication for considering these NSAID combinations.

There are two general methods for combining an NSAID with an opioid for treating these rare cases of moderate-to-

---

Box 18-3   **CONSIDERATIONS FOR EFFECTIVE "3-D" PAIN CONTROL**

1. Diagnosis
2. Definitive dental treatment
3. Drugs
   a. Pretreat with NSAIDs or acetaminophen when appropriate
   b. Use long-acting local anesthetics when indicated
   c. Use a flexible-prescription plan
   d. Prescribe "by the clock" rather than prn

severe pain. The first method achieves the analgesic advantages of both an NSAID and an opioid by prescribing an alternating regimen consisting of an NSAID followed by an acetaminophen and opioid combination.[6,28] For example, the emergency pain patient could take ibuprofen 400 mg (or an NSAID of choice) at the office. Then, the patient could take an acetaminophen and opioid combination 2 hours later (see Table 18-7 for examples). The patient would then take each treatment every 4 hours, taking each drug on an alternating 2-hour schedule. In most cases, this treatment need not be continued beyond 24 hours.[6,28,37]

Aspirin and opioid combinations are not, of course, used in this alternating schedule because of the potential for NSAID and aspirin interactions. Recent studies have shown that combining an NSAID with acetaminophen 1,000 mg alone (i.e., no opioid) produces nearly twice the analgesic response, compared with patients treated with just the NSAID.[16] In addition, studies have shown that the concurrent administration of an NSAID with an acetaminophen and opioid combination drug provided significantly greater analgesia as compared with the NSAID alone.[16,149] The concurrent administration of acetaminophen and NSAIDs appears to be well tolerated without an apparent increase in side effects or alterations in pharmacokinetics.[16,91,149,173]

The second method for combining an NSAID with an opioid for treating rare cases of moderate-to-severe pain achieves the analgesic advantages of both an NSAID and an opioid by administering a single combination drug consisting of an NSAID and opioid combination. For example, Vicoprofen contains ibuprofen 200 mg and hydrocodone 7.5

mg in one tablet. Postoperative pain studies have shown that this combination was about 80% more effective for analgesia as compared with ibuprofen 200 mg alone, with about the same incidence of side effects.[166] Doubling the dose (to ibuprofen 400 mg and hydrocodone 15 mg) produced greater levels of analgesia with a concomitant increase in side effects.[152,166] Data are not currently available comparing Vicoprofen alone to the combination of Vicoprofen and an additional 200 to 400 mg of ibuprofen. Other opioids can also be added to an NSAID for increased analgesia. For example, ibuprofen 400 mg with a 10 mg oxycodone tablet produces significantly greater analgesia than ibuprofen 400 mg alone.[34] A recent study on postendodontic pain demonstrated short-term benefits of the combination of flurbiprofen and tramadol.[37] Other NSAID and opioid combinations have also been evaluated.[35]

Of course, not all patients require concurrent use of NSAIDs with acetaminophen and opioid combinations or combinations of an NSAID and opioid. Indeed, this is the basic premise of a flexible prescription plan—that the analgesic prescribed should be matched to the patient's need. The major advantage of a flexible plan is that the clinician is prepared for those rare cases when additional pharmacotherapy is indicated, which increases both the efficiency and efficacy of pain control. As described previously, the presence of preoperative hyperalgesia may serve as an indication for more comprehensive pharmacotherapy.

The information and recommendations provided in this chapter were selected to aid the clinician in the management of acute endodontic pain. However, clinical judgment must

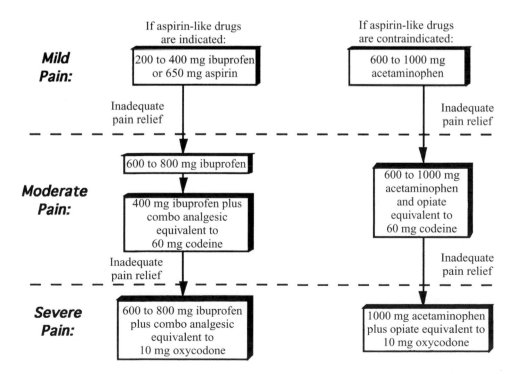

Fig. 18-3 A flexible analgesic strategy.

also take into account other sources of information, including patient history, concurrent medications, nature of the pain, and the treatment plan to provide the best plan for managing the individual pain problem of each patient. Integrating these general principles of pain mechanisms and management with the clinician's assessment of each individual patient provides an effective approach for the successful management of endodontic pain.

References

1. Abbott AA et al: A prospective randomized trial on efficacy of antibiotic prophylaxis in asymptomatic teeth with pulpal necrosis and associated periapical pathosis, *Oral Surg* 66:722, 1988.

2. Abbott PV: Factors associated with continuing pain in endodontics, *Aust Dent J* 39:157, 1994.

3. Akopian A et al: The tetrodotoxin-resistant sodium channel SNS has a specialized function in pain pathways, *Nat Neursci* 2:541, 1999.

4. Albashaireh ZS, Alnegrish AS: Postobturation pain after single- and multiple-visit endodontic therapy. A prospective study, *J Dent* 26:227, 1998

5. American Association of Endodontists: *1999-2000 Membership Roster*, Chicago, 1999, The Association.

6. American Association of Endodontists: *Endodontics: colleagues for excellence,* Chicago, 1995, The Association.

7. Arbuckle JB, Docherty RJ: Expression of tetrodotoxin-resistant sodium channels in capsaicin-sensitive dorsal root ganglion neurons of adult rats, *Neurosci Lett* 85:70, 1995.

8. Arnold J, Salom I, Berger A: Comparison of gastrointestinal microbleeding associated with use of etodolac, ibuprofen, indomethacin, and naproxen in normal subjects, *Curr Ther Res* 37:730, 1985.

9. Bacsik, C, Swift J, Hargreaves KM: Toxic systemic reactions of bupivacaine and etidocaine: review of the literature, *Oral Surg. Oral Med Oral Pathol* 79:18, 1995.

10. Balaban FS, Skidmore AE, Griffin JA: Acute exacerbations following initial treatment of necrotic pulps, *J Endod* 10:78, 1984.

11. Barnett F, Tronstad L: The incidence of flare-ups following endodontic treatment, *J Dent Res* 68(special issue):1253, 1989.

12. Basbaum A, Fields H: Endogenous pain control systems: brainstem spinal pathways and endorphin circuitry, *Ann Rev Neurosci* 7:309, 1984.

13. Beaver W: Mild analgesics. A review of their clinical pharmacology, *Am J Med Sci* 251:576, 1966.

14. Beck P, Handwerker HO: Bradykinin and serotonin effects on various types of cutaneous nerve fibers, *Pflugers Arch* 347:209, 1974.

15. Bisgaard H, Kristensen J: Leukotriene B4 produces hyperalgesia in humans, *Prostaglandins* 30:791, 1985.

16. Breivik E, Barkvoll P, Skovlund E: Combining diclofenac with acetaminophen or acetaminophen-codeine after oral surgery: a randomized, double-blind, single oral dose study, *Clin Pharmacol Ther* 54:(in press), 2000.

17. Brown A et al: Spatial summation of pre-pain and pain in human teeth, *Pain* 21:1, 1985.

18. Buck S, Reese K, Hargreaves KM: Pulpal exposure alters neuropeptide levels in inflamed dental pulp: evaluation of axonal transport, *J Endod* 25:718, 1999.

19. Bunczak-Reeh M, Hargreaves KM: Effect of inflammation on delivery of drugs to dental pulp, *J Endod* 24:822, 1998.

20. Byers M et al: Effects of injury and inflammation on pulpal and periapical nerves, *J Endod* 16:78, 1990.

21. Byers MR: Dynamic plasticity of dental sensory nerve structure and cytochemistry, *Arch Oral Biol* 39(suppl):13S, 1994.

22. Byers MR, Narhi MVO: Dental injury models: experimental tools for understanding neuroinflammatory nociceptor functions, *Crit Rev Oral Biol Med* 10:4, 1999.

23. Chance K, Lin L, Shovlin FE, Skribner J: Clinical trial of intracanal corticosteroid in root canal therapy, *J Endod* 13:466, 1987.

24. Chiang C et al: NMDA receptor mechanisms contribute to neuroplasticity induced in caudalis nociceptive neurons by tooth pulp stimulation, *J Neurophysiol* 80:2621, 1998.

25. Clem WH: Post-treatment endodontic pain, *J Am Dent Assoc* 81:1166, 1970.

26. Cooper SA, Berrie R, Cohn P: The analgesic efficacy of ketoprofen compared to ibuprofen and placebo, *Adv Ther* 5:43, 1988.

27. Cooper SA: New peripherally acting oral analgesics, *Ann Rev Pharmacol Toxicol* 23:617, 1983.

28. Cooper SA: Treating acute dental pain, *Postgraduate Dentistry* 2:7, 1995.

29. Creech J, Walton RE, Kaltenbach R: Effect of occlusal relief on endodontic pain, *J Am Dent Assoc* 109:64, 1984.

30. Crout R, Koraido G, Moore P: A clinical trial of long-acting local anesthetics for periodontal surgery, *Anesth Preog* 37:194, 1990.

31. Dionne R et al: Suppression of postoperative pain by preoperative administration of ibuprofen in comparison to placebo, acetaminophen and acetaminophen plus codeine, *J Clin Pharmacol* 23:37, 1983.

32. Dionne R: Suppression of dental pain by the preoperative administration of flurbiprofen, *Am J Med Sci* 80:41, 1986.

33. Dionne RA: COX-2 inhibitors: better than ibuprofen for dental pain? *Compendium* 20:518, 1999.

34. Dionne RA: Additive analgesic effects of oxycodone and ibuprofen in the oral surgery model, *J Oral Maxillofac Surg* 57:673, 1999.

35. Dionne RA, Berthold C: Therapeutic uses of non-steroidal anti-inflammatory drugs in dentistry, *Crit Rev Oral Biol Med,* 2000 (in press).

36. Dionne RA et al: Analgesic effects of peripherally administered opioids in clinical models of acute and chronic in inflammation, *Pain,* 2000 (in press).

37. Doroshak A, Bowles W, Hargreaves KM: Evaluation of the combination of flurbiprofen and tramadol for management of endodontic pain, *J Endod* 25:660, 1999.

38. Draisci, G, Iadarola, M: Temporal analysis of increases in c-fos, preprodynorphin and preproenkephalin mRNAs in rat spinal cord, *Brain Res Mol Brain Res* 6:31, 1989.

39. *Drug Facts and Comparisons*, St Louis, 2000, Facts and Comparisons Inc.

40. Dubner R, Basbaum AI: Spinal dorsal horn plasticity following tissue or nerve injury. In Wall PD and Melzack R, editors: *Textbook of pain,* Edinburgh, 1996, Churchill-Livingston.

41. Dubner R, Bennett G: Spinal and trigeminal mechanisms of nociception, *Ann Rev Neurosci* 6:381, 1983.

42. Dubner R, Ruda MA: Activity-dependent neuronal plasticity following tissue injury and inflammation, *Trends Neurosci* 15:96, 1992.

43. Eglen R, Hunter J, Dray A: Ions in the fire: recent ion-channel research and approaches to pain therapy, *Trends Pharmacol Sci* 20:337, 1999.

44. Ehrich E et al: Characterization of rofecoxib as a cyclooxygenase inhibitor and demonstration of analgesia in the dental pain model, *Clin Pharmacol Ther* 65:336, 1999.

45. Eleazer PD, Eleazer KR: Flare-up rate in pulpally necrotic molars in one-visit versus two-visit endodontic treatment, *J Endod* 24:614, 1998.

46. Fava LR: A comparison of one versus two appointment endodontic therapy in teeth with non-vital pulps, *Int Endod J* 22:179, 1989.

47. Fields H: *Pain,* New York, 1987, McGraw-Hill.

48. Flath RK et al: Pain suppression after pulpectomy with preoperative flurbiprofen, *J Endod* 13:339, 1987.

49. Follenfant R et al: Inhibition by neuropeptides of interleukin-1ß-induced, prostaglandin-independent hyperalgesia, *Br J Pharmacol* 98:41, 1989.

50. Fouad AF, Rivera EM, Walton RE: Penicillin as a supplement in resolving the localized acute apical abscess, *Oral Surg Oral Med Oral Pathol* 81:590, 1996.

51. Fox J et al: Incidence of pain following one-visit endodontic treatment, *Oral Surg Oral Med Oral Pathol* 30:123, 1970.

52. Frank AL et al: The intracanal use of sulfathiazole in endodontics to reduce pain, *J Am Dent Assoc* 77:102, 1968.

53. Gage T, Pickett F: *Mosby's Dental Drug Reference,* ed 4, St Louis, 2000 Mosby.

54. Galeazza M, Stucky C, Seybold V: Changes in [125I] h-CGRP binding in rat spinal cord in an experimental model of acute, peripheral inflammation, *Brain Res* 591:198, 1992.

55. Garry MG, Hargreaves KM: Enhanced release of immunoreactive CGRP and substance P from spinal dorsal horn slices occurs during carrageenan inflammation, *Brain Res* 582:139, 1992.

56. Garry MG, Durnett-Richardson J, Hargreaves KM: Carrageenan-induced inflammation alters levels of i-cGMP and i-cAMP in the dorsal horn of the spinal cord, *Brain Res* 646:135, 1994.

57. Gear R et al: Kappa-opioids produce significantly greater analgesia in women than in men, *Nat Med* 2:1248, 1996.

58. Genet JM et al: Preoperative and operative factors associated with pain after the first endodontic visit, *Int Endod J* 20:53, 1987.

59. Georgopoulou M, Anastassiadis P, Sykaras S: Pain after chemomechanical preparation, *Int Endod J* 19:309, 1986.

60. Glassman G et al: A prospective randomized double-blind trial on efficacy of dexamethasone for endodontic interappointment pain in teeth with asymptomatic inflamed pulps, *Oral Surg Oral Med Oral Pathol* 67:96, 1989.

61. Gold M et al: Hyperalgesic agents increase a tetrodotoxin-resistant Na+ current in nociceptors, *Proc Natl Acad Sci U S A* 93:1108, 1996.

62. Gold M: Tetrodotoxin-resistant Na currents and inflammatory hyperalgesia, *Proc Natl Acad Sci U S A* 96:7645, 1999.

63. Gordon S et al: Blockade of peripheral neuronal barrage reduces postoperative pain, *Pain* 70:209, 1997.

64. Gracely R et al: Placebo and naloxone can alter post-surgical pain by separate mechanisms, *Nature* 306:264, 1983.

65. Hagermark O, Hokfelt T, Pernow B: Flare and itch produced by substance P in human skin, *J Invest Dermatol* 71:233, 1979.

66. Hargreaves KM et al: Naloxone, fentanyl and diazepam modify plasma beta-endorphin levels during surgery, *Clin Pharmacol Ther* 40:165, 1986.

67. Hargreaves KM, Dubner R: Mechanisms of pain and analgesia. In Dionne R and Phero J, editors: *Management of pain and anxiety in dental practice,* New York, 1992, Elsevier Press.

68. Hargreaves KM, Joris J: The peripheral analgesic effects of opioids, *J Am Pain Soc* 2:51, 1993.

69. Hargreaves KM et al: Pharmacology of peripheral neuropeptide and inflammatory mediator release, *Oral Surg Oral Med Oral Pathol* 78:503, 1994.

70. Hargreaves KM et al: Neuroendocrine and immune responses to injury, degeneration and repair. In Sessle B, Dionne R, and Bryant P, editors: *Temporomandibular disorders and related pain conditions,* Seattle, WA, 1995, IASP Press.

71. Hargreaves KM, Troullos E, Dionne R, Pharmacologic rationale for the treatment of acute pain, *Dent Clin North Am* 31:675, 1987.

72. Hargreaves KM: Neurochemical factors in injury and inflammation in orofacial tissues. In Lavigne G, Lund J, Sessle B, and Dubner R, editors: *Orofacial pain: basic sciences to clinical management,* Chicago, 2000, Quintessence Publishers.

73. Harrison JW, Bellizzi R, Osetek EM: The clinical toxicity of endodontic medicaments, *J Endod* 5:42, 1979.

74. Harrison JW, Baumgartner CJ, Zielke DR: Analysis of interappointment pain associated with the combined use of endodontic irrigants and medicaments, *J Endod* 7:272, 1981.

75. Harrison JW, Baumgartner JC, Svec TA: Incidence of pain associated with clinical factors during and after root canal therapy. I. Interappointment pain, *J Endod* 9:384, 1983.

76. Harrison JW, Baumgartner JC, Svec TA: Incidence of pain associated with clinical factors during and after root canal therapy. II. Postobturation pain, *J Endod* 9:434, 1983.

77. Hasselgren G, Reit C: Emergency pulpotomy: pain relieving effect with and without the use of sedative dressings, *J Endod* 15:254, 1989.

78. Hohmann AG, Herkenham M: Cannabinoid receptors undergo axonal flow in sensory nerves, *Neurosci* 92:1171, 1999.

79. Hylden J, Nahin R, Traub R, Dubner R: Expansion of receptor fields of spinal lamina I projection neurons in rats with unilateral adjuvant-induced inflammation, *Pain* 37:229, 1989.

80. Imura N, Zuolo ML: Factors associated with endodontic flare-ups: a prospective study, *Int Endod J* 28:261, 1995.

81. Jackson D, Moore P, Hargreaves KM: Preoperative nonsteroidal anti-inflammatory medication for the prevention of postoperative dental pain, *J Am Dent Assoc* 119:641, 1989.

82. Janig W, Kollman W: The involvement of the sympathetic nervous system in pain, *Arzneim Forsch Drug Res* 34:1066, 1984.

83. Jebeles J et al: Tonsillectomy and adenoidectomy pain reduction by local bupivacaine infiltration in children, *Int J Pediatr Otorhinolaryngol* 25:149, 1993.

84. Johnson D, Harshbarger J, Rymer H: Quantitative assessment of neural development in human premolars, *Anat Rec* 205:421, 1983.

85. Jostes JL, Holland GR: The effect of occlusal reduction after canal preparation on patient comfort, *J Endod* 10:34, 1984.

86. Juan H, Lembeck F: Action of peptides and other analgesic agents on paravascular pain receptors of the isolated perfused rabbit ear, *Naunyn Schmiedebergs Arch Pharmacol* 283:151, 1974.

87. Kaufman E et al: Intraligamentary injection of slow-release methylprednisolone for the prevention of pain after endodontic treatment, *Oral Surg Oral Med Oral Pathol* 77:651, 1994.

88. Kimberly C, Byers M: Inflammation of rat molar pulp and periodontium causes increased calcitonin gene related peptide and axonal sprouting, *Anat Rec* 222:289, 1988.

89. Krasner P, Jackson E: Management of posttreatment endodontic pain with oral dexamethasone: a double-blind study, *Oral Surg Oral Med Oral Pathol* 62:187, 1986.

90. Kumazawa T, Mizumura K: Thin-fiber receptors responding to mechanical, chemical and thermal stimulation in the skeletal muscle of the dog, *Am J Physiol* 273:179, 1977.

91. Lanza F et al: Effect of acetaminophen on human gastric mucosal injury caused by ibuprofen, *Gut* 27:440, 1986.

92. Levine J, Gordon N, Fields H: The mechanism of placebo analgesia, *Lancet* ii:654, 1978.

93. Levine J, Taiwo Y: Inflammatory pain. In Wall P and Melzack R, editors: *Textbook of pain,* Edinburgh, 1994, Churchill-Livingston.

94. Levine J, Moskowitz M, Basbaum A: The contribution of neurogenic inflammation in experimental arthritis, *J Immunol* 135:843, 1985.

95. Lewin G, Rueff A, Mendell L: Peripheral and central mechanisms of NGF-induced hyperalgesia, *Eur J Neurosci* 6:1903, 1994.

96. Liesinger A, Marshall F, Marshall J: Effect of variable doses of dexamethasone on posttreatment endodontic pain, *J Endod* 19:35, 1993.

97. Light AR: *The initial processing of pain and its descending control: spinal and trigeminal systems,* Basel, Switzerland, 1992, Karger.

98. Lindahl O: Pain—a chemical explanation, *Acta Rheumatol Scand* 8:161, 1962.

99. Maddox D, Walton R, Davis C: Influence of posttreatment endodontic pain related to medicaments and other factors, *J Endod* 3:447, 1977.

100. Madison S et al: Sensitizing effects of leukotriene B4 on intradental primary afferents, *Pain* 49:99, 1992.

101. Maixner W et al: Responses of monkey medullary dorsal horn neurons during the detection of noxious heat stimuli, *J Neurophysiol* 62:437, 1989.

102. Malmberg A, Yaksh T: Antinociceptive actions of spinal nonsteroidal anti-inflammatory agents on the formalin test in rats, *J Pharmacol Exp Ther* 263:136, 1992.

103. Marshall J, Liesinger A: Factors associated with endodontic posttreatment pain, *J Endod* 19:573, 1993.

104. Marshall J, Walton R: The effect of intramuscular injection of steroid on posttreatment endodontic pain, *J Endod* 10:584, 1984.

105. Marshall J, Walton R: The effect of intramuscular injection of steroid on posttreatment endodontic pain, *J Endod* 19:573, 1993.

106. Martin H et al: Leukotriene and prostaglandin sensitization of cutaneous high-threshold C- and A-delta mechanoreceptors in the hairy skin of rat hindlimbs, *Neurosci* 22:651, 1987.

107. Meller S, Gebhart G: Nitric oxide (NO) and nociceptive processing in the spinal cord, *Pain* 52:127, 1993.

108. Meyer R, Campbell J: Myelinated nociceptive afferents account for the hyperalgesia that follows a burn to the hand, *Science* 213:1527, 1981.

109. Moore P et al: Analgesic regimens for third molar surgery: pharmacologic and behavioral considerations, *J Am Dent Assoc* 113:739, 1986.

110. Moore PA: Long-acting local anesthetics: a review of clinical efficacy in dentistry, *Compendium* 11:24, 1990.

111. Mor C, Rotstein I, Friedman S: Incidence of interappointment emergency associated with endodontic therapy, *J Endod* 18:509, 1992.

112. Morse DR et al: Infectious flare-ups and serious sequelae following endodontic treatment: a prospective randomized trial on efficacy of antibiotic prophylaxis in cases of asymptomatic pulpal-periapical lesions, *Oral Surg Oral Med Oral Pathol* 64:96, 1987.

113. Morse D, Koren L, Esposito J: Infection flare-ups: reduction and prevention, *Int J Psychosom* 33:5, 1988.

114. Morse D et al: Prophylactic penicillin versus erythromycin taken at the first sign of swelling in cases of asymptomatic pulpal-periapical lesions: a comparative analysis, *Oral Surg Oral Med Oral Pathol* 65:228, 1988.

115. Morse D et al: A comparison of erythromycin and cepadroxil in the prevention of flare-ups from asymptomatic teeth with pulpal necrosis and associated periapical pathosis, *Oral Surg Oral Med Oral Pathol* 69:619, 1990.

116. Moskow A et al: Intracanal use of a corticosteroid solution as an endodontic anodyne, *Oral Surg Oral Med Oral Pathol* 58:600, 1984.

117. Mulhern J et al: Incidence of postoperative pain after one-appointment endodontic treatment of asymptomatic pulpal necrosis in single-rooted teeth, *J Endod* 8:370, 1982.

118. Nakanishi T, Shimuzu H, Matsuo T: Immunohistochemical analysis of cyclooxygenase-2 in human dental pulp, *J Dent Res* 78:142, 1999 (abstract).

119. Narhi M: Activation of dental pulp nerves of the cat and the dog with hydrostatic pressure, *Proc Finn Dent Soc* 74(suppl V):1, 1978.

120. Narhi M et al: Role of intradental A and C type nerve fibers in dental pain mechanisms, *Proc Finn Dent Soc* 88(suppl 1):507, 1992.

121. Narhi M: The characteristics of intradental sensory units and their responses to stimulation, *J Dent Res* 64:564, 1985.

122. Neumann S et al: Inflammatory pain hypersensitivity mediated by phenotype switch in myelinated primary sensory neurons, *Nature* 384:360, 1996.

123. Niv D: Intraoperative treatment of postoperative pain. In Campbell J, editor: *Pain 1996- an updated review,* Seattle, 1996, IASP Press.

124. Nobuhara WK, Carnes DL, Gilles JA: Anti-inflammatory effects of dexamethasone on periapical tissues following endodontic overinstrumentation, *J Endod* 19:501, 1993.

125. O'Keefe EM: Pain in endodontic therapy: preliminary study, *J Endod* 2:315, 1976.

126. Okeson J: *Bell's orofacial pains,* ed 5, Chicago, 1995, Quintessence Publishers.

127. Oliet S: Single-visit endodontics: a clinical study, *J Endod* 9:147, 1983.
128. Pekruhn RB: Single-visit endodontic therapy: a preliminary clinical study, *J Am Dent Assoc* 103:875, 1981.
129. Penniston S, Hargreaves KM: Evaluation of periapical injection of ketorolac for management of endodontic pain, *J Endod* 22:55, 1996.
130. Perl E: Causalgia, pathological pain and adrenergic receptors, *Proc Natl Acad Sci U S A* 96:7664, 1999.
131. Petty B et al: The effect of systemically administered recombinant human nerve growth factor in healthy human subjects, *Ann Neurol* 36:244, 1994.
132. Porreca F et al: A comparison of the potential role of the tetrodotoxin-insensitive sodium channels, PN3/SNS and NaN/SNS2, in rat models of chronic pain, *Proc Natl Acad Sci U S A* 96:7640, 1999.
133. Rang H, Bevan S, Dray A: Nociceptive peripheral neurons: cellular properties. In Wall PD and Melzack R, editors: *Textbook of pain,* Edinburgh, 1996, Churchill-Livingston.
134. Ren K, Iadarola M, Dubner R: An isobolographic analysis of the effects of N-methyl-D-aspartate and NK1 tachykinin receptor antagonists on inflammatory hyperalgesia in the rat, *Br J Pharmacol* 117:196, 1996.
135. Richardson JD, Aanonsen L, Hargreaves KM: Hypoactivity of the spinal cannabinoid system results in an NMDA-dependent hyperalgesia, *J Neurosci* 18:451, 1998.
136. Richardson JD, Aanonsen L, Hargreaves KM: Antihyperalgesic effect of spinal cannabinoids, *Eur J Pharmacol* 345:145, 1998.
137. Richardson JD, Kilo S, Hargreaves KM: Cannabinoids reduce hyperalgesia and inflammation via interaction with peripheral CB1 receptors, *Pain* 75:111, 1998.
138. Roane JB, Dryden JA, Grimes EW: Incidence of postoperative pain after single- and multiple-visit endodontic procedures, *Oral Surg Oral Med Oral Pathol* 55:68, 1983.
139. Roszkowski M, Swift J, Hargreaves KM: Effect of NSAID administration on tissue levels of immunoreactive prostaglandin E2, leukotriene B4 and (S)-flurbiprofen following extraction of impacted third molars, *Pain* 73:339, 1997.
140. Roy M, Narahashi T: Differential properties of tetrodotoxin-sensitive and tetrodotoxin-resistant sodium channels in rat dorsal root ganglion neurons, *J Neurosci* 12:2104, 1992.
141. Rowe N et al: Control of pain resulting from endodontic therapy: a double-blind, placebo-controlled study, *Oral Surg Oral Med Oral Pathol* 50:257, 1980.
142. Schaible H, Schmidt R: Discharge characteristics of receptors with fine afferents from normal and inflamed joints: influence of analgesics and prostaglandins, *Agents Actions* 19(suppl):99, 1986.
143. Seltzer S et al: The intracanal use of sulfathiazole in endodontics to reduce pain, *J Am Dent Assoc* 77:102, 1968.
144. Sessle B: Neurophysiology of orofacial pain, *Dent Clin North Am* 31:595, 1987.
145. Sessle BJ et al: Convergence of cutaneous, tooth pulp, visceral, neck and muscle afferents onto nociceptive and non-nociceptive neurons in trigeminal subnucleus caudalis (medullary dorsal horn) and its implications for referred pain, *Pain* 27:219, 1986.
146. Sessle BJ: Dental deafferentation can lead to the development of chronic pain. In Klineberg I and Sessle B, editors: *Oro-facial pain and neuromuscular dysfunction. Mechanisms and clinical correlates,* Oxford, 1985, Pergamon Press.
147. Sessle BJ: Recent developments in pain research: central mechanisms of orofacial pain and its control, *J Endod* 12:435, 1986.
148. Soltanoff W: A comparative study of the single-visit and the multiple-visit endodontic procedure, *J Endod* 4:278, 1978.
149. Stambaugh J, Drew J: The combination of ibuprofen and oxycodone/acetaminophen in the management of chronic cancer pain, *Clin Pharmacol Ther* 44:665, 1988.
150. Steen K et al: Protons selectively induce lasting excitation and sensitization to mechanical stimulation of nociceptors in rat skin in vitro, *J Neurosci* 21:86, 1992.
151. Sugimoto T, Bennett G, Kajander K: Transsynaptic degeneration in the superficial dorsal horn after sciatic nerve injury: effects of a chronic constriction injury, transection and styrchnine, *Pain* 42:205, 1990.
152. Sunshine A et al: Analgesic efficacy of a hydrocodone with ibuprofen combination compared with ibuprofen alone for the treatment of acute postoperative pain, *J Clin Pharmacol* 37:908, 1997.
153. Torabinejad M et al: Factors associated with endodontic interappointment emergencies of teeth with necrotic pulps, *J Endod* 14:261, 1988.
154. Torabinejad M et al: Effectiveness of various medications on postoperative pain following complete instrumentation, *J Endod* 20:345, 1994.
155. Torabinejad M et al: Effectiveness of various medications on postoperative pain following root canal obturation, *J Endod* 20:427, 1994.
156. Trope M: Relationship of intracanal medicaments to endodontic flare-ups, *Endod Dent Traumatol* 6:226, 1990.
157. Trope M: Flare-up rate of single-visit endodontics, *Int Endod J* 24:24, 1991.
158. Troullos E, Freeman R, Dionne R: The scientific basis for analgesic use in dentistry, *Anesth Prog* 33:123, 1986.
159. Trowbridge H: Review of dental pain—histology and physiology, *J Endod* 12:445, 1986.
160. Wagner R, Myers R: Endoneurial injection of TNF-alpha produces neuropathic pain behaviors, *Neuroreport* 7:2897, 1996.
161. Wall P, Woolf C: Muscle but not cutaneous C-afferent input produces prolonged increases in the excitability of the flexion reflex in the rat, *Am J Physiol* 356:443, 1984.
162. Wallace J: Selective COX-2 inhibitors: is the water becoming muddy? *Trends Pharmacol Sci* 20:4, 1999.
163. Walton R, Fouad A: Endodontic interappointment flare-ups: a prospective study of incidence and related factors, *J Endod* 18:172, 1992.
164. Walton R, Chiappinelli J: Prophylactic penicillin: effect on posttreatment symptoms following root canal treatment of asymptomatic periapical pathosis, *J Endod* 19:466, 1993.
165. Waxman S et al: Sodium channels and pain, *Proc Natl Acad Sci U S A* 96:7635, 1999.
166. Wideman G et al: Analgesic efficacy of a combination of hydrocodone with ibuprofen in postoperative pain, *Clin Pharm Therap* 65:66, 1999.
167. Willis W: *Hyperalgesia and allodynia,* New York, 1992, Raven Press.
168. Willis W: *The pain system,* Basel, Switzerland, 1985, Karger.

169. Wolf M, Lichtenstein D, Singh G: Gastrointestinal toxicity of nonsteroidal antiinflammatory drugs, *New Eng J Med* 340: 1888, 1999.

170. Woolf C: Evidence for a central component of post-injury pain hypersensitivity, *Nature* 306:686, 1983.

171. Woolf C: Windup and central sensitization are not equivalent, *Pain* 66:105, 1996.

172. Woolf C: Transcriptional and posttranslational plasticity and the generation of inflammatory pain, *Proc Natl Acad Sci U S A* 96:7723, 1999.

173. Wright C et al: Ibuprofen and acetaminophen kinetics when taken concurrently, *Clin Pharm Therap* 34:707, 1983.

174. Wurm C et al: Evaluation of functional G-protein coupled receptors in dental pulp, *J Endod* 77:160, 1998 (abstract).

175. Wynn R, Meiller T, Crossley H: *Drug information handbook for dentistry*, Hudson, Ohio, 2000, Lexi-Comp Inc.

176. Xiao W-H et al: TNF-*alpha applied to the sciatic nerve trunk elicits background firing in nociceptive primary afferent fibers. Abstracts 8th world congress on pain*, Seattle, 1996, IASP Press.

177. Zhou Q et al: Persistent Fos protein expression after orofacial deep or cutaneous tissue inflammation in rats: implications for persistent orofacial pain, *J Comp Neurol* 412:276, 1999.

Chapter 19

 # Endodontic Microsurgery

Syngcuk Kim

Chapter Outline

BENEFITS OF ENDODONTIC MICROSURGERY

Microsurgery is limited to a surgical procedure on exceptionally small and complex structures with the aid of an operation microscope. The microscope allows the surgeon to assess pathologic changes more precisely and to remove pathologic lesions with far greater precision, thus minimizing tissue damage during the surgery.

If one examines the way endodontic surgery was performed with the traditional nonmicroscopic method, pathologic lesions were grossly curetted but the microscopic causes of the lesions were often missed; furthermore, there was avoidable damage to healthy tissues during the surgery.

Thus modern dental surgeons who perform this surgery must have indepth knowledge, not only in surgical principles, but also in the use of the microscope and microinstruments.

PROBLEMS WITH TRADITIONAL ENDODONTIC SURGERY

Endodontic surgery is often perceived as difficult because of restricted access (especially in posterior teeth), small operating field, and anatomic structures (e.g., such as large neurovascular bundles). When operating on posterior teeth, the mental nerve and the maxillary sinus are often proximate to the operation site. Another reason for skepticism is the limited success rate of earlier periapical surgery.[25,35] In addition, endodontic surgery is usually carried out under local anesthesia, so there is the further challenge of working on a conscious, often nervous patient. For all these reasons endodontic surgery is viewed as the last resort when nonsurgical endodontic therapy or endodontic retreatment is impossible or unsuccessful.

IMPLICATION OF MICROSURGERY IN ENDODONTICS

In medicine, incorporation of the concept of microsurgery began in the late 1950s. The surgical operating microscope was used for the first time in neurosurgery and opthalmology in 1960. Currently, most surgical procedures in medicine are routinely performed under the operating microscope. Thus it would only be a matter of time until other fields, including endodontics, would recognize the advantages the microscope offers.

Precision is a key element in endodontic microsurgery because of the restricted access to the surgical field. To achieve precision, the surgical area must be well illuminated and magnified. The standard operating light and 2 × or 3.5 × loupes, which are sufficient for simple operative procedures on larger structures, are not sufficient to observe and treat the microstructures and defects common in and around the tooth apex. The surgical operating microscope, which has long been a standard instrument in medical surgery, provides the necessary illumination with a bright, focused light and magnification up to 32×. This enhanced visibility allows the surgeons to locate and treat anatomic variations that previously would have escaped their attention. These include the partial or complete isthmus, multiple foramina, C-shaped canals, and apical root fractures. These variations often cannot be treated by nonsurgical means.

INDICATIONS

The late Dr. Irving J. Naidorf said, "A good surgeon knows *how* to cut, and an excellent surgeon knows *when* to cut."

When faced with an apparent endodontic failure, the quality of the nonsurgical endodontic treatment must be carefully considered. Eccentric-angle periapical radiographs, for instance, may show a missed canal or an inadequate filling (Fig. 19-1). The microsurgical approach is indicated *only when* the clinician has determined that nonsurgical retreatment is not possible or will not correct the problem.

The definitions of endodontic success and failure remain controversial: the clinical definition of success is an asymptomatic tooth; the radiographic definition is the remineralization of a periapical radiolucency; and the histologic definition is the reestablishment of normal periapical cell structures in the absence any inflammatory cells. Even successfully treated asymptomatic teeth show histologic evidence of inflammatory cells in the periapical region[9] and cell disruption; the clinical and radiographic definitions are generally accepted criteria for success in clinical practice.

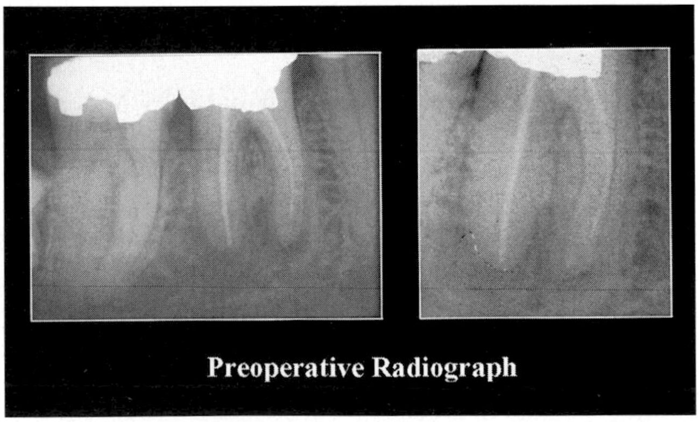

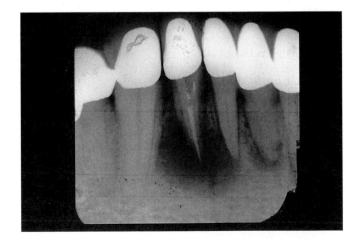

Fig. 19-1 Failed endodontic therapy. Surgery was not needed because an untreated mesiobuccal canal found on an eccentric angle radiograph was identified and treated nonsurgically. Due to poor shaping and obturation, the other root canals were retreated.

Fig. 19-2 Numerous retreatments of this anterior tooth failed necessitating endodontic microsurgery. The cause of the failure was an elongated facial-lingual canal, which was only partially filled.

Failure of Previous Nonsurgical Endodontic Therapy

The following cases illustrate two frequent situations in clinical practice.

Case 1 A nonsurgically endodontically retreated tooth, asymptomatic and without swelling or a sinus tract, may have a persistent or enlarging periapical radiolucency (Fig. 19-2). The cause of the repeated failure was a long buccolingual root with a ribbon-shaped apex that was never completely cleaned and obturated. Some anterior teeth have similar ribbon-shaped apices. Such cases illustrate that complex apical canal systems cannot always be completely accessed, cleaned, and obturated by good, nonsurgical, endodontic techniques.

Case 2 After endodontic therapy a periapical rarefaction persists or enlarges and the tooth has a permanent post-and-crown restoration (Fig. 19-3). When endodontic treatment fails, nonsurgical retreatment of the tooth may be possible. However, the procedure is often very difficult and may lead to irreparable damage to the tooth. Root fractures and root perforations are constant risks during attempts to remove a post with a nonsurgical bur or post remover or both. Such retreatments are more successful now (as described in Chapter 25), partly because the microscope minimizes the need for canal enlargement, thus reducing the chances of perforation or fracture. When one encounters this type of case the clinician must consider the surgical approach and retreatment. In fact, in some cases the surgical approach is the more conservative treatment option.[15] Furthermore, even if a post or core or both are successfully removed, the post, core, and crown restoration will have to be redone at considerable expense of time and money.

Failure of Previous Endodontic Surgery

The causes of failed endodontic surgery are numerous, but the most common cause is apical leakage. Failing cases that had been treated with traditional surgical techniques must be retreated microsurgically; this approach can correct the deficiencies. For instance, notice the round, radiopaque amalgam fillings on the mesiobuccal (MB) and mesiolingual (ML) apices of the mandibular first molar (Fig. 19-4). Not only were these fillings loose (allowing leakage), but the isthmus was not treated and a large osteotomy caused the iatrogenic loss of the buccal plate.

Anatomic Deviations

Many teeth have some form of anatomic deviation from the norm. Tortuous roots, severe S- and C-shaped canals, sharp-angled bifurcations, pulp stones, calcifications, and other elements that complicate the complete débridement and subsequent obturation of the root canal system are more common than previously thought (Fig. 19-5). Many of these teeth are treated by endodontic therapy first, and the lesion is observed at intervals for signs of resolution. If the lesion heals and the patient has no symptoms, the treatment is considered successful; otherwise microsurgery should be considered.

Procedural Errors

Clinicians may ledge, block, or perforate canals during instrumentation; they may also break an instrument inside the canal (Fig. 19-6) and overfill (Fig. 19-7) or underfill the canal because of apical blockage (Fig. 19-8). The consequence of a procedural error is usually an incomplete filling or an insufficient apical seal, which eventually enables periapical pathologic conditions to develop. If the procedural error occurred in the apical third of the root (Fig. 19-9), the favorable crown/root ratio favors an apicoectomy as a relatively simple surgical correction of the problem, while still offering a good prognosis. A broken instrument in a canal or root perforation does not automatically indicate the need for endodontic surgery. For example, if an instrument is broken

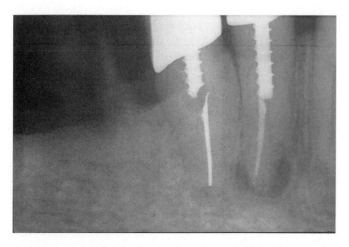

Fig. 19-3 A maxillary anterior tooth shows a post restoration and an enlarging periapical lesion.

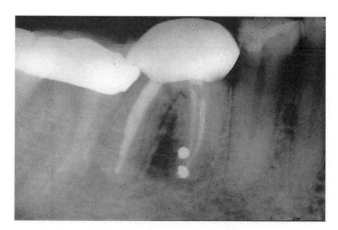

Fig. 19-4 Failed surgeries performed with premicrosurgical techniques. Note the round amalgam "dots" at the apices. The angle of the root resection was too acute, resulting in the loss of buccal cortical plate.

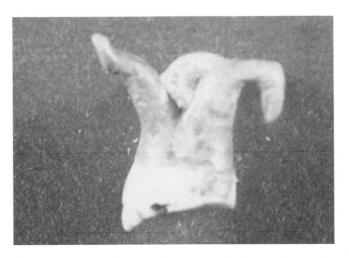

Fig. 19-5 Example of an extremely tortuous molar tooth. (Courtesy Dr. A. Moreinis.)

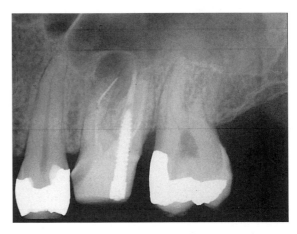

Fig. 19-6 A broken file lodged in the apical third of the mesiobuccal root of tooth no. 14. The root is very close to or in the sinus, but carefully performed endodontic microsurgery remains a reasonable choice.

where it can be bypassed or a perforation can be nonsurgically repaired and the canal can be properly cleaned and filled, nonsurgical endodontics is the treatment of choice.

Exploratory Surgery

Occasionally, despite careful radiographic evaluations, thorough clinical examination, and a complete gathering of history, a confident diagnosis is difficult to make. An experienced surgeon may decide to follow up an educated "guess" about the problem with exploratory surgery, which usually provides the missing information for a definitive diagnosis. Of course, once the tissue flap is raised, the surgeon should be prepared to do whatever is necessary to correct the problem. If a root fracture is identified, for instance, the surgeon should decide to either resect or hemisect the root or to extract the tooth (Figs. 19-10 and 19-11).

Potential Contraindications

Some dentists decide to extract a tooth rather than attempt endodontic surgery because of anatomic factors, such as proximity to the mental foramen, maxillary sinus, or molars with limited access. These concerns were certainly justified before the availability of the microscope. Currently, microsurgical techniques have greatly reduced some of these concerns. Nevertheless, several anatomic factors should be discussed further for the purposes of comparison.

Proximity to Neurovascular Bundles   The mental neurovascular bundle is usually found close to the apices of the mandibular second premolars and first molars. Also, the inferior alveolar neurovascular bundle must always be identified radiographically before initiating apical surgery on a posterior tooth. In most situations this does not present undue difficulty to the experienced surgeon, especially if the surgeon works with a microscope and uses the cortical-groove technique to prevent accidental slippage of an instrument into the nerve bundle. Under the intense illumination provided by the microscope, subtle color differences identifying the location of the mandibular canal and mental foramen can be detected and serve as guides for the osteotomy. However, unless the surgeon is experienced and works with a microscope, this operation could increase the risk of the undesirable outcome of permanent nerve damage. Only experienced dental surgeons should perform apical surgery in the posterior region.

Second Mandibular Molar Area   In most patients the second mandibular molar has the following characteristics: the buccal plate is too thick, the roots are inclined lingually, and the apices are very close to the mandibular canal. In addition, the more restricted access often makes a routine surgical approach difficult if not impossible. In this situation, extraction and replantation after treating the tooth extraorally is usually a more prudent choice.

Maxillary Sinus   The proximity of the sinus is not a factor in determining whether surgery should be performed. Many roots of the maxillary premolars and molars are in close proximity to the sinus or even into the sinus, separated only by a thin layer of cortical bone and the Schneiderian membrane (Fig. 19-12). A close examination of the radiographic image of the roots and careful dissection under the microscope usually prevents a sinus perforation during surgery. However, even if the sinus is accidentally perforated, the outcome of the surgery is not necessarily compromised (Fig. 19-13).[78]

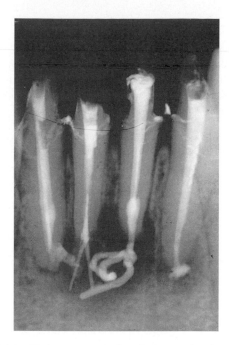

Fig. 19-7 Mandibular anterior teeth with periapical pathosis and gross overextensions. (Courtesy Dr. G. Pecora.)

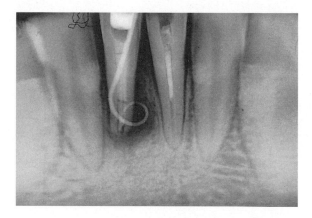

Fig. 19-10 A gutta-percha cone inserted into the sinus tract. The root has a demineralized "halo" appearance, strongly suggesting a vertical root fracture.

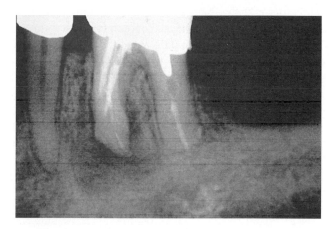

Fig. 19-8 Tooth no. 19 with poor endodontic treatment, a large periapical demineralized area, total canal calcification in the apical half, and a separated instrument at the apex. (Courtesy Dr. G. Pecora.)

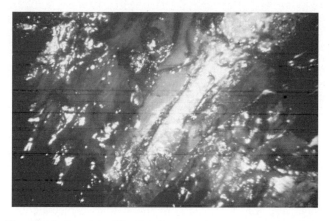

Fig. 19-11 Elevation of the flap during exploratory surgery revealed a vertical fracture. The tooth was extracted.

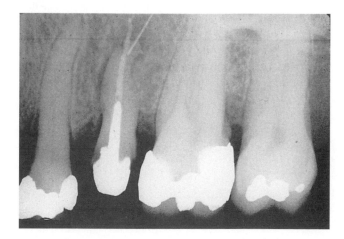

Fig. 19-9 Tooth no. 13 with separated and overextended instruments, along with a post restoration.

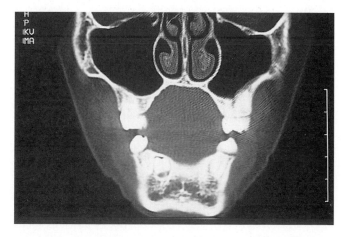

Fig. 19-12 A computer tomographic image of the lower head, showing that molar roots and the sinus cavities are separated by a thin Schneiderian (i.e., sinus) membrane.

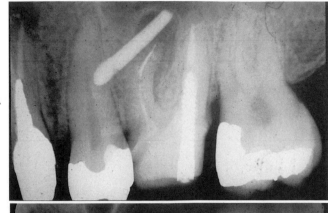

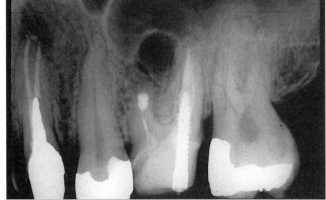

Fig. 19-13 **A**, A sinus tract (gutta-percha point) leads to the apex of the mesiobuccal root of tooth no. 14 that is very close to or in the sinus. **B**, The sinus membrane was perforated during the surgery; nevertheless, the case had a successful outcome.

CONTRAINDICATIONS

There are very few true contraindications for endodontic microsurgery. Many conditions that would eliminate surgery as a treatment option are temporary and, once corrected, can be performed. Nevertheless, three contraindications to endodontic surgery remain:

1. Periodontal health of the tooth
2. Patient health considerations
3. Surgeon's skill and ability

In the following sections, each of these factors are examined.

Periodontal Health of the Tooth

When considering endodontic surgery, the periodontal health of the tooth is the most important factor. Tooth mobility and periodontal pockets are the two key elements the surgeon must consider. It has been shown that endodontic surgery can have over 96% short-term success (1 year) and 91% long-term success (5 to 7 years), provided that the cases have no periodontal involvement (Class A, B, and C).[61] Because periodontal defects are common in the adult popu-

lation, surgeons have to be careful in assessing the periodontal condition before surgery. A compromised attachment apparatus reduces the chances of endodontic surgical success, especially if the surgery results in an endodontic and periodontic communication.

Patient Health Considerations

In most cases the patient's medical condition does not preclude endodontic surgery. It is uncommon for patients with leukemia or neutropenia in the active state, uncontrolled diabetes, or recent serious cardiac or cancer surgery, as well as patients who are very old and infirmed to be candidates for endodontic surgery. However, the clinician should remember that older patients should not automatically be eliminated as candidates for the surgical procedure. The decision for endodontic surgery should be based on considered judgment and, if needed, on consultation with the patient's primary physician.

Surgery should be postponed if a patient is recuperating from a myocardial infarction or is taking anticoagulant medicines (e.g., Coumadin). A consultation with the patient's physician is essential before the surgery so that medications taken by the patient can be titrated or temporarily terminated. The risk of temporarily stopping an anticoagulant in preparation for surgery has recently been reported at a negligible 0.5%.[81] Surgery should also be avoided (if possible) when a patient has had radiation treatment of the jaw, because the radiation reduces the blood supply to the area, thereby enabling osteoradionecrosis. It is also advisable to postpone endodontic surgery for patients who are in the first trimester of pregnancy.[67]

When diabetes is controlled, endodontic surgery does not pose an undue health risk, provided the patient is premedicated and maintained on proper antibiotics; however, opinions vary on this issue.[65,84] Therefore the surgeon should consult the treating physician before proceeding with the surgery.

Surgeon's Skill and Ability

Clinicians must be completely honest about their surgical skill and knowledge. When clinicians encounter a case beyond their abilities, these cases should be referred to an endodontist (or oral surgeon) who has microsurgical training and experience with complex cases involving periapical surgery.

PREPARING FOR ENDODONTIC MICROSURGERY

Preparing for endodontic microsurgery encompasses strong magnification, high illumination, and precise instrumentation (Fig. 19-14).[40] Strong illumination and magnification are provided by the surgical microscope. With bright, focused magnification ranging from 4 × to 32 ×, the surgeon

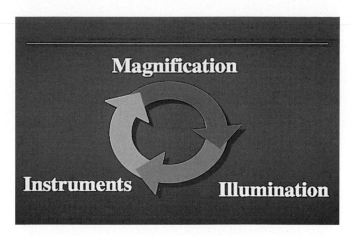

Fig. 19-14 The triad of magnification, illumination, and microinstruments provides greater accuracy in apical surgery.

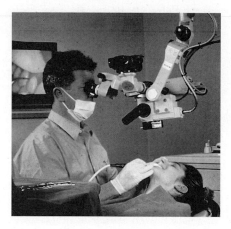

Fig. 19-15 Incorporation of the microscope in endodontic practice.

Table 19-1   TRADITIONAL ENDODONTIC SURGERY VERSUS MICROSURGERY

Procedure	Traditional Surgery	Microsurgery
Identification of the apex	Sometimes difficult	Precise
Osteotomy	Large (= >10 mm)	Small (= <5 mm)
Root surface inspection	Imprecise	Precise
Bevel angle	Large (45 degrees)	Small (<10 degrees)
Isthmus identification	Nearly impossible	Customary
Retro-preparation	Approximate	Precise
Root end filling	Imprecise	Precise

can observe every detail of the apical structures, thus allowing precision during surgery (Fig. 19-15). As an additional benefit the magnification allows smaller osteotomies. More discrete removal of healthy bone to gain access to root apices has resulted in less patient discomfort and faster healing. Magnification and illumination with the microscope have fundamentally changed the way endodontic surgery is performed. Working in a magnified surgical site requires a different set of surgical instruments. Dr. Gary Carr originally designed the basic microsurgical instruments in endodontic microsurgery in the late 1980s; since then many variations and improvements have been made.

The standard endodontic surgical instruments are too large for microsurgery (everything but the instrument handles had to be reduced in size). Ultrasonic tips, compactors, pluggers, curettes, mirrors, and other instruments have been reduced in size to comfortably fit into an osteotomy no larger than 5 mm to gain access to the canals. Earlier, osteotomies of 10 mm or larger were routinely made to gain access to root apices with standard endodontic instruments using the traditional method. With the microscope, ultrasonics, and microinstruments, today's surgeons can execute apical surgery with confidence and accuracy (see Fig. 19-15). The entire surgical field is visible, accessible, and nothing is left to guesswork.

Comparing Traditional and Modern Endodontic Microsurgery

Endodontic microsurgery can be performed with precision and predictability, eliminating the assumptions inherent in traditional endodontic surgery. Table 19-1 summarizes the differences between traditional endodontic surgery and microsurgery.[40]

The main advantages of the microsurgical approach are easier identification of the root apex, smaller osteotomies, and shallow resection angles, which conserve cortical bone and root structure. In addition, a resected root surface under high illumination and magnification readily reveals anatomic details, such as isthmuses, canal fins, microfractures, and lateral canals. Ultrasonics permit conservative, root end preparations parallel to the long axis of the root and precise root end fillings, satisfying mechanical and biologic principles of endodontic surgery. Comparison of the radiographic appearances of amalgam retrofilling material using traditional surgery and microsurgery with Super ethoxybenzoic acid (EBA) as the retrofilling material is presented in Fig. 19-16. The amalgam retrofilling looks like a highly opaque dot at the apex, whereas a retrofilling made with the new techniques and biocompatible materials looks like an elongated filling 3 mm into the canal.

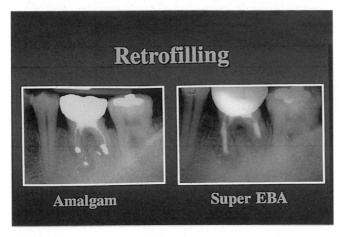

Fig. 19-16 Small, round amalgam retrofillngs with the traditional technique (*left*), which only seal part of the elongated apices, thus enabling leakage. Super EBA retrofillings (3 mm) in the buccal canals (*right*). Even the elongated isthmus was prepared and filled easily with the proper application of the endodontic microscope.

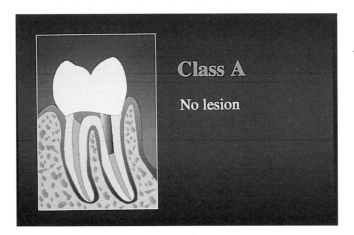

Fig. 19-17 Class A tooth with no periapical lesion, but the tooth is symptomatic.

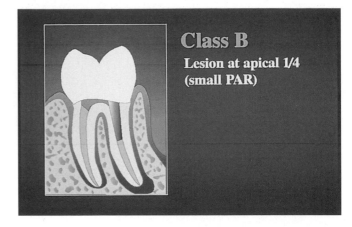

Fig. 19-18 Class B tooth with a small periapical lesion.

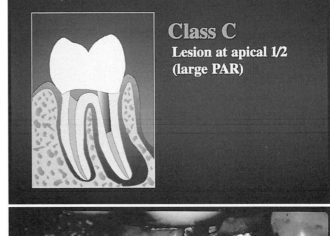

A

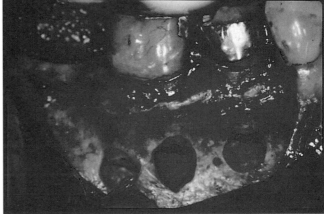

B

Fig. 19-19 A, Class C tooth with a periapical lesion covering approximately one half of the root. B, Clinical view of Class C tooth.

Classification of Endodontic Microsurgical Cases

Endodontic surgery can be classified as follows:

- Class A represents the absence of a periapical lesion, but unresolved symptoms after nonsurgical approaches have been exhausted. The symptoms are the only reason for the surgery (Fig. 19-17).
- Class B represents the presence of a small periapical lesion and no periodontal pockets (Fig. 19-18).
- Class C represents the presence of a large periapical lesion progressing coronally but without periodontal pocket (Fig. 19-19, *A* and *B*).
- Class D represents a clinical picture similar to Class C with a periodontal pocket (Fig. 19-20).

- Class E classifies a periapical lesion with an endodontic and periodontal communication but no root fracture (Fig. 19-21, *A* and *B*).
- Class F represents a tooth with an apical lesion and complete denudement of the buccal plate (Fig. 19-22, *A* and *B*).

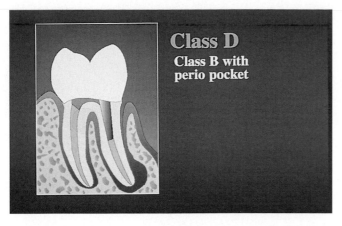

Fig. 19-20 Class D tooth. Class B or C along with a periodontal pocket.

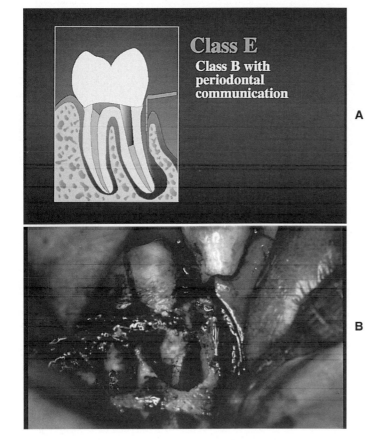

Fig. 19-21 **A**, Class E tooth. Class B or C along with periodontal communication to the apex. **B**, Clinical view of Class E tooth showing periodontal communication on the buccal surface of the mesial root.

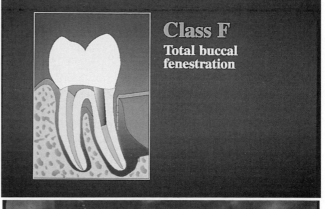

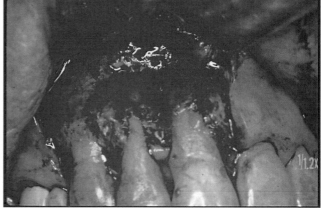

Fig. 19-22 **A**, Class F tooth. Total buccal fenestration (i.e., dihisence). **B**, Clinical view of Class F tooth shows complete loss of the cortical plate.

Classes A, B, and C present no significant treatment problems and do not adversely affect the successful treatment outcomes. However, cases in the D, E, and F categories present serious difficulties. Although these cases are in the endodontic domain, proper and successful treatment requires not only endodontic microsurgical techniques but also cur-

rent periodontal surgical techniques (e.g., the membrane barrier technique). Endodontic surgeons are faced with these challenges.

PRESURGICAL PREPARATIONS

Patient Interview

The patient interview is an important part of the diagnostic work-up. Some patients react with apprehension, anxiety, or outright fear to the prospect of endodontic surgery. Therefore it is important to establish a rapport with the patient and to explain in layperson's terms the reason for the surgery, the procedure itself, the postoperative instructions, and the prognosis. The interview gives the surgeon the opportunity to assess the patient's state of mind and physical conditions; it also presents the patient with the opportunity to develop trust in the doctor. This is extremely important because most surgeries are done under local anesthesia so the patient's confidence in the surgeon allays anxiety. The surgeon should also explain the microscope and microsurgical methods. For most patients this is the first experience with a microscope; therefore having it come to within a few inches of the face can be intimidating.

Medical Evaluation

A systematic approach to determine the patient's medical condition is essential. (The reader is referred to Chapters 2 and 18 for more information on this subject.)

Because endodontic surgical procedures produce a transient bacteremia, antibiotics must be given prophylactically for patients with a history of rheumatic fever, endocarditis, abnormal or damaged heart valves, organ transplants, or placement of an implant prosthesis, such as a hip or knee replacement.[1,17] It is important that the patient be treated in consultation with the patient's physician; the most recent guidelines of the American Heart Association (AHA) should be observed.

Oral Examination

The oral examination should be conducted in a systematic manner and in a specific sequence. The patient's complaint or complaints and chronologic history of the problem should guide the line of inquiry to identify the etiology and source of the problem.

Pain and swelling are the most common symptoms that patients report before endodontic surgery. At this first visit the patient may report a history of pain, and some will complain of referred pain, such as an earache and heaviness or tightness of the jaw or muscles. An earache is usually indicative of radiating pain from an infected ipsilateral mandibular molar tooth.

Extraoral swelling indicates that surgery should be postponed until the swelling is reduced with oral antibiotics (as described in Chapter 18). If a sinus tract has developed, it should be traced with a gutta-percha point (as described in Chapter 1). The tooth should also be evaluated for its periodontal integrity and for fractures. For instance, in cases designated Class E or F, the success of surgical endodontics becomes questionable.

Clinically or radiographically complete vertical fractures can be detected (see Fig. 19-10 and Chapter 1). A vertical fracture was confirmed upon elevation of the flap (see Fig. 19-11). Exploratory surgery should be considered to confirm suspicions of vertical root fracture.

Radiographic Evaluation

Valuable information can be obtained from periapical radiographs in the evaluation of a case for periapical surgery. Anatomic deviations, fractures, periradicular pathosis, evidence of traumatic injuries, root resorption, periodontal disease, changes in bone patterns, and the success or failure of prior endodontic therapy are some of the salient pieces of information obtained from radiographs. Comparison of previous and current radiographs determines whether an area of periradicular pathosis is new, recurrent, or enlarged and will indicate the necessity for periradicular surgery.

At least two periapical radiographs taken from different angles are needed to ascertain root length, long axis, mor-

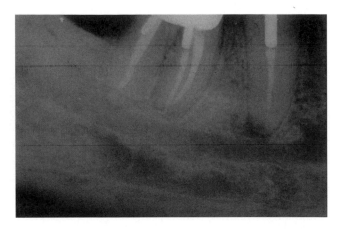

Fig. 19-23 Note proximity of the apices of the second premolar and the first molar to the inferior alveolar and mental neurovascular bundles.

phology, and proximity to the mental foramen, inferior alveolar nerve bundle,[40] (Fig. 19-23) or the antrum. In most cases a definitive decision for either surgical endodontics or nonsurgical endodontic therapy can be made after gathering radiographic evidence from two interpretable films; this allows the clinician to visualize the three-dimensional (3-D) space.

It is important to view the radiograph systematically. The following is one way to interpret radiographs before surgery (Fig. 19-24). Two radiographs are taken, one straight on and the other 25 to 30 degrees mesially or distally.

These radiographs will help the clinician to determine the following:

- Approximate root length
- Number of roots and their configurations (e.g., fused, separate)
- Long axis of the root and degree of root curvature
- Size and type of lesion (e.g., Class B, C)
- Proximity of anatomic structures to the root apex (e.g., mental foramen, sinus)
- Distance from the root apex to the inferior alveolar nerve cortical housing
- Distance between root tips, especially in anterior teeth

PREMEDICATION

Each case presents certain conditions that must be considered in the aggregate. The following are drugs used in endodontic practices that are recommended before and after endodontic surgery[20,34,66]:

- Antiinflammatory analgesics. It is recommended that the patient (average weight of 150 lbs) take ibuprofen (400 mg) *just before* surgery to minimize the postsurgical inflammatory response. To minimize bleeding problems during surgery the dose should not be taken sooner. The postsurgery to reduce pain and swelling. With this regimen most patients will not require narcotic pain medica-

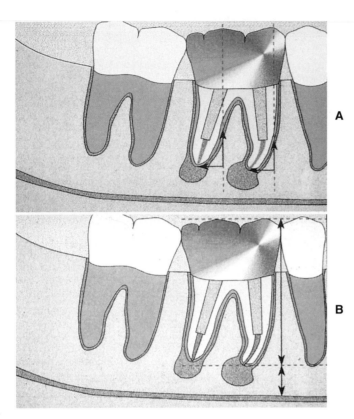

Fig. 19-24 **A** and **B**, Schematic diagram illustrates the systematic examination of the radiograph before surgery. Features such as the apical curvature, length of the roots, and proximity to the inferior alveolar canal or mental foramen or both are mentally noted.

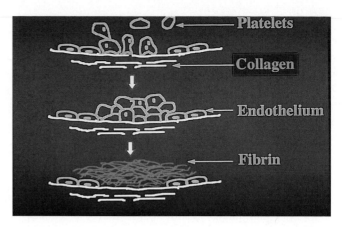

Fig. 19-25 Schematic diagram illustrates formation of fibrin plug from the platelets initiating hemostasis.

tion.[18] (See Chapter 18 for more information about this subject.)

- Tranquilizers. If a patient is very anxious about the surgery, sublingual triazolam taken 15 to 30 minutes before the surgery provides relief. (See Chapter 2 for more information on this issue.)
- Antibiotics. As stated previously, patients in poor health (e.g., with advanced diabetes, heart valve problems) must be premedicated in accordance with the most recent AHA recommendations. (See Chapter 18 for further information on this subject.)
- Antibacterial rinses. To reduce oral microflora, the patient should be instructed to rinse with a 0.12% chlorhexidine gluconate mouth rinse (e.g., Peridex, Perioguard) the night before surgery, the morning of surgery, and 1 hour before surgery. Rinsing continued after the surgery for 1 week reduces microorganisms in the oral cavity and promotes better healing.

LOCAL ANESTHESIA AND HEMOSTASIS

Adequate hemostasis is a prerequisite for microsurgery.[43] Achieving effective hemostasis was a challenge. Earlier, some surgeons performed endodontic surgery in a pool of blood, guessing at anatomic landmarks and structures. For endodontic microsurgery, effective hemostasis is essential because the bone crypt and resected root surfaces have to be examined at high magnification. If continuous bleeding obscures the view, the benefit of microsurgery is negated.

Mechanisms and Stages of Hemostasis

Hemostasis of a severed vessel is achieved by a sequence of events. Immediately after a blood vessel is cut, the stimulus of the trauma to the vessel causes the wall of the vessel to contract; this instantaneously reduces the flow of blood from the transected vessel. This local vascular spasm can last for many minutes or even hours, during which time the ensuing processes of platelet plugging and coagulation can take place.

The second stage in hemostasis is the formation of a platelet plug. Platelet repair of vascular openings is based on several important functions of the platelet itself. When platelets come in contact with a damaged vascular surface, such as the collagen fibers in the vascular walls, they immediately change their characteristics. They begin to swell and become sticky so that they adhere to the collagen fibers. This begins a cycle of activation with successively increasing numbers of platelets that themselves attract additional platelets, thus forming a platelet plug (Fig. 19-25).

The third step for hemostasis is formation of the blood clot. Activator substances or clotting factors both from the traumatized vascular wall and from platelets and blood proteins adhering to the traumatized vascular wall initiate the clotting process.

Clotting takes place in three essential steps:

1. In response to rupture of the vessel or damage to the blood itself, a complex cascade of chemical reactions occurs in the blood involving more than a dozen blood coagulation factors. The net result is formation of a complex of activated substances collectively called *prothrombin activator*.

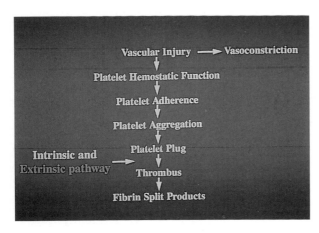

Fig. 19-26 Summary of events that leads to hemostasis from vascular injury.

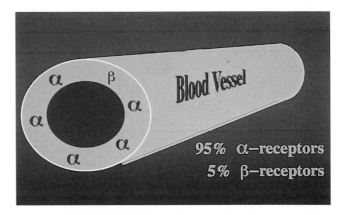

Fig. 19-27 Note that 95% of the receptors in the oral mucosa are α-receptors; their activation causes vasoconstriction.

2. The prothrombin activator catalyzes the conversion of prothrombin to thrombin.
3. The thrombin acts as an enzyme to convert fibrinogen into fibrin fibers that enmesh platelets, blood cells, and plasma to form the clot (Fig. 19-26).

Hemostasis in a surgical procedure can be considered in three phases: (1) presurgical , (2) surgical, and (3) post-surgical.

Presurgical Phase

Local Anesthesia
In surgical endodontics local anesthesia has two prime purposes: (1) anesthesia and (2) hemostasis. Profound anesthesia of the surgical site is essential for the comfort of the patient and the working efficiency of the surgeon. Assurance that everything will be done to keep the patient completely comfortable is the first step. Next, a good topical anesthetic ointment or transoral lidocaine patch (e.g., DentiPatch) is left in place for a minimum of 2 minutes to take effect. Then a generous amount of a vasoconstrictor containing local anesthetic should be injected slowly to ensure profound anesthesia throughout the surgery. An inadequately anesthetized patient produces considerably more endogenous catecholamine in response to pain than the concentration of vasoconstrictor contained in the anesthetic solution. Inadequate hemostasis leads to a prolonged and difficult procedure to control.

A cardiovascular disorder, unless it is severe, does not automatically contraindicate the use of epinephrine-containing anesthetics. Consultation with the physician should verify this issue and should allay any concerns the patient may have. On occasion, patients may state that they are "allergic to novocaine," "allergic to epinephrine," or that they had heart palpitation after an epinephrine-containing anesthetic was used. These patients often request that such an anesthetic not be used. Although the patient's concerns should be acknowledged, it is strongly recommended that the surgery should be done only if vasoconstrictor-containing

anesthetics are used. The patient should be informed of the reason for this choice, and a consultation with the patient's physician before the surgery is advisable to ensure that there are no unexpected complications from an unknown health factor. Cardiologists generally agree that locally injected epinephrine-containing anesthetics are safe.

The anesthetic solution of choice for endodontic surgery is lidocaine 2% HCl with 1:50,000 epinephrine.[14, 43] The high concentration of 1:50,000 epinephrine is preferred for surgery, because it produces effective-and-lasting vasoconstriction via the a-adrenergic receptors in the smooth muscle of the arterioles. This prevents the anesthetic from being dissipated prematurely by the microcirculation.

Epinephrine Connection
Epinephrine binds α-1, α-2 and β-1, and β-2 adrenergic receptors. Epinephrine causes vasoconstriction by stimulating the membrane-bound a receptors on vascular smooth muscle.[41,51] α-1 receptors are located adjacent to sympathetic nerves innervating blood vessels, whereas α-2 receptors are distributed throughout the vascular system and are generally bound by circulating catecholamines. When epinephrine binds to the adrenergic β-1 receptors located in the heart muscle, it causes increases in heart rate, cardiac contractility, and peripheral resistance, whereas epinephrine bound β-2 receptors, located in the peripheral vasculature, result in vasodilation. These receptors are prevalent in blood vessels supplying skeletal muscle and certain viscera, but they are relatively rare in mucous membranes, oral tissues, and skin.

Ideally, for the purposes of endodontic microsurgery, an adrenergic vasoconstrictor would be a pure α agonist. Fortunately, the predominant receptor in the oral tissues is an α receptor, and the number of colocated β-2 receptors is very small.[43] Thus the drug's predominant effect in the oral mucosa, submucosa, and periodontium is that of vasoconstriction (Fig. 19-27).

A source of enduring controversy in dentistry is the potential of epinephrine for causing systemic effects when

Table 19-2 EPINEPHRINE DOSES FOR LOCAL ANESTHESIA

Epinephrine mg/ml	Maximum Doses parts/thousand	mg	ml	# Cartridges
0.02	1:50,000	0.20	10	5.5
0.01	1:100,000	0.20	20	11
0.005	1:200,000	0.20	40	22

(The maximum allowable dose of epinephrine 1:50,000 for an adult is 5.5 carpules.)

used in relatively small amounts for local anesthesia. It has been shown that epinephrine given submucosally and slowly, elicits little-or-no response from the cardiovascular system.* However, when an identical dose is injected directly into the blood vessel, heart rate and stroke volume increase and therefore cardiac output. At the same time, simultaneous β-receptor activation causes mean arterial blood pressure to decrease, lowering peripheral resistance through skeletal muscle vasodilatation. To avoid such an occurrence, an aspirating syringe ensures that epinephrine is not accidentally injected into the blood stream. *Virtually all effects associated with epinephrine in dentistry are dose- and route-dependent.* The current recommended maximum doses of epinephrine in local anesthetics are shown in Table 19-2.

Clinical Reasons for Using 1:50,000 Epinephrine

Buckley and co-workers[10] provided strong evidence of the need for the higher concentration in a clinical study of 10 patients requiring bilateral, posterior segment periodontal-flap surgery. Almost twice as much blood loss occurred when patients were anesthetized with 1:100,000 epinephrine as compared to 1:50,000 epinephrine. These investigators further observed that the reduced blood loss with 1:50,000 epinephrine kept the surgical site drier, thus reducing the operating time. In addition, postsurgical hemostasis was also improved.

In a study using a clinic population there was no correlation between the administration of epinephrine, blood pressure, and pulse rate during periapical surgery using 1:50,000 epinephrine. The majority of patients had transitory, statistically insignificant increases in pulse rate 2 minutes after the injection. Pulse rates returned to normal within 4 minutes.

Local Anesthetic Injection Techniques

It is essential that the administration of 2% lidocaine with 1:50,000 of epinephrine provide profound-and-prolonged anesthesia and hemostasis. Hemostasis, unlike anesthesia, cannot be established effectively by injection into sites other than the surgical site. Although an inferior alveolar nerve block using the epinephrine-containing lidocaine has been shown to reduce blood flow to the jaw by 90%,[42] this has to be supplemented with buccal or lingual infiltration to enhance the vasoconstrictive effect at the surgical site. Whatever the injection technique used for anesthesia, infiltration into the surgical site is essential for hemostasis.

The infiltration sites for the anesthesia are in the loose connective tissue of the alveolar mucosa near the root apices. Injection into the deeper supraperiosteal tissues over the basal bone, rather than the alveolar bone, may not provide hemostatic control in the surgical site but may instead deposit anesthetic into the skeletal muscle. As skeletal muscle has a predominance of β-2 receptors, the injection of epinephrine into muscle will produce vasodilation rather than vasoconstriction and therefore must be avoided. If the anesthetic is injected into the muscle, not only is hemostasis inadequate, but a more rapid uptake of the anesthetic and vasoconstrictor occurs, increasing the potential for substantial bleeding during surgery.[14]

Anesthesia should be deposited into numerous infiltration sites to ensure distribution of the solution throughout the entire surgical field. The rate of injection should be no faster than 1 or 2 mm/min.[49] Rapid injection produces localized pooling of solution in the injected tissues, resulting in delayed and limited diffusion into adjacent tissues, minimal surface contact with microvascular and neural channels, and less than optimal hemostasis. The initial incision should be delayed for at least 15 minutes after the injection until the soft tissues throughout the surgical site have blanched.

Maxillary Anesthesia

Infiltration anesthesia in the mucobuccal fold over the apex of the root and in the adjacent mesial and distal areas is the most effective anesthesia for maxillary teeth. In addition, for surgery on anterior teeth, a supplemental nerve block should be injected near the incisive foramen to block the nasopalatine nerve (Fig. 19-28). For surgery in the posterior quadrant, the anesthetic is injected near the greater palatine foramen to block the greater palatine nerve. If a patient has a large swelling in the cuspid and premolar region, an infraorbital block injection can be very effective to attain profound anesthesia in this area. The choice for the supplemental anesthetic is also a 2%

*References 7,14,43,68,82

lidocaine HCL (e.g., Xylocaine) solution with 1:50,000 epinephrine. The sequence and doses of the injections are as follows:

- The anesthesia is best injected in three intervals, beginning about 15 minutes before the surgery.
- After the topical anesthesia, a full carpule (1.8 ml) is injected into the apical area of the tooth and half of a carpule (0.9 ml) is injected into the adjacent apical areas.
- An aspirating syringe with a 30 gauge, short, 1-inch needle is used to prevent the anesthetic solution from being injected into a blood vessel.
- Ten minutes after the initial infiltration, about half a carpule (0.9 ml) is injected into the palate. When expressed slowly and adroitly, patients will have very little discomfort with palatal anesthesia.
- After profound anesthesia on the facial side, an ultrashort, 30-gauge needle can inject 0.2 ml of the anesthetic through the base of the interdental papilla toward the palatal side of the papilla; this begins virtually painless anesthesia of the palatal side.
- Next, on the now-blanched palatal side of the papilla, using the same 30-gauge, ultrashort needle, the clinician injects 0.4 ml of the anesthetic with the needle inserted parallel to the palatal plate. The palatal tissue will now appear completely blanched.
- An additional 0.4 ml of the anesthetic can now be injected perpendicular to the palate to complete profound anesthesia of the palatal side.

Mandibular Anesthesia   For surgery in the mandible a mandibular and long buccal nerve block with a supplemental infiltration injection in the mucobuccal fold and lingual mucosa in the apical area is the most effective method. One carpule of 2% lidocaine HCl (i.e., Xylocaine) solution with 1:50,000 epinephrine is also preferred for the mandibular block administered with a 27 gauge, 1 1-inch needle in an aspirating syringe. After the mandibular block, another carpule is injected into the mucobuccal fold, mesial and distal to the tooth. After 10 minutes, another infiltration injection of one-half carpule is made into the lingual aspect of the tooth (Fig. 19-29).

Hemostatic Control During Surgery

The next challenge is to control minor local bleeding during the surgery. Local hemostasis can be achieved by the pressure technique of pressing cotton pellets or gauze into the bone crypt for a few minutes. However, if the bleeding persists, topical hemostats should be considered.

Topical Hemostats   Many topical hemostatic agents are available. The agents listed in Box 19-1 are broadly classified by their mode of action.

Epinephrine pellets.   Racellets are cotton pellets containing racemic epinephrine HCl, first suggested by Grossman.[29] The amount of epinephrine in each pellet varies according to the number on the label. For example, Racellet no. 3 pellets contain an average of 0.55 mg racemic epinephrine, and Racellet no. 2 pellets contain 0.2 mg. Racellet no. 2 pellets do not seem to change the pulse rate of patients when pressed into the bone cavity for 4 minutes. This is plausible because topically applied epinephrine causes immediate local vasoconstriction, thus there is minimal absorption into the systemic circulation.

The following procedure is most effective to achieve local hemostasis quickly during apical surgery:

- A small epinephrine-saturated cotton pellet is first placed in the bone crypt and packed solidly against the lingual wall of the bony crypt.
- In quick succession, small sterile cotton pellets are packed in over the first pellet, filling until the entire bone crypt (Fig. 19-30).
- Pressure is applied on these pellets and all but the last pellet is removed after 2 to 4 minutes. At this time even

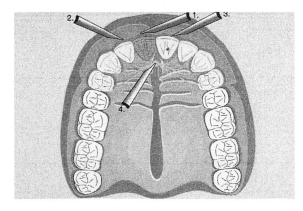

Fig. 19-28 For the maxillary anterior region, one carpule of anesthetic is injected at the apex of the tooth (*shaded*) (*1*), followed by half a carpule both mesial and distal of the apex. Finally, half a carpule is injected into the palate over the apex (*4*).

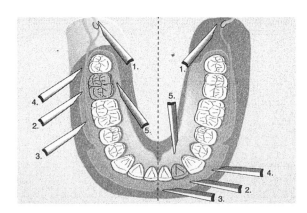

Fig. 19-29 For mandibular surgery, one carpule of anesthetic is injected as a mandibular block (*1*), followed by half a carpule at the apex and half a carpule both mesial and distal of the apex. Finally, half a carpule is injected lingually (*5*).

the most persistent bleeding should have stopped (Fig. 19-31).[6]

Care should be taken to leave the epinephrine-saturated cotton pellet inside the osteotomy to avoid reopening of the ruptured vessels. The combination of both epinephrine and pressure has a synergistic effect, which results in good hemostasis in the bone crypt. As described at the beginning of this chapter, epinephrine causes local vasoconstriction by acting on the α-1 receptors in the membranes of the blood vessels, and the pressure takes advantage of body's clotting mechanism. The epinephrine and cotton pellet should, of course, be removed before the final irrigation and closure of the surgical site. This epinephrine pellet technique is the most efficient and economic technique for hemostatic management in the bone crypt.

Ferric sulfate solution.   Another chemical agent used in hemostasis is ferric sulfate (FS). FS is a hemostatic agent that has been used for a long time in restorative dentistry.[22] Even though its mechanism is still unclear, it is believed that hemostasis occurs by agglutination of blood proteins from the reaction of blood with both ferric and sulfate ions and the acidic pH (0.21) of the solution. The agglutinated proteins form plugs that occlude the capillary orifices. Thus unlike other hemostatic agents, FS affects hemostasis through a chemical reaction with blood. Ferric sulfate is an excellent surface hemostatic agent on the buccal plate for small-and-slow bleeders and is readily applied and easily removed by irrigation. The yellowish FS fluid turns into a dark-brown or greenish-brown coagulum immediately upon contact with blood and epinephrine. The color differences are useful for identification of the source of any persistent bleeders. There

are many commercially available FS solutions. Cutrol has 50% FS, Monsel sol has 70% FS, and Stasis has 21% FS.

FS is known to be cytotoxic and to cause tissue necrosis, but systemic absorption of FS solution is unlikely because the coagulum isolates it from the vascular bed. FS has also been found to damage bone and to delay healing when used in maximum amounts and when left in situ.[45] However, when the FS coagulum is completely removed and the surgical site is thoroughly irrigated with saline immediately after the hemostasis and before closure, there is no adverse reaction.

Because the epinephrine-saturated cotton pellet technique is very effective in bone crypt management, clinicians seldom use FS solution first. However, when there is a persis-

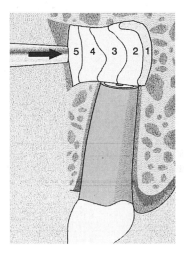

Fig. 19-30 In the epinephrine-saturated cotton pellet technique, one Racellet pellet is placed into the bone crypt, followed by sterile cotton pellets. These pellets must be pressed hard with a blunt instrument (e.g., back of mirror handle) for about 3 minutes.

Box 19-1   Topical Hemostats

Mechanical agents
  Bone Wax (Ethicon, Somerville, NJ)
Chemical agents
  Epinephrine-saturated cotton pellets and other
    vasoconstrictors
  Ferric sulfate solution
Biologic agents
  Thrombin USP (Thrombostat, Thrombogen)
Absorbable hemostatic agents
  Intrinsic action
    1. Gelfoam (The Upjohn Co., Kalamazoo, MI)
    2. Absorbable collagen
    3. Microfibrillar collagen hemostats
  Extrinsic action
    1. Surgicel (Johnson & Johnson, New Brunswick,
      NJ)
  Mechanical action
    1. Calcium sulphate

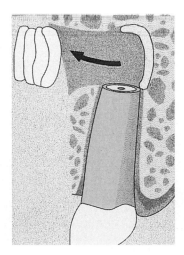

Fig. 19-31 After 3 minutes, cotton pellets are removed one by one, leaving the epinephrine-saturated cotton pellet in place. Ultrasonic retropreparation can begin once hemostasis is established.

tent bleeding despite of the epinephrine and cotton pellet technique, FS solution is applied to the bone crypt. The most frequent use of FS solution is the bone surface hemostasis for small bleeders around the bone crypt on the buccal plate. Brushing FS solution onto the buccal surface around the bone crypt just before retrofilling ensures hemostasis during this important procedure.

Calcium sulfate paste. Hemihydrate medical grade calcium sulfate (CS) is not designed as a topical hemostat. However, CS paste functions well as an effective hemostat by mechanically blocking open vessels (i.e., tamponade effect). Initially developed as a bone-inductive agent, it is absorbed by the body after approximately 2 to 3 weeks. CS comes as a powder and a mixing solution, which can be mixed to make a thick, pasty pellet the size of the osteotomy. After placing the pellet into the bone it is tamped down with a moist cotton pellet. CS paste hardens quickly and the excess is removed, exposing the root apex for further surgery. After the surgery the CS is left in the bone cavity, where it acts as a barrier to the faster-growing soft tissue and potentially aids bone regeneration by providing a matrix for the osteoblasts.[69,70] CS is an excellent agent for a large bone crypt that does not respond to the other methods of hemostasis.

Other commercially available hemostats. Inexpensive epinephrine-saturated cotton pellets, FS solution, and CS paste have been found to provide excellent local hemostasis during surgery. Many other commercially available topical hemostats include bone wax, Thrombin, Gelfoam, Collagen, microfibrillar collagen, Hemostat (MCH), and Surgicel. These hemostats are no more effective than the ones described earlier, but they are considerably more costly. Instead of describing the detailed mechanisms of these agents, Fig. 19-32 illustrates the main point of action in the hemostasis cascade. Calcium sulfate paste, bone wax, and Surgicel achieve hemostasis through a tamponade effect by mechanically blocking open vessels, whereas epinephrine

causes vasoconstriction by activating a-adrenergic receptors. Gelfoam, made of animal skin gelatin, acts intrinsically by promoting the disintegration of platelets, causing a subsequent release of thromboplastin. Collagen is known to aggregate platelets, which then release coagulation factors.[81] These and plasma factors help form fibrin and subsequently a clot. Thrombin is a protein that acts rapidly in an intrinsic fashion, combining with fibrinogen to form blood clots. One product worth mentioning is MCH. It is prepared from bovine corium, which promotes rapid hemostasis by attracting platelets.

Benefits of the cotton pellet technique. The topical hemostats, FS, and epinephrine are applied with a cotton pellet matrix. There are several other materials, such as the Telfa pad (Kendall Co., Mansfield, MA) and CollaCote (Cal-Citek, Plainsboro, NJ), and other hemostats, such as Avitene (Johnson & Johnson, New Brunswick, NJ). The hemostat's active ingredient is collagen, which promotes clotting. None of these products are problem free. A concern is that any cotton fibers that remain in the bone crypt may cause inflammation and, therefore, retard healing.[14] The Telfa pad and CollaCote also have loose fibers, and the collagen preparations are only marginally effective. In addition, all of the brand name products are costly. Although the cotton pellets are not perfect, they are a convenient, inexpensive, and an effective means to apply hemostats. With the aid of the microscope any loose fibers are easily removed from the bone crypt before closure.

Recommended Hemostatic Technique for Endodontic Microsurgery

The most important method of achieving good hemostasis begins with effective local anesthesia and vasoconstriction (as described earlier). When using local hemostats the clinician should wait 2 to 3 minutes for the body-clotting mechanisms to become fully effective. If the anesthesia is profound, achieving local hemostasis

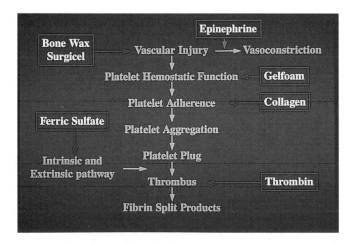

Fig. 19-32 Summary of events in hemostasis and the action of topical hemostats.

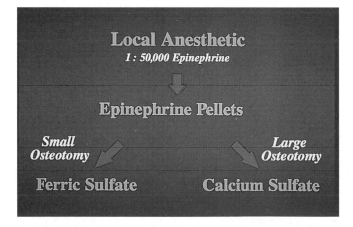

Fig. 19-33 Recommended hemostatic techniques for endodontic microsurgery.

during the surgery is ensured. Fig. 19-33 demonstrates the following recommended steps:

1. Local anesthetic technique using 2% lidocaine with 1:50,000 epinephrine
2. Epinephrine-saturated cotton pellets for additional hemostatic control in the osteotomy
3. FS solution application for osteotomies smaller than 5 mm
4. CS paste application in osteotomies larger than 5 mm

Postsurgical Hemostasis

To avoid postsurgical bleeding, it is important that hemostasis be maintained after the flap is sutured. An ice-cold, wet, sterilized gauze placed over the sutures helps stabilize the flap and control oozing of the blood from the surgical sites. The gauze should be placed into the mucobuccal fold for about 1 hour and an ice pack should be applied to the cheek 10 minutes on, 5 minutes off, for 1 to 2 days.

SOFT-TISSUE MANAGEMENT

The soft-tissue management consists of flap design, incision, elevation, retraction, repositioning, and suturing.

At least two reasons exist for properly managing soft tissues when performing endodontic surgery: (1) to gain adequate access to the surgical site and (2) to ensure good post-surgery healing. To achieve these goals the surgeon must be able to choose the proper flap design, make a precise incision, elevate and retract the flap with minimum trauma to the tissue, and reposition and suture the flap precisely into its original position.

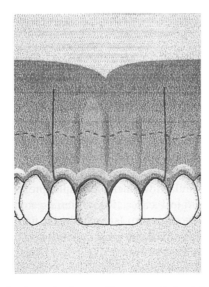

Fig. 19-34 A schematic diagram illustrates sulcular full-thickness flap design. The *shaded* tooth is the problem tooth, the *solid line alone* represents the incision line for a triangular flap; the *dotted line with the solid line* represents the incision line for a rectangular flap.

FLAP DESIGNS

The two major categories of flap designs are (1) sulcular full-thickness flap (or full mucoperiosteal flap) and (2) mucogingival flap design (or limited mucoperiosteal flap).[14,32,58] Two different terminologies may confuse some readers. The sulcular full-thickness flap (i.e., full mucoperiosteal flap) design calls for reflecting the entire soft tissues, attached gingiva, midcol and mucosa, and overlying the cortical plate with the horizontal incision being an intrasulcular incision. The mucogingival flap design or limited mucoperiosteal flap design calls for reflecting one half of the attached gingiva close to the mucobuccal fold, leaving the remaining one half of the attached gingiva intact around the root and the sulcus.

Sulcular Full-Thickness Flap

This flap design involves horizontal and vertical incisions. The horizontal incision extends from the gingival sulcus, through the fibers of the periodontal ligament to the crestal bone (Fig. 19-34). The incision should pass through the midcol area separating the buccal and lingual papillae (Fig. 19-35). The vertical incision should be firmly against cortical bone between the root eminences, because the mucoperiosteum is thin over the root eminence and tears easily.

This flap design provides the best access to all surgical sites in the oral cavity and can be a triangular flap with one vertical releasing incision or a rectangular flap with two vertical releasing incisions (Figs. 19-36 and 19-37).

The rectangular design may be better for anterior teeth than the triangular design because it provides better access to the root apex, especially when the root is long (Fig. 19-38). When the rectangular design is used, the base of the flap should be as wide as the top so that the incision follows the direction of the tissue fibers and blood vessels. In this manner the least number of fibers and blood vessels are severed, thus the sutured incisions will heal quickly with virtually no

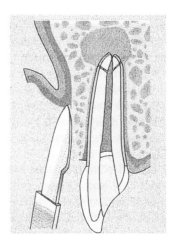

Fig. 19-35 Sagittal view of the sulcular full-thickness flap design. Note that no attached gingiva remains around the neck of the crown.

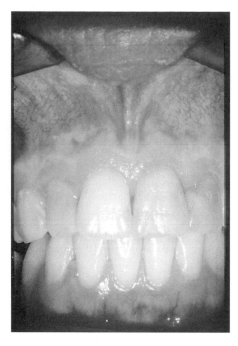

Fig. 19-44 At the 6-month checkup hardly any scar of the mucogingival flap is present.

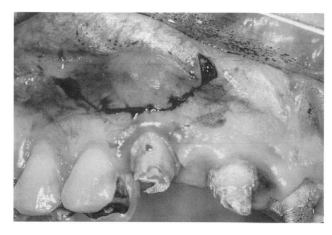

Fig. 19-45 Semilunar incision (if used at all) is used only for incision and drainage.

Semilunar Flap

This flap design was used widely in the past; however, it is not generally recommended now. Some limited value may exist in uncommon situations (e.g., for incision and drainage) (Fig. 19-45). The semilunar flap is rarely used because it does not allow for adequate access to the surgical site and often leaves a noticeable scar (Fig. 19-46).

INCISION

When making a full-thickness flap, the clinician begins the vertical-releasing incision at the line angle (see Fig. 19-36), pressing firmly enough to ensure the scalpel is cutting down to the cortical bone. A 15C Bard-Parker blade makes this incision efficiently and precisely, tracing the fiber lines in the mucosa. The base of the flap should be as wide as the top of the flap so that the majority of the blood vessels, also distributed vertically along the fiber lines, can adequately perfuse the flap. For the sulcular incision the gingival margin must also be incised fully and carefully, tracing the contours of the margin. The interproximal papillae must be cut sharply toward the lingual extension, tracing the root contour. Failure to follow the tooth neck contour closely causes blunting of the papillae after healing, which raises esthetic concerns, especially in the anterior region. For these reasons miniblades (e.g., Beaver blades) are recommended because their size permits a more precise incision in the tight interproximal spaces. However, the miniblade is not recommended for

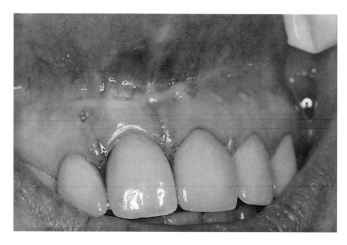

Fig. 19-46 A permanent mucosal scar resulting from a semilunar flap incision is esthetically unacceptable. This flap design should not be used in endodontic surgery.

a vertical releasing incision because it is too small; the Bard-Parker 15C blade is better choice for this purpose.

FLAP ELEVATION

Once the horizontal and releasing incision or incisions have been made, the mucoperiosteum is elevated and reflected with a sharp elevator. The elevators P 14S or P 9HM (G Hartzell & Son Co.) are placed underneath the gingiva at the line angle. The mucoperiosteum is lifted away from the alveolar bone by gently lifting the elevator toward the apex while it is under the flap (Fig. 19-47). The sharp, wide end of the elevator is placed at a 45-degree angle to the cortical bone surface; the mucoperiosteum is reflected apically with a slow, firm, controlled peeling motion *closely tracing the cortical bone contours*. The surfaces of the buccal cortical plates are

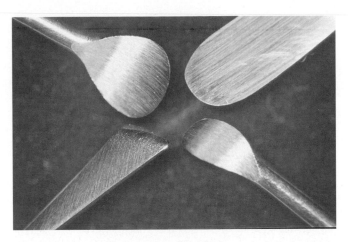

Fig. 19-47 An enlarged view of various soft-tissue elevator tips. They are sharp and thin, with different shapes and sizes.

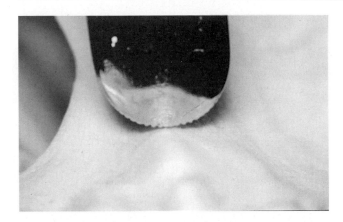

Fig. 19-48 Problems with using a retractor on a convex bone. It does not follow the contour of the buccal bone.

not flat and smooth; there are many irregularities including bone eminences, concavities, and fenestrations. These irregularities, if not carefully negotiated, can easily contribute to tearing or perforating the flap during the reflection. Elevation of the flap with a sudden or uncontrolled force, such as accidental slippage, will damage the tissue; great care should be taken to avoid this. Normally, a flap shrinks a certain degree while it is separated from the bone. In addition to shrinking, a traumatized flap will also swell, making it difficult to place it back to its original position without additional trauma. A perforated or torn flap will be difficult to suture. Therefore during flap elevation experienced surgeons will place a piece of moist gauze underneath the initially reflected flap and gently push at the gauze with an elevator for smooth flap elevation. A properly elevated flap will show minimal bleeding.

FLAP RETRACTION

Flap retraction, usually performed by an assistant, must be done adroitly to maintain a clear view and unimpeded access to the operating site. Frequent slippage and repositioning of the retractor causes tearing and traumatizes the retracted flap.[33] Improper retraction interrupts the surgeon's concentration, compromising a smooth execution of the surgical procedure. This becomes more important during microscopic surgery, because readjustment of the microscope will prolong the surgery.

The retractor should be chosen for the specific purpose and to fit the anatomy of the cortical plate. None of the retractors available today are completely satisfactory. Currently available retractors are too narrow at the tip, causing the retracted tissue to overhang into the surgical site, thus hindering access. The second major problem is that all retractor tips are convex. Where the cortical bone protrudes the convex retractor is an unstable anchor, because the only

point of contact with the bone is the small area at the top of the curve (Fig. 19-48).

Retractors in Endodontic Microsurgery

These new retractors, called KP retractors, (Figs. 19-49 and 19-50) have wider (15 mm) and thinner (0.5 mm) serrated working ends. Some are concave and some are convex to accommodate the irregular contours of the buccal plate (Fig. 19-51). The serrated tips provide better anchorage on the bone and prevent accidental slipping (see Fig. 19-50). In addition, the surfaces of the retractors are matte so that the light from the microscope is not reflected. The KP-1 retractor has a V-shaped working end to fit the bone eminences in the maxillary molar and mandibular incisor regions. The KP-2 retractor has a slight concavity in the center and is curved gently inward to accommodate the slight bone eminences found in the maxillary canine region. The KP-3 retractor tip has a slight convexity that is well suited for the mandibular premolar and molar bone anatomy. These retractors have greatly eased the assistant's job of retracting, resulting in less fatigue, less tissue trauma, and less operating time. However, even with these stable retractors, apicoectomy on a mandibular premolar or molar brings the edge of the retractor dangerously close to the mental foramen. This danger has been overcome by a simple procedure, the groove technique. Recently other manufacturers have designed retractors that are every bit as good as the KP retractors (and may be less expensive). The reader is urged to become familiar with all brands.

Repositioning of the Flap

At the completion of the surgical procedure the retracted tissue is carefully repositioned with tissue forceps. Occasionally, inexperienced surgeons may suture the flap in the wrong position. Care should be taken to confirm the proper position before suturing. After repositioning the flap, a

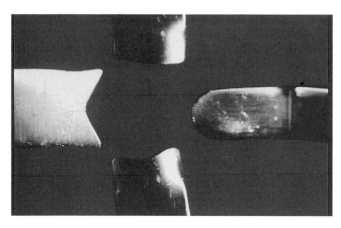

Fig. 19-49 KP-endodontic retractor series. The blades are 15 mm wide; they are thin and convex or concave to follow the contours of the buccal cortical plate.

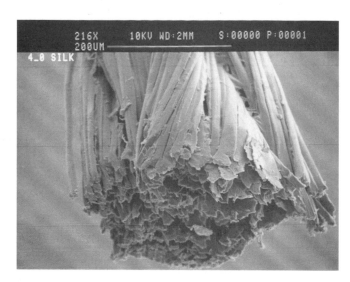

Fig. 19-52 SEM shows wicking effect of silk sutures.

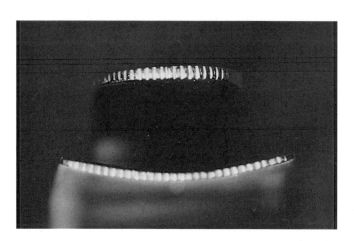

Fig. 19-50 Close view of the KP retractors that have a thin, serrated blades for a firmer grip.

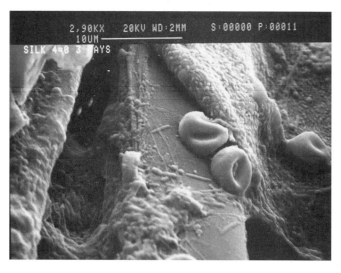

Fig. 19-53 SEM shows bacterial colonization of a silk suture.

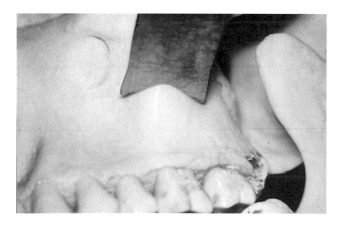

Fig. 19-51 The KP-2 follows the contour of the convex maxillary posterior region for more secure tissue retraction.

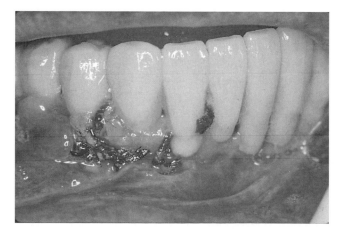

Fig. 19-54 A 4-0 silk suture is braided; thus it easily collects plaques and bacteria.

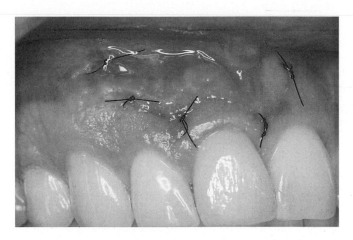

Fig. 19-55 Little or no plaque accumulation can be found around the 5-0 monofilament synthetic suture for microsurgery.

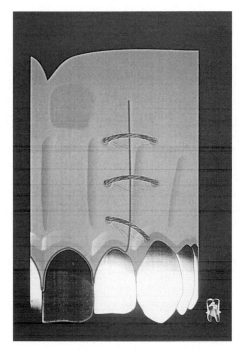

Fig. 19-56 A schematic drawing of the interrupted suturing technique used in a vertical-releasing incision.

chilled (with ice water), damp gauze pad is placed firmly on the flap with finger pressure to remove accumulated blood and fluids from underneath the flap. A clean, bloodless surgical site will aid in the accurate repositioning of the flap. As the flap shrinks during the surgery, especially if the surgery lasts a long time, it may have to be stretched for proper adaptation and first be sutured at strategic points. The first strategic suture is placed into the free ends of the triangular or rectangular flap. Another suture is placed just above the free ends to reduce the tension on the free ends. The third strategic suture is a sling suture around the tooth central to the

flap. After the flap has reassumed its original size, the remaining sutures can be placed.

SUTURE MATERIALS AND SUTURING TECHNIQUES

A variety of suture materials is on the market today. Although silk is still most commonly used, the newer synthetic nonfilament sutures are strongly recommended. Silk sutures are braided and exhibit a wicking effect that accumulates bacterial plaques (Fig. 19-52).[47] Silk sutures cause severe inflammation in the incision site (Figs. 19-53 and 19-54).[14,46,48]

Synthetic monofilament sutures, such as Supramid and Monocryl, have no wicking effect, resulting in a better, more predictable postoperative outcome (Fig. 19-55). The preferred suture size is 5-0 or 6-0. Monofilament sutures have the same working characteristics (e.g., smoothness, flexibility) as 4-0 silk sutures without the risk of causing inflammation.

Resorbable gut sutures are not recommended, except when the patient cannot return for suture removal. In the past, sutures were removed in 4 to 7 days after the surgery. Currently, removal of the sutures is recommended within 48 hours.[14] Regardless of the suture materials, the patient must keep the surgical site as clean as possible by frequent rinsing with warm salt water and chlorhexidine to prevent any plaque accumulation after the surgery.

Clinicians should be familiar with two simple suturing techniques: interrupted (Fig. 19-56) and sling. The vertical-releasing incision is sutured with interrupted sutures; the interproximal and sulcular incisions are sutured with sling sutures. In the sling-suturing technique the buccal gingival papilla is pierced with a ⅜-inch circle or straight 5-0 suture needle that is then brought through the interproximal space of the tooth. The suture is then led around the lingual and interproximal aspects of the tooth to go through the adjacent buccal papilla. The path is now reversed to arrive at the first buccal papilla, where a knot is made to secure the suture.

The value of using a microscope with this procedure is marginal, because the site for suturing is readily seen by with 3.5 × to 4.5 × telescopes (see Chapter 5). Suturing under the microscope provides negligible added advantage, except when a 6-0 or smaller sutures are used. The 6-0 sutures are generally used for crowned maxillary anterior teeth where gingival esthetics and crown margins are always a concern.

OSTEOTOMY

Osteotomy (i.e., the removal of the facial cortical plate to expose the root end) must be approached with a visualized 3-D mental image to ensure it is made exactly over the apices. The first step is to expose periapical radiographic images perpendicular to the roots from two different horizontal angles. This is done to ascertain the length and curvature of the roots, the position of the apices in relation to the crown, and the number of roots. Additionally, the proximity of each apex to the apices of adjacent teeth, the mental foramen, the inferior alveolar nerve, and the antrum can be ascertained. Once the flap has been raised, the clinician should superimpose the visualized mental image gained from the radiographs and clinical examination onto the cortical plate.

If unsure of the exact location of the apex, the surgeon should do the following:

1. Mark the probable apex position on the buccal plate using the radiograph as a guide.
2. Make a 1-mm deep indentation with a no. 1 round, high-speed bur and fill it with a small amount of radiopaque material, such as gutta-percha. A radiograph exposed with this marker in place will show the marker in relation to the root apex.

Only when the surgeon is certain of the exact location of the apex (cortical topography is an excellent guide in the anterior region) is the cortical bone removed slowly and carefully with copious water spray under low magnification (2.5 × to 6 ×). The H 161 Lindemann bone cutter and the Impact Air 45 hand piece are best suited for making an osteotomy (Fig. 19-57). The bone cutter bur is specially designed to remove the bone while keeping the frictional heat to a minimum. It has fewer flutes than conventional burs, which results in less clogging and more efficient cutting. The advantage of the Impact Air 45 hand piece is that water is directed along the bur shaft, while air is ejected out of the back of the hand piece (see Fig. 19-57). This creates less splatter than conventional hand pieces and decreases the chance of tissue emphysema and pyemia.

The microscope clearly distinguishes the root tip from the surrounding bone. The root has a darker, yellowish color and is hard, whereas the bone is white, soft, and bleeds when scraped with a probe. When the root tip cannot be distinguished from its surroundings, the osteotomy site is stained with methylene blue, which preferentially stains the periodontal ligament. The absence of a distinct periodontal liga-

ment (PDL) stain at midmagnification (10 × to 12 ×) indicates that the root tip has not yet been exposed. Because the apex is generally small in relation to the osteotomy, the surgeon must be very observant of even the smallest color-and-texture change within the bone.

Optimal Osteotomy Size

Because even a small osteotomy looks large at the higher magnifications of 8 × to 16 ×, a tendency exists to want to make the osteotomy even smaller. With the availability of microsurgical instruments, the new criteria for the size of an osteotomy is "just large enough to manipulate ultrasonic tips freely within the bone crypt." Because the length of an ultrasonic tip is 3 mm, the ideal diameter of an osteotomy is about 4 to 5 mm, leaving just enough space to manipulate the ultrasonic tip and microinstruments within its confines (Fig. 19-58).

Periradicular Curettage

Periradicular curettage does not eliminate the origin of the lesion—it only relieves the symptoms temporarily. Nevertheless, the granulomatous soft tissue must be removed completely before the apex is resected. Once the lesion and the root tip are exposed, Columbia no. 13 and no. 14 curettes or Molt or Jaquette 34/35 curettes are used to remove the granulation (or cystic) tissue completely under medium magnification (10 × to 16 ×).

APICAL RESECTION

Apical resection (root end resection or apicoectomy) is a straightforward procedure. Once the bone crypt is free of granulation tissue and the root tip is clearly identified, 3 mm of the root tip is resected perpendicular to the long axis of the root. This is best done at low magnification of 4 × to 8 × with

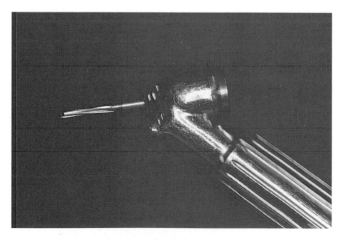

Fig. 19-57 An Impact Air 45-degree hand piece with a Lindenmann bone-cutting bur. These are ideal instruments for osteotomy.

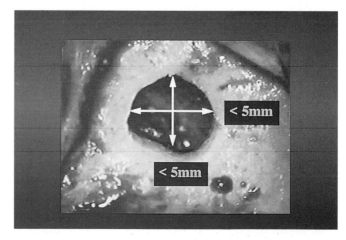

Fig. 19-58 Optimal osteotomy size of 4 to 5 mm in diameter for free movement of 3 mm long, ultrasonic tips.

the Lindemann bur in an Impact Air 45 hand piece using copious water spray. The only caveat here is to try to resect perpendicular to the long axis of the root, especially with lingually inclined roots. After the resection the root surface is examined at midmagnification (10× to 12×) for the presence of the periodontal ligament. This is done to verify that the entire root tip has been removed. If the PDL is not clearly visible as a complete circle around the root surface, a methylene blue stain is helpful to identify the ligament. If the stained PDL is visible only around the buccal aspect, the resection must be extended deeper lingually.

There are two important elements to consider with this procedure: (1) extent of apical resection, and (2) bevel angle.

Extent of Apical Resection (Apicoectomy)

The amount of root tip to resect depends on the incidence of lateral canals and apical ramifications at the root end. The author examined this question using the Hess model of root anatomy. Using a computer system the roots of the Hess models were resected 1, 2, 3, and 4 mm from the apex, counting the incidence of lateral canals and apical ramifications at each level. (Fig. 19-59 illustrates the results.)

Only when 3 mm of the apex is resected are lateral canals reduced by 93%. Additional resection reduced the percentage insignificantly.[76] A root resection of 3 mm at a 0-degree bevel angle removes the majority of anatomic entities that are potential causes of failure. Any remaining lateral canals are sealed during retrograde filling of the canal. Therefore removing the apex beyond 3 mm is of marginal value and compromises a sound crown/root ratio.

Bevel Angle

Until the early 1990s a bevel angle of 45 degrees would be found in all endodontic textbook illustrations. No biologic basis for this practice existed; the only reasons for its use were to enable the surgeon to (1) gain visual and operating

access for root tip resection, (2) place retrofilling materials, and (3) inspect. These reasons were especially true for operating on lingually inclined roots (e.g., mesiolingual root of mandibular molars). In this process the mesiobuccal root surface was significantly reduced, occasionally causing untreatable periodontic and endodontic communications.

The root resection must be done perpendicular to the long axis of the root whenever possible. Resections not made at 90 degrees result in an uneven or incomplete resection of the apex. The buccal aspect is resected but the lingual part is partially or not resected at all, leaving leaky lateral canals. As shown in Fig. 19-60, resecting along lines 1 and 2 misses some lateral canals and apical ramifications. Only when the resection follows line 3 (i.e., perpendicular to the long axis of the root) are 98% of the apical ramifications and 93% of the lateral canals removed. Because the apices of many teeth (especially maxillary anterior teeth) are tilted slightly lingually, surgeons must approach the resection with this lingual inclination in mind.

The cause of some failed surgeries is a large osteotomy along with an acute bevel angle leading to endodontic and periodontic communications. In some situations (e.g., in the mesiolingual root of the mandibular first molar) a perpendicular bevel may not possible. In such a case, the clinician should use a 10-degree bevel and tilt the patient's head to the side, away from the microscope, for optimal viewing of the apex. (For comparison, a 10-degree bevel and a 45-degree bevel are shown in Fig. 19-61.)

Wide Lingual Root Extensions

Many roots, especially maxillary premolars and the mesial roots of mandibular molars, extend rather deep lingually (Fig. 19-62). One cause of surgical failure in these teeth is a root resection that does not extend deeply enough (i.e., lingually), thereby leaving the lingual aspect of the root unresected.[12,14] With extreme lingual anatomy it is difficult to see the lingual border of the resected root end, even at high mag-

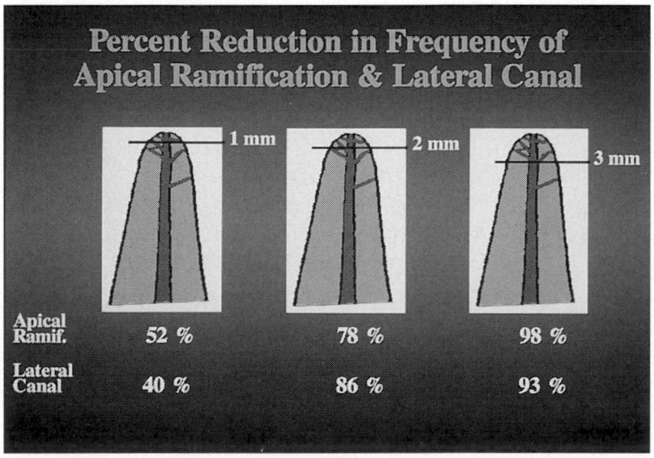

Fig. 19-59 A schematic diagram illustrates percent reduction in frequency of apical ramification and lateral canals.

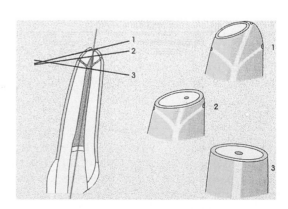

Fig. 19-60 Apical resections must be performed perpendicular to the long axis of the roots when possible. Section level no. 1 and no. 2 result in incomplete root resection; only section level no. 3 eliminates all accessory canals.

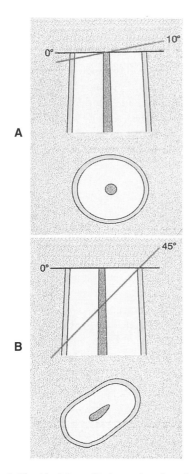

Fig. 19-61 **A**, The ideal 0- to 10-degree bevel angles used in microsurgery. **B**, The 45-degree (or more) bevel angles advocated in traditional surgery is biologically undesirable and structurally destructive.

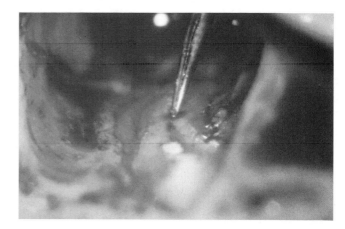

Fig. 19-62 Long buccolingual extension of a posterior tooth. After 3 mm of apical resection, the remaining root will have an ovoid appearance.

nification. Under these conditions, the root surface should be stained with methylene blue and reexamined at midmagnification of 10 × to 12 ×. The stained PDL should clearly outline the most lingual aspect of the root.

Cleaning and Drying the Apical Preparation

Before the introduction of the Stropko air/water syringe tip (designed by Dr. John Stropko), it was difficult to clean the apical preparation of blood and tissue debris (Fig. 19-63). The Stropko air/water syringe tip permits the controlled introduction of air, water, or saline into the apical preparation, so it can be rinsed and dried easily and effectively (Fig. 19-64). When microscopic amounts of water are left in the line, an atomized droplet of water may be sprayed in the preparation when the air button is pressed. The option of two Stropko irrigators and dryers, one for rinsing only and the second for drying only, eliminates this minor problem and adds versatility and precision to the surgical armamentarium.

The irrigator and drier replaces the standard three-way tip on most air-and-water syringes and accepts most Luer-Loc needle attachments. For example, the Stropko air/water

syringe tip is compatible with the following: Ultradent tips, Monojet endodontic irrigating needles, Monojet 27-gauge needles, and Maxiprobe 30-gauge needles.

Is Apical Root Resection Really Necessary?

Because the major cause of periapical lesions is a leaky apical seal allowing the egress of microorganisms and their toxins, periradicular curettage only eliminates the effect of the leakage, not the cause. Periradicular curettage alone (without apical resection) will invite the recurrence of the lesion. Apical surgery, therefore, entails not just the removal of the diseased tissue or the root tip, but most importantly, the retrofilling and resealing of the root canal system. If the entire root canal system could be cleaned and totally sealed every time, the endodontic success rate would be 100% and endodontic surgery would not be required. In reality, however, the complexity of the root canal system, especially in the apical region, prevents a 100% success for nonsurgical endodontic therapy. Thus when treating such failures surgically, periradicular curettage *must* be followed by a root end resection and retrograde sealing with a biocompatible material.

Microinspection of the Resected Root Surface

One of the most important advantages of using the microscope in endodontic surgery is the ability to inspect the resected root surface under high magnification (16 × to 25 ×) with a CX-1 microexplorer.[36] To enhance the anatomic structures, the resected root surface is stained with a methylene blue–soaked cotton swab.[14,36] After removing the excess stain with saline, the periodontal ligament and leaky areas are clearly defined by the blue stain. Frequently seen anatomic details are isthmuses, C-shaped canals, accessory

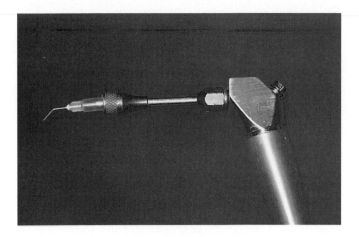

Fig. 19-63 The Stropko drier is designed to dry the bone crypt, resected root surface, and retropreparation with precision.

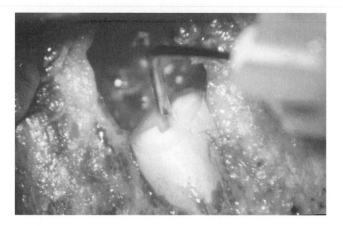

Fig. 19-64 The Stropko drier applied at the retroprepared cavity. (Courtesy Dr. R. Rubinstein.)

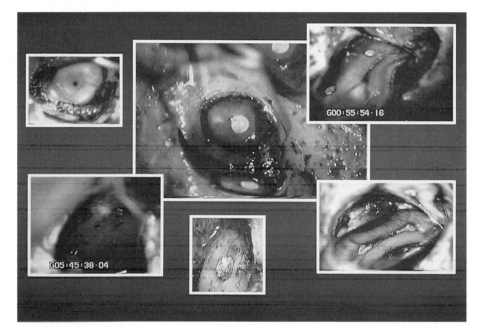

Fig. 19-65 Composite picture of the resected root surfaces stained with methylene blue dye and reflected in a micromirror under the microscope. All pictures are 16 × to 24 × . They show microleakage, four apices, and a microfracture.

canals, canal fins, apical microfractures, and leaky canals with partial seals of gutta-percha (Fig. 19-65).Careful examination of the resected root surface at high magnifications (16 × to 25 ×) is essential. Once the defects, anatomic or iatrogenic, are identified they can be treated.

Benefits of the Methylene Blue Staining Technique

Methylene blue is applied to the dry, resected root surface with a microapplicator tip (Fig. 19-66). After a few seconds the root and the bone crypt are rinsed with isotonic saline to remove the excess stain. This is followed by drying with a Stropko drier. The stained area can then be examined under the microscope at 10 × to 12 × magnification. If the entire root tip has been resected, the PDL can be identified as an unbroken line around the root surface (see Fig. 19-65, *middle*). A partial line indicates that only part of the root has been resected. If there is no definable line, it probably means that only bone has been stained. The staining also helps to distinguish craze lines from microfractures. Microfractures stain; craze lines do not. A microfracture can also be confirmed with a microexplorer. If the explorer tip catches, it is a fracture; if it does not, it is a craze line.

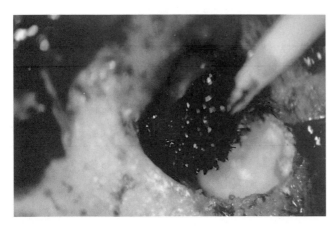

Fig. 19-66 Clinic view of methylene blue application with a microapplicator on a dried, resected root surface (16 ×).

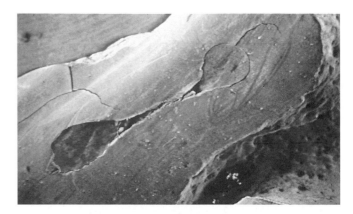

Fig. 19-67 SEM showing an isthmus. (Courtesy Dr. G. Carr.)

ISTHMUS

A common finding of resected root surfaces of posterior teeth is an isthmus,[36] which is a narrow connection between two root canals usually containing pulp tissue (Fig. 19-67). The isthmus has been called a "corridor" by Green,[28] a "lateral connection" by Pineda,[60] and an anastomosis by Vertucci.[76] In many teeth with a fused root there is a weblike connection between two canals called an isthmus, which can be either complete or incomplete. At 3 mm from the apex, isthmuses are often found to merge two canals in one root.[28,36,60] Thus the isthmus is a part of the canal system and not a separate entity; accordingly, it must be cleaned, shaped, and retrosealed.

Isthmus Characteristics

Examination of many resected root surfaces during endodontic microsurgery and careful *in vitro* microscope examinations of resected root surfaces of extracted human teeth reveal many different isthmus forms:

- Type 1, classified as an incomplete isthmus, is a barely traceable communication between two canals.
- Type 2 is a definite connection between the two main canals. A Type 2 complete isthmus can be a straight line between two canals or a C-shaped connection.
- Type 3 is a complete but very short connection between two canals. A Type 3 isthmus sometimes looks like one elongated canal.
- Type 4 can be either complete or incomplete, but it connects three or more canals instead of two. Incomplete isthmuses connecting three canals in a C-shape are also included in this category.
- Type 5 isthmuses include two or three canal openings on an elongated ovoid root surface, which do not have any visible connections even after being stained. The dilemma with a root surface of this type is whether to treat it as

though an isthmus connected the canals or to treat the canal orifices only. The absolute absence of any visible staining between the canals examined at high magnification (16 × to 25 ×) indicates the absence of an isthmus, so only the canal orifices need to be treated.

Sometimes seemingly separate canal orifices are connected microscopically when examined under scanning electron microscopy (SEM); therefore some endodontic surgeons treat this microscopic connection as an isthmus. In the absence of controlled clinical study results regarding the healing outcome of treated versus untreated microscopic connections between apical canals, the issue whether to treat or not to treat remains unresolved.

Isthmus Frequency

The incidence of isthmuses in mandibular anterior teeth appear to be relatively low at 15%.[79,83] In the maxillary premolar group, the incidence of isthmuses increases as the resections are made (progressing coronally). This variability is not the same in mandibular premolars where the isthmus frequency is constant at approximately 30%, beginning with 2 mm from the apex.[79] In the maxillary first molar, over 60% of the mesiobuccal roots have two canals.[78] In a 1994 study, 50 maxillary first molar mesiobuccal roots of extracted teeth were randomly selected, cut into 1 mm cross sections (beginning at the apex), and examined at 25 × magnification.[79]

Two types of isthmuses were found: (1) complete (i.e., Type 2) and (2) incomplete (i.e., Type 1). The incidence of these isthmuses (combining Types 1 and 2) accounted for over 45% at 3 mm from the apex and 50% at 4 mm from the apex (Fig. 19-68). A frequency of isthmus in premolars of both arches was almost 30% at 3 to 4 mm level. In the mesial root of the mandibular first molar, approximately 70% of the 3 to 4 mm sections contain isthmuses (Fig. 19-69). By contrast only 15% of the distal roots have isthmuses at the 3 mm level (Fig. 19-70).

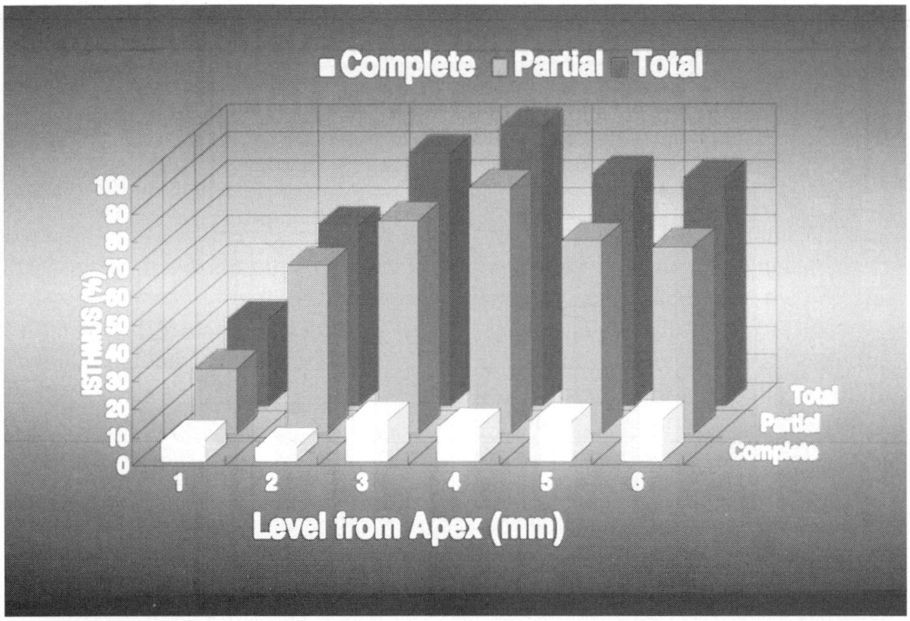

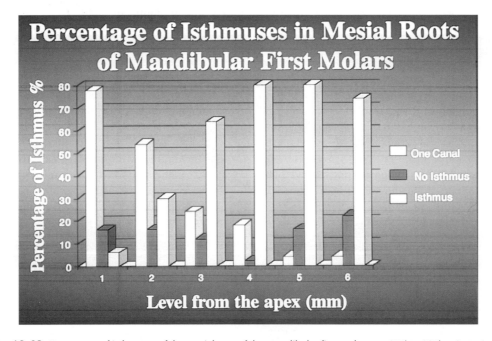

Fig. 19-68 Diagram illustrates over 45% of MB-roots of the maxillary first molar at 3- to 4-mm level have isthmuses.

Fig. 19-69 Frequency of isthmuses of the mesial root of the mandibular first molar was 65% to 80% at 3- to 4-mm level.

Isthmus Preparation with Ultrasonic Tips

Ultrasonic tip preparation is the only way to carve an isthmus.[13,14,21,36] This requires a careful and delicate approach, because the isthmus is located in the thinner portion of the root, which can easily be perforated or stripped. The ultrasonic tip with a diameter of less than 0.2 mm is the best tip to treat the isthmus without causing procedural mishaps.

Occasionally, the dental surgeon encounters an incomplete isthmus (Fig. 19-71, *A*). It is helpful in this case to provide a guideline for the ultrasonic tip by creating a shallow groove along the isthmus line with a microexplorer (Fig. 19-71, *B*). This is called a tracking groove.[14] The ultrasonic tip is first activated without water coolant to make a tracking groove connecting the two canals, which are

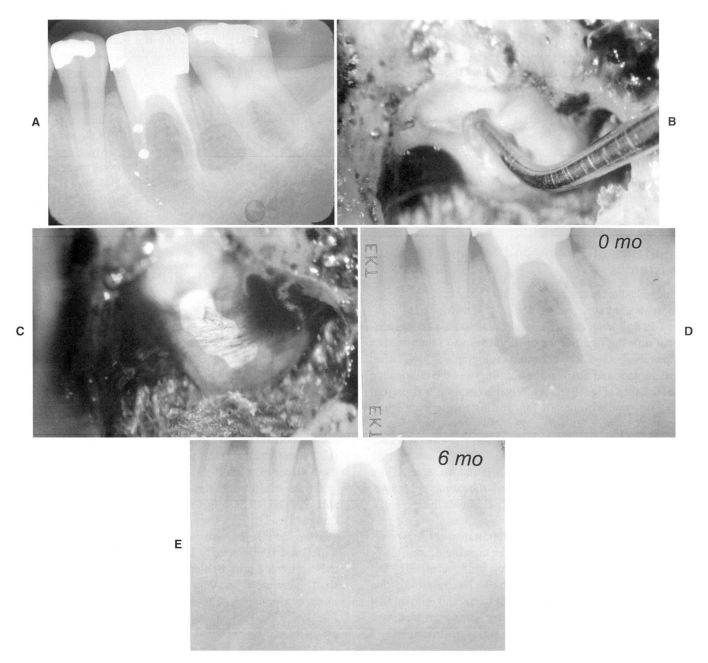

Fig. 19-72 **A**, The first molar had apical surgery 1 year earlier; now it is failing. Two round amalgam retrofillings are visualized in the mesial root with a PAR. **B**, High magnification (16 ×) of isthmus retropreparation with an ultrasonic instrument. The cause of the failure was missing an isthmus. **C**, Retrofilling of the isthmus in **B** with Super EBA (16 × magnification). Note the elongated retrofilling covering two apices and connecting isthmus. **D**, Immediately postoperative. **E**, Six months later, significant healing with no symptoms is observed.

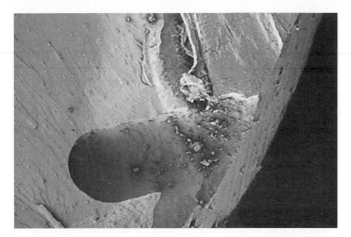

Fig. 19-73 Sectioned longitudinal view demonstrates how the axial wall of the preparation (instead of the pulpal floor of the preparation) seals off the canal.

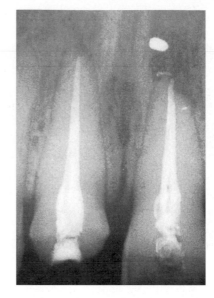

Fig. 19-76 A floating amalgam retrofilling.

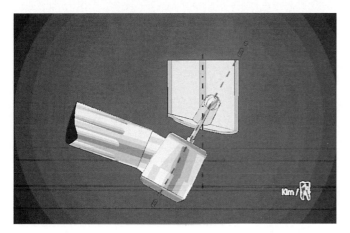

Fig. 19-74 Schematic diagram illustrates retropreparation with a bur; the preparation does not predictably follow the long axis of the canal, thus risking lingual perforations.

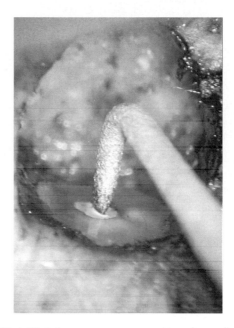

Fig. 19-77 A KiS-1 tip retroprepares a root. Note the small osteotomy and the cutting end of the 3 mm KiS-1 tip.

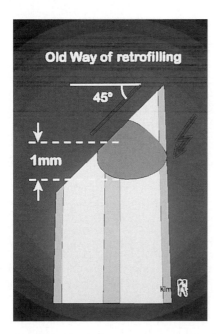

Old Way of retrofilling

45°

1mm

Fig. 19-75 Schematic diagram illustrates 45-degree bevel with the bur preparation; this unnecessarily removes root structure and risks perforation.

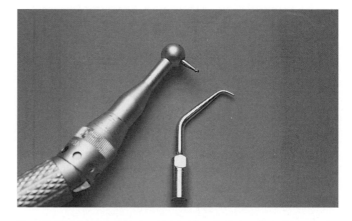

Fig. 19-78 Size comparison of a microhandpiece and an ultrasonic tip.

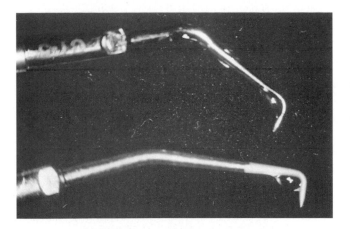

Fig. 19-79 CT/KiS tip comparison.

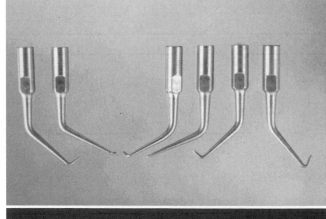

A

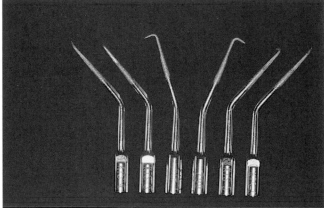

B

Fig. 19-81 **A,** Full set of CT-1, 2, 3, 4, and 5 tips (*left to right*) and CK-back action tip (*far right*). **B,** KiS-1, 2, 3, 4, 5, 6 tips (*left to right*).

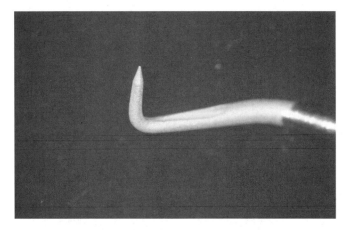

Fig. 19-80 A KiS tip shows zirconium nitride coating (*gold*) and the irrigation port near the tip.

Ultrasonic Root End Preparation

This procedure is accomplished under the microscope at low-to-mid magnifications (4 × 16 ×). First, a number of appropriate tips are preselected, depending upon the location of each apex. Second, the resected root surface, stained with methylene blue, must be critically examined at high magnification (16 × to 25 ×) to see the microanatomy. Third, at low magnification (4 × to 6 ×), the selected ultrasonic tip is positioned at the apex. It is important at this stage that the tip is positioned parallel with the long axis of the root. To accomplish this the surgeon must examine the position of entire tooth at low magnification (4 ×), including the crown and root eminence and compare this with the position of the ultrasonic tip. Failure to make this comparison will risk an off-angle root end preparation or perforation. Fourth, the ultrasonic tip is activated and the apical canal is retroprepared with copious water coolant to a depth of 3 mm. If an ultrasonic tip is pressed too firmly it is dampened to deactivation, thus a light sweeping motion using short forward-

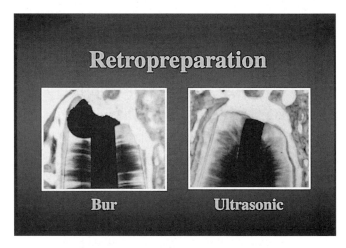

Fig. 19-82 Histologic picture of the bur preparation (*left*) and ultrasonic preparation.

and-backward and up-and-down strokes is all that is needed for effective cutting action. Depending on the canal configuration, a typical 3 mm retropreparation should take less than 1 minute with KiS tips.

Once the retropreparation is completed, the cavity preparation is inspected with a micromirror at high magnification

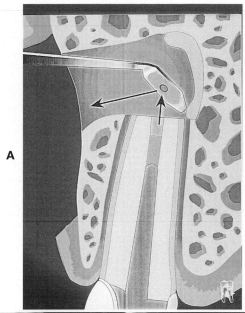

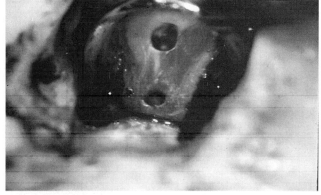

Fig. 19-83 **A**, Schematic diagram illustrates the way inspection of the retropreparation is performed. **B**, Retroprepared two apices reflected on the micromirror at 16 × viewed through the microscope. (Courtesy Dr. R. Rubinstein.)

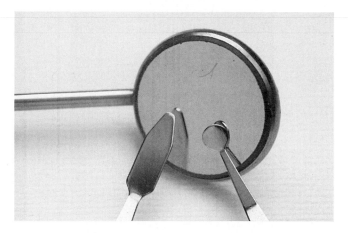

Fig. 19-84 Size comparison of a dental mirror with two most useful micromirrors (3-mm diameter; round and elongated, rectangular).

of 16 × to 25 × (Fig. 19-83, *A* and *B*). A thorough inspection should include the interior canal walls for remnants of gutta-percha, especially on the difficult-to-reach facial wall, and confirmation that the parallel walls are sharply defined and smooth.

Micromirrors

One of the key instruments in microsurgery is the micromirror[12,14] (Fig. 19-84). The reflective surface is made of either highly polished stainless steel or sapphire. The mirrors are small enough to fit into an osteotomy measuring no larger than 4 to 5 mm in diameter. Inspection of root ends cannot be performed thoroughly without the aid of micromirrors. The anatomy of the root surface is reflected in the micromirror into the viewing range of the microscope before and after the retropreparation (see Fig. 19-83, *B*).

INSPECTION OF THE ROOT END PREPARATION

For depth of field purposes, the root end is best prepared at low-to-mid magnification (8 × to 12 ×). However, the preparation must be inspected at high magnification (16 × to 25 ×). Uncommonly, retropreparations can also be inspected by direct view. In addition to examining the completed preparation for clean, sharply defined walls, it should also be examined one last time for important anatomic structures (e.g., accessory canals, microfracture) that may have escaped detection during the initial inspection.

DEPTH OF THE ROOT END PREPARATION

The optimal depth of the root end preparation should be 3 mm; however, depths of 1, 2, and 4 mm have also been studied.[27] Using the Hess model slides provided by Dr. N. Perrini, the incidence of lateral canals and apical ramifications in the natural apex have been studied; over 95% of these anatomic entities are found within the apical 3 mm (see Fig. 19-59). Although a retropreparation deeper than 3 mm does not provide any greater benefits, a retropreparation shorter than 3 mm may jeopardize the long-term success of the apical seal. Fig. 19-85 illustrates the management of the apical 6 mm:3 mm root resection perpendicular to the long axis of the root and retropreparation and retrofilling of 3 mm parallel the long axis of the root. Each is essential to ensure an adequate seal of the root apex.

COMPACTION OF GUTTA-PERCHA IN THE RETROPREPARED CAVITY

Ultrasonic vibrations generate heat that may thermoplasticize gutta-percha. The remnants of gutta-percha have to be

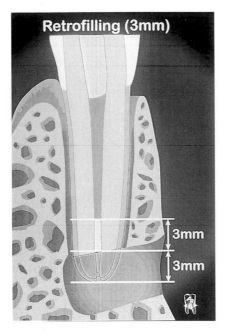

Fig. 19-85 Schematic diagram illustrates the principles involving the retropreparation and retrofilling.

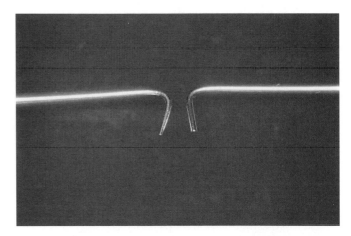

Fig. 19-86 Working tips of the microcondensers; diameter is 0.2 mm, length is 0.3 mm.

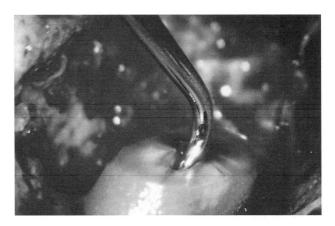

Fig. 19-87 A microcondenser compacting gutta-percha.

compacted well to a 3 mm depth with microcondensers. There are many different types of microcondensers with different handles, but their working tips are basically the same, with a 0.2 mm diameter and a 3 mm length (Figs. 19-86 and 19-87). The retroprepared canals must be void of any gutta-percha or debris for the final filling.

PROPERTIES FOR AN IDEAL RETROFILLING MATERIAL

The purpose of placing a retrograde filling is to provide a tight, biocompatible apical seal, which prevents the leakage of potential irritants from the root canal into the periradicular tissues. Numerous publications support various materials as ideal retrofilling materials.[81,82] Box 19-2 is a revised outline of the ideal properties for retrofilling materials originally proposed by Dr. L.I. Grossman.[29]

Throughout dental history a wide variety of materials have been used for retrograde fillings. Box 19-3 lists of some of the materials that have been or are currently being used as retrograde fillings. Although a plethora of materials is available, no material has been found that fulfills all or most of the properties for the ideal retrograde filling material.

Amalgam had been the most popular and widely used retrograde filling material since the last century. It is easy to manipulate, readily available, well tolerated by soft tissues, radiopaque, and initially provides a tight apical seal. However, its disadvantages are significant: it is slow setting, dimensionally unstable, eventually leaks from corrosion, and stains overlying soft tissues causing a tattoo.

Thus other (and better) materials, such as intermediate restorative material (IRM), Super EBA, or mineral trioxide aggregate (MTA) are replacing amalgam. Most recently, MTA has shown great promise as a retrofilling material. Histologic examination of bone response to MTA showed remarkable bone regeneration not seen with other retrograde filling materials.[74]

Only retrofilling materials that have been found to be acceptable, based upon what is known today, will be considered. These materials include Super EBA, IRM, MTA, and some composite resins.

ZINC OXIDE–EUGENOL CEMENTS

As early as 1962, Nicholls[53] showed preference for zinc oxide–eugenol cement over amalgam. The original zinc oxide–eugenol cements were weak and had a long setting

Box 19-2 IDEAL PROPERTIES FOR RETROFILLING MATERIALS

Ideal retrograde filling materials:
- Should be well tolerated by periapical tissues
- Should adhere (i.e., ideally bond) to the tooth structure
- Should be dimensionally stable
- Should be resistant to dissolution
- Should promote cementogenesis
- Should be bacteriocidal or bacteriostatic
- Should be noncorrosive
- Should be electrochemically inactive
- Should not stain tooth or periradicular tissue
- Should be readily available and easy to handle
- Should allow adequate working time, then set quickly
- Should be radiopaque

Box 19-3 RETROGRADE FILLING MATERIALS

- *Amalgam
- *Gutta-percha
- *Gold foil
- *Titanium screws
- Glass ionomers
- Ketac silver
- Zinc oxide–eugenol
- *Cavit
- Composite resins
- *Polycarboxylate cement
- PolyHEMA
- Bone cements
- IRM
- Super EBA
- Mineral Trioxide Aggregate (MTA)

* No longer recommended based on what the literature shows in 2001.

time. When used as a retrograde filling, the cement tended to be absorbed over time because of its high water solubility.

When zinc oxide–eugenol cement is in contact with water or tissue fluids, it is hydrolyzed to produce zinc hydroxide and eugenol. The eugenol will continue to be removed by leaching until all the original zinc eugenolate is converted to zinc hydroxide. After this hydrolysis, the free eugenol may have several undesirable effects depending on its concentration. Eugenol can competitively inhibit prostaglandin synthetase by preventing the biosynthesis of cyclooxygenase. It inhibits sensory nerve activity, inhibits mitochondrial respiration, kills a range of native oral microorganisms, and can be an allergen. To overcome some of these problems, zinc oxide–eugenol cements were modified.

Intermediate Restorative Material IRM is zinc oxide–eugenol cement reinforced by the addition of 20% polymethacrylate by weight to the powder.[39] The reinforcement eliminated the problem of absorbability; IRM was found to have a milder reaction than unmodified zinc oxide–eugenol cement. In a tissue tolerance study it was found that IRM elicited a mild-to-zero inflammatory effect after 80 days.[8] The conclusion was that oral tissue is just as tolerant to IRM as to any other retrograde filling material. Because IRM was found to be relatively biocompatible it has been used as an endodontic retrograde filling. In a retrospective study on retrograde filling materials, IRM was found to have a statistically significant higher success rate compared to amalgam.[19]

To further improve IRM as a retrograde filling material, hydroxyapatite was added because of its biocompatibility with bone.[56] The addition of 10% and 20% hydroxyapatite to IRM produced a significantly better seal than amalgam; however, it was not significantly different from plain IRM. The addition of hydroxyapatite to IRM increased its disintegration rate; this is a distinct disadvantage. Its disintegration may allow leakage of potential irritants from the root canal

into the periapical tissues. Because unmodified IRM does not disintegrate it can be used as a retrograde filling material.

Super Ethoxybenzoic Acid Super EBA is a zinc oxide–eugenol cement modified with EBA[39] to alter the setting time and increase the strength of the mixture. The cement was modified by the partial substitution of eugenol liquid with ortho-ethoxybenzoic acid and the addition of fused quartz or alumina to the powder. Stailine Super EBA (Stailine, Staident, Middlesex, England) contains 60% zinc oxide, 34% silicone dioxide, and 6% natural resin in the powder component, along with 62.5% EBA and 37.5% eugenol in the liquid. In the United States, the most similar formulation is Bosworth's Super EBA cement, which has the same contents except for silicone dioxide that is substituted by 37% aluminum oxide (i.e., alumina), making the cement stronger. Stailine Super EBA has a neutral pH, low solubility, and is radiopaque. EBA is the strongest and least soluble of all zinc oxide–eugenol formulations. It yields a high compressive and tensional strength.

Tissue tolerance studies show that the Super EBA and eugenol cements produce similarly mild reactions. It has been demonstrated *in vitro* that EBA cement produces a tight seal compared with amalgam, glass ionomer cement, and hot-burnished gutta-percha.[26] Leakage studies demonstrated that Super EBA allowed significantly less leakage than amalgam.[5,54] Oynick and Oynick[57] reported that Super EBA is nonresorbable and radiopaque.

Super EBA cement has a very good adaptation to the canal walls compared to amalgam. However, Super EBA is a difficult material to manipulate because the setting time is short and greatly affected by humidity. It tends to adhere to all surfaces, so there may be difficulty in placing and compacting. To date there is little data regarding the most effective method of manipulating Super EBA to achieve a tight seal.

Preparation and placement of IRM. IRM (a good alternative to super-EBA) is comparatively easy to handle. A thicker mix than usual is placed into the prepared cavity using a carrier; it is packed with a microball burnisher under 10 × magnification. Burnishing is followed by a deeper compaction using microcondensers. More IRM is added and burnished a second time to complete the retroseal.

Preparation and placement of Super EBA. Super EBA is comparatively difficult to mix and handle. The liquid and powder are mixed in a 1:4 ratio (Fig. 19-88). The powder is mixed into the liquid slowly in small increments. When the mixture is thick but still shiny, additional powder has to be added. When the rolled Super EBA mixture loses its shine and the tip does not droop when picked up by an EBA carrier (Fig. 19-89), the mixture has the right consistency. A small portion is picked up and placed directly into the dried, retro-

prepared cavity at 10 × magnification (Fig. 19-90, *A*). Now the Super EBA is packed with the microball burnisher on the other end of the carrier (Fig. 19-90, *B*), followed by deeper compaction using microcondensers of appropriate sizes. Placement and packing are repeated two to three times; excess Super EBA is carved away with excavators. The retrosealed root surface may be polished with a fine-diamond bur under copious water spray for a smooth finish (Fig. 19-90, *C*). In view of the recent report[24] that burnishing Super EBA without polishing provides a better seal, the pol-

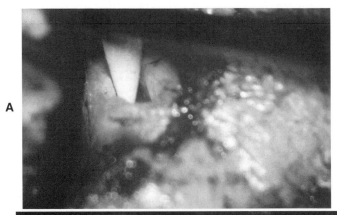

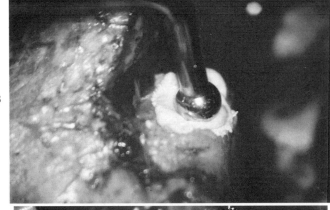

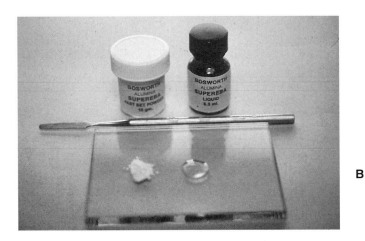

Fig. 19-88 Super EBA cement: liquid and powder on a glass slab. Proper mixing of the material requires practice.

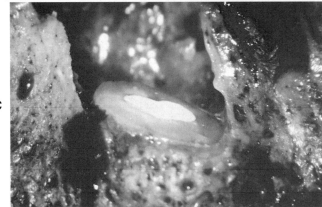

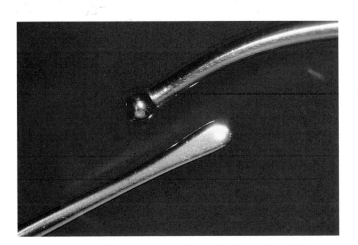

Fig. 19-89 Enlarged view of a retrofilling carrier; one end has a flat surface (*bottom*); the other end has a burnisher (0.4 mm diameter).

Fig. 19-90 **A**, A small portion of rolled Super EBA is picked up and placed directly into the retroprepared cavity. **B**, Super EBA is packed with a microball burnisher at 10 ×. **C**, Polished Super EBA surface is examined carefully for defects under mid- to high-magnification. (Courtesy Dr. R. Rubinstein.)

ished surface should be reexamined under high magnification to ensure that the seal remained intact.

Mineral Trioxide Aggregate

Based on many well-designed studies, MTA was introduced as a retrograde filling material.[71,72,73,74,75] MTA powder consists of fine hydrophilic particles. The principle compounds present in this material are tricalcium silicate, tricalcium aluminate, tricalcium oxide, and silicate oxide. In addition, small amounts of other mineral oxides exist that are responsible for the chemical and physical properties of this aggregate. Bismuth oxide powder has been added to make the aggregate radiopaque. Electron probe microanalysis of MTA powder showed that calcium and phosphorous are the main ions present in this material. Because MTA has a high pH similar to calcium hydroxide cement, it is not surprising that induction of hard-tissue formation often occurs after the use of this substance as a retrograde filling material.

The sealing ability of MTA has been shown to be *superior* to that of amalgam or even Super EBA[75]; it is not adversely affected by blood contamination. MTA in contact with periradicular tissue forms fibrous connective tissue and cementum, causing only low levels of inflammation. The regeneration of *new cementum* over MTA is a *unique phenomenon* that has not been reported with other root end fillings.[72,74] The mechanism for the formation of cementum over MTA is unclear. MTA possibly activates cementoblasts to produce a matrix for cementum formation. This might be caused by its sealing ability, its high pH, or the release of substances that activate cementoblasts to lay down a matrix for cementogenesis.

The use of MTA has many advantages:
1. Least toxic of all the filling materials
2. Excellent biocompatibility
3. Hydrophilic
4. Reasonably radiopaque.[71,72,74,75]

The disadvantages of MTA are that it is more difficult to manipulate and has a long setting time.

MTA placement technique. The ultrasonic cavity preparation remains the same. The bone crypt should be packed with a sterile cotton pellet or similar materials, exposing only the resected root surface; this allows easy removal of excess MTA after compaction. The bone crypt must not be irrigated after placing the MTA to avoid washing it out.

To prepare the MTA a small amount of liquid and powder are mixed to putty consistency. Because the MTA mixture is a loose granular aggregate (it has been likened to concrete cement), it does not stick very well to itself or to any instrument (Fig. 19-91, *A*). MTA cannot be carried to the cavity using a normal cement carrier; it has to be carried with a Messing gun, amalgam carrier, or other specially designed carrier. Once the MTA is placed into the retropreparation, microball burnishers and microplugger are used to gently compact it (Fig. 19-91, *B* and *C*). Unless compacted very gently the loosely bound aggregate will be pushed out of the cavity. Next, a small damp cotton pellet is used to gently clean the resected surface and to remove any excess MTA from the cavity (Fig. 19-91, *D*). Finally, the retrofilled area is reexamined under 16 × magnification (Fig. 19-91, *E*).

Composite Resins

Since 1990, certain composite resins have been advocated as the retrofilling material of choice.[50,62,63] Studies on the long-term success and physical properties of composites are impressive.[50,62,63] However, for maximum performance of the composites, the bone crypt and the retroprepared cavities must be absolutely dry; composites are very technique sensitive. Although the microsurgical techniques (including the use of the Stropko drier) have greatly improved drying within the surgical site, the majority of clinicians have difficulty in obtaining and maintaining a totally dry bone crypt. Composite resins (e.g., Geristore) can be an alternative to Super EBA, IRM, or MTA; however, because they are so technique sensitive, they have not been widely adopted by endodontic surgeons.

POSTOPERATIVE SEQUELAE

Surgical sequelae include pain, swelling, ecchymosis, laceration, premature separation of sutures, infection, maxillary sinus perforation, and transient paraesthesia. Calling the patient at home the evening after surgery and the next day is always deeply appreciated. To minimize postsurgical sequelae, oral and written postoperative instructions must be given to the patient and the person accompanying the patient. Because of anxiety and nervousness, patients sometimes misunderstand or simply do not remember the verbal instructions; for this reason written instructions allay confusion or further anxiety.

Pain

Pain is usually not a serious problem. Long-acting anesthetic agents, such as bupivacaine (i.e., Marcaine) or etidocaine (i.e., Duranest), can be injected postoperatively into the surgical site to control pain for a period of up to 8 hours. The reader is referred to Chapter 18 for the preventive ibuprofen or acetaminophen regimen that almost always ensures that any pain will be minimal and transient. Rarely are narcotic analgesics required.

Hemorrhage

Postoperative hemorrhage is rare. To prevent it from occurring, two 2 × 2 sterile gauze pads are folded in half and moistened with chilled, sterile water. This pack is placed over the sutured flap in the buccal fold and pressed by the surgeon with moderate pressure for several minutes. The patient is provided an ice pack to press lightly against the cheek or jaw for at least 30 minutes to constrict the cut microvasculature, minimizes swelling and promotes initial coagulation.

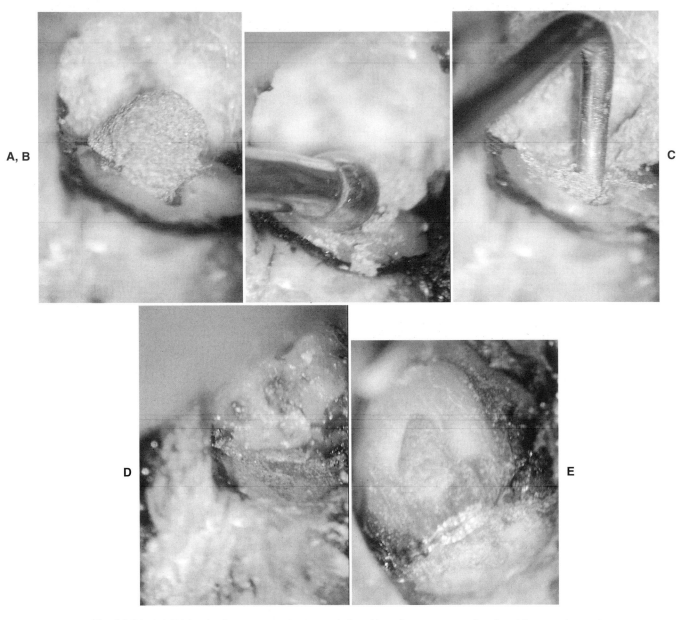

Fig. 19-91 **A**, MTA is mixed to putty consistency and placed into the retroprepared cavity with an amalgam carrier (16 ×). **B**, Packing the MTA with a ball burnisher. **C**, Microplugger (16 ×). **D**, Wiping the resected root surface with a damp cotton pellet eliminates excess MTA. **E**, Final examination of the MTA filling under 16 × magnification to ensure a good seal.

Swelling

Swelling is a common surgical sequelae and is a major concern for the patient. Patients must be informed that the surgical site and face may swell regardless of the home care. Also, patients must be assured that the degree of swelling is not an indication of the success or failure of the surgery or the severity of the case. Intermittent application of ice packs, 10 minutes on and 5 minutes off, for the first 2 days almost always minimizes swelling.

Ecchymosis

Ecchymosis is the discoloration of facial and oral soft tissues because of the extravasation and subsequent breakdown of blood in the interstitial subcutaneous tissues (Fig. 19-92). This is basically an esthetic problem. It is more prevalent in elderly patients with capillary fragility and patients with fair skin.[55,59] Frequently, ecchymosis occurs below the surgical site because of gravity. For instance, the surgical site may be a maxillary premolar, but the ecchymosis may be found in

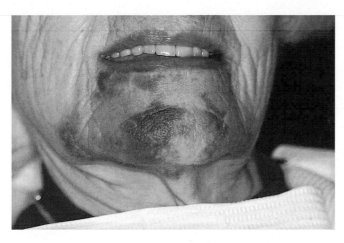

Fig. 19-92   Patient with ecchymosis.

the neck area. The patient should be assured that the ecchymosis has no bearing on the success or severity of case.

Paresthesia

When paresthesia occurs, it is when the mental nerve presents near the second premolar and first molar. However, transient paresthesia may occur even if the surgical site is far from the nerve. Inflammatory swelling of the surgical site may cause temporary impingement on the mandibular nerve causing transient paresthesia. If the nerve has not been severed, normal sensation generally returns within a few weeks. In rare instances, however, it may take a few months to regain normal sensation.[44] The patient should be assured of the probable return of sensation in the affected side; however, on rare occasions paresthesia can be permanent.

Maxillary Sinus Perforation

Perforation of the Schneiderian membrane covering the sinuses may occur. If perforation of the sinus occurs, utmost care should be taken to *prevent any material from entering the sinus.*

The patient should be cautioned not to blow his or her nose and should be instructed to elevate the head during the night. Prophylactic antibiotic therapy with Augmentin 500 mg every 6 hours along with Sudafed for 1 week should be prescribed. The patient should return for a postsurgical checkup in 1 week.

References

1. American Dental Association & American Academy of Orthopedic Surgeons: Advisory statement. Antibiotic prophylaxis for dental patients with total joint replacements, *J Am Dent Assoc* 128(7):1004, 1997.
2. Arens D et al: *Endodontic surgery*, Philadelphia, 1981, Harper and Row.
3. Barkhordar R et al: Cyanoacrylate as a retrofilling material, *Oral Surg* 65:468, 1988.
4. Barnes I: *Surgical endodontics: Color manual*, Boston, 1991, Wright.
5. Bates C, Carnes DL, del Rio CE: Longitudinal sealing ability of mineral trioxide aggregate as root-end filling material, *J Endod* 22(11):575, 1996.
6. Beer R, Baumann M: *Color atlas of dental medicine*, Stuttgart, 1999, Geor Thieme Verlag.
7. Bennett C: *Monheim's local anesthesia and pain control in dental practice, ed 7*, St Louis, 1984, Mosby.
8. Blackman R, Gross M, Seltzer S: An evaluation of the biocompatibility of a glass ionomer-silver cement in rat connective tissue, *J Endod* 15(2):76, 1989.
9. Brynoff I: A histological and roentgenological study of the periapical region of human upper incisors, *Odontol Revy* 18:1, 1967.
10. Buckley J, Ciancio S, McMullen J: Efficacy of epinephrine concentration on local anesthesia during periodontal surgery, *Va Dent J* 49:9, 1972.
11. Cambruzzi J, Marshall F: Molar endodontic surgery, *J Can Dent Assoc* 1:61, 1983.
12. Carr G: Common errors in periradicular surgery, *Endod Rep* 8:12, 1993.
13. Carr G: Ultrasonic root end preparation, *Dent Clin North Am* 41:541, 1997.
14. Carr G, Bentkover S: Surgical endodontics. In Cohen S, Burns RC, editors: *Pathways of pulp*, ed 7, St Louis, 1994, Mosby.
15. Chivian N: Surgical endodontics: conservative approach, *J NJ State Dent Soc* 40:234, 1969.
16. Cutright DE, Hunsuck EE: Microcirculation of the perioral regions in the Macaca rhesus: part 1, *Oral Surg* 29:776,1970.
17. Dajani AS et al: Prevention of bacterial endocarditis. Recommendations by the American Heart Association, *JAMA* 277(22):1794, 1997.
18. Dionne R et al: Suppression of postoperative administration of ibuprofen in comparison to placebo, acetaminophen and acetaminophen plus codeine, *J Clinic Pharmacol* 23:37, 1983.
19. Dorn SO, Gartner AH: Retrograde filling materials; a retrospective success-failure study of amalgam, EBA and IRM, *J Endod* 8:391, 1990.
20. Ehrich DG et al: Comparison of triazolam, diazepam and placebo as outpatient oral premedication for endodontic patients, *J Endod* 23(3):181, 1997.
21. Engle T, Steiman H: Preliminary investigation of ultrasonic root end preparation, *J Endod* 21:443, 1995.
22. Evans B: Local hemostatic agents, *N Y State Dent J* 47:109, 1977.
23. Flanders D, James G, Burch B, Dockum N: Comparative histopathologic study of zinc-free amalgam and Cavit in connective tissue of the rat, *J Endod* 1:56, 1975.
24. Forte SG, Hauser MJ, Hahn C, Hartwell GR: Microleakage of super-EBA with and without finishing as determined by the fluid filtration method, *J Endod* 24(12):799, 1998.
25. Frank A, Glick D, Patterson S, Weine F: Long-term evaluation of surgically placed amalgam fillings, *J Endod* 18(8):391, 1992.

26. Gartner AH, Dorn SO: Advances in endodontic surgery, *Dent Clin North Am* 36:357, 1992.

27. Gilheany P, Figdor D, Tyas M: Apical dentin permeability and microleakage associated with root end resection and retrograde filling, *J Endod* 20:22, 1994.

28. Green D: Double canals in single roots, *Oral Surg* 35:689, 1973.

29. Grossman L: *Endodontic practice,* ed 7, Philadelphia, 1970, Lea & Febiger.

30. Grossman L: Intentional replantation of teeth: a clinical evaluation, *J Am Dent Assoc* 104:633, 1966.

31. Grossman L, Oliet S, Del Rio C: *Endodontics,* ed 11, Lea & Febiger, 1988.

32. Gutmann JL, Harrison JW: *Surgical endodontics,* St Louis-Tokyo, 1994, Ishiyaku EuroAmerica.

33. Harrison J, Jurosky K: Wound healing in the tissues of the periodontium following periradicular surgery. II. The dissectional wound, *J Endod* 17:544, 1991.

34. Hersh EV et al: Single dose and multidose analgesic study of ibuprofen and meclofenamate sodium after third molar surgery, *Oral Surg Oral Med Oral Pathol* 76(6):680, 1993.

35. Hirsh J et al: Periapical surgery, *Int J Oral Surg* 8:173, 1979.

36. Hsu YY, Kim S: The resected root surface. The issue of canal isthmuses, *Dent Clin North Am* 41(3):529, 1997.

37. Jesslen P, Zetterqvist L, Heimdahl A: Long-term results of amalgam versus glass ionomer cement as apical sealant after apicoectomy, *Oral Pathol* 79:101, 1995.

38. Johnson J, Anderson R, Pashley D: Evaluation of the seal of various amalgam products used for root-end fillings, *J Endod* 21:505, 1995.

39. Jou Y, Pertl C: Is there a best retrograde filling material? *Dent Clin North Am* 41:555, 1997.

40. Kim S: Principles of endodontic surgery, *Dent Clin North Am* 41(3):481, 1997.

41. Kim S: *Regulation of blood flow of the dental pulp: macrocirculation and microcirculation studies, doctoral dissertation,* New York, 1981, Columbia University.

42. Kim S, Edwall L, Trowbridge H, Chien S: Effects of local anesthetics on pulpal blood flow, *J Dent Res* 63:650, 1984.

43. Kim S, Rethnam S: Hemostasis in endodontic microsurgery, *Dent Clin North Am* 41(3):499, 1997.

44. Kohn MW, Chase DC, Marciani RD: Surgical misadventures, *Dent Clin North Am* 17:533, 1973.

45. Lemon R, Steel P, Jeansonne B: Ferric sulfate hemostasis: effect on osseous wound healing: I. Left in situ for maximum exposure, *J Endod* 19:170, 1993.

46. Lilly G, Amstrong J, Cutcher J: Reaction of oral tissues to suture materials. Part III. *Oral Surg* 28:432, 1969.

47. Lilly G et al: Reaction of oral tissues to suture materials. II. *Oral Surg* 26:592, 1968.

48. Lilly G et al: Reaction of oral tissues to suture materials. Part IV, *Oral Surg* 33:152, 1972.

49. Malamed S: *Handbook of local anesthesia,* ed 4, St Louis, 1996, Mosby.

50. McDonald N, Dumsha T: A comparative retrofill leakage study utilizing a dentin bonding material, *J Endod* 13:224, 1987.

51. Mountcastle VB: *Medical physiology,* ed 12, St Louis, 1968, Mosby.

52. Nelson L, Mahler D: Factors influencing the sealing behavior of retrograde amalgam fillings, *Oral Surg* 69:356, 1990.

53. Nicholls E: Retrograde filling of root canal, *Oral Surg* 15:463, 1962.

54. O'Connor R, Hutter J, Roahen J: Leakage of amalgam and super-EBA root-end fillings using two preparation techniques and surgical microscopy, *J Endod* 21:74, 1995.

55. Osbon DB: Post-operative complications following dentoalveolar surgery, *Dent Clin North Am* 17:483, 1973.

56. Owadally ID, Chong BS, Pitt-Ford TR, Wilson RF: Biological properties of IRM with the addition of hydroxyapatite as a retrograde root filling material, *Endod Dent Traumatol* 10(5):228, 1994.

57. Oynick J, Oynick T: A study of a new material for retrograde fillings, *J Endod* 4:203, 1978.

58. Peters L, Wesselink P: Soft tissue management in endodontic surgery, *Dent Clin North Am* 41(3):513, 1997.

59. Peterson L: Prevention and management of surgical complications. In Peterson L, Ellis E, Hupp JR, Tucker MR, editors, *Contemporary oral and maxillofacial surgery,* ed 3, St Louis, 1998, Mosby.

60. Pineda F: Roentgenographic investigation of the mesiobuccal root of the maxillary first molar, *Oral Surg* 36:253, 1973.

61. Rubinstein R, Kim S: Short-term observation of the results of endodontic surgery with the use of a surgical operation microscope and Super EBA as root-end filling material, *J Endod* 25:43, 1999.

62. Rud J et al: Retrograde root filling with composite and a dentin-bonding agent: part 1, *Endod Dent Traumatol* 7:118, 1991.

63. Rud J, Rud V, Munksgaard EC: Retrograde root filling with dentin-bonded modified resin composite, *J Endod* 22:477, 1996.

64. Rud J, Rud V, Munksgarrd EC: Long-term evaluation of retrograde root filling with dentin-bonded resin composite, *J Endod* 22:90, 1996.

65. Schade DS: Surgery and diabetes, *Med Clin North Am* 72(6):1531, 1988.

66. Seymour RA et al: The comparative efficacy of aceclofenac and ibuprofen in postoperative pain after third molar surgery, *Br J Oral Maxillofac Surg* 36(5):375, 1998.

67. Silverton SF: Endocrine disease and dysfunction. In Lynch MA, Brightman VJ, Greenberg MS, editors: *Burket's oral medicine: diagnosis and treatment,* ed 9, New York-Philadelphia, 1997, Lippincot-Raven Publishers.

68. Smith G, Pashley D: Periodontal ligamental injection: evaluation of systemic effects, *Oral Surg* 56:232, 1983.

69. Sottosanti J: Calcium sulfate: an aid to periodontal, implant and restorative therapy, *J Calif Dent Assoc* 20(4):45, 1992.

70. Sottosanti J: Calcium sulfate: a biodegradable and biocompatible barrier for guided tissue regeneration, *Compendium* 13(3):226, 1992.

71. Torabinejad M, Hong CU, Pitt-Ford TR, Kettering JD: Cytotoxicity of four root end filling materials, *J Endod* 21(10):489, 1995.

72. Torabinejad M et al: Histological assessment of MTA as root-end filling in monkeys, *J Endod* 23:225, 1997.

73. Trobinejad M, Pitt-Ford TR: Root end filling materials: a review, *Endod Dent Traumatol* 12:161, 1996.

74. Torabinejad M et al: Tissue reaction to implanted root-end filling materials in the tibia and mandible of guinea pigs, *J Endod* 24(7):468, 1998.

75. Torabinejad M, Higa RK, McKendry DJ, Pitt-Ford TR: Dye leakage of four root end filling materials: effects of blood contamination, *J Endod* 20(4):159, 1994.

76. Vertucci F: Root canal anatomy of human permanent teeth, *Oral Surg* 58:589, 1984.

77. Watzek G, Bernhart T, Ulm C: Complications of sinus perforation and their management in endodontics, *Dent Clin North Am* 41:563, 1997.

78. Weine F et al: Canal configuration in the mesiobuccal root of the maxillary first molar and its endodontic significance, *Oral Surg* 28:419, 1969.

79. Weller RN, Niemczyk SP, Kim S: Incidence and position of the canal isthmus. Part 1. Mesiobuccal root of the maxillary first molar, *J Endod* 21(7):380, 1995.

80. Whal M: Myths of dental surgery in patients receiving anticoagulant therapy, *J Am Dent Assoc* 131:77, 2000.

81. Witherspoon DE, Gutmann JL: Hemostasis in periradicular surgery, *Int Endod J* 29:135, 1996.

82. Yagiela J: Vasoconstrictor agents for local anesthesia, *Anesth Progr* 42:116, 1995.

83. Yu DC, Tam A, Chen MH: The significance of locating and filling the canal isthmus in multiple root canal systems. A scanning electron microscopy study of the mesiobuccal root of maxillary first permanent molars, *Micron* 29(4):261, 1998.

84. Zimmerman BR, Service FJ: Management of noninsulin-dependent diabetes mellitus, *Med Clin North Am* 72(6):1355, 1998.

Chapter 20

 # Management of Pain and Anxiety

Stanley F. Malamed

Chapter Outline

PAIN CONTROL
  Local Anesthetics: How They Work
  "Pulpally Involved" Tooth
  Local Anesthetics: Drugs
  Local Anesthetics: Techniques
  Pain Control: Additional Considerations
ANXIETY CONTROL
  Recognition of Anxiety
  Management of Anxiety

In dental practice, clinicians must manage their patients' pain and anxiety. Studies have demonstrated that fear of pain is one of the major reasons that over 50% of adult Americans do not routinely seek dental care.[32] From interviews with many of these patients it becomes clear that although they may not be in pain when they visit the dentist, a large majority believe that they will experience pain during the dental appointment (and the person most likely to be responsible for the pain is the dentist).

Fear keeps some patients from visiting the dentist until they experience excruciating dental pain. This pain they experience has been shown to be a significant factor in increasing the incidence of life-threatening medical emergencies arising during dental treatment, because it is clinically more difficult to obtain profound pulpal anesthesia when pain or infection has been present for a prolonged period of time.

Table 20-1 presents data obtained from 4309 dentists in independent surveys by Fast[11] and Malamed.[23] These dentists reported an array of 30,608 emergency situations arising in their practices over a 10-year period. Emergencies ranged from benign (e.g., syncope) to the catastrophic (e.g., cardiac arrest). Although specific details of these clinical situations are not available, it can be presumed that as many as 23,105 (75.5%) of the emergencies listed may have been precipitated, in part, by the increased stress (fear or pain) that is so frequently associated with dental treatment. Syncope alone accounted for 50.34% of the reported emergencies. Other potentially "stress-induced" problems included angina pectoris, seizures, acute asthmatic attacks, hyperventilation, car-

diac arrest, myocardial infarction, acute pulmonary edema, cerebrovascular accident, acute adrenal insufficiency, and thyroid storm.

Fear and pain are associated with an increased occurrence of emergency situations, as was further confirmed by Matsuura,[30] who reported that 77.8% of life-threatening systemic complications in the dental office developed either during or immediately after the administration of local anesthesia or during the ensuing dental treatment (Table 20-2). Of those emergencies arising during dental treatment, 38.9% developed during the extraction of teeth and 26.9% occurred during pulpal extirpation (two procedures where adequate pain control is frequently difficult to obtain) (Table 20-3).

In studying which teeth are most difficult to anesthetize, Walton and Abbott[45] found that mandibular molars were implicated in 47% of clinical situations. Malamed,[22] repeating this study at the University of Southern California, found mandibular molars to be "the problem" in 91% of cases of inability to obtain adequate pulpal anesthesia. Table 20-4 compares these two studies.

It appears that the occurrence of sudden and unexpected pain can induce profound changes in the cardiovascular, respiratory, endocrine, and central nervous systems, which may lead (in certain situations) to a potentially significant medical emergency.

The problems of the management of pain and anxiety are closely related. Pain produced by dental treatment can usually be minimized or entirely prevented through thoughtful patient management and judicious use of the techniques of pain control, especially local anesthesia. Anxiety can also be managed effectively in almost all situations; however, before anxiety can be managed, it must first be recognized. Discovery of the cause of a patient's anxiety is *the* major factor in managing the problem. Once aware of a patient's fears, there are many techniques that the dentist can use to care for the patient.

In most areas of dental care the problem of anxiety control is greater than the management of pain. Pain control is almost always obtainable through the administration of local anesthetics. Once adequate pain control is achieved, anxiety control is usually more readily achievable. However, in endodontics (more than in any other dental specialty) pain control often proves to be a more difficult problem than the manage-

Table 20-1 **REPORTED INCIDENCE OF EMERGENCY SITUATIONS BY PRIVATE-PRACTICE DENTISTS DURING A 10-YEAR PERIOD**

	Total
Syncope	15,407
Mild allergic reaction	2,583
Angina pectoris	2,552
Postural hypotension	2,475
Seizures	1,595
Asthmatic attack (bronchospasm)	1,392
Hyperventilation	1,326
"Epinephrine reaction"	913
Insulin shock (hypoglycemia)	890
Cardiac arrest	331
Anaphylactic reaction	304
Myocardial infarction	289
Local anesthetic overdose	204
Acute pulmonary edema (heart failure)	141
Diabetic coma	109
Cerebrovascular accident	68
Adrenal insufficiency	25
Thyroid storm	4

Data from Fast TB, Martin MD, Ellis TM: Emergency preparedness: a survey of dental practitioners, *J Am Dent Assoc* 112:499, 1986; and Malamed SF: Managing medical emergencies, *J Am Dent Assoc* 124:40-53, 1993.

Table 20-2 **TIME OF OCCURRENCE OF REPORTED SYSTEMIC COMPLICATIONS**

Complication	Percentage
Just before treatment	1.5%
During/after local anesthesia	54.9%
During treatment	22.9%
After treatment	15.2%
After leaving dental office	5.5%

Data from Matsuura H: Analysis of systemic complications and deaths during dental treatment in Japan, *Anesth Prog* 36:219-228, 1990.

ment of anxiety. Because of this difficulty in providing effective pain control, the patient undergoing endodontic treatment often anticipates the experience with a great deal of apprehension.

The following discussion covers the dual problems of pain control and anxiety control, with special emphasis on the pulpally involved tooth.

Table 20-3 **TYPE OF DENTAL TREATMENT DURING OCCURRENCE OF COMPLICATIONS**

Treatment	Percentage
Tooth extraction	38.9%
Pulp extirpation	26.9%
Unknown	12.3%
Other treatment	9.0%
Preparation	7.3%
Filling	2.3%
Incision	1.7%
Apicoectomy	0.7%
Removal of fillings	0.7%
Alveolar plastics	0.3%

Data from Matsuura H: Analysis of systemic complications and deaths during dental treatment in Japan, *Anesth Prog* 36:219-228, 1990.

Table 20-4 **INABILITY TO ACHIEVE ADEQUATE PULPAL ANESTHESIA**

	Maxillary		Mandibular	
	Walton and Abbott	Malamed	Walton and Abbott	Malamed
Molars	12%	5%	47%	91%
Premolars	18%	2%	12%	0%
Anteriors	2%	2%	9%	0%

Data from Malamed SF: *Handbook of local anesthesia*, ed 4, St Louis, 1997, Mosby; and Walton RE, Abbott BJ: Periodontal ligament injection: a clinical evaluation, *J Am Dent Assoc* 103:571, 1981.

PAIN CONTROL

Although achieving adequate pain control for endodontic care is not usually difficult, there are all too many instances when a satisfactory result eludes the dentist. Indeed, many of the queries posted in dental discussion groups on the Internet deal with exactly this problem: the patient with the "hot" tooth and the dentist's inability to provide satisfactory pain control. The most likely explanation for the greater number of anesthetic failures in endodontics than in other areas of dental care lies in the tissue changes that commonly develop in and around pulpally involved teeth.

Table 20-5   DISSOCIATION CONSTANTS (PK$_a$) OF LOCAL ANESTHETICS

Agent	pK$_a$	Base (RN) at pH 7.4 (%)	Approximate Onset of Action (min)
Mepivacaine	7.6	40	2–4
Etidocaine	7.7	33	2–4
Articaine	7.8	29	2–4
Lidocaine	7.9	25	2–4
Prilocaine	7.9	25	2–4
Bupivacaine	8.1	18	5–8
Tetracaine	8.5	8	10–15
Chloroprocaine	8.7	6	10–15
Procaine	9.1	2	14–18

RN, unchanged molecule.

Table 20-6   LIPID SOLUBILITY OF LOCAL ANESTHETICS

Agent	Approximate Lipid Solubility	Usual Effective Concentration (%)
Procaine	1	2–4
Mepivacaine	1	2–3
Prilocaine	1.5	4
Lidocaine	4	2
Bupivacaine	30	0.5–0.75
Tetracaine	80	0.15
Etidocaine	140	0.5–0.75
Articaine	—	—
Chloroprocaine	—	—

Local Anesthetics: How They Work

Injectable local anesthetics are acid salts; the weakly alkaline and poorly water-soluble local anesthetic being combined with hydrochloric acid to form the hydrochloride salt (e.g., lidocaine HCl), which is quite soluble in water and slightly acidic.

In solution, local anesthetic exists in two ionic forms: (1) an uncharged anion (RN) and (2) a positively charged cation (RNH$^+$). The relative proportions of each ionic form depend on the pH of the anesthetic solution and the tissue, and on the pK$_a$ of the specific local anesthetic. The pK$_a$ is that pH value at which the local anesthetic solution contains 50% of each ionic form. The pK$_a$ for a given local anesthetic is a constant (pK$_a$s for commonly used local anesthetics are presented in Table 20-5). Because pK$_a$ is a constant, the relative proportion of RN and RNH$^+$ ionic forms will depend on the pH of the anesthetic solution.

$$RNH^+ \longleftrightarrow RN + H^+$$

As the pH of the local anesthetic decreases (becomes more acidic), H$^+$ ion concentrations increase and the equilibrium shifts toward the charged cationic form. Proportionally more cation is present than free base. Conversely, as the pH of a local anesthetic solution becomes more basic (pH increases), the H$^+$ concentration decreases, and a proportionally greater percentage of local anesthetic exists in the RN form.

At the normal tissue pH of approximately 7.4 there exists a greater proportion of local anesthetic cation (RNH$^+$) (see Table 20-5). Both ionic forms of the local anesthetic are essential for its anesthetic activity.[41,42]

Several factors are responsible for the ultimate anesthetic profile of a local anesthetic. These include (1) diffusion of the local anesthetic through the lipid-rich nerve sheath (i.e., pK$_a$ and lipid solubility) and (2) binding of the local anesthetic at the receptor site (i.e., protein binding, nonnervous tissue diffusibility, intrinsic vasodilator activity).[9] The lipid-soluble RN ionic form is able to diffuse more readily through the lipoid-rich nerve sheath than does the water-soluble RNH$^+$ ionic form. Indeed, (clinically) local anesthetics with a lower pK$_a$ (more RN ionic forms) possess a more rapid onset of action than do local anesthetics with higher pK$_a$'s (see Table 20-5).

The degree of lipid solubility appears to be important in determining the intrinsic potency of a local anesthetic (Table 20-6). Increased lipid solubility permits the anesthetic to penetrate the nerve sheath (which is 90% lipid) more easily.[4] This is reflected clinically as increased potency. Local anesthetics with greater lipid solubility produce more effective conduction blockade at lower concentrations (e.g., 2% vs. 4%) than do less lipid-soluble anesthetics.

After penetration of the lipid-rich nerve sheath by the RN ions, a reequilibrium occurs between the RN and RNH$^+$ ionic forms, both outside and within the nerve sheath. Within the nerve itself, the RNH$^+$ ions bind to the (protein) drug receptor site located within the sodium channel. Binding of the anesthetic molecule to this receptor site is responsible for (1) suppression of the electrophysiologic events occurring in propagation of a nerve impulse and (2) the duration of anesthetic activity of the drug. Proteins comprise approximately 10% of the nerve membrane. Local anesthetics (e.g., bupivacaine, etidocaine) possessing greater degrees of protein binding (Table 20-7) than others (e.g., procaine) attach more firmly to protein drug receptor sites and provide longer durations of anesthesia.

Fig. 20-1 illustrates the sequence of events involved in peripheral nerve block in normal tissues. At a pH of 7.4, an anesthetic with a pK$_a$ of 7.9 reaches equilibrium in the tissues with approximately 75% of its molecules in the RNH$^+$ ionic form and 25% in the RN ionic form. The RN molecules are able to pass through the barrier to diffusion represented

Table 20-7   PROTEIN-BINDING CHARACTERISTICS AND DURATION OF ACTION OF LOCAL ANESTHETICS

Agent	Protein Binding	Approximate Duration of Action (min) (Soft Tissue)
Procaine	5	60–90
Prilocaine	55	100–240
Lidocaine	65	90–200
Mepivacaine	75	120–240
Tetracaine	85	180–600
Etidocaine	94	180–600
Bupivacaine	95	180–600
Articaine	95	120–480
Chloroprocaine	—	—

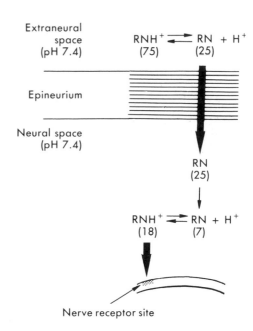

Fig. 20-1 Mode of action of a local anesthetic in normal tissue (pH 7.4). The anesthetic (pK$_a$ = 7.9) is deposited in the extraneural tissues. Equilibrium occurs with approximately 75% of the molecules in the charged cationic form and 25% in base form. (Numbers in parentheses represent the proportion of anesthetic cation and base in extracellular and neural compartments.)

by the lipid nerve sheath much more readily than the RNH$^+$ ionic form. Once these RN ions enter into the nerve, they encounter an intraneural pH of 7.4. The pH of the tissues within the nerve itself remains quite uniform, even in the presence of marked changes in the pH of extracellular tissues. The pH of extracellular fluid may, therefore, differ from the pH within the nerve membrane, and similarly the ratio of RNH$^+$ to RN at these sites may differ. In this internal environment (pH of 7.4) ionic reequilibration occurs with approximately 75% of the RN reverting to the RNH$^+$ ionic form, which attaches to the drug receptor site within the sodium channel, producing neural blockade.

Anesthesia will persist for as long as the concentration of local anesthetic within the nerve remains great enough to prevent nerve conduction. However, once equilibrium of local anesthetic (LA) concentration is reached within and without the nerve, the diffusion gradient reverses and anesthetic molecules begin to diffuse out of the nerve (carried away from the injection site in the capillaries and lymphatics). The patient will perceive sensation again when the concentration of the LA within the nerve falls below that which is necessary to block nerve conduction effectively.

"Pulpally Involved" Tooth

The problem of inadequate pain control during endodontics may be explained, in part, through changes occurring in periapical tissues. Pulpal and apical pathologic inflammation or infection decreases tissue pH in the region surrounding the involved tooth. The degree to which this decrease in pH develops varies significantly with the study cited.[38] The pH of inflamed tissues is decreased below that of "normal" tissues. In the presence of this decreased pH, dissociation of the local anesthetic favors formation of a larger proportion of

RNH$^+$ to RN (Fig. 20-2). Ninety-nine percent of a local anesthetic with a pK$_a$ of 7.9 will be in the RNH$^+$ ionic form, which is unable to migrate through the neural sheath. The relative absence of RN ions leads to fewer anesthetic molecules entering the nerve sheath and reaching the nerve membrane, where intracellular pH remains 7.4 and reequilibration between RN and RNH$^+$ can occur. Fewer RNH$^+$ molecules are present intracellularly, decreasing the likelihood of complete anesthesia developing.

Additional factors that may be involved in producing this difficulty in achieving adequate pulpal anesthesia include increased local dilution at the site of injection, increased absorption of the local anesthetic away from the site of administration (secondary to localized hyperemia), and peripheral nerve sensitization.[39,40]

Solutions   One method of obtaining more intense anesthesia in an area of infection would be to deposit a greater volume of anesthetic into the region. A greater number of RN molecules would be liberated, with greater diffusion through the nerve sheath and a somewhat greater likelihood of achieving adequate pain control. Although this procedure is somewhat effective, injection of anesthetics into infected areas is undesirable because of the possibility of the spread of infection into a previously uncontaminated area. Deposition of the anesthetic into an area at a distance from the involved tooth is more likely to provide adequate pain control because of the normal tissue conditions existing there.

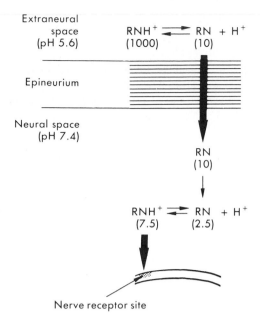

Extraneural space (pH 5.6)

$$RNH^+ \rightleftharpoons RN + H^+$$
$$(1000) \qquad (10)$$

Epineurium

Neural space (pH 7.4)

RN
(10)

$$RNH^+ \rightleftharpoons RN + H^+$$
$$(7.5) \qquad (2.5)$$

Nerve receptor site

Fig. 20-2 Mode of action of a local anesthetic in an inflamed or infected area. The anesthetic ($pK_a = 7.9$) is deposited in the extraneural tissues (pH of 5.6). Equilibrium develops with approximately 99% of solution in the cationic form. Fewer anesthetic molecules pass through the epineurium to the neural space. The pH in the neural space is 7.4, and molecules re-equilibriate. However, an insufficient number of molecules may be present, leading to a failure to produce profound clinical anesthesia.

Therefore regional nerve block anesthesia is a major factor in pain control for pulpally involved teeth.

There are occasions, fortunately rare, when even regional nerve block anesthesia at a distance from the infected tooth fails to provide adequate pain control. Omitting for a moment the most likely cause of this situation (i.e., faulty injection technique), Najjar[33] has proposed that inadequate pain control may be due to the fact that morphologic changes (e.g., neurodegenerative changes in the axon or the presence of inflammatory mediators) are developing. He further states that morphologic changes in inflamed nerve, even at a distance from the actual inflammatory site, appear to be a significant barrier for normal electrolyte exchange at membrane level. The net result is reinforcement of a nerve fiber's ability to generate action potentials. Studies[5,43] have demonstrated that inflammation potentiates peripheral nerve excitability.

In addition, when the inflamed tooth is anesthetized it becomes asymptomatic; however, on attempts to gain access to the pulp chamber and canals it becomes exquisitely sensitive to manipulation. Although no entirely satisfactory explanation exists for this circumstance, it may be explainable on the basis of an increase in the rate of stimulation of the nerve endings that occurs with use of the high- or low-speed hand piece. The degree of neural blockade may be adequate for a lower level of stimulation before preparation, yet prove inadequate to block completely the rapid flood of impulses arising with the use of the hand piece.

Local Anesthetics: Drugs

Although many drugs are classified as local anesthetics and find use within the health professions, only a few of them are currently used in dentistry. Six local anesthetics are available in dental-cartridge form in North America:

1. Lidocaine
2. Mepivacaine
3. Prilocaine
4. Bupivacaine
5. Etidocaine
6. Articaine

With this availability of local anesthetics in various combinations (with and without vasopressors), it is now possible to select a drug possessing the specific properties required by the patient for a given dental procedure.

Duration of Anesthesia: Considerations
The duration of pulpal (i.e., hard-tissue) and soft-tissue (i.e., total) anesthesia for each drug discussed in the following sections is an approximation. Factors exist that affect both the depth and the duration of a drug's anesthetic action, either prolonging or (much more commonly) decreasing it. These include the following:

1. Individual variation in response to the drug administered
2. Accuracy in administration of the drug
3. Status of the tissues at the site of drug deposition (i.e., vascularity, pH)
4. Anatomic variation
5. Type of injection administered (i.e., supraperiosteal ["infiltration"], nerve block)

The duration of anesthesia (pulpal and soft tissue) is presented as a range (e.g., 40 to 60 minutes). This attempts to take into account the previously mentioned factors that influence drug action.

Variation in individual response to a drug is quite common and is depicted in the so-called "bell" or normal distribution curve. A majority of patients (~70%) respond in a predictable manner to a drug's actions (i.e., 40 to 60 minutes). However, some patients (with none of the other factors that influence drug action obviously present) will demonstrate either a shorter (~15% [hyporesponders]) or a longer duration (~15% [hyperresponders]) of anesthesia. *This is to be expected and is entirely normal.*

Accuracy in the administration of the injected local anesthetic is an influencing factor. Although not as significant in certain techniques (e.g., supraperiosteal), accuracy in deposition is a major factor in many nerve blocks in which a considerable thickness of soft tissue must be penetrated to access the nerve to be blocked. The inferior alveolar nerve block (IANB) is a prime example of a technique in which the duration of anesthesia is greatly influenced by accuracy of injection. Deposition of the anesthetic close to a nerve provides greater depth and duration of anesthesia, compared with an anesthetic deposited at a greater distance from the nerve to be blocked.

The *status of the tissues* into which a local anesthetic is deposited influences the observed duration of anesthetic action and is of greater significance in endodontic procedures. The presence of normal healthy tissue at the site of drug deposition is assumed. Inflammation, infection, or pain (acute or chronic) usually leads to a decrease in the anticipated duration of action. Increased vascularity at an injection site results in a more rapid absorption (i.e., redistribution) of the local anesthetic and to a decreased depth and duration of anesthesia. This is most notable in areas of infection and inflammation but is also a consideration in "normal" anatomy. For example, the neck of the mandibular condyle, the target for local anesthetic deposition in the Gow-Gates mandibular nerve block, is considerably less vascular than the target area for the IANB. The expected duration of anesthesia for *any* local anesthetic is greater in a less vascular region.

Anatomic variation also influences the duration of clinical anesthesia. If anything, the most notable aspect of "normal" anatomy is the presence of extreme variation (e.g., in size and shape of the head) from person to person. The techniques described in this chapter assume a patient in the middle of the bell curve, the so-called "normal responder." Anatomic variations away from this "norm" usually adversely influence the duration of clinical drug action. Although most obvious in the mandible (e.g., height of the mandibular foramen, width of the ramus), such variation may also be noted in the maxilla. Supraperiosteal infiltration, usually quite effective in providing pulpal anesthesia for maxillary teeth, provides shorter than expected or inadequate anesthesia where the alveolar bone is more dense than usual. Where the zygomatic arch is lower than "normal" (primarily in children but occasionally in adults), infiltration anesthesia of the maxillary first and second molars may provide a shorter duration or even fail to provide adequate pulpal anesthesia. In other cases the palatal root of maxillary molars may not be adequately anesthetized, even in the presence of a normal alveolar bony thickness, when that root flares more than usual toward the midline of the palate.

Finally, and of potentially great importance, the duration of clinical anesthesia is influenced by the *type of injection administered*. For all the drugs presented, administration of a nerve block provides a longer duration of both pulpal and soft-tissue anesthesia than supraperiosteal injection. This assumes that the recommended minimal volume of anesthetic is injected. For example, a duration of 40 minutes pulpal anesthesia may be expected after a supraperiosteal injection, whereas a 60-minute duration is to be expected with a nerve block. Less than recommended volumes of anesthetic decrease the duration of action. Greater than recommended doses do *not* provide any increase in duration.

Two major classes of injectable local anesthetics, (1) esters and (2) amides, are recognized, distinguished by the type of linkage joining the two ends of the drug. Early local anesthetics, such as cocaine and procaine, were esters, whereas most local anesthetics introduced since the mid-1940s have been amides.

The use of injectable local anesthetics in dentistry in North America is limited to amide type of drugs. In fact, no ester local anesthetic is currently being marketed in dental-cartridge form in North America. Given the number of local anesthetic injections administered in dentistry (conservatively estimated at more than 300 million cartridges in the United States annually), a drug with minimal risk of allergy is desirable. The risk of allergy to amide anesthetics is significantly less than that with esters. Conversely, the risk of systemic toxicity with amides is somewhat greater than that with esters. However, as toxic reactions are usually dose related, adherence to proper injection techniques, including the use of minimal volumes of anesthetic, minimizes this risk. Amide formulations have also proved more effective than their ester counterparts in achieving intraoral anesthesia. Comparison of risk-to-benefit ratios for local anesthetics as used in dentistry greatly favors amide formulations.

The selection of a local anesthetic for use in a dental procedure should be based on the following criteria:
1. Duration of the dental procedure
2. Requirement for hemostasis
3. Requirement for post-surgical pain control
4. Contraindication to the selected anesthetic drug or vasoconstrictor

Local anesthetic formulations available in dentistry may be categorized broadly by their expected duration of pulpal anesthesia into short-, intermediate-, and long-acting drugs. Box 20-1 lists local anesthetics, the various combinations in which they are currently available in North America, and their expected duration of pulpal anesthesia.

Box 20-1   EXPECTED DURATION OF PULPAL ANESTHESIA

Short-Duration Pulpal Anesthesia (<30 Minutes)
- Mepivacaine 3% (20-40 minutes)
- Prilocaine 4% (5-10 minutes via infiltration)

Intermediate-Duration Pulpal Anesthesia (About 60 Minutes)
- Articaine 4% + epinephrine 1:1000,000 and 1:200,000
- Lidocaine 2% + epinephrine 1:50,000, 1:100,000
- Mepivacaine 2% + levonordefrin 1:20,000
- Prilocaine 4% (40-60 minutes via nerve block)
- Prilocaine 4% + epinephrine 1:200,000 (60-90 minutes)

Long-Duration Pulpal Anesthesia (>90 Minutes)
- Bupivacaine 0.5% + epinephrine 1:200,000
- Etidocaine 1.5% + epinephrine 1:200,000 (via nerve block)

Local Anesthetics: Techniques

Fortunately, many techniques are available to aid in obtaining clinically adequate pain control during virtually all endodontic procedures, even in the presence of acute or chronic localized tissue changes.

Supraperiosteal Injection (Local Infiltration)   Supraperiosteal anesthesia is described as a technique in which anesthetic is deposited *into* the area of treatment.[21] Small, terminal nerve endings in the area are rendered incapable of transmitting impulses. Infiltration anesthesia is commonly used in maxillary teeth. Because of the ability of the anesthetic solution to diffuse through periosteum and the relatively thin cancellous bone of the maxilla, this technique provides effective pain control in maxillary endodontic procedures in the absence of infection. Very often, however, where infection *is* present at the onset of an endodontic case, infiltration proves ineffective and other anesthetic techniques must be relied on initially. Infiltration anesthesia may prove effective at subsequent visits, provided cleaning and shaping of the root canals has been accomplished and infection and inflammatory responses are resolved.

Infiltration anesthesia is rarely effective in the adult mandible because of the inability of the anesthetic to penetrate the more dense cortical plate of bone. In pediatric dentistry, however, infiltration anesthesia of the mandible is more successful. As a general rule, infiltration anesthesia in the pediatric mandible is successful when a primary tooth is being treated. Once replaced by a permanent tooth, the success rate of mandibular infiltration anesthesia decreases dramatically. Regional nerve block anesthesia or accessory techniques, such as the periodontal ligament (PDL) injection or intraosseous (IO) injection, should receive primary consideration for permanent mandibular teeth.

Supraperiosteal ("Infiltration")

Teeth anesthetized	Volume of anesthetic	Recommended needle
One maxillary tooth	0.6 ml	27-gauge, short

In infiltration anesthesia the target area for deposition of the anesthetic is the apex of the tooth to be treated. Only 0.6 ml of anesthetic need be administered for adequate pain control, using a 27-gauge, short dental needle. Approximately 3 to 5 minutes are allowed to elapse before starting the procedure (e.g., placement of rubber dam). On rare occasion adequate pulpal anesthesia, even on nonpulpally involved teeth, is not achieved after infiltration. From clinical experience it appears that the most common cause of this is the failure to deposit the anesthetic solution at or above the apex of the tooth. The maxillary canine is most often the culprit, with the maxillary central incisor also frequently involved. Maxillary first and second molars may, on rare occasion, have buccal root apexes located beneath the thicker bone of the zygoma or may have palatal roots that flare considerably toward the midline. In either case, infiltration anesthesia may prove ineffective. Therefore nerve block anesthesia *is* the answer.

Regional Nerve Block   In the event that infiltration anesthesia proves ineffective in providing clinically adequate pain control, regional nerve block anesthesia is recommended. Nerve block is defined as a method of achieving regional anesthesia by depositing a suitable local anesthetic close to a main nerve trunk, preventing afferent impulses from traveling centrally beyond that point.[21] Nerve block anesthesia is more likely to be effective in cases where infiltration has failed, because the nerve is being blocked at some distance from the inflamed or infected tissue (where tissue pH and other factors are more nearly normal).

Several nerve blocks are beneficial in dentistry. A brief summary of major intraoral maxillary and mandibular nerve blocks follows.

Maxillary anesthesia.   Maxillary nerves that can be anesthetized and are of importance in endodontic procedures are the maxillary (V_2), posterior superior alveolar (PSA), anterior superior alveolar (ASA), greater palatine, and nasopalatine nerves.

The PSA nerve block provides pulpal anesthesia to the three maxillary molars and their overlying buccal soft tissues and bone. Anesthetic is deposited into the pterygomaxillary space located superior, distal, and medial to the maxillary tuberosity. In 28% of patients the mesiobuccal root of the first molar receives innervation from the middle superior alveolar nerve, in which case an additional volume of 0.6 ml of anesthetic should be infiltrated high into the buccal fold, just anterior to the first maxillary molar. In addition, palatal infiltration may be required for anesthesia of the palatal soft tissues for placement of the rubber dam clamp.

PSA Nerve Block

Teeth anesthetized	Volume of anesthetic	Recommended needle
Maxillary molars	0.9 ml	27-gauge, short

The ASA nerve block is an easy injection to administer, providing anesthesia of the infraorbital, ASA, and middle superior alveolar nerves in virtually all patients. By depositing local anesthetic outside the infraorbital foramen and then pressing it into the foramen, anesthesia of the maxillary premolars, anterior teeth, and their overlying buccal soft tissues and bone is obtained. Palatal infiltration may be necessary for placement of a rubber dam clamp. Additionally, the soft tissues of the lower eyelid, lateral portion of the nose, and the upper lip are anesthetized (i.e., the infraorbital nerve). An important requirement for successful ASA nerve block is the application of finger pressure over the injection site for a minimum of 2 minutes after deposition of the anesthetic. This converts the infraorbital nerve block (soft tissue only) into the ASA nerve block (i.e., teeth, soft tissues, and bone).

ASA Nerve Block

Teeth anesthetized	Volume of anesthetic	Recommended needle
Maxillary incisors, canine, premolars	0.9 ml	27-gauge, long

Palatal anesthesia is frequently required during endodontic procedures and is also needed around the gingival margins of the tooth to be clamped. Deposition of 0.3 ml of anesthetic by infiltration into the palatal gingiva 3 to 5 mm below the gingival margin provides adequate anesthesia. Larger areas of the palate rarely need to be anesthetized for endodontic procedures, but when necessary two nerve blocks are available: (1) the greater palatine and (2) nasopalatine.

The *greater* (i.e., anterior) *palatine nerve block* provides anesthesia to both the palatal hard and soft tissues, ranging from the distal of the third molar as far anterior as the medial aspect of the first premolar. At the first premolar, soft-tissue anesthesia may only be partial because of overlap from the nasopalatine nerve.

Greater Palatine Nerve Block

Area anesthetized (soft tissue palatal to teeth)	Volume of anesthetic	Recommended needle
Maxillary premolars and molars	0.45 ml	27-gauge, long

The *nasopalatine nerves* enter the palate through the incisive foramen, located in the midline just palatal to the central incisors and directly beneath the incisive papilla. They provide sensory innervation to the hard and soft tissues of the premaxilla as far distal as the mesial aspect of the first premolar, where fibers from the greater palatine nerve may be encountered.

Nasopalatine Nerve Block

Area anesthetized (soft tissue palatal to teeth)	Volume of anesthetic	Recommended needle
Maxillary incisors, canine	0.45 ml	27-gauge, long

Because of the density of palatal soft tissues and their firm attachment to bone, especially in the anterior palatal region, palatal injections are considered potentially traumatic both by patients and dentists. Palatal anesthesia *can* be achieved with a minimum of discomfort if care is taken throughout the procedure to ensure the following:

- Adequate topical anesthesia
- Adequate pressure anesthesia
- Slow penetration of tissues
- Continual, slow deposition of anesthetic
- Injection of not more than 0.45 ml of solution

Although rarely necessary, *a maxillary, or second-division, nerve block should be considered when other techniques of pain control prove ineffective* because of infection accompanied by inflammation. The second-division nerve block provides anesthesia of the entire maxillary nerve peripheral to the site of injection: pulps of all maxillary teeth on the side of injection; their overlying buccal soft tissues and bone; palatal hard and soft tissues on the injection side; and the upper lip, cheek, side of the nose, and lower eyelid.

Maxillary Nerve Block (High-Tuberosity or Greater Palatine Approach)

Teeth anesthetized	Volume of anesthetic	Recommended needle
Maxillary incisors, canine, premolars, molars	1.8 ml	27-gauge, long

Two intraoral approaches are available for the maxillary nerve block[28,37]:

1. The *high-tuberosity approach* follows the same path as the PSA nerve block except that the depth of needle penetration is greater (i.e., 30 mm versus 16 mm in the PSA).
2. The *greater palatine canal* approach involves entering the greater palatine foramen, usually located palatally between the second and third maxillary molars at the junction of the alveolar process and palatal bone. A 27-gauge, long needle is carefully inserted into the greater palatine foramen to a depth of 30 mm before 1.8 ml of anesthetic is deposited.

Recently a new maxillary anesthetic technique has been described by Friedman and Hochman that they call the *anterior middle superior alveolar nerve block* (AMSA).[12] Although the authors strongly advocate the AMSA injection be administered with a computer-controlled local anesthesia delivery system (e.g., the Wand) the injection can be administered successfully with the traditional syringe-and-needle system.

AMSA Nerve Block

Teeth anesthetized	Volume of anesthetic	Recommended needle
Maxillary incisors, canine, premolars	1.35 ml	27-gauge, short

The AMSA nerve block provides, with one injection, pulpal anesthesia of the central incisor through the second premolar, along with the adjacent buccal *and* palatal soft tissues and bone. Of greatest interest to patients is the fact that the AMSA does not produce anesthesia of the face and muscles of expression. Administered on the palate at a point midway between the two premolars and the midline of the palate, this injection can be delivered easily, consistently, and virtually imperceptibly with a computer-controlled local-anesthesia delivery system. With a traditional syringe-and-needle system the AMSA can be administered relatively comfortably if the administrator observes the basic rules of atraumatic palatal anesthesia presented earlier. The AMSA nerve block has proved to be successful when periapical infection has made infiltration and anterior superior alveolar nerve block ineffective. In addition, the palatal anesthesia provided in this injection allows for the atraumatic placement of rubber dam clamps.

Mandibular anesthesia
Inferior alveolar nerve block (IANB)   Pulpal anesthesia of mandibular teeth is traditionally obtained through the

IANB. Additionally, anesthesia of the buccal soft tissues and bone anterior to the mental foramen is provided. If anesthesia of the buccal soft tissues overlying the mandibular molars is needed, the buccal nerve must be blocked. The anterior two thirds of the lingual nerve is usually blocked along with the inferior alveolar nerve, the floor of the mouth, and the mucous membrane and mucoperiosteum on the lingual side of the mandible. A 25- or 27-gauge, long needle is recommended; after multiple negative aspirations, 1.5 ml of anesthetic is deposited. To block the buccal nerve the same needle used for IANB is placed into the buccal fold distal and buccal to the last mandibular molar in the quadrant, and the remaining 0.3 ml of anesthetic deposited.

In the absence of pulpal or periapical pathosis, IANB provides clinically adequate anesthesia 85% to 90% of the time. Its rate of success diminishes where periapical disease exists. Because of the density of bone in the adult mandible, infiltration anesthesia is of little value. When IANB proves ineffective, fewer alternatives are available. However, other nerve blocks and alternative techniques may succeed in the mandible.

IANB

Teeth anesthetized	Volume of anesthetic	Recommended needle
Mandibular incisors, canine, premolars, molars	1.5 ml	25- or 27-gauge, long

Incisive nerve block   The incisive and mental nerves are terminal branches of the inferior alveolar nerve arising at the mental foramen. The *mental nerve,* exiting the mental foramen, provides sensory innervation to the skin of the lower lip and chin regions and the mucous membrane lining the lower lip; the *incisive nerve,* remaining within the mandibular canal, provides sensory innervation to the pulps of the premolars, canine, incisors, and the bone anterior to the mental foramen. Pulpal anesthesia of the region served by the incisive nerve should be considered when endodontic treatment is contemplated on premolars or other anterior teeth. Anesthetic is placed *outside* the mental foramen, with finger pressure applied at the injection site for a minimum of 1 minute (2 minutes is preferred) to ensure entry of anesthetic into the mental foramen and mandibular canal.

Incisive Nerve Block

Teeth anesthetized	Volume of anesthetic	Recommended needle
Mandibular incisors, canine, premolars	0.6 ml	27-gauge, short

Infiltration anesthesia   As mentioned previously, infiltration anesthesia is rarely effective in the adult mandible. The sole exceptions to this are (1) the lateral incisor, where up to 1 ml of anesthetic may be deposited into the mucobuccal fold at the level of the apex of the tooth, and (2) the mandibular molars, where (in *a few* patients) deposition of 0.9 ml

on the *lingual* aspect of the mandible may provide successful anesthesia.

Occasionally after IANB, adequate pain control is achieved in the mandible, except in isolated areas (most often in the mesial root of the first molar). Successful pulpal anesthesia of third molars is frequently difficult to achieve because of the multiplicity of accessory innervations that are thought to exist in some situations. Indeed, adequate anesthesia is easier to obtain for third molar extraction than for restorative or endodontic procedures.

The mesial root of the mandibular first molar is occasionally sensitive to noxious stimuli when all other portions of the same tooth and adjacent structures are insensitive. Although many theories (involving cervical accessory and transverse neck nerves) have been put forward to explain this situation, the mylohyoid nerve (a branch of the posterior division of the mandibular division) appears to be the culprit.[13] The mylohyoid nerve branches off the inferior alveolar nerve well above the inferior alveolar nerve's entry into the mandibular foramen. It passes along the lingual border of the mandible in the mylohyoid groove, sending motor fibers to the anterior belly of the digastric muscle. On occasion the mylohyoid nerve has been shown to contain sensory fibers that branch off and enter into the body of the mandible through small foramina on the lingual side of the mandible in the area of the second molar. These fibers presumably pass anteriorly through the body of the mandible to the mesial root of the first molar.

Regardless of the nerve responsible for this phenomenon, the problem of mesial root sensitivity in the inflamed first molar pulp can usually be alleviated with a 27-gauge, short needle and 0.6 ml of anesthetic deposited against the lingual side of the mandible at the level of the apex of the mandibular *second* molar. Within 2 to 3 minutes adequate anesthesia should develop. Although usually observed with the first molar, the problem of partial anesthesia can also occur with other teeth. Management consists of depositing 0.6 ml of solution at the apex of the tooth immediately *distal* to the involved tooth (on the lingual of the mandible). PDL or IO anesthesia also resolves this problem.

Mandibular block: Gow-Gates technique   A true mandibular (V_3) block injection, one that provides adequate anesthesia of all sensory portions of the mandibular nerve (i.e., buccal, inferior alveolar, lingual, mylohyoid), can be obtained through the Gow-Gates mandibular block.[15,20] The target area is higher than in the traditional IANB technique: the lateral aspect of the neck of the condyle below the insertion of the lateral pterygoid muscle (Fig. 20-3).[15]

For this reason alone the success rate with the Gow-Gates mandibular block can be expected to be greater than that of the traditional approach *once the dentist learns the technique.* In one study, 97.25% of patients receiving the Gow-Gates block did not require supplemental anesthesia.[20] Another advantage is a low positive aspiration rate (1.8%, compared with approximately 10% in IANB). A 25-gauge, long needle is recommended in the Gow-Gates technique.

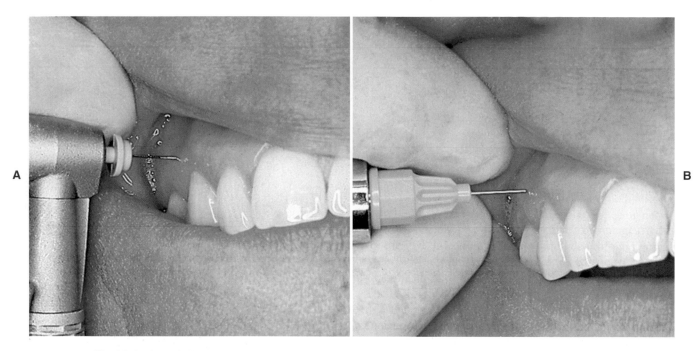

Fig. 20-6   The Stabident System consists of a perforator, a solid needle that perforates the cortical plate of bone (**A**) with a conventional slow-speed contraangle handpiece, and an 8-mm long, 27-gauge needle that is inserted into this predrilled hole for anesthetic administration (**B**). (Courtesy Fairfax Dental Inc., Miami, Fla.)

When periapical or periodontal infection is present on the tooth to be treated, the PDL and intraseptal injections are not recommended. IO anesthesia may still be administered, the perforation site being moved distal to the tooth to be treated (e.g., a perforation site distal to the mandibular second molar, if the injection site for the involved first molar is unusable because of infection).

IO Injection

Teeth anesthetized	Volume of anesthetic	Recommended needle
1 or 2 teeth	0.45 to 0.6 ml	27- gauge, short

The most vexing aspect of administering IO anesthesia has been the difficulty of locating the hole made by the perforator with the needle. With clinical experience several solutions have been forthcoming:

1. When the hand piece is removed, clinicians should not take their eyes off the perforation site until the needle has been inserted into the hole.
2. After perforating the cortical plate of bone, clinicians can stop the hand piece, detach the perforator, and leave it in the hole until the syringe and needle are lined up for insertion.

In an attempt to make location of the hole somewhat easier, the manufacturer of the Stabident has recently introduced blunt-ended needles that are easier to insert into the hole. More recently the X-Tip (X-Tip Technologies, LLC, Lakewood, N.J.) has been developed (Fig. 20-7) The perforation is made in the cortical plate of bone and, when the needle is withdrawn, a cannula remains in the hole. The needle is simply inserted into the canula, which guides it directly into the perforation.

Intrapulpal injection.   When the pulp chamber of a tooth has been exposed pathologically or while making an access opening, the intrapulpal injection may be used in addition to local infiltration or block anesthesia to achieve adequate pain control.

A 27-gauge, short needle is inserted into the pulp chamber or specific root canal as needed. Ideally, the needle is firmly wedged into the chamber or canal (Fig. 20-8). On injection, significant resistance is encountered and the solution must be inserted under pressure. Anesthesia is produced both by the action of the local anesthetic and the applied pressure. There may be a very brief moment of pain as the injection is started; however, anesthesia usually occurs immediately thereafter instrumentation can proceed painlessly. When a snug fit of the needle is not possible, two procedures are used:

1. With the needle in the canal, warm baseplate gutta-percha is inserted around it. After cooling, injection under pressure may proceed.
2. The anesthetic solution can be deposited into the chamber or canal, with anesthesia being produced by the chemical actions of the solution only. At least 30 seconds should elapse before an attempt is made to proceed with instrumentation.

The former technique is preferred whenever possible.[29]

Intrapulpal Injection

Teeth anesthetized	Volume of anesthetic	Recommended needle
1 tooth	0.2 to 0.3 ml	27-gauge, short

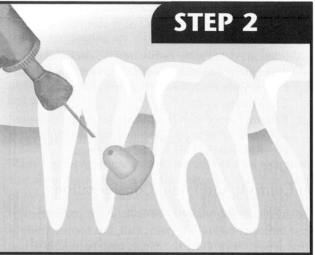

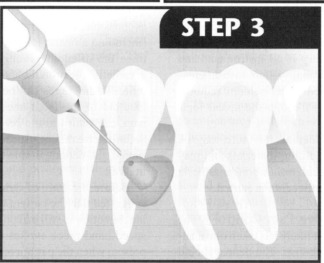

Fig. 20-7 The X-Tip intraosseous system inserts a cannula into the bone, making needle insertion easier. *Step 1*, Insert the X-Tip using a slow speed handpiece. *Step 2,* Withdraw drill leaving the special guide sleeve X-Tip in place. *Step 3*, Insert included 27-gauge ultra short needle into guide sleeve; slowly inject into cancellous bone. Profound anesthesia is instant; dental treatment may begin immediately (without lip and tongue numbness). (Courtesy X-Tip Technologies, LLC, Lakewood, N.J.)

The PDL, IO, and intrapulpal injections are the only injections where it may be necessary to bend the local anesthetic needle to gain access to the injection site and to obtain successful anesthesia. With the reintroduction of IO anesthesia, it has become considerably easier to obtain consistently reliable pulpal anesthesia, even in previously difficult to manage situations, such as the mandibular molars. The IO technique should become an integral part of the pain control armamentarium of all endodontists and other dentists who frequently treat emergency pain patients.

There are occasions, happily rare, when all of the previously described techniques fail to provide clinically acceptable pain control and pulpal anesthesia cannot be attained until the pulp chamber is exposed. The following sequence of treatment may then be considered:

1. Use IO anesthesia.

2. If high-speed instrumentation proves highly traumatic, use of slow-speed high-torque instrumentation is usually less traumatic.

3. Use conscious sedation (which does not prevent pain but helps to moderate a patient's response to painful stimuli). Inhalation sedation (N_2O-O_2) or intravenous (IV) sedation or both are readily available, safe, and highly effective methods of allaying anxiety and of elevating a patient's pain reaction threshold.

4. When the pulp chamber has been opened, direct intrapulpal anesthesia usually can be administered and proves effective.

5. If a high level of pain persists and it is still not possible to enter into the pulp chamber, the following sequence should be considered:

ration, despite effective air-conditioning. Patients may even complain about the warmth of the room.

When these methods of recognizing anxiety in the dental patient are used, the situation takes on the aspect of a game: Can the dentist detect the patient's anxiety? Will the patient successfully keep his or her fears hidden from the dentist so as not to appear "childish?" Unfortunately, on many occasions the patient wins. Then the dentist, unaware of the patient's fears, proceeds with the dental treatment only to discover, all too late, that the patient was indeed apprehensive and faints at the sight of the local anesthetic syringe or pushes the dentist's hand away at a critical time during the procedure. Anxiety is obvious at this point, but the ideal time to detect it is *before* dental treatment begins.

The *medical history questionnaire* may be used to assist in fear recognition before the start of dental treatment. Corah[7] and Gale[14] devised an anxiety questionnaire to help determine the degree of a patient's anxiety. The University of Southern California School of Dentistry has included several of these questions in its medical history questionnaire[31]:

- Do you feel very nervous about having dental treatment?
- Have you ever had an upsetting experience in the dental office?
- Has a dentist ever behaved badly toward you?
- Is there anything else about having dental treatment that bothers you? If so, please explain.

These questions permit patients to express their feelings about dentistry, perhaps for the very first time. Many patients who would never verbally admit to anxiety answer these questions honestly.

Management of Anxiety

A variety of techniques for the management of anxiety in dentistry are available. Together these techniques are termed a spectrum of pain and anxiety control (Fig. 20-9). They represent a wide range, from nondrug techniques through general anesthesia. Although general anesthesia has a useful place in this spectrum, its use today is quite limited outside the specialty of oral and maxillofacial surgery (and even within that specialty) and dental anesthesiology. Two reasons for the decreased reliance on general anesthesia as a means of anxiety control have been the introduction and acceptance of the concept of conscious sedation in dentistry and the development in the past two decades of more highly effective drugs for the management of anxiety.

From a practical viewpoint, conscious sedation techniques present relatively safe, reliable, and effective methods of controlling anxiety with little or no added risk to the patient. *Conscious sedation* is defined as "a minimally depressed level of consciousness that retains the patient's ability to independently and continuously maintain an airway and respond appropriately to physical stimulation and verbal command and that is produced by a pharmacologic or nonpharmacologic method or combination thereof."[8] There are two major types of sedation:

1. Iatrosedation—Techniques that do not necessitate the administration of drugs for the control of anxiety (e.g., hypnosis, biofeedback, acupuncture, electroanesthesia, and the critically important "chair side manner"). This term, introduced by Dr. Nathan Friedman of the Univer-

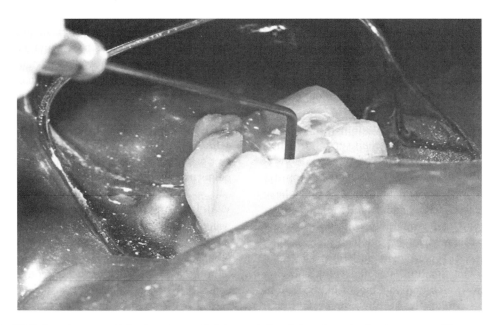

Fig. 20-8 In an intrapulpal injection, the needle is inserted directly into the pulp chamber or a specific root canal. Ideally, resistance is met and the solution is expressed under pressure. With the advent of intraligamentary anesthesia, this technique is seldom necessary.

sity of Southern California School of Dentistry, is defined as "relaxing the patient through the doctor's behavior."

2. Pharmacosedation—Techniques that require drug administration.

Iatrosedation   Before discussing pharmacosedation, nondrug techniques should be considered. The techniques of iatrosedation form the building blocks from which all pharmacosedative techniques arise. A relaxed dentist-patient relationship favorably influences the action of sedative drugs. Patients who are comfortable with their dentist either require a smaller dose of a given drug to achieve a desired effect or respond more intensely to the usual dose. This is in contrast to patients who are uncomfortable with their dentist. Their greater anxieties or fears cause them, either knowingly or unknowingly, to fight the effect of the drug, the result being poor sedation and an unpleasant experience for both the dentist and the patient. Therefore a determined effort must be made by all members of the dental office staff to help allay the anxieties of the patient.

Pharmacosedation   Although iatrosedation is the starting point for all sedative procedures in the dental office, the level of anxiety present in many patients may prove too great to allow dental care to proceed without pharmacologic intervention. Fortunately, several effective techniques are available to aid in relaxing the apprehensive patient.

The following goals are to be sought whenever pharmacosedation is considered[3]:
- Patient's mood must be altered.
- Patient must remain conscious.
- Patient must be cooperative.
- All protective reflexes must remain intact and active.
- Vital signs must be stable and within normal limits.
- Patient's pain threshold should be elevated.

- Amnesia may be present.

A second component to ideal sedation must always be considered:

The level of sedation must never reach beyond the level at which the dentist remains relaxed and capable of completing the dental procedure with uncompromised quality.

Indeed, the quality of the same treatment on that patient should be at least as high as, if not higher than, the quality of the same treatment on that patient without the use of pharmacosedation. Drug administration in dentistry must never become an excuse for inferior-quality dentistry.

Oral sedation.   The oral route is the most frequently used technique of pharmacosedation. The oral route offers some definite advantages and possesses some definite disadvantages, compared with other techniques (Table 20-8).

The disadvantages of oral sedation tend to overshadow its advantages. Because of this the goals of oral sedation should be kept within certain well-defined limits of safety. It is recommended that oral sedation not be used to achieve deep levels of sedation. Other, more controllable (i.e., titratable), techniques should be used to achieve these levels.

There are two recommended uses of the oral route of conscious sedation:

1. If anxiety is severe the evening before dental treatment, the patient should take an oral sedative 1 hour before going to sleep.
2. If anxiety is severe the day of dental treatment, the patient should take an oral sedative 1 hour before the scheduled appointment to lessen preoperative anxiety.

Many drugs are available for oral administration. It is strongly recommended that before prescribing any oral sedative to a patient the clinician consult the drug package insert or a textbook[25] to determine correct dose, contraindications, precautions, and other important information. In clinical experience the following drugs have proven to be the most effective in reaching the goals just enumerated: benzodi-

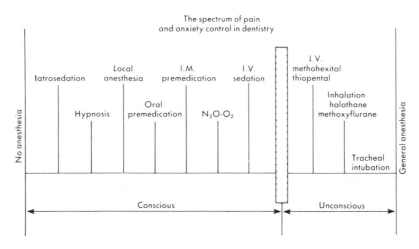

Fig. 20-9 Spectrum of pain and anxiety control in dentistry. Vertical bar represents the loss of consciousness. (From Malamed SF: *Sedation: A guide to patient management*, ed 4, St Louis, 2001, Mosby.)

Table 20-8   **ADVANTAGES AND DISADVANTAGES OF ORAL SEDATION**

Advantages	Disadvantages
Practically universally accepted	Slow onset of action (15-30 min)
Increased safety	Maximal clinical action in ~60 min
Adverse reactions less frequent	Inability to titrate patient to ideal level of sedation
Adverse reactions less severe	Long duration of action (3-4 hr)
	Inability to rapidly increase or decrease sedation level
	Impaired status of patient at conclusion of procedure, requiring escort from office

Table 20-9   **COMMONLY USED ORAL SEDATIVE DRUGS**

Drug Group	Proprietary Name (US)	Dose* (mg)
Benzodiazepines		
Alprazolam	Xanax	0.25-0.50
Diazepam	Valium	2-10
Flurazepam	Dalmane	15-30
Lorazepam	Ativan	1-3
Midazolam	Versed	2-5
Oxazepam	Serax	10-30
Triazolam	Halcion	0.125-0.250
Chloral hydrate	Noctec	500-1500
Hydroxyzine	Atarax, Vistaril	50-100

*For a normal, healthy 70-kg man. Patient response to these doses may vary; therefore the reader is advised to consult the drug package insert for specific prescribing information before prescribing any drug.

azepines (e.g., diazepam, oxazepam, triazolam, flurazepam, midazolam).

Triazolam and flurazepam are recommended to aid in sleep the evening before scheduled dental treatment, whereas diazepam, midazolam, and oxazepam are recommended for preoperative anxiety management.

An additional advantage to oral midazolam is the occurrence of amnesia (i.e., lack of recall of events) in a significant percentage of patients. With the availability of benzodiazepines, the continued use of oral barbiturates can no longer be recommended. Other benzodiazepines are available for oral administration and prove to be equally effective. Textbooks must be consulted for their doses and other important prescribing information. Table 20-9 lists commonly used oral antianxiety and sedative-hypnotic drugs. (Additional information regarding drugs for oral sedation may be found in Chapter 2.) Clinicians must remember that patients receiving oral sedatives must not be permitted to drive a motor vehicle to or from the dental office.

Oral sedation may be required, especially at the first endodontic appointment, because of the preconceived ideas patients maintain about endodontic care. Proper use of iatrosedation and pain control usually obviate the need for oral sedation at subsequent visits.

The use of oral sedation in patients under the age of 13 years has been shown to be associated with an increased risk.[27] Three states, Ohio, Florida, and California, have recently passed legislation mandating that doctors administering oral conscious sedation to patients who are minors receive a special permit. It behooves endodontists contemplating treating children to determine the specific requirements established by the Board of Dental Examiners in their locality.

Intramuscular sedation. Intramuscular (IM) sedation is infrequently used in dental practices; however, it remains an effective method of anxiety control in certain situations. Advantages and disadvantages of intramuscular drug administration (compared with the oral route) appear in Table 20-10.

Like the oral route the IM route lacks a degree of control that would be desirable. Therefore the level of sedation sought with IM sedation should remain light to moderate. Only doctors trained in this technique of drug administration and in airway management should consider sedation via the IM route. Indeed, all 50 states in the United States require the doctor to obtain a parenteral sedation permit to use IM conscious sedation.

The most effective IM sedative has proven to be the water-soluble benzodiazepine, midazolam (e.g., Versed, Hypnovel, Dormicum). Its IM use is frequently associated with the occurrence of amnesia, which is a welcome happenstance because the patient has a lack of recall of events occurring during the dental procedure.[10,26]

Opioid agonists, such as meperidine (i.e., Demerol) are often used for IM sedation. These drugs are not recommended for use for conscious sedation (the benzodiazepines being significantly more effective in this regard). Respiratory depression and the incidence of nausea and vomiting are increased when opioids are used. Increased vigilance, requir-

Table 20-10   **ADVANTAGES AND DISADVANTAGES OF INTRAMUSCULAR DRUG ADMINISTRATION**

Advantages	Disadvantages
More rapid onset of action (10-15 minutes)	Inability to titrate to ideal level of sedation
Increased safety	Maximal clinical effect in ~30 minutes
Adverse reactions less frequent	Inability to rapidly increase or decrease sedation level
Adverse reactions less severe	Long duration of action (3-4 hours)
More reliable absorption	Need for an injection
	Impaired status of patient at conclusion of procedure, requiring escort from office

Table 20-11   **ADVANTAGES AND DISADVANTAGES OF INHALATION SEDATION**

Advantages	Disadvantages
Rapid onset of action (20 seconds, although 3 to 5 minutes may be required for titration)	Cost and size of equipment
	Requirement for education in proper use of inhalation sedation
Ability to titrate to ideal level of sedation	Potential complications:
Ability to rapidly increase or decrease sedation level	Chronic exposure to low levels of nitrous oxide
Total clinical recovery within 3 to 5 minutes (in virtually all patients)	Abuse potential of nitrous oxide
	Sexual phenomena and nitrous oxide (and all other forms of sedation)
Ability to discharge most patients without need for adult escort	

ing the use of pulse oximetry and automatic vital-sign monitors, is necessary when IM opioids are used.

IM sedation is not contraindicated in endodontics; however, if a radiograph unit is not readily available chair side, the clinician should remember that the patient will need to walk to the radiograph unit (perhaps several times) during the appointment. Patients who receive an IM injection may require assistance doing this; those receiving any IM central nervous system (CNS) depressant must have an adult available to escort them home after their treatment.

Inhalation sedation. Nitrous oxide and oxygen inhalation sedation is a remarkably controllable technique of pharmacosedation used by approximately 35% of dentists practicing in the United States.[17] Because of its advantages over other routes of drug administration, inhalation sedation is usually the method of choice when sedation is required (Table 20-11).

Because of the degree of control maintained over inhalation sedation by the dentist, any level of conscious sedation compatible with the dentist's degree of experience can be achieved. Although nitrous oxide and oxygen inhalation sedation seems to be a nearly perfect technique, as with all drugs there are times when the desired actions do not develop. Approximately 70% of patients receiving nitrous oxide and oxygen are ideally sedated between 30% and 40% nitrous oxide. Fifteen percent require less than 30% nitrous oxide, whereas 15% require in excess of 40%. Of this last

15%, it may be said that some 5% to 10% are unsedatable with any level of nitrous oxide less than 70%.

Inhalation sedation units have a number of safety devices incorporated into them that prevent a patient from ever receiving less than 20% oxygen. Therefore it is probable that approximately 5% of patients receiving inhalation sedation never become adequately sedated. If we add to this other patients who are unable to breathe through their nose and those with a very high anxiety level, it is entirely possible that a failure rate of 10% to 15% could occur with nitrous oxide and oxygen inhalation sedation.

These comments are not meant to denigrate nitrous oxide and oxygen. The purpose in stressing the possibility of failures is to illustrate that no technique of conscious sedation, even inhalation sedation, is universally successful. Failures can and will occur whenever drugs are administered to patients. The drug administrator must know when to stop the administration. Nitrous oxide does not possess significant analgesic properties, although a degree of soft-tissue analgesia does develop in most patients at about 35% nitrous oxide. Local anesthesia must always be administered as it would if inhalation sedation were not being used.

Inhalation sedation is entirely compatible with endodontic treatment. Indeed, use of rubber dam converts most patients into nose breathers, facilitating the administration of nitrous oxide and oxygen. Inhalation sedation with nitrous oxide and oxygen is a highly effective, easy-to-use, and safe

Table 20-12   **ADVANTAGES AND DISADVANTAGES OF IV-DRUG ADMINISTRATION**

Advantages	Disadvantages
Rapid onset of action (9 to 30 seconds, although several minutes may be required for titration)	Potential complications due to rapidity of drug effect mandates increased monitoring (e.g., pulse oximetry, vital signs)
Ability to titrate to ideal level of sedation	Requirement for education in proper use of IV sedation
Ability to rapidly increase sedation level	Inability to easily lighten level of sedation
Ability to reverse the clinical actions of many IV drugs	Inability to reverse the clinical actions of all IV drugs
Ability to discharge most patients without need for adult escort	Impaired status of patient at conclusion of procedure, requiring escort from office
	Need for venipuncture
	Increase in liability insurance costs

IV, Intravenous.

technique of pharmacosedation. It is most effective for patients with mild-to-moderate levels of anxiety. Failures may be noted in unusually apprehensive patients, but for these, other techniques are available (e.g., IM, IV, general anesthesia). Nitrous oxide and oxygen is administered along with the other drugs in these techniques (e.g., IM plus nitrous oxide and oxygen; IV plus nitrous oxide and oxygen).

In recent years, three concerns have arisen relative to use of nitrous oxide and oxygen in dentistry. The first involves potential health effects of long-term exposure of dental personnel to low levels of nitrous oxide. The use of a scavenger type of device to remove exhaled nitrous oxide from the clinical environment is strongly recommended, despite the continued absence of definitive evidence of danger to dental personnel.[6] A second concern is the abuse of nitrous oxide by dental personnel. This has led to devastating effects, including peripheral sensory nerve deprivation.[19] Nitrous oxide is a potent anesthetic drug, not an innocuous vapor, and it must not be abused. A third concern involves the administration of any CNS depressant drug, including nitrous oxide, on a patient of the opposite sex from the doctor. Many cases have been reported in which the dentist was accused of sexual improprieties, sexual misconduct, or rape while the patient received nitrous oxide and oxygen.[16] Most cases have involved nitrous oxide and oxygen because it is the most commonly used of these techniques of conscious sedation.

Two common threads appear in many of these cases: (1) the patient received high concentrations of nitrous oxide (in excess of 50% to 60%), and (2) the dentist treated the patient without the benefit of a second person (i.e., auxiliary) present in the treatment room. Accusations of sexual misconduct or worse may be prevented by titrating nitrous oxide to the ideal sedation level and by having an auxiliary (preferably of the same sex as the patient) present in the treatment room at all times.

IV sedation.   The goal in the administration of any drug (except obviously, local anesthetics) is to achieve a therapeutic level of that drug in the bloodstream. The delays in onset of action noted with other techniques were caused by slow absorption of drugs from the gastrointestinal tract or from muscle into the blood. The direct administration of a drug into the venous circulation results in a much more rapid onset of action and a greater degree of control than are found with other pharmacosedative techniques.

Only inhalation sedation (in which the inhaled gases rapidly reach the alveoli and capillaries) has an onset of action approaching that of IV sedation. A drop of blood requires between 9 and 30 seconds to travel from the hand to the heart and then to the cerebral circulation. Titration is possible with IV-drug administration. The time required to achieve ideal sedation varies with the drug technique: IV diazepam or midazolam may require up to 4 minutes, whereas the Jorgensen technique may require up to 10 minutes. Advantages and disadvantages of IV-drug administration are summarized in Table 20-12.

Venipuncture, a learned skill, requires practice and continued repetition if it is to be performed atraumatically. Once venipuncture is accomplished, IV-drug administration is quite simple. Because of the degree of control maintained by the dentist, the level of sedation sought can vary from light to moderate to deep; it is entirely dependent on the experience of the dentist and team and the clinical requirements of the patient.

Many techniques of IV sedation are available. Most involve sedative drugs administered alone or in conjunction with opioids. Although many drugs have been successfully used IV, several techniques have become more popular, primarily because of their relative simplicity, their effectiveness, and the degree of safety associated with their proper administration. These include the administration of a benzodiazepine, either midazolam or diazepam, or in some cases, both a benzodiazepine and an opioid analgesic. The use of propofol, a rapid-acting, short-duration nonbarbiturate sedative-hypnotic, or ketamine, a dissociative anesthetic, should not be considered for IV conscious sedation use by dentists not trained in and permitted to use general anesthesia.

Guidelines for teaching IV conscious sedation have been enacted into dental practice acts in all 50 states (January

Table 20-13   **COMMON ROUTES OF SEDATION IN THE DENTAL OFFICE**

Route of Administration	Control		Recommended Safe Sedative Levels
	Titrate	Rapid Reversal	
Oral	No	No	Light only
Intramuscular	No	No	Adults: light, moderate; Children: light, moderate, deep
Intravenous	Yes	Yes (most drugs)	Children*: light, moderate, deep; Adults: light, moderate, deep
Inhalation	Yes	Yes	Any level of sedation

*There is little need for intravenous sedation in healthy children. Most children who permit a venipuncture also permit a local anesthetic to be administered intraorally. Intravenous sedation is of great benefit, however, in management of handicapped children or precooperative or uncooperative children.
(From Malamed SF: *Medical emergencies in the dental office*, ed 5, St Louis, 2000, Mosby.)

2001). Most require an intensive didactic (approximately 60 hours) and clinical program (20 patients treated with IV sedation under supervision) and an in-office evaluation program.

IV conscious sedation, particularly with the short-acting benzodiazepines, midazolam and diazepam, or either in combination with an opioid, such as meperidine or fentanyl, are ideally suited for endodontic therapy. However, if the radiograph unit is located at a distance from the patient, it may be both difficult and inconvenient to move the patient to the unit. During the early phase of the procedure, immediately after administration of the IV drugs, the patient may also have difficulty maintaining an open mouth. Bite blocks should be available for use at this time. Table 20-13 summarizes the recommended levels of sedation for the techniques discussed in this chapter.

Combined techniques. On occasion it may be necessary to consider combining several of the techniques just described. Therefore some words of caution are in order.

Quite frequently the patient who requires either inhalation or IV sedation is apprehensive enough to also need oral sedation, either the night before or the day of the dental appointment. There is no contraindication to this practice, provided the level of oral sedation is not excessive *and* the inhalation or IV drugs are carefully titrated. Because a blood level of oral sedative already exists, the requirement for other CNS depressants is usually decreased. If "average" doses of inhalation or IV drugs are used without titration, an overdose is more likely to develop. Titration is an important safety factor (it is foolhardy not to titrate a drug when possible to do so).

The combination of inhalation and IV sedation should be avoided by all but the most experienced dentists. Too frequently reports are forthcoming of significant morbidity and, on occasion, mortality, resulting from the ill-conceived conjoint use of these two potent techniques. Levels of sedation can vary rapidly; unless constant effective monitoring is maintained, unconsciousness may develop with attendant airway problems before the dentist ever becomes aware of it.

Nitrous oxide and oxygen may be used successfully at the same appointment when a patient requiring IV sedation is apprehensive about venipuncture. Nitrous oxide and oxygen may be used to aid in establishing the IV infusion. Benefits of nitrous oxide and oxygen during venipuncture include (1) a vasodilating effect, (2) anxiety-reducing actions, and (3) some analgesic properties. After the venipuncture is established, the patient should be administered 100% oxygen and returned to the presedative state before any IV drug is administered.

References

1. Acute Pain Management Guideline Panel: *Acute pain management: operative or medical procedures and trauma: clinical practice guidelines*, Rockville, MD, 1992, Agency for Health Care Policy and Research, Public Health Service, US Department of Health and Human Resources.
2. Akinosi JO: A new approach to the mandibular nerve block, *Br J Oral Surg* 15:83, 1977.
3. Bennett CR: *Conscious sedation in dental practice*, ed 2, St Louis, 1978, Mosby.
4. Camejo G et al: Characterization of two different membrane fractions isolated from the first stellar nerves of the squid *Dosidicus gigas, Biochim Biophys Acta* 193:247, 1969.
5. Chapman LF, Goodell H, Wolff HG: Tissue vulnerability, inflammation, and the nervous system. Paper presented at the American Academy of Neurology, April, 1959.
6. Cohen F et al: Occupational disease in dentistry and chronic exposure to trace anesthetic gases, *J Am Dent Assoc* 101:21, 1980.
7. Corah N: Development of dental anxiety scale, *J Dent Res* 48:596, 1969.
8. Council on Dental Education, American Dental Association: Guidelines for teaching the comprehensive control of pain and anxiety in dentistry, *J Dent Educ* 36:62, 1972.
9. Covino BJ: Physiology and pharmacology of local anesthetic agents, *Anesth Prog* 28:98, 1981.
10. Dormauer D, Aston R: Update: midazolam maleate, a new water-soluble benzodiazepine, *J Am Dent Assoc* 106:650, 1983.
11. Fast TB, Martin MD, Ellis TM: Emergency preparedness: a survey of dental practitioners, *J Am Dent Assoc* 112:499, 1986.
12. Friedman MJ, Hochman MN: The AMSA injection: a new concept for local anesthesia of maxillary teeth using a computer-controlled injection system, *Quintessence Int* 29(5):297, 1998.
13. Frommer J, Mele FA, Monroe CW: The possible role of the mylohyoid nerve in mandibular posterior tooth sensation, *J Am Dent Assoc* 85:113, 1972.

14. Gale E: Fears of the dental situation, *J Dent Res* 51:964, 1972.

15. Gow-Gates GAE: Mandibular conduction anesthesia: a new technique using extraoral landmarks, *Oral Surg Oral Med Oral Pathol* 36:321, 1973.

16. Jastak JT, Malamed SF: Nitrous oxide and sexual phenomena, *J Am Dent Assoc* 101:38, 1980.

17. Jones TW, Greenfield W: Position paper of the ADA ad hoc committee on trace anesthetics as a potential health hazard in dentistry, *J Am Dent Assoc* 95:751, 1977.

18. Leonard M: The efficacy of an intraosseous injection system of delivering local anesthetic, *J Am Dent Assoc* 126(1):81, 1995.

19. Malamed SF: The recreational abuse of nitrous oxide by health professionals, *J Calif Dent Assoc* 8:38, 1980.

20. Malamed SF: The Gow-Gates mandibular block: evaluation after 4275 cases, *Oral Surg Oral Med Oral Pathol* 51:463, 1981.

21. Malamed SF: *Handbook of local anesthesia,* ed 4, St Louis, 1997, Mosby.

22. Malamed SF: Local anesthetics: dentistry's most important drugs, *J Am Dent Assoc* 125:1571, 1994.

23. Malamed SF: Managing medical emergencies, *J Am Dent Assoc* 124:40, 1993.

24. Malamed SF: The periodontal ligament injection: an alternative to mandibular block, *Oral Surg Oral Med Oral Pathol* 53:118, 1982.

25. Malamed SF: *Sedation: a guide to patient management,* ed 3, St Louis, 1995, Mosby.

26. Malamed SF, Quinn CL, Hatch HG: Pediatric sedation with intramuscular and intravenous midazolam, *Anesth Prog* 36:155, 1989.

27. Malamed SF, Reggiardo P: Pediatric oral conscious sedation: changes to come, *J Calif Dent Assoc,* 1999 (in press).

28. Malamed SF, Trieger NT: Intraoral maxillary nerve block: an anatomical and clinical study, *Anesth Prog* 30:44, 1983.

29. Malamed SF, Weine F: *Profound pulpal anesthesia,* Chicago, 1988, American Association of Endodontists (audiotape).

30. Matsuura H: Analysis of systemic complications and deaths during dental treatment in Japan, *Anesth Prog* 36:219, 1990.

31. McCarthy FM, Pallasch TJ, Gates R: Documenting safe treatment of the medical-risk patient, *J Am Dent Assoc* 119:383, 1989.

32. Milgrom P, Getz T, Weinstein P: Recognizing and treating fears in general practice, *Dent Clin North Am* 32(4):657, 1988

33. Najjar TA: Why you can't achieve adequate regional anesthesia in the presence of infection, *Oral Surg* 44:7, 1977.

34. Nelson PW: Injection system, *J Am Dent Assoc* 103:692, 1981 (letter).

35. Nusstein J, Reader A, Nist R, Beck M, Meyers WJ: Anesthetic efficacy of the supplemental intraosseous injection of 2% lidocaine with 1:100,000 epinephrine in irreversible pulpitis, *J Endod* 24(7):487, 1998.

36. Parente SA, Anderson RW, Herman WW, Kimbrough WF, Weller RN: Anesthetic efficacy of the supplemental intraosseous injection for teeth with irreversible pulpitis, *J Endod* 24 (12):826, 1998.

37. Poore TE, Carney FMT: Maxillary nerve block: a useful technique, *J Oral Surg* 31:749, 1973.

38. Punnia-Moorthy A: Buffering capacity of normal and inflamed tissues following injection of local anaesthetic solutions, *Br J Anaesth* 61:154, 1988.

39. Punnia-Moorthy A: Evaluation of pH changes in inflammation of the subcutaneous air pouch lining in the rat, induced by carrageenan, dextran and staphylococcus aureus, *J Oral Pathol* 16:36, 1987.

40. Punnia-Moorthy A: Personal communication, March 1999.

41. Ritchie JM, Ritchie B, Greengard P: Active structure of local anesthetics, *J Pharmacol Exp Ther* 150:152, 1965.

42. Ritchie JM, Ritchie B, Greengard P: The effect of the nerve sheath on the action of local anesthetics, *J Pharmacol Exp Ther* 150:160, 1965.

43. Rood JP, Pateromichelakis S: Inflammation and peripheral nerve sensitization, *Br J Oral Surg* 19:67, 1981.

44. Saadoun AP, Malamed SF: Intraseptal anesthesia in periodontal surgery, *J Am Dent Assoc* 111:249, 1985.

45. Walton RE, Abbott BJ: Periodontal ligament injection: a clinical evaluation, *J Am Dent Assoc* 103:571, 1981.

46. Weisman G: Electronic anesthesia: expanding applications are its future, *Dent Prod Rep* 30(5):88, 1996.

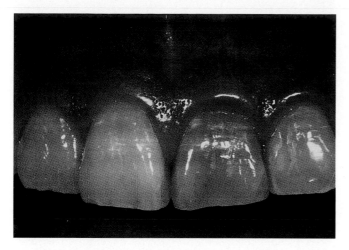

Plate 21-1 Left central incisor illustrating discolorations, post trauma, and endodontic treatment.

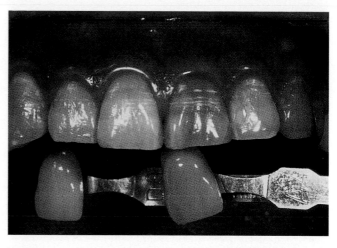

Plate 21-2 Pretreatment shade photograph documents extent of darkening.

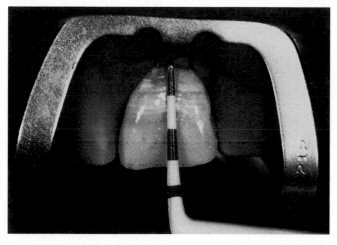

Plate 21-3 Proper preparation of the nonvital tooth before instituting the bleaching process.

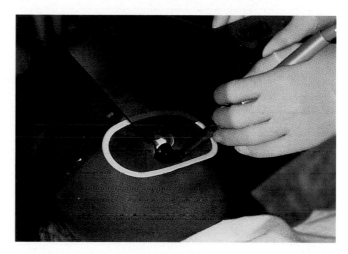

Plate 21-4 Patient during the nonvital tooth bleaching process. Various heat or light sources can be used to intensify and accelerate the bleaching process.

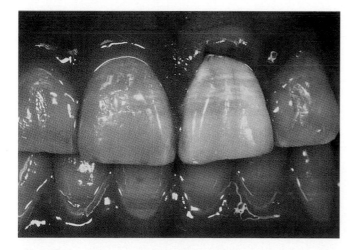

Plate 21-5 Patient in Plates 21-1 through 21-4 immediately after rubber dam removal from second bleaching session in a 24-hour time period. Rehydration of the bleached tooth will idealize the final result.

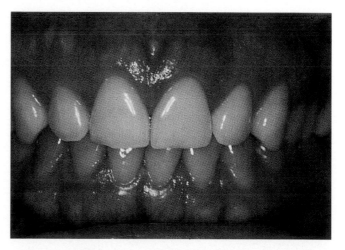

Plate 21-6 Maxillary arch bleached with a take home tray. Mandibular arch was a control to illustrate potential color change to patient.

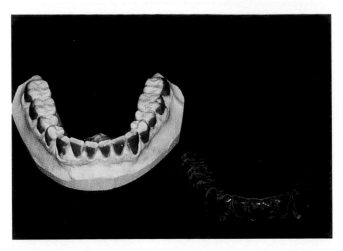

Plate 21-7 Typical custom home tray fabrication. Spacer material placed on facial surfaces of cast before fabrication of tray is optional.

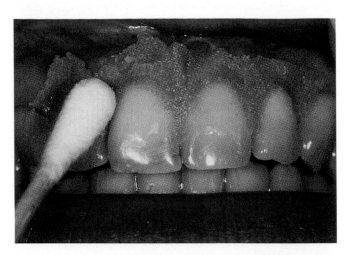

Plate 21-8 Technique depicted places Kenalog in Orabase at dried-tissue interface before rubber dam placement in order to protect gingival tissues from the bleaching agent.

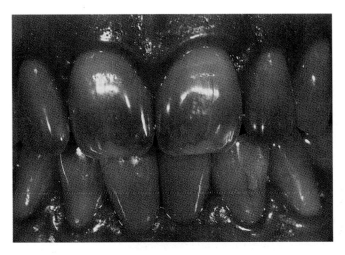

Plate 21-9 Pretreatment photograph of patient illustrating a combination of intrinsic and extrinsic stains.

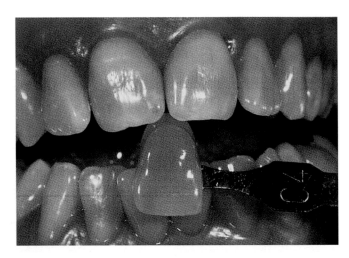

Plate 21-10 Two-week posttreatment of patient in Plate 21-9. Original shades of C4 and A4 have lightened significantly. Patient was treated with a combination of patient-administered take home bleaching trays and dentist-administered, in-office spot bleaching for excessively stained areas.

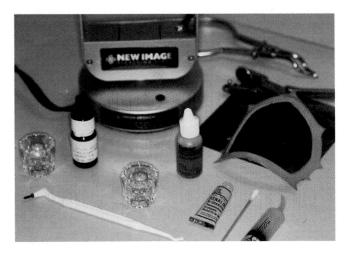

Plate 21-11 Typical armamentarium used for in-office, doctor administered, high-intensity bleaching. A variety of additional systems are available today.

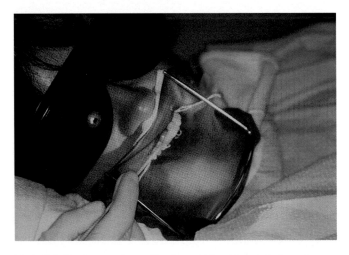

Plate 21-12 Cotton tip application of bleaching solution allows a controlled delivery of bleach. Patient's eyes are protected. Wet gauze placed over lip and above and below the rubber dam helps dissipate heat on facial tissues.

Chapter 21

 # Tooth-Whitening Modalities for Pulpless and Discolored Teeth

Cherilyn G. Sheets, Jacinthe M. Paquette, Robert S. Wright

Chapter Outline

Currently, the general population relates modern dentistry to improved facial aesthetics, health, and social success.[27,29] The traditional work of the endodontist (i.e., relief of pain and treatment of infection), has broadened to include membership on the restorative dental team. If the endodontist of tomorrow is to build and maintain a referral base, sensitivity to the patients' aesthetic desires and a comprehensive understanding of the aesthetic challenges that face other team members is required. A lighter dentition is associated with health, youth, and vigor. A recent survey of American women showed that 55% of those between 34 and 55 years would have their teeth whitened or straightened to create a more youthful appearance.[19] Tooth whitening is now the most commonly requested elective cosmetic service in the dental office.[65]

It has been predicted that dental professionals with the highest skills and corresponding reputations will benefit from the billions of dollars being spent in health care over the next 10 years.[75] According to patients seeking elective health care services, the first group of health care "specialists" that they are interested in seeing are "dentists providing cosmetic dentistry, including bleaching, bonding, veneers, invisible braces, etc." Approximately 90% of all practicing U.S. dentists now administer tooth-whitening treatments; 30% of those perform in-office bleaching. This trend will continue, with patients seeking an ever-increasing level of aesthetic restorative treatment.[11,38] Along with this trend comes an increase in productivity and professional satisfaction for all members of the team.[40]

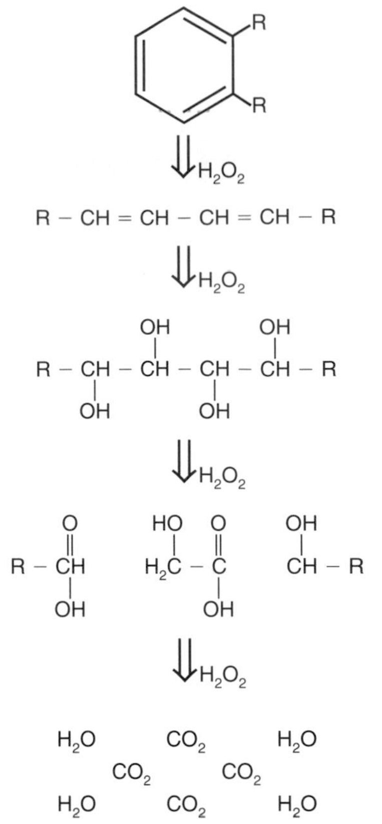

Fig. 21-1 The chemistry of tooth whitening.

CHEMISTRY OF BLEACHING

Tooth whitening continues to be an evolving science; therefore the endodontic specialist has a professional obligation to remain current with developments in the field and the supporting literature. Nathoo has developed three classifications of extrinsic dental stain[63]:

1. N1 type dental stain or direct dental stain: Colored material (chromogen) binds to the tooth's surface and causes discoloration. The color of the chromogen is similar to that of dental stain.

2. N2 type dental stain or direct dental stain: Colored material changes color after binding to the tooth.

3. N3 type dental stain or indirect dental stain: Colorless material or a pre-chromogen binds to the tooth and undergoes a chemical reaction to cause a stain.

The whitening mechanism of bleaching is believed to be linked to the degradation of high molecular weight and complex organic molecules that reflect a specific wavelength of light that is responsible for the color of the stain.[24,25,63] The resulting degradation products are of lower molecular weight and composed of less complex molecules that reflect less light, resulting in a reduction or elimination of discoloration. Darkly pigmented organic material responsible for enamel discoloration is composed of carbon ring structures with unsaturated, double-carbon bonds.

With further oxidation these products are modified to hydrophilic, nonpigmented carbon structures with saturated carbon bonds (i.e., the saturation point). Ideally, this is the point at which whitening should be terminated. If the degradation process continues, however, there is a further decomposition of organic matrix, which can lead to complete oxidation with generation of carbon dioxide and water, resulting in a total loss of enamel matrix protein (Fig. 21-1).*

Bleaching to improve the appearance of teeth has been documented for over 100 years[9,28,63]: oxalic acid (Chappell, 1887); hydrogen peroxide (Harlan, 1884); chlorine (Taft and Atkinson, 1989); heated hydrogen peroxide (Pearson, 1950); "walking bleach technique" (i.e., 35% hydrogen peroxide and sodium perborate) (Nutting and Poe, 1976); nightguard vital bleaching (i.e., 10% carbamide peroxide) (Haywood and Haymann, 1989); whitening toothpaste and the introduction of enzyme-based dentifrices (Rembrandt, 1992); manufacturing standards established (ADA, 1994); light-activated bleaching agents (1994); Argon, CO_2 laser and plasma arc activated chemicals (1994 to 1997); and, finally, Diode laser as a vector in tooth whitening (1999). From 1995 to 1998 a variety of concentrations of bleaching gels containing remineralizing agents, fluorides, and peroxide-free chemicals have been available. In 1996 an international symposium concluded that there were no significant adverse effects of dentist-monitored, "at home" bleaching agents on the oral tissues.[3,21,40,56]

Peroxides and oxygen free radicals are reactive oxygen agents that are formed as natural products in all living systems that use oxygen. Reactive oxygen is usually only at very low concentrations, because natural antioxidant protective systems prevent their accumulation.[10,55] Reactive oxygen in the presence of free metal ions, such as Fe or Cu, combine to cause oxidative damage to the tissue.[21] The safe use of peroxides in dentistry requires adherence to practices that minimize oxidative damage to oral cavity tissue.[12,69] Hydrogen peroxide is more stable; thus it has a longer shelf life in acidic solutions. However, it is more effective as a bleaching agent at pH values closer to the dissociation constant.[25] Also, solubility factors suggest that alkaline solutions would be less likely to penetrate the pulp than acidic solutions.

Alkaline solutions cause less demineralization of tooth surfaces than acidic agents.[24,25] The active ingredients in the bleaching agents must be quickly reactive with stains, nonreactive with dental or oral tissues, pleasant to use, and stable over long periods of shelf storage. Hydrogen peroxide readily breaks down to oxygen and water and is often accelerated by enzymes, such as peroxidase. Carbamide peroxide and hydrogen peroxide are most common and have been used in dentistry for decades. Other names for carbamide peroxide are urea peroxide, carbamyl peroxide, and perhydrol urea.

Carbamide peroxide converts to carbamide and hydrogen peroxide.[63] The carbamide portion is urea, a substance well tolerated by the human body.[70] Sodium perborate comes in a variety of preparations (i.e., monohydrate, trihydrate, tetrahydrate), with a varying content of oxygen. Sodium perborate solutions contain 95% perborate, providing 10% of the available oxygen. In the presence of acid, water, or heat it produces sodium metaborate, hydrogen peroxide, and nascent oxygen. Sodium perborate solutions are alkaline. Because they tend to be easier to control and safer to work with than Superoxyl, they are more popular for intracoronal bleaching.

Historically, internal bleaching treatments of nonvital teeth using 35% hydrogen peroxide (e.g., Superoxol) resulted in an incidence of cervical root resorption of 6% to 8%; combined with the application of heat, the rate rose to 18% to 25%.[22,23,72] The etiology of bleach-related external root resorption is complex.[31,34,50,51] For resorption to occur, there must be a combination of deficiency in the cementum (exposing the dentin), injury to the periodontal ligament (triggering an inflammatory response), or an infection (sustaining the inflammation).[73,82] The cementum deficiencies may be caused by a prior traumatic injury or by an incomplete cementoenamel junction (CEJ).[57,61] Such deficiencies expose permeable dentine that can allow toxic substances and bacteria from within the coronal pulp chamber and root canal to emerge at the root surface, where they may cause an inflammatory process in the periodontal ligament.[62]

Hydrogen peroxide is capable of generating a hydroxyl radical, an oxygen-derived free radical, in the presence of ferrous salts. Hydroxyl radicals are extremely reactive and have been shown to degrade components of connective tissue, particularly collagen and hyaluronic acid. Dahlstrom et al showed that there was a significant association between the production of hydroxyl radicals and the presence of tooth discoloration caused by blood components.[17]

Greatest yields of hydroxyl radicals occurred in teeth in which ethylenediaminetetracitic acid (EDTA) had been used to clean the pulp chamber before bleaching. It was concluded that hydroxyl radicals are generated during the thermocatalytic bleaching of root-filled teeth. Dahlstrom postulated that the generation of these toxic chemical by-products may be one mechanism underlying periodontal tissue destruction and root resorption after intracoronal bleaching.[17] Internal bleaching may be accomplished using sodium perborate mixed with water.[66] The aesthetic outcome is still acceptable, and the potential for resorption may be minimized.

Carbamyl peroxide has a slower rate of reaction than hydrogen peroxide, especially at room and oral temperatures.[40] Hydrogen peroxide releases oxygen within the first few seconds of contacting tooth surfaces, whereas carbamyl peroxide remains active for 40 to 90 minutes after tissue contact.[63] Oxygen combines with stain molecules in enamel to make stains more soluble. They are dissolved into the saliva or an oral rinse. The higher the concentration of the active ingredient, the faster the decoloration.

On the other hand, very high concentrations of carbamyl peroxide are more likely to irritate periodontal tissues.[48] Scherer et al found that nightguard bleaching actually had a therapeutic effect on inflamed gingival tissues. Leonard et al found that the ratio of tooth sensitivity and gingival irritation is related to the frequency of changing the solution.

Improving the chemistry of the bleaching agent is one way to improve its effectiveness; another may be modifying it to be initiated and catalyzed by the use of high-powered curing lights, ultraviolet lights, plasma arc lights, or laser lights.[19,26,83]

It is always wise to question claims made by manufacturers that have not been backed up by independent research. Both of these chemical modifications must be tempered with the potential for an increased incidence of thermal trauma. The balance of this chapter will review the cause of tooth discoloration and address the traditional and the contemporary treatment modalities for tooth whitening.

ETIOLOGY OF TOOTH DISCOLORATION

The etiology of tooth discoloration may be extrinsic or intrinsic or both; it may affect dentin, enamel, pulp, or any such combination of these tissues. Iatrogenic discoloration is a consequence of dentist or physician therapy, or it is the result of dietary, environmental, habitual, or age-related factors. The condition may be recent, temporary or permanent, and of local or systemic origin. The cause of the condition influences the potential outcome of the bleaching treatment and its lasting prognosis.[30] Therefore it is crucial that a thorough patient history is taken before the clinician makes a diagnosis and embarks on remedial treatment. Any concerns should be discussed with both the patient and the referring or restorative dentist. The clinical examination of the patient's dentition should include an assessment of plaque control; dental caries; surface texture; presence of external staining; type, quality, and extent of existing restorations; dental sensitivity; and pulpal status. Transillumination may reveal dental caries and assist in determining the comparative levels of calcification. The diode laser caries detector (Diagnodent, KaVo), a recent adjunct to the clinician's armamentarium, provides a more objective assessment of calcification. A complete series of periapical radiographs is essential for diagnosis and individual tooth assessment.

Discoloration Associated with Pulpal Involvement

Pulpal injury may be a consequence of bleaching; bacteria; physical, mechanical, thermal, or chemical trauma; orthodontic tooth movement; erosion; abrasion; attrition; or destructive patient habits.[64]

Intrapulpal Hemorrhage

After acute trauma, intrapulpal hemorrhage will give the tooth a reddish tinge. Occasionally, in the younger patient, the color may return to normal as the inflammation subsides.

More often, the discoloration changes to gray-brown in a matter of days as the pulp becomes necrotic. In other cases, especially where the trauma was not as marked, the pulp may accelerate the process of secondary dentin formation and pulpal fibrosis, resulting in reduction or obliteration of the pulp chamber. This process may span several years and result in a characteristic yellowing of the tooth. Rarer still, but with greater potential for disaster, is the initiation of internal resorption (i.e., pink spot), with the eventual loss of the tooth. The dentist should provide endodontic treatment as soon as this is discovered before the hemosiderin or necrotic pulpal toxins stain the dentin. Endodontic treatment and its sequelae must be balanced by the aesthetic compromise posed by it and that of delayed calcification. When making treatment decisions the clinician must also consider the eventual difficulty of performing latent endodontics in a calcified canal.

DENTIN AND ENAMEL DISCOLORATION

Developmental Defects in Enamel Formation

Amelogenesis Imperfecta   Amelogenesis Imperfecta (AI) encompasses a complicated group of conditions that demonstrate developmental alterations in the structure of the enamel in the absence of a systemic disorder. There are also numerous systemic diseases with associated enamel disorders that are not considered isolated AI. A vast number of rare disorders have been described in which dental anomalies have been observed. Some of these syndromes show enamel defects as the sole dental anomaly (Box 21-1); others affect enamel and other dental tissues. Enamel agenesis demonstrates a total lack of enamel formation. At least 14 different hereditary subtypes of AI exist, with numerous patterns of inheritance and a wide variety of clinical manifestations. As proof of the complicated nature of the process, several different classifications exist. The most likely accepted is that

---

Box 21-1   DEFECTS IN ENAMEL FORMATION

- Amelogenesis Imperfecta
- Endemic Fluorosis
- Ricketts
- Chromosomal Anomalies
- Inherited Diseases
- Lead
- Thalidomide, Tetracyline
- Childhood Illnesses
- Malnutrition
- Metabolic Disorders
- Neurologic Disorders

---

developed by Witkop. The formation of enamel is a multistep process, and problems may arise in any one of the steps.

Generally the development of enamel can be divided into three major stages:

1. Elaboration of the organic matrix
2. Mineralization of the matrix
3. Maturation of the enamel

The hereditary defects of the formation of the enamel also are divided along these lines: hypoplastic, hypocalcified, and hypomaturation. The estimated frequency of AI in the population varies between 1:700 and 1:14,000. As in any hereditary disorder, clustering in certain geographic areas may occur, resulting in a wide range of reported prevalence. In general, both deciduous and permanent dentitions are diffusely affected.

Developmentally, AI in its various forms can be linked to these types of genes: autosomal dominant, autosomal recessive, x-linked dominant, and x-linked recessive. For most situations this classification is academic, because bleaching of AI dentitions is merely an adjunct to comprehensive restorative treatment.

Endemic Fluorosis   The optimum concentration of fluoride in the drinking water for dental development is one part per million. When the level of fluoride intake approaches two parts per million, noticeable white patches occur in the enamel. Such teeth are more resistant to dental caries but may be aesthetically unappealing. When the levels exceed three parts per million, patchy brown discoloration of the enamel occur. Higher concentrations than this in the drinking water can result in pitting and anomalies in enamel formation. Black and McKay first reported this condition in the literature in 1916.[9]

An excessive amount of fluoride can be ingested by children or absorbed through the mucous membrane, resulting in mottling of the enamel. The type and extent of fluorosis is related to the age of the patient and the duration and quantum of the exposure. Genetic disposition may also play a part. The excess fluoride induces a metabolic change in the ameloblasts. The resultant enamel has a defective matrix and an irregular, poorly mineralized structure. Simple cases of white or brown spot fluorosis can be successfully bleached. In cases where the enamel is more opaque, bleaching may cause the white spots to become more pronounced. Preceding the bleaching with microabrasion can sometimes improve the aesthetic outcome.

Vitamin and Mineral Deficiencies   Ricketts, a vitamin D deficiency, results in osteomalacia, developmental anomalies in the bones, and as characteristic white-patch hypoplasia in teeth. Scurvy, a vitamin C deficiency, together with deficiencies in vitamin A or phosphorous uptake during the formative period of the dentition, may result in enamel hypoplasias.

A variety of other chromosomal anomalies and inherited conditions exist that result in malformation of the enamel too numerous to mention. In these cases, a clinical assessment of the condition of the enamel is more important than determining the genetic cause.

Childhood Illness   A common childhood illness or condition of jaundice can result in blue-gray or yellow-brown dentin discoloration from the circulating bilirubin and biliverdin. Congenital erythropoietic porphyria is an autosomal recessive disorder of porphyrin metabolism that results in the increased synthesis and excretion of porphyrins and their related precursors. These teeth demonstrate an unsightly deep purplish brown pigmentation of the dentin and fluoresce under UV light. Erythroblastosis fetalis, an Rh factor incompatibility of the mother's and infant's blood, induces jaundicelike conditions and associated dentin discoloration.

Malnutrition   Before malformations in the dentition are evident, malnutrition has to be severe and prolonged. Metabolic disorders occurring shortly after birth or extended periods during the early years of life will be displayed chronologically on the developing teeth as linear areas of hypoplasia. This may follow infection or kidney damage.

Neurologic Disorders   Neurologic disorders can result in developmental retardation and anomalies in dental development.

Dental Caries

Dental caries is the most common cause of external and internal discoloration of enamel and dentin. The shade is related to the rate of the carious destruction, with the darkness being indirectly proportionate to the rate.

Extrinsic Enamel Stain

Diet-Related Stains   The consumption of strong tea or coffee, especially when immediately preceded by orange or grapefruit juice, is a common dietary cause of external discoloration. Blackcurrant juice or cola drinks act by both etching and staining the tooth structure simultaneously (Box 21-2).

Bacterial Stains   Chromophilic bacteria frequently seen in the deciduous or mixed dentition can cause a dotted or black-line stain. It has been documented that this type of bacteria is associated with lower-than-normal caries rates and that removal may result in recolonization of the oral cavity by a more cariogenic flora.

Gingival Hemorrhage   Chronic gingivitis may induce staining from the breakdown of blood in the gingival sulcus.

Chlorhexidene   Chlorhexidene acts in reducing plaque formation by altering the chemistry of the primary pellicle by disturbing matrix formation. This altered pellicle does, however, attract more extrinsic stain not readily removed by tooth brushing.

Marijuana and Tobacco   Smoking marijuana may produce characteristic linear, green, circumferential rings at the cervical margins. Smoking tobacco produces a yellow-brown discoloration, especially on the lingual aspects of the teeth. Chewing tobacco causes a black-brown stain that is most noticeable on the buccal surfaces of the mandibular posterior teeth. This can be unilateral, depending upon the habit (e.g., chewing tobacco).

Age-Related Discoloration

Age-related discoloration (Box 21-3) is a natural process resulting from secondary dentin formation and thinning of the enamel layer. Bleaching is particularly effective in older adults whose yellowed teeth have smaller pulps and greater dentin. These teeth generally tend to be less sensitive and can withstand higher bleaching temperatures.

Defects in Dentin Formation

Dentinogenesis Imperfecta   Dentinogenesis imperfecta (DI) is a hereditary developmental disturbance of the dentin that may be seen alone or in conjunction with its related systemic hereditary disorder of bone, osteogenesis imperfecta. Most cases can be traced to Caucasians (especially people of English or French ancestry) from communities close to the English Channel. The disorder is autosomal dominant and occurs in about 1:8000 in the United States (Box 21-4).

Box 21-2   **EXTRINSIC ENAMEL STAIN**

- Dental Caries
- Bacterial
- Dietary
- Gingival Hemorrhage
- Chlorhexidene
- Marijuana, Chewing Tobacco, Beetle Nut, etc.

Box 21-3   **AGE-RELATED DISCOLORATION**

- Secondary Dentin Formation
- Thinning of Enamel
- Chipping and Microfractures

Box 21-4   DEFECTS IN DENTIN FORMATION

- Dentinogenesis Imperfecta
- Erythropoetic Porphyria
- Tetracycline and Minocycline
- Genetic Anomalies
- Hyperbilirubinemia
- Osteogenesis Imperfecta

Witkop outlined three descriptive classifications of this disorder:

- Dentinogenesis imperfecta
- Hereditary with opalescent dentin
- Brandywine isolate

Both permanent and deciduous dentitions are affected. The teeth have a blue-brown discoloration, often with a distinctive translucence. The enamel frequently separates from the underlying dentin. Once exposed, the dentin often demonstrates significant accelerated attrition. Key radiographic features are bulbous crowns, cervical constriction, thin roots, and early obliteration of root canals and pulp chambers. Shell teeth have normal thickness enamel but extremely thin dentin with enlarged pulps.

Other dentinal defects in dentin formation include the following:

- Erythropoetic porphyria
- Tetracycline and minocycline staining
- Hyperbilirubinemia
- A variety of other genetic anomalies

Systemic Medications

Tetracycline Family   Tetracycline is a chelating agent for calcium, forming tetracycline orthophosphate. Consequently, tetracycline, when consumed during the developmental period of the teeth, will result in a characteristic blue-gray or yellow-brown opalescent discoloration of the dentin. This is thought to be a photo-initiated reaction, explaining why the incisors tend to be more affected than the molars.

Jordan and Boksman have proposed three categories of discoloration of the dentin:

1. Light yellow or gray stain
2. Yellow-brown or deeper gray stain
3. Brownish-yellow or blue-gray stain with distinctive banding

The first two categories normally respond well to bleaching. The third category is less amenable to bleaching, and the teeth usually have residual banding. These teeth will require veneers and, in some cases, full coverage crowns to achieve a satisfactory aesthetic improvement. Either treatment modality can induce life-changing benefits for such patients.

Tetracycline, a bacteriostatic antimicrobial, was commonly used for the treatment of chronic middle ear infections in children and long-term therapy for acne vulgaris. Fortu-nately this drug is rarely prescribed now for pregnant women or young children. It is still used, however, in the treatment of cystic fibrosis and Rocky Mountain spotted fever. Minocy-cline is a semisynthetic derivative of tetracycline. Unlike tetracycline, minocycline is poorly absorbed from the gastrointestinal tract and does not combine readily with calcium; however, it does combine readily with iron, forming a yellow-gray discoloration of varying severity. Success of bleaching is similar to that of tetracycline staining.

Iatrogenic Discoloration   A variety of restorative materials and procedures (e.g., residual or recurrent dental caries; silver and mercury alloy stain; corroded steel pins, silver points, metal posts; degrading restorative materials and cements; endodontic obturation materials and sealers), together with unremoved pulpal remnants, can all lead to discoloration of the dentin.

CONTRAINDICATIONS TO BLEACHING

Patient Selection

Careful assessment of the patient may prevent subsequent difficulties.[11,27,37,40,48] Those with emotional or psychologic problems or those with unrealistic goals do not make good candidates for bleaching.

Case Selection

It should be determined at the consultation stage whether bleaching will improve the aesthetic appearance of the patients dentition; whether white spots may become more visible; or where orthodontics, periodontics, or restorative treatment (or any combination) is necessary to obtain the desired result.[9,32,49,58] Both dentist and patient may be able to "test the waters" by using computer imaging. The general dentist or specialist should not hesitate in declining to treat a patient should his or her professional opinion dictate that bleaching is not in the patient's best interest.

Dentin Hypersensitivity

These symptoms may be associated with severe cases of attrition, abrasion, erosion, or abfraction. Sometimes the most severe cases of hypersensitivity are associated with the early stages of the foregoing when there is recent exposure of the DEJ. This can be hard to control when using home care bleaching trays.[72] When the bleaching is conducted by the dentist, the clinician can isolate the cervical areas with a rubber dam or protect the dentin with a bonding agent.

Suspected or Confirmed Bulimia

Application of bleaching agents with such patients may result in acute pulpitis. It is unwise for obvious professional reasons to embark on any irreversible dental procedure other than relief of pain until such a time that the patient's psychologic problems have been adequately addressed. Bulimic patients usually require a comprehensive course of restorative treatment involving veneers or crowns.

Generalized Dental Caries and Leaking Restorations

Use of bleaching agents for patients who fall into this category may lead to severe, generalized hypersensitivity. This is one reason contraindicating the use of "do-it-yourself, over-the-counter," home bleaching kits. All carious lesions and clinically unserviceable restorations should be retreated before prescribing dental bleaching.

Heavily Restored Teeth

Teeth with visible, tooth-colored restorations respond poorly to bleaching because the composite restorations do not lighten and, hence, become more evident after bleaching the tooth structure. The patient should be informed before treatment that a replacement of the preexisting restorations may be required after the bleaching treatment.

Teeth with Opaque White Spots

Application of bleaching agents to such teeth are likely to enhance the contrast between the good and hypocalcified enamel.[4] Either microabrasion or selected ameloplasty and composite resin bonding may be required in conjunction with the bleaching treatments.*

Teeth Slated for Bonded Restorations or Orthodontic Bracketing

The oxygen produced during bleaching remains in the enamel and dentin for up to 2 weeks. Oxygen interferes with the chemistry of bonding agents and will induce bonding failure.[79,80] Such treatment should be delayed 2 to 3 weeks to allow complete dissipation of residual oxygen.[5,77]

ALTERNATIVES TO BLEACHING

Microabrasion

Microabrasion is a technique for removing about 25 microns of the enamel surface.[13,14] It is particularly useful for eliminating white or brown spots or surface roughness. The original protocol called for the use of 18% hydrochloric acid and pumice. Proprietary products, such as Prema (Premier Dental Products), consist of a water-soluble gel containing a dilute concentration of hydrochloric acid and an abrasive compound. The gel is applied to the enamel surface with special rubber cups in a contraangle hand piece. The application

time is short, about 10 seconds per tooth, and teeth must be rinsed well with water. An assessment is made of color change and degree of tooth removal, and the process is repeated as required. When the desired result has been achieved, teeth are rinsed thoroughly with water and the residual solution is neutralized with sodium bicarbonate. The teeth are rinsed again with water, dried, and polished with a fine, fluoride-containing prophy paste.

The McInnes Microabrasion Technique

A solution of 5 parts 30% hydrogen peroxide, 5 parts 36% hydrochloric acid, and 1 part diethyl ether is applied directly to the discolored areas for 1 to 2 minutes.[59] Fine cuttle discs are used over the enamel surface for 15 seconds to remove the softened enamel surface.

INTERNAL BLEACHING OF PULPLESS TEETH

Darkening and loss of translucency may follow loss of vitality, both before and subsequent to endodontic therapy. In the case of acute trauma this can be related to internal hemorrhage within the dentin. Other causes include seepage of toxins from a necrotic pulp or staining from medicaments, cements, metal posts, or the optical effects of dehydration.[63] In the case of a single incisor tooth, most clinicians would be reluctant to violate the tooth by preparing it for a full-coverage restoration. Bleaching unsightly, discolored teeth has been documented for over 100 years; Superoxol in concentrations of 30% to 35% have commonly been used.

Superoxol is a strong oxidizing agent and can readily burn soft tissue. The operator and assistant must take great care not to spill the solution, causing needless injury to the patient or themselves. Heating Superoxol solution placed in the access cavity of the endodontically treated tooth initiates the release of oxygen. The oxygen breaks down the darkly pigmented macromolecules into smaller, lighter-colored molecules. An alternative treatment is to seal a pledget of cotton wool soaked in a mixture of Superoxol and sodium perborate in the access cavity of the tooth for a period of 4 to 7 days. This has been termed the "walking bleach" technique.*

Early internal bleaching of nonvital teeth using 30% hydrogen peroxide (e.g., Superoxol) resulted in an incidence of cervical root resorption of 6% to 8%; when combined with the application of heat the rate rises to 18% to 25%. As explained earlier in the chapter, the cause of bleaching-related external root resorption is complex.

Protocol for Internal Bleaching

With proper case selection, internal bleaching remains an excellent treatment choice.

---

*References 13,14,15,76,77,78

*References 22,23,70,71,72

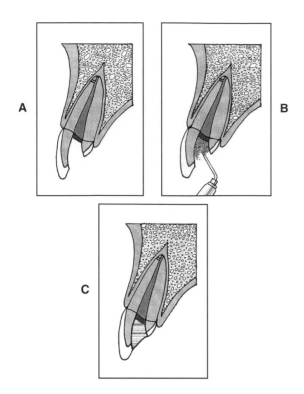

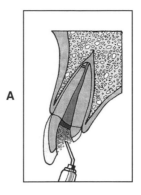
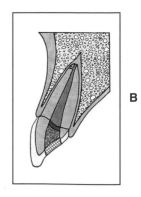

Fig. 21-3 "Walking bleach" technique. **A**, Infusion of Superoxyl into cotton pledget reservoir in access cavity protected with a glass ionomer cement base. **B**, Mixture of Superoxyl and sodium perborate in cotton pledget reservoir sealed in access cavity with Cavit.

Fig. 21-2 "Chair side" internal bleaching. **A**, Access cavity in maxillary incisor with barrier layer of glass ionomer cement. **B**, Infusion of Superoxyl into access cavity. **C**, Closure of access cavity with Cavit.

- Examine the tooth clinically and radiographically, using all customary adjunctive diagnostic aids to determine whether the tooth requires retreatment (Fig. 21-2, *A-C*) (Plate 21-1).
- Take an intraoral photograph of the tooth to be bleached with a corresponding tab from a ceramic shade guide placed next to it to record initial shade (Plate 21-2).
- Perform prophylaxis of the objective and neighboring teeth.
- Probe circumferentially to determine the outline of the CEJ.
- Place a well-fitting rubber dam (exposing at least the adjacent teeth for shade comparison), and ligate the treatment tooth at the gingiva with dental floss.
- Prepare the access cavity in a conservative and meticulous manner. Remove all endodontic obturation material, sealer, cement, and necessary restorative material; however, remove no more dentin than is necessary. Ensure that all pulpal remnants and debris (a common source for discoloration) is eliminated from the pulp horns.
- Remove 2 to 3 mm of obturating material from the root canal.
- Irrigate the access cavity with copious amount of water and dry well without desiccating.
- Introduce resin-modified glass ionomer cement (in a Centrix syringe or with a lentulo spiral) into the canal and access cavity.

- Contour the base so that it follows the outline of the CEJ and about 1 mm incisal to it. The barrier material should be a minimum of 2 mm in thickness (Plate 21-3).
- Place a cotton pellet against the internal labial aspect of the tooth. Introduce Superoxol to the access cavity carefully from a syringe with a metal needle.
- Heat the solution with a bleaching wand at a low-to-medium setting or with a dry endosonic spreader. The temperature should be no higher than 15° F above body temperature. Repeat as required (Plate 21-4).
- Rinse the tooth with copious amounts of water. Place a fresh, dry cotton pellet in the access cavity and seal with Cavit.
- Photograph tooth with corresponding shade guide (Plate 21-5).
- Recall the patient in 1 week to assess the color after rehydration.
- Repeat the procedure as necessary. If color change is satisfactory seal with glass ionomer cement.
- Recall patient in 2 weeks to place permanent, bonded, composite-resin restoration in the access cavity. This will allow dissipation of residual oxygen that would otherwise have interfered with the efficacy of the bonding agent.

"Walking Bleach" Technique

The "walking bleach" technique (Fig. 21-3) is advocated where the results of chair side internal bleaching have been inadequate.

Years ago, "walking bleach" was the most common technique used by dentists. With careful case selection, it still can be quite successful.

- Depending upon the severity of the residual discoloration and the age of the patient, the clinician can use either sodium perborate and water or a mixture of sodium perborate and Superoxyl. The majority of cases of external resorption appear in patients under the age of 25 years. It has been speculated that this is related to the fact that younger patients have a greater number of more patent dentinal tubules.

- Etching of the dentin opens up the tubules, permitting more of the bleaching agent to penetrate (increasing the risk of root resorption). Because this does not appear to increase the effectiveness of the tooth whitening, etching should not be performed.
- The clinician should pack the paste into the access cavity and seal it with a 2 mm thick layer of Cavit to prevent intraoral leakage.
- The mixture should be left in place for up to 1 week, with instructions that the patient return to the dental office when the tooth appears lighter than the adjacent ones. This treatment may have to be repeated several times.
- The shelf life of bleaching agents is short, and their effectiveness is reduced by 50% after 6 months.
- Similar directions apply for placement of a final restoration.

Note that increasing the amount of bleaching increases the risk of cervical resorption,* which should be minimal provided that the barrier layer is well placed. It has been documented that bleaching teeth may result in a reduction in fracture toughness.†

Recall Appointments

Evidence of cervical root resorption does not usually manifest for at least 6 months postoperatively. Lesions detected 2 years later are usually too advanced for the tooth to be salvaged. Early detection and repair enhances the prognosis.

Repair of Cervical Resorptive Lesions

Cases of initial resorptive lesions can sometimes be arrested using calcium hydroxide. In more severe cases, orthodontic extrusion or crown-lengthening procedures may be necessary to access the lesion and avoid violating the biologic width.[52,53]

Where aesthetics is not of primary importance, silver alloy is often the simplest and most predictable restorative material. Composite resin can provide an aesthetic restoration but when dependent solely upon dentine bonding, the prognosis is limited.

Dumfahrt and Moschen have described a technique for restoring cervical resorptive lesions with indirect porcelain inlays after clinical crown-lengthening procedures.[18] The shortfall of this technique would again be the dependence upon dentin bonding. Preventing cervical root resorption with proper restorative materials in the coronal third of the canal is always the most prudent choice.

VITAL BLEACHING

This category includes over-the-counter tooth-whitening products, nightguard matrix bleaching, and dentist- or hygienist-administered power bleaching (Plates 21-6 and 21-7). Regardless of the technique being used it is essential that a thorough clinical examination and prophylaxis be performed before applying tooth whitening agents. Any soft tissue problems, defective restorations, and carious lesions should be corrected. It is good practice to record the shade of the patient's teeth in a photograph with a tab from a shade guide.

Patients with visible ceramic or composite restorations should be informed that these will not be lightened by bleaching and may become more evident as a consequence. Patients should be further advised that they should not proceed with the treatment unless they plan to replace the existing restorations after bleaching. Patients who are planning to have veneers or all-ceramic restorations placed on their teeth but who had not contemplated vital bleaching should be advised that such treatment will reduce the amount of opacifier required to mask out the underlying tooth color.[5] This will permit the ceramist to fabricate more translucent and vital-looking restorations. Tooth preparation should be delayed for 2 to 3 weeks after bleaching to allow for rehydration and rebound, and to permit the dissipation of residual oxygen that would interfere with the bonding agents.

Bleaching Agents

Hydrogen peroxide, although now available in a variety of gels and pastes, is still the most effective bleaching agent. It is available in concentrations from 30% to 50%. The gels used for nightguard bleaching are 5% to 22% sodium perborate that effectively produces the equivalent oxygen as 2% to 5% hydrogen peroxide (but over a slower time period). It has been shown that the delivery of hydrogen peroxide in an alkaline rather than an acid medium will significantly improve its oxidizing efficiency.

Patient Preparation

- The patient should be draped with a protective cape to prevent spillage of the bleaching agent on hands, skin, or clothing.
- The patient should be supplied with protective eyewear.
- No local anesthesia should be administered that could otherwise inhibit patient feedback about pain or discomfort.
- Before application of the rubber dam, Oraseal (a light-cured resin) or Orabase paste can be applied liberally to protect the labial and lingual tissues (Plate 21-8).
- Next the clinician should place a heavy gauge rubber dam, ligating the individual teeth with floss. Oraseal can also be applied to any amalgam restorations, reducing the build up of heat from the light source. The punched holes should be smaller than normal, rendering them further apart to ensure adequate coverage of the proximal gingiva.
- Vaseline should be applied to the patients' lips before mounting the rubber dam frame. Wet gauze can also be placed over the patients' lips to prevent thermal trauma

---

*References 16,22,31,34,51,57
†References 7,8,54,74,81,84

from the heat lamp. It is important to keep rewetting the gauze during the procedure.

Tooth Preparation

Most authorities agree that there is little or no advantage in etching the enamel before bleaching; it results in a roughening and loss of surface enamel tissue (i.e., 10 µm from the pumice and 20 µm from the etchant). This enamel must then be polished with diamond paste after bleaching to bring back the surface luster, which removes approximately 20 to 30 µm of fluoride-rich enamel. There are situations where the enamel fails to bleach in the absence of etching. Before applying the bleaching agent the clinician should be sure to remove all excess Orabase, Vaseline, or varnish. Next the clinician should pumice the teeth to be bleached and rinse thoroughly. Areas of cervical erosion, abfraction, or attrition into the dentin can be protected with a bonding agent.

In most situations, clinicians should follow the manufacturer's directions and apply the gel or paste liberally, 3 to 4 mm thick. In cases of hypoplasia or fluorosis where there could be spots or banding, the clinician should modify the application accordingly. Some teeth may be more discolored than others. As a rule, yellow-brown stains respond better than blue-gray stains, and the incisal half lightens more readily than the cervical portion of the crown because of the varying degrees of thickness of the dentin (Plates 21-9 and 21-10).

Traditional Vital Bleaching

The traditional bleaching protocol called for the use of a special bleaching lamp (Plates 21-11 and 21-12). Upon application of the hydrogen peroxide solution to the teeth, the lamp was placed 12 to 14 inches from the patient's face and left there for 20 to 30 minutes. This had the advantage of not requiring the dentist or assistant to move the light source from tooth to tooth.

Although the heat source is set at a temperature not to cause thermal trauma to the pulp, many patients complain that it becomes uncomfortably hot on the skin surface. After isolating the teeth with a rubber dam, a layer of single ply gauze is applied to the surface of the teeth. Because the Superoxol solution is a liquid, the gauze acts as a wick and reservoir to retain the solution in close proximity to the teeth. Double-thickness gauze is correspondingly applied over the rubber dam, covering the lower lip to catch the excess solution and protect the mucosa. Other devices for getting into grooves and hollows, such rheostat-controlled heating devices, are available with special metal tips of various shapes and sizes.

Intentional Endodontics and Intracoronal Bleaching

In 1982 Abou-Raas suggested performing intentional endodontics and intracoronal bleaching for patients with severe tetracycline staining.[1] This was proposed as being a "more conservative" treatment to full coverage crowns. At that time, porcelain laminate veneers were in their infancy and tended to be rather opaque and monochromatic. In addition, bonding agents did not have the predictability that they have at the present time. Today tetracycline-staining cases will normally be treated by power bleaching and restored with veneers. In severe cases, however, a satisfactory aesthetic result can only be achieved with full coverage crowns. Abou-Raas published a follow-up report in 1998 claiming that excellent, permanent, aesthetic results were obtained with no side effects for some 112 teeth in 20 patients.[2]

CONTEMPORARY TOOTH-WHITENING MODALITIES

Tungsten-Halogen Curing Lamp

The new wave of vital bleaching in the 1980s started with Fuji HiLite dual-cure material (35% hydrogen peroxide). The paste was mixed (turning a green-blue color) and activated with a standard, composite-curing light. As the chemical reaction progressed the paste changed to white, at which point no more oxygen was being produced.

Nightguard Vital Bleaching

This form of slow release custom matrix delivery is also known as the "dentist-prescribed, patient-administered" technique.* The advantage of this technique is that it does not tie up the dental chair. The disadvantage is that it takes 2 to 6 weeks; some patients find this inconvenient, and there tends to be more sensitivity. Originally when these products came on the market, the patient had a choice of either sleeping with the bleach-filled trays during the night (for 4 to 6 weeks) or wearing them during the day (for 2 to 3 weeks). Today varieties of tooth-whitening gels are on the market in a range of concentrations. Success of treatment depends upon patient cooperation, but it is essentially dose and time related. Understandably, patient-administered bleaching is potentially open to abuse; the dentist should have the patient return to the practice once a week to monitor the progress.

Since the introduction of nightguard vital bleaching in the late 1980s, a multitude of articles have been written on the subject, many by Haywood. They conclude that dentist-supervised nightguard vital bleaching has no detrimental effect on the teeth or tissues. Common side effects, such as blanching of the gingival papilla or crest and occasional thermal sensitivity, are transient. The color change will remain stable for a minimum of 1 to 3 years.[47]

Fabrication of the Bleaching Trays

Alginate impressions are taken of the patient's maxillary and mandibular arches. Care must be taken to avoid incorpo-

---

*References 11,35,36,37,39,41-47

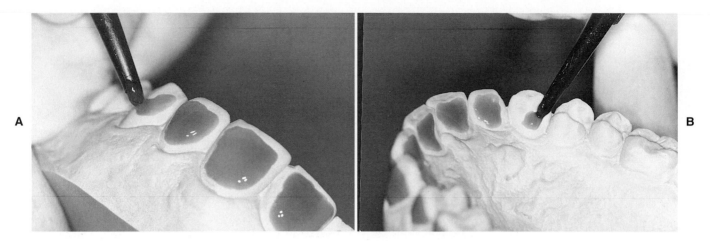

Fig. 21-4   Fabrication of a bleaching tray starts with an accurate cast. Light-cured resin is placed on the labial (**A**) and lingual (**B**) surfaces to create a reservoir for the bleaching solution.

rating voids or drags in the impression. After disinfecting the impressions and thoroughly rinsing them, casts are poured in stone. The casts are then prepared for the vacuum-forming machine by removing the palate and vestibule. It is customary to treat one arch at a time, allowing one to act as a control for the other. Reservoirs are placed on the labial surface of the teeth to be bleached just shy of the gingival margin as shown (Figs. 21-4, 21-5, 21-6, and 21-7). A soft, clear, plastic sheet (approximately 0.3 mm thick) is placed in the vacuum former, softened by heating, and then sucked down over the cast (Figs. 21-8 and 21-9). Upon cooling, the plastic matrix is trimmed with a scalpel or electric knife approximately 3 mm apically from the gingival margin facially and lingually in a scalloped manner (Figs. 21-10 and 21-11). A rubber wheel in a micromotor can then be used to smooth the rough edges (Fig. 21-12).

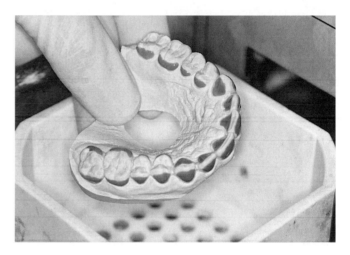

Fig. 21-5   The cast is placed in a light-curing oven to harden the resin.

Delivery of the Bleaching Trays

The matrix is tried in the patient's mouth and relieved where there is tissue blanching or occlusal interference. The patient should be instructed to place a couple of drops of the gel into each tooth slot and then place the matrix gently over the teeth. If the nightguard is to be worn while sleeping, only one application is required and the gel concentration should not exceed 16%. For daytime uses the gel should be replaced every 2 hours.

Patients should be cautioned about the antiseptic taste and the possibility of tissue irritation and thermal sensitivity. This should be transient. However, should patients feel that this is excessive, they should discontinue use and return to the dentist for evaluation. Daytime wearers should be instructed to return once a week for 3 weeks; nighttime wearers should be told to return once every 2 weeks for a 6-week period.

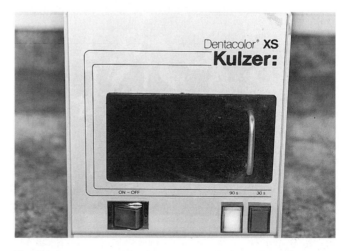

Fig. 21-6   Ninety seconds of exposure in a high-intensity light oven is required.

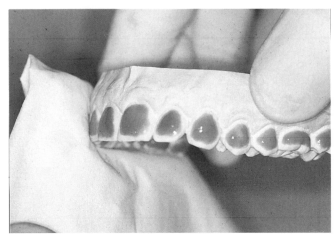

Fig. 21-7 Nonpolymerized resin on the surface is gently wiped off with a tissue.

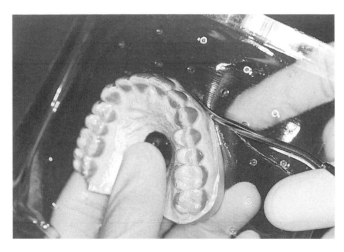

Fig. 21-10 The excess tray material is grossly trimmed from the cast.

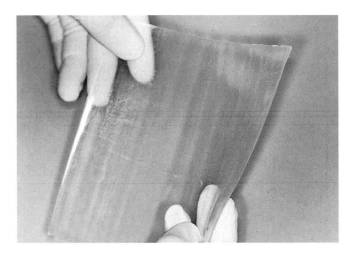

Fig. 21-8 A sheet of SofTray vinyl is chosen for final tray fabrication.

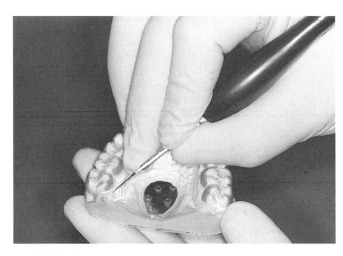

Fig. 21-11 A sharp knife is used for fine trimming; edges are further refined with a finishing bur and smoothed with a warm instrument.

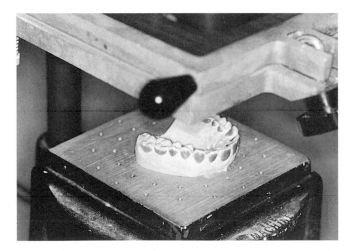

Fig. 21-9 The cast is placed in a vacuum-former unit, ready to heat and "shrink fit" the resin tray to the patient's cast.

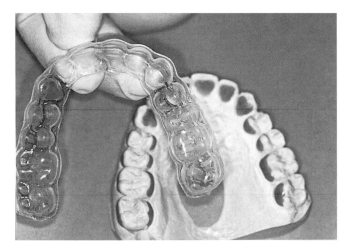

Fig. 21-12 The finished tray ready for the patient to use with a doctor-prescribed bleaching solution.

Power Bleaching

Power bleaching is the term given to accelerated, in-office, tooth-whitening procedures using either a xenon plasma arc–curing light or a laser. The plasma arc lamp was introduced in 1993. Shortly afterwards came the "liquid rubber dam." This is a light-cured resin gel that can be painted on the gingivae and areas of the teeth that you do not wish to bleach. The advantages being that it is much quicker to apply but does have a tendency to flow up onto the cervical area of the teeth under mouth temperature if you delay the curing. More care has to be exerted when applying the bleaching gel as, unlike the rubber dam, the lips and soft tissues are not protected. In most states the dental hygienist can use a plasma arc light but not an Argon laser. Hygienists in some states are permitted to use the recently introduced diode laser–curing light.

Advantages of Power Bleaching Delegating the power bleaching to a dental auxiliary will generate more revenue for the practice, freeing up more time for the dentist to perform more skillful procedures. Most patients, given the choice, would rather have their teeth bleached in one visit rather than spend several weeks of tedious efforts with home-bleaching trays. The dentist has the ability to isolate areas, such as abfractions or erosions, with bonding agents to prevent sensitivity.

Power-Bleaching Protocol By following a precise power bleaching protocol, treatment success is improved from the perspective of patient satisfaction and clinical results. The following outlines an accepted protocol:
- Arrange all materials for easy access to the operator and the patient, allowing for a delivery of materials that does not pass over the patient's face.
- Operator, assistant, and patient should wear protective yellow-lensed eyewear.
- The patient should be instructed to raise a hand should a tingling sensation in the gums, lips, or teeth be felt or if the temperature feels uncomfortably hot.
- Two Vitamin E capsules should be cut open and the oil expressed onto a glass slab; a number of cotton pellets should be placed in the oil and a pair of cotton pliers should be at hand. Vitamin E is a powerful antioxidant. If the clinician notices blanching of the tissues caused by the hydrogen peroxide (which can burn soft tissue), the vitamin E oil should be immediately applied to the area. If response is quick, the oxidation process can be reversed before any damage occurs.

Power-Bleaching Technique Once the patient and operator are prepared for the bleaching appointment, the operator can commence the bleaching process. The recommended protocol is as follows:
- Pumice the teeth.
- Isolate the teeth using bilateral cheek retractors and cotton rolls.

- Use a ligated rubber dam or apply a light-cured resin dam extending from the gingival crevice.
- Mix power bleach solution (e.g., Qasar-Brite, Apollo Secret) following the manufacturer's directions.
- Apply the gel 2 to 3 mm thick over the labial surface of the teeth using a disposable brush.
- Expose one tooth at a time for 10 seconds. When arch is complete, repeat twice for a total exposure of 30 seconds per tooth.
- Leave the gel on the teeth for an additional 5 minutes.
- Remove gel with wet gauze, then irrigate with copious amounts of water.
- Pumice teeth to remove residual exposed gel from enamel surface. Repeat process 2 to 4 times until desired result is achieved.
- Remove gel and irrigate thoroughly.
- Polish teeth with diamond paste and a prophylaxis with neutral-pH sodium fluoride gel.
- Instruct patients to avoid coffee, tea, and cola drinks for 2 weeks (they may stain the newly bleached teeth).

REVIEW OF AVAILABLE LIGHT SOURCES

Conventional Bleaching Light

The conventionally used bleaching light supplied energy to enhance the bleaching action of hydrogen peroxide simply by adding heat. The heat caused a more vigorous release of oxygen and facilitated the dissolution of the pigments. It was slow and often uncomfortable for the patient.

Tungsten-Halogen Curing Light

The standard curing light provides heat and stimulates the initiation of the chemical reaction by activating the light-sensitive chemicals in the bleaching agent. This is a time-consuming process (i.e., 40 to 60 seconds per application per tooth).

Argon Laser

A true laser light is delivered to the chemical agent. Argon laser wavelengths are not attracted to water. The action is to stimulate the catalyst in the chemical. There is no thermal effect; therefore there will be less dehydration of the enamel and subsequent rebound effect. The rapid treatment time of 10 seconds per application per tooth is an advantage for clinician and patient.

Xenon Plasma Arc Light

This nonlaser, high-intensity light (Fig. 21-13) produces a great deal of heat; therefore it can only be applied for brief, 3-second periods to the tooth. The action is thermal and stimulates the catalyst in the chemical. Although it is very fast,

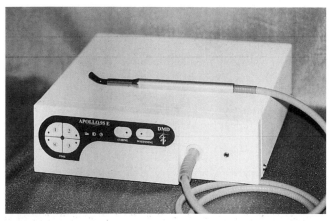

Fig. 21-13 Nonlaser, high-intensity light (used in 3 second bursts) is very fast, but it has greater potential for thermal trauma.

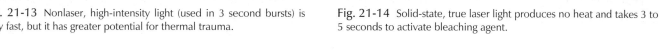

Fig. 21-14 Solid-state, true laser light produces no heat and takes 3 to 5 seconds to activate bleaching agent.

there is a greater potential for thermal trauma to the pulp and surrounding soft tissues than with other light sources.

Diode Laser Light

A true laser light produced from a solid-state source. It is ultrafast, taking 3 to 5 seconds to activate the bleaching agent. This type of laser produces no heat (Fig. 21-14).

References

1. Abou-Raas M: The elimination of tetracycline discoloration by intentional endodontics and internal bleaching, *J Endod* 8:101, 1982.
2. Abou-Raas M: Long-term prognosis of intentional endodontics and internal bleaching of tetracycline-stained teeth, *Compend Contin Educ Dent* 19(10):1034, 1998.
3. ADA Council on Dental Therapeutics: Guidelines for the acceptance of peroxide-containing oral hygiene products, *J Am Dent Assoc* 125:1140, 1994.
4. Bailey RW, Christen AG: Bleaching of vital teeth stained with endemic dental fluorosis, *J Dent Res* 49:168, 1970.
5. Barghi N: Making a clinical decision for vital tooth bleaching: at-home or in-office? *Compend Contin Educ Dent*: 19(8):831, 1998.
6. Ben-mar A et al: Effect of mouthguard bleaching on enamel surface, *Am J Dent* 8:29, 1995.
7. Bitter NC: A scanning electron microscopy study of the effect of bleaching on enamel: a preliminary report, *J Prosthet Dent* 67:852, 1992.
8. Bitter NC, Sanders JL: The effect of four bleaching agents on the enamel surface. A scanning electron microscopic study, *Quintessence Int* 24:817, 1993.
9. Black GV, McKay FS: Mottled teeth: an endemic developmental imperfection of the enamel of the teeth heretofore unknown in the literature of dentistry, *Dent Cosmos* 58:129, 1916.
10. Carlsson J: Salivary peroxidase: an important part of our defense against oxygen toxicity, *J Oral Pathol* 16:412, 1987.

11. Christensen GJ: Bleaching teeth: report of a survey, 1997, *J Esthet Dent* 10(1):16, 1998.
12. Costas FL, Wong M: Intraoral isolating barriers: effect of location on root leakage and effectiveness of bleaching agents, *J Endod* 17:365, 1991.
13. Croll T: Enamel microabrasion: observations after 10 years, *JADA* (128):45, 1997.
14. Croll T: Enamel microabrasion: the technique, *Quintessence Int* 89(20):395, June 1989.
15. Croll T, Cavanaugh RR: Enamel color modification by controlled hydrochloric acid-pumice abrasion, *Quintessence Int* 17:81, 1986.
16. Cvek M, Lindvall AM: External root resorption following bleaching of pulpless teeth with hydrogen peroxide, *Endod Dent Traumatol* 1:56, 1985.
17. Dahlstrom SW, Heithersay GS, Bridges TE: Hydroxyl radical activity in thermo-catalytically bleached root-filled teeth, *Endod Dent Traumatol* 13(3):119, 1997.
18. Dumfahrt H, Moschen I: A new approach in restorative treatment of external root resorption. A case report, *J Periodontol* 69(8):941, 1998.
19. Engelhardt D: Power bleaching, *Cont Esthet Rest Prac* 9:22, 1999.
20. Fasanara TS: Bleaching teeth: history, chemicals and methods used for common tooth discolorations, *J Esthet Dent* 4(3):71, 1991.
21. Floyd RA: The effect of peroxides and free radicals on body tissues, *JADA* 128: 37S, 1997.
22. Friedman S et al: Incidence of external root resorption in 58 bleached pulpless teeth, *Endod Dent Traumatol* 4:23, 1988.
23. Friedman S: Internal bleaching: long-term outcomes and complications, *J Am Dent Assoc* 128:51S, 1997.
24. Frysch H et al: Effect of pH on hydrogen peroxide bleaching agents, *J Esthet Dent* 7(3):130, 1995.
25. Frysh H, Bowles W, Baker F, Rivera-Hidalgo G: Effect of pH on bleaching efficiency, *J Dent Res* 72:384, 1993 (abstract).
26. Garber DA: Dentist-monitored bleaching: a discussion of combination and laser bleaching, *J Am Dent Assoc* 128:26S, 1997.
27. Goldstein RE: *Changing your smile*, ed 3, Chicago, 1997, Quintessence Publishers.

28. Goldstein RE: In-office bleaching: where we came from, where we are today, *J Am Dent Assoc* 128:11S, 1997.

29. Goldstein RE et al: Bleaching of vital and non-vital teeth. In Cohen S and Burns R, editors: *Pathways of the pulp*, ed 6, St Louis, 1994, Mosby.

30. Goldstein RE, Lancaster J: Survey of patient attitudes toward current esthetic procedures, *J Prosthet Dent* 2:775, 1984.

31. Goon WWY, Cohen S, Borer RF: External cervical root resorption following bleaching, *J Endod* 12:414, 1986.

32. Griffin RE, Grower MF: Effects of solutions to treat dental fluorosis on permeability of teeth, *J Endod* 11:391, 1977.

33. Hammel S: Do-it-yourself tooth-whitening can be risky, *US News World Rep,* April 20, 1998.

34. Harrington GW, Natkin E: External resorption associated with bleaching of pulpless teeth, *J Endod* 5:344, 1979.

35. Haywood VB: Achieving, maintaining and recovering successful tooth bleaching, *J Esthet Dent* 8:31, 1996.

36. Haywood VB: Bleaching of vital and non-vital teeth, *Curr Opin Dent* 3:142, 1992.

37. Haywood VB: Considerations and variations of dentist-prescribed, home-applied vital tooth-bleaching techniques, *Compend Contin Educ Dent* (suppl):S616-626, 1994.

38. Haywood VB: History, safety, and effectiveness of current bleaching techniques and the application of the nightguard vital bleaching technique, *Quintessence Int* 23:471, 1992.

39. Haywood VB: Nightguard vital bleaching, *Quintessence Int* 20:173,1989.

40. Haywood VB: Nightguard vital bleaching: current concepts and research, *J Am Dent Assoc* 128: 19S, 1997.

41. Haywood VB: Nightguard vital bleaching: current information and research, *Esthet Dent Update* 1(20):20, 1990.

42. Haywood VB: Nightguard vital bleaching: a history and products update, part 2, *Esthet Dent Update* 2(5):82, 1991.

43. Haywood VB, Heymann HO: Nightguard vital bleaching: How safe is it? *Quintessence Int* 22:515, 1991.

44. Haywood VB, Houck VM, Heymann HO: Effect of various nightguard bleaching solutions on enamel surfaces and color changes, *J Dent Res* 70:377, 1991 (abstract).

45. Haywood VB, Leech T: Nightguard vital bleaching. Effect on enamel surface texture and diffusion, *Quintessence Int* 21:801, 1990.

46. Haywood VB, Leonard RH, Dickinson GL: Efficacy of six months of nightguard vital bleaching of tetracycline-stained teeth, *J Esthet Dent* 9:13, 1997.

47. Haywood VB, Leonard RH, Nelson CF, Brunson WD: Effectiveness, side effects and long-term status of nightguard vital bleaching, *J Am Dent Assoc* 125:1219, 1994.

48. Herrin JR, Squier CA, Rubright WC: Development of erosive gingival lesions after use of a home care technique, *J Periodontol* 58:785, 1987.

49. Kendell RL: Hydrochloric acid removal of brown fluorosis stains: clinical and scanning electron micrograph observations, *Quintessence Int* 20:837, 1989.

50. Kravitz LH, Tyndal DA, Bagnell CP, Dove SB: Assessment of external root resorption using digital subtraction radiography, *J Endod* 18(6):275, 1992.

51. Lado EA, Stanley HR, Weismann MI: Cervical resorption in bleached teeth, *Oral Surg* 55:78, 1983.

52. Latcham NL: Management of a patient with post-bleaching cervical resorption. A clinical report, *J Prosthet Dent* 65:603, 1991.

53. Latcham NL: Post-bleaching cervical resorption, *J Endod* 12: 262, 1986.

54. Lewenstein I, Hirschfield Z, Stabholz A, Rotstein I: Effect of hydrogen peroxide and sodium perborate on the microhardness of human enamel and dentin, *J Endod* 20(2):61, 1994.

55. Li Y: Toxicological considerations of tooth bleaching using peroxide-containing agents, *JADA* 128:31S, 1997.

56. Li Y, Noblitt T, Zhang A, Origel A, Kaftaway A, Tookey K: Effects of long-term exposure to a tooth whitener, *J Dent Res* 72:246, 1993 (abstract).

57. Madison S, Walton RE: Cervical root resorption following bleaching of endodontically treated teeth, *J Endod* 16:570, 1990.

58. McCloskey RJ: A technique for removal of fluorosis stain, *J Am Dent Assoc* 109:64, 1984.

59. McEvoy S: Chemical agents for removing intrinsic stains from vital teeth, *Quintessence Int* 20:323, 1989.

60. McGuikin RS, Babin JF, Meyer BJ: Alterations in human enamel surface morphology following vital bleaching, *J Prosthet Dent* 68:754, 1992.

61. Montgomery S: External cervical resorption after bleaching a pulpless tooth, *Oral Surg* 57:203, 1984.

62. Muller CJF, Van Wyk CW: The amelocemental junction, *J Dent Assoc S Afr* 39: 799, 1984.

63. Nathoo SA: The chemistry and mechanisms of extrinsic and intrinsic discoloration, *JADA* 128:6S, 1997.

64. Neville BW, Damm DD, Allen CM, Bouquot JE: *Oral and Maxillofacial Pathology,* Philadelphia, 1995, WB Saunders Co.

65. Reise-Schmidt T: Trends in dentistry. Longer, whiter, brighter: trends in tooth-whitening products and procedures, *Dental Products Report,* July 1996.

66. Rotstein I et al: In vitro efficacy of sodium perborate preparations used for intracoronal bleaching of discolored non-vital teeth, *Endod Dent Traumatol* 7:177, 1991.

67. Rotstein I, Danker E, Goldman A, Heling I, Stabholz A, Zalkind M: Histochemical analysis of hard tissues following bleaching, *J Endod* 22:23, 1996.

68. Rotstein I, Lehr T, Gedalia I: Effects of bleaching agents on the inorganic components of human dentine and cementum, *J Endod* 18:290, 1992.

69. Rotstein I, Lewenstein I, Zuwabi O, Stabholz A, Friedman M: Effect of cervical coating of ethyl cellulose polymer and metacrylic acid copolymer on the radicular penetration of hydrogen peroxide during bleaching, *Endod Dent Traumatol* 8:202, 1992.

70. Rotstein I, Mor C, Friedman S: Prognosis for intra-coronal bleaching with sodium perborate preparations in vitro: 1-year study, *J Endod* 19:10, 1993.

71. Rotstein I, Torek Y, Lewinstein I: Effect of bleaching time and temperature on the radicular penetration of hydrogen peroxide, *Endod Dent Traumatol* 4:32, 1988.

72. Rotstein I, Torek Y, Misgav R: Effect of cementum defects on radicular penetration of 30% hydrogen peroxide during intracoronal bleaching, *J Endod* 17:230, 1991.

73. Schroeder HE, Scherle WF: Cemento-enamel junction revisited, *J Periodontal Res* 23:53, 1988.

74. Shannon H, Spencer P, Gross K, Tira D: Characterization of enamel exposed to 10% carbamide peroxide bleaching agents, *Quintessence Int* 24:39, 1993.

75. Stanley TJ, Danko WD: *The millionaire next door,* Marietta, GA, 1996, Longstreet Press.

76. Swift EJ: A method for bleaching discolored teeth, *Quintessence Int* 19:607, 1988.

77. Swift EJ: Restorative considerations with vital tooth bleaching, *JADA* 128:60S, 1997.

78. Swift EJ Jr, Perdigai J: Effect of bleaching on teeth and restorations, *Compendium* 19(8):815, 1998.

79. Titley K, Torneck CD, Ruse ND: The effect of carbamide-peroxide gel on the shear bond strength of a microfil resin to bovine enamel, *J Dent Res* 71:20, 1992.

80. Titley K, Torneck CD, Ruse ND, Krmec D: Adhesion of resin composite to bleached and unbleached enamel, *J Endod* 19:112, 1993.

81. Titley K, Torneck CD, Smith DC: Effect of concentrated hydrogen solution on the surface morphology of cut human dentine, *Endod Dent Traumatol* 4:32, 1988.

82. Trope M: Cervical root resorption, *J Am Dent Assoc* 128:56S, 1997.

83. Whitening products and fluorides, *The Dental Advisor* 3:(4):1, 1996.

84. Zalkind M, Arwaz JR, Goldman A, Rotstein I: Surface morphology changes in enamel, dentine and cementum following bleaching: a scanning electron microscopic study, *Endod Dent Traumatol* 12:82, 1996.

Chapter 22

 # Restoration of the Endodontically Treated Tooth

Galen W. Wagnild, Kathy I. Mueller

Chapter Outline

RESTORATIVE DENTISTRY AND THE VITAL TOOTH

Effect of Restorative Procedures and Materials on the Pulp

Teeth that require extensive restorations suffer pulpal injury from both dental disease and treatment procedures. A number of precautions are listed that can help to reduce the harmful consequences of dental procedures on the pulp. (See Chapter 15 for a discussion of the effect of restorative techniques and materials on the living pulp.)

Risk of Postrestorative Endodontic Complications

Adverse effects on the pulp are an inherent risk of restorative procedures. Despite precautions, damage to the pulp cannot be entirely eliminated from restorative dentistry.[5] Intact dentin provides biologic resistance to dental pain and sensitivity, caries, tooth fracture, and pulpal breakdown.[2] As increasing amounts of structural dentin are removed during tooth preparation, the number of exposed dentin tubules increases dramatically. At the surface of the dentin, or the dentin and enamel junction (DEJ), dentin tubules range between 15,000 and 20,000 per square millimeter. At the pulpal surface the number of dentin tubules increases threefold to 45,000 to 60,000/mm², and the tubule diameter increases. Therefore deep preparations expose a large number of wide dentin tubules to trauma, dental materials, and bacterial products. Dentin permeability is greatest on thin axial surfaces, particularly mesial surfaces. These surfaces are often extensively reduced during preparation for full veneer crowns, and especially for fixed partial dentures involving mesially tipped abutments. Pulpal irritation becomes significant when the dentin thickness is reduced to 0.3 mm.[47]

The process of tooth preparation and restoration is irritating to the pulp; occasionally the injury can be irreversible. Dental procedures are considered to be responsible for those endodontic complications that develop in restored teeth for no other known reason. Abutment teeth have a higher risk of developing subsequent pulpal necrosis than vital teeth restored with single crowns. This is undoubtedly due to the increased preparation required for parallelism. In a study of endodontic complications in restored teeth, approximately 0.3% of crowned teeth and 4.0% of abutment teeth became endodontically involved when no caries, fracture, or other causative factors were present. When known cause was also present, pulpal necrosis significantly increased. The combined effect of dental procedures and recurrent dental disease nearly quadrupled the rate of endodontic involvement for abutment teeth, and it increased the rate for teeth with single crowns more than tenfold.[6]

Endodontic involvement increases in proportion to the degree of dental destruction and the complexity of the restoration. Teeth treated with a buildup and a full veneer crown became necrotic roughly 30 times more frequently than unrestored teeth.[17] In complex cases requiring periodontal and prosthetic reconstruction, twice as many teeth with advanced periodontal disease developed endodontic complications, compared with teeth with moderate periodontal disease. This reflects a complicated interplay between multiple disease processes, more extensive tooth preparation, and the cumulative effects of previous dental breakdown and restoration.

Pulpal degeneration also increases with time after the insertion of the restorations. The pulpal insult initiated by preparation and restoration procedures can continue undetected for many years. Among restored teeth that became endodontically involved for no known reason, 12% deteriorated in the first 3 years after the restorative treatment. The necrosis rate tripled by year 7, and it increased to 50% of the restored teeth by year 12.[6]

The clear risks of endodontic involvement in teeth that require restorations mandate a careful prerestorative evaluation, particularly as the case size and complexity increases. Endodontic intervention should be planned and integrated into a logical treatment sequence before any therapy is started. Both the patient and the clinician must be aware of the interdisciplinary nature of this approach.

Indications for Prerestorative Endodontic Therapy

The evaluation of teeth to be restored should include three considerations:

1. The health of the pulp
2. The impact of planned restorative procedures on the pulp
3. The magnitude of the restorative effort

Cases in which restorative requirements will significantly decrease predictability of pulpal health should be managed with preventive endodontics.

Prophylactic Endodontics   Teeth to be restored are candidates for prophylactic endodontic therapy when restorative procedures requiring significant dentin removal are likely to endanger pulpal integrity. For example, vital teeth with minimal remaining tooth structure often require auxiliary retention for restorations. Retentive grooves, boxes, and pins are all placed at the expense of the dentin; this can ultimately compromise vitality. Judicious endodontic therapy can be crucial to the success of the restoration when substantial tooth structure is missing. A tooth that has lost pivotal coronal dentin to caries, fracture, or old restorations may remain vital but exhibit insufficient supragingival tooth structure for retention of a new restoration. In this case the root canal system may be considered an extension of the restorative zone and the tooth devitalized to allow placement of a dowel, core, and crown restoration.

Substantial tooth preparation is common in cases with missing or malposed teeth, and this can jeopardize pulpal health. Preparation of nonparallel abutment teeth for fixed restorations entails extensive dentin removal from axial walls that can encroach upon the pulp. Intracoronal attachments are also used to solve problems of missing or malposed teeth. However, the additional preparation needed for placement of the attachment within the confines of the crown can result in irreversible pulpal injury.[50]

Periodontally involved teeth are at risk for pulpal involvement when crown margins are placed considerably apical to the cementoenamel junction (CEJ) (Fig. 22-1). The narrow circumference of the root dictates increased dentin removal to prepare tapered axial walls. The remaining layer of tooth structure overlying the pulp may be too thin to protect against irreversible degeneration from the combined effects of the tooth preparation process and potentially irritating restorative materials.

Prerestorative endodontic therapy is also prescribed before restoration of periodontally involved vital teeth when root amputation or hemisection is planned to salvage portions of guarded teeth. Similarly, teeth with significant periodontal bone loss can be endodontically treated and the roots retained to provide needed support for an overdenture.

Major occlusal correction of vital teeth may also dictate endodontic treatment before crown placement. Decreasing the occlusal height of a hypererupted tooth to restore a proper occlusal plane may require devitalizing the tooth. Similarly, correction of an unfavorable crown-to-root ratio is accomplished by decreasing the clinical crown height through substantial coronal reduction. Prophylactic endodontics should be considered to avoid access preparation through the crown at a later date.

Endodontic therapy should be planned in advance for teeth with fragile pulpal systems that require a cast restoration. Treatment of chronic pulpitis is more efficient and effective when the tooth is endodontically treated before placement of a crown or bridge retainer. The dental history of a tooth must be considered before crown preparation. Teeth that have undergone multiple episodes of dental disease or trauma and multiple dental procedures develop a "stressed pulp" syndrome and have an increased risk of subsequent pulpal breakdown.[1] Vital teeth should first be endodontically treated if they have a guarded pulpal prognosis and would be difficult to treat endodontically after completion of the planned restoration.

Magnitude of the restorative treatment.   As the size and complexity of the restorative effort increases, the need for prerestorative endodontics also increases. The hazards associated with retroactive treatment are a serious and dangerous risk. Endodontic access through an existing restoration can remove a significant portion of the underlying dentin core and vertical walls of the underlying preparation. This can disrupt the cement integrity and compromise retention and resistance of the restoration. Loss of cement seal and ensuing leakage at the crown margins can result in severe caries of

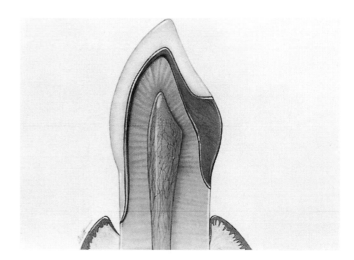

Fig. 22-1 Attachment loss often results in elongated clinical crowns. Restorative procedures require additional dentin removal from the axial walls and may be detrimental to pulpal vitality.

the dentin core inside the crown. Core caries of a nonvital tooth is difficult to detect with radiographs or symptoms until the damage is severe (Fig. 22-2). Extensive caries extending into the root may require periodontal crown-lengthening surgery to expose the carious dentin for repair. Root caries is sometimes not restorable, resulting in a need for extraction and possible loss of a multitooth, fixed restoration.

Creation of an access opening through an all-ceramic or a porcelain fused-to-metal crown also structurally weakens the restoration. Simply perforating the glazed porcelain surface reduces porcelain strength significantly. Perforation of the occlusal porcelain and the metal coping can weaken the porcelain bond strength enough to cause separation of the porcelain veneer from the metal substructure. Clearly, although it is possible to perform endodontic procedures after restorations are complete, postrestorative endodontics should be avoided whenever possible.

In more compromised dentitions occlusal requirements may alter the normal relationship of root anatomy to clinical crown in the restored dentition. The disorientation of crown morphology and underlying root form can lead to difficulty in endodontic access and result in excessive removal of coronal tooth structure. In the severe case this disorientation can contribute to a mechanical perforation of the root (Fig. 22-3). These clinical realities may not greatly impact a treatment plan for the tooth requiring a single crown, but they may cause rapid destruction of the larger, more fragile, more complex restoration. These cases require prerestorative endodontic evaluation and the definitive treatment of strategic teeth with questionable pulpal prognosis.

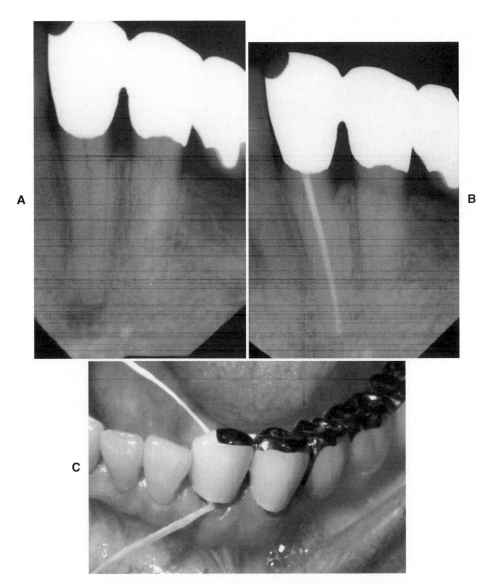

Fig. 22-2 **A**, Existing fixed partial denture with periapical lesion. **B**, After endodontic therapy. **C**, Rapid loss of cement seal with resultant carious destruction of anterior abutment. (Courtesy Dr. George Gara.)

Pretreatment Evaluation   Before initiation of restorative therapy the tooth must be thoroughly evaluated to ensure success of all ultimate treatment goals. The tooth should be examined individually and in the context of its contribution to the overall treatment plan. The prognosis of the tooth, adjacent teeth, opposing teeth, and patient desires for treatment should all be considered. This survey includes endodontic, periodontal, restorative, and esthetic evaluations.

Endodontic evaluation.   In addition to identification of nonvital teeth and the endodontic evaluation of vital teeth described previously, the prerestorative examination should include an inspection of the quality of existing endodontic treatment. New restorations, particularly complex restorations, should not be placed on abutment teeth with a questionable endodontic prognosis. Endodontic retreatment may

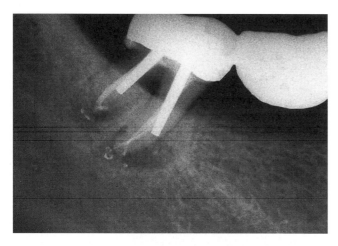

Fig. 22-3 Root anatomy dictates dowel location and dimension. The occlusal surface anatomy of this molar was used to project root location. Long axis dislocation of the restored crown and the root can result in dramatic clinical errors.

be indicated for teeth that exhibit radiographic periapical pathology or clinical symptoms of inflammation (see Chapter 24). Restorations that require a dowel will need a dowel space, which is prepared by removal of gutta-percha from the canal. Canals obturated with a silver cone or other inappropriate filling materials should be identified and endodontically retreated before the start of restorative therapy.

Periodontal evaluation.   Maintenance of periodontal health is critical to the long-term success of teeth that have been endodontically treated and restored. The periodontal condition of the tooth must be determined before initiation of endodontic therapy, and the effect of the planned restoration on the attachment apparatus must be considered. Many teeth suffer from significant structural defects that jeopardize coronal reconstruction. Extensive caries, tooth fracture, previous restorations, perforations, and external resorption can destroy tooth structure at the level of the periodontal attachment. An attempt to place restorative margins on solid tooth structure beyond these defects further invades the biologic attachment zone. Violation of the biologic width can cause failure of the clinical results (Fig. 22-4). A mutilated tooth in which restorative treatment would compromise the junctional epithelium or connective tissue attachment levels should be considered for periodontal crown-lengthening surgery or orthodontic extrusion, in addition to endodontic and restorative procedures. Further, teeth mutilated from caries or fracture often have excellent bone support; extraction of weak teeth and replacement with dental implants should be included in treatment options.

Restorative evaluation.   It is essential to determine if the tooth is restorable before endodontic treatment is performed; a restorative evaluation should be made before any definitive therapy. Successful endodontic treatment is of no value if a tooth is too extensively damaged from caries, fracture, previous restorations, or periodontal disease to be reliably restored.

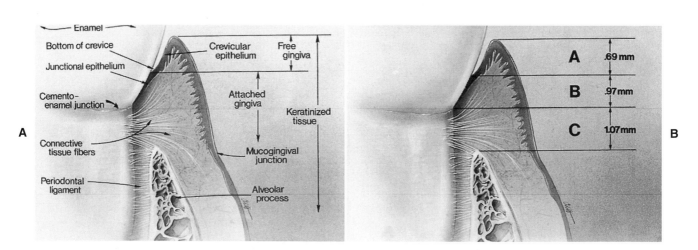

Fig. 22-4 **A,** Anatomy of the healthy attachment apparatus. **B,** Defective tooth structure, necessitating margin placement into zones *B* and *C*, is an indication of the need for crown-lengthening surgery or orthodontic extrusion. These zones contain the junctional epithelium and the connective tissue attachments.

The strategic importance of a tooth should be determined before a final plan is formulated. The success of a large restoration may depend on the availability of a strategic tooth, such as an intermediate abutment. The distal-most tooth in a quadrant can be critical to avoid a distal extension removable partial denture. Teeth with strategic importance to an overall treatment plan require predictable endodontic and restorative procedures to optimize their longevity. Conversely, mutilated teeth may not warrant extensive treatment if adjacent healthy teeth are available as abutments or if dental implants are appropriate. Extraction of an extensively damaged tooth may be indicated.

The reliability and prognosis of a tooth should be considered before inclusion in a final treatment plan. The tooth to be retained must be able to withstand the functional forces placed upon it after reconstruction. Missing tooth structure can be replaced with a cast restoration, a core, and a dowel. However, the risk of root fracture increases with the amount of missing coronal or internal radicular tooth structure. A critical amount of solid coronal dentin is required, which must be encased in a coronal restoration for structural integrity of the restored tooth. This ferrule (i.e., a band that encircles the external dimension of the residual tooth, similar to the metal bands around a barrel) has been shown to significantly reduce the incidence of fracture in the root canal–treated tooth.* If sufficient solid tooth structure to accommodate a restoration with a ferrule is not available, the tooth should first be treated periodontally, orthodontically, or it should be extracted.

Esthetic evaluation. Potential esthetic complications should be investigated before initiation of endodontic therapy. Thin gingiva may transmit a shadow of dark root color through the tissue. Metal or dark, carbon fiber dowels or amalgam placed in the canal can result in unacceptable gingival discoloration from the underlying root. The translucency of all-ceramic crowns must be considered in the selection of dowel and buildup materials. Tooth-colored carbon core, fiberglass-reinforced composite resin, or zirconia dowels can be used in esthetic areas.[30,35,48,60] Similarly, tooth-colored, rather than opaque, composite core material should be selected for the esthetic case.

An esthetic tooth that will not need a crown after endodontic treatment requires critical control of endodontic filling materials in the coronal third of the canal and the pulp chamber (Fig. 22-5). The color and translucency of most uncrowned teeth will be adversely affected by opaque substances. Similarly, discoloration from gutta-percha can be visible in the coronal aspect of an endodontically treated tooth and should be limited to an apical level in the root. Endodontic and restorative materials in these esthetically critical cases must be selected to provide the best health service with the minimum of esthetic compromise.

The evaluation of clinical problems should be completed before any definitive therapy is started. When endodontic

---

*References 4,23,33,43,59

treatment is initiated by an acute pulpitis, treatment should be restricted to emergency care. After stabilization, the clinician should complete the entire evaluation before continuation of treatment. Accurate assimilation of endodontic, periodontal, restorative, and esthetic variables will contribute to a rational, successful treatment outcome.

There will be instances in which endodontic therapy could succeed, whereas failure would occur in other dental disciplines. These conditions should be detected and treated with an interdisciplinary approach to maximize success. Extraction may be indicated for teeth where endodontics could succeed but total completion of the treatment plan is impossible because of periodontal or restorative deficiencies that cannot be corrected. These cases must be identified in the planning stage, and replacement of the condemned teeth must then be included in the overall treatment plan.

RESTORATIVE DENTISTRY AND THE NONVITAL TOOTH

Effect of Endodontics on the Tooth

Changes in Endodontically Treated Teeth   The disease processes and restorative procedures that create the need for endodontic therapy affect much more than the pulp vitality. The tooth structure that remains after endodontic treatment has been undermined and weakened by all of the previous episodes of caries, fracture, tooth preparation, and restoration. Endodontic manipulation further removes important intracoronal and intraradicular dentin. Finally, the endodontic treatment changes the actual composition of the remaining tooth structure. The combined result of these changes is the common clinical finding of increased fracture susceptibility and decreased translucency in nonvital teeth. Because restorations for endodontically treated teeth are designed to compensate for these changes, it is important to understand the effects of endodontics on the tooth and the significance of each factor. The major changes in the endodontically treated tooth include the following:

- Loss of tooth structure
- Altered physical characteristics
- Altered esthetic characteristics of the residual tooth

Loss of tooth structure.   The decreased strength seen in endodontically treated teeth is primarily because of the loss of coronal tooth structure; it is not a direct result of the endodontic treatment. Endodontic procedures have been shown to reduce tooth stiffness by only 5%, whereas a mesial-occlusal-distal (MOD) preparation reduces stiffness by 60%.[49] Endodontic access into the pulp chamber destroys the structural integrity provided by the coronal dentin of the pulpal roof and allows greater flexing of the tooth under function.[27] In cases with significantly reduced remaining tooth structure, normal functional forces may fracture undermined cusps or fracture the tooth in the area of the smallest circumference, frequently at the CEJ. The decreased volume of tooth structure from the combined effect of prior dental

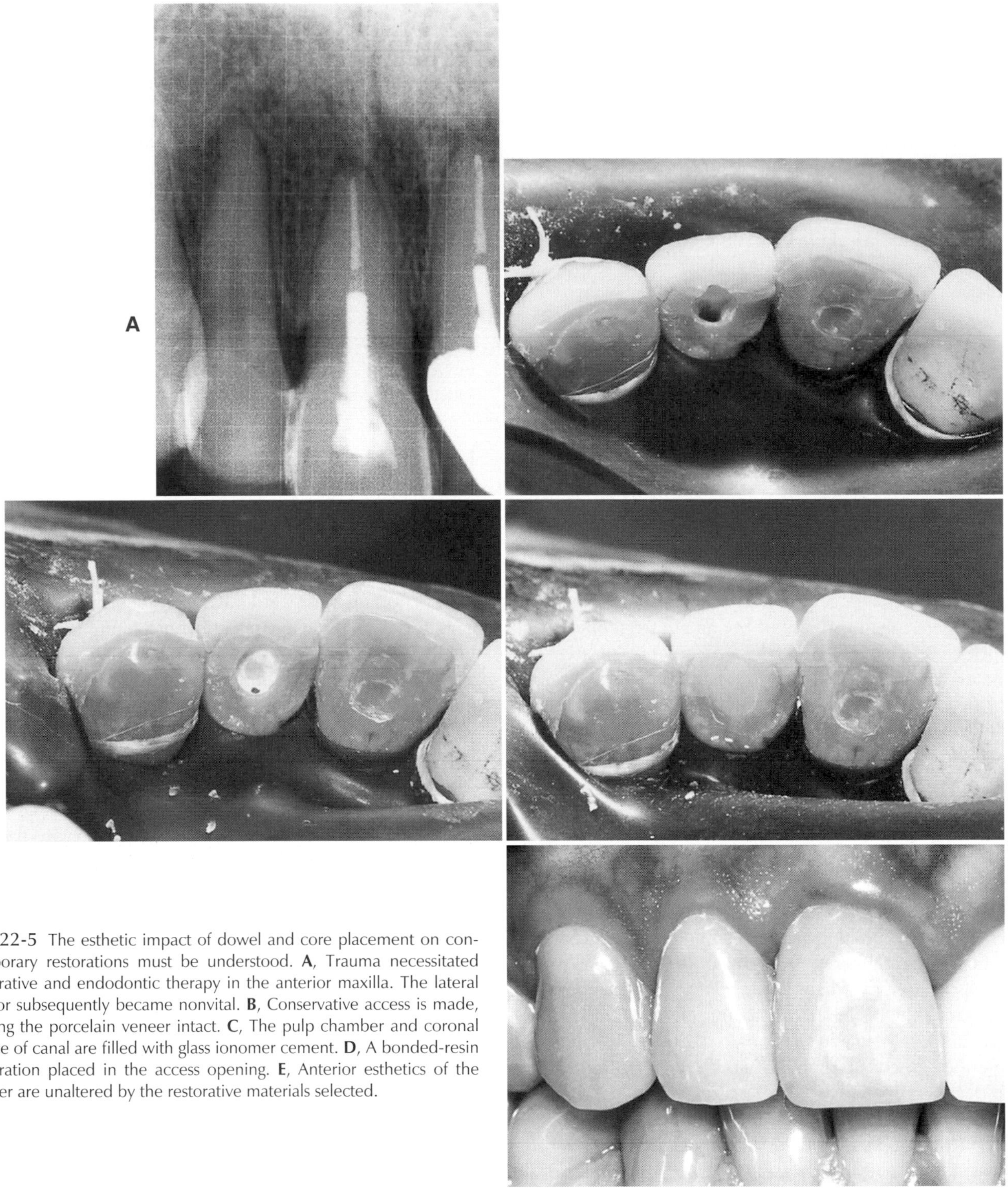

Fig. 22-5 The esthetic impact of dowel and core placement on contemporary restorations must be understood. **A**, Trauma necessitated restorative and endodontic therapy in the anterior maxilla. The lateral incisor subsequently became nonvital. **B**, Conservative access is made, leaving the porcelain veneer intact. **C**, The pulp chamber and coronal orifice of canal are filled with glass ionomer cement. **D**, A bonded-resin restoration placed in the access opening. **E**, Anterior esthetics of the veneer are unaltered by the restorative materials selected.

procedures creates a significant potential for fracture of the endodontically treated tooth.

Altered physical characteristics. The tooth structure remaining after endodontic therapy also exhibits irreversibly altered physical properties. Changes in collagen cross-linking and dehydration of the dentin result in a 14% reduction in strength and toughness of endodontically treated molars. Maxillary teeth are stronger than mandibular teeth, and mandibular incisors are the weakest.[27] The combined loss of structural integrity, loss of moisture, and loss of dentin toughness compromise endodontically treated teeth and requires special care in the restoration of pulpless teeth.

Altered esthetic characteristics. Esthetic changes also occur in endodontically treated teeth. Biochemically altered dentin modifies light refraction through the tooth and modifies its appearance. The darkening of nonvital anterior teeth is a well-known phenomenon. Inadequate endodontic cleaning and shaping of the coronal area also contribute to this discoloration by staining the dentin from degradation of vital tissue left in the pulp horns. Medicaments used in dental treatment and remnants of root canal–filling material can affect the appearance of endodontically treated teeth. Endodontic treatment and restoration of teeth in the esthetic zone require careful control of procedures and materials to retain a translucent, natural appearance.

Treatment Planning for Restoration of Nonvital Teeth

All of the changes that accompany root canal therapy influence the selection of restorative procedures for endodontically treated teeth. Important considerations include the following:

- The amount of remaining tooth structure
- The anatomic position of the tooth
- The functional load on the tooth
- The esthetic requirements for the tooth

The various combinations of these factors will determine whether dowels, cores, or crowns are indicated and aid in the selection of each. Teeth, of course, do not fall neatly into separate categories, and no single restorative system can be used for all situations.

The amount of remaining tooth structure. Tooth structure loss can range from minimal access preparations in intact teeth to extensive damage that endangers the longevity of the tooth itself. The amount of tooth structure damage is one of the most important aspects in restoration of the endodontically treated tooth (and the one in which the clinician has the least control). Teeth with more than half of the tooth structure intact are inherently stronger than damaged teeth and can be restored conservatively with coronal restorations and without dowels inside the roots.[10] Conversely, extensive tooth structure loss from caries, fracture, and previous restorations significantly weakens the remaining tooth, making dowels, cores, and crowns necessary.

Teeth with minimal remaining tooth structure present several clinical problems. These include the following:

- An increased root fracture risk
- A greater potential for devastating recurrent caries after restoration
- A higher occurrence of final restoration dislodgement or loss
- An increased incidence of biologic width invasion during preparation[46,66,72]

The amount of remaining dentin is far more significant to the long-term prognosis of the restored tooth than is the selection of artificial dowel, core, or crown materials. The difference between an effective, long-term restoration and a failure can be as small as 1 mm of additional tooth structure at the marginal area. This extra dentin, when encased by the crown margin or ferrule, provides greater protection than any of the following dowel and core considerations. Treatment

planning requires use of all dental specialties to obtain the necessary sound tooth structure, to design the dowel-core-crown complex for atraumatic retention, and also to recognize when the prognosis is poor. When a long-lasting, functional restoration cannot be predictably created, tooth extraction should be considered.

The anatomic position of the tooth

Anterior teeth   Intact, nonvital, anterior teeth that have not lost tooth structure beyond the endodontic access preparation are at minimal risk for fracture. Generally they do not require a crown, core, or dowel. Restorative treatment is limited to sealing of the access cavity. A nonvital, anterior tooth that has lost significant tooth structure requires a crown. The crown is supported and retained by the dowel and core. Desired physical properties of dowels will determine the selection of materials for the crown, core, and dowel. Esthetic dowels are available in zirconia, with high radiopacity and high modulus of elasticity (i.e., stiffness). They are also available in fiberglass-reinforced composite materials with low radiopacity and low stiffness.

Posterior teeth   Posterior teeth carry greater occlusal loads than anterior teeth, and restorations must be planned to protect posterior teeth against fracture (Fig. 22-6). Teeth with significant remaining natural tooth structure after endodontic treatment must be considered separately from those with extensive missing tooth structure. The functional forces against molars require crown or onlay protection; the need for dowels and cores depends on the amount of remaining tooth structure. When there is sufficient tooth structure to retain the core and crown, dowels are not needed. Ceramic or metal crowns or onlays provide the best cuspal protection against tooth fracture and should be used for posterior teeth (except in unusual cases of minimal functional force). Although in vitro research suggests that premolars with access openings or conservative MOD preparations can be restored to near normal cusp fracture values with current dentin bonding and composite resin systems,[2,65] this strengthening may be only temporary.[14]

Functional load of the tooth   The horizontal and torquing forces endured by abutments for fixed or removable partial dentures dictate more extensive protective and retentive features in the restoration. Abutment teeth for long-span, fixed bridges and distal extension, removable, partial dentures absorb greater transverse loads and require more protection than do abutments of smaller bridges or tooth-supported, removable, partial dentures. Similarly, teeth that exhibit extensive wear from bruxism, heavy occlusion, or heavy lateral function require the full complement of dowel, core, and crown.[10]

Esthetic requirements of the tooth   Anterior teeth, premolars, and often the maxillary first molar inhabit the esthetic zone of the mouth. These teeth are framed by the gingiva and lips to create an esthetically pleasing smile. Alterations to the color or translucency of the visible hard tissue and soft tissue negatively impact the esthetics of this zone. Teeth in the esthetic zone require careful selection of

Clinical Fracture Rate for Tooth Types

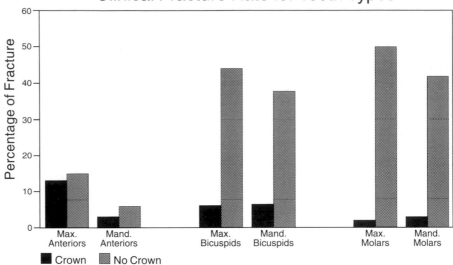

Fig. 22-6 Fracture of nonvital teeth increases in the posterior dentition when a coronal coverage restoration is not used.[70]

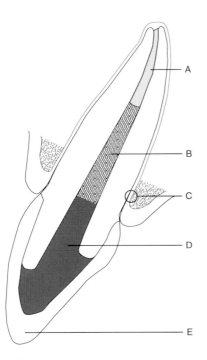

Fig. 22-7 The final configuration of the restored, endodontically treated tooth. The apical endodontic seal is preserved with 3 to 5 mm of gutta-percha (*A*). The dowel (*B*) is the restorative material within the root. The core (*D*) replaces missing coronal tooth structure and retains the final coronal restoration (*E*). Restorative and endodontic therapy must preserve the residual root and its attachment mechanism (*C*).

restorative materials, careful handling of the tissues, and timely endodontic intervention to prevent darkening of the root as the tooth loses vitality. Current restorative materials for these teeth include tooth-colored dowels; tooth-colored, composite resin or ceramic cores; tooth-colored cements; and various porcelain or ceramic crown materials.

Basic Components Used in Restoration of Nonvital Teeth

Restorations for endodontically treated teeth are designed to protect the remaining tooth from fracture and to replace the missing tooth structure. The final restoration will include some combination of (1) dowel, (2) core, and (3) coronal restoration. The selection of the individual components for the restoration will depend on whether the nonvital tooth is an anterior or posterior tooth and whether significant coronal tooth structure is missing (Table 22-1). Not every endodontically treated tooth needs a crown or a dowel; some need all three components and some need only an access seal for the coronal restoration.

When a nonvital anterior or posterior tooth has lost significant tooth structure, a coronal restoration is required. The dowel and core is used to support and retain the crown. The final configuration of the restored tooth includes four parts (Fig. 22-7):

1. Residual tooth structure and periodontal attachment apparatus
2. Dowel material located within the root
3. Core material located in the coronal area of the tooth
4. Definitive coronal restoration

The dowel, core, and crown function together and should be considered as a whole. The core replaces lost coronal

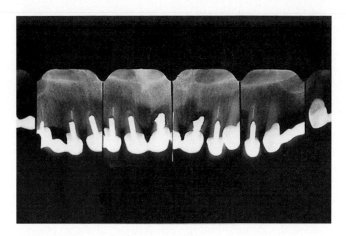

Fig. 22-8 Excessive dentin removal for the placement of large dowels results in weakened tooth structure.

tooth structure and provides retention for the crown. The dowel provides retention for the core and must be designed to minimize the potential for root fracture from functional forces. The crown restores function and esthetics and protects the remaining root and coronal structure from fracture. The specific design of each dowel and core is determined by the relative clinical need for each of these functions.

Dowel (Post)

The dowel (see Fig. 22-7) is a post or other relatively rigid, restorative material placed in the root of a nonvital tooth. Dowels can be fabricated from metal or a variety of newer nonmetallic substances. The dowel is especially important in restoration of nonvital teeth that have suffered significant damage and have insufficient sound tooth structure remaining above the periodontal attachment to secure a coronal restoration. The dowel within the residual root extends apically to anchor the core materials that support the crown. The foremost purpose of the dowel is to provide retention for the core and coronal restoration. It should do so without increasing the risk of root fracture. Thus the dowel has both a retentive and protective function: the dowel functions primarily to aid in the retention of the restoration and to protect the tooth by dissipating or disbursing forces along the length of the root. The dowel itself does not strengthen a tooth. To the contrary, the tooth is weakened if dentin is sacrificed to place a large diameter dowel. This is an important distinction, because significant damage can result from misplaced efforts to fortify roots with large dowels (Fig. 22-8).

Ideal properties of the dowel. Dowels should have as many of the following clinical features as possible:

- Maximum protection of the root
- Adequate retention within the root
- Maximum retention of the core and crown
- Maximum protection of the crown margin cement seal
- Pleasing esthetics, when indicated
- High radiographic visibility

- Retrievability
- Biocompatibility

These clinical features reflect the underlying physical properties of the dowel. The physical properties result from each dowel system's unique combination of composition, shape, size, and surface configuration. In addition, cements, dowel space preparation techniques, additional restorative antirotational features, and internal adaptation to the walls of the root canal all directly affect the clinical results. Discussion of dowel systems must focus primarily on the desired clinical outcome, supported by an understanding of the underlying physical properties of dowels and restorative materials.

It is important to understand that dowel research is largely conducted as in vitro studies of dowels in teeth without crown restorations that are subjected to forces that may or may not occur clinically. These conditions are designed to elucidate and sharpen differences among dowels or other studied components and, thus, provide valuable information. However, the clinician must then consider this data in relation to specific clinical conditions, including final restoration with a crown. In vivo and in vitro studies repeatedly show that the presence of a crown causes the differences between various dowel systems to disappear.[1,58,61]

Dowel classification. Endodontic dowels have been classified in various ways, including preformed and custom cast, metallic and nonmetallic, stiff and flexible, and esthetic and nonesthetic. Dowels, however, exhibit important physical properties that cross over between these obvious categories, making any simple classification system incomplete. Traditionally, dowels were metal and were either preformed or custom-cast dowels and cores. These broad categories are no longer useful because technology continues to provide new materials and concepts for endodontic dowels. Because many dowels exhibit features of more than one category, classification by desired clinical properties is more clinically meaningful. Three clinically significant features can be categorized as follows:

1. Retentive qualities of dowels
2. Protective qualities of dowels
3. Esthetic qualities of dowels

These qualities are interrelated and are significantly affected by the amount of remaining tooth structure and by the presence and design of the crown.

Retentive qualities: dowel-to-root and dowel-to-core retention. Retention must be clinically sufficient to anchor the dowel into the root and to anchor the core to the residual tooth structure. The optimal amount of dowel-to-root retention is that amount that is enough to reliably retain the dowel during clinical function. However, excessive retention of metal or zirconia dowels may preclude conventional endodontic retreatment if dowels cannot be atraumatically removed. Dowel retention varies with dowel design, dowel composition, and cement type.

Dowel design and dowel retention. Classic studies of metal dowels in vitro found retention to be increased in dowels with parallel sides, serrated surfaces, and longer lengths. Parallel sided dowels are more retentive than tapered dowels, and they distribute functional loads to the root more passively than tapered dowels. Serrated surfaces of metal dowels increase retention over smooth metal surfaces by providing mechanical undercuts for cement. However, carbon fiber and fiber-reinforced, composite resin dowels are smooth (to preserve the integrity of the fiber bundles).[39] Because these dowels are commonly cemented with resin cements, retention is achieved with chemical bonding, not mechanical undercuts. Dowel retention is also proportional to dowel length in traditional dowels; increasing the length of metal dowels increases the retention (when measuring retention of metal dowels and nonadhesive cement). Dowel designs that achieve retention by active engagement of the root wall with screw threads are highly retentive but have been shown to increase the risk of root fracture.[8,18,60] There is little clinical indication for active root engagement. Carbon fiber, carbon core, and fiberglass-reinforced composite dowels with bonded retention may not need to be as long as traditional dowels. A 1:1 ratio between the dowel length and the replacement crown is sufficient.[10]

The dowel's ability to anchor the core is clinically important for successful reconstruction of the endodontically treated tooth. Loss of core retention results in loss of the crown. Core retention can be achieved by creating a one-piece dowel and core that has no interface between the dowel and the core. Indirect, custom-cast, metal dowel and cores and zirconia dowels with laboratory processed ceramic cores use this integrated dowel and core concept. Direct dowels designed with mechanical locking features in the heads show increased retention of the core, as compared with smaller heads.[12] Although a large, retentive dowel head is beneficial for a large tooth and a large core, large dowel heads can occupy most of the space available in a small, anterior tooth for the crown preparation, resulting in a thin layer of core buildup material that can fracture.

Dowel composition and dowel retention. Dowels are fabricated from a variety of materials and, therefore, exhibit a variety of physical properties. Dowel retention is a clinical quality that is related to the underlying physical properties of the dowel material. The inherent strength of the dowel affects the dowel retention to the root and to the core. If a dowel fractures, the coronal-most portion is no longer retained in the root and can no longer anchor the core. Metal dowels were more fracture resistant and, therefore, more retentive than carbon fiber dowels in experimental pull out tests. The carbon fiber dowels all fractured and retention could not be measured; no metal dowels fractured.[15] However, pure tensile forces are rare in clinical function.

Dowels and their associated core-to-crown complex experience repeated lateral forces in clinical function, and dowels can fracture at the mouth of the canal. This is particularly true in damaged teeth with little protection from intact, coronal, dentin and crown ferrule. As less and less tooth structure and ferrule remain, more and more force is transferred to the dowel and concentrated at the point of dowel flexure. Fracture toughness, flexural strength, and brittleness

are physical properties that describe the ability of dowels to resist clinical failure from excessive deformation, permanent bending, or fracture of the dowel. Excessively narrow metal dowels in damaged anterior teeth under heavy protrusive forces can bend or break in function. In all cases, dowel selection and dowel physical properties are most important in teeth that are structurally weak. For teeth that have largely intact tooth structure, all mainstream dowels in use today have sufficient strength and retention for clinical function; other factors will influence dowel selection.

Dowels composed of fiber-reinforced composite resin are retained by dentin-bonding materials; retention of the dowel reflects the interaction of the dowel material, the effectiveness of the dentin-bonding procedures, and the physical properties of the resin cement. Similarly, most metal dowels, carbon fiber and carbon core dowels, and ceramic and zirconia dowels chemically bond to resin cement.

The composition of the dowel also affects the dowel's ability to retain the core. Stainless steel (SS) dowels are more retentive of composite resin cores than are carbon fiber dowels.[39] Any dowel that mechanically retains a core of another material, however, is at risk for separation of the core from the dowel, especially in damaged teeth in which the dowel and core combination absorbs significant functional force. Integrated dowel and core systems in which both the dowel and the core are formed simultaneously from the same material eliminate the dowel and core interface. One-piece dowel and cores traditionally were custom-cast metal, but now include zirconia and ceramic and fiber-reinforced composite systems. The direct composite dowel and core combinations have been termed "monoblock" or "monocore" techniques. A study comparing a variety of metallic and nonmetallic dowels supporting composite cores reports that the buildups fractured off from the dowels in systems using dissimilar materials for the dowel and the core. In addition, 33% to 47% of the roots fractured. Those with a homogenous dowel and core unit of reinforced composite resin failed cohesively, but they did so without damage to the root.[10]

Dowel cementation and dowel retention. Retention for all types of dowels is affected by the cement selection. Traditional cements, such as zinc phosphate, provide retention through mechanical means. These cements have no chemical bond to the dowel or dentin but provide clinically sufficient retention for dowels in teeth with adequate tooth structure. The lack of chemical bond becomes advantageous if removal of the dowel becomes necessary, because most traditional cements can be dissolved with ultrasonic vibration. Glass ionomer cements bond to dentin but not to the dowel. However, in an in vitro comparison of retention of identical dowels, glass ionomer cements achieved retention levels similar to resin cements. Both glass ionomer and resin cements were statistically more retentive than resin-modified, glass ionomer cements.[40] Resin-modified, glass ionomer cements also exhibit hygroscopic expansion, which can damage or fracture roots.[10] Except for specific, low-expansion formulations, resin-modified, glass ionomer cements are not indicated for dowel cementation.

As the available dentin surface decreases, cement retention becomes increasingly important and can be achieved with chemically adhesive resin cements. Resin cements bond to dentin within the root and residual tooth and to most dowel materials. Thus they achieve very high retention. For example, parallel dowels cemented with an adhesive cement are equal in retention to active or screw-type dowels, without the inherent risk from screw threads in dentin. This cement-mediated, maximum retention is not risk free: 80% of the roots fractured when dowels were dislodged by force.[63]

Cement manipulation procedures and ease of use also affect clinical retention of cements to the dowel. Maximum retention requires complete coverage of dentin and dowel surfaces. Cement flow properties and consistency may affect the completeness of cement coverage inside the canal. Some resin-modified, glass ionomer cements do not spread out or flow easily, which could result in voids. Similarly, dentin-bonding agents must penetrate dentin deep inside visually inaccessible canals to provide the chemical bond and the levels of retention achievable in the laboratory. The strength and retention of resin cements also depends on complete setting. Eugenol is a common component of many restorative materials, including temporary cements, endodontic sealers, and temporary access–filling materials. Eugenol inhibits polymerization of resins. Although the eugenol-containing endodontic sealer did not affect retention of resin-cemented dowels in an in vitro study,[53] high concentration eugenol restorative materials should probably be avoided if resin cements or composite resin cores are planned.

Protective qualities of dowels: resistance to root fracture and to microleakage.   The dowel must furnish maximum resistance to root fracture while providing retention between the root and the core. Root fracture is a significant problem in endodontically treated teeth, resulting in tooth loss. In a clinical evaluation of dowels and cores beneath existing crowns, 10% of all failures were due to root fracture.[24,28] In an earlier clinical study, 40% of self-threaded dowels failed by angular and vertical root fracture.[64] Cast dowel and cores also exhibit a high rate of root fracture because of rigidity, taper, and close adaptation to dentin walls.[21,31,42,57] Dowels that resist deformation or permanent bending also protect the integrity of crown margins and cement seal, particularly in teeth with minimal tooth structure remaining for an ample ferrule; fatigue of the dowel, core, and dentin complex can distort and open crown margins and increase the risk of dowel or core fracture.[22] This can result in loss of the restoration or potentially devastating caries.

Dowel design and resistance to root fracture

Dowel shape   Parallel metal dowels distribute functional loads to the root more passively than tapered dowels. Classic photoelastic studies of metal dowels demonstrated that tapered dowels act like a wedge to exert significant lateral forces on the tooth structure that can result in vertical root fracture. Clinically, tapered dowels (including the custom-cast dowel and core) that are closely adapted to the internal shape of the root canal are more likely to result in root fracture than are parallel-sided dowels.[21,31,42,57,58]

Because canals are tapered, dowels have been designed to take advantage of the safety of parallel sides while maintaining dentin integrity in narrow apical portions of the canal. Dowels with a parallel coronal portion and a conical apical portion, or dowels that increase in coronal diameter with series of parallel-sided steps, provide stability and address the tapered nature of the canal.[36]

It is not necessary to have intimate tooth-to-dowel contact in all areas of the restoration. This means that conservative, parallel dowels in funnel-shaped canals will not contact the coronal aspect of the canal wall and will be surrounded by layer of cement. This internal layer of composite resin or resin cement can reinforce weak teeth and provide an elastic layer between the elastic dentin and the dowel that may have a higher modulus of elasticity. Some newer, composite resin–based direct dowels do not require dowel space preparation and therefore preserve dentin integrity and strength. Once cured these dowels reflect the internal shape of the canal but do not increase the risk of root fracture because of their more elastic physical properties (compared with earlier studies of tapered-metal dowels).

Dowel diameter   The dowel must be of sufficient diameter (but no larger) to resist distortion or permanent bending under functional forces. A larger diameter gives no improvement in the dowel-to-root retention but will significantly increase the risk of root fracture (Fig. 22-9). Instrumentation of the radicular dentin walls during dowel space preparation should be very conservative to preserve tooth structure. The minimum diameter a given dowel can have and still resist

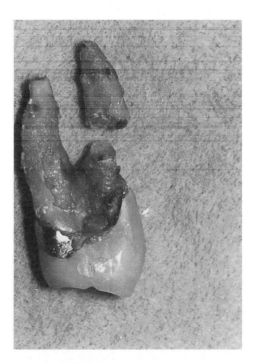

Fig. 22-9 Large dowel diameter in the buccal root resulted in a functional fracture of this premolar. Coronal to the fracture, the dowel can be seen through the thinned root surface. Excessive radicular dentin removal weakened the tooth.

distortion depends on the dowel's composition. Parallel-metal dowels are available in narrower diameters than nonmetallic dowels. Nonmetallic dowels are designed either with an overall tapered configuration or with two parallel steps containing a narrower parallel apical portion. This allows a greater bulk of coronal dowel material but requires more dentin removal to accommodate the wider coronal segment of the dowel in narrow canals.

Dowel length   The length of metal dowels affects their ability to transfer stresses along the length of the root. Metal dowels should be long enough to extend below the crest of alveolar bone root to reduce concentration of force in an area of root that is not embedded in alveolar bone. The greatest protection against root fracture, however, comes from the coronal restoration. In a recent study, increasing dowel length from 5 to 10 mm did not increase fracture resistance in teeth protected by crowns designed with adequate ferrule. [32]

Dowel composition and resistance to root fracture Historically, a key criteria for dowels was rigidity to resist bending under function. Today there are also dowels with physical properties that resemble those of dentin, in addition to addressing all other clinical retention, esthetic, and radiographic issues. Occlusal forces are transferred through the core to the dowel and ultimately disbursed along the length of the root. The more similarly dowels, cements, and restorative materials behave in comparison to dentin, the less force is concentrated among the components and the root during function. In general, metal and zirconia dowels are stiffer than dentin. Fiberglass-reinforced composite matrix; woven-fiber, ribbon-reinforced composite resin; and carbon fiber or carbon core dowels approximate the stiffness (i.e., modulus of elasticity) of dentin. Among metal dowels, SS is stiffer than titanium alloy, which is stiffer than pure titanium. Metal dowels (preformed and cast) are reported to have a greater risk of root fracture in in vitro studies of uncrowned teeth.[13,33,42,55,70] Carbon fiber; carbon core; and fiberglass-reinforced, composite matrix dowels have a lower modulus of elasticity than metal dowels and are considered to have elasticity similar to dentin. This provides them with a greater ability to dissipate force, which reduces the risk of root fracture. However, successful restoration of endodontically treated teeth includes more than root fracture resistance. Function and esthetics must be restored, and this restored dentin dowel core and cement-crown complex must remain intact and resist microleakage and recurrent caries over time.

Many different materials are used in the restoration of a single tooth, all with different degrees of stiffness and different responses to functional forces. Stiff dowels historically have been recommended to reinforce the cervical area of teeth against flexion and possible disruption of the cement seal. Very little has been published about the ability of newer dowel materials, with their more dentinlike modulus of elasticity, to protect the integrity of the cement seal.[62] This is especially critical in damaged teeth that have little remaining tooth structure at the margin. Dowel selection will be a continuing challenge for clinicians in restoration of devastated teeth, balancing root fracture resistance with marginal seal integrity and possibly with esthetic concerns.

Dowel design for the damaged root   Composite resin technology can be used to unify the radicular dentin and dowel and core structures in damaged roots. Minimal radicular dentin can be found in teeth with extensive caries, in roots with excessive endodontic instrumentation, in roots with excessive dowel preparation, and in the roots of immature anterior teeth. Retention of dowels in these thin, flared canals has traditionally been achieved with custom-cast dowel and cores that reflect the internal canal shape but risk failure from root fracture. Composite resin, coupled with a central metal dowel, can be valuable in reinforcing internal radicular walls of roots thinned by caries or other dentin loss. The resultant dentin and composite dowel complex is up to 50% stronger than roots restored conventionally.[51] Rather than removing scarce dentin during dowel space preparation, internal canal walls can be built up to form the appropriate shape for the dowel. With this concept, a light-transmitting dowel is used to mold and cure the internal composite resin, creating a customized composite matrix. This composite matrix contains a standardized dowel space for metal dowel cementation. Composite resin and dentin bonding systems can also be reinforced with a woven polyethylene fiber system to create an entirely custom dowel and integrated core.

The most important aspect of fracture prevention, however, is not the dowel design but the amount of remaining tooth structure and the design of the final crown. Teeth with coronal tooth structure replaced with a composite core and a variety of posts all fractured with lower force than teeth with endodontic treatment, access seal, and crown preparation.[13] Fracture resistance increases significantly with increasing length of the ferrule on sound-tooth structure.[4,23,32,43] It is important to understand the basis of in vitro studies, which are designed to amplify the differences between materials. However, in considering clinical application of this information it is important to remember that test conditions are often not found clinically, including those using force against dowels or cores in teeth without crowns.

Esthetic qualities of the dowel   Current restorative procedures allow fabrication of highly esthetic, ceramic, coronal restorations that contain no metal substructure. These restorations can have remarkable depth of lifelike color and vitality, with no unnatural opacity, shadows, gray colorations, or artificial brightness from underlying metal or metal-masking agents. Esthetic restoration of nonvital teeth is also possible today, with the development of white or tooth-colored, dowel and core materials.

Carbon core, zirconia, or fiberglass-reinforced composite resin dowel systems are all clinically esthetic. Dowel selection for the esthetic case will depend on evaluation of desired physical properties of the esthetic dowels in relation to the amount of remaining tooth structure and on an estimation of the potential need for future endodontic retreatment. Carbon core dowels and fiber-reinforced, composite resin dowel systems have a modulus of elasticity similar to dentin and can be removed from the canal with special burs. However, these dowels are not radiographically obvious; a faint outline from the cement is all that delineates their presence (Fig. 22-10). Zirconia dowels are highly radiopaque and visible on radiographic films (Fig. 22-11), but they are stiffer than dentin. Zirconium can, therefore, be considered an esthetic equivalent to preformed metal dowels. They are highly bondable to the root structure but can also be cemented with traditional cement if future retrievability is desired. Zirconium is extremely hard and cannot be cut from a canal; the length must be trimmed before cementation.

Carbon fiber and metal dowels are not esthetic and should not be used for esthetically critical restorations. These dowels are black or metallic in color, which can reflect through gingiva, tooth structure, or ceramic restorations. They are appropriate for teeth to be restored with gold or porcelain fused-to-metal crowns. Dowel selection will also depend on the desired physical properties previously discussed, as well as radiopacity, retrievability, and biocompatibility.

SS, cast metal, and zirconia dowels are highly radiopaque. The radiopacity of titanium dowels is similar to gutta-percha; they are difficult to distinguish in radiographs with densely condensed, gutta percha–filled canal[26] (Fig. 22-12). Carbon fiber, carbon core, and fiberglass-reinforced composite matrix dowels are only faintly visible inside the root as an "empty" cement outline of radiopaque cement (Fig. 22-13).

Retrievability of metal and zirconia dowels is dependent on the cementing medium. Traditional cements may allow dowel removal with ultrasonic vibration. Adhesive-resin cements render dowels virtually unremovable. Carbon fiber and fiberglass-reinforced composite dowels are easily removed by cutting with special burs.

SS dowels contain nickel and may present an allergic potential in some patients. Carbon fiber, titanium, and cast metal dowels are all biocompatible. Cytotoxicity tests of carbon fiber dowels found no cytotoxic effects.[70] Dowel materials should be inert to the corrosive effects of oral fluids because no dowel and cement combination has been shown to form a liquid proof seal against microleakage.[3,19,20] Corrosion is not an issue with nonmetallic dowels or with custom-cast dowel and cores if the cast dowel and core are fabricated completely from nonreactive gold alloys. The most significant corrosion occurs in SS dowels when a custom core is cast onto a preformed metal dowel.

Dowel space preparation   The dowel should be long enough to satisfy clinical requirements without jeopardizing the root integrity. The standard parameters for dowel length in a tooth with normal periodontal support[25] range between:

1. Two thirds the length of the canal
2. An amount equal to the coronal length of the tooth
3. One half the bone-supported length of the root

The final length of the dowel in the periodontally healthy tooth will be limited by two major variables: (1) the root morphology and (2) the need for sufficient apical seal in the root canal system.

Root morphology plays a great role in determination of dowel length. The total root length is the most obvious factor in dowel length design. Equally important are root taper, root curvature, and cross-sectional root form. The root should have greater than 1 mm of tooth structure remaining circumferentially around the apical end of the dowel to avoid perforation and resist fracture (Fig. 22-14). This dictates a shorter dowel in a tapered root so that the apical extent of the dowel does not impinge on converging root walls. A longer dowel can safely be placed in a parallel-sided root of equal length. Root curvature reduces dowel length; the greater the curve of the root and the more coronally located the curve, the shorter will be the dowel. Cross-sectional root form cannot be determined by radiographs, because root concavities are not readily visible in a two-dimensional film. Thorough knowledge of root morphology for each tooth is mandatory for dowel placement. Furcations, both faciolingual and mesiodistal, along with developmental depressions are present in predictable locations in the dentition (Fig. 22-15). Maxillary first molars have deep concavities on the furcal surface of 94% of the mesial buccal roots, 31% of distal buccal roots, and 17% of palatal roots. Mandibular first molars have root concavities on the furcal surface of 100% of mesial root and 99% of distal roots.[7] Maxillary first premolars have deep mesial concavities and slender roots with thin dentin. Endodontically treated teeth with these root concavities will require alteration of the length and placement of dowel materials to eliminate thin dentinal walls or outright root perforations.

The need to maintain adequate obturation is the second major limiting factor in dowel length. Retaining the last 3 to 5 mm of filling material at the apex is sufficient for the endodontic seal. A dowel placed closer to the apex than this distance, even when surrounded by adequate tooth structure, risks failure of the seal and, thus, of the restorative effort (Fig. 22-16). Alveolar bone height also influences dowel length. Occlusal forces generate the least risk to the remaining tooth structure and surrounding bone when a dowel extends apical to the alveolar crest. Short, stiff dowels transfer forces to the unsupported root extending above the alveolus and can cause root fracture.

When dowels are indicated they should be placed in roots that are husky, straight, and long. Root anatomy of multirooted teeth is most suitable in the palatal roots of maxillary molars, palatal roots of maxillary premolars,[16] and distal roots of mandibular molars.

In summary, conventional dowels should be passive and cemented into place. The residual dentin should undergo minimal alteration to accept the dowel. Length and diameter should be the minimum dimension needed to withstand functional loading.

Dowels should be fabricated from materials that exhibit physical properties for long-term success and materials that will not corrode. The dowel should be an extension into the conservatively shaped root canal system, not an intrusion into the radicular dentin. The goal of dowel design is clini-

Text continued on p. 782

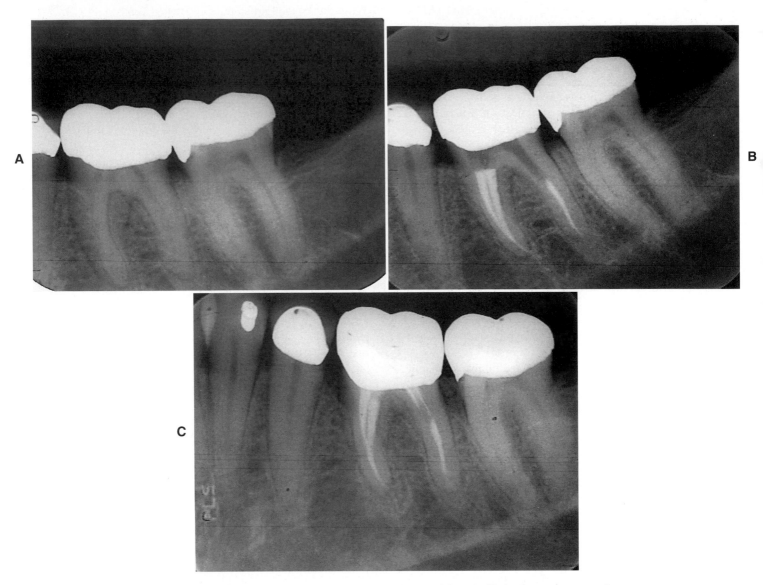

Fig. 22-10 Radiograph of carbon fiber dowel in the distal root of the mandibular first molar. Nonradiopaque carbon fiber dowels are delineated by the cement outline and are more difficult to detect on a radiograph than SS or zirconia dowels. **A**, Pretreatment. **B**, Dowel space prepared. **C**, Carbon fiber dowel cemented.

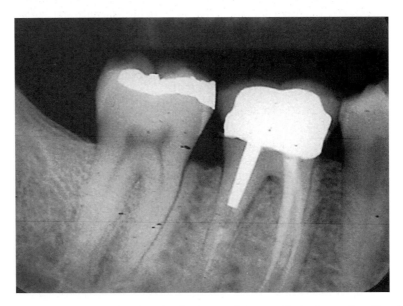

Fig. 22-11 Radiograph of zirconia dowel in the distal root of the mandibular first molar. Zirconia dowels are radiopaque and are highly visible on radiographic film. (Courtesy Dr. James Gregory.)

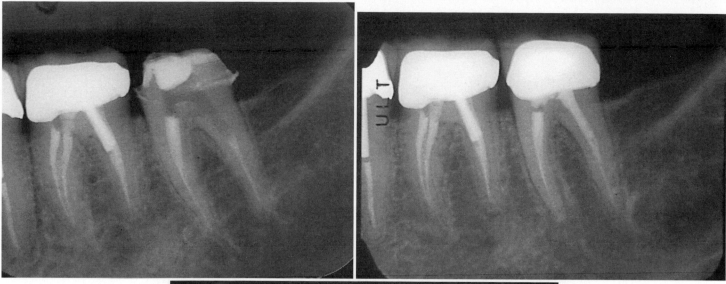

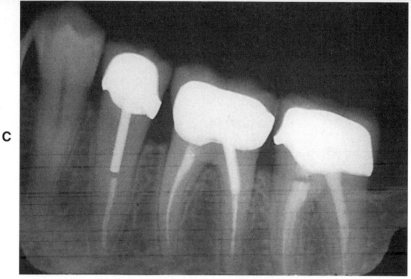

Fig. 22-12 Radiograph of a titanium dowel in the distal root of the mandibular second molar. This material is more difficult to detect on radiographs than SS cast dowels. **A,** Dowel space prepared. **B,** Titanium dowel cemented. **C,** Note differences in radiopacity between the SS dowel in the mandibular premolar and the titanium dowel in the mandibular second molar.

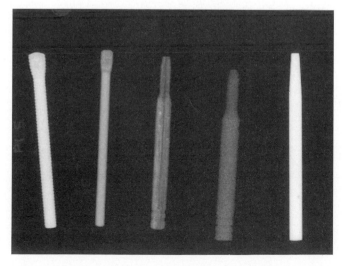

Fig. 22-13 Radiographic visibility of dowels is greater without the presence of soft tissue, alveolar bone, or tooth structure. *Left to right:* Zirconium, white carbon fiber, black carbon fiber, titanium, SS.

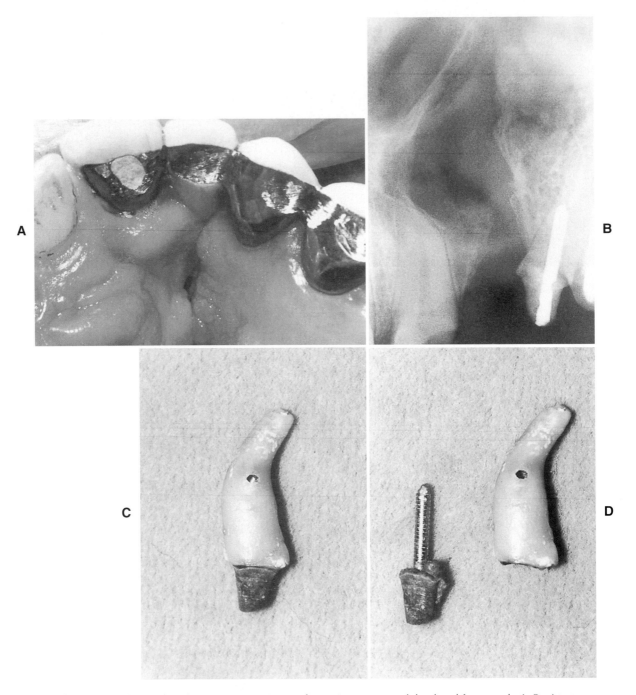

Fig. 22-14 Substantial tooth structure (a minimum of 1 mm) must surround the dowel for strength. **A,** Persistent symptoms in the treated cuspid adjacent to the cleft were diagnosed as a root perforation. **B,** The radiograph appears to demonstrate an intact root surface. **C,** The extracted tooth reveals the dowel visible through the perforation. **D,** Dowel and core separation from the root verify that the perforation occurred at the apex of the dowel.

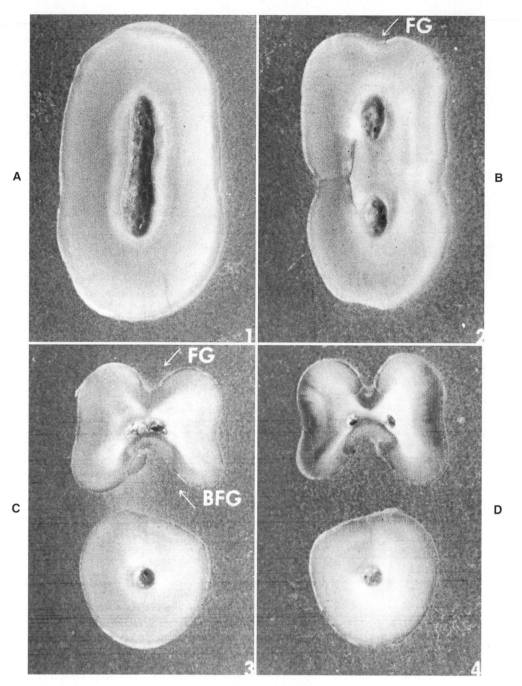

Fig. 22-15 Root anatomy has significant influence over dowel placement. **A,** The cross section of a maxillary first premolar at the CEJ; the buccal surface faces the top of the section. **B,** 2 mm apical to the CEJ, root irregularities and developmental depressions become apparent. **C,** 4 mm apical to the CEJ, the root has separated into buccal (*top*), and the palatal roots and developmental grooves have deepened. **D,** 6 mm apical to the CEJ, the buccal root continues to demonstrate more accentuated depressions. Placement of a dowel in the buccal root risks perforation into the furcation of this tooth. The palatal root is a better choice for dowel placement. (From Gher ME, Vernino AR: *Int J Periodont Rest Dent* 1[5]:52, 1981.)

cally sufficient retention of the dowel and maximum fracture resistance of the root, not the converse (Fig. 22-17)

Core

The core (Fig. 22-18) consists of restorative material placed in the coronal area of a tooth. This material replaces carious, fractured, or otherwise missing coronal structure and retains the final crown. The core is anchored to

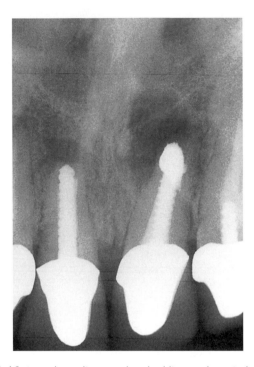

Fig. 22-16 Long, large-diameter dowels obliterate the apical seal and cause endodontic failure of two central incisors. A 3- to 5-mm intact endodontic seal must be retained at the apex.

the tooth by extending into the coronal aspect of the canal or through the endodontic dowel. The attachment between tooth, dowel, and core are mechanical or chemical or both, because the core and dowel are usually fabricated of different materials.

The remaining tooth structure can also be altered to augment retention of the core. Although pins, grooves, and channels can be placed in the dentin, these modifications all increase the core retention and resistance to rotation at the expense of tooth structure. In most cases the irregular nature of the residual, coronal tooth structure and the normal morphology of the pulp chamber and canal orifices eliminate the need for these tooth alterations. Using restorative materials that bond to tooth structure enhances retention and resistance without the need to remove valuable dentin. Therefore if additional retentive or antirotation form for the core is deemed necessary, dentin removal should be kept to a minimum. Desirable physical characteristics of a core include the following:

- High compressive strength
- Dimensional stability
- Ease of manipulation
- Short setting time for cement
- An ability to bond to both tooth and dowel

Contemporary cores include cast metal or ceramic, amalgam, composite resin and (sometimes) glass ionomer resin materials.

Cast core. A cast metal dowel and core (Fig. 22-19) is a traditional way to restore endodontically treated teeth. The core is an integral extension of the dowel, and the cast core does not depend on mechanical means for retention to the dowel. This construction avoids dislodgement of the core and crown from the dowel and root when minimal tooth structure remains. Noble metals are noncorrosive. Ceramic cores can

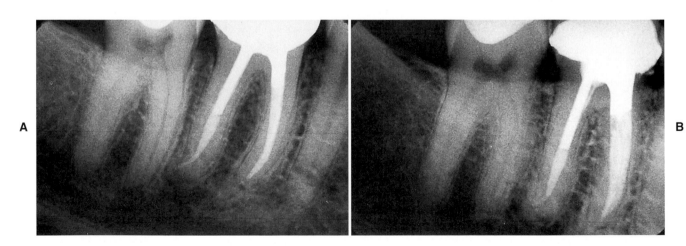

Fig. 22-17 Components of a successful restoration can be seen in these two radiographs of the same tooth. **A**, The gutta-percha seal is intact. Minimal dowel space instrumentation allows the dowel to be an extension of the canal system in the distal root. Cementing medium is evident in the larger, coronal opening of the distal canal. **B**, The mesial roots contain alloy condensed into the first 2 to 4 mm of the canal. The coronal restoration provides protection, function, and (if needed) esthetics. (Courtesy Dr. Frank Casanova.)

also be integrated with zirconia dowels in similar laboratory procedures.[29,62]

The disadvantages of the cast dowel and core system, however, are considerable. Most importantly, cast dowel and cores have been shown to have a higher rate of root fracture than preformed dowels.[13,57] Secondly, the financial cost of providing this service is high (i.e., two appointments are needed and laboratory expense may be significant). The laboratory phase is technique sensitive. Casting a pattern with a large core and a small diameter dowel can result in porosity in the gold at the dowel and core interface. Fracture of the metal at this interface under function will result in the failure of the restoration. Attempts to circumvent this problem by casting a core to a preformed dowel made of SS degrade the physical characteristics of the SS, resulting in a dowel and core restoration that is not sufficiently strong or inert to withstand clinical forces.[59]

Amalgam core. Dental amalgam is a traditional core buildup material with a long history of clinical success. Amalgam has high compressive strength, high tensile strength, and high modulus of elasticity. It is stable to thermal and functional stress and, therefore, transmits minimal stress to the residual tooth structure and cement and crown margins. Bonded amalgam procedures can improve

the seal at the tooth and alloy junction.[52] Amalgam is easily manipulated and can have a rapid setting time.

Placement of a fast-setting, high-copper alloy core permits final crown preparation at the initial operative appointment, although the early strength is low. Amalgam cores are highly retentive when used as coronal and radicular restorations or with a preformed SS dowel in posterior teeth; they require more force to dislodge than cast-dowel cores.[34,44] A significant disadvantage of amalgam cores is the potential for corrosion and subsequent discoloration of the gingiva or remaining dentin. Amalgam use is declining worldwide, because of legislative, safety, and environmental issues.

Composite resin core. Composite resin exhibits favorable ease of manipulation, very rapid set, and strong compressive strength.[9] Preparation for the final restoration is readily accomplished during the core placement appointment. Additional retention and antirotation mechanisms are also easily achieved with auxiliary pins.

Composite resin properties pertaining to microleakage and retention to tooth structure are dependent on the dentin-bonding agent. Early composites preceded the development of dentin-bonding agents and suffered from polymerization shrinkage and contraction away from the tooth structure, resulting in marginal core and tooth opening, microcracks,

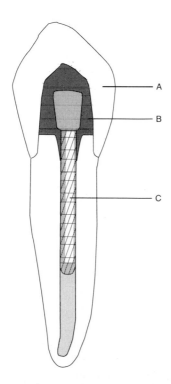

Fig. 22-18 The preformed dowel and core restoration. The preformed metal dowel (C) is cemented into the prepared dowel space. The core material (B) is retained by the dowel by bonding to the tooth structure; by undercuts in the pulp chamber; and, occasionally, by auxiliary retentive pins, grooves, or boxes. The coronal restoration (A) provides the ferrule and restores esthetics and function.

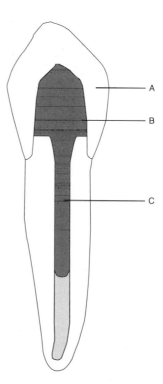

Fig. 22-19 The cast dowel and core restoration. The dowel (C) and the core (B) are cast of the same material and cemented to the tooth as a single unit. The coronal restoration (A) provides the ferrule and restores esthetics and function.

and microleakage. These openings can still occur if dentin-bonding procedures are not meticulously performed. They can be potential avenues of extensive invasion for oral fluids after a break in the cement seal or marginal integrity of the crown. No bonding agent, however, has been shown to entirely eliminate microleakage.[19,69,71,74] Therefore as with all buildup materials for decimated teeth, more than 2 mm of sound tooth structure should remain at the margin for optimum composite resin core function. In addition, the composite-resin core and the bonding agent must be compatible to achieve retention of the core. Recent reports indicate inadequate bonding between light-cured bonding agents and chemical-cured composite core materials.[11]

Glass ionomer core. Glass ionomer and glass ionomer silver are adhesive materials useful for small buildups or to fill undercuts in prepared teeth. The major benefit of glass ionomer materials is an anticariogenic quality resulting from the presence of fluoride in the chemical composition.[67]

Glass ionomer materials are limited to small restorations in which core strength is not required. Low strength and fracture toughness results in brittleness, which contraindicates the use of glass ionomer buildups in thin, anterior teeth or to replace unsupported cusps. Glass ionomer cores also exhibit low retention to preformed metal dowels.[44] Glass ionomer is soluble and sensitive to moisture. Adhesive failure can result from contamination of the tooth surface with cutting debris, saliva, blood, or protein. Glass ionomer is not strong enough for a core for an abutment tooth. It is indicated in posterior teeth in which (1) a bulk of core material is possible, (2) significant sound dentin remains, (3) additional retention is available with pins or dentin preparations, (4) moisture control is assured, and (5) caries control is indicated.

Resin-modified glass ionomer core. Resin-modified glass ionomer materials are a combination of glass ionomer and composite resin technologies; they exhibit properties of both materials. Resin-modified glass ionomer exhibits moderate strength, greater than glass ionomer and less than composite resin. As a core material it is adequate for moderate-size buildups. However, hygroscopic expansion can cause fracture of ceramic crowns.[56] Solubility is between that of glass ionomer and composite resin. Fluoride release is equal to glass ionomer, and far more than composite resin. The bond to dentin is close to that of dentin-bonded composite resin, and it is significantly higher than traditional glass ionomer. Resin-modified glass ionomer exhibits minimal microleakage.

Coronal Coverage
The final component of the endodontic reconstruction is the coronal restoration (see Fig. 22-7). All coronal restorations reestablish function and isolate the dentin and endodontic fill materials from microleakage. Cast crowns are coronal restorations that fulfill all of these requirements and also distribute functional forces and protect the tooth against fracture. High strength and highly esthetic ceramic crowns on onlays achieve the same purpose.

As a general rule most endodontically treated posterior teeth and all structurally damaged anterior or posterior teeth should be restored with a crown. Crowns prevent a significant number of fractures in posterior teeth but do not similarly protect anterior teeth (see Fig. 22-6). In a large clinical study, the fracture rate for uncrowned bicuspids and molars was double that for those restored with crowns. The success rate for maxillary molars dropped from 97.8% for those with crowns to 50.0% for those without crowns. Anterior teeth are less at risk for fracture than posterior teeth and showed no further improvement when restored with a crown. Maxillary anterior teeth exhibited a success rate of 87.5% for crowned teeth and 85.4% for uncrowned teeth. Therefore endodontically treated anterior teeth do not require a crown or dowel unless extensive tooth structure is missing and integrity, function, and esthetics must be restored. The coronal restoration for endodontically treated, intact anterior teeth consists of sealing the lingual access cavity. Posterior teeth generally need coronal coverage to protect against fracture from occlusal forces.

When a coronal restoration is indicated, the amount of tooth structure remaining after final preparation has the greatest importance in determining the design of the dowel and core. Tooth structure that appears adequate before the crown preparation may be grossly unsatisfactory after occlusal and axial reductions. Therefore the initial crown preparation is first completed and the bulk and position of the prepared tooth structure is evaluated for dowel and core selection. Crown preparation for endodontically treated teeth is identical to that of vital teeth when substantial tooth structure remains. Once restored with a crown, the underlying sound tooth structure provides greater resistance to fracture than any dowel type or design. Natural tooth structure should be carefully preserved during all phases of dowel space and crown preparation.

The crown preparation design for extensively damaged nonvital teeth is critical. The minimal remaining tooth structure must be used effectively so that the crown can restore function without harm to the remaining root or to the periodontal attachment. The residual tooth between the core and the gingival sulcus must be structurally sound and a minimum of 2 mm in height for the crown ferrule and margin. Because caries, fracture, and other endodontic precedents can decimate the tooth to the tissue level, this amount of unaffected tooth structure is often not available and adjunctive procedures are indicated to first obtain the necessary length.

The final crown provides added security by consolidating the remaining cusps and prepared tooth structure and by creating a ferrule effect (Fig. 22-20). It is formed by the walls and margins of the crown (Fig. 22-21) or cast telescopic coping (Fig. 22-22) encasing the gingival 2 mm of the axial walls of the preparation above the crown margin. A properly executed ferrule significantly reduces the incidence of fracture in the nonvital tooth by reinforcing the tooth at its external surface and dissipating force that concentrates at the narrowest circumference of the tooth.[38,73] Fracture resistance is increased significantly with increasing ferrule length.[32] The ferrule also resists lateral forces from dowels and leverage from the crown in function, and it increases the retention and resistance of the restoration. Crown preparations with as little as 1 mm coronal extension of dentin above the margin exhibit double the fracture resistance, compared with preparations with the core terminating on a flat surface immediately above the margin.[37,45,58]

To be successful the ferrule must encircle a vertical wall of sound tooth structure above the margin and must not terminate on restorative material. Both the crown and crown preparation must meet five requirements:

1. A minimum of 2 mm dentin axial wall height
2. Parallel axial walls
3. The metal must totally encircle the tooth
4. It must be on solid tooth structure
5. It must not invade the attachment apparatus.

This means that a 4 to 5 mm height and 1 mm thickness of sound suprabony tooth structure should be available to accommodate the periodontal biologic width and the restorative ferrule.[43] A tooth with remaining structure that is insufficient to construct a ferrule as described should be evaluated for periodontal crown lengthening surgery or orthodontic extrusion to gain access to additional root surface. The lack of sufficient ferrule in the final restoration forces the core, the dowel, and the root to accept high functional stresses, often resulting in fracture (Fig. 22-23).

Crown cementation.   Cement selection for luting of final crowns is especially important in the case of compromised teeth. Functional forces cause strain against crown margins, resulting in possible failure of the cement bond. The type of cement affects the rate of microleakage (more than the core material) under crowns[68] and along posts.[3] It also affects the ability of the crown and tooth to resist failure. This preliminary failure is undetectable, but it allows microleakage that may lead to dental caries. A pulpless tooth will not

exhibit symptoms; caries hidden from clinical and radiographic view by the crown can increase to unrestorable levels.

Resin-modified glass ionomer cements have been shown to expand hygroscopically and can cause cracking or fracture of lower strength, ceramic crowns.[56] Crowns cemented with resin cements are more resistant to force-related failure than

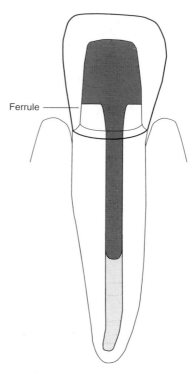

Fig. 22-20 The ferrule is an encircling band of metal, usually provided by the coronal restoration. It greatly increases the resistance of a tooth to fracture. A ferrule should (1) be a minimum of 1 to 2 mm in height, (2) have parallel axial walls, (3) completely encircle the tooth, (4) end on sound tooth structure, and (5) not invade the attachment apparatus of the tooth.

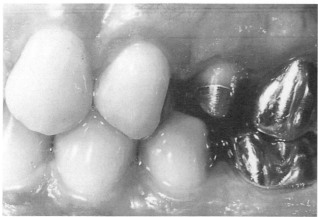
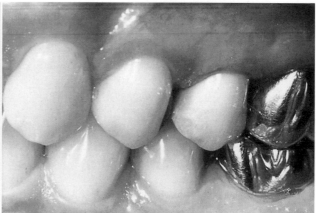

Fig. 22-21 The ferrule effect is provided by the coronal restoration. **A,** The second premolar with a preformed dowel and alloy core. **B,** The coping of the porcelain and metal crown supplies the ferrule. This encirclement significantly increases the fracture resistance of the tooth.

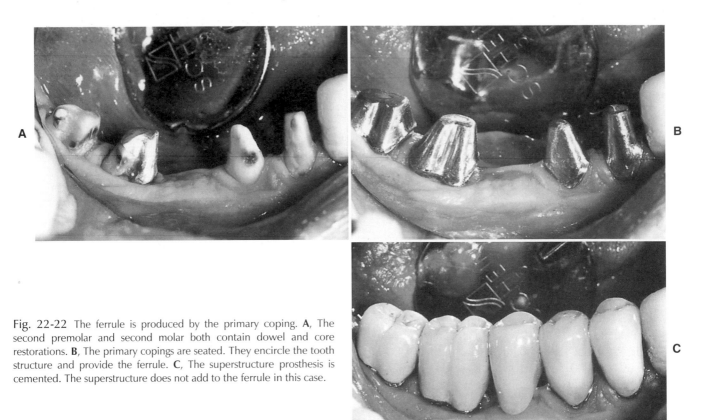

Fig. 22-22 The ferrule is produced by the primary coping. **A**, The second premolar and second molar both contain dowel and core restorations. **B**, The primary copings are seated. They encircle the tooth structure and provide the ferrule. **C**, The superstructure prosthesis is cemented. The superstructure does not add to the ferrule in this case.

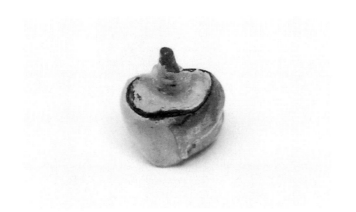

Fig. 22-23 A failed restoration with inadequate ferrule. The level of the core material is coincident with the restorative margin; functional forces were not resisted by adequate axial walls of sound tooth structure.

resin-modified glass ionomer or zinc phosphate cements. However, it should be noted that excess resin cement, once set, is nearly impossible to remove from root surfaces, substituting a periodontal problem for a restorative problem. Dual cure resin cements address this issue by allowing brief, light cure of excess cement for ease of removal, while the internal cement cures chemically.

Provisional restorations. The true extent of caries or other damage in a broken down tooth can be difficult to determine before tooth preparation. Placement of a provisional restoration allows total evaluation of the tooth and supporting structures before committing the patient to definitive endodontics. As discussed previously, although endodontic therapy can be successful, structural, occlusal, and periodontal findings may condemn a tooth to extraction. It is prudent for the clinician to discover these facts before the canals are treated. Once the decision to retain a tooth is made, crown preparation and provisional restoration in advance of endodontic treatment can assist the endodontic endeavor. Removal of this temporary crown at the endodontic appointment allows structural evaluation of the remaining coronal dentin and facilitates access to the chamber.

Preendodontic preparation and provisionalization may assist in differential diagnosis. Diagnosis can be difficult when multiple clinical problems are present on the same tooth or on adjacent teeth. Clarification of the true cause of the patient's problem is aided by the removal of potential symptomatic variables, including caries, defective restorations, and cracked cusps. Decisions about the restorability of the tooth can be made and the tooth returned to temporary esthetics and function before scheduling definitive endodontic treatment or extraction of the tooth. After endodontic treatment (if a cast dowel and core is planned) a provisional

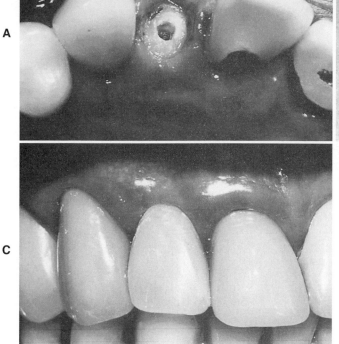

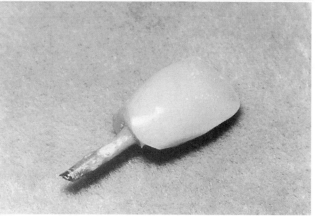

Fig. 22-24 Provisional crowns may be retained by temporary dowels until definitive therapy can be provided. **A,** A lateral incisor fractured below the level of the free gingival margin. **B,** Endodontic therapy was completed, and a provisional crown fabricated with an aluminum dowel. **C,** The provisional restoration in place. This procedure allowed time for orthodontic extrusion of the root. A final dowel, core, and coronal restoration were placed after sufficient tooth structure was present above the periodontal attachment.

crown with attached, temporary dowel can be fabricated for a tooth with limited supragingival tooth structure (Fig. 22-24). Proprietary dowel systems include temporary dowels. The final dowel and core and crown should be fabricated as soon as possible, because microleakage can contaminate the post space and endodontic fill.[20,74]

Provisional crowns for endodontically treated teeth must be used with extreme caution, because a partial loss of cement seal will not provoke symptoms in the tooth and may go undetected for some time. This leakage can lead to severe carious invasion and loss of the tooth. This is especially true when the combination provisional crown and temporary dowel are used. The lack of tooth structure necessitating this combination predisposes the cement seal to breakdown and places these teeth at risk. In addition to caries formation, leakage of the postobturation, temporary restoration can jeopardize success of the endodontic treatment.

Dowel and core fabrication techniques. The first step for all types of dowel and core restorations is the removal of the gutta-percha from the dowel space. The amount of gutta-percha to be removed is dictated by the desired dowel length, the bone height, and the root morphology, as discussed earlier. The procedure is generally best accomplished by the clinician providing the endodontic service (because that clinician has clear knowledge of the canal system size and form).

The initial dowel space preparation procedure is similar for most standardized dowel and core systems. The space (cleared of gutta-percha) has the form of the canal after cleaning and shaping and must be refined to the correct dimension and shape for the dowel space. All of the proprietary systems are supplied with a series of drills to prepare the internal surface of the canal. With a minimum of dentin wall alteration, the drills gradually increase the size of the canal, remove natural undercuts, and shape the canal to correspond with the dowel. Intimate contact of the dowel and dentin surface is not indicated for the passive dowel systems; adequate depth and proper cementation provide sufficient retention for these restorations. Correct depth can be measured by a periodontal probe or other small measuring device. Direct composite reinforcement systems require little or no dowel space preparation.

Cast dowel and core fabrication technique Cast dowel and core restorations can be fabricated with either direct or indirect techniques. In the direct technique, a castable dowel and core pattern is fabricated directly in the mouth on the prepared tooth. The indirect technique uses an impression and stone die of the tooth for the pattern fabrication. The pattern is then invested and cast with gold or crown and bridge alloy. Using the direct technique, a preformed plastic dowel pattern is seated in the dowel space. Any necessary antirotation pins or dentin preparations are added,

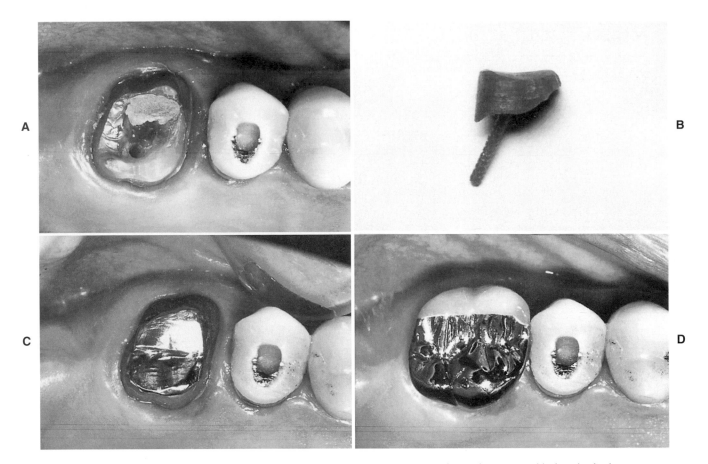

Fig. 22-25 The cast dowel and core restoration (i.e., direct technique). **A**, The tooth is prepared before the final selection of a dowel and core system. The buccal canal undercuts are blocked out to form a path of withdrawal for the pattern without additional dentin removal. A plastic burnout dowel is fit to the refined dowel space in the palatal root and resin is added to form the core portion of the pattern. **B**, The one-piece pattern is removed from the tooth and cast. **C**, Cast dowel and core is cemented in the preparation. **D**, The final coronal restoration is fabricated.

ensuring that they are parallel to the path of withdrawal. Undercuts are blocked out with glass ionomer cement, rather than removing valuable dentin. Acrylic resin is added to create a core attached to the dowel pattern and is prepared with a dental hand piece. The finished pattern is removed from the tooth to be cast in the laboratory (Fig. 22-25).

Using the indirect technique, a final impression of the prepared tooth and dowel space is made and the final pattern will be fabricated on a die from this impression. The crown margins need not be accurately reproduced at this stage. Proprietary systems provide matched drills, impression dowels, and laboratory casting patterns of various diameters. An impression dowel is selected and fit to the dowel space. Adhesive is applied to the coronal portion of the impression dowel, and a final impression is made that captures the form of the coronal tooth structure and picks up the impression dowel. In the laboratory, a die reproduces the dowel space and the residual coronal tooth structure for fabrication of the dowel and core pattern. Esthetic dowel and cores can also be fabricated indirectly in the laboratory, using a ceramic ingot cast onto a zirconia dowel. At a second appointment, the cast

dowel and core is seated in the dowel space of the tooth. Obstructions are detected with a paint-disclosing medium and removed. The cast dowel and core is now ready for cementation. It is important to note that total marginal integrity between the casting and the tooth is not mandatory, except as an indication of complete seating. This is an internal restoration; the entire cast dowel and core (along with the tooth structure) will be encapsulated by the final crown, which must have marginal integrity.

Preformed dowel and core fabrication technique.
Preformed dowel and core combinations are the restoration of choice for most clinical situations. They make up the vast majority of intermediary restorations placed in dental practices today. These systems contain preformed dowels corresponding to the instrumentation used in refining the dowel space. Once the dowel space is prepared, the matching dowel is placed. Resistance to seating should be removed by refining the dowel space. Total seating is assessed by measuring the length of the dowel space from a fixed, coronal landmark with a periodontal probe. This measurement is transferred to the preformed dowel.

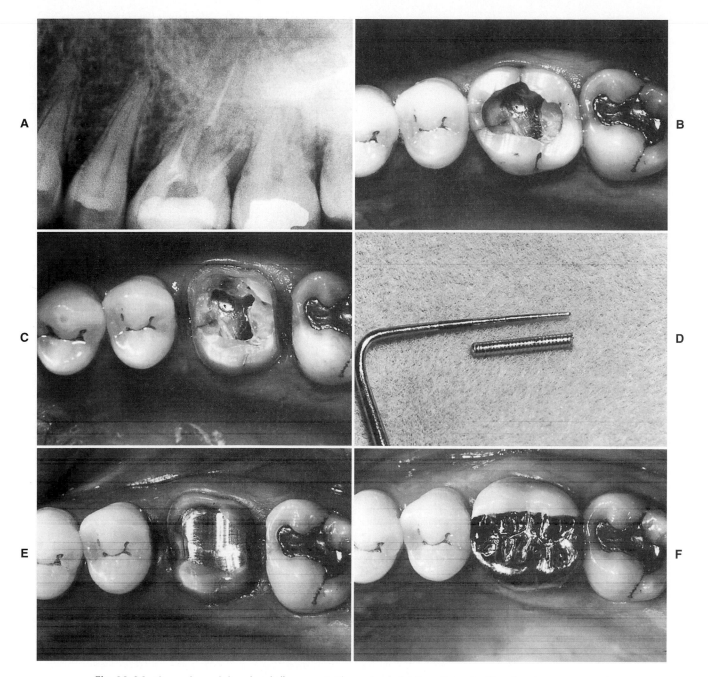

Fig. 22-26 The preformed dowel and alloy core. **A,** The postendodontic radiograph with a dowel space prepared in the palatal root. **B,** Occlusal view before preparation. The dowel and core system has not yet been selected. **C,** Final coronal preparation with sufficient tooth structure for a preformed dowel and alloy core. **D,** The dowel is cut to size before cementation using a periodontal probe to measure from a fixed coronal landmark to the base of the dowel space. **E,** Final preparation with the core in place. **F,** Final coronal restoration.

Complete seating may also be confirmed by radiograph. After achieving a passive fit within the root, the dowel is shortened coronally to an appropriate length. The dowel should be short of the internal occlusal surface of the final coronal restoration but must be long enough to retain the core. This adjustment must be completed before the dowel is cemented when using metal or zirconia dowels. Cutting these dowels after final cementation causes vibration, cement deg-radation, decreased retention, and possible microleakage into the canal space (Fig. 22-26).

Root-reinforcing dowel techniques. Composite resin can be used to reinforce the internal walls of roots thinned by caries. Composite resin is injected into the primed and bonded dentin canal, and a light-transmitting dowel is used to shape and set the composite. The light-transmitting dowel is removed, and a conventional metal dowel is cemented into the prepared space.

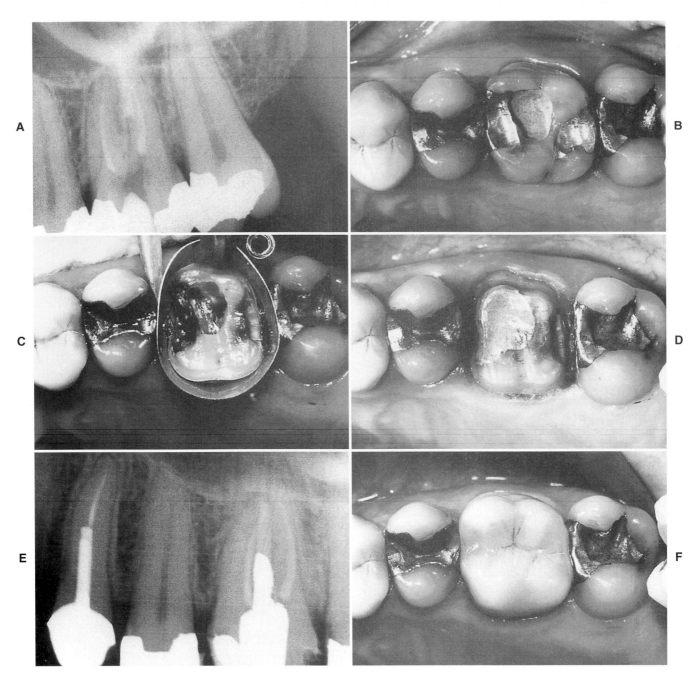

Fig. 22-27 The coronal radicular alloy. **A**, Postendodontic radiograph of maxillary first molar. **B**, Occlusal view before preparation. The dowel and core system has not yet been selected. **C**, Final coronal preparation with sufficient tooth structure for a bonded coronal radicular alloy. A matrix is used when condensing the alloy. **D**, Final preparation with core in place. **E**, Radiograph before final restoration. **F**, Final coronal restoration.

Core Fabrication Technique   After the dowel is luted to the root, any necessary retentive and antirotation mechanisms are added. A minimal number of additional retentive devices should be used, because these pins, grooves, and other dentin preparations remove tooth structure. Often the undercut nature of the remaining pulp chamber, the irregularity of the residual coronal tooth structure, and the angle at which the dowel exits the tooth are adequate to ensure core retention. The core material is then placed around the dowel, into the remaining pulp chamber, and built up to form the coronal area

(a suitable matrix may be necessary). After the core material is set, it can be prepared for the final coronal restoration.

Coronal radicular restoration technique.   When posterior teeth are largely intact, a coronal radicular restoration may be used (Fig. 22-27). This restoration consists of a core that extends 2 to 4 mm into the coronal portion of the canals. The core is retained by a combination of the divergence of the canals in a multirooted tooth, the natural undercuts in the pulp chamber, and adhesion with dentin-bonding agents, rather than with a dowel. A single, homogenous

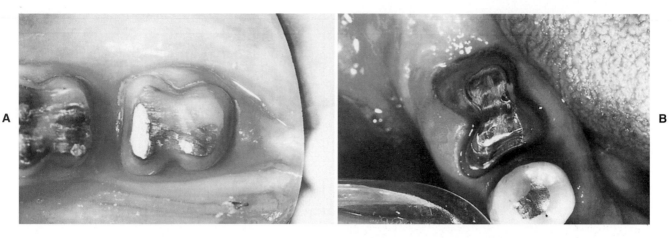

Fig. 22-28 Tooth preparation advantageous to the periodontium can prove deleterious to the pulp. **A,** Dentin reduction to decrease furcation invasions will bring the preparation and restoration in close proximity to the pulp chamber. **B,** Increased osseous destruction in the furcation results in exaggerated preparation designs.

material is used for the entire restoration, as opposed to the dual phases of a conventional, preformed dowel and core. The coronal radicular core is indicated for posterior teeth that have large pulp chambers and multiple canals for retention. The physical characteristics of alloy and composite resin allow this restoration to function well when up to 50% of the coronal tooth structure has been lost. Greater amounts of tooth structure must be present if glass ionomer is used because of its low tensile strength.

The technique for coronal, radicular buildup of the nonvital tooth is straightforward. Gutta-percha is removed from 2 to 4 mm of the canals. Undercuts and irregularities found in the canal walls increase retention of the restoration. Restorative materials should be bonded to the available tooth structure to increase retention, decrease microleakage, and increase fracture resistance of the tooth. The tooth is now ready for the final coronal restoration.

The Compromised Tooth   Restoration of endodontically treated teeth becomes more complex as the teeth or supporting structures become increasingly diseased. The compromises created by extensive loss of tooth structure alter the restorative procedures and affect the longevity of the tooth and the prosthesis. Mechanical requirements for structural integrity of the restoration and biologic requirements for the periodontal attachment apparatus often conflict. The narrow band of tooth structure that remains after severe breakdown is needed by both the restoration for a ferrule and by the tissue for periodontal health. Adjunctive dental procedures from other specialties may be needed before endodontic restoration of the severely damaged tooth.

Endodontic treatment can also become a form of adjunctive therapy to facilitate treatment of periodontally compromised teeth. Portions of teeth that otherwise may be candidates for extraction can sometimes be retained with hemisection or root amputation procedures. Periodontally guarded anterior teeth can be shortened and roots used as overdenture abutments. Endodontic treatment is needed for these periodontal procedures. Dowel, core, and coronal restorations must also be designed for the new shape and function of the altered, endodontic teeth. Lastly, the compromised tooth may not be a candidate for rehabilitation. In some circumstances, endodontic, restorative, and periodontal therapy will not add predictably to the prognosis of a tooth or teeth. Inclusion of implant dentistry into treatment planning options will make heroic attempts to salvage some compromised teeth unnecessary.

Posterior dentition.   Teeth with diminished periodontal support may require integrated periodontal, endodontic, and restorative treatment. Moderate-to-severe attachment loss results in a significant alteration of crown-to-root ratio. The complexity of diminished periodontal attachment is increased with multirooted teeth. The furcation involvement is common in the posterior dentition. Additionally, the loss of supporting tissues and periodontal therapy used to correct these problems often compromise restorative options.

Coronal preparation for both a path of withdrawal and reduction of the horizontal furcation invasion usually results in severe diminution of tooth structure. Establishment of a satisfactory taper for these teeth requires aggressive tooth preparation. The axial walls begin on the root surface, which has a smaller circumference than the CEJ. The axial walls must converge throughout the elongated clinical crown. This dentin removal brings the operative procedure, as well as the final restoration, in close proximity to the root canal system. The problem is exacerbated in the multirooted tooth when restorative procedures attempt to diminish furcation invasions. Teeth that exhibit attachment loss apical to the root trunk have horizontal defects into the furcation area. Tooth preparation to minimize this dimension requires removal of significant tooth structure coronal to the furcation. The resultant "fluted" preparation will be seen throughout the full length of the axial wall (Fig. 22-28). This procedure decreases the horizontal dimension of the furcation invasion

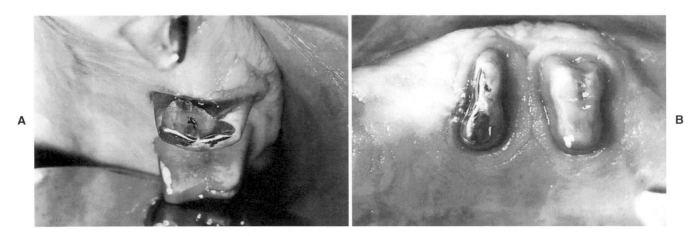

Fig. 22-29 A sectioned maxillary first molar with a preformed dowel and alloy core in place. **A,** The mesial view shows the core after removal of the mesiobuccal root. The alloy obliterates the pulp chamber and is separated from the attachment by the thin chamber floor. **B,** The root morphology and degree of periodontal attachment loss dictate margin geometry. Ultimate tooth reduction and preparation form converge from this level.

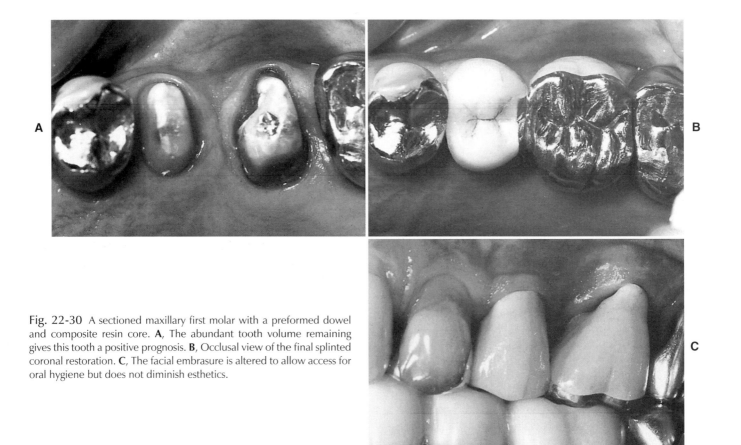

Fig. 22-30 A sectioned maxillary first molar with a preformed dowel and composite resin core. **A,** The abundant tooth volume remaining gives this tooth a positive prognosis. **B,** Occlusal view of the final splinted coronal restoration. **C,** The facial embrasure is altered to allow access for oral hygiene but does not diminish esthetics.

but also increases pulpal morbidity. As previously discussed, preventive endodontics is indicated in cases with a strong suspicion of future pulpal involvement, because the probability of pulpal degeneration in these teeth is statistically high.

When prerestorative root canal therapy is indicated for elongated, periodontally involved teeth, it is extremely important to retain as much radicular dentin as possible. These teeth are subject to fracture because of increased leverage caused by greater crown length and the smaller diameter of root structure at the alveolar crest. Dowel placement may be needed for retention of the core. However, conventional dowel guidelines do not apply in the restoration of

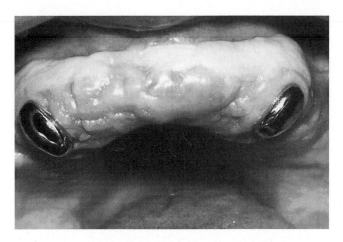

Fig. 22-31 Conventional overdenture teeth do not require dowels for stress distribution. Endodontic therapy is completed to allow reduction of the crown-to-root ratio. This case has cast gold copings for root coverage. In cases with sound tooth structure and low caries potential, bonded amalgam in the coronal segment of the canal is sufficient restoration.

the severely periodontally compromised tooth. The dowel is rarely as long as the clinical crown and often will not reach to the alveolar crest. Narrowing root morphology further limits the apical extension. The apical end of the dowel should not be at the level of the alveolar crest; it should terminate above or below the alveolus. The bony crest and dowel terminus are both stress concentrators and coincident placement increases fracture potential.

Root amputation or tooth sectioning may be included in periodontal treatment of the multirooted tooth. The root structure just coronal to the attachment level dictates the geometry of the restorative finish line. Thus the morphology of the remaining root structure at the attachment level dictates the preparation design in the amputated or sectioned tooth (Figs. 22-29 and 22-30). Concern for long-term structural integrity of the tooth is always heightened by this finding. Predictably, studies of these teeth reveal the major cause of failure over time is root fracture, followed by recurrent periodontal disease, endodontic failure, caries, or loss of cement seal. As with periodontally sound teeth, the endodontic, periodontal, and initial restorative preparation should be completed before selection of a dowel and core system. Maintenance of dentin is again the primary goal. Adequate ferrule and exquisite control of occlusion is critical for longevity of these teeth.

Anterior dentition. The same caution in restoration of the periodontally compromised posterior dentition is present in the anterior dentition. Single-root formation is an anatomic advantage in this area because it eliminates the need for the furcation. However, esthetic demands are a compounding issue. Margin location coronal to the free gingiva or minimal axial tooth reduction can lessen pulpal embarrassment in the posterior preparation. Heightened esthetic demands in the anterior dentition may not allow these com-

promises. Margin placement in the gingival crevice and full-depth facial reduction for veneering material may be esthetic requirements. The anterior dentition may also require connection to some or all of the posterior dentition. Paralleling these abutments usually mandates additional (or increased) dentin removal in the anterior segment. The cumulative effects of these insults on the anterior teeth may require preventive root canal therapy.

Anterior teeth with significant periodontal attachment loss may be retained as overdenture abutments. Functional forces to these abutments are directed mainly through the long axis of the tooth. A preparation depth of approximately 3 mm is sufficient to retain the restoration and protect the root canal system. Coverage of the entire dome-shaped overdenture abutment is occasionally indicated for caries control and restoration (Fig. 22-31). A short dowel may be used in such a case to retain the coronal restoration. Only when the overdenture abutment is used for active retention of the prosthesis should guidelines for full-length dowels be followed. In addition to supplying support in the direction of the tissue, these abutments also provide lateral stability and retain the prosthesis. Dowel placement distributes the functional load to the residual root and retains the precision attachment.

SUMMARY

The interrelationship between endodontics and restorative dentistry has been reviewed in this chapter. This connection is complex and requires a thorough understanding to produce consistent, successful clinical results. Treatment planning considerations were presented for the vital and the nonvital tooth. They included endodontic, periodontal, restorative, and esthetic evaluations. Guidelines for restoration of the nonvital tooth and clinical techniques for this treatment were outlined. It is clear that recent advances have had a significant impact on the restoration of the endodontically treated tooth. In the future, the ability to bond multiple restorative materials to each other and to tooth structure will continue to revolutionize this relationship.

References

1. Assif D, Avraham B, Pilo R: Effect of post design on resistance to fracture of endodontically treated teeth with complete crowns, *J Prosthet Dent* 69:36, 1993.
2. Ausiello P, De Gee AJ, Rengo S, Davidson CL: Fracture resistance of endodontically-treated premolars adhesively restored, *Am J Dent* 10:237, 1997.
3. Bachicha WS et al: Microleakage of endodontically treated teeth restored with posts, *J Endod* 24:703, 1998.
4. Barkhodar RA, Radke R, Abbasi J: Effect of metal collars on resistance of endodontically treated teeth to root fracture, *J Prosthet Dent* 61:676, 1989.
5. Barnett F: Pulpal response to restorative procedures and materials, *Curr Opin Dent* 2:93, 1992.

6. Bergenholtz G, Nyman S: Endodontic complications following periodontal and prosthetic treatment of patients with advanced periodontal disease, *J Periodontol* 50:366, 1979.

7. Bower RC: Furcation morphology relative to periodontal treatment, *J Periodontol* 50:366, 1979.

8. Burns DA, Drause WR, Douglas HB, Burns DR: Stress distribution surrounding endodontic posts, *J Prosthet Dent* 64:412, 1990.

9. Cho GC, Kaneko LM, Donovovan TE, White SN: Diametral and compressive strength of dental core materials, *J Prosthet Dent* 82:272, 1999.

10. Christensen G: Posts and cores: state of the art, *J Am Dent Assoc* 129:96, 1998.

11. Christensen G: Core buildup and adhesive incompatibility, *Clinical Research Associates Newsletter* 24:6, 2000.

12. Cohen BI, Condos S, Deutsch AS, Musikant BL: Fracture strength of three different core materials in combination with three different endodontic posts, *Int J Prosthodont* 7:178, 1994.

13. Dean JP, Jeansonne BG, Sarkar N: In vitro evaluation of a carbon fiber post, *J Endod* 24:807, 1998.

14. Donovan TE, Cho GC: Contemporary evaluation of dental cements, *Compendium* 20:197, 1999.

15. Drummond JL, Toepke TR, King TJ: Thermal and cyclic loading of endodontic posts, *Eur J Oral Sci* 107:220, 1999.

16. Fan P, Nicholls JI, Kois JC: Load fatigue of five restoration modalities in structurally compromised premolars, *Int J Prosthodont* 8:213, 1995.

17. Felton D: Long-term effects of crown preparation on pulp vitality, *J Dent Res* 68:1009, 1989.

18. Felton DA, Bebb EL, Kanoy BE, Dugoni J: Threaded endodontic dowels: effect of post design on incidence of root fracture, *J Prosthet Dent* 64:179, 1991.

19. Fogel HM: Microleakage of posts used to restore endodontically treated teeth, *J Endod* 21:376, 1995.

20. Fox K, Gutteridge DL: An in vitro study of coronal microleakage in root-canal-treated teeth restored by the post and core technique, *Int Endod J* 30:361, 1997.

21. Fraga RC, Chaves BT, Mello GS, Siqueira JF Jr: Fracture resistance of endodontically treated roots after restoration, *J Oral Rehabil* 25:809, 1998.

22. Freeman MA, Nicholls JI, Kydd WL, Harrington GW: Leakage associated with load fatigue-induced preliminary failure of full crowns placed over three different post and core systems, *J Endod* 24:26, 1998.

23. Gluskin AH, Radke RA, Frost SL, Watanabe LG: The mandibular incisor: rethinking guidelines for post and core design, *J Endod* 21:33, 1995.

24. Goodacre CJ, Spolnik KJ: The prosthodontic management of endodontically treated teeth: a literature review. Part I. Success and failure data, treatment concepts, *J Prosthodont* 3:243, 1994.

25. Goodacre CJ, Spolnik KJ: The prosthodontic management of endodontically treated teeth: a literature review. Part II. Maintaining the apical seal, *J Prosthodont* 4:51, 1995.

26. Goss JM, Wright WJ, Bowles WF: Radiographic appearance of titanium alloy prefabricated posts cemented with different luting materials, *J Prosthet Dent* 67:632, 1992.

27. Gutmann JL: The dentin-root complex: anatomic and biologic considerations in restoring endodontically treated teeth, *J Prosthet Dent* 67:458, 1992.

28. Hatzikyriakos AH, Reisis GE, Tsingos N: A 3-year postoperative clinical evaluation of posts and cores beneath existing crowns, *J Prosthet Dent* 67:454, 1992.

29. Holloway JA, Miller RB: The effect of core translucency on the aesthetics of all-ceramic restorations, *Pract Periodontics Aesthet Dent* 9:567, 1997.

30. Hornbrook DS, Hastings JH: Use of bondable reinforcement fiber for post and core build-up in an endodontically treated tooth: maximizing strength and aesthetics, *Pract Periodontics Aesthet Dent* 7:33, 1995.

31. Isidor F, Brondum K: Intermittent loading of teeth with tapered, individually cast or prefabricated, parallel-sided posts, *Int J Prosthodont* 5:257, 1992.

32. Isidor F, Brondum K, Ravnholt G: The influence of post length and crown ferrule length on the resistance of cyclic loading of bovine teeth with prefabricated titanium posts, *Int J Prosthodont* 12:78, 1999.

33. Isidor F, Odman P, Brondum K: Intermittent loading of teeth restored using prefabricated carbon fiber posts, *Int J Prosthodont* 9:131, 1996.

34. Kane JJ, Burgess JO, Summitt J: Fracture resistance of amalgam coronal-radicular restorations, *J Prosthet Dent* 63:607, 1990.

35. Koutayas SO, Kern M: All-ceramic posts and cores: the state of the art, *Quintessence Int* 30:383, 1999.

36. Lambjerg-Hansen H, Asmussen E: Mechanical properties of endodontic posts, *J Oral Rehabil* 24:882, 1997.

37. Lenchner NH: Restoring endodontically treated teeth: ferrule effect and biologic width, *Pract Periodontics Aesthet Dent* 1:19, 1989.

38. Libman WJ, Nicholls JI: Load fatigue of teeth restored with cast posts and cores and complete crowns, *Int J Prosthodont* 8:155, 1995.

39. Love RM, Purton DG: The effect of serrations on carbon fiber posts-retention within the root canal, core retention, and post rigidity, *Int J Prosthodont* 9:484, 1996.

40. Love RM, Purton DG: Retention of posts with resin, glass ionomer and hybrid cements, *J Dent* 26:599, 1998.

41. Marshall, GW: Dentin: microstructure and characterization, *Quintessence Int* 24:606, 1993.

42. Martinez-Insua A, da Silva L, Rilo B, Santana U: Comparison of the fracture resistances of pulpless teeth restored with a cast post and core or carbon-fiber post with a composite core, *J Prosthet Dent* 80:527, 1998.

43. McLean A: Criteria for the predictably restorable endodontically treated tooth, *J Can Dent Assoc* 64:652, 1998.

44. Millstein PL, Ho J, Nathanson D: Retention between a serrated steel dowel and different core materials, *J Prosthet Dent* 65: 480, 1991.

45. Milot P, Stein RS: Root fracture in endodontically treated teeth related to post selection and crown design, *J Prosthet Dent* 68: 428, 1992.

46. Nicopoulou-Karayianni K, Bragger U, Lang NP: Patterns of periodontal destruction associated with incomplete root fractures, *Dentomaxillofac Radiol* 26:321, 1997.

47. Pashley DH: Clinical correlations of dentin structure and function, *J Prosthet Dent* 66:777, 1991.

48. Paul SJ, Scharer P: Post and core reconstruction for fixed prosthodontic restoration, *Pract Periodontics Aesthet Dent* 9:513, 1997.

49. Reeh ES, Messer HH, Douglas WH: Reduction in tooth stiffness as a result of endodontic and restorative procedures, *J Endod* 15:512, 1989.
50. Rosenberg MM, Kay HB, Keough BE, Holt RL: *Periodontal and prosthetic management for advanced cases*, Chicago, 1988, Quintessence Publishing Co.
51. Saupe, WA, Gluskin AH, Radke RA Jr: A comparative study of fracture resistance between morphologic dowel and cores and a resin-reinforced dowel system in the intraradicular restoration of structurally compromised roots, *Quintessence Int* 27:483, 1996.
52. Scherer W et al: Bonding amalgam to tooth structure: a scanning electron microscope study, *J Esthet Dent* 4(6):199, 1992.
53. Schwartz RS, Murchison DF, Walker WA III: Effects of eugenol and noneugenol endodontic sealer cements on post retention, *J Endod* 24:564, 1998.
54. Sidhu SK, Watson TF: Resin-modified glass ionomer materials, *Am J Dent* 8:59, 1995.
55. Sidoli GE, King PA, Setchell DJ: An in vitro evaluation of a carbon fiber-based post and core system, *J Prosthet Dent* 78:5, 1997.
56. Sindel J, Frandenberger R, Kramer N, Petschelt A: Crack formation of all-ceramic crowns dependent on different core build-up and luting materials, *J Dent* 27:175, 1999.
57. Sirimai S, Riis DN, Morgano SM: An in vitro study of the fracture resistance and the incidence of vertical root fracture of pulpless teeth restored with six post-and-core systems, *J Prosthet Dent* 81:262, 1999.
58. Sorensen JA, Engelman MJ: Ferrule design and fracture resistance of endodontically treated teeth, *J Prosthet Dent* 63:529, 1990.
59. Sorensen JA, Engelman MJ, Daher T, Caputo AA: Altered corrosion resistance from casting to stainless steel posts, *J Prosthet Dent* 63:630, 1990.
60. Sorensen JA, Martinoff JT: Clinically significant factors in dowel design, *J Prosthet Dent* 52:28, 1984.
61. Sorensen JA, Martinoff JT: Endodontically treated teeth as abutments, *J Prosthet Dent* 53:631, 1985.
62. Sorensen JA, Mito WT: Rationale and clinical technique for esthetic restoration of endodontically treated teeth with the CosmoPost and IPS Empress Post System, *QDT* 81, 1998.
63. Standlee JP, Caputo AA: Endodontic dowel retention with resinous cements, *J Prosthet Dent* 68:913, 1992.
64. Standlee JP, Caputo AA: The retentive and stress distributing properties of split threaded endodontic dowels, *J Prosthet Dent* 68:436, 1992.
65. Steele A, Johnson BR: In vitro fracture strength of endodontically treated premolars, *J Endod* 25:6, 1999.
66. Sundh B, Odman P: A study of fixed prosthodontics performed at a university clinic 18 years after insertion, *Int J Prothsodont* 10:513, 1997.
67. Thakur A, Johnston WM: Fluoride release of resin-based luting cements, *J Dent Res* 75:68, 1996 (abstract).
68. Tjan AH, Chiu J: Microleakage of core materials for complete cast gold crowns, *J Prosthet Dent* 61:659, 1989.
69. Tjan AH, Grant BE, Dunn JR: Microleakage of composite resin cores treated with various dentin bonding systems, *J Prosthet Dent* 66:24, 1991.
70. Torbjorner A, Karlsson S, Syverud M, Hensten-Pettersen A: Carbon fiber reinforced root canal posts. Mechanical and cytotoxic properties, *Eur J Oral Sci* 104:605,1996.
71. Van Meerbeek B, Vanherle G, Lambrechts P, Braem M: Dentin and enamel bonding agents, *Curr Opin Dent* 2:117, 1992.
72. Vire DE: Failure of endodontically treated teeth: classification and evaluation, *J Endod* 17:338, 1991.
73. Wiskott HW, Nicholls JI, Belser UC: The effect of tooth preparation height and diameter on the resistance of complete crowns to fatigue loading, *Int J Prosthodont* 10:207, 1997.
74. Wu MK, Pehlivan Y, Kontakiotis EG, Wesselink PR: Microleakage along apical root fillings and cemented posts, *J Prosthet Dent* 79:264, 1998.

Chapter 23

Pediatric Endodontics: Endodontic Treatment for the Primary and Young, Permanent Dentition

Joseph H. Camp, Edward J. Barrett, Franklin Pulver

Chapter Outline

The premature loss of primary and young, permanent teeth continues despite the emphasis that the dental profession has placed on prevention. Because neither dental caries nor dental traumas have been eliminated, procedures that preserve the primary and young, permanent teeth continue to be an integral part of dental practice. This chapter deals with preservation of the primary and young, permanent teeth that are pulpally involved.

Preservation of arch space is one of the primary objectives of pediatric dentistry. Premature loss of primary teeth may cause aberration of the arch length, resulting in mesial drift of the permanent teeth and consequent malocclusion. Whenever possible, the pulpally involved tooth should be maintained in the dental arch free of disease (provided that it can be restored to function).

Other objectives of preserving primary teeth are to enhance aesthetics and mastication, prevent aberrant tongue habits, aid in speech, and prevent the psychologic effects associated with tooth loss. Premature loss of the maxillary incisors before age 3 has been shown to cause speech impairment that may persist in later years.[168]

Loss of pulpal vitality in the young, permanent tooth creates special problems. Because the pulp is necessary for the formation of dentin, if the pulp is lost before root length is completed the tooth will have a poor crown-to-root ratio. Pulpal necrosis before the completion of dentin deposition within the root leaves a thin root more prone to fracture in the event of trauma. This situation also creates special problems in endodontic treatment, because endodontic techniques are usually not adequate to obturate the large blunderbuss canals. Additional procedures of apexification or apical surgery often become necessary to maintain the pulpless, immature, permanent tooth; the prognosis for permanent retention of the tooth is poorer than for the completely formed tooth.

In this chapter, emphasis is on maintenance of pulpal vitality in the primary and young, permanent teeth (whenever possible) to avoid many of the problems discussed elsewhere in this text.

Successful pulpal therapy in the primary dentition requires a thorough understanding of primary pulp morphology, root formation, and the special problems associated with resorption of primary tooth roots. Differences in the morphology of the primary and permanent pulps, root formation, and primary root resorption are discussed later in this chapter. (See Chapter 11 for a complete description of pulp and dentin formation.)

DIFFERENCES IN PRIMARY AND PERMANENT TOOTH MORPHOLOGY

According to Finn[50] and Ash[8] there are 12 basic differences between the primary and the permanent teeth (Fig. 23-1):

1. Primary teeth are smaller in all dimensions than corresponding permanent teeth.
2. Primary crowns are wider in the mesial-to-distal dimension in comparison to their crown length than are permanent crowns.
3. Primary teeth have narrower and longer roots in comparison with crown length and width in permanent teeth.
4. The facial and lingual cervical thirds of the crowns of anterior, primary teeth are much more prominent than those of permanent teeth.
5. Primary teeth are markedly more constricted at the dentin and enamel junction (DEJ) than are permanent teeth.
6. The facial and lingual surfaces of primary molars converge occlusally so that the occlusal surface is much narrower in the faciolingual than the cervical width.
7. The roots of primary molars are comparatively more slender and longer than the roots of permanent molars.
8. The roots of primary molars flare out nearer the cervix and more at the apex than do the roots of permanent molars.

9. The enamel is thinner, about 1 mm, on primary teeth than it is on permanent teeth, and it has a more consistent depth.
10. The thickness of the dentin between the pulp chambers and the enamel in primary teeth is less than that in permanent teeth.
11. The pulp chambers in primary teeth are comparatively larger than those in permanent teeth.
12. The pulp horns, especially the mesial horns, are higher in primary molars than they are in permanent molars.

Root Formation

According to Orban[149] development of the roots begins after enamel and dentin formation has reached the future cementoenamel junction (CEJ). The epithelial dental organ forms Hertwig's epithelial root sheath, which initiates formation and molds the shape of the roots. Hertwig's sheath takes the form of one or more epithelial tubes (depending on the number of roots of the tooth, one tube for each root). During root formation the apical foramen of each root has a wide opening limited by the epithelial diaphragm. The dentinal walls diverge apically, and the shape of the pulp canal is like a wide-open tube. Each root contains one canal at this time, and the number of canals is the same as the number of roots (Fig. 23-2, *A*). When root length is established, the sheath disappears but dentin deposition continues internally within the roots.

Differentiation of a root into separate canals, as in the mesial root of the mandibular molars, occurs by continued deposition of dentin; this narrows the isthmus between the walls of the canals and continues until there is formation of dentin islands within the root canal and eventual division of the root into separate canals. During the process, communications exist between the canals as an isthmus, then as fins connecting the canals (Fig. 23-2, *B*). (See Chapter 11 for a complete description of pulp and dentin formation.)

As growth proceeds, the root canal is narrowed by continued deposition of dentin and the pulp tissue is compressed. Additional deposition of dentin and cementum

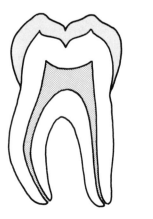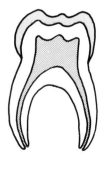

Fig. 23-1 Cross section of primary and permanent molars.

closes the apex of the tooth and creates the apical convergence of the root canals common to the completely formed tooth (Fig. 23-2, *C*).

Root length is not completed until 1 to 4 years after a tooth erupts into the oral cavity. In the primary teeth the root length is completed in a shorter period of time than in the permanent tooth because of the shorter length of the primary roots.

The root-to-crown length of the primary teeth is greater than that of the permanent teeth. The primary roots are narrower than the permanent roots. The roots of the primary molars diverge more than those of the permanent teeth. This feature allows more room for the development of the crown of the succeeding premolar[8] (see Fig. 23-1).

The primary tooth is unique insofar as resorption of the roots begins soon after formation of the root length has been completed. At this time the form and shape of the root canals roughly correspond to the form and shape of the external anatomy of the teeth. Root resorption and the deposition of additional dentin within the root canal system, however, significantly change the number, size, and shape of the root canals within the primary tooth.

It should be noted that most of the variations within the root canals of primary and permanent teeth are in the faciolingual plane and that dental radiographs do not visualize this plane but show the mesiodistal plane. Therefore when reviewing radiographs of teeth, many of the variations that are present are not visible.

Primary Root Canal Anatomy

To treat the pulps of primary teeth successfully, the clinician must have a thorough knowledge of the anatomy of the primary root canal systems and the variations that normally exist in these systems. To understand some of the variations in the primary root canal systems requires an understanding of root formation (see previous discussion).

Primary Anterior Teeth

The form and shape of the root canals of the primary anterior teeth (Figs. 23-3 and 23-4) resemble the form and shape of the roots of the teeth. The permanent tooth bud lies lingual and apical to the primary, anterior tooth. Owing to the position of the permanent tooth bud, resorption of the primary incisors and canines is initiated on the lingual surface in the apical third of the roots (see Fig. 23-3, *A*).

Maxillary Incisors

The root canals of the primary maxillary, central, and lateral incisors are almost round but somewhat compressed. Normally these teeth have one canal without bifurcations. Apical ramifications or accessory canals and lateral canals are rare, but they do occur[227] (see Fig. 23-3).

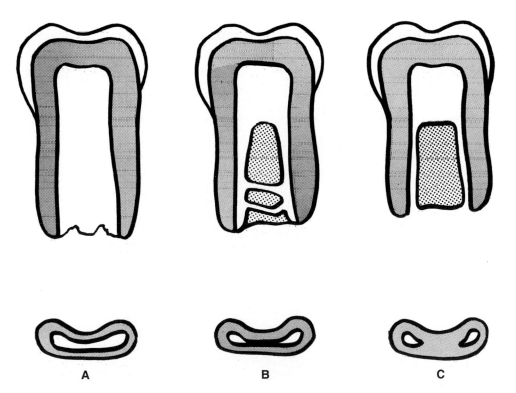

A   **B**   **C**

Fig. 23-2 Faciolingual cross section of the mesial root of a mandibular primary molar. **A**, Formation of the root at the time the root length is completed and only one canal is present. **B**, Differentiation of the root into separate canals by the continued deposition of dentin *(shaded areas)*. Small fins and connecting branches are present between the two canals. **C**, Canals are completely divided, and root resorption has begun.

Mandibular Incisors

The root canals of the primary mandibular, central, and lateral incisors are flattened on the mesial and distal surfaces and sometimes grooved, pointing to an eventual division into two canals. The presence of two canals is seen less than 10% of the time. Occasionally lateral or accessory canals are observed.[227]

Maxillary and Mandibular Canines

The root canals of the maxillary and mandibular canines correspond to the exterior root shape, a rounded, triangular shape with the base toward the facial surface. Sometimes the lumen of the root canal is compressed in the mesiodistal direction. The canines have the simplest root canal systems of all the primary teeth and offer few problems when being treated endodontically. Bifurcation of the canal does not normally occur. Lateral canals and accessory canals are rare[227] (see Fig. 23-4).

Primary Molars

Normally the primary molars (Fig. 23-5, *A-E*) have the same number and position of roots as the corresponding permanent molars. The maxillary molars have three roots: two facial and one palatal; the mandibular have two roots: mesial

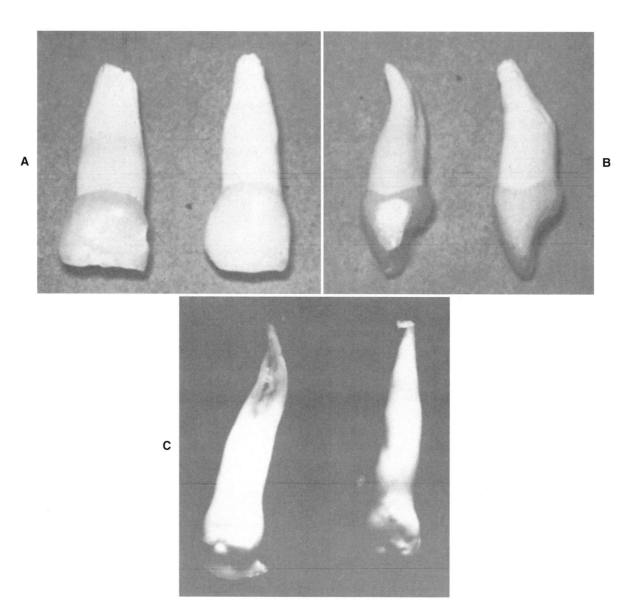

Fig. 23-3 Primary central incisors and silicone models of the pulp canals. **A**, Facial surfaces. **B**, Beginning resorption of the roots on the apical third of the lingual surfaces. **C**, Models. The pulp canals were injected with silicone and the tooth structure decalcified away, leaving a model of the root canal systems. Note the division of the canal on the right.

and distal. The roots of the primary molars are long and slender compared with crown length and width, and they diverge to allow for permanent tooth bud formation.

When full length of the roots of the primary molars has just been completed, only one root canal is present in each of the roots. The continued deposition of dentin internally may divide the root into two or more canals. During this process, communications exist between the canals and may remain in the fully developed primary tooth as isthmuses or fins connecting the canals (see Fig. 23-2, *B*).

The deposition of secondary dentin in primary teeth has been reported.[13,79,83] After root formation the basic morphologic pattern of the root canals may change, producing variations and alterations in the number and size of the root canals caused by the deposition of secondary dentin. This deposition begins at about the time root resorption begins. Variations in form are more pronounced in teeth that show evidence of root resorption.[79]

The most variation in the morphology of the root canals is found in the mesial roots of maxillary and mandibular, primary molars. This variation originates in the apical region as a thinning of the narrow isthmus between the facial and lingual extremities of the apical pulp canals. Subsequent deposition of secondary dentin may produce a complete separation of the root canal into two or more individual canals. Many fine-connecting branches or lateral fibrils form a connecting network between the facial and lingual aspects of the root canals.

The variations found in the mesial roots of the primary molars are also found in the distal and lingual roots but to a lesser degree. Accessory canals, lateral canals, and apical ramifications of the pulp are common in primary molars—occurring in 10% to 20%.[79,227]

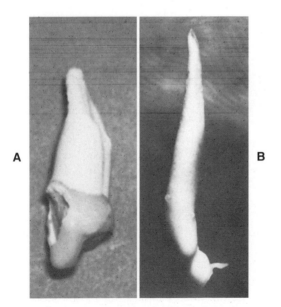

Fig. 23-4 Maxillary primary canine and silicone model of the root canal. **A**, Mesial surface. **B**, Model of the root canal.

In the primary molars, resorption usually begins on the inner surfaces of the roots next to the interradicular septum. The effects of resorption on canal anatomy and root canal–filling on the primary teeth are discussed in detail later in this chapter.

Maxillary First Primary Molar

The maxillary first primary molar has two to four canals that roughly correspond to the exterior root form with much variation. The palatal root is often round; it is often longer than the two facial roots. Bifurcation of the mesiofacial root into two canals occurs in approximately 75% of maxillary, first, primary molars.[79,227]

Fusion of the palatal and distofacial roots occurs in approximately one third of the maxillary primary first molars. In most of these teeth two separate canals are present, with a very narrow isthmus connecting them. Islands of dentin may exist between the canals, with many connecting branches and fibrils (see Fig. 23-5, *A*).

Maxillary Second Primary Molar

The maxillary second primary molar has two to five canals roughly corresponding to the exterior root shape. The mesiofacial root usually bifurcates or contains two distinct canals. This occurs in approximately 85% to 95% of maxillary second primary molars[79,227] (see Fig. 23-5, *B*).

Fusion of the palatal and distofacial roots may occur. These fused roots may have a common canal, two distinct canals, or two canals with a narrow connecting isthmus of dentin islands between them and many connecting branches or fibrils.

Mandibular First Primary Molar

The mandibular first primary molar usually has three canals roughly corresponding to the external root anatomy, but it may have two to four canals. It is reported that approximately 75% of the mesial roots contain two canals, whereas only 25% of the distal roots contain more than one canal[79,227] (see Fig. 23-5, *C* and *D*).

Mandibular Second Primary Molar

The mandibular, second, primary molar may have two to five canals, but it usually has three. The mesial root has two canals approximately 85% of the time, whereas the distal root contains more than one canal only 25% of the time[79,227] (see Fig. 23-5, *E*).

Diagnosis

Before the initiation of restorative procedures on a tooth, a thorough clinical and radiographic examination must be conducted. In addition, the case history and any pertinent med-

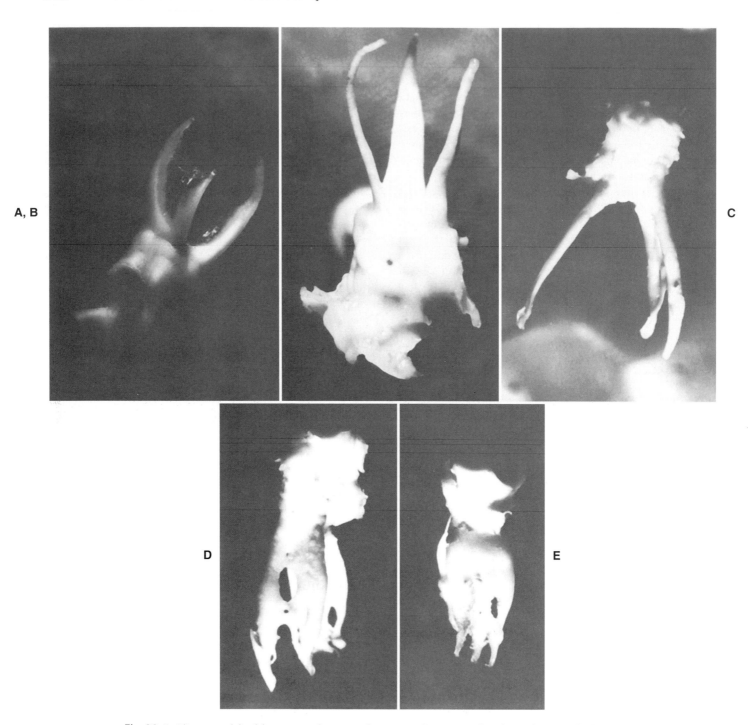

Fig. 23-5 Silicone models of the root canal systems of primary molars. **A,** Maxillary first molar. Note the fused distal and palatal roots. Note the thin fin connecting the roots. **B,** Maxillary second molar: facial surface. **C,** Mandibular first molar: facial view. **D,** Same tooth from the mesial surface. Note the connecting fibrils between the facial and lingual canals. **E,** Mandibular second molar: distal view. Three canals are present.

ical history must be thoroughly reviewed. (See Chapter 1 for a comprehensive discussion of diagnostic procedures.)

Periapical and bite-wing radiographs are essential to complete the diagnosis. Examination of the soft and hard tissues for any apparent pathosis is a routine part of the examination.

In the event that pulpal therapy is required, the preoperative diagnosis is of utmost importance and should dictate the type of treatment to be carried out. If the pulpal status is not determined before operative procedures are begun and pulp therapy becomes necessary during the treatment, an adequate diagnosis may be impossible.

There are no reliable clinical diagnostic tools for accurately evaluating the status of the pulp that has become inflamed. An accurate determination of the extent of inflammation within the pulp cannot be made short of histologic examination.[195] Diagnosis of pulpal health in the exposed pulp of children is difficult, and the correlation between clinical symptoms and histopathologic conditions is poor.[124]

Although the diagnostic tests are admittedly poor for evaluating the degree of inflammation within the primary and young, permanent pulp, they must always be performed to obtain as much information as possible to aid in the diagnosis before treatment is rendered. (The recommended diagnostic tests for use in primary and young, permanent teeth are discussed in the next section.)

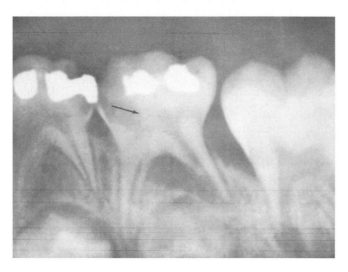

Fig. 23-6 Calcified mass in the pulp chamber. There is internal and external root resorption. Calcified mass *(arrow)* is an attempt to block a massive carious lesion. Because of resorption, this tooth should be extracted. Note the bone loss in the bifurcation area.

Radiographs

Current radiographs are essential to examining for caries and periapical changes. Interpretation of radiographs is complicated in children by physiologic root resorption of primary teeth and by incompletely formed roots of permanent teeth. If the clinician is not familiar with diagnosing radiographs of children or does not have radiographs of good quality, these normally occurring circumstances can easily lead to misinterpretation of normal anatomy for pathologic changes.

The radiograph does not always demonstrate periapical pathosis, nor can the proximity of caries to the pulp always be accurately determined. What may appear as an intact barrier of secondary dentin overlying the pulp may actually be a perforated mass of irregularly calcified and carious dentin overlying a pulp with extensive inflammation.[124]

The presence of calcified masses within the pulp is important to making a diagnosis of pulpal status (Fig. 23-6). Mild, chronic irritation to the pulp stimulates secondary dentin formation. When the irritation is acute and of rapid onset, the defense mechanism may not have a chance to lay down secondary dentin. When the disease process reaches the pulp, the pulp may form calcified masses away from the exposure site. These calcified masses are always associated with advanced pulpal degeneration in the pulp chamber and inflammation of the pulp tissue in the canals.[124]

Pathologic changes in the periapical tissues surrounding primary molars are most often apparent in the bifurcation or trifurcation areas, rather than at the apexes (such as in permanent teeth) (Fig. 23-7, *A*). Pathologic bone and root resorption are indicative of advanced pulpal degeneration that has spread into the periapical tissues. The pulpal tissue may remain vital even with such advanced degenerative changes.

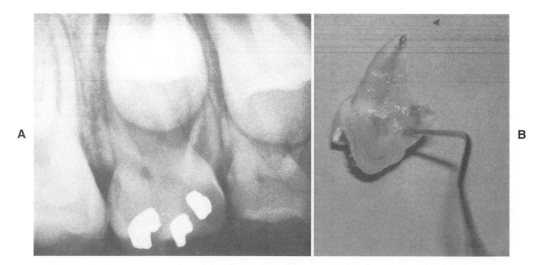

A   B

Fig. 23-7 Internal resorption caused by inflammation from carious pulp exposure. **A,** Note the bone loss in the trifurcation and the internal resorption in the mesial root. **B,** Extracted tooth. Note the perforation of internal resorption. Probe is extended through the resorption defect.

Internal resorption occurs frequently in the primary dentition after pulpal involvement. It is always associated with extensive inflammation,[68] and it usually occurs in the molar root canals adjacent to the bifurcation or trifurcation area. Because of the thinness of primary molar roots, once the internal resorption has become advanced enough to be seen radiographically there is usually a perforation of the root by the resorption (Fig. 23-7, *B*). After the occurrence of perforation of the primary tooth root by internal resorption, all forms of pulpal therapy are contraindicated. The treatment of choice is extraction.

Pulp Tests

The electrical pulp tester is of little value in the primary dentition or in young permanent teeth with incompletely developed apices. Although the tester may indicate vitality, it will not give reliable data as to the extent of inflammation within the pulp. Many children with perfectly normal teeth do not respond to the electrical pulp tester even at the higher settings. Added to these factors is the unreliability of the response in the young child because of apprehension, fear, or management problems.

Thermal tests are also generally unreliable in the primary dentition for determining pulpal status.

Percussion and Mobility

Teeth with extensive pulpal inflammation usually exhibit tenderness to percussion; however, this test is not very reliable in primary teeth of young children because of the psychologic aspects involved.

Tooth mobility is also not a reliable test of pulpal pathosis in primary teeth. During phases of active physiologic root resorption, primary teeth with normal pulps may have varying degrees of mobility. Furthermore, teeth with varying degrees of pulpal inflammation may have very little mobility.

Pulpal Exposures and Hemorrhage

It has been reported that the size of the exposure, the appearance of the pulp, and the amount of hemorrhage are important factors in diagnosing the extent of inflammation in a cariously exposed pulp. A true carious exposure is always accompanied by pulpal inflammation[124,195] (see Chapter 15). The pinpoint carious exposure may have pulpal inflammation varying from minimal to extensive to complete necrosis. However, the massive exposure always has widespread inflammation or necrosis and is not a candidate for any form of vital pulp therapy except in young, permanent teeth with incomplete root development. Excessive hemorrhage at an exposure site or during pulp amputation is evidence of extensive inflammation. These teeth should be considered candidates for pulpectomy or extraction.

History of Pain

A history of spontaneous toothache is usually associated with extensive degenerative changes in the pulp of a primary tooth[68]; nevertheless, absence of pain cannot be used to judge pulpal status because varying degrees of degeneration (or even complete necrosis) of the pulp are seen without any history of pain.

Guthrie et al[68] attempted to use the first drop of hemorrhage from an exposed pulp site as a diagnostic aid for determining the extent of degeneration within the pulp. A white blood cell differential count (i.e., hemogram) was made for each of 53 teeth included in the study. A detailed history, including percussion, electrical pulp test, thermal tests, mobility, and history of pain, was obtained. The teeth were extracted and histologically examined. On correlation of the histologic findings with the hemogram and a detailed history, it was determined that percussion, electrical, and thermal pulp tests, and mobility were *unreliable* in establishing the degree of pulpal inflammation. The hemogram did not give reliable evidence of pulpal degeneration, although teeth with advanced degeneration of the pulp involving the root canals did have an elevated neutrophil count. A consistent finding of the study, however, was advanced degeneration of pulpal tissue in teeth with a history of spontaneous toothache.

Primary teeth with a history of spontaneous, unprovoked toothache should not be considered for any form of pulp therapy short of pulpectomy or extraction.

VITAL PULPAL THERAPY

Indirect Pulp Therapy

Indirect pulp therapy is a technique for avoiding pulp exposure in the treatment of teeth with deep carious lesions in which there exists no clinical evidence of pulpal degeneration or periapical disease. The ultimate objective is to arrest the carious process by promoting dentinal sclerosis and stimulating promotion of reparative dentin with remineralization of the carious dentin while preserving pulpal vitality. The procedure allows the tooth to use the natural protective mechanisms of the pulp against caries. It is based on the theory that a zone of affected, demineralized dentin exists between the outer infected layer of dentin and the pulp. When the infected dentin is removed, *the affected dentin can remineralize and the odontoblasts form reparative dentin,* thus avoiding a pulp exposure.

Studies[93,127,203] have shown that physiologic remineralization can occur only if the inner carious layer contains sound collagen fibers and living odontoblastic processes. The sound collagen fibers function as a base to which apatite crystals attach.[104,146] The living odontoblastic processes supply calcium phosphate from the vital pulp for physiologic remineralization.[225]

Tatsumi et al[203] produced an artificially demineralized dentin with an outer layer stainable with a caries detector stain and an inner transparent layer, which was not stainable. The teeth were restored with bonded, composite restoration after acid etching with 40% phosphoric acid. After a study period of 4 months, complete remineralization was established by hardness tests and calcium concentration equal to that of normal dentin.

Disagreement exists as to whether the deep layers of the carious dentin are infected. Several studies[97,105] showed deep, carious lesions to be infected, whereas another[60] reported an area of softened and discolored dentin far in advance of bacterial contamination in acute caries. Still others[185,223] found that most organisms had been removed after the removal of the softened dentin, although the incidence of bacterial contamination was higher in primary teeth than in permanent teeth; however, some dentinal tubules still contained small numbers of bacteria.

Kopel[102] summarized the results of various studies of the carious process and identified three distinct layers in active caries: (1) necrotic, soft dentin not painful to stimulation and grossly infected with bacteria; (2) firm but softened dentin, painful to stimulation but containing fewer bacteria; and (3) slightly discolored, hard, sound dentin containing few bacteria and painful to stimulation.

In indirect pulp therapy the outer layers of carious dentin are removed. Thus most of the bacteria are eliminated from the lesion. When the lesion is sealed, the substrate on which the bacteria act to produce acid is also removed. Exposure of the pulp occurs when the carious process advances faster than the reparative mechanism of the pulp. With the arrest of the carious process, the reparative mechanism is able to lay down additional dentin and avoid a pulp exposure.

Although carious dentin left in the tooth probably contains some bacteria, the number of organisms can be greatly diminished when this layer is covered with zinc oxide eugenol (ZOE) or calcium hydroxide[47,97] (Fig. 23-8).

Although these have traditionally been the materials placed over the remaining affected dentin, numerous reports* of the use of acid-etched and bonded composites have shown equally favorable results. These studies have demonstrated that it is not the material that is applied; it is an adequate seal to prevent bacterial microleakage that allows healing to occur.

Dimaggio and Hawes[38,39] selected primary and permanent teeth that were free of clinical signs of pulpal degeneration and periapical pathosis and that appeared radiographically to have a pulp exposure if all the decay were removed. On removal of all decay, pulp exposure occurred in 75% of the teeth. In another group of teeth judged clinically to be the same as the first group, the authors achieved 99% success in avoiding pulp exposures with indirect pulp therapy. Reporting on an expanded number of teeth observed from 2 weeks to 4 years, their success rate remained at 97% for the indirect pulp therapy technique.[72]

*References 23,24,26,93,188,203.

Indirect pulp therapy has proved to be a very successful technique when cases are properly selected. Reports[96,144,210] show successes ranging from 74% to 99%. Differences in case selection, length of study, and type of investigation are responsible for the variations in success. Frankel's report[53] of pulp therapy in pediatric dentistry provides a complete review of the earlier literature on indirect pulp therapy.

Indirect Pulp Therapy Technique

Indirect pulp therapy is used when pulpal inflammation has been judged minimal, and complete removal of caries would probably cause a pulp exposure (see Fig. 23-8, *A*). Careful diagnosis of the pulpal status is completed before the treatment is initiated. Any tooth judged to have widespread inflammation or evidence of periapical pathosis is not a candidate to be treated with indirect pulp therapy.

The tooth is anesthetized and isolated with a rubber dam. Care must be taken to eliminate all the caries at the DEJ. Because of its closeness to the surface, caries left in this area will likely cause failure. If there is communication of the caries with the oral cavity, the carious process will continue, resulting in failure.

Care must also be taken in removing the caries to avoid exposure of the pulp. Caries indicators can help in determining the extent of the outer infected layers of caries. All stained dentin must be removed, although the unstained inner transparent layer is left intact. A large, round bur is best to remove the caries. The use of spoon excavators when approaching the pulp may cause an exposure by removal of a large segment of decay. Nevertheless, if used judiciously, a spoon excavator is not contraindicated for removing caries near the DEJ. All undermined enamel is not removed, because it will help retain the temporary filling.

After all caries (except that just overlying the pulp) has been removed, a sedative filling of either ZOE or calcium hydroxide is placed over the remaining carious dentin and areas of deep excavation. Studies have shown both materials to be effective, and no compelling evidence has been presented that either is superior.[43,96] The tooth is then sealed externally with a hard-setting ZOE (e.g., IRM), or amalgam may be placed (see Fig. 23-8, *C* and *D*). The external seal is achieved with an acid-etched, bonded composite when only calcium hydroxide liner is used. Composite resins will not set properly in the presence of ZOE.

An alternative, although still somewhat controversial procedure, involves placing an acid-etched, bonded composite directly over the remaining affected dentin and deep areas of excavation to seal the tooth against microleakage of bacteria.[203]

If the remaining tooth structure is insufficient to retain the temporary filling, a stainless steel (SS) band or temporary crown must be adapted to the tooth to maintain the dressing within the tooth. If the dressing is lost and the remaining

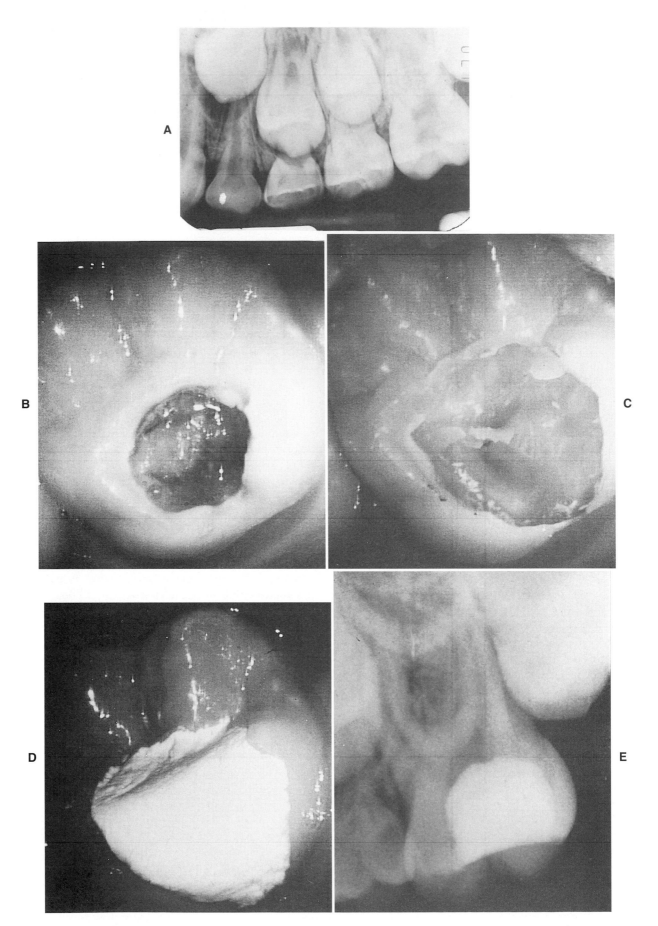

Fig. 23-8 Indirect pulp therapy. **A**, Preoperative radiograph of maxillary first permanent molar showing deep occlusal caries that appears to be into the pulp. **B**, Tooth showing caries. **C**, All caries removed except that immediately overlying the pulp. **D**, IRM sealing the tooth. **E**, Postoperative radiograph 1 year later. The IRM was removed after 12 weeks and a bonded composite resin was placed. Note the caries in the second primary molar.

caries reexposed to the oral fluids, the desired effects cannot be achieved and a failure will occur.

If this preliminary caries removal is successful, the inflammation will be resolved and deposition of reparative dentin beneath the caries will allow subsequent eradication of the remaining caries without pulpal exposure (see Fig. 23-8, *E*).

The treated tooth is reentered in 6 to 8 weeks, and the remaining caries are removed. The rate of reparative dentin deposition has been shown to average 1.4 μm/day after cavity preparations in dentin of human teeth. The rate of reparative dentin formation decreases markedly after 48 days.[192] Dentin is laid down fastest during the first month after indirect pulp therapy, and the rate then diminishes steadily with time. Pulpal floor depth reportedly has little effect on the amount of reparative dentin formed.[210] By contrast, another report[176] states that dentin formation occurs with longer treatment times, and that greater dentin formation is observed in primary teeth than it is in permanent teeth.

If the initial treatment is successful, when the tooth is reentered the caries appears to be arrested. The color changes from a deep red rose to light gray or light brown. The texture changes from spongy and wet to hard, and the caries appears dehydrated. *Practically all bacteria are destroyed under ZOE and calcium hydroxide dressing sealed in deep carious lesions.*[6,97] After removal of the remaining caries, the tooth may be permanently restored (see Fig. 23-8, *E*).

DIRECT PULP CAPPING AND PULPOTOMY

Direct pulp capping and pulpotomy involve the application of a medicament, dressing or dental material to the exposed pulp in an attempt to preserve its vitality. Pulpotomy differs from pulp capping only in that a portion of the remaining pulp is removed before application of the capping material. These procedures have been used for carious, mechanical, and traumatic exposures of the pulp—with reported high incidence of success as judged radiographically and by the absence of clinical signs and symptoms. Histologic examinations, however, have shown chronic inflammation under many carious pulp caps and diminished success rates.

Orban[148] described the histopathologic condition of the pulp and concluded that the cells of the pulp were the same as those of loose connective tissue. He believed these cells could differentiate and healing could occur in the dental pulp. In subsequent years much experimentation has taken place, with advocates both for and against pulp capping and pulpotomy procedures.

Although disagreement exists concerning pulp capping and pulpotomy as permanent procedures in mature, secondary teeth, it is universally accepted that vital technique must be employed in teeth with incompletely formed roots with exposed pulps. Once root formation has been completed, routine endodontic treatment may be performed, if necessary.

Cvek[28,30,31] has reported that pulp capping and partial pulpotomy with calcium hydroxide on *traumatically exposed*

permanent pulps are successful 96% of the time. He found that the time between the accident and treatment was not critical as long as the superficially inflamed pulp tissue was removed before capping. The size of the exposure had no bearing on success or failure. The study included both mature teeth and teeth with incompletely formed roots. Continued calcification of the pulp after pulp capping was not a consistent finding; when it occurred it was usually within the first year. These findings have been substantiated by subsequent studies.[57,76,100]

Because of the normal aging of the dental pulp, chances of successful pulp capping diminish with age. Increases in fibrous and calcific deposits and a reduction in pulpal volume may be observed in older pulps. With age the fibroblast proliferation observed in the teeth of young animals is significantly reduced.[180]

Teeth with calcifications of the pulp chamber and root canals are not candidates for pulp capping procedures. These calcifications are indicative of previous inflammatory responses or trauma and render the pulp less responsive to vital therapy.[29]

Agreement generally exists concerning pulp caps in young, permanent teeth with blunderbuss apices, but there is disagreement as to whether mature, permanent teeth should be pulp capped after a carious pulp exposure. Pulp capping after carious pulp exposure is widely accepted as the treatment of choice. Many clinicians believe that to obtain good results teeth must be carefully selected; pulp capping should be done only in the absence of a history of pain and when there is little or no bleeding at the exposure site.[124] However, other clinicians recommend extirpation of all cariously exposed pulps except those with incompletely formed apexes (the rationale being that although there may be no pain, enough toxic products remain in the pulp to maintain the inflammation).[106]

These long-standing inflammations with circulatory disturbances are frequently accompanied by apposition and resorption of the canal walls and calcification in the pulp. The inflammation, calcification, apposition, and resorption may thrive under pulp caps, regardless of which material is used as the pulp capping agent. In teeth with blunderbuss apices, some clinicians recommend pulp extirpation and filling of the canals after a pulp cap as soon as the apical foramen has closed because continued calcification may eventually render the canals unnegotiable.[106]

Few disagree that the ideal treatment for all carious pulp exposures on mature, permanent teeth should be pulpal extirpation and endodontic treatment. It is unrealistic, however, to believe that this can be achieved in all cases. Extirpating the pulp is economically unfeasible in many cases and is time consuming and difficult to accomplish in certain teeth. If vital pulp therapy fails, the clinician still has the option (in most cases) of endodontic treatment.

Agreement exists that exposed caries on primary teeth should *not* be pulp capped. *Pulp capping procedures in primary teeth should be reserved for teeth with mechanical exposures.* The pulpotomy procedure for primary teeth (see the following section) has been shown to be much more successful than pulp capping, and the time requirements for performing the procedures are similar. Therefore *it is recommended that carious pulp exposures on primary teeth should not be pulp capped.*[194,195]

According to Seltzer and Bender[180] pulp capping should be discouraged for carious pulp exposures, because microorganisms and inflammation are invariably associated. Macroscopic examination of such exposures is difficult, and areas of liquefaction necrosis may be overlooked. Because of accelerated aging processes in carious teeth and teeth having undergone operative procedures, they are poorer candidates for pulp caps than noncarious teeth; because of diminished blood supply, periodontally involved teeth are poor risks for pulp capping.

There is general agreement[34,124,180] that the larger the area of carious exposure the poorer the prognosis for pulp capping. With a larger exposure more pulpal tissue is inflamed, and there is greater chance for contamination by microorganisms. There is also greater damage from crushing of tissues and hemorrhage, causing a more severe inflammation. However, when exposure occurs as a result of traumatic or mechanical injury to a healthy pulp, the size of the exposure does not influence healing.[28,154]

Location of the pulp exposure may be an important consideration in the prognosis. If the exposure is on the axial wall and the remaining pulp tissue coronal to the exposure site is deprived of its blood supply, it will undergo necrosis. In such cases, a pulpotomy or pulpectomy should be performed rather than a pulp cap.[190]

If pulp capping or pulpotomy is to be done, care must be exercised in removal of caries or dentin over the exposure site to keep to a minimum the pushing of dentin chips into the remaining pulp tissue. Decreased success has been shown when dentin fragments are forced into the underlying pulp tissue.[89] Inflammatory reaction and formation of dentin matrix are stimulated around these dentin chips.[128] In addition, microorganisms may be forced into the tissue. The resulting inflammatory reaction can be so severe as to cause failure.

After mechanical exposure of the pulp, an acute inflammation occurs at the exposure site. Blood vessels dilate, edema occurs, and polymorphonuclear leukocytes accumulate at the injury site. If the initial tissue damage is too severe, the pulp becomes chronically inflamed, with eventual necrosis of the pulp. It has been shown, however, that repair can occur after pulp exposure. Mechanical exposures have a much better prognosis than do carious exposures because of the lack of previous inflammation and infection associated with the carious exposures. Repair depends on the amount of tissue destruction, the presence of hemorrhage, the patient's age, the resistance of the host, and other factors involved in connective tissue repair.[180]

After pulpal injury, reparative dentin is formed as part of the repair process. Although formation of a dentin bridge has been used as one of the criteria for judging successful pulp capping or pulpotomy procedures, bridge formation can occur in teeth with irreversible inflammation. Moreover, successful pulp capping has been reported without the presence of a reparative dentin bridge over the exposure site.[177,218]

Experiments on germ-free animals have shown the importance of microorganisms in the healing of exposed pulp tissues; injured pulp tissue contaminated by microorganisms did not heal, whereas tissue in germ-free animals did heal regardless of the severity of the exposure.[88,153] Pulp procedures should always be carried out with rubber dam isolation and aseptic conditions to prevent introduction of microorganisms into the pulp tissue.

Marginal seal over the pulp-capping or pulpotomy procedure is of prime importance. In deep cavities without pulp exposure, Kanka[90] has hypothesized that pulpal inflammation is a consequence of bacterial microleakage, rather than acid etching of dentin. In a follow-up study[222] it was shown that healing after acid etching was better with composite resin adhesives than with controls of ZOE cement when placed in deep dentinal preparations. Leakage of bacteria in the controls was associated with severe pulpal inflammation. Thus it was concluded that bacterial leakage, rather than acid etching, impairs pulpal healing in deep dentinal cavities. Healing and the formation of secondary dentin are inherent properties of the pulp. If allowed to do so, the pulp, like any connective tissue, will heal itself. Healing after pulp amputation has been shown to be essentially the same as initial calcification events that occur in other normal and diseased, calcified tissues.[73] Factors promoting healing are conditions of the pulp at the time of amputation, removal of irritants, and proper postoperative care, such as proper sealing of the margins.

The ideal treatment for all carious exposures, except those in teeth with incompletely formed roots, might be pulp extirpation and root canal filling; nevertheless, there are still indications for direct pulp capping. Economics, time, and difficulty of achieving root canal filling in certain teeth are a few of the reasons a clinician may choose pulp capping over another form of pulp therapy. If pulp capping is considered, the clinician must consider all the factors discussed in this section to determine the prognosis of each case. In the event of failure of direct pulp capping, there is usually the option of endodontic therapy.

Traditional Pulp-Capping Agents

Many materials and drugs have been used as pulp capping agents. Materials, medicaments, antiseptics, antiinflammatory agents, antibiotics, and enzymes have been used as pulp capping agents, but *calcium hydroxide* has been the standard by which all others were judged and generally accepted as the agent of choice.[29,124,180] However, in recent years acid etching and direct bonding over pulpal exposures has gained wide acceptance and popularity. (Direct bonding of pulpal exposures is discussed later in this section.)

Before 1930 when Hermann[77] introduced calcium hydroxide as a successful pulp-capping agent, pulp therapy had consisted of devitalization with arsenic and other fixative agents. Hermann demonstrated the formation of secondary dentin over the amputation sides of vital pulps capped with calcium hydroxide.

In 1938 Teuscher and Zander[205] introduced calcium hydroxide in the United States; they histologically confirmed complete dentinal bridging with healthy radicular pulp under calcium hydroxide dressings. Further reports firmly established calcium hydroxide as the pulp-capping agent of choice. After these early works many studies have reported various forms of calcium hydroxide used, with success rates ranging from 30% to 98%.[53] The dissimilar success rates are attributed to many factors, including selection of teeth, criteria for success and failure, differences in responses among different animals, length of study, area of pulp to which the medicament was applied (i.e., coronally or cervically), and the type of calcium hydroxide used.

When calcium hydroxide is applied directly to pulp tissue, there is necrosis of the adjacent pulp tissue and an inflammation of the contiguous tissue. Dentin bridge formation occurs at the junction of the necrotic tissue and the vital, inflamed tissue. Although calcium hydroxide works effectively, the exact mechanisms are not understood. Compounds of similar alkalinity (i.e., a pH of 11) cause liquefaction necrosis when applied to pulp tissue. Calcium hydroxide maintains a local state of alkalinity that is necessary for bone or dentin formation. Beneath the region of coagulation necrosis, cells of the underlying pulp tissue differentiate into odontoblasts and elaborate dentin matrix.[180]

Occasionally (in spite of successful bridge formation) the pulp remains chronically inflamed or becomes necrotic. Internal resorption may occur after pulp exposure and capping with calcium hydroxide. In other cases complete dentin mineralization of the remaining pulp tissue occludes the canals to the extent that they cannot be penetrated for endodontic therapy, if necessary. For these reasons pulpal extirpation and canal filling have been recommended as soon as root formation is completed after the use of calcium hydroxide[106,180] (Fig. 23-9). However, in view of the low incidence of this occurrence, it does not seem to be routinely justified unless necessary for restorative purposes.

It was postulated[226] that calcium would diffuse from a calcium hydroxide dressing into the pulp and participate in the formation of reparative dentin. Experiments with radioactive ions, however, have shown that calcium ions from the calcium hydroxide do *not* enter into the formation of new dentin. Radioactive calcium ions injected intravenously were identified in the dentin bridge. Thus it was established that *the calcium for the dentin bridge comes from the bloodstream.*[9,157,179] The action of calcium hydroxide to form a dentin bridge appears to be a result of the low-grade irritation in the underlying pulpal tissue after application. This theory was supported by the demonstration of successful dentin bridging after application of calcium

hydroxide for short periods of time, followed by removal of the material.[32]

Different forms of calcium hydroxide have produced marked difference when applied to a pulp exposure.[156,201,212]

Commercially available compounds of calcium hydroxide in modified forms are known to be less alkaline and, thus, less caustic on the pulp. The reactions to Dycal, Prisma VLC Dycal, Life, and Nu-Cap have been shown to be similar.[190,191,201] The chemically altered tissue created by application of these compounds is resorbed first, and the bridge is then formed in contact with the capping material.[211,212] With calcium hydroxide powder (i.e., Pulpdent) the bridge forms at the junction of the chemically altered tissue and the remaining, subjacent, vital, pulp tissue. The altered tissue degenerates and disappears, leaving a void between the capping material and the dentin bridge. For this reason a bridge can be visualized better radiographically with calcium hydroxide powder or Pulpdent than with the other commercial compounds. The quality of the dentin bridging was equally good with either material (see Fig. 23-6).

Direct Bonding of Pulp Exposures

Although a controversial procedure, direct bonding of pulp exposures has been advocated by numerous researchers.[26,147] Cox et al[21,25] demonstrated that healing of dental pulp exposures is not exclusively dependent on the stimulatory effects of a particular type of medicament. Healing is directly related to the capacity of the capping agent and the definitive restorative material to provide a biologic seal against immediate and long-term, bacterial microleakage along the entire surface interface with tooth structure.[21] In experiments[24,25] to determine the effects of various materials when applied directly to exposed pulps, composite, silicate cement, zinc phosphate cement, and amalgam were used as direct pulp-capping agents. In half the cases the entire cavity was filled

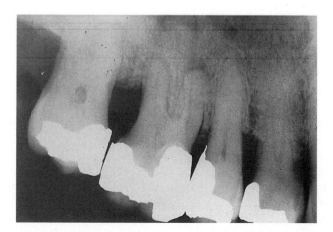

Fig. 23-9 Calcification of pulp chamber and root canals of maxillary first permanent molar after calcium hydroxide pulp capping. The pulp chamber and canal are almost obliterated after the pulp capping, making location and negotiation of the root canals extremely difficult.

with the material, whereas the other half were sealed externally with ZOE. Calcium hydroxide was used as a control. In the cases unsealed with ZOE, bacterial contamination with severe inflammatory responses and degeneration was observed as contrasted to normal healing (similar to that of calcium hydroxide) in the externally sealed specimens. Adequate sealing to prevent bacterial microleakage allowed cell reorganization and dentin bridge formation under the acid cements and composite. Although healing occurred beneath amalgam when sealed, there was no evidence of bridge formation. The data suggests that although the pulp has an inherent healing capacity when bacterial microleakage is excluded, a low-grade irritation is needed to encourage hard tissue repair. They concluded that neither calcium hydroxide nor any particular restorative material or specific pH is specifically responsible for stimulation of pulpal healing or dentin bridging, but that it appears to be an inherent genetic response when exposed to a low-grade irritation. Their findings are in agreement with experiments[88,153] on germ-free animals that showed pulpal healing in the absence of bacterial contamination, whereas the introduction of bacteria prevented healing.

Numerous bonding materials and composite resin systems have been tested as pulp capping agents with reported* healing of the pulp and deposition of hard tissue at the exposure site. Unanimity exists among these researchers that healing is not dependent on the material but upon its capacity to provide a biologic seal.

Nakabayashi et al[141] introduced the term *hybrid layer* to describe the morphologic impregnation of vital dentin with resin that provides the biologic seal at the dentin and resin interface. The hydrophilic resins infiltrate the collagen fibers left after acid etching has demineralized the dentin surface and result in a strong, hybrid linkage between the dentin and the bonding agent. It is this hybrid layer of resin surrounding odontoblastic processes, which increases the bond strength and provides a long-term biologic seal against bacterial microleakage.

A study[22] of dentin bridging underneath hard-setting calcium hydroxide was shown (in 95% of cases) to contain multiple tunnel defects that were patent to the underlying pulp. These morphologic disruptions of the dentin bridge failed to provide a permanent barrier and, thus, a long-term seal against bacterial microleakage. They further demonstrated long-term evidence that calcium hydroxide becomes softened and allows leakage, resulting in recurrent pulpal inflammation and necrosis after 1 to 2 years.

Although direct bonding of pulp exposures has gained wide popularity, it should be noted that no long range, histologic studies have been published. Also unfavorable effects with direct bonding have been reported. In a comparison of acid-etched, bonded, composite pulp capping to Dycal, one researcher[151] found 45% pulpal necrosis and only 25% dentin bridging (compared with 7% necrosis and 82% bridging

---

*References 2,23,24,25,69,98,147,222.

respectively). Another report[74] comparing All Bond 2 with calcium hydroxide (i.e., Dycal) showed persistent inflammatory reactions and hyaline alteration of extracellular matrix inhibiting complete pulpal repair or bridge formation in the bonded specimens. Conversely, the calcium hydroxide specimens produced complete dentin bridge formation. These results led the authors to conclude that direct bonding is not recommended for human pulp capping.

Mineral Trioxide Aggregate

Excellent results have been reported[1,86,140,158] with the use of a new, biocompatible pulp capping agent, mineral trioxide aggregate (MTA). When compared with calcium hydroxide, MTA produced significantly more dentinal bridging in a shorter period of time with significantly less inflammation. Dentin deposition also began earlier with MTA. The disadvantage of this technique is that 3 to 4 hours is needed for setting of the MTA after placement. The procedure involves placing MTA directly over the exposure site and sealing the tooth temporarily to allow the cement to harden. The tooth is later reentered and permanently sealed over the set MTA with an etched, dentinal bonding agent and composite resin to prevent future bacterial microleakage. Although this approach requires an additional appointment the results seem to justify the added time when pulp capping is the treatment of choice.

The ideal treatment for all carious exposures (except those in teeth with incompletely formed roots), might be pulp extirpation and root canal filling; nevertheless, there are still indications for direct pulp capping. Economics, time, and difficulty of achieving root canal filling in certain teeth are a few of the reasons clinicians may choose pulp capping over another form of pulp therapy. If pulp capping is considered, clinicians must consider all the factors discussed in this section to determine the prognosis of each case. In the event of failure of direct pulp capping, there is usually the option of endodontic therapy.

Pulp capping should *not* be considered for primary, carious pulp exposures or for permanent teeth with a history of spontaneous toothache, radiographic evidence of pulpal or periapical pathosis, calcifications of the pulp chamber or root canals, excessive hemorrhage at the exposure site, or exposures with purulent or serous exudates.

Direct Pulp Capping in Primary Teeth

Because the life span of the average primary tooth is only approximately 12 to 14 years from the beginnings of development to exfoliation, primary teeth undergo dramatic physiologic and physical changes over a relatively short period of time. The clinician should keep in mind that they are not dealing with pulp tissue that is static in nature and, therefore, outcomes for the same procedure may differ depending on the age of the patient. Furthermore, because of the aging of the dental pulp, the likelihood of successful pulp capping diminishes with age. This may be explained by the increase in fibrous and calcific deposits. Also a reduction in pulpal volume may be observed in older pulps. With age the fibroblast proliferation observed in the teeth of young animals is significantly reduced.[180]

Exposures from caries on primary teeth should *not* be pulp capped. *Guidelines developed by the American Academy of Pediatric Dentistry (AAPD) recommend that direct pulp capping should be reserved for small mechanical or traumatic exposures in primary teeth.* Under these circumstances it is presumed that the conditions for a favorable response are optimal. *The AAPD Guidelines recommend that carious pulp exposures on primary teeth not be pulp capped.*[194,195]

Pulpotomy in Primary Teeth

The 1996 AAPD guidelines[67] for pulp therapy for primary and young, permanent teeth describes the pulpotomy procedure in primary teeth as the amputation of the affected or infected, coronal portion of the dental pulp, preserving the vitality and function of all or part of the remaining radicular pulp. Evidence of success in therapy includes:

- Vitality of the majority of the radicular pulp
- No prolonged adverse clinical signs or symptoms, such as prolonged sensitivity, pain, or swelling
- No radiographic evidence of internal resorption or abnormal canal calcification
- No breakdown of periradicular tissue
- No harm to succedaneous teeth

Many pharmacotherapeutic agents have been employed to achieve the previously mentioned criteria. Formocresol has been the most popular agent, mainly because of its ease in use and excellent clinical success. Yet despite its good clinical results, formocresol has come under close scrutiny because of concerns regarding the systemic distribution of this agent and its potential for toxicity, allergenicity, carcinogenicity, and mutagenicity. Other medicaments (e.g., glutaraldehyde, calcium hydroxide, collagen, ferric sulfate) have been suggested as possible replacements. However, varying success rates and concerns regarding the safety of these materials make it clear that additional research on the use of these and other pharmacotherapeutic agents is required.

Nonpharmacologic, hemostatic techniques have been recommended, including electrosurgery* and laser therapy.[184] Research on both of these techniques is sparse; nevertheless, electrosurgical pulpotomy is currently being taught in several dental schools. Ranley[163] provides a thorough review of pulpotomy agents and discusses new modalities for possible future use. (The formocresol, glutaraldehyde, electrosurgical, and laser pulpotomy techniques are discussed further in this section.)

*References 117,159,172,182,183.

Formocresol Pulpotomy on Primary Teeth

The use of formocresol in dentistry has become a controversial issue because of reports of wide distribution of the medicament after systemic injection[135] and the demonstration of an immune response to formocresol-fixed, autologous tissue implanted in connective tissues or injected into root canals.[14,206] However, the formocresol pulpotomy continues to be one treatment of choice for primary teeth with vital, carious exposures of the pulp in which inflammation or degeneration are judged to be confined to the coronal pulp. The last reported worldwide survey of dental schools (in 1987[10]) showed a majority of pediatric dentistry departments and practicing pediatric dentists advocated the formocresol pulpotomy technique; it is still widely taught and used in clinical practice. The current formocresol pulpotomy technique is a modification of that reported by Sweet in 1930.[200]

Histologic studies[119,122] have demonstrated the effects of formocresol on pulps of primary and permanent, human teeth. Formocresol-saturated cotton pellets caused the surface of the pulp to become fibrous and acidophilic within a few minutes. After exposure to the formocresol for a period of 7 to 14 days, three distinct zones became evident:

1. A broad, acidophilic zone of fixation
2. A broad, pale-staining zone with diminished cellular and fiber definition (i.e., atrophy)
3. A broad zone of inflammatory cells concentrated at the pale-staining zone junction and diffusing apically into normal pulp tissue

There was no evidence of an attempt to wall off the inflammatory zone by fibrous tissue or calcific barrier. After 60 days to 1 year, the pulp was progressively fixed and the entire pulp ultimately became fibrous. Subsequent investigations[45] showed that the effect of formocresol on the pulp varied, depending on the length of time the drug was in contact with the tissue. After 5 minutes there was a surface fixation blending into normal pulp tissue apically. Formocresol sealed in contact with the pulp for 3 days caused calcific degeneration, and the technique was termed vital or nonvital, according to the length of time of the application. As a part of this report, the clinical data from Sweet's files were compiled and showed a 97% success rate.

The ingrowth of fibroblasts in tissue underlying formocresol-pulpotomized, noncarious, human, primary canines have been reported.[36] At 16 weeks the entire pulp had degenerated and was being replaced with granulation tissue. Mild inflammation, in addition to some calcific degeneration, was noted.

Doyle et al[40] compared calcium hydroxide and formocresol pulpotomies on mechanically exposed, healthy, primary, dental pulps. A formocresol pellet was sealed in place for 4 to 7 days, and the histologic study was conducted from 4 to 388 days. Of the 18 teeth in the calcium hydroxide group, only 50% were judged histologically to be successful; of the 14 teeth treated with formocresol, 92% were histologically successful. Radiographically, the success rates were 64% and 93%, whereas the clinical success rates were 71%

and 100% (calcium hydroxide versus formocresol pulpotomy). The authors were able to identify vital tissue in the apical third of the root canals after treatment with formocresol pulpotomies.

Studies of the effect of adding formocresol to the ZOE filling over the 5-minute, formocresol-pulpotomized primary tooth[216] have shown no appreciable differences between cases in which formocresol was included in the cement and those in which it was not; and histologic investigations[189,216] have reported no significant differences between two- and one-appointment (i.e., 5-minute) formocresol pulpotomies.

Accumulation of formocresol has been demonstrated in the pulp, dentin, periodontal ligament, and bone surrounding the apexes of pulpotomized teeth.[59,134] Formaldehyde was shown to be the component of formocresol that interacts with the protein portion of cells. The addition of cresol to formaldehyde appears to potentiate the effect of formaldehyde on protein.[142] In a study using human pulp fibroblast cultures, formaldehyde was shown to be the major component of formocresol that caused cytotoxic effects and to be 40 times more toxic than cresol.[84]

Application of radioactive formocresol to amputated pulp sites has been shown to result in immediate absorption of the material. The systemic absorption was limited to about 1% of the applied dose, regardless of the amount of time the drug was applied. It was shown that formocresol compromised the microcirculation, causing vessel thrombosis, which limited further systemic accumulation.[134]

Animal experiments[14,206] have demonstrated that in vivo, formocresol-fixed, autologous tissue produced an immune response when implanted into connective tissues or injected into root canals. The tissue became antigenically altered by formocresol and activated a specific, cell-mediated lymphocyte response.

Other studies have demonstrated no evidence of this response in nonpresensitized animals,[187] and presensitized animals showed only a weak allergic potential.[215] This is in agreement with researchers[37] who have shown that formaldehyde demonstrated a low level of antigenicity in rabbits and, as such, would be an acceptable pulp medicament in regard to immunoreactive potential. Other investigators[112] studied lymphocyte transformation induced by formocresol treated and untreated extracts of homologous pulp tissue in children with varying past experience with formocresol pulpotomies. Significant transformation responses were noted in over half of the children, but they were unrelated to a clinical history of formocresol pulpotomy. Sensitization to pulp-related antigens was a common finding in the study. The authors concluded that formocresol pulpotomy does not induce significant immunologic sensitization to extracted antigens of homologous pulp or to pulp antigen altered by treatment with formocresol, and therefore it does not support other animal studies in which intense immunization schedules were used.[112] Clinical use of formocresol (for many years without reports of allergic reaction) has only anecdotally substantiated this finding.

Concerns regarding the systemic effects of formocresol have also led to investigations concerning its possible embryotoxic and teratogenic effects.[54] In a study using injections of 25% and 50% formocresol into chick embryos, significant increases were noted in mortality, structural defects, and retarded development.

After systemic administration of formocresol in experimental animals, formocresol is distributed throughout the body. Metabolism and excretion of a portion of the absorbed formocresol occur in the kidneys and lungs. The remaining drug is bound to tissue predominantly in the kidneys, liver, and lungs. When administered systemically in large doses, acute toxic effects (e.g., cardiovascular changes, plasma and urinary enzyme changes, histologic evidence of cellular injury to the vital organs) were noted. The degree of tissue injury appeared to be closely related, with some of the changes being reversible in the early stages. The authors[135] were careful to point out that the administered doses were far in excess of those used clinically in humans and should not be extrapolated to clinical dental practice. In another study the same authors emphasized that the quantities of formaldehyde absorbs systemically via the pulpotomy route were small and did not contraindicate the use of formocresol.[152]

A subsequent study[136] in which 16 pulpotomies (i.e., 5-minute application of full-strength formocresol) were performed on a dog that displayed early tissue injury to the kidneys and liver. However, cellular recovery could be expected because there was no evidence of the onset of an inflammatory reaction. In animals subjected to only one to four pulpotomies, there was no injury to the kidneys or liver. The heart and lungs of all the animals were normal. The authors pointed out that 16 pulpotomies expose a small dog to a much higher systemic level of formocresol than would several pulpotomies in a human. They further concluded that no clinical implications regarding the toxicity of absorbed formocresol should be drawn from this study. Other investigators[61] have shown that the effect of formocresol on pulp tissue is controlled by the quantity that diffuses into the tissue, and the quantity can be controlled by the length of time of application, the concentration used, the method of application, or a combination of all of these factors.

With the use of isotope-labeled, 19% formaldehyde, the presence of the drug was demonstrated in the lung, liver, kidney, muscle, serum, urine, and carbon dioxide after a 5-minute application to pulpotomy sites. The concentrations achieved in the tissues were equivalent to those found after an infusion of 30% of the amount placed in the pulp chamber.[162]

Another study using C-labeled formocresol showed that 12% of the material used in a 5-minute, full-strength pulpotomy was recovered after 36 hours, chiefly from the teeth, plasma, urine, and also from the liver, kidneys, lungs, heart, and spleen.[71]

Implantation of undiluted, formocresol-fixed tissue in animals causes necrosis of the surrounding connective tissues,[15] and dilution of the formocresol decreases the tissue irritation potential.[63] Investigations using one-fifth concentration formocresol for pulpotomies have noted little difference as related to the initial effects on tissue fixation; however, earlier recovery of enzyme activity was apparent with the diluted formocresol than with the undiluted formocresol. Postoperative complications were reduced, and there was an improvement in the rate of recovery from the cytotoxic effects for formocresol when diluted.[113,114,199] It has been reported clinically that the same success is achieved with the diluted formocresol as with the undiluted formocresol.[55,129,130] *Therefore it is recommended that, if formocresol is to be used at all, only one-fifth concentration formocresol be used for pulpotomy procedures because it is as effective as and less damaging than the traditional preparation.*

One-fifth concentration formocresol is prepared in the following manner:
- The dilute solution is prepared by mixing three parts glycerin with one part distilled water.
- One part formocresol is then thoroughly mixed with four parts diluent.

A histologic study[95] on teeth with induced pulpal and periapical pathosis showed no resolution of inflammation or periapical pathosis after a 5-minute pulpotomy procedure. Canals with vital tissue exhibited more internal resorption than was reported by other researchers, and more apical resorption was seen in teeth with periapical and furcal involvement than was seen in teeth with vital pulps. Ingrowth of tissue was not observed in canals with necrotic tissue. Also noted was the lack of evidence of formocresol fixation of either apical or furcal lesions. Despite extensive inflammatory reactions around the apexes of primary teeth close to the permanent tooth germs, no ill effects were observed on any tooth germs from the formocresol. Formocresol fixation was confined within the canals in all instances. Because the authors[95] concluded that the formocresol pulpotomy is an unacceptable procedure for teeth with pulpal and periapical pathosis, this study points out the importance of *confining formocresol pulpotomies to primary teeth containing vital tissue in the root canals.* Clinically, these results have also been substantiated.[204]

The fear of damage to the succedaneous tooth has been offered as an argument against formocresol pulpotomy on primary teeth. Studies have shown conflicting findings, ranging from the same incidence of enamel defects in treated and untreated, contralateral teeth[131,171] to an increase in defects and positional alterations of the underlying permanent tooth.[126] It should be pointed out that studies of this nature are follow-up studies long after treatment, without knowledge of the existing status of the pulp before pulpotomy. Nor has anyone devised a study to ascertain the effects of the condition that necessitated the pulpotomy procedure. (If the strict criteria outlined in this section are followed, the incidence of defects to the permanent teeth does not increase after formocresol pulpotomy.)

Studies have shown that the exfoliation time of primary molars after formocresol pulpotomy is not affected.[131,214]

Indications and Contraindications   The formocresol pulpotomy is indicated for pulp exposure on primary teeth in which the inflammation or infection is judged to be confined to the coronal pulp. If inflammation has spread into the tissues within the root canals, the tooth should be considered a candidate for pulpectomy and root canal filling or extraction. There are eight contraindications for formocresol pulpotomy on a primary tooth:
1. A nonrestorable tooth
2. A tooth nearing exfoliation or with no bone overlying the permanent tooth crown
3. A history of spontaneous toothache
4. Evidence of periapical or furcal pathology
5. A pulp that does not hemorrhage
6. Inability to control hemorrhage after a coronal pulp amputation
7. A pulp with serous or purulent drainage
8. The presence of a fistula

Technique   The formocresol pulpotomy is used on primary teeth with roots judged to be free of inflammation and infection. Compromise on this principle leads to a diminished success rate and possible damage to the succedaneous tooth. Therefore the importance of a proper diagnosis cannot be overstressed (Fig. 23-10).

After the diagnosis has been completed, the primary tooth is anesthetized and isolated with a rubber dam. All caries is removed, and the entire roof of the pulp chamber is cut away with a high-speed bur and copious water spray. All the coronal pulp is removed with a bur or spoon excavator. Care must be exercised to extirpate all filaments of the coronal pulp. If any filaments remain in the pulp chamber, hemorrhage will be impossible to control. The pulp chamber is thoroughly washed with water to remove all debris. The water is removed by vacuum and cotton pellets.

Hemorrhage is controlled by slightly moistened cotton pellets (wetted and blotted almost dry) placed against the stumps of the pulp at the openings of the root canals. Completely dry cotton pellets should not be used, because fibers of the cotton will be incorporated into the clot and, when removed, will cause hemorrhage. Dry cotton pellets are placed over the moist pellets, and pressure is exerted on the mass to control the hemorrhage. Hemorrhage should be controlled in this manner within several minutes. It may be necessary to change the pellets to control all hemorrhage. If hemorrhage occurs, the clinician should carefully check to be sure that all filaments of the pulp were removed from the pulp chamber and that the amputation site is clean.

If hemorrhage cannot be controlled within 5 minutes, the pulp tissue within the canals is probably inflamed and the tooth is not a candidate for a formocresol pulpotomy. The clinician should then proceed with pulpectomy, or the tooth should be extracted.

When the hemorrhage has been controlled, one-fifth dilution formocresol on a cotton pellet is placed in direct contact with the pulp stumps. Fixation does not occur unless

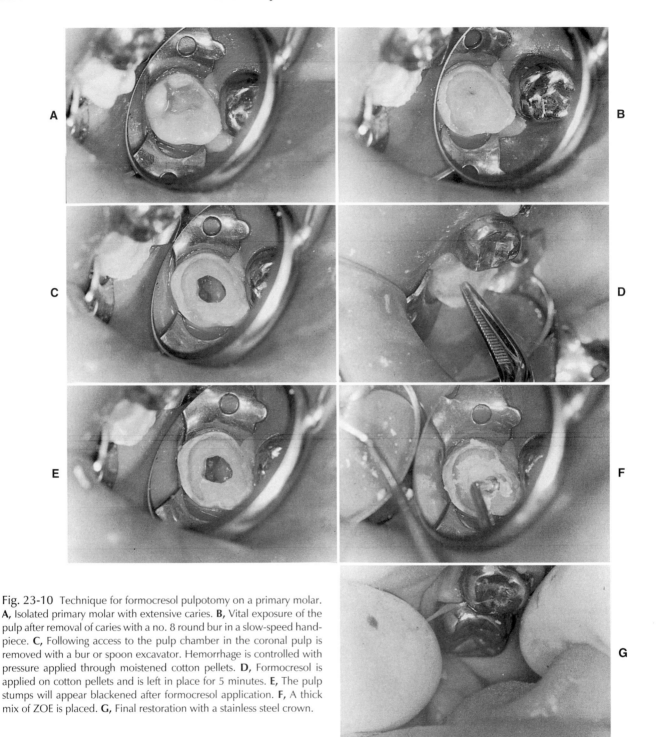

Fig. 23-10 Technique for formocresol pulpotomy on a primary molar. **A,** Isolated primary molar with extensive caries. **B,** Vital exposure of the pulp after removal of caries with a no. 8 round bur in a slow-speed handpiece. **C,** Following access to the pulp chamber in the coronal pulp is removed with a bur or spoon excavator. Hemorrhage is controlled with pressure applied through moistened cotton pellets. **D,** Formocresol is applied on cotton pellets and is left in place for 5 minutes. **E,** The pulp stumps will appear blackened after formocresol application. **F,** A thick mix of ZOE is placed. **G,** Final restoration with a stainless steel crown.

the formocresol is in contact with the stumps. The cotton pellet is blotted to remove excess formocresol after saturation and before the tooth is entered. Formocresol is caustic and creates a severe tissue burn if allowed to contact the gingiva.

The formocresol is left in contact with the pulp stumps for 5 minutes. When it is removed, the tissue appears brown and no hemorrhage should be present. If an area of the pulp was not contacting the medication, the procedure must be repeated for that tissue. Small cotton pellets for applying the medication usually work best, because they allow closer approximation of the material to the pulp.

A cement base of ZOE is placed over the pulp stumps and allowed to set. The tooth may then be restored permanently. The restoration of choice is a SS crown for primary molars. On anterior, primary teeth a composite, tooth-colored resto-

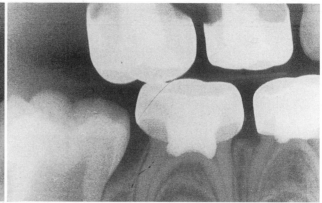
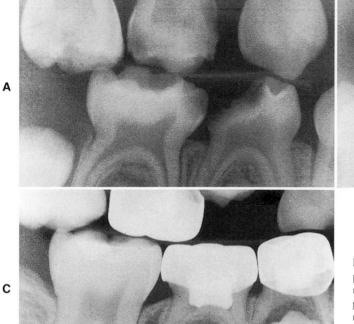

Fig. 23-11 Five-year follow-up of a primary tooth with a formocresol pulpotomy. **A,** Pre-treatment radiograph showing deep caries on lower right first and second primary molars. **B,** One-year post-treatment radiograph. **C,** Five-year follow-up radiograph. Note the eruption of the lower right first permanent molar and first bicuspid.

ration is the treatment of choice unless the tooth is so badly broken down that it requires a crown.

With the formocresol, no dentin bridge formation occurs as with the calcium hydroxide pulpotomy (Fig. 23-11). However, narrowing of the root canal through the deposition of dentin may be observed in some cases (Fig. 23-12).

Criteria for Success   Failure of a formocresol pulpotomy is usually detected radiographically (Fig. 23-13). The first signs of failure are often internal resorption of the root adjacent to the area where the formocresol was applied. This may be accompanied by external resorption, especially as the failure progresses. In the primary molars a radiolucency develops in the bifurcation or trifurcation area. In the anterior teeth a radiolucency may develop at the apexes or lateral to the roots. With more destruction the tooth becomes excessively mobile; a fistula usually develops. It is rare for pain to occur with the failure of a formocresol pulpotomy. Consequently, unless patients receive follow-up checks after a formocresol pulpotomy, failure may be undetected. When the tooth loosens and is eventually exfoliated, the parents and child may consider the circumstances normal.

The development of cystic lesions after pulp therapy in primary molars has been reported.[16,175] An amorphous, eosinophilic material shown to contain phenolic grouping similar to those present in medicaments was found in the lesions. Other researchers[138] have observed furcal lesions in untreated, pulpally involved, primary molars containing granulomatous tissue with stratified squamous epithelium, suggesting the potential for cyst formation. In a subsequent study involving failed, pulpotomized, primary molars, most specimens were diagnosed as furcation cysts.[139] These findings emphasize the importance of periodic follow-up to endodontic treatment on primary teeth.

Glutaraldehyde Pulpotomy

A body of evidence has accumulated that has led some investigators to suggest that glutaraldehyde should replace formocresol as the medicament of choice for chemical pulpotomy procedures on primary teeth. Numerous studies[37,202,219] have shown that the application of 2% to 4% aqueous glutaraldehyde produces rapid surface fixation of the underlying pulpal tissue, although its depth of penetration is limited. Unlike the varied response to formocresol, a large percentage of the underlying pulp tissue remains vital and is free of inflammation. A narrow zone of eosinophilic, stained and compressed, fixed tissue is found directly beneath the area of application that blends into vital, normal-appearing tissue apically. With time, the glutaraldehyde-fixed zone is replaced through macrophagic action with dense collagenous tissue; thus the entire root canal tissue is vital.[103]

Glutaraldehyde is absorbed from vital pulpotomy sites. However, unlike formocresol, which is absorbed and dis-

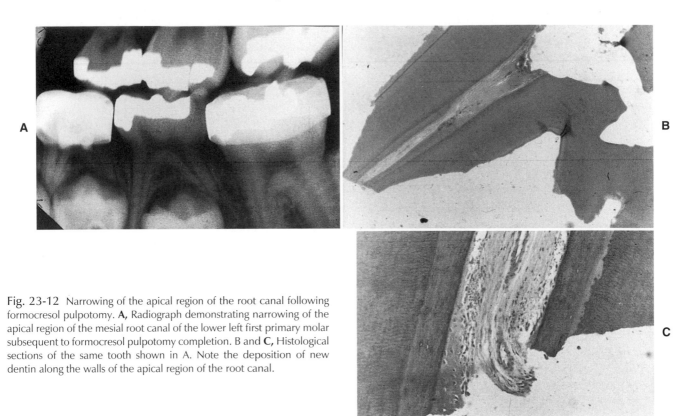

Fig. 23-12 Narrowing of the apical region of the root canal following formocresol pulpotomy. **A,** Radiograph demonstrating narrowing of the apical region of the mesial root canal of the lower left first primary molar subsequent to formocresol pulpotomy completion. B and **C,** Histological sections of the same tooth shown in A. Note the deposition of new dentin along the walls of the apical region of the root canal.

tributed throughout the body within minutes of placement,[152] glutaraldehyde does not perfuse the pulp tissue to the apex and demonstrates less systemic distribution immediately after application.[35,109,220] Autoradiographs of isotope-labeled glutaraldehyde show that the drug is limited largely to the pulp space, with little evidence of escape outside the tooth after pulpotomy.[137] No differences have been reported in the incidence of enamel defects on succedaneous teeth with the use of formocresol- or glutaraldehyde-based pulpotomy techniques.[3]

Also unlike formaldehyde, which is mostly tissue bound with only a small fraction being metabolized, glutaraldehyde exhibits very low-tissue binding and is readily metabolized. Glutaraldehyde is metabolized mostly in the kidney and lungs but is also found in liver, heart, and muscle tissues.[91,137] Glutaraldehyde is eliminated primarily in urine and expired in gases; 90% of the drug is gone within 3 days.[165]

Virtually no toxic effects have been shown after glutaraldehyde administration (either via pulpotomy or systemic application). Large doses (i.e., up to 500 times the amount applied in a pulpotomy procedure) caused little toxic effect.[165] Cytotoxicity studies in human pulp fibroblasts showed 2.5% glutaraldehyde to be 15 to 20 times less toxic than formocresol or 19% formaldehyde.[84]

Although glutaraldehyde has been shown to produce antigenic products in much the same manner as formocresol,[167] it has a relatively low antigenicity[166] compared with formo-cresol. Unfortunately, purified solutions of glutaraldehyde have been shown to be unstable.[161]

The indications, contraindications, and technique for the glutaraldehyde pulpotomy are the same as for the formocresol pulpotomy, except that glutaraldehyde is substituted for formocresol. Unfortunately, neither the optimal concentration of glutaraldehyde nor the amount of time of application has been conclusively established.

Investigators[62,111,164] have reported the effects of various concentrations and lengths of application of glutaraldehyde. Application of the glutaraldehyde through incorporation in ZOE led to a high failure rate, thus contraindicating this route of administration.[62] Buffering glutaraldehyde, increasing its concentration, and applying it for longer periods enhance the degree of fixation. Only stronger solutions increase the depth of fixation. Increased fixation gives greater resistance to removal and replacement of the fixed tissue. Weak concentrations and short application times lead to more severe inflammatory responses in the underlying pulp tissue and to eventual failure.[111]

Their research has led Ranley et al[164] to recommend 4% buffered glutaraldehyde with a 4-minute application time or 8% for 2 minutes.

In a 24-month follow-up of pulpotomies performed with 2% glutaraldehyde, the failure rate rose to 18% after 2 years, and the authors could not justify its use over formocresol.[58] Other authors have examined the evidence with regard to

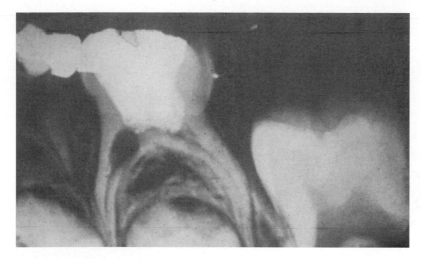

Fig. 23-13   Formocresol pulpotomy failure. Note the internal resorption in the mesial root and the radiolucency in the bifurcation.

toxicity, mutagenicity, and systemic distribution, and they do not recommend the substitution of glutaraldehyde for formocresol in pulpotomy technique.[48] The majority of training institutions continue to teach the formocresol technique, and a large majority of practicing pediatric dentists employ formocresol.[10]

In a recent article,[16] 2% buffered glutaraldehyde was used for three minutes and then covered with a dressing of either a single drop of 2% buffered glutaraldehyde plus ZOE or a single drop of 2% buffered glutaraldehyde plus calcium hydroxide (i.e., Dycal). Both showed similar clinical and radiographic success rates. The authors concluded that neither protocol, however, was as successful as formocresol pulpotomy.

Given comparable success rates and the undesirable effects of formocresol and glutaraldehyde, it has been suggested to substitute the pulpectomy technique for the pulpotomy in primary teeth.[224]

Electrosurgical Pulpotomy

Although electrocoagulation on the pulps of teeth was reported in 1957,[108] it was a decade later that Mack[116] became the first U.S. dentist routinely to perform electrosurgical pulpotomies. Oringer[150] also strongly advocated this technique in his 1975 text on electrosurgery. Several clinical studies[172,183] have produced results comparable to those found with the use of formocresol. Conflicting results have been reported from histologic studies, ranging from comparable results to formocresol pulpotomy[182] to pathologic root resorption with periapical and furcal involvement.[186] A retrospective human study by Mack and Dean[117] in 1993 showed a success rate of 99% for primary molars undergoing electrosurgical pulpotomies. Compared with a formocresol pulpotomy study of similar design, the success rate of the electrosurgery technique was shown to be significantly higher. A

more recent clinical study[159] showed success rates of 95% and 87% respectively for electrosurgical pulpotomies and formocresol pulpotomies.

The steps in the electrosurgical pulpotomy technique (Fig. 23-14) are basically the same as those for the formocresol technique through the removal of the coronal pulp tissue. Large sterile cotton pellets are placed in contact with the pulp and pressure is applied to obtain hemostasis. The Hyfrecator Plus 7-797 (Birtcher Medical Systems, Irvine, CA) is set at 40% power (high at 12W), and the 705A dental electrode is used to deliver the electrical arc. The cotton pellets are quickly removed, and the electrode is placed 1 to 2 mm above the pulpal stump (see Fig. 23-14, *C*). The electrical arc is allowed to bridge the gap to the pulpal stump for 1 second, followed by a cool down period of 5 seconds. Thus heat and electrical transfer are minimized by keeping the electrode as far away from the pulpal stump and tooth structure as possible while still allowing electrical arcing to occur. If necessary this procedure may be repeated up to a maximum of three times. The procedure is then repeated for the next pulpal stump. When the procedure is properly performed, the pulpal stumps appear dry and completely blackened (see Fig. 23-14, *D*). The chamber is filled with ZOE placed directly against the pulpal stumps. Research[51] has shown no difference between ZOE or calcium hydroxide as the dressing. The tooth should then be restored with a SS crown (see Fig. 23-14, *E* and *F*).

Lasers

Recently, several reports have appeared in the literature on the use of the carbon dioxide laser for performing vital pulpotomies on primary teeth.[44,110] Elliot et al[44] compared the use of the laser with formocresol in caries-free, primary, cuspid teeth that were scheduled for extraction in children between 6 and 10 years of age. Thirty teeth were included in the study.

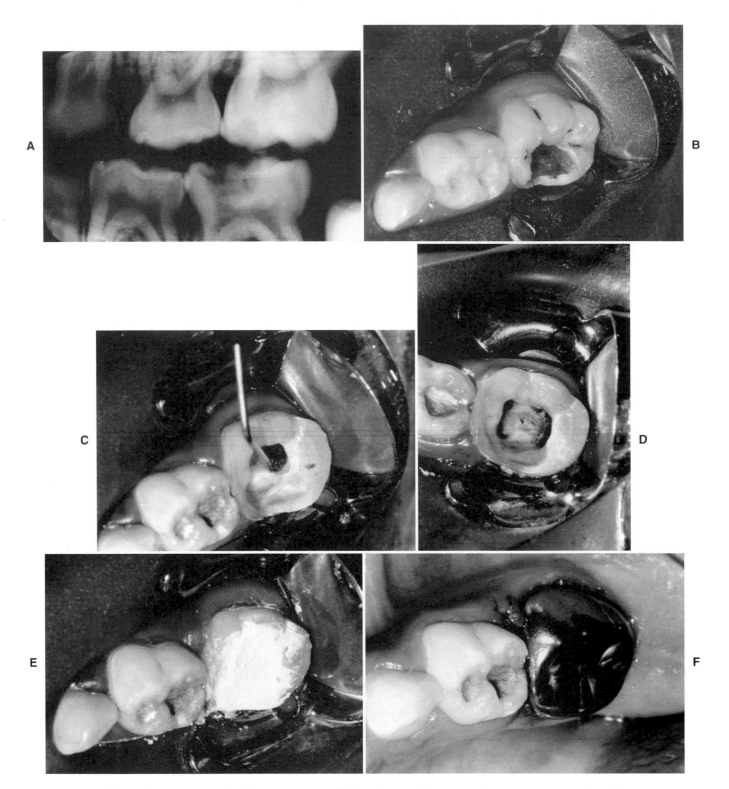

Fig. 23-14 Electrosurgical pulpotomy on a mandibular right second primary molar. **A**, Preoperative radiograph showing caries into the pulp. **B**, Tooth isolated with the rubber dam. **C**, The 705A dental electrode in the Hyfrecator Plus 7-797 is activated over each pulpal stump for 1 second. **D**, Pulpal stumps appear dry and completely blackened after the electrosurgery pulpotomy. **E**, Pulp chamber is filled with ZOE placed directly against the pulpal stumps. **F**, Tooth is restored with a SS crown. (Courtesy Dr. Ronald B. Mack.)

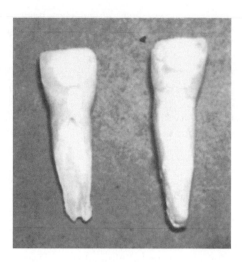

Fig. 23-15 These two primary mandibular incisors have lingual and apical resorption. Note that the left incisor has the apical foramen just beneath the cervical line, whereas the right one has its apical foramen at the apex of the root.

The authors found no significant differences between the formocresol and laser-treated groups. Areas of isolated internal resorption were identified in one of the formocresol-treated teeth and two of the laser-treated teeth. They were concerned about energy threshold necessary to create conditions to minimize the initial inflammatory response. They concluded that, on the basis of symptomatic, clinical, and histologic findings, the carbon dioxide laser appears to compare favorably to formocresol treatment. They also felt that additional studies should be conducted to establish the ideal applied laser energy to maximize optimum, residual, pulpal response and to explore the effects of laser treatment to pulps previously exposed by carious lesions.

Liu et al[110] reported on the use of the laser on primary teeth with pulpal exposures caused by carious lesions. Thirty-three teeth, which included 21 primary molars and 12 primary canines, were treated and followed for 12 to 27 months. All were clinically successful and only one showed evidence of internal resorption at the 6-month, follow-up visit. The author observed complete calcification radiographically after 9 months in about half of the treated teeth.

On the basis of these early studies the use of the carbon dioxide laser should be considered as a viable alternative to other methods that show possible toxic side effects. However, the considerable cost of the laser may not make this method cost effective.

NONVITAL PULP THERAPY ON PRIMARY TEETH

Pulpectomy in Primary Teeth

Role of Resorption on Canal Anatomy and Apical Foramina   In the newly completed roots of the primary teeth the apical foramina are located near the anatomic apexes of the roots. After the deposition of additional dentin and cementum, there are multiple apical ramifications of the pulp as it exits the root, just as in the mature permanent tooth.

Because of the position of the permanent tooth bud, physiologic resorption of the roots of the primary incisors and canines is initiated on the lingual surfaces in the apical third of the roots. In the primary molars, resorption usually begins on the inner surfaces of the roots near the interradicular septum.

As resorption progresses, the apical foramen may not correspond to the anatomic apex of the root but be coronal to it. Therefore radiographic establishment of the root canal length may be erroneous. Resorption may extend through the roots and into the root canals, creating additional communications with the periapical tissues other than through the apical foramina or lateral and accessory canals (Fig. 23-15). This has been shown to occur at all levels of the root.[169]

Permanent Tooth Bud   The effects of primary endodontic therapy on the developing, permanent tooth bud should be of paramount concern to the clinician. Manipulation through the apex of the primary tooth is contraindicated, because the permanent tooth bud lies immediately adjacent to the apex of the primary tooth. Overextension of root canal instruments and filling materials must be avoided. If signs of resorption are visible radiographically, it is advisable to establish the working length of endodontic instruments 2 or 3 mm short of the radiographic apex. The use of the radiographic paralleling technique with a long cone for maximal accuracy when measuring canal lengths is recommended.

Anesthesia is usually necessary for pulp extirpation and enlargement of the canals but is rarely needed when primary teeth are filled at a subsequent appointment. The response of the patient can sometimes be used as a guide to the approach to the apex and as a check to the length of the canal that was previously established radiographically. Hemorrhage after pulp removal indicates overextension into the periapical tissues.

The filling material used to obliterate the root canals on primary teeth must be absorbable so that it can be absorbed as the tooth resorbs and so that it offers no resistance or deflection to the eruption of the permanent tooth. *Materials, such as gutta-percha or silver points, are contraindicated in root canals of primary teeth.*

Pulpectomy   Pulpectomy and root canal filling procedures on primary teeth have been the subject of much controversy. Fear of damage to developing permanent tooth buds and a belief that the tortuous root canals of primary teeth could not be adequately negotiated, cleaned, shaped, and filled have led to the needless sacrifice of many pulpally involved, primary teeth.

Much has been written regarding potential damage to the developing, permanent tooth bud from root canal fillings. While magnifying these dangers, many authors have advocated extraction of pulpally involved, primary teeth and placement of space maintainers. However, there is no better space maintainer than the primary tooth. Also nothing has been written concerning the damage of space maintainers on existing teeth in the mouth. For many space maintainers that are placed, adequate follow-up is not achieved because of the carelessness of either the patient or the clinician.

Decalcification and rampant caries are frequent sequelae of loosened bands retained for extended periods of time. Poor oral hygiene around space maintainers contributes to increased decay and gingival problems. Deflection of erupting permanent teeth caused by prolonged retention of space maintainers is sometimes encountered. Loss of space maintainers with resulting space loss can occur if the patient delays returning for treatment. These are a few of the problems that may be avoided by retention of the pulpally involved, primary tooth when possible.

It has been reported[82] that although severe hypoplasia and disturbances in root development do not intensify, minor hypoplasia is increased in succedaneous teeth after root canal treatment of the primary precursors. Others[19] have reported the same amount of defects on the untreated side and concluded that there are no effects from primary pulpectomy on the succedaneous teeth. Enamel defects increased as the amount of preoperative, primary root resorption increased. It was summarized that defects result from the infection existing before the pulpectomy and not the procedure itself. It should be pointed out that all such studies are retrospective, involving erupted permanent teeth and, as such, cannot ascertain the causes of defects.

Economics has been advanced as an argument against endodontic treatment of primary teeth, but it is not a reasonable argument when compared with the cost of space maintainers, including the required follow-up treatment. In fact, endodontic treatment is probably the less expensive alternative when the entire treatment sequence is considered.

Success of endodontic treatment on primary teeth is judged by the same criteria that are used for permanent teeth. The treated primary tooth must remain firmly attached in function without pain or infection. Radiographic signs of furcal and periapical infection should be resolved with a normal periodontal attachment. The primary tooth should resorb normally and in no way interfere with the formation or eruption of the permanent tooth.

Success rates ranging from 75% to 96% have been reported.[4,81,107,224] The usual means of studying root canal filling on primary teeth have been clinical and radiographic. There exists a great need for histologic study in this area.

Early reports of endodontic treatment on primary teeth usually involved devitalization with arsenic in vital teeth and the use of creosote, formocresol, or paraformaldehyde pastes in nonvital teeth. The canals were filled with a variety of materials, usually consisting of zinc oxide and numerous additives.[42,64,85,193]

Rabinowitch published the first well-documented, scientific report of endodontic procedures on primary teeth in 1953.[160] A 13-year study of 1363 cases of partially or totally nonvital, primary molars was reported. Only seven cases were failures; most patients were followed for 1 or 2 years clinically and radiographically. Fillings of ZOE and silver nitrate were placed only after a negative culture result was obtained for each tooth. Periapically involved teeth required an average of 7.7 visits to complete treatment; teeth with no periapical involvement required an average of 5.5 visits. Rabinowitch listed internal resorption and gross pathologic external resorption as contraindications to primary root canal fillings.

Another well-documented study reported a success rate of 95% in vital and infected teeth using a filling material of thymol, cresol, iodoform, and zinc oxide.[4] (See Bennett[11] for a review of the techniques of partial and total pulpectomy.)

In a well-controlled, clinical study of primary root canals using Oxpara paste as the filling material,[107] five preexisting factors were reported to render the prognosis less favorable:

1. Perforation of the furcation
2. Excessive external resorption of roots
3. Internal resorption
4. Extensive bone loss
5. Periodontal involvement of the furcation.

When teeth with these factors were eliminated, a clinical success rate of 96% was achieved. When all symptoms of residual infection were resolved before filling of the canals, the success rate improved. No radiographic evidence of damage to the permanent teeth was noted.

After reviewing the literature on root canal fillings on primary teeth, it is clear that there is a lack of histologic material in this area. There exists a great need for further research on the subject.

Contraindications for Primary Root Canal Fillings

Except for the following six situations, all primary teeth with pulpal involvement that has spread beyond the coronal pulp are candidates for root canal fillings, whether they are vital or nonvital.

1. A nonrestorable tooth
2. Radiographically visible, internal resorption in the roots
3. Teeth with mechanical or carious perforations of the floor of the pulp chamber
4. Excessive pathologic root resorption involving more than one third of the root
5. Excessive pathologic loss of bone support with loss of the normal periodontal attachment
6. The presence of a dentigerous or follicular cyst

Internal resorption usually begins just inside the root canals near the furcation area. Because of the thinness of the roots of the primary teeth, once internal resorption has become visible radiographically, there is invariably a perforation of the root by the resorption (see Fig. 23-7). The short, furcal surface area of the primary teeth leads to rapid communication between the inflammatory process and the oral cavity through the periodontal attachment. The end result is loss of the periodontal attachment of the tooth and, ultimately, further resorption and loss of the tooth. Mechanical or carious perforations of the floor of the pulp chamber fail for the same reasons. It has been shown that root length is the most reliable criterion of root integrity, and at least 4 mm of root length is necessary for the primary tooth to be treatable.[169]

Access Openings for Pulpectomy on Primary Teeth

Access openings for endodontic treatment on primary or permanent, anterior teeth have traditionally been through the lingual surface. This continues to be the surface of choice (except for the maxillary, primary incisors); it has been recommended that the clinician use a facial approach followed by an acid-etched, composite restoration to improve aesthetics

(Fig. 23-16).[118] Bleaching techniques that are quite successful in permanent teeth are unsuccessful in primary teeth.

Many maxillary, primary incisors requiring pulpectomy have discoloration caused by the escape of hemosiderin pigments into the dentinal tubules after a previous traumatic injury. Subsequent to pulpectomy and root canal filling, most primary incisors discolor.

The anatomy of the maxillary, primary incisors is such that access may successfully be made from the facial surface. The only variation to the opening is more extension to the incisal edge than with the normal lingual access to give as straight an approach as possible into the root canal.

The root canal is filled with ZOE (see the following section); then the ZOE is carefully removed to near the cervical

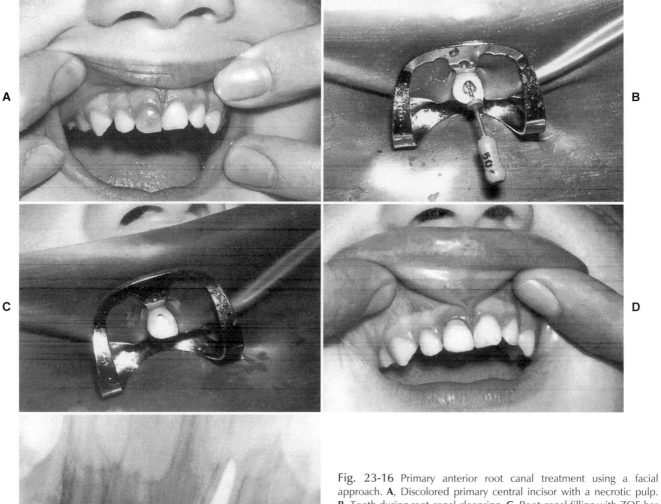

Fig. 23-16 Primary anterior root canal treatment using a facial approach. **A,** Discolored primary central incisor with a necrotic pulp. **B,** Tooth during root canal cleansing. **C,** Root canal filling with ZOE has been completed. ZOE was removed to the cervical line and a Dycal liner was placed over the dentin. Tooth has been acid etched. **D,** Composite resin has been bonded over the facial surface to achieve esthetics. **E,** Postoperative radiograph showing the completed procedures.

line. A liner of Dycal or Life is placed over the ZOE to serve as a barrier between the composite resin and the root canal filling. The liner is extended over the darkly stained, lingual dentin to serve as an opaquer. The access opening and entire facial surface are acid etched and restored with composite resin (see Fig. 23-16, *C,D*).

Unlike posterior primary teeth, anterior primary teeth have one canal without ramifications and lateral or accessory canals. Therefore primary, anterior root canals may be filled immediately after cleaning, provided the canal can be dried.

Posterior Teeth   Access openings into the posterior, primary root canals are essentially the same as those for the permanent teeth (see Chapter 7). Important differences between the primary and permanent teeth are the length of the crowns, the bulbous shape of the crowns, and the very thin dentinal walls of the pulpal floors and roots. The depth necessary to penetrate into the pulpal chamber is much less than that in the permanent teeth. Likewise, the distance from the occlusal surface to the pulpal floor of the pulp chamber is much less than in permanent teeth. In the primary molars, care must be taken not to grind on the pulpal floor because perforation is likely (Fig. 23-17).

When the roof of the pulp chamber is perforated and the pulp chamber identified, the entire roof should be removed with the bur. Because the crowns of the primary teeth are more bulbous, less extension toward the exterior of the tooth

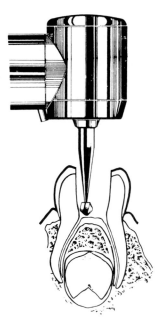

Fig. 23-17 Access opening in primary molar. A no. 4 round bur has been used to remove the root of the pulp chamber and the dentin ledges over the canal orifices. Note the minimal length of the bur needed to penetrate to the pulpal floor. Caution must be exercised to avoid perforation of the pulpal floor. (From Goerig AC, Camp JH: Root canal treatment in primary teeth-a review, *Pediatr Dent* 5:33, 1983.)

is necessary to uncover the openings of the root canals than in the permanent teeth.

As in permanent endodontic therapy, canal cleaning and shaping is one of the most important phases of primary root canal treatment. The main objective of the chemical and mechanical preparation of the primary tooth is débridement of the canals. Although an apical taper is desirable, it is not necessary to have an exact shape to the canals, because the filling is with an absorbable paste rather than gutta-percha. As with any endodontic procedure, use of the rubber dam is mandatory.

A preliminary working length is determined by measurement of a radiograph taken with a paralleling technique. The working length is then determined from a radiograph with an endodontic file in the canal. The use of apex locators may be unreliable because root resorption may create lateral openings into the periodontal tissues at any level.[169] To prevent overextension through the apical foramen, it is advisable that the working length be shortened to 2 to 3 mm short of the radiographic length, especially in teeth exhibiting signs of apical root resorption.

After establishment of the working length, the canal is cleaned and shaped (as described in Chapter 8). Because of the thin walls of the roots, sonic and ultrasonic cleaning devices should not be used to prepare the canals of primary teeth. Also the use of Gates-Glidden (GG) or Peeso drills is contraindicated because of the danger of perforation or stripping of the roots.

Because of their greater flexibility, nickel-titanium (NiTi) instruments are recommended rather than SS. Hand or rotary techniques are ideal for primary teeth. If SS files are used, the instruments must be gently curved to help negotiate the canals. Shaping of the canals proceeds in much the same manner as is done to receive a gutta-percha filling. Care must be taken not to perforate the thin roots during cleaning and shaping procedures. The canals are enlarged several sizes past the first file that fits snugly in the canal, with a minimal size of 30 to 35.

Because many of the pulpal ramifications cannot be reached mechanically, copious irrigation during cleaning and shaping must be maintained (see Chapter 8). Débridement of the primary root canal is more often accomplished by chemical means than by mechanical means.[102] This statement should not be misinterpreted as a deemphasis of the importance of thorough débridement and disinfection of the canal. The use of sodium hypochlorite to dissolve organic debris and RC-Prep to produce effervescence must play an important part in removal of tissue from the inaccessible areas of the root canal system.

After canal débridement the canals are again copiously flushed with sodium hypochlorite and are then dried with sterile paper points; a pellet of cotton is barely moistened with camphorated parachlorophenol (CMCP) and sealed into the pulp chamber with a temporary cement.

At a subsequent appointment the rubber dam is placed and the canals reentered. As long as the patient is free of all signs and symptoms of inflammation, the canals are again irrigated with sodium hypochloride and dried before filling. If signs or symptoms of inflammation are present, the canals are recleaned and remedicated and the filling procedure delayed until a later time.

Filling of the Primary Root Canals

The filling material for primary root canals must be absorbable so that it absorbs as the roots resorb and does not interfere with the eruption of the permanent tooth. Most reports in the U.S. literature have advocated the use of ZOE as the filler, whereas other parts of the world have used iodoform paste[81] (KRI paste, Pharmachemic AG, Zurich, Switzerland) or ZOE. The antibacterial activity of KRI paste has been shown to be less than ZOE, whereas its cytotoxicity in direct and indirect contact with cells is equal to and greater (respectively) than ZOE. *The filling material of choice is ZOE without a catalyst.* The lack of a catalyst is necessary to allow adequate working time for filling the canals. *The use of gutta-percha or silver points as primary root canal fillers is contraindicated.*

The filling of the primary tooth is usually performed without a local anesthetic. This is preferable, if possible, so the patient's response can be used to indicate approach to the apical foramen. It is, however, sometimes necessary to anesthetize the gingiva with a drop of anesthetic solution to place the rubber dam clamp without pain.

The ZOE is mixed to a thick consistency and is carried into the pulp chamber with a plastic instrument or on a lentulo spiral. The material may be packed into the canals with pluggers or the lentulo spiral. A cotton pellet held in cotton pliers and acting as a piston within the pulp chambers is quite effective in forcing the ZOE into the canals. The endodontic pressure syringe[12,66] is also effective for placing the ZOE in root canals. In a study of apical seal and quality of filling evaluated radiographically, no statistically significant differences were determined when the canal was filled with the lentulo spiral, pressure syringe, or incrementally with a plugger.[33]

Regardless of the method used to fill the canals, care should be taken to prevent extrusion of the material into the periapical tissues. It is reported that a significantly greater failure rate occurs with overfilling of ZOE than with filling just to the apex or slightly underfilling.[19,81] The adequacy of the obturation is checked by radiographs (Figs. 23-18, 23-19, and 23-20).

In the event a small amount of the ZOE is inadvertently forced through the apical foramen, it is left alone (because the material is absorbable). It has been reported that defects on succedaneous teeth have no relationship to length of the ZOE filling.[19]

When the canals are satisfactorily obturated, a fast-setting, temporary cement is placed in the pulp chamber to seal over the ZOE canal filling. The tooth may then be restored permanently. In the primary molars it is advisable to place an SS crown as the permanent restoration to prevent possible fracture of the tooth.

When the succedaneous, permanent tooth is missing and the retained primary tooth becomes pulpally involved, the canals are filled with gutta-percha after pulpectomy. Because eruption of the permanent tooth is not a factor in these cases, gutta-percha is substituted for ZOE as the filling material of choice (Fig. 23-21).

Follow-Up After Primary Pulpectomy

As previously stated, the rate of success after primary pulpectomy is high. However, these teeth should be periodically recalled to check for success of the treatment and to intercept any problem associated with a failure. Although resorbing normally without interference with the eruption of the permanent tooth, the primary tooth should remain asymptomatic, firm in the alveolus, and free of pathosis. If evidence of pathosis is detected, extraction and conventional space maintenance are recommended.

It has been pointed out[19,196] that pulpally treated primary teeth may occasionally present a problem of overretention. One study[19] reported 20% incidence of crossbites or palatal eruption of permanent incisors after pulpectomy on primary incisors. In the posterior, teeth extraction was required in 22% of cases because of ectopic eruption of the premolars or difficulty in exfoliation of the treated primary molar.[19] After normal physiologic resorption of the roots reaches the pulp chamber, the large amount of ZOE present may impair the absorption and lead to prolonged retention of the crown. Treatment usually consists of simply removing the crown and allowing the permanent tooth to complete its eruption.

Retention of ZOE in the tissues is a common sequela to primary pulpectomy. One long-term study reported that after loss of the tooth 50% of cases had retained ZOE. Teeth filled short of the apices had significantly less retained filler. In time most showed complete absorption or reducing amounts. Retention of filler was not related to success and caused no pathology.[173] Therefore no attempt is made to remove retained filler from the tissues (see Fig. 23-18, *E* and *G*; and Fig. 23-19, *D,E*).

PULPAL THERAPY FOR THE YOUNG, PERMANENT DENTITION

Pulpotomy

The pulpotomy procedure involves removing pulp tissue that has inflammatory or degenerative changes, leaving intact the remaining vital tissue, which is then covered with a pulp-capping agent to promote healing at the amputation site. (Pulp capping is discussed earlier in this chapter.) The only difference between pulpotomy and pulp capping is that in pulpotomy additional tissue is removed from the exposed pulp. Traditionally, the term *pulpotomy* has implied removal of pulp tissue to the cervical line. However, the depth to

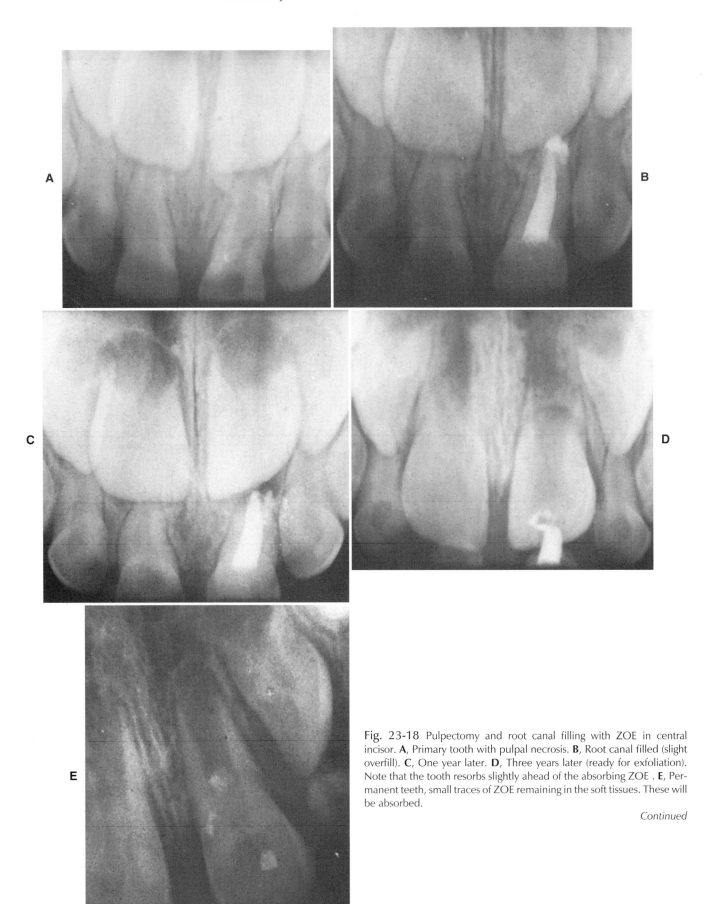

Fig. 23-18 Pulpectomy and root canal filling with ZOE in central incisor. **A**, Primary tooth with pulpal necrosis. **B**, Root canal filled (slight overfill). **C**, One year later. **D**, Three years later (ready for exfoliation). Note that the tooth resorbs slightly ahead of the absorbing ZOE. **E**, Permanent teeth, small traces of ZOE remaining in the soft tissues. These will be absorbed.

Continued

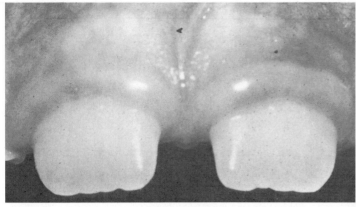

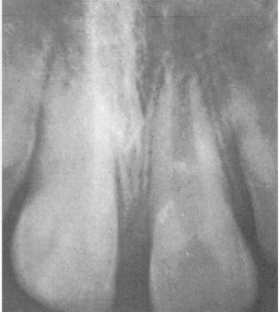

Fig. 23-18, cont'd **F**, Permanent central incisors newly erupted. Note that no defects are present on the crown even though there was a slight overfill of the primary root canal filling. **G**, Five years after pulpectomy and root canal filling. Note the normal apical closure and the almost total absorption of the ZOE remnants.

which tissue is removed is determined by clinical judgment. All tissue judged to be inflamed should be removed to place the dressing on healthy, uninflamed pulp tissue. Better results are obtained if the amputation level is shallow because of better visualization of the working area. In multirooted teeth the procedure may be simplified by removing tissue to the orifices of the root canals.

The difficulties of assessing the extent of inflammation in cariously exposed pulps have been previously discussed. However, several studies[31,75,76] have shown that inflammation is confined to the surface 2 to 3 mm of the pulp when traumatically exposed and left untreated for up to 168 hours. In experimental animals the results were the same whether the crowns were fractured or ground off. Direct invasion of vital pulp tissue by bacteria did not occur, although the pulps were left exposed to the saliva. Under the same circumstances with cavity preparations into the teeth that left areas to impact food, debris, and bacteria in contact with the pulp, the inflammation ranged from 1 to 9 mm with abscess and pus formation.[31,75] The same results have been obtained in permanent teeth with incompletely formed roots and teeth with mature roots. (Pulpotomy procedures for primary teeth were discussed earlier in this chapter.)

The Cvek Pulpotomy on Young, Immature, Permanent Teeth

Despite the fact that vital pulp-capping and pulpotomy procedures for cariously exposed pulps in teeth with developed apices remain controversial, it is universally accepted that vital techniques be employed in those teeth with incompletely developed apexes. Although many materials and drugs have been used as pulp-capping agents, the application of calcium hydroxide to stimulate dentin bridge formation in accidentally or cariously exposed pulps of young, permanent teeth has traditionally been the treatment of choice. (See the previous sections on pulp-capping agents for discussion of other materials and techniques.)

The indirect pulp therapy technique should be used whenever possible with deep carious lesions to avoid exposure of the pulp. Every attempt should be made to maintain the vitality of these immature teeth until their full-root development has been completed. Loss of vitality before root completion leaves a weak root more prone to fracture. Loss of vitality before completion of root length may leave a poor crown-to-root ratio and a tooth more susceptible to periodontal breakdown because of excessive mobility. If necessary, the remaining pulp tissue can be extirpated and conventional endodontic therapy completed when root formation has been accomplished.

Endodontic treatment is greatly complicated in teeth with necrotic pulps and open apices. Although apexification procedures have been perfected for these teeth, the treatment is extensive and costly for the patient and the resulting root structure is weaker than in teeth with fully developed roots. If the pulpotomy is not successful, the apexification procedure or surgical endodontics may still be performed.

Technique   After the diagnosis is completed, the tooth is anesthetized. If possible, pulpal procedures should always be performed under rubber dam isolation and aseptic conditions to prevent further introduction of microorganisms into the pulp tissues. Care must be taken when placing the rubber dam on a traumatized tooth. If any loosening of the tooth has occurred, the rubber dam clamps must be applied to adjacent uninjured teeth. If this is impossible because of lack of adja-
Text continued on p. 829

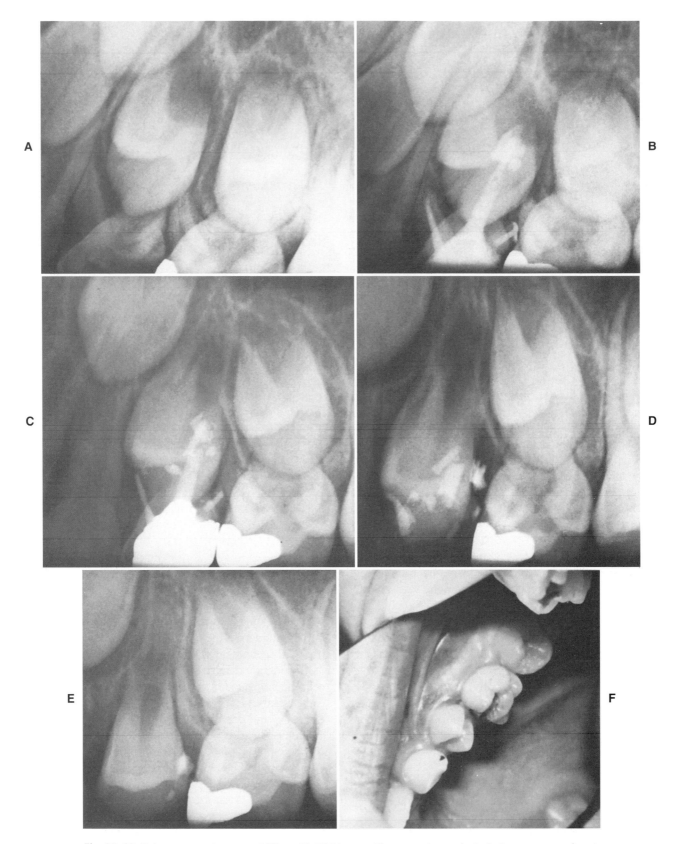

Fig. 23-19 Pulpectomy and root canal filling with ZOE in a maxillary posterior tooth. **A**, Carious exposure of a primary first molar. **B**, Root canals filled with ZOE. **C**, One year later. **D**, Two and one half years later. Tooth is ready to exfoliate. **E**, Erupted permanent premolar. Note the slight amount of ZOE retained in the soft tissue. ZOE will undergo absorption. **F**, Note the permanent crown that is free of defects.

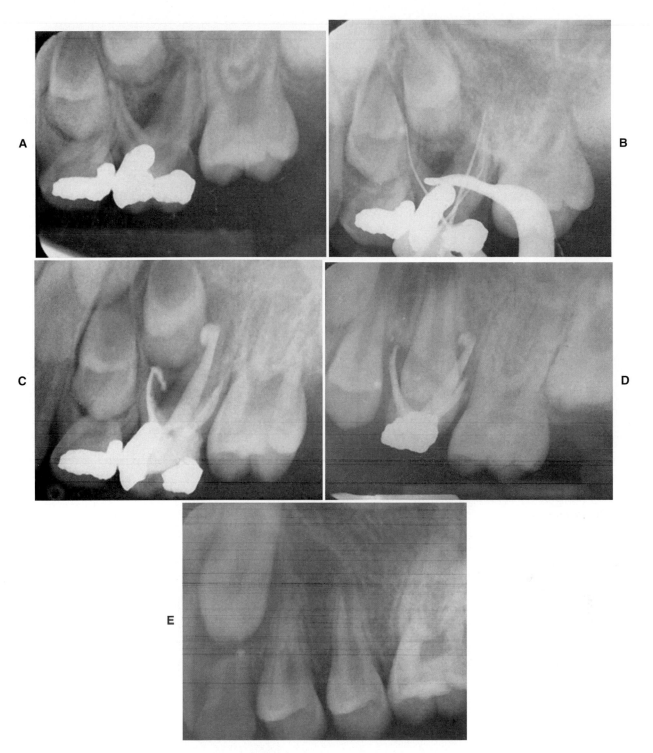

Fig. 23-20 Pulpectomy and root canal filling with ZOE in a maxillary primary second molar. **A,** Carious pulp exposure with a chronic abscess. Note the furcal and periapical radiolucencies. **B,** Instruments in place establishing the working length. **C,** Root canal filled with ZOE. **D,** Four and one half years after root canal treatment. Tooth is near exfoliation. **E,** One year later. Premolar is fully erupted and all traces of the ZOE have been resorbed.

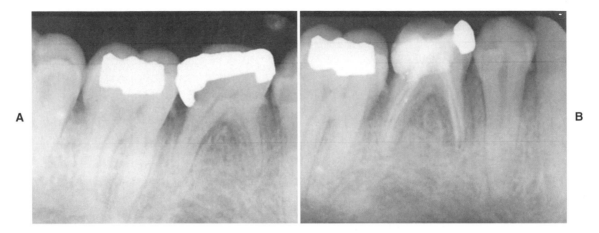

Fig. 23-21 Pulpectomy and root canal filling with gutta-percha in a retained mandibular primary second molar with no succedaneous permanent tooth. **A,** Carious exposure of pulp. **B,** Because the permanent premolar is absent, the root canals of the primary tooth were filled with gutta-percha rather than ZOE.

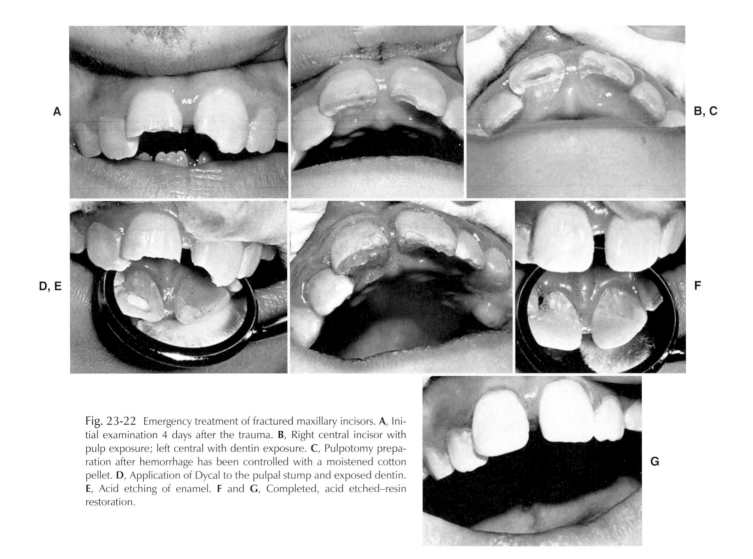

Fig. 23-22 Emergency treatment of fractured maxillary incisors. **A,** Initial examination 4 days after the trauma. **B,** Right central incisor with pulp exposure; left central with dentin exposure. **C,** Pulpotomy preparation after hemorrhage has been controlled with a moistened cotton pellet. **D,** Application of Dycal to the pulpal stump and exposed dentin. **E,** Acid etching of enamel. **F** and **G,** Completed, acid etched–resin restoration.

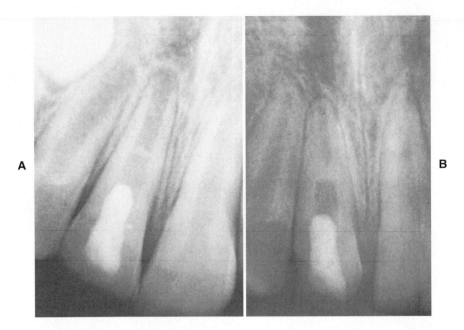

Fig. 23-23 Deep calcium hydroxide pulpotomy. **A**, Central incisor with an immature apex 10 weeks after a traumatic exposure of the pulp and a calcium hydroxide pulpotomy. Note the dentin bridge. **B**, Three years after pulpotomy. Note the thickening of the dentin bridge and the completion of root development. Tooth remained asymptomatic. No further endodontic treatment is indicated at this time.

cent teeth or partially erupted ones that cannot be clamped, careful isolation with cotton rolls and constant aspiration by the dental assistant may be used to maintain a dry field (Fig. 23-22).

In traumatically exposed pulps, only tissue judged to be inflamed is removed. Cvek[28] has shown that with pulp exposures resulting from traumatic injuries, regardless of the size of the exposure or the amount of lapsed time, pulpal changes are characterized by a proliferative response with inflammation extending only a few millimeters into the pulp. When this hyperplastic, inflamed tissue is removed, healthy pulp tissue is encountered.[28] In teeth with carious exposure of the pulp, it may be necessary to remove pulp tissue to a greater depth to reach uninflamed tissue.

The instrument of choice for tissue removal in the pulpotomy procedure is an abrasive diamond bur, using high-speed, adequate water cooling. This technique has been shown to create the least damage to the underlying tissue.[65] Care must be exercised to ensure removal of all filaments of the pulp tissue coronal to the amputation site; otherwise, hemorrhage will be impossible to control. After pulpal amputation, the preparation is thoroughly washed with physiologic saline or sterile water to remove all debris; the water is removed by vacuum and cotton pellets. Air should not be blown on the exposed pulp, because it will cause desiccation and tissue damage.

Hemorrhage is controlled by cotton pellets slightly moistened with saline (i.e., wetted and blotted almost dry) placed against the stumps of the pulp. Completely dry cotton pellets should not be used, because fibers of the dry cotton will be incorporated into the clot and, when removed, will cause hemorrhage. Dry cotton pellets are placed over the moist pellets, and slight pressure is exerted on the mass to control the hemorrhage. Hemorrhage should be controlled in this manner within several minutes (see Fig. 23-22, *C*). It may be necessary to change the pellets to control all hemorrhage. If hemorrhage continues, the clinician must carefully check to be sure that all filaments of the pulp coronal to the amputation site were removed and that the site is clean.

The use of sodium hydrochloride (NaOCl) to control pulpal hemorrhage before pulp capping has been reported. According to these researchers,[2,23] 2.5% NaOCl is placed on the exposure site to cause hemostasis. It also has the beneficial effect of killing bacteria. It was reported that when used as a hemostatic agent there was no damage to pulpal cells and it did not inhibit pulpal healing, odontoblastic cell formation, or dentinal bridging.

If hemorrhage cannot be controlled, amputation should be performed at a more apical level. Should it become necessary to extend into the root canals, a small endodontic spoon or round, abrasive, diamond bur may be used to remove the tissue on anterior teeth with single canals (Fig. 23-23). On posterior teeth the use of endodontic files or reamers may be necessary if tissue is being amputated within the canals. *Obviously, extension of the amputation site is carried into the root canals only in teeth with blunderbuss apices* (Fig. 23-24).

On teeth with blunderbuss apices, if tissue removal has been extended several millimeters into the root canals and hemorrhage continues, a compromise treatment should be

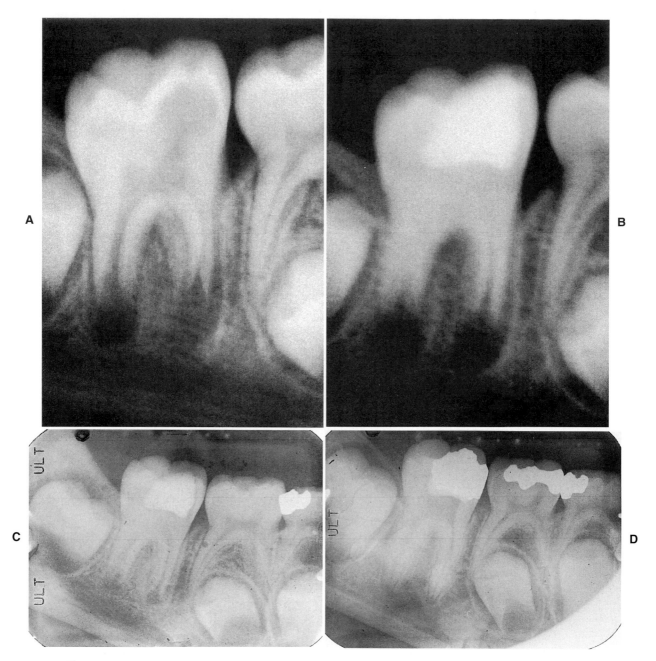

Fig. 23-24 Apexogenesis following a deep calcium hydroxide pulpotomy on a mandibular permanent first molar. **A,** Pre-operative radiograph showing extensive caries, incomplete root development, and possible periapical involvement. The tooth was symptomatic. **B,** Upon entry into the pulp chamber, vital tissue was encountered. Pulpal tissue was removed several millimeters into the canals, hemorrhage controlled, and calcium hydroxide placed on the pulp stumps. **C,** One year later the periapical lesion is healed and root formation is continuing. **D,** Two years later root formation is completed.

considered. The hemorrhage is controlled with chemicals, such as aluminum chloride or other hemostatic agents. Once the hemorrhage is controlled, calcium hydroxide is placed in the canal against the pulp stump and the tooth is sealed. These compromised teeth must be closely monitored for development of pathologic conditions. If necrosis of the remaining pulp tissue occurs, apexification procedures are instituted. If vitality is maintained, further root development

with dystrophic calcification usually occurs. In these compromised cases (once the apex has formed) the tooth is reentered and conventional endodontic therapy is completed with gutta-percha obliteration.

In the normal pulpotomy procedure (once the hemorrhage has been controlled) a dressing of calcium hydroxide is placed over the amputation site (Fig. 23-25). If the pulpal amputation extends into the tooth only a few millimeters, the

Fig. 23-25 Calcium hydroxide pulpotomy on a maxillary permanent incisor with an immature apex. **A,** Pre-operative radiograph following traumatic exposures of the pulp. Calcium hydroxide was placed following a Cvek pulpotomy. **B,** Four months later a dentin bridge is seen beneath the calcium hydroxide. **C,** Three years later the root formation has been completed. Note the dentin bridge has not thickened.

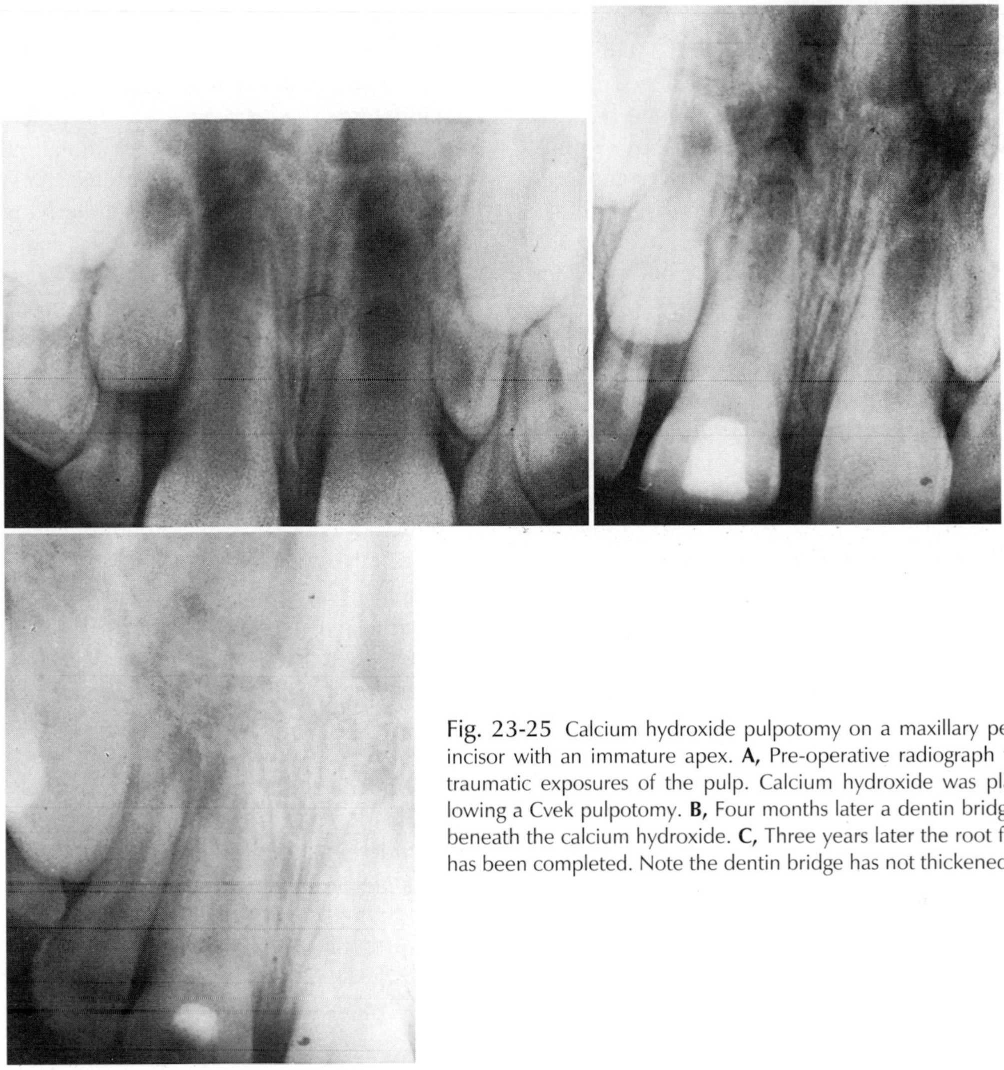

use of a hard-setting material (e.g., Dycal or Life) is usually easiest. However, for deeper amputation, calcium hydroxide powder carried to the tooth in an amalgam carrier is the easiest method of application. The amalgam carried is tightly packed with powder, then all but one fourth to one third of the pellet is expressed from the carrier and discarded. The remaining calcium hydroxide in the carrier is then expressed into the preparation side. The pellet of calcium hydroxide powder is carefully teased against the pulp stump with a rounded-end, plastic instrument. The entire pulp stump must be covered with a thin layer of calcium hydroxide. Care must be taken not to pack the calcium hydroxide into the pulp tissue, because this causes greater inflammation and increases the changes of failure or, if pulpotomy is successful, there is increased calcification of the remaining pulp tissues around the particles of calcium hydroxide.[213]

Pulpdent (i.e., calcium hydroxide in a methylcellulose base) may also be used for the pulpotomy procedure. If commercial preparations of calcium hydroxide are used, care must be taken to avoid trapping air bubbles when applying the material. If Pulpdent or another nonhard-setting material is applied to the pulp stumps, a hard-setting material (e.g., Dycal, Life, a glass ionomer[29]) must be flowed over this and allowed to set completely. When a composite resin restoration is to be used, eugenol-containing compounds must be avoided because they interfere with the setting reaction of the composite.

A permanent type of restoration should always be placed in the tooth to ensure the retention of the pulp-capping material. Unless a crown is necessary the material of choice is usually a bonded composite restoration.

PARTIAL PULPOTOMY FOR YOUNG, PERMANENT, POSTERIOR TEETH

A technique termed *partial pulpotomy for the management of vital carious pulp exposure on young permanent molars* has been reported by several researchers.[120,121,125,145] The procedure is usually reserved for teeth with little or no history of pain; absence of radiographic signs of periapical pathosis or resorption; and lack of percussion sensitivity, swelling, or mobility.

The procedure involves the removal of pulp tissue beneath the exposure site judged to be inflamed (usually 1 to 3 mm) to reach healthy tissue below. After hemorrhage is controlled, the exposure site is covered with calcium hydroxide and the tooth sealed with ZOE and a permanent restoration. The use of MTA as the capping agent has successfully been used by the authors.

Mejare and Cvek[125] reported a success rate of 91% in cases with no clinical or radiographic signs of pathology. Of the 31 cases, 29 were successful when followed 24 to 140 months. The same study reported that four of six cases with temporary pain and radiographic signs of minor periapical involvement responded successfully. Another study[120] reported a success rate of 91.4% in 35 cases followed between 12 to 48 months. Exposures exceeding 2 mm, or those in which bleeding was not controlled in 1 to 2 minutes, were excluded from the study.

Before initiating treatment it is critical to evaluate the degree of pulp inflammation in an attempt to distinguish between reversible and irreversible pulpitis. Although the correlation between clinical and histologic evaluation is poor, young, permanent teeth are good candidates for this conservative treatment because of their rich blood supply that enhances the healing ability. Because the loss of the pulp in teeth with immature apexes is so devastating, it seems advisable to attempt the partial pulpotomy procedure. If failure occurs, apexification can always be performed.

Follow-Up After Pulp Capping and Pulpotomy

After pulp capping and pulpotomy, the patient should be recalled periodically for 2 to 4 years to determine success. Although the normal vitality tests (e.g., electrical and thermal sensitivity tests) are reliable after pulp capping, they are usually not helpful in the pulpotomized tooth. Although histologic success cannot be determined, clinical success is judged by the absence of any clinical or radiographic signs of pathosis, the verification of a dentin bridge (both radiographically and clinically), and the presence of continued root development in teeth with incompletely formed roots.

Controversy exists as to whether the pulp should be reentered after the completion of root development in the pulpotomized tooth. Some researchers[106,180] believe that pulp capping and pulpotomy procedures invariably lead to progressive calcification of the root canals. After successful root development, they advocate extirpation of the remaining pulp tissue and endodontic treatment. They recommend endodontic therapy because of the high incidence of continued calcification, which would render the canals nonnegotiable at some future time when (because of disease)

endodontic therapy might be required. However, it has been the experience of others[30,57,76] that (with good case selection) progressive calcification of the pulp is an infrequent sequela of pulpotomy if a gentle technique is used in removing pulp tissue, care is taken to avoid contamination of the pulp with bacteria and dentin chips, and the dressing of calcium hydroxide is not packed into the underlying pulp tissue (see Fig. 23-23).

In a follow-up study of clinically successful pulpotomies previously reported,[28] researchers[30] removed the pulps 1 to 5 years later for restorative reasons and found histologically normal pulps. They concluded that changes seen in the pulps do not represent sufficient histologic evidence to support routine pulpectomy after pulpotomy in accidentally fractured teeth with pulp exposures. Thus the routine reentry to remove the pulp and place a root canal filling after completion of root development is contraindicated unless dictated by restorative considerations, such as the necessity for retentive post placement. Nevertheless, canal calcification, internal resorption, and pulp necrosis are potential sequelae of pulp-capping and pulpotomy procedures. Although unlikely, they are possible, and the patient should be clearly informed.

In posterior teeth where surgical endodontics is difficult, if continued calcification of the canal is observed after root closure, reentry of the tooth for endodontic therapy is recommended. In anterior teeth, if calcification of the canal has made conventional endodontics impossible, surgical endodontics may be performed with relative ease. Therefore in anterior teeth, routine endodontic therapy after completion of root development is contraindicated unless clinical signs and symptoms of pathosis are present or unless such therapy is necessary for restorative procedures (e.g., placement of a post for retention of a crown because of missing tooth structure) (Fig. 23-26).

Formocresol Pulpotomy on Young, Permanent Teeth

Because of the reported clinical and histologic success with the formocresol pulpotomy on primary teeth, there has been much interest in this technique on young, permanent teeth. Evidence of continued apical development after formocresol pulpotomy procedures on young, permanent teeth with incompletely developed apexes has been reported.[49,133,174,216] Several authors have reported better results with diluted formocresol. However, they reported a high incidence of internal resorption, which increased in severity with longer periods of time.[56,155]

The formocresol procedure has appeal because there is a lack of calcification of the remaining pulp tissue, as may be seen with calcium hydroxide pulpotomy. After root completion the tooth can easily be reentered, the pulp extirpated, and routine endodontic therapy performed. Contrary to these findings, one group of researchers[7] has shown calcification of

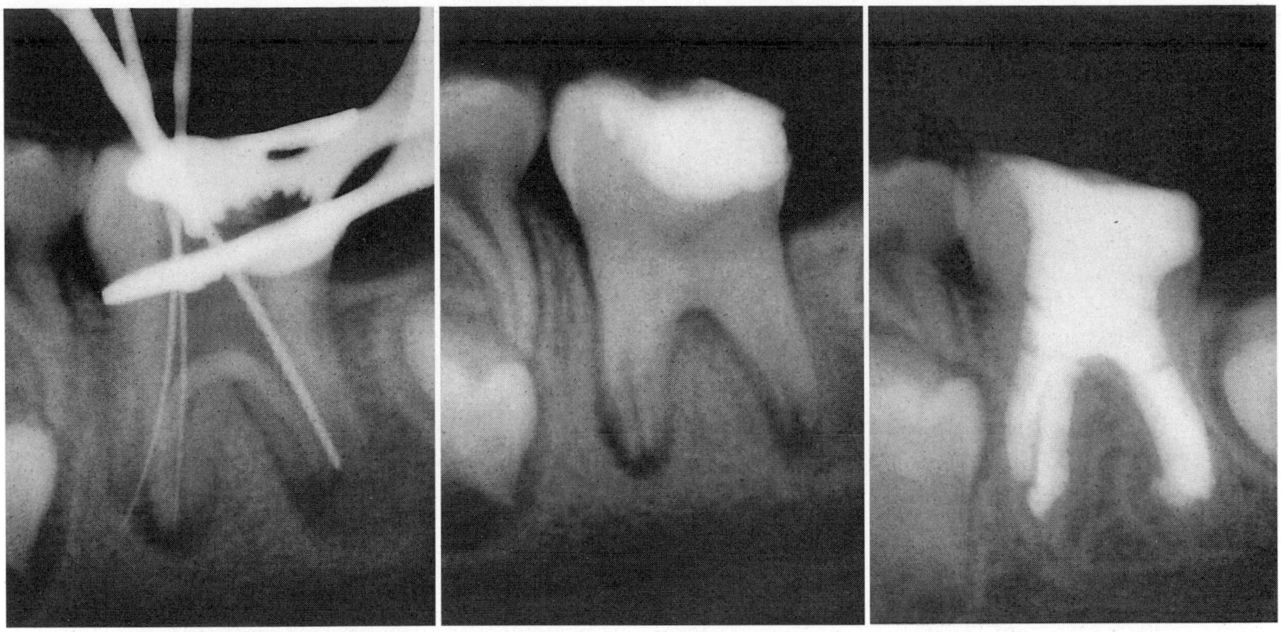

Fig. 23-26 Apexification on a mandibular permanent molar. **A,** Radiograph of endodontic files in canals establishing the length. Calcium hydroxide was placed in the canals. **B,** Radiograph 1 year later shows the apices closing. **C,** Apexification is completed 2 years after initiation of treatment, and the canals have been obliterated with gutta percha.

the canals by continuous apposition of dentin on the lateral walls with equal frequency whether using calcium hydroxide or formocresol. The only common denominator to this reaction was the presence of dentin chips that had accidentally been pushed into the radicular pulp tissue.

A retrospective study using clinical and radiographic criteria reported successful results; however, there was a high degree of root canal obliteration by calcification, which might preclude future root canal treatment.[204]

Other studies[94,132] have shown complete replacement of the pulp tissue with granulation tissue and the formation of osteodentin along the walls of the canals in permanent teeth after formocresol pulpotomies. The reaction was described as a healing rather than a destructive process, but persistent, chronic inflammation was noted.

Although this treatment has been reported to be partly successful, it cannot be routinely recommended until further research showing the technique to be successful (i.e., safe and effective) has been completed.

Formocresol pulpotomy procedures have been reported as temporary treatments on permanent teeth with necrotic pulps. Clinical success after 3 years has been reported.[209] The formocresol pulpotomy was performed rather than extraction when routine endodontic therapy could not be completed because of financial considerations. Complete endodontic treatment was advocated at a later date, with the formocresol pulpotomy used only as a *temporary* treatment.

APEXIFICATION

A thorough knowledge of normal root formation is necessary to help the clinician understand the processes involved in treatment of the pulpless, permanent tooth with a wide open immature apex.

Endodontic management of the pulpless, permanent tooth with a wide-open blunderbuss apex has long presented a challenge to dentistry. Before the introduction of apical closure techniques, the usual approach to this problem was surgical. Although the surgical approach was successful, the mechanical and psychologic aspects offered many contraindications. In the pulpless tooth with an incompletely formed apex, the thin, fragile dentinal walls made it difficult to achieve an apical seal. When a portion of the root was removed to obtain a seal, the crown-to-root ratio was poor. Because this situation was usually present in the child patient, a less traumatic approach was desirable.

Many techniques have been advocated to manage the pulpless, permanent tooth with an incompletely developed apex. The most widely accepted technique involves cleaning and filling the canal with a temporary paste to stimulate the formation of calcified tissue at the apex. The temporary paste is later removed after radiographic evidence of apical closure has been obtained, and a permanent filling of gutta-percha is placed in the canal. The term *apexification* is used to describe this procedure (see Figs. 23-26) (Fig. 23-27).[197]

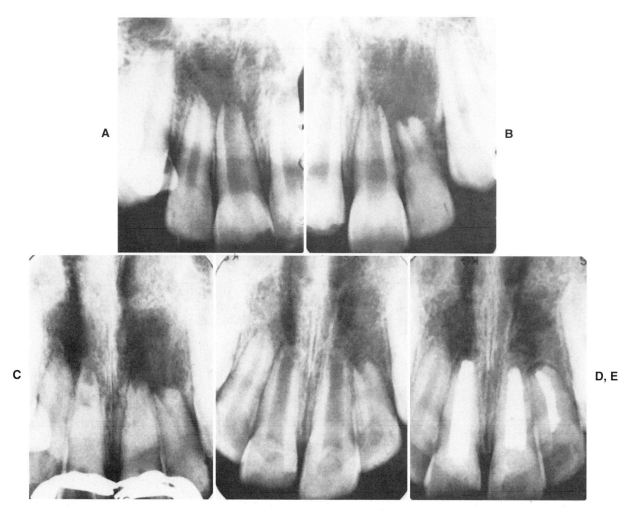

Fig. 23-27 Apexification in three permanent incisors, using calcium hydroxide–camphorated parachlorophenol filling material. **A** and **B,** Open apices of the three incisors with periapical pathosis. Note the calcification that has occurred in the lateral incisor before pulpal necrosis. **C,** Calcium hydroxide–camphorated parachlorophenol filling placed in two teeth. Note the void in the left incisor requiring further filling. **D,** Radiographic appearance of apexification one year later. **E,** Permanent root canal filling of gutta-percha after apexification.

An alternate approach in which a material is packed into the apical 2 to 4 mm of the blunderbuss canal to act as a barrier against which gutta-percha is condensed is becoming accepted as the treatment of choice. (Materials and techniques for this method to achieve apexification will be discussed later in this section.)

Diagnosis of pulpal necrosis in the tooth with an incompletely formed apex is sometimes difficult unless a frank exposure of the pulp chamber exists.

The usual cause of endodontic involvement in a tooth with an incompletely developed root is trauma. A detailed history and documentation of any injury (for insurance and dental and legal reasons) is of prime importance from both a diagnostic and a treatment point of view.

Radiographic diagnosis of disease is complicated in these teeth because of the normal radiolucency occurring at the apex as the root matures. Comparison of root formation with that in contralateral teeth should always be considered.

The electrical pulp tester usually does not provide meaningful data in teeth with incompletely formed roots. Thermal tests are more reliable for ascertaining vitality but may be complicated by the reliability of the response in the young child.

The presence of acute or chronic pain, percussion sensitivity, mobility, and any discoloration of the crown should be considered in the diagnosis.

In the tooth without a pulp exposure—if any doubt persists after all the foregoing tests have been completed—the clinician should take a watch-and-wait approach before entering the tooth endodontically to be certain that conclusive evidence of pulpal necrosis exists. If dentin exposure is present, the tooth must be restored in such a manner as to prevent any further pulpal irritation.

Although highly successful, apexification should be the treatment of last resort in a tooth that has incompletely formed roots. Attention should be focused on the mainte-

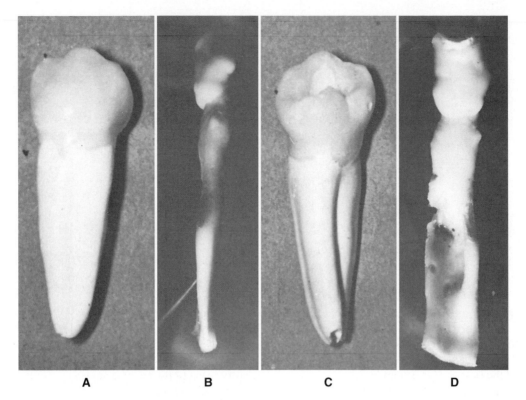

Fig. 23-28 Extracted mandibular premolar and silicone model of the root system. **A**, Facial view. **B**, Model from the facial surface. Note that the root canal diverges apically, which would correspond to the radiographic view of the tooth in the mouth. **C**, Lingual view. **D**, Model from the proximal view (apically divergent canal). With further development the root canal system will divide into two canals.

nance of vitality in these teeth so that as much root length and dentin formation as possible can occur in the root. Indirect pulp therapy and vital pulp-capping and pulpotomy techniques have proved to be successful, aided by the tremendous blood supply present with the open apex. These procedures should be the treatment of choice if there is the possibility of success with any of them. When the tooth with an incompletely formed apex becomes pulpless or periapical disease has developed, apexification is the preferred treatment.

Apexification has been reported in an adult after failed conventional endodontic treatment and apicoectomy performed in childhood.[221] It has also been achieved during active orthodontic treatment.[5]

Determination of the extent of apical closure is many times more difficult to ascertain. Radiographic interpretation of apical closure is often misleading. It must always be remembered that the dental radiograph is a two-dimensional picture of a three-dimensional object. Under normal conditions, the dental radiograph shows the mesiodistal plane of the tooth, rather than the faciolingual plane. The faciolingual aspect of the root canal, however, is usually the last to become convergent apically as the root develops. Therefore it is possible to have a dental radiograph showing an apically convergent root canal, whereas in the faciolingual plane the root canal is divergent (Fig. 23-28).

In teeth with vital tissue remaining in the root canal, techniques to maintain the vitality, rather then pulpectomy, should be used until complete root formation has occurred.

Many materials have been reported to successfully stimulate apexification. The use of calcium hydroxide for apexification in the pulpless tooth was first reported by Kaiser in 1964.[87] The technique was popularized by the work of Frank.[52] Since that time, calcium hydroxide alone or in combination with other drugs has become the most widely accepted material to promote apexification.

The calcium hydroxide powder has been mixed with CMCP, metacresyl acetate, Cresanol (i.e., a mixture of CMCP and metacresyl acetate), physiologic saline, Ringer's solutions, distilled water, and anesthetic solution. Although some of these materials appear to enhance the action of the calcium hydroxide better than others, all have been reported to stimulate apexification. Most reports in the U.S. literature [17,70,198] have advocated mixing the calcium hydroxide with CMCP or Cresanol, whereas reports from other parts of the world[27,123] show the same success using distilled water or physiologic saline as the vehicle with which the calcium hydroxide is mixed. The addition of barium sulfate to calcium hydroxide to enhance radiopacity has been shown to produce apexification. The recommended ratio of barium sulfate is one part added to eight parts calcium hydroxide.[217]

In the teeth of humans and animals, tricalcium phosphate,[101,170] collagen calcium phosphate,[143] osteogenic protein-1,[181] bone growth factors,[207] and MTA[181,207] have been reported to promote apexification similar to that found with calcium hydroxide.

Numerous other materials to promote apexification have been studied with mixed results. Webber[217] provides expanded data on these materials. Although apexification occurs with many materials, it has been reported even without the presence of canal-filling material after removal of the necrotic pulp tissue.[46] The most important factors in achieving apexification seem to be thorough débridement of the root canal (to remove all necrotic pulp tissue) and sealing of the tooth (to prevent the ingress of bacteria and substrate). Apexification does not occur when the apex of the tooth penetrates the cortical plate. To be successful, the apex must be completely within the confines of the cortical plates.

Calcium Hydroxide Technique

In the apexification technique the canal is cleaned and disinfected (as described in Chapter 8). As in any endodontic procedure, the use of the rubber dam is mandatory.

The access opening is made as usual but may require some extension, especially in the anterior teeth, to accommodate the larger instruments necessary to clean the root canals.

The length of the canal is established radiographically, and the canal is cleaned as thoroughly as possible. Frequent irrigation with sodium hypochlorite helps remove debris from the canal. Because the coronal half of the root canal is of smaller diameter than the apical half, root canal instruments that are smaller than the canal space must be used. Thus while mechanically cleaning and reshaping the canal, the clinician should lean the instruments toward each surface of the tooth to contact all surfaces of the root because the canal diverges apically. Sonic and ultrasonic devices are extremely helpful in débriding the canal.

After thorough débridement the canal is dried and just *minimally* medicated with CMCP or some other suitable intracanal medicament. The canal is then sealed with a temporary cement.

If symptoms persist or any signs of infection are present at a subsequent appointment or if the canal cannot be dried, the débridement phase is repeated and the canal is medicated with a slurry of calcium hydroxide paste and sealed.

When the tooth is free of signs and symptoms of infection, the canal is dried and filled with a stiff mix of calcium hydroxide and CMCP. The filling procedure is usually performed without the use of local anesthetic. This is preferable if possible so that the patient's response can be used to indicate the approach to the apical foramen.

The material should be spatulated as little possible, because spatulation decreased the working time and may cause the material to set into a semihard mass before the filling procedure is completed. If this happens, the canal may contain voids and should be recleaned; the filling procedure is then repeated.

The paste may be carried into the canal with an amalgam carrier, lentulo spiral, disposable syringe, or endodontic pressure syringe. Pluggers are helpful for packing the material to the apex. The addition of some dry calcium hydroxide powder within the canal by means of an amalgam carrier aids in condensing the paste of the apex. The canal should ideally be completely filled with the paste but should not be overfilled. The response of the patient is used as a guide in approaching the apex; however, because of differences in patient response, this method is not wholly reliable. Radiographic checks of the depth of the filling are essential to verify an adequate filling. The addition of small amounts of barium sulfate to the paste aids in radiographic interpretation without altering the response of the material.

Commercial pastes of calcium hydroxide (e.g., Calasept, Pulpdent, Hypo-cal, Calyxl) may be used to fill the canals. In this technique, the paste is placed in the canal via the sterile needle supplied with the paste. The liquid portion of the paste is then absorbed with paper points placed into the canal. Injection and absorption of the liquid are repeated until filling of the canal is achieved. Compaction of the dried paste with pluggers is necessary to completely obliterate the canal space.

It has been reported that successful apexification can occur with an overfill of material; in fact it has been reported that an overfill is preferable to an underfill.[17] In the event of an overfill, the material (being absorbable) is not removed from the apical tissues. The presence of an overfill rarely causes postoperative pain.

After the canal is filled, the access opening must be sealed with a permanent filling material. If the outer seal is defective, the calcium hydroxide paste is lost and recontamination of the canal results. For this reason, a temporary type of cement should never be used to seal the tooth after the filling procedure. Composite resin or silicate cement is recommended for anterior teeth and amalgam for posterior teeth.

Periodic Recall with Calcium Hydroxide Technique

The usual time required to achieve apexification is 6 to 24 months (average 1 year ± 7 months).[99] Factors that lead to increased time are the presence of a radiolucent lesion, interappointment symptoms, and loss of the external seal with reinfection of the canal.

During this time the patient is recalled at 3-month intervals for monitoring of the tooth. It has been reported[18] that following the initial root filling with calcium hydroxide, nothing is gained by repeated filling (either monthly or after 3 months for at least 6 months).

If any signs or symptoms of reinfection or pathology occur at any time during this phase of treatment, the canal is recleaned and refilled with the calcium hydroxide paste. The

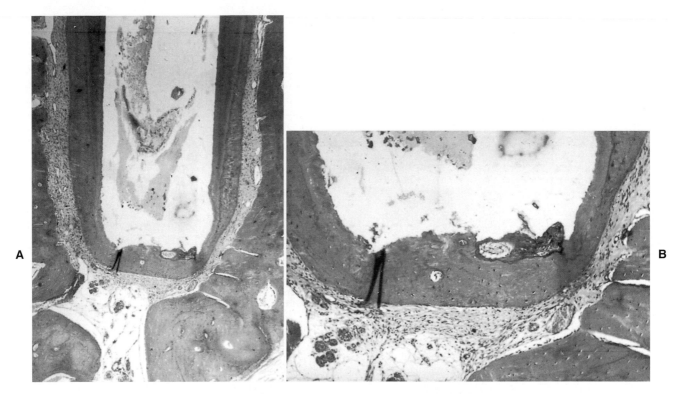

Fig. 23-29 Histologic sections of a dog's tooth after apexification. **A,** Cementumlike calcified tissue is closing the wide open apical foramen. Note the presence of debris within the canal because of inadequate cleaning of the canal before filling. **B,** Higher magnification showing cellular detail. Periodontal ligament is free of inflammation. Filling material, calcium hydroxide–camphorated parachlorophenol, was lost during processing. Note the presence of tissue communication through the calcified tissue. (Stain: H & E).

patient is recalled until radiographic evidence of apexification has become apparent. Then the tooth is reentered and clinical verification of apexification is made by the failure of a small instrument to penetrate through the apex after removal of the calcium hydroxide paste. The canal is then obturated with gutta-percha in the usual manner. Because of the large size of the canal, it may be necessary to prepare a customized gutta-percha point (see Chapter 9).

If apexification is incomplete, the canal is repacked with the calcium hydroxide paste, and the periodic recall continues.

Histology of Apexification with Calcium Hydroxide

The calcified material that forms over the apical foramen has been histologically identified as an osteoid (i.e., bonelike) or cementoid (i.e., cementumlike) material by investigators who have done apexification after periapical involvement of the treated teeth.[17,70,197] The formation of osetodentin after the placement of calcium hydroxide paste immediately on conclusion of a vital pulpectomy has also been reported.[41]

Histologic studies consistently report the absence of Hertwig's epithelial root sheath. Normal root formation usually does not occur after apexification. Instead, there appears to be a differentiation of adjacent connective tissue cells into specialized cells; there is also deposition of calcified tissue adjacent to the filling material. The calcified material is continuous with the lateral root surfaces. The closure of the apex may be partial or complete but consistently has minute communications with the periapical tissues (Fig. 23-29). For this reason, apexification must always be followed by filling of the canal with a permanent root canal filling of gutta-percha.

Various types of apical closure have been reported in clinical studies of apexification. In view of the histologic evidence of subsequent studies, it would appear that these types of apical closure simply relate to the level to which the filling material was placed within or beyond the apical foramen.

Many of the failures of apexification have been shown histologically to arise from the difficulty of adequately cleaning and sanitizing the wide-open canals. The tooth with an apically divergent root canal is much more difficult to clean thoroughly than is the mature tooth, which becomes increasingly smaller as the apex is approached.

Although the formation of calcified tissue was noted in the presence of mild inflammation,[17] the results were consistently better in specimens that were free of inflammation. It is recommended, therefore, that the cleaning and filling pro-

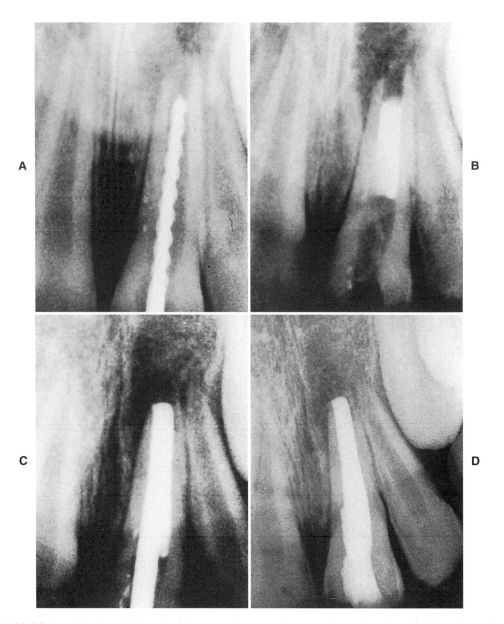

Fig. 23-30 Apexification with the apical barrier technique. **A,** Pre-operative radiograph establishing the working length. **B,** Radiograph of MTA placed slightly short of apex. After calculating the remaining distance to the apex, the MTA is forced to the root end. **C,** Filling the canal with gutta percha after the MTA has hardened. **D,** The incisal half of the canal and crown have been restored with a bonded composite restoration to strengthen the root.

cedure be done at separate appointments, rather than in a single appointment. Likewise, ideally all signs and symptoms of infection and inflammation should be absent before the calcium hydroxide paste is placed.

Apical Barrier Technique

Although apexification with pastes has been highly successful, an alternative treatment is the use of an artificial apical barrier that allows immediate obturation of the canal.

Thus some of the inherent disadvantages of calcium hydroxide therapy, including increased cost and patient compliance with the multiple appointments over the 6 to 24 months of treatment, can be eliminated. Also, during this extended period root fractures are a common sequel because of the thin roots and increased incidence of traumatic injuries in children.

In 1979 Coviello and Brilliant[20] reported the use of tricalcium phosphate as an apical barrier. The material was packed into the apical 2 mm of the canal against which gutta-percha

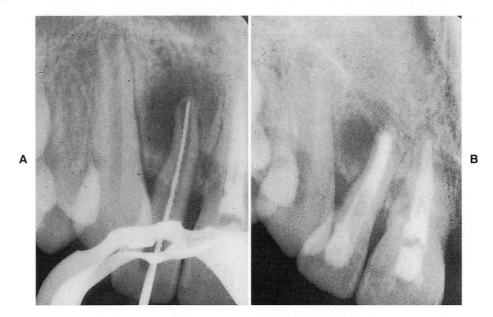

Fig. 23-31 Restoration following apexification with a bonded composite utilizing a clear plastic (Luminex) post. **A,** Radiograph of a maxillary lateral incisor with a successful apexification in which the canal was not filled following the treatment and has become reinfected. Note the resorption on the central incisor, which had been replanted several years ago. **B,** Radiograph several months after obliteration of the canal with gutta percha. A Luminex post was used to transmit light into the canal to cure a bonded composite. The plastic post can be seen in the center of the composite restoration.

was condensed. The treatment was achieved in one appointment. Using radiographic assessment, the authors reported successful apexification comparable to that achieved with calcium hydroxide.

Calcium hydroxide has also been used successfully as an apical barrier against which to pack gutta-percha.[178] MTA has recently been advocated as a material to serve as an apical barrier for root end induction.[208] MTA was reported to produce equivalent amounts of apical hard tissue with no more inflammation than calcium hydroxide or osteogenic protein-1.[181] Bone, cementum, and uninflamed periodontal tissue was demonstrated in direct opposition to MTA. Because of its good sealing ability and high degree of biocompatability, MTA would seem to be the material of choice for an apical barrier.

In the MTA apical barrier technique the canal is thoroughly cleaned and medicated with calcium hydroxide for 1 week. On reentry into the canal, it is cleansed and rinsed with NaOCl. After drying, a 3 to 4 mm plug of MTA is packed into the apical end of the canal. A moist cotton pellet is placed against the MTA and the access sealed for at least 4 to 6 hours to allow a hardening of the material. The canal is then obturated with gutta-percha or a bonded composite (Fig. 23-30).

Restoration After Apexification

Because of the thin dentinal walls there is a high percentage of root fractures in teeth after apexification. Restoration of the immature tooth after obturation with gutta-percha must be designed to strengthen the tooth as much as possible. The use of newer dentinal bonding techniques has been shown to strengthen endodontically treated teeth to levels close to that of intact teeth.[78,92]

Placement of an autocuring composite may be difficult because of the short working time. Light curing composites allow sufficient time for proper placement in the canal but have the disadvantage of incomplete polymerization in the deeper depths of the canal because of limited transmission of light through the material. Clear plastic posts (the Luminex System, Dentatus USA, New York, NY) have been developed to allow light transmission throughout the canal, curing the entire mass of composite.

After obturation, all gutta-percha except a plug of 5 to 6 mm in the apical end is removed. A Luminex post is selected. The dentin is acid etched, and a dentin bonding agent is applied to the internal surfaces of the canal. Light curing composite is placed in the canal, and care is taken not to trap bubbles. The Luminex post is placed to the depth of the preparation and the composite cured by transmitting light through the post. After curing, the plastic post may be trimmed to the cervical line and the incisal opening is restored. If a crown is needed, an appropriate, corresponding, metal post may be placed (Fig. 23-31).[92]

In the barrier technique using MTA, it is not necessary to place gutta-percha in the canal. Instead, the entire remaining canal is obliterated with the bonded composite resin.

References

1. Abedi HR, Torabinejad M, Pitt-Ford TR, Bakland LK: The use of mineral tri-oxide aggregate cement (MTA) as a direct pulp-capping agent, *J Endod* 22:199, 1996 (abstract).

2. Akimoto N et al: Biocompatability of Clearfil linear bond 2 and Clearfil AP-X system on nonexposed and exposed primate teeth, *Quintessence Int* 22:177, 1998.

3. Alacam A: Long-term effects of primary teeth pulpotomies with formocresol, glutaraldehyde-calcium hydroxide and glutaraldehyde-zinc oxide-eugenol on succedaneous teeth, *J Peridontol* 13:307, 1989.

4. Andrew P: The treatment of infected pulps in deciduous teeth, *Br Dent J* 98:122, 1955.

5. Anthony DR: Apexification during active orthodontic movement, *J Endod* 12:419, 1986.

6. Aponte AJ, Hartsook JT, Crowley MC: Indirect pulp capping success verified, *J Dent Child* 33:164, 1966.

7. Armstrong RL et al: Comparison of Dycal and formocresol pulpotomies in young permanent teeth in monkeys, *Oral Surg* 48:160, 1979.

8. Ash M: *Wheeler's dental anatomy, physiology and occlusion*, ed 7, Philadelphia, 1992, WB Saunders.

9. Attala MN, Noujaim AA: Role of calcium hydroxide in the formation of reparative dentin, *J Can Dent Assoc* 35:267, 1969.

10. Avram DC, Pulver F: Pulpotomy medicaments for vital primary teeth: surveys to determine use and attitudes in pediatric dental practice and in dental schools throughout the world, *J Dent Child* 56:426, 1989.

11. Bennett CG: Pulpal management of deciduous teeth, *Pract Dent Monogr,* p 1, May-June, 1965.

12. Berk H, Krakow AA: Endodontic treatment in primary teeth. In Goldman HM et al, editors: *Current therapy in dentistry,* vol 5, St Louis, 1974, Mosby.

13. Bevelander G, Benzer D: Morphology and incidence in secondary dentin in human teeth, *J Am Dent Assoc* 30:1079, 1943.

14. Block RM et al: Cell-mediated immune response to dog pulp tissue altered by formocresol within the root canal, *J Endod* 3:424, 1977.

15. Brian JD et al: Reaction of rat connective tissue to unfixed and formaldehyde-fixed autogenous implants enclosed in tubes, *J Endod* 6:628, 1980.

16. Caldwell RE, Freilich MM, Sandor GKB: Two radicular cysts associated with endodontically treated primary teeth. Rationale for long-term follow-up, *Ont Dent* 76:29, 1999.

17. Camp JH: Continued apical development of pulpless permanent teeth after endodontic therapy, master's thesis, Bloomington, 1968, Indiana University School of Dentistry.

18. Chosack A, Cleaton-Jones P: A histological and quantitative histomorphometric study of apexification of nonvital permanent incisors of vervet monkeys after repeated root fillings with a calcium hydroxide paste, *Endod Dent Traumatol* 13:211, 1997.

19. Coll JA, Sadrian R: Predicting pulpectomy success and its relationship to exfoliation and succedaneous dentition, *Pediatr Dent* 18:57, 1996.

20. Coviello J, Brilliant JD: A preliminary clinical study of the use of tricalcium phosphate as an apical barrier, *J Endod* 5:6, 1979.

21. Cox CF et al: Capping of the dental pulp mechanically exposed to the oral microflora: a 5-week observation of wound healing in the monkey, *J Oral Pathol* 11:327, 1982.

22. Cox CF et al: Pulp-capping of dental pulp mechanically exposed to oral microflora: a 1-to-2-year observation of wound healing in the monkey, *J Oral Pathol* 14:156, 1985.

23. Cox CF et al: Biocompatability of primer, adhesive and resin composite systems on non-exposed and exposed pulps of non-human primate teeth, *Am J Dent* 11:55, 1998 (special issue).

24. Cox CF et al: Biocompatability of surface-sealed dental materials against exposed pulp, *J Prosthet Dent* 57:1, 1987.

25. Cox CF et al: Biocompatability of various dental materials: pulp healing with a surface seal, *Int J Periodont Restorative Dent* 16:241, 1996.

26. Cox CF, Suzuki S: Re-evaluating pulpal protection: calcium hydroxide liners vs cohesive hybridization, *J Amer Dent* 125:823, 1994.

27. Cvek M: Treatment of non-vital permanent incisors with calcium hydroxide, *Odontol Rev* 23:27, 1972.

28. Cvek M: A clinical report on partial pulpotomy and capping with calcium hydroxide in permanent incisors with complicated crown fractures, *J Endod* 4:232, 1978.

29. Cvek M: Endodontic treatment of traumatized teeth. In Andreasen JO: *Traumatic injuries of the teeth,* ed 2, Philadelphia, 1981, WB Saunders.

30. Cvek M, Lundberg M: Histological appearance of pulps after exposure by a crown fracture, partial pulpotomy, and clinical diagnosis of healing, *J Endod* 9:8, 1983.

31. Cvek M et al: Pulp reactions to exposure after experimental crown fracture or grinding in adult monkey, *J Endod* 8:391, 1982.

32. Cvek M et al: Hard tissue barrier formation in pulpotomized monkey teeth capped with cyanoacrylate or calcium hydroxide for 10 and 60 minutes, *J Dent Res* 66:1166, 1987.

33. Dandashi MB et al: An in vitro comparison of three endodontic techniques for primary incisors, *Pediatr Dent* 15:254, 1993.

34. Dannenberg JL: Pedodontic-endodontics, *Dent Clin North Am* 18:367, 1974.

35. Davis MJ, Myers R, Switkes MD: Glutaraldehyde: an alternative to formocresol for vital pulp therapy, *J Dent Child* 49:176, 1982.

36. Dietz D: A histological study of the effects of formocresol on normal primary pulpal tissue, master's thesis, Seattle, 1961, School of Dentistry, University of Washington.

37. Dilley GJ, Courts FJ: Immunological response to four pulpal medicaments, *Pediatr Dent* 3:179, 1981.

38. Dimaggio JJ, Hawes RR: Evaluation of direct and indirect pulp capping, *J Dent Res* 40:24, 1962 (abstract).

39. Dimaggio JJ, Hawes RR: Continued evaluation of direct and indirect pulp capping, *J Dent Res* 41:38, 1963 (abstract).

40. Doyle WA, McDonald RE, Mitchell DF: Formocresol versus calcium hydroxide in pulpotomy, *J Dent Child* 29:86, 1962.

41. Dylewski JJ: Apical closure of non-vital teeth, *Oral Surg* 32:82, 1971.

42. Easlick KA: Operative procedures in management of deciduous molars, *Int J Orthod* 20:585, 1934.

43. Ehrenreich DW: A comparison of the effects of zinc oxide and eugenol and calcium hydroxide on carious dentin in human primary molars, *J Dent Child* 35:451, 1968.

44. Elloit RD et al: Evaluation of the carbon dioxide laser on vital human primary pulp tissue, *J Pediatr Dent* 21:327, 1999.

45. Emmerson C et al: Pulpal changes following formocresol applications on rat molars and human primary teeth, *J South Calif Dent Assoc* 27:309, 1959.

46. England MC, Best E: Noninduced apical closure in immature roots of dogs' teeth, *J Endod* 3:411, 1977.

47. Fairbourn DR, Charbeneau GT, Loesche WJ: Effect of improved Dycal and I.R.M. on bacteria in deep carious lesions, *J Am Dent Assoc* 100:547, 1980.

48. Feigal RJ, Messer HH: A critical look at glutaraldehyde, *Pediatr Dent* 12:69, 1990.

49. Feltman EM: A comparison of the formocresol pulpotomy techniques and Dycal pulpotomy technique in young permanent teeth, master's thesis, Bloomington, 1972, School of Dentistry, Indiana University.

50. Finn SB: Morphology of the primary teeth. In Finn SB et al, editors: *Clinical pedodontics,* ed 3, Philadelphia, 1967, WB Saunders.

51. Fishman SA et al: Success of electrofulguration pulpotomies covered by zinc oxide and eugenol, *Pediatr Dent* 18:385, 1996.

52. Frank AL: Therapy for the divergent pulpless tooth by continued apical formation, *J Am Dent Assoc* 72:87, 1966.

53. Frankel SN: Pulp therapy in pedodontics, *Oral Surg* 34:293, 1972.

54. Friedberg BH, Gartner LP: Embryotoxicity and teratogenicity of formocresol on developing chick embryos, *J Endod* 16:434, 1990.

55. Fuks AB, Bimstein EC: Clinical evaluation of diluted formocresol pulpotomies in primary teeth of school children, *Pediatr Dent* 3:321, 1981.

56. Fuks AB, Bimstein E, Bruchimn A: Radiographic and histologic evaluation of the effect of two concentrations of formocresol on pulpotomized primary and young permanent teeth in monkeys, *Pediatr Dent* 5:9, 1983.

57. Fuks AB et al: Partial pulpotomy as a treatment alternative for exposed pulps in crown-fractured permanent incisors, *Endod Dent Traumatol* 3:100, 1987.

58. Fuks AB et al: Assessment of a 2 percent buffered glutaraldehyde solution in pulpotomized primary teeth of school children, *J Dent Child* 57:371, 1990.

59. Fulton R, Ranly DM: An autoradiographic study of formocresol pulpotomies in rat molars using ^{3}H-formaldehyde, *J Endod* 5:71, 1979.

60. Fusayama T, Okuse K, Hosoda H: Relationship between hardness, discoloration and microbial invasion in carious dentin, *J Dent Res* 45:1033, 1966.

61. Garcia-Godoy F, Novakovic DP, Carvajal IN: Pulpal response to different application times of formocresol, *J Peridontol* 6:176, 1982.

62. Garcia-Godoy F, Ranly D: Clinical evaluation of pulpotomies with ZOE as the vehicle for glutaraldehyde, *Pediatr Dent* 9:144, 1987.

63. Gazi HA, Nayak RG, Bhat KS: Tissue-irritation potential of dilute formocresol, *Oral Surg* 51:74, 1981.

64. Gerlach E: Root canal therapeutics in deciduous teeth, *Dent Surv* 8:68, 1932.

65. Granath LE, Hagman G: Experimental pulpotomy in human bicuspids with reference to cutting technique, *Acta Odontol Scand* 29:155, 1971.

66. Greenberg M: Filling root canals of deciduous teeth by an injection technique, *Dent Dig* 67:574, 1964.

67. Guidelines for pulp therapy for primary and young permanent teeth: *American Academy of Pediatric Dentistry reference manual, Pediatr Dent* 18:44, 1996.

68. Guthrie TJ, McDonald RE, Mitchell DF: Dental hemogram, *J Dent Res* 44:678, 1965.

69. Gwinnett AJ, Tay FR: Early and intermediate time response of the dental pulp to an acid etch technique in vivo, *Am J Dent* 11:S35, 1998 (special issue).

70. Ham JW, Patterson SS, Mitchell DF: Induced apical closure of immature pulpless teeth in monkeys, *Oral Surg* 33:438, 1972.

71. Hata G et al: Systemic distribution of ^{14}C-labeled formaldehyde applied in the root canal following pulpectomy, *J Endod* 15:539, 1989.

72. Hawes RR, Dimaggio JJ, Sayegh F: Evaluation of direct and indirect pulp capping, *J Dent Res* 43:808, 1964 (abstract).

73. Hayashi Y: Ultrastructure of initial calcification in wound healing following pulpotomy, *J Oral Pathol* 11:174, 1982.

74. Hebling J, Giro EMA, deSouza Costa CA: Biocompatability of an adhesive system applied to exposed human dental pulp, *J Endod* 25:676, 1999.

75. Heide S: Pulp reactions to exposure for 4, 24 and 168 hours, *J Dent Res* 59:1910, 1980.

76. Heide S, Kerekes K: Delayed partial pulpotomy in permanent incisors of monkeys, *Int Endod J* 19:78, 1986.

77. Hermann BW: Dentinobliteran der Wurzelkanalc nach der Behandlung mit Kalzium, *Zahaerizl Rund* 39:888, 1930.

78. Hernandez R, Bader S, Boston D, Trope M: Resistance to fracture of endodontically treated premolars restored with new generation dentin bonding systems, *Int Endod J* 27:281, 1994.

79. Hibbard ED, Ireland RL: Morphology of the root canals of the primary molar teeth, *J Dent Child* 24:250, 1957.

80. Hill S et al: Comparison of antimicrobial and cytotoxic effects of glutaraldehyde and formocresol, *Oral Surg Oral Med Oral Pathol* 71:89, 1991.

81. Holan G, Fuks AB: A comparison of pulpectomies using ZOE and KRI paste in primary molars: a retrospective study, *Pediatr Dent* 15:403, 1993.

82. Holan G, Topf J, Fuks AB: Effect of root canal infection and treatment of traumatized primary incisors on their permanent successors, *Endod Dent Traumatol* 8:12, 1992.

83. Ireland RL: Secondary dentin formation in deciduous teeth, *J Am Dent Assoc* 28:1626, 1941.

84. Jeng HW, Feigal RJ, Messer HH: Comparison of the cytotoxicity of formocresol, formaldehyde, cresol, and glutaraldehyde using human pulp fibroblast cultures, *Pediatr Dent* 9:295, 1987.

85. Jordon ME: *Operative dentistry for children,* New York, 1925, Dental Items of Interest Publishing Co.

86. Junn DJ, McMillan P, Bakland LK, Torabinejad M: Quantitative assessment of dentin bridge formation following pulpcapping with mineral trioxide aggregate (MTA), *J Endod* 24:278, 1998 (abstract).

87. Kaiser JH: Management of wide-open canals with calcium hydroxide. Paper presented at the meeting of the American Association of Endodontics, Washington, DC, April 17, 1964. Cited by Steiner JC, Dow PR, Cathey GM: Inducing root end closure of nonvital permanent teeth, *J Dent Child* 35:47, 1968.

88. Kakehashi S, Stanley HR, Fitzgerald RT: The effects of surgical exposures of dental pulps in germ-free and conventional laboratory rats, *Oral Surg* 20:340, 1965.

89. Kalnins V, Frisbie HE: Effect of dentin fragments on the healing of the exposed pulp, *Arch Oral Biol* 2:96, 1960.

90. Kanka J III: An alternative hypothesis to the cause of pulpal inflammation in teeth treated with phosphoric acid on the dentin, *Quintessence Int* 21:83, 1990.

91. Karp WB, Korb P, Pashley D: The oxidation of glutaraldehyde by rat tissues, *Pediatr Dent* 9:301, 1987.

92. Katebzadeh N, Dalton BC, Trope M: Strengthening immature teeth during and after apexification, *J Endod* 24:256, 1998.

93. Kato S, Fusayama T: Recalcification of artificially decalcified dentin in Vivo, *J Dent Res* 49:1060, 1970.

94. Kelley MA, Bugg JL, Skjonsby HS: Histologic evaluation of formocresol and oxpara pulpotomies in rhesus monkeys, *J Am Dent Assoc* 86:123, 1973.

95. Kennedy DB et al: Formocresol pulpotomy in teeth of dogs with induced pulpal and periapical pathosis, *J Dent Child* 40:44, 1973.

96. Kerkhove BC et al: A clinical and television densitometric evaluation of the indirect pulp capping technique, *J Dent Child* 34:192, 1967.

97. King JB, Crawford JJ, Lindahl RL: Indirect pulp capping: a bacteriologic study of deep carious dentine in human teeth, *Oral Surg* 20:663, 1965.

98. Kitasako Y, Inokoshi S, Tagami J: Effects of direct resin pulp capping techniques on short-term response of mechanically exposed pulps, *J Dent* 27:257, 1999.

99. Kleier DJ, Barr ES: A study of endodontically apexified teeth, *Endod Dent Traumatol* 7:112, 1991.

100. Klein H et al: Partial pulpotomy following complicated crown fracture in permanent incisors: a clinical and radiographic study, *J Pedodontol* 9:142, 1985.

101. Koenigs JF et al: Induced apical closure of permanent teeth in adult primates using a resorbable form of tricalcium phosphate ceramic, *J Endod* 1:102, 1975.

102. Kopel HM: Pediatric endodontics. In Ingle H, Beveridge EE, editors: *Endodontics,* ed 2, Philadelphia, 1976, Lea & Febiger.

103. Kopel HM et al: The effects of glutaraldehyde on primary pulp tissue following coronal amputation: an in vivo histologic study, *J Dent Child* 47:425, 1980.

104. Kuboki Y, Ohgushi K, Fusayama T: Collagen biochemistry of the two layers of carious dentin, *J Dent Res* 56:1233, 1977.

105. Langeland K: Management of the inflamed pulp associated with deep carious lesion, *J Endod* 7:169, 1981.

106. Langeland K et al: Human pulp changes of iatrogenic origin, *Oral Surg* 32:943, 1971.

107. Laurence RP: A method of root canal therapy for primary teeth, master's thesis, Atlanta, GA, 1966, School of Dentistry, Emory University.

108. Laws AJ: Pulpotomy by electro-coagulation, *N Z Dent J* 53:68, 1957.

109. Lekka M, Hume WR, Wolinsky LE: Comparison between formaldehyde and glutaraldehyde diffusion through the root tissues of pulpotomy-treated teeth, *J Pedodontol* 8:185, 1984.

110. Liu J et al: Laser pulpotomy of primary teeth, *J Pediatr Dent* 21:128, 1999.

111. Lloyd JM, Scale NS, Wilson CFG: The effects of various concentrations and lengths of application of glutaraldehyde on monkey pulp tissue, *Pediatr Dent* 10:115, 1988.

112. Longwill DG, Marshall FJ, Creamer HR: Reactivity of human lymphocytes to pulp antigens, *J Endod* 8:27, 1982.

113. Loos PJ, Han SS: An enzyme histochemical study of the effect of various concentrations of formocresol on connective tissues, *Oral Surg* 31:571, 1971.

114. Loos PJ, Straffon LH, Han SS: Biological effects of formocresol, *J Dent Child* 40:193, 1973.

115. Lui JL: Depth of composite polymerization within simulated root canals using light-transmitting posts, *Oper Dent* 19:165, 1994.

116. Mack ES: Personal communication, 1967.

117. Mack RB, Dean JA: Electrosurgical pulpotomy: a retrospective human study, *ASDC J Dent Child* 60:107, 1993.

118. Mack RB, Halterman CW: Labial pulpectomy access followed by esthetic composite resin restoration for nonvital maxillary deciduous incisors, *J Am Dent Assoc* 100:374, 1980.

119. Mansukhani N: Pulpal reactions to formocresol, master's thesis, Urbana, 1959, College of Dentistry, University of Illinois.

120. Mass E, Zilberman U: Clinical and radiographic evaluation of partial pulpotomy in carious exposures of permanent molars, *Pediatr Dent* 15:257, 1993.

121. Mass E, Zilberman U, Fuks AB: Partial pulpotomy: another treatment option for cariously exposed permanent molars, *J Dent Child* 62:342, 1995.

122. Massler M, Mansukhani H: Effects of formocresol on the dental pulp, *J Dent Child* 26:277, 1959.

123. Matsumiya S, Susuki A, Takuma S: *Atlas of clinical pathology,* vol 1, Tokyo, 1962, Tokyo Dental College Press.

124. McDonald RE, Avery DR: Treatment of deep caries, vital pulp exposure, and pulpless teeth in children. In McDonald RE, Avery DR, editors: *Dentistry for the child and adolescent,* ed 7, St Louis, 1999, Mosby.

125. Mejare I, Cvek M: Partial pulpotomy in young permanent teeth with deep carious lesions, *Endod Dent Traumatol* 9:238, 1993.

126. Messer LB, Cline JT, Korf NW: Long-term effects of primary molar pulpotomies on succedaneous bicuspids, *J Dent Res* 59:116, 1980.

127. Miyauchi H, Iwaku M, Fusayama T: Physiological recalcification of carious dentin, *Bull Tokyo Med Dent Univ* 25:169, 1978.

128. MjörI A, Dahl E, Cox CF: Healing of pulp exposures: an ultrastructural study, *J Oral Pathol Med* 20:496, 1991.

129. Morawa AP et al: Clinical studies of human primary teeth following dilute formocresol pulpotomies, *J Dent Res* 53:269, 1974, (abstract).

130. Morawa AP et al: Clinical evaluation of pulpotomies using dilute formocresol, *J Dent Child* 42:360, 1975.

131. Mulder GR, van Amerongen WE, Vingerling PA: Consequences of endodontic treatment of primary teeth. II. A clinical investigation into the influence of formocresol pulpotomy on the permanent successor, *J Dent Child* 54:35, 1987.

132. Mniz MA, Keszler A, Dominiguez FV: The formocresol technique in young permanent teeth, *Oral Surg* 55:611, 1983.

133. Myers DR: Effects of formocresol on pulps of cariously exposed permanent molars, master's thesis, 1972, College of Dentistry, University of Tennessee.

134. Myers DR et al: Distribution of ^{14}C-formaldehyde after pulpotomy with formocresol, *J Am Dent Assoc* 96:805, 1978.

135. Myers DR et al: Acute toxicity of high doses of systemically administered formocresol in dogs, *Pediatr Dent* 3:37, 1981.

136. Myers DR et al: Tissue changes induced by the absorption of formocresol from pulpotomy sites in dogs, *Pediatr Dent* 5:6, 1983.

137. Myers DR et al: Systemic absorption of ^{14}C-glutaraldehyde from glutaraldehyde-treated pulpotomy sites, *Pediatr Dent* 8:134, 1986.

138. Myers DR et al: Histopathology of furcation lesions associated with pulp degeneration in primary molars, *Pediatr Dent* 9:279, 1987.

139. Myers DR et al: Histopathology of radiolucent furcation lesions associated with pulpotomy-treated primary molars, *Pediatr Dent* 10:291, 1988.

140. Myers K, Kaminski E, Lautenschlater E: The effects of mineral trioxide aggregate on the dog pulp, *J Endod* 22:198, 1996.

141. Nakabayashi N, Kojima K, Masuhara E: The promotion of adhesion by the infiltration of monomers into tooth substrates, *J Biomed Mater Res* 16:265, 1982.

142. Nelson JR et al: Biochemical effects of tissue fixatives on bovine pulp, *J Endod* 5:139, 1979.

143. Nevins A et al: Induction of hard tissue into pulpless open-apex teeth using collagen-calcium phosphate gel, *J Endod* 4:76, 1978.

144. Nirschl RF, Avery DR: Evaluation of new pulp capping agent in indirect pulp therapy, *J Dent Child* 50:25, 1983.

145. Nosrat IV, Nosrat CA: Reparative hard tissue formation following calcium hydroxide application after partial pulpotomy in cariously exposed pulps of permanent teeth, *Int Endod J* 31:221, 1998.

146. Ogushi K, Fusayama T: Electron microscopic structure of the two layers of carious dentin, *J Dent Res* 54:1019, 1975.

147. Olmez A, Oztas N, Basak F et al: A histopathologic study of direct pulp-capping with adhesive resins, *Oral Surg Oral Med Oral Pathol Oral Radiol Endod* 86:98, 1998.

148. Orban B: Contribution to the histology of the dental pulp and periodontal membrane with special reference to the cells of defense of these tissues, *J Am Dent Assoc* 16:965, 1929.

149. Orban BJ, editor: *Oral histology and embryology,* ed 4, St Louis, 1957, Mosby.

150. Oringer MJ: *Electrosurgery in dentistry,* ed 2, Philadelphia, 1975, WB Saunders.

151. Pameijer CH, Stanley HR: The disastrous effects of the "total etch" technique in vital pulp capping in primates, *Am J Dent* 11:S45, 1998.

152. Pashley EL et al: Systemic distribution of ^{14}C-formaldehyde from formocresol-treated pulpotomy sites, *J Dent Res* 59:603, 1980.

153. Paterson RC, Watts A: Further studies on the exposed germ-free dental pulp, *Int Endod J* 20:112, 1987.

154. Pereira JC, Stanley HR: Pulp capping: influence of the exposure site on pulp healing—histologic and radiographic study in dogs' pulp, *J Endod* 7:213, 1981.

155. Peron LC, Burkes EJ, Gregory WB: Vital pulpotomy utilizing variable concentrations of paraformaldehyde in rhesus monkeys, *J Dent Res* 55:B129, 1976 (abstract 269).

156. Phancuf RA, Frankl SN, Ruben M: A comparative histological evaluation of three calcium hydroxide preparations on the human primary dental pulp, *J Dent Child* 35:61, 1968.

157. Pisanti S, Sciaky I: Origin of calcium in the repair wall after pulp exposure in the dog, *J Dent Res* 43:641, 1964.

158. Pitt-Ford TR, Torabinejad M, Abedi HR et al: Mineral trioxide aggregate as a pulp-capping material, *J Amer Dent Assoc* 127:1491, 1996.

159. Rabbach VP et al: Comparison of the effectiveness of electrosurgery versus formocresol in the pulpotomy procedure for primary teeth: a prospective human study, (in press).

160. Rabinowitch BZ: Pulp management in primary teeth, *Oral Surg* 6:542, 1953.

161. Ranley DM: Glutaraldehyde purity and stability: implications for preparation, storage, and use as a pulpotomy agent, *Pediatr Dent* 6:83, 1984.

162. Ranley DM: Assessment of the systemic distribution and toxicity of formaldehyde following pulpotomy treatment. I, *J Dent Child* 52:431, 1985.

163. Ranley DM: Pulpotomy therapy in primary teeth: new modalities for old rationals, *Pediatr Dent* 16:403, 1994.

164. Ranley DM, Garcia-Godoy F, Horn D: Time, concentration, and pH parameters for the use of glutaraldehyde as a pulpotomy agent: an in vivo study, *Pediatr Dent* 9:199, 1987.

165. Ranley DM, Horn D, Zislis T: The effect of alternatives to formocresol on antigencity of protein, *J Dent Res* 64:1225, 1985.

166. Ranley DM, Amstutz L, Horn D: Subcellular localization of glutaraldehyde, *Endod Dent Traumatol* 6:251, 1990.

167. Ranley DM, Horn D: Distribution, metabolism, and excretin of (^{14}C) glutaraldehyde, *J Endod* 16:135, 1990.

168. Rickman GA, Elbadrawy HE: Effect of premature loss of primary incisors on speech, *Pediatr Dent* 7:119, 1985.

169. Rimondini L, Baroni C: Morphologic criteria for root canal treatment of primary molars undergoing resorption, *Endod Dent Traumatol* 11:136, 1995.

170. Roberts SC Jr, Brilliant JD: Tricalcium phosphate as an adjunct to apical closure in pulpless permanent teeth, *J Endod* 1:263, 1975.

171. Rolling I, Poulsen S: Formocresol pulpotomy of primary teeth and occurrence of enamel defects on the permanent successors, *Acta Odontol Scand* 36:243, 1978.

172. Ruemping DR, Morton TH Jr, Anderson MW: Electrosurgical pulpotomy in primates—a comparison with formocresol pulpotomy, *Pediatr Dent* 5:14, 1983.

173. Sadrian R, Coll JA: A long-term follow-up on the retention of zinc oxide eugenol filler after primary tooth pulpectomy, *Pediatr Dent* 15:249, 1993.

174. Sanchez ZMC: Effects of formocresol on pulp-capped and pulpotomized permanent teeth of rhesus monkeys, master's thesis, Ann Arbor, 1971, University of Michigan.

175. Savage NW et al: A histological study of cystic lesions following pulp therapy in deciduous molars, *J Oral Pathol* 15:209, 1986.

176. Sayegh FS: Qualitative and quantitative evaluation of new dentin in pulp capped teeth, *J Dent Child* 35:7, 1968.

177. Sayegh FS: The dentinal bridge in pulp-involved teeth. I, *Oral Surg* 28:579, 1969.

178. Schumacher JW, Rutledge RE: An alternative to apexification, *J Endod* 19:529, 1993.

179. Sciaky I, Pisanti S: Localization of calcium placed over amputated pulps in dogs' teeth, *J Dent Res* 39:1128, 1960.

180. Seltzer S, Bender IB: Pulp capping and pulpotomy. In Seltzer S, Bender IB, editors: *The dental pulp, biologic considerations in dental procedures,* ed 2, Philadelphia, 1975, JB Lippincott.

181. Shabahang S et al: A comparative study of root-end induction using osteogenic protein-I, calcium hydroxide, and mineral trioxide aggregate in dogs, *J Endod* 25:1, 1999.

182. Shaw DW et al: Electrosurgical pulpotomy—a 6-month study in primates, *J Endod* 13:500, 1987.
183. Sheller B, Morton TH Jr: Electrosurgical pulpotomy: a pilot study in humans, *J Endod* 13:69, 1987.
184. Shoji S, Nakamura M, Horluchi H: Histopathological changes in dental pulps irradiated by CO_2 laser: a preliminary report on laser pulpotomy, *J Endod* 11:379, 1985.
185. Shovelton DS: A study of deep carious dentin, *Int Dent J* 18:392, 1968.
186. Shulman ER, Melver FF, Burkes EJ Jr: Comparison of electrosurgery and formocresol as pulpotomy techniques in monkey primary teeth, *Pediatr Dent* 9:189, 1987.
187. Simon M, van Mullem PJ, Lamers AC: Formocresol: no allergic effect after root canal disinfection in non-presensitized guinea pigs, *J Endod* 8:269, 1982.
188. Snuggs HM, Cox CF, Powell CF et al: Pulp healing and dentinal bridge formation in an acidic environment, *Quintessence Int* 24:501, 1993.
189. Spedding RH: The one-appointment formocresol pulpotomy for primary teeth, *J Tenn Dent Assoc* 48:263, 1968.
190. Stanley HR, Lundy T: Dycal therapy for pulp exposure, *Oral Surg* 34:818, 1972.
191. Stanley HR, Pameijer CH: Pulp capping with a new visible-light-curing calcium hydroxide composition (Prisma VLC Dycal), *Oper Dent* 10:156, 1985.
192. Stanley HR, White CL, McCray L: The rate of tertiary (reparative) dentine formation in the human tooth, *Oral Surg* 21:180, 1966.
193. Stanton WG: The non-vital deciduous tooth, *Int J Orthod* 21:181, 1935.
194. Starkey PE: Methods of preserving primary teeth which have exposed pulps, *J Dent Child* 30:219, 1963.
195. Starkey PE: Management of deep caries of pulpally involved teeth in children. In Goldman HM et al, editors: *Current therapy in dentistry,* vol 3, St Louis, 1968, Mosby.
196. Starkey PE: Treatment of pulpally involved primary molars. In McDonald RE et al, editors: *Current therapy in dentistry,* vol 7, St Louis, 1980, Mosby.
197. Steiner JC, Dow PR, Cathey GM: Inducing root end closure of nonvital permanent teeth, *J Dent Child* 35:47, 1968.
198. Steiner JC, Van Hassel HJ: Experimental root apexification in primates, *Oral Surg* 31:409, 1971.
199. Straffon LH, Han SS: Effects of varying concentrations of formocresol on RNA synthesis of connective tissue in sponge implants, *Oral Surg* 29:915, 1970.
200. Sweet CA: Procedure for the treatment of exposed and pulpless deciduous teeth, *J Am Dent Assoc* 17:1150, 1930.
201. Tagger M, Tagger E: Pulp capping in monkeys with Reolite and Life, two calcium hydroxide bases with different pH, *J Endod* 11:394, 1985.
202. Tagger E, Tagger M, Sarnat H: Pulpal reaction for glutaraldehyde and paraformaldehyde pulpotomy dressings in monkey primary teeth, *Endod Dent Traumatol* 2:237, 1986.
203. Tatsumi T et al: Remineralization of etched dentin, *J Prosthet Dent* 67:617, 1992.
204. Teplitsky PE: Formocresol pulpotomies on posterior permanent teeth, *J Can Dent Assoc* 50:623, 1984.
205. Teuscher GW, Zander HA: A preliminary report on pulpotomy, *Northwest Univ Dent Res Grad Q Bull* 39:4, 1938.
206. Thoden van Velzen SK, Feltkamp-Vroom TM: Immunologic consequences of formaldehyde fixation of autologous tissue implants, *J Endod* 3:179, 1977.
207. Tittle KW, Farley J, Linkhardt T et al: Apical closure induction using bone growth factors and mineral trioxide aggregate, *J Endod* 22:198, 1996 (abstract no. 41).
208. Torabinejad M, Chivian N: Clinical applications of mineral trioxide aggregate, *J Endod* 25:197, 1999.
209. Trask PA: Formocresol pulpotomy on (young) permanent teeth, *J Am Dent Assoc* 85:1316, 1972.
210. Traubman L: A critical clinical and television radiographic evaluation of indirect pulp capping, master's thesis, Bloomington, 1967, Indiana University School of Dentistry.
211. Tronstad L: Reaction of the exposed pulp to Dycal treatment, *Oral Surg* 38:945, 1974.
212. Turner C, Courts FJ, Stanley HR: A histological comparison of direct pulp capping agents in primary canines, *J Dent Child* 54:423, 1987.
213. Tziafas D, Molyvdas I: The tissue reaction after capping of dog teeth with calcium hydroxide experimentally crammed into the pulp space, *Oral Surg Oral Med Oral Pathol* 65:604, 1988.
214. van Amerongen WE, Mulder GR, Vingerling PA: Consequences of endodontic treatment in primary teeth. I. A clinical and radiographic investigation into the influence of the formocresol pulpotomy on the life-span of primary molars, *J Dent Child* 53:364, 1986.
215. van Mullen PJ, Simon M, Lamers AC: Formocresol: a root canal disinfectant provoking allergic skin reactions in presensitized guinea pigs, *J Endod* 9:25, 1983.
216. Venham LL: *Pulpal responses to variations in the formocresol pulpotomy technique: a histologic study,* master's thesis, Columbus, 1967, College of Dentistry, Ohio State University.
217. Webber RT: Apexogenesis versus apexification, *Dent Clin North Am* 28:669, 1984.
218. Weiss MB, Bjorvatn K: Pulp capping in deciduous and newly erupted permanent teeth of monkeys, *Oral Surg* 29:769, 1970.
219. Wemes JC et al: Histologic evaluation of the effect of formocresol and glutaraldehyde on the periapical tissues after endodontic treatment, *Oral Surg* 54:329, 1982.
220. Wemes JC et al: Diffusion of carbon-14-labeled formocresol and glutaraldehyde in tooth structures, *Oral Surg* 54:341, 1982.
221. West NM, Lieb RJ: Biologic root-end closure on a traumatized and surgically resected maxillary central incisor: an alternative method of treatment, *Endod Dent Traumatol* 1:146, 1985.
222. White KC et al: Pulpal response to adhesive resin systems applied to acid-etched vital dentin: damp versus dry primer application, *Quintessence Int* 25:259, 1991.
223. Whitehead FI, MacGregor AB, Marsland EA: The relationship of bacterial invasions of softening of the dentin in permanent and deciduous teeth, *Br Dent J* 108:261, 1960.
224. Yacobi R et al: Evolving primary pulp therapy techniques, *J Am Dent Assoc* 122:83, 1991.
225. Yamada T et al: The extent of the odontoblast process in normal and carious human dentin, *J Dent Res* 62:798, 1983.
226. Zander HA: Reaction of the pulp to calcium hydroxide, *J Dent Res* 18:373, 1939.
227. Zurcher E: *The anatomy of the root canals of the teeth of the deciduous dentition and of the first permanent molars,* New York, 1925, William Wood & Co.

Chapter 24

 # Geriatric Endodontics

Carl W. Newton, David Clifford Brown

Chapter Outline

Dental service requirements are determined by four demographic and epidemiologic factors:

1. The population at risk
2. The incidence and prevalence of dental diseases
3. The accepted standards of care
4. The perceived need and expectations toward dental health by the public[13]

These factors are changing as a result of the aging of the population.

AN AGING SOCIETY

According to the U.S. Census Bureau, America's population age 65 or older grew by 82% between 1965 and 1995. Between 1980 and 1995, this same population grew by 28% to an historic high of 33.5 million people. The "oldest old" is defined as people who are at least 85 years old. This group is the fastest growing segment of America's senior citizen population. The number of people age 85 and older has more than doubled since 1965 and has grown by 40% since 1980.

The 75 million people born in the United States between 1946 and 1964 constitute the baby boom generation. In 1994 baby boomers represented nearly one third of the U.S. population. Soon these people will enter the 65-years-and-older category. As the baby boomers begin to age, the United States will see an unparalleled increase in the absolute number of older persons. Although one in eight Americans was 65 years of age or older in 1994, in a little more than 30 years about one in five is expected to be in this group[2] (Fig. 24-1).

Information available from the U.S. Census Bureau and National Institute on Aging indicates that America's older population is unevenly distributed between geographic locations. The most populous states have the largest number of older adults; Florida and Midwestern states currently have the highest proportions of older adults. Florida was the only state where the population of older adults was greater than 16% of its population in 1993; however, it is predicted that 32 states will fall in this category by 2020.

Increased longevity of the dentition with expanding fields of advanced restorative procedures and periodontology lend support that dentistry will see a substantial growth in the number of older patients. Until 1983, persons age 65 and older made an average of 1.5 dental visits annually, a lower utilization rate than that of any other age group.[49] Between 1983 and 1986 a 29% increase in visits by those 65 years and older was noted by the National Health Survey.[48] According to this survey, older adults currently make more visits per year, on average, than those in the "all ages combined" category. In the future, general dentists will routinely serve a growing number of older persons, who will account for one third to two thirds of their workload.[24,25]

Future dental services (including root canal procedures) for older patients are anticipated to be of two general types:

1. Services for relatively healthy older adults who are functionally independent
2. Services for older patients with complex conditions and problems who are functionally dependent[29]

The latter group will require care from dentists who have advanced training in geriatric dentistry. This age group is being targeted in dental education programs and advanced training through improved curriculum, research, and publications on aging. The National Institute on Aging stated that all dental professionals should receive education concerning treatment of older adults as part of basic professional education.[12,29]

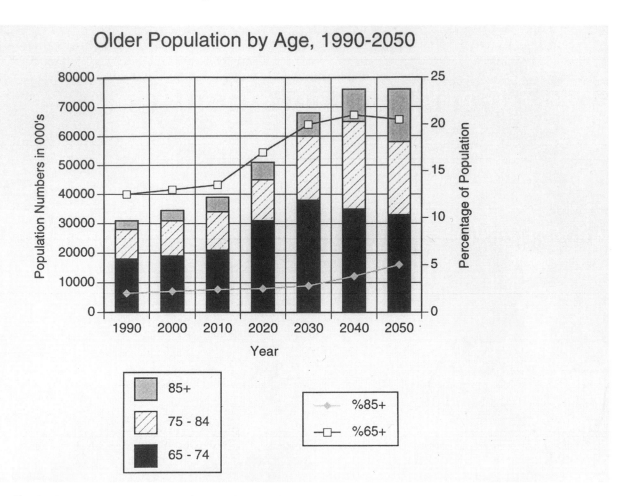

Fig. 24-1 Projected percentage growth rates of U.S. adults age 65+ and 85+ from 1990 to 2050. (U.S. Census Bureau.)

The purpose of this chapter is to discuss the effect of aging on the diagnosis of pulpal and periapical disease and successful root canal treatment. The quality of life for older patients can be significantly improved by saving teeth through endodontic treatment and can have a large and impressive value to overall dental, physical, and mental health.

With age the simple pleasure of being able to eat what one wishes often becomes an issue, as does the increased need for proper diet and nourishment. Every tooth may be strategic, and old age is no time to be forced to replace sound teeth with removable appliances or dentures. Consultation with older patients should help them overcome what may be a very limited knowledge of root canal treatment and lack of appreciation for regular dental care. Well-meaning friends and spouses who contend that their dentures are as good or better than their natural teeth may have had a lifetime of poor dental experiences or have forgotten what it is like to enjoy natural dentition.

Negative social attitudes toward older adults tend to carry over into their care. Older patients are in danger of being dismissed as hopeless or not worth the effort. At times, clinicians shy away from providing care for seniors because of the perceived difficulty or cost of certain treatment procedures or because of complicated medical conditions. Clinicians sometimes consider older patients less able to pay for treatment because of their age and appearance. However, most older adults engage in normal activity and can recognize and afford the value of good dentistry.[5]

It should be considered that most older patients have had active, productive lives; they are very interested in maintaining their dignity and do not consider themselves a bad investment. As with any age group, older patients must be considered as individuals. This may prove difficult in the face of the tendency of many health care professionals to assign any person older than 65 to the classification *geriatric* and to stereotype patients (e.g., confusion, dementia, poor treatment response). Each older adult patient comes with unique psychologic and social life history, with a set of values, needs, and with resources unlike those of any other patient the provider will see. Most seniors are more concerned with maintaining control of their lives than they are about being old.[36]

Because the primary function of teeth is mastication, it is presumed that loss of teeth leads to detrimental food changes and reduction in health.[18] However, this may not be the driving force when seniors are seeking treatment. Many times social issues are the motivation for a senior to visit a dentist. After suggesting a mandibular anterior tooth extraction to a 93-year-old man, one clinician was told, "I can't, Doctor. You see, I go dancing every Saturday night, and I need that tooth. I can't look like that."

Dentists should not presume that they know what is best for senior patients or what they can afford without the patient's full awareness. The needs, expectations, desires, and demands of older people may exceed those of any age group, and the gratitude shown by older patients is among the most satisfying of professional experiences.

The desire for root canal treatment among aging patients has increased considerably in recent years. Older patients are aware that treatment can be performed comfortably and that age is *not* a factor in predicting success.[3,44,46] Obtaining informed consent also requires that root canal treatment be offered as a favorable alternative to the trauma of extraction and the cost of replacement. The distribution of specialists and the improved endodontic training of all dentists have broadened the availability of most endodontic procedures to everyone, regardless of age. Expanded dental insurance benefits for retirees and a heightened awareness of the benefits of saving teeth have encouraged many older patients to seek endodontia rather than extraction.[51]

This chapter compares the typical geriatric patient's endodontic needs with those of the general population. (Pulp changes attributed to age are discussed in Chapter 12; their effects on clinical treatment are also discussed in this chapter.)

MEDICAL HISTORY

It is important to focus on those factors that will truly indicate the risks undertaken in treating the older patient. Clinicians must recognize that the biologic or functional age of an individual is far more important than chronologic age. A medical history should be taken before the patient is brought into the treatment room, and a standardized form (see Fig. 1-2) should be used to identify any disease or therapy that would alter treatment or its outcome. In general, aging causes dramatic changes to the cardiovascular, respiratory, and central nervous system (CNS) that result in most drug therapy needs. However, the decline in renal and liver function in older patients should also be considered when predicting behavior and interaction of drugs (e.g., anesthetics, analgesics, antibiotics) that may be used in dental treatment.

The review of the patients' medical history is the first opportunity for the dentist to talk with the patient. The time and consideration taken at the outset will set the tone for the entire treatment process. This first impression should reflect a warm, caring practitioner, who is highly trained and able to help patients with complex treatments. Some older patients may need assistance in filling out the forms and may not be fully aware of their conditions or history. Some patients may withhold their date of birth to conceal their age for reasons of vanity or even fear of ageism. Vision deficits caused by outdated glasses or cataracts can adversely affect a patient's ability to read the small print on many history forms. Consultation with the patient's family, guardian, or physician may be necessary to complete the history; however, the dentist is ultimately responsible for the treatment.

An updated history, including information on compliance with any prescribed treatment and sensitivity to medications, must be obtained at each visit and reviewed. In general, older adults use more drugs than younger patients, and most of these medications are potentially important to the dentist.[26] *The Physicians' Desk Reference* should be consulted and any precaution or side effect of medication noted.

Although geriatric patients are usually knowledgeable about their medical history, some may not understand the implications of their medical conditions in relation to dentistry or may be reluctant to let the clinician into their confidence. Their perceptions of their illnesses may not be accurate, so any clue to a patient's conditions should be investigated.

Symptoms of undiagnosed illnesses may present the dentist with a screening opportunity that can disclose a condition that might otherwise go untreated or lead to an emergency. Management of medical emergencies in the dental office is best directed toward prevention rather than treatment.

Few families are without at least one member whose life has been extended as a result of medical progress. A great number have had diseases or disabilities controlled with therapies that may alter the clinician's case selection. Root canal treatment is certainly far less traumatic in the extremes of age or health than is extraction.

Chief Complaint

Most patients who are experiencing dental pain have a pulpal or periapical problem that requires root canal treatment or extraction. Dental needs are often manifested initially in the form of a complaint, which usually contains the information necessary to make a diagnosis. The diagnostic process is directed toward determining whether pulpal or periapical disease is present, whether palliative or root canal therapy is indicated, the vitality of the pulp, and which tooth is the source (see Chapter 1).

The clinician should, without leading, allow the patient to explain the problem in his or her own way. This gives the examiner an opportunity to observe the patient's level of dental knowledge and ability to communicate. Visual and auditory handicaps may become evident at this time.

Patiently encouraging the patient to talk about problems may lead into areas of only peripheral interest to the dentist, but it establishes a needed rapport and demonstrates sincere interest. A patient may exhibit some feelings of distrust if there is a history of failed treatments or if well-meaning, denture-wearing friends or relatives have claimed normal function and freedom from the need for dental treatment. The effect of the "focal infection" theory is still evident when other aches and pains cannot be adequately explained and loss of teeth is accepted as inevitable. The best patients are those who have already had successful endodontic treatment. Older patients are more likely to have already had root canal treatment and have a more realistic perception about treatment comfort.

Most geriatric patients do not complain readily about signs or symptoms of pulpal and periapical disease and may consider them to be minor compared with other health concerns and discomfort. A disease process usually arises as an acute problem in children, but assumes a more chronic or less dramatic form in the older adult. The *mere presence* of teeth indicates proper maintenance or resistance to disease. A lifetime of experiencing pains puts a different perspective on interpreting dental pain.

Pain associated with vital pulps (i.e., referred pain; pain caused by heat, cold, or sweets) seems to be reduced with age, and severity seems to diminish over time. Heat sensitivity that occurs as the only symptom suggests a reduced pulp volume, such as that occurring in the older pulps.[19] Pulpal-healing capacity is also reduced, and necrosis may occur quickly after microbial invasion, again with reduced symptoms.

Although complaints are fewer, they are usually more conclusive evidence of disease. The complaint should isolate the problem sufficiently to allow the clinician to take a periapical radiograph before proceeding. Studying radiographs before an examination can prejudice rather than focus attention; accordingly, they should be reviewed *after* the clinical examination has been completed.

DENTAL HISTORY

The clinician should search patients' records and explore their memories to determine the history of involved teeth or surrounding areas. The history may be as obvious as a recent pulp exposure and restoration, or it may be as subtle as a routine crown preparation 15 or 20 years ago. Any history of pain before or after treatments may establish the beginning of a degenerative process. Subclinical injuries caused by repeated episodes of decay and its treatment may accumulate and approach a clinically significant threshold that can be later exceeded after additional routine procedures. Multiple restorations on the same tooth are common (Fig. 24-2).

Recording information at the time of treatment may seem to be unnecessary "busy work," but it could prove to be helpful in identifying the source of a complaint or disease many years later. A patient's recall of dental treatments is usually limited to a few years, but the presence of certain materials or appliances, such as silver points, can sometimes date a procedure. Aging patients' dental histories are rarely complete and may indicate treatment by several dentists at different locations. They likely have outlived at least one dentist and been forced to establish a relationship with a new, younger dentist. This new dentist may find dental needs that require an updated treatment plan.

Subjective Symptoms

The examiner can pursue responses to questions about the patient's complaint, the stimulus or irritant that causes pain, the nature of the pain, and its relationship to the stimulus or irritant. This information is most useful in determining whether the source is pulpal disease, whether inflammation or infection has extended to the apical tissues, and whether these problems are reversible. Thus the dentist can determine

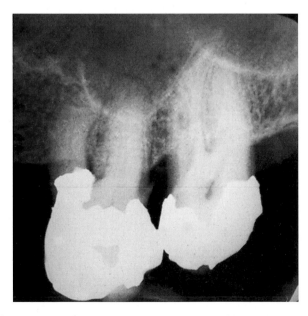

Fig. 24-2 Multiple restorations on this 74-year-old patient suggest repeated episodes of caries and restorative procedures with pulpal effects that accumulated in the form of subclinical inflammation and calcification.

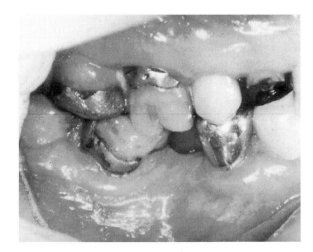

Fig. 24-3 Missing teeth and the subsequent tilt, rotation, and supereruption of adjacent and opposing teeth contribute to reduced functional ability and increased susceptibility to caries and periodontal disease.

what types of tests are necessary to confirm findings or suspicions. (For further information see Chapter 1.)

Diagnostic Procedures   It is important to remember that pulpal symptoms are usually chronic in older patients, and other sources of orofacial pain should be ruled out when pain is not soon localized. Much of the information to be obtained from the complaint, history, and description of subjective symptoms can be gathered in a screening interview by the clinician's assistant or over the phone by the receptionist. The need for treatment can be established and can provide a focus for the examination.

Objective Signs

The intraoral and extraoral clinical examination provides valuable first-hand information about disease and previous treatment. The overall oral condition should not be overlooked while centering on the patient's complaint, and all abnormal conditions should be recorded and investigated. Exposures to factors that contribute to oral cancers accumulate with age, and many systemic diseases may initially manifest prodromal oral signs or symptoms.

Missing teeth contribute to reduced functional ability (Fig. 24-3). The resultant loss of chewing efficiency leads to a higher carbohydrate diet of softer, more cariogenic foods. Increased sugar intake to compensate for loss of taste[17,28] and xerostomia[4] (often induced by medication[40]) are also factors in the renewed susceptibility to decay.

Gingival recession, which creates sensitivity and is hard to control, exposes cementum and dentin that are less resistant to decay. A clinical study of 600 patients older than age 60 showed that 70% had root caries and 100% had some degree of gingival recession.[50] The removal of root caries is irritating to the pulp and often results in pulp exposures or reparative dentin formation that affect the negotiation of the

canal, should root canal treatment later be needed[16] (Fig. 24-4). Asymptomatic pulp exposures on one root surface of a multirooted tooth can result in the uncommon clinical situation of the presence of both vital and nonvital pulp tissue in the same tooth (Fig. 24-5).

Interproximal root caries is difficult to restore, and restoration failure as a result of continued decay is common (Fig. 24-6). Although the microbiology of diseases is not substantially different in different age groups, the altered host response during aging may modify the progression of these diseases.[47]

Attrition (see Fig. 23-6), abrasion, and erosion (Fig. 24-7) also expose dentin through a slower process that allows the pulp to respond with dentinal sclerosis and reparative dentin.[42] Secondary dentin formation occurs throughout life and may eventually result in almost complete pulp obliteration. In maxillary anterior teeth, the secondary dentin is formed on the lingual wall of the pulp chamber[33]; in molar teeth the greatest deposition occurs on the floor of the chamber.[8] Although this pulp may appear to recede, small pulpal remnants can remain or leave a less calcific tract that may lead to a pulp exposure.

In general, canal and chamber volume is inversely proportional to age: as age increases, canal size decreases (Fig. 24-8). Reparative dentin resulting from restorative procedures, trauma, attrition, and recurrent caries also contributes to diminution of canal and chamber size. In addition, the cementodentinal junction (CDJ) moves farther from the radiographic apex with continued cementum deposition (Fig. 24-9).[21] The thickness of young apical cementum[38] is 100 to 200 μm and increases with age to two or three times that thickness.[55]

The calcification process associated with aging appears clinically to be of a more linear type than that which occurs in a younger tooth in response to caries, pulpotomy, or trauma (Fig. 24-10). Dentinal tubules become more occluded with

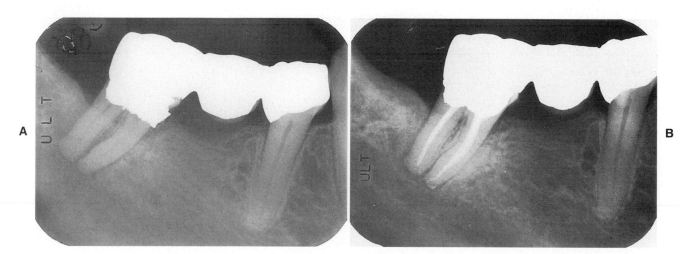

Fig. 24-4   Gingival recession exposes cementum and dentin, which are less resistant to caries. Root caries (**A**) often results in pulp exposures (**B**) that require endodontic treatment.

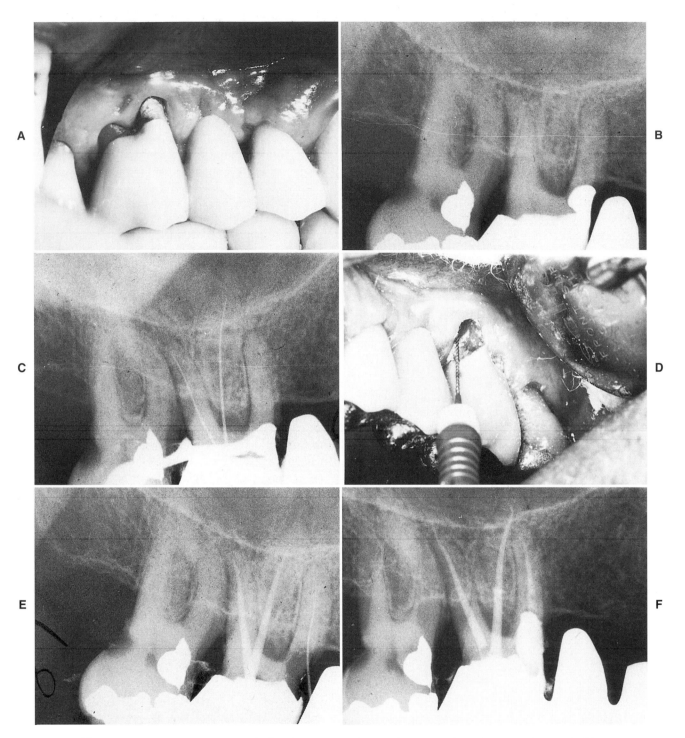

Fig. 24-5 **A**, Root caries repaired with alloy that appears to be into the (**B**) mesiobuccal (MB) canal on a valuable abutment to a long, fixed bridge. **C**, The palatal and distal canals are negotiated and treated through an occlusal access opening. **D**, The MB canal is negotiated and treated after the alloy is removed (**E**). **F**, Treatment is completed and the bridge is saved.

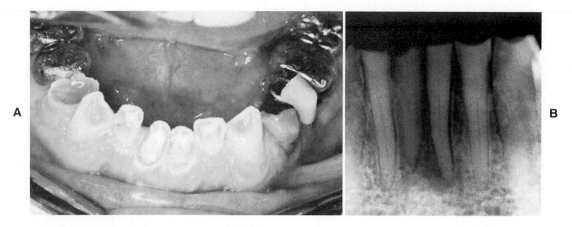

Fig. 24-6 **A**, Attrition exposes dentin through a slow process that allows the pulp to respond with reparative dentin, but pulp exposure eventually becomes clinically evident (**B**).

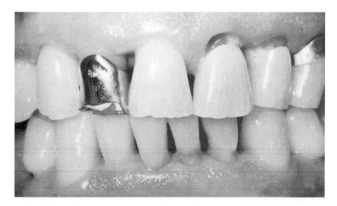

Fig. 24-7 Gingival recession also exposes cementum and dentin that are less resistant to abrasion and erosion, which can expose pulp or require restorative procedures that could result in pulp irritation.

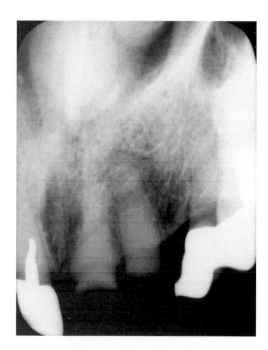

Fig. 24-8 In general, canal and chamber volume is inversely proportional to age: as age increases, canal size decreases. These maxillary incisors illustrate reduced canal and chamber volume in an older patient.

advancing age, decreasing tubular permeability.[27] Lateral and accessory canals can calcify, thus decreasing their clinical significance.

The compensating bite produced by missing and tilted teeth (or attrition) can cause temporomandibular joint (TMJ) dysfunction (less common in older adults) or loss of vertical dimension. The authors have observed diminished eruptive forces with age, reducing the amount of mesial drift and super eruption. Any limitation in opening reduces available working time and the space needed for instrumentation.

The presence of multiple restorations indicates a history of repeated insults and an accumulation of irritants. Marginal leakage and microbial contamination of cavity walls is a major cause of pulpal injury.[9] Violating principles of cavity design combines with the loss of resiliency that results from a reduced organic component to the dentin to increase susceptibility to cracks and cuspal fractures. In any further restorative procedures on such teeth, the clinician should consider the effect on the pulp and the effect on accessing and negotiating canals through such restorations if root canal therapy is indicated later.

Many cracks or craze lines (see Fig. 24-7) may be evident as a result of staining, but they do not indicate dentin penetration or pulp exposure. Pulp exposures caused by cracks are less likely to present acute problems in older patients and often penetrate the sulcus to create a periodontal defect, as well as a periapical one. If incomplete cracks are not detected early, the prognosis for cracked teeth in older patients is questionable (Fig. 24-11).

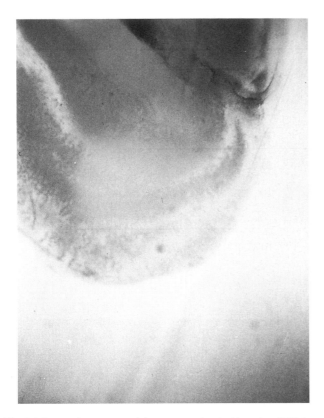

Fig. 24-9 Histologic image of the cementodentinal junction (CDJ) in an older tooth illustrates increased cementum deposition with age and increased distance from the apex. (Courtesy Dr. Thomas Stein.)

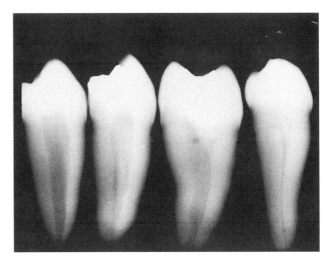

Fig. 24-10 This radiograph illustrates pulp volume changes in mandibular premolars. Viewed from left to right: a normal pulp, reparative dentin adjacent to a shallow restoration, more extensive reparative dentin adjacent to a more extensive restoration, and the overall reduced volume that occurs during aging.

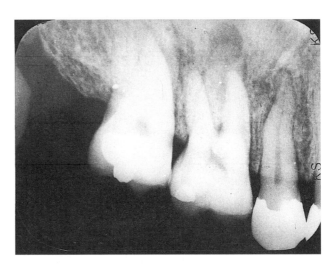

Fig. 24-11 A split tooth should always be considered when a nonvital pulp and chronic apical periodontitis are evident on a nonrestored tooth. The crack usually extends into the periodontium, and the prognosis is generally poor.

Periodontal disease may be the principal problem for dentate seniors.[14] The relationship between pulpal and periodontal disease can be expected to be more significant with age. Retention of teeth alone demonstrates some resistance to periodontal disease. The increase in disease prevalence is largely attributable to an increase in the proportional size of the population who have retained their teeth.[23] The periodontal tissues must be considered a pathway for sinus tracts (Fig. 24-12). Narrow, bony-walled pockets associated with nonvital pulps are usually sinus tracts, but they can be resistant to root canal therapy alone when, with time, they become chronic periodontal pockets.

Periodontal treatment can produce root sensitivity, disease, and pulp death.[22] In developing a successful treatment plan it is important to determine the effects of periodontal disease and its treatment on the pulp (Fig. 24-13). The mere increase in incidence and severity of periodontal disease with age increases the need for combined therapy. The chronic nature of pulp disease demonstrated with sinus tracts can often be manifested in a periodontal pocket. Root canal treatment is commonly indicated before root amputations are performed. With age, the size and number of apical and accessory foramen are actually reduced as pathways of communication,[37] as is the permeability of dentinal tubules.

Examination of sinus tracts should include tracing with gutta-percha cones to establish the tracts' origin (Fig. 24-14). Sinus tracts may have long clinical histories and usually indicate the presence of chronic periapical inflammation. Their disappearance after treatment is an excellent indicator of healing. The presence of a sinus tract reduces the risk of interappointment or postoperative pain, although drainage may follow canal débridement or filling.

Pulp Testing   Information collected from the patient's complaint, history, and examination may be adequate to

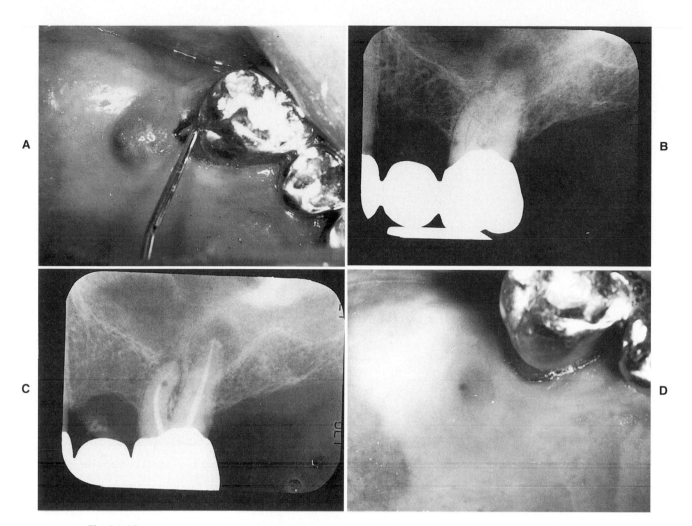

Fig. 24-12 **A**, A periodontal pocket is probed and a sinus tract is evident on this maxillary molar abutment (**B**); this could indicate pulpal or periodontal disease or both. **C**, Root canal treatment results in (**D**) healing that confirms the pulpal cause of this periradicular lesion.

establish pulp vitality and to direct the clinician toward the techniques that are most useful in determining which tooth or teeth are the object of the complaint. Slow and gentle testing should be done to determine pulp and periapical status and whether palliative or definitive therapy is indicated. Vitality responses must correlate with clinical and radiographic findings and be interpreted as a supplement in developing clinical judgment. (Techniques for clinical pulp-testing procedures are discussed in Chapter 1.)

Transilluminating[34] and staining have been advocated as means to detect cracks, but the presence of cracks is of little significance in the absence of complaints because most older teeth, especially molars, demonstrate some cracks. Vertically cracked teeth should always be considered when pulpal or periapical disease is observed and little or no cause for pulpal irritation can be observed clinically or radiographically. The high magnification available with microscopes during access opening and canal exploration permits visualization of the extent of cracks in determining prognosis. Cracks that are

detected while the pulp is still vital can offer a reasonable prognosis if immediately restored with full cuspal coverage. The chronic nature of any periapical pathologic condition caused by vertically cracked teeth indicates that it is long-standing, and the prognosis is questionable (even when pocket depths appear normal). Periodontal pockets associated with cracks indicate a hopeless prognosis.

The reduced neural and vascular components of aged pulps,[7] the overall reduced pulp volume, and the change in character of the ground substance[41] create an environment that responds differently to both stimuli and irritants than that of younger pulps (Fig. 24-15).

There are fewer nerve branches in older pulps. This may be due to retrogressive changes resulting from mineralization of the nerve and nerve sheath (Fig. 24-16).[6] Consequently, the response to stimuli may be weaker than in the more highly innervated younger pulp.

No correlation exists between the degree of response to electric pulp testing and the degree of inflammation. The

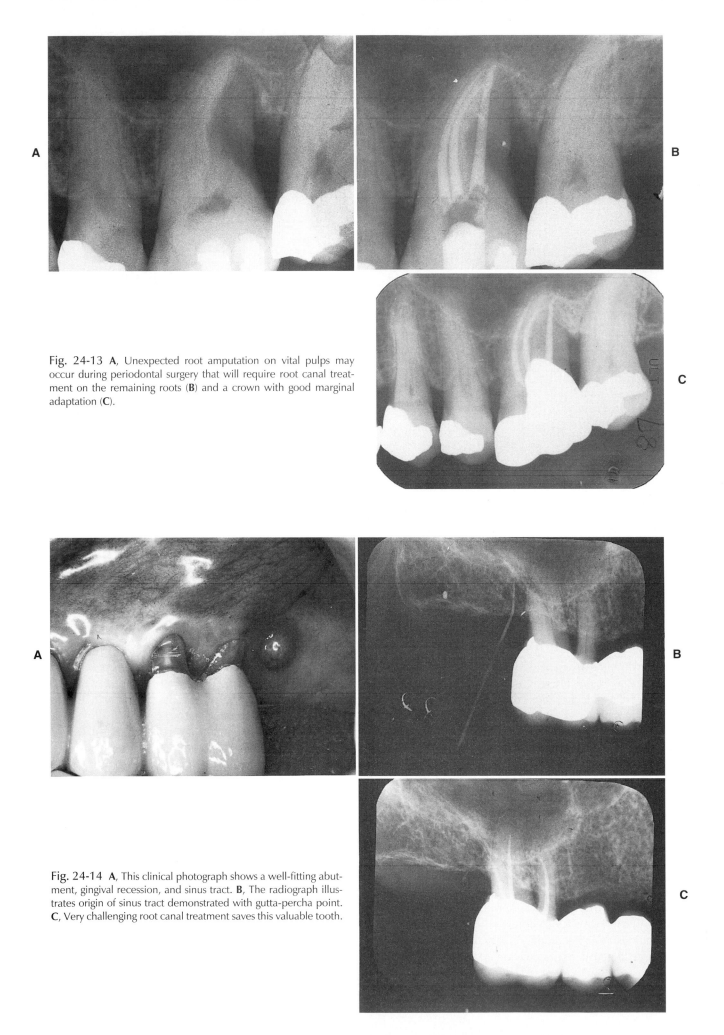

Fig. 24-13 **A**, Unexpected root amputation on vital pulps may occur during periodontal surgery that will require root canal treatment on the remaining roots (**B**) and a crown with good marginal adaptation (**C**).

Fig. 24-14 **A**, This clinical photograph shows a well-fitting abutment, gingival recession, and sinus tract. **B**, The radiograph illustrates origin of sinus tract demonstrated with gutta-percha point. **C**, Very challenging root canal treatment saves this valuable tooth.

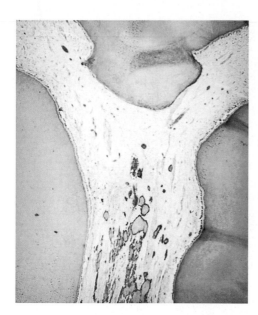

Fig. 24-15 There is a gradual decrease in the cellularity of older pulp tissue, and the odontoblasts decrease in size and number and may disappear altogether in certain areas, particularly on the pulpal floor in multirooted teeth.

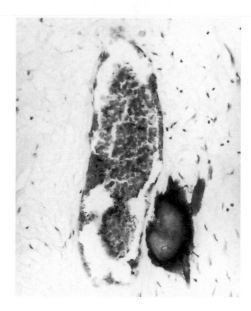

Fig. 24-16 Fibrosis appears to occur along the pathways of degenerated vessels and may serve as foci for pulpal calcification.

presence or absence of response is of limited value and must be correlated with other tests, examination findings, and radiographs. Extensive restorations, pulp recession, and excessive calcifications are limitations in both performing and interpreting results of electric and thermal pulp testing. Attachments that reduce the amount of surface contact necessary to conduct the electric stimulus are available (Analytic Technology, Orange County, Calif.) and bridging the tip to a small area of tooth structure with an explorer has been suggested.[31] Use of even this small electric stimulus in patients with pacemakers[52] is not recommended; any such risk would outweigh the benefit. The same caution holds true for electrosurgical units.

A test cavity is generally less useful as the test of last resort because of reduced dentin innervation. Vital pulps can sometimes be exposed and even negotiated with a file with minimal pain (Fig. 24-17); then the root canal treatment becomes part of the diagnostic procedure. Test cavities should be used only when other findings are suggestive but not conclusive.

Diffuse pain of vague origin is also uncommon in older pulps and limits the need for selective anesthesia. Pulpal disease is progressive and produces diagnostic signs or symptoms in a relatively short time. Nonodontogenic sources should be considered when factors associated with pulpal disease are not readily identified or when acute pain does not localize within a short time.

Discoloration of single teeth may indicate pulp death, but this is a less likely cause of discoloration with advanced age. Dentin thickness is greater and the tubules are less permeable to blood or breakdown products from the pulp. Dentin

deposition produces a yellow, opaque color that would indicate progressive calcification in a younger pulp; however, this is common in older teeth.

Radiographs   Indications for and techniques of taking radiographs do not differ much among adult age groups. However, several physiologic, anatomic changes can significantly affect their interpretation. Film placement may be adversely affected by tori but can be assisted by the apical position of muscle attachments that increase the depth of the vestibule. Older patients may be less capable of assisting in film placement, and holders that secure the position should be considered. The presence of tori, exostoses, and denser bone (Fig. 24-18) may require increased exposure times for proper diagnostic contrast. The subjective nature of interpretation can be reduced with correct processing, proper illumination, and magnification.

The periapical area must be included in the diagnostic radiograph, which should be studied from the crown toward the apex. Angled radiographs should be ordered only after the original diagnostic radiograph suggests that more information is needed for diagnosis or to determine the degree of difficulty of treatment. RadioVisioGraphy (RVG) may be more useful than conventional radiography in detecting early bone changes.[54]

In older patients, pulp recession is accelerated by reparative dentin and complicated by pulp stones and dystrophic calcification. Deep proximal or root decay and restorations may cause calcification between the observable chamber and root canal.

The depth of the chamber should be measured from the occlusal surface and its mesiodistal position noted.

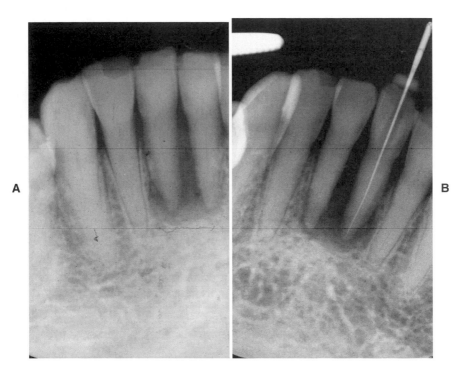

Fig. 24-17   Vital pulp testing was inconclusive (**A**), and the canal was negotiated (**B**) with little discomfort, although this was primarily periodontal disease. The rubber dam was secured with wedgets rather than a clamp.

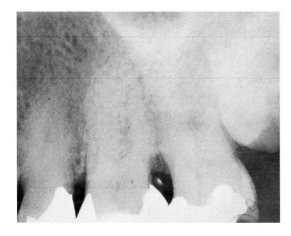

Fig. 24-18   Dense bone may indicate the need for increased exposure times to improve contrast needed to see the canal and root anatomy.

Receding pulp horns that are apparent on a radiograph may remain microscopically much higher. Deep restorations or extensive occlusal crown reduction may produce pulp exposures that were not expected. The axial inclinations of crowns may not correlate with the clinical observation when tilted teeth have been crowned or become abutments for fixed or removable appliances. Access to the root canals is the most limiting condition in root canal treatment of older patients.

Canals should be examined for their number, size, shape, and curvature. Comparisons to adjacent teeth should be made. Small canals are the rule in older patients. A midroot disappearance of a detectable canal may indicate bifurcation rather than calcification. Canals calcify evenly throughout their length unless an irritant (e.g., decay, restoration, cervical abrasion) has separated the chamber from the root canal. Root end fillings during apicoectomies (more common during retreatment of older patients) indicate missed canals and roots as a common cause of failure.[1]

The lamina dura should be examined in its entirety and anatomic landmarks distinguished from periapical radiolucencies and radiopacities. The incidence of some odontogenic and nonodontogenic cysts and tumors characteristically increases with age, and this should be considered when vitality tests do not correlate with radiographic findings. However, the incidence of osteosclerosis and condensing osteitis decreases with age.

Resorption associated with chronic apical periodontitis may significantly alter the shape of the apex and the anatomy of the foramen through inflammatory osteoclastic activity (Fig. 24-19).[11] The narrowest point in the canal may be difficult to determine; it is positioned farther from the radiographic apex because of continued cementum deposition.

A continued normal rate of cementum formation may be demonstrated by a canal or foramen that appears to end or exit short of the radiographic apex, and hypercementosis (Fig. 24-20) may completely obscure the apical anatomy.

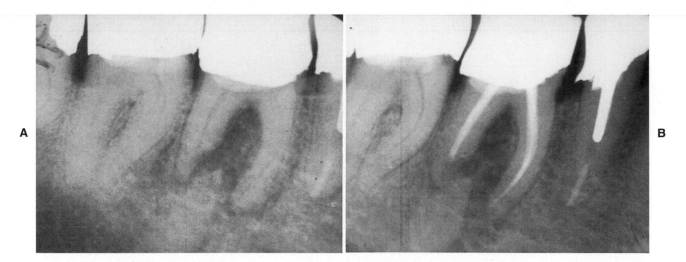

Fig. 24-19 **A**, Resorption associated with chronic apical periodontitis may alter the shape and position of the foramen through osteoclastic activity. **B**, The narrowest point in the canal is now positioned further from the radiographic apex.

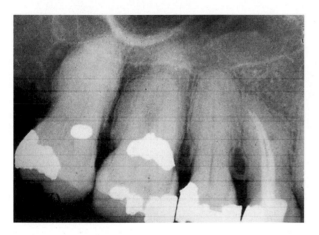

Fig. 24-20 Hypercementosis may completely obscure the apical anatomy and result in a constriction farther from the radiographic apex.

DIAGNOSIS AND TREATMENT PLAN

A clinical classification that accurately reflects the histologic status of the pulp and periapical tissues is not possible and not necessary beyond determining whether root canal treatment is indicated. A clinical judgment can be made, based on the patient's complaint, history, signs, symptoms, testing, and radiographs, as to the vitality of the pulp and the presence or absence of periapical pathologic conditions. This classification has not been shown to be a factor in predicting success, interappointment or postoperative pain, or the number of visits necessary to complete treatment when the objectives of cleansing, shaping, and filling are clearly understood and consistently met. Of great clinical significance in treatment procedures is the assessment of pulp status to deter-

mine the depth of anesthesia necessary to perform the treatment comfortably.

One appointment procedures offer obvious advantages to older patients. The length of a dental appointment does not usually cause inconvenience, as may more numerous appointments, especially if a patient must rely on another person for transportation or needs physical assistance to get into the office or operatory.

Root canal treatment as a restorative expediency on teeth with normal pulps must be considered when cusps have fractured or when supraerupted or malaligned teeth, intracoronal attachments, guide planes for partial abutments, rest seats, or overdentures require significant tooth reduction (Fig. 24-21). Predicting the need for future root canal treatment and a clinician's ability to perform treatment later is even more important, because the risk of losing the restoration during later access preparation increases with the thickness of the restoration and the reduction in canal size (Fig. 24-22). Because of a reduced blood supply, pulp capping is not as successful in older teeth as in younger ones; therefore it is not recommended. Any risk to the patient's future health and the effect that health may have on his or her ability to withstand future procedures should also be considered. Endodontic surgery at a later time is not as viable an alternative as for a younger patient.

Consultation and Consent

Good communication should be established and maintained with all patients, regardless of whether they are physically impaired or unable to make treatment decisions for themselves. Relatives or trusted friends should be included in consultations if their judgment is valued by the patient or needed for consent; however, the clinician should direct the discussion toward the patient (Fig. 24-23).

Clinicians should explain procedures in a way that is completely comprehensible and provides an opportunity for questions from the patient. "Patient friendly" pamphlets are available from the American Association of Endodontists (AAE) that thoroughly explain and illustrate most endodontic procedures. Obtaining signed consent to outlined treatment is encouraged and may be especially useful if the patient is forgetful.

Determining the patient's desires is as important as determining his or her needs, and it is required in obtaining informed consent. Priorities in treating pain and infection to properly and anesthetically restore teeth to health and function should be unaffected by age (Fig. 24-24). A patient's limited life expectancy should not appreciably alter treatment plans and is no excuse for extractions or poor root canal treatment. It is important that all older patients be well informed of risks and alternatives (Fig. 24-25).

Acceptance of the eventual loss of teeth has been replaced by an understanding of the psychologic and functional importance of maintaining dentition. Older patients whose

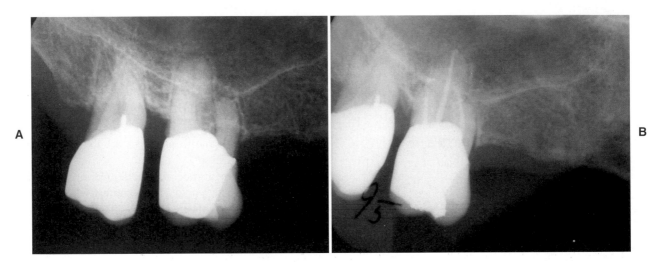

Fig. 24-21 **A**, Valuable maxillary first- and second-molar abutments in an 85-year-old patient. **B**, Later need for endodontic therapy was made very challenging because of access difficulties.

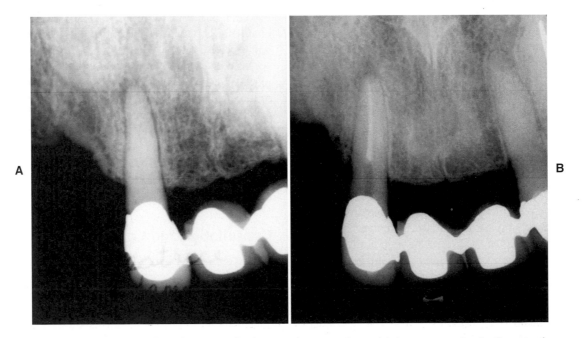

Fig. 24-22 **A**, Intracoronal attachments, guide planes, and rest seats for partial abutments require significant tooth reduction and a bulk of metal that makes endodontic treatment more likely and difficult. **B**, Successful treatment and preservation of the restoration when the canal is small are challenges to the most skilled clinician.

lives have been changed for the worse by a previous surgical procedure may readily recognize the implications of the loss of teeth.

The capability of the clinician and the availability of endodontic specialists should also be considered. The obligation to offer root canal treatment as an alternative to extraction may exceed a clinician's ability to perform the

procedure efficiently or successfully, and referral may be indicated. Older patients are more likely to be aware that there are specialists in performing root canals but will trust and do what their dentist recommends. In advance of the scheduled visit, referring dentists should provide the endodontist with as much information about the patient as possible (and thoroughly explain the reason for referral to the patient). Dentists should consider making the referral appointment for the patient while they are in the dentist's office to confirm compliance and understanding.

Obtaining informed consent before dental procedures usually is not a problem. However, medically compromised or cognitively impaired patients may make it difficult to acquire

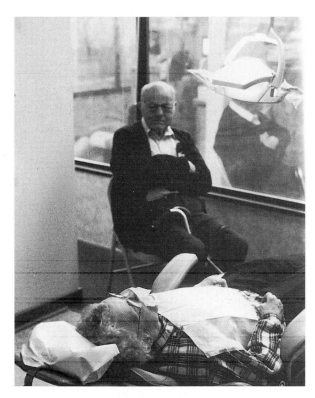

Fig. 24-23 Some patients may request or require that a family member be present during consultation or treatment.

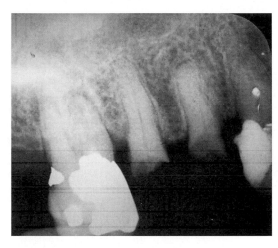

Fig. 24-24 This 84-year-old patient was pleased to find that all these teeth could be saved with endodontic therapy and crowns; she was eager to make the investment in time and money in spite of her limited life expectancy. Her concern focused on why these procedures had not been recommended by her previous dentist, whom she visited regularly.

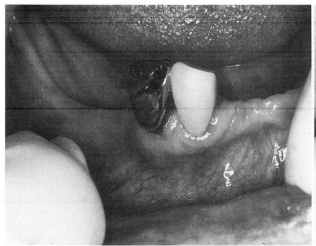

A

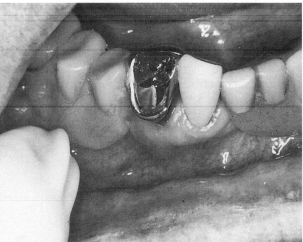

B

Fig. 24-25 **A**, These two remaining abutments were the only teeth this 99-year-old patient needed to retain a removable prostheses (**B**).

valid informed consent. Neuropsychiatric impairment may result in gross manifestations and indicate a reduced level of competency. Physicians or mental health experts should be consulted as needed, and no elective procedures performed until valid consent is established. Fortunately, acute pulpal and periapical episodes in which immediate treatment is indicated for pain or infection are less common than the low-grade signs and symptoms of chronic disease.

TREATMENT

The vast majority of geriatric patients who need and demand endodontic therapy are ambulatory and not institutionalized. Institutionalized and nonambulatory patients require clinicians trained in those environments and facilities designed for access to dental health care (Fig. 24-26). Such access is a benefit required in most institutions, but alternatives to root canal therapy may be the only services available. Extended health care facilities are now required to have dentists on staff before Medicare certification can be obtained. The dental office building, including both the interior design and the exterior approach, must be able to accommodate people with special needs.[30] Access for those who use ambulation aids (e.g., canes, walkers, wheelchairs) should include comfort and safety in the parking lot, reception room, operatory, and rest room.

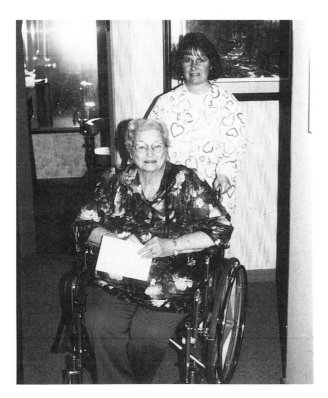

Fig. 24-26 Office design should consider access for wheelchairs and walkers. Staff should be experienced in assisting patients into and out of the operatory and chair.

A physical and mental evaluation of the patient should determine the ideal time of day and length of time necessary to schedule treatment. A patient's daily personal, eating, and resting habits should be considered, as well as any medication schedule. Morning appointments are preferable for some older patients, and their comfort, which varies with the procedure indicated, dictates the length of the appointment. Some patients prefer late morning or early afternoon visits, to allow "morning stiffness" to dissipate.[15]

Older patients are more likely to tolerate long appointments, although chair positioning and comfort may be more important for older adults than for younger patients. Patients should be offered assistance into the operatory and into or out of the chair, and chair adjustments should be made slowly (and the ideal position established and used, if possible). Pillows should be offered, as well as assistance in positioning them comfortably. Every effort should be made to accommodate the ideal position, even at some expense to the clinician's comfort or access.

The patient's eyes should be shielded from the intensity of the clinician's light. If the temperature selected for the comfort of the office staff is too cool for the patient, a blanket should be available. As much work as possible should be performed at each visit and a rest room break offered at intervals as the patient's needs indicate. Jaw fatigue is readily recognizable and may be the most limiting factor in a long procedure, requiring periods of rest; however, once such fatigue is evident, the procedure should be terminated as soon as possible. Bite blocks are useful in comfortably maintaining freeway space and reducing jaw fatigue.

Retired persons may rely on rides from friends or relatives or public transportation to get to the dental office. Although they often arrive early for appointments, most older patients are in no hurry once they arrive. Enough time should be scheduled to allow some social exchange, and a sincere personal interest should be demonstrated before proceeding. Endodontic specialists need to consider separate consultations for making this initial social contact and evaluating the degree of difficulty that will determine the chair time needed to perform treatment. Staff should allow patients to initiate handshakes, which may be very uncomfortable to arthritic joints. From a behavioral and management standpoint, geriatric patients are among the most cooperative, available, and appreciative.

Older, medically compromised patients are at no more risk of complications than those in any other age group, and the chronicity of their diseases can alert the clinician to necessary precautions. Once again, clinicians should recognize that root canal therapy is far less traumatic than extraction for older patients.

The pulp vitality status and the cervical positioning of the rubber dam clamp determine the need for anesthesia. Older patients more readily accept treatment without anesthesia, and sometimes they must be convinced that anesthesia is necessary for root canal treatment if their routine operative procedures have been performed without it. Generally older patients demonstrate less anxiety about dental treatment and may have previous experience with root canal treatment.

The cutting of dentin does not produce the same level of response in an older patient for the same reason that a test cavity is not as revealing during examination. The number of low threshold, high conduction velocity nerve endings in dentin is reduced or absent, and they do not extend as far into the dentin. In addition, the dentinal tubules are more calcified.[7,41] A painful response may not be encountered until actual pulp exposure has occurred.

Anatomic landmarks that are used as guides to needle placement during block and infiltration injections are usually more distinguishable in older patients. The effects of epinephrine should be considered when selecting anesthetics for routine endodontic procedures. Anesthetics should be deposited very slowly (and skeletal muscle avoided) if epinephrine is the vasoconstrictor.

The reduced width of the periodontal ligament[20] makes needle placement for supplementary intraligamentary injections more difficult. Placing an anesthetic under pressure produces an intraosseous anesthesia that extends to the apex and to adjacent teeth, but it also distributes small amounts of solution systemically.[39] Smaller amounts of anesthetic should be deposited during intraosseous injections, and the depth of anesthesia should be checked before repeating the procedure. Like intrapulpal anesthesia, intraosseous anesthesia is not prolonged; therefore the pulp tissue must be removed within 20 minutes. The majority of patients receiving an intraosseous injection of 2% lidocaine with 100,000 epinephrine solution experience a transient increase in heart rate. This would not be clinically significant in most healthy patients. However, in the older patient whose medical condition, drug therapies, or epinephrine sensitivity suggests caution, 3% mepivacaine is a good alternative for intraosseous injections.[35]

The reduced volume of the pulp chamber makes intrapulpal anesthesia difficult in single rooted teeth and almost impossible in multirooted teeth. Initial pulp exposures are also hard to identify. Wedging a small needle into each canal to produce the necessary pressure for anesthesia is the method of last resort. Every effort should be made to produce profound anesthesia. Patients should be encouraged to report any unpleasant sensation, and a prompt response should be made to any complaint. Patients should never be expected to tolerate pulpal pain.

Isolation

Single tooth rubber dam isolation should be used whenever possible. Badly broken-down teeth may not provide an adequate purchase point for the rubber dam clamp, and alternate rubber dam isolation methods should be considered (see Chapter 5). Multiple-tooth isolation may be used if adjacent teeth can be clamped and saliva output is low or a well-placed saliva ejector can be tolerated (Fig. 24-27). A petroleum-based lubricant for the lips and gingiva reduces chafing from saliva or perspiration beneath the rubber dam. Reduction in salivary flow and gag reflex reduces the need for a saliva ejector. Artificial saliva is available and should be used just before isolation because it is difficult to apply after the dam is in place.

Canals should be identified and their access maintained if restorative procedures are indicated for isolation. The clinician should not attempt isolation and access in a tooth with questionable marginal integrity of its restorations. Fluid-tight isolation cannot be compromised when sodium hypochlorite is used as an irrigant. Difficult-to-isolate defects produced by root decay present a good indication, in initial preparation, for the use of sonic hand pieces that use flow-through water as an irrigant.

The many merits of single visit root canal procedures should again be considered when isolation is compromised (see Chapter 4). The few minor benefits of multiple visit treatment are further reduced if an interappointment seal is difficult to obtain.

Access

Adequate access and identification of canal orifices are probably the most difficult parts of providing root canal treatment for older patients. Although the effects of aging and multiple restorations may reduce the volume and coronal extent of the chamber or canal orifice, its buccolingual and mesiodistal positions remain the same and can be predicted from radiographs and clinical examination. Canal position, root curvature, and axial inclinations of roots and crowns should be considered during the examination (Fig. 24-28). The effects of access on existing restorations and the possible need for actual removal of the restoration should be discussed with the patient before proceeding (Fig. 24-29). Coronal tooth structure or restorations should be sacrificed when they com-

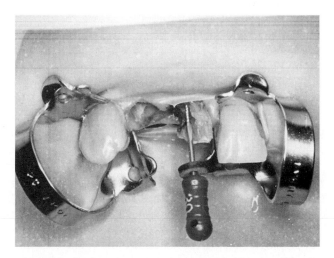

Fig. 24-27 Multiple tooth isolation techniques protect the patient from instruments but do not provide the fluid-tight environment preferred for the safe use of sodium hypochlorite.

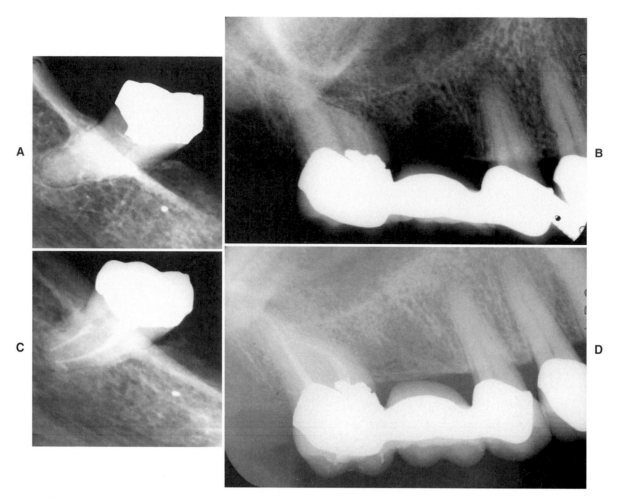

Fig. 24-28 **A**, This mandibular third molar in a 78-year-old patient has tilted mesially and has been restored with a full crown, upright to allow a path of insertion for a removable partial denture. **B**, Successful root canal treatment is the primary objective; retaining the crown, when possible, also represents significant savings to the patient. This crown will be replaced; a post space has been prepared. **C**, This maxillary third molar on the same patient is tilted mesially and rotated, making access (**D**) the most difficult part of this treatment.

promise access for preparation or filling (Fig. 24-30). (See Chapter 7 for more details on proper access openings.)

Magnification in the range of 2.5 × to 4.5 × (Designs for Vision, Ronkonkoma, N.Y.) has become a common tool and can be designed to fit the clinician's most comfortable working distance. The growing acceptance and availability of endodontic microscopes offers clear magnification of up to 25 × or greater and has obvious advantages in treating smaller geriatric canals (see Fig. 6-4).

Location and penetration of the canal orifice is often difficult and time consuming in calcified canals. The most important instrument for initial penetration is the DG 16 explorer. The explorer will not stick in solid dentin; however, it will resist dislodgment in the canal. Once the canal has been distinguished, negotiation is attempted with a stainless steel (SS) 21 mm, no. 8 or no. 0 K-file. The no. 6 file lacks stiffness in its shaft and easily bends and curls under gentle apical pressure. Nickel and titanium (NiTi) files lack strength in the long axis and are contraindicated for initial negotiation. The canal can be negotiated using a watch-winding action with slight apical pressure. Chelating agents are seldom of value in locating the orifice but can be useful during canal negotiation. Dyes may distinguish an orifice from the surrounding dentin.

Pain, bleeding, disorientation of the probing instruments, or an unfamiliar feel to the canal may indicate a perforation (Fig. 24-31). The size of the perforation and the extent of contamination determine the success of repair (which should be done immediately) and do not necessarily indicate failure (Fig. 24-32). Supererupted teeth can be easily perforated (Fig. 24-33) if the reduced distance to the furcation is not noted.

A lengthy, unproductive search for canals is fatiguing and frustrating to both the clinician and the patient. Scheduling a second attempt at this procedure is often productive. Personal clinical experiences and judgment determine when the search for the canals must be terminated and referral or alter-

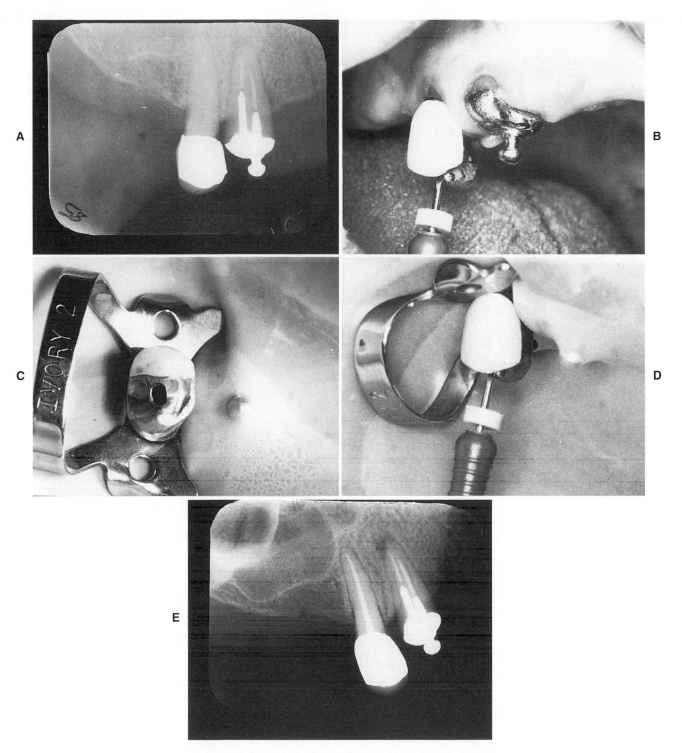

Fig. 24-29 **A**, Radiograph of strategic abutment and calcified canal. **B**, Access is initiated before isolation to increase visibility and alignment. **C**, An access opening that conserves tooth structure and provides straight-line access is then isolated with the rubber dam (**D**) and treated (**E**).

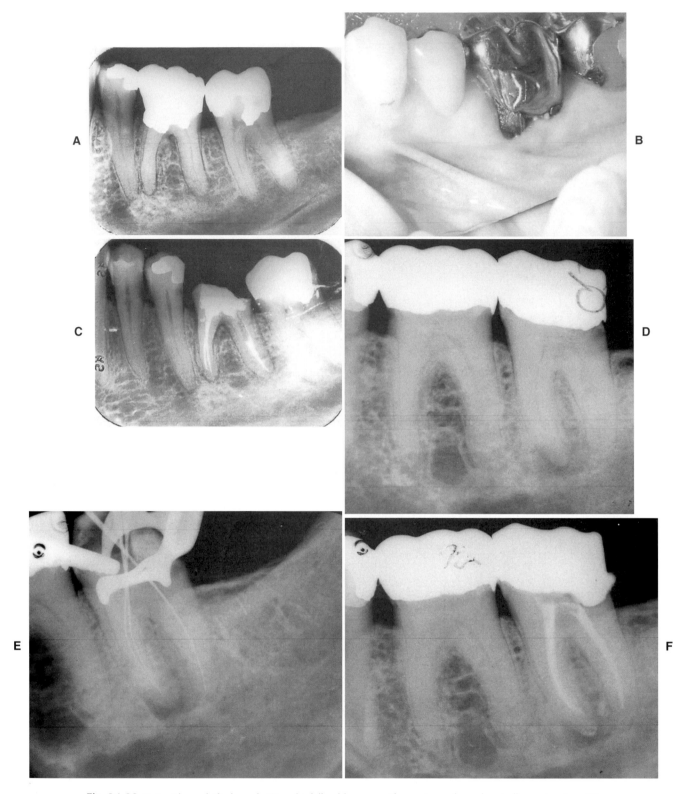

Fig. 24-30 Patient has calcified canals (**A**) and a full-gold crown with margins on buccal root alloy restorations (**B**). **C**, Access to all canals required crown removal. **D**, Caries under this crown would make isolation impossible. Crown was removed for isolation and caries removal (**E**) and endodontic treatment was completed in one visit (**F**).

natives to nonsurgical root canal treatment considered (Fig. 24-34).

Modifications to enhance access vary from widening the axial walls to increasing visibility or light to complete removal of the crown. Alterations may be indicated after canal penetration to the apex if tooth structure interferes with instrumentation or filling procedures.

Teeth with chronic apical periodontitis will usually have patent canals (Fig. 24-35). Surgical access (Fig. 24-36) may be preferred if the risk of deviation from the long axis exists when canals are calcified and the tooth is heavily restored (Fig. 24-37).

Very few canals of older teeth, even maxillary anterior teeth, have adequate diameter to allow the safe and effective uses of broaches. Older pulps may give a clinical appearance that reflects their calcified, atrophic state with the stiffened, fibrous consistency of a wet toothpick. Any broached canals should be thoroughly instrumented at the same appointment.

Preparation

The calcified appearance of the canals resulting from the aging process presents a much different clinical situation than that of a younger pulp in which trauma, pulpotomy, decay, or restorative procedures have induced premature canal obliteration. Unless further complicated by reparative dentin formation, this calcification appears to be much more concentric and linear. This allows easier penetration of canals once they are found. An older tooth is more likely to have a history of earlier treatments, with a combination of calcifications present. (For a description of cleaning and shaping root canals, see Chapter 8.)

The length of the canal from the actual anatomic foramen to the CDJ increases with the deposition of cementum throughout life.[21] The advantage of this situation in the treatment of teeth with vital pulps is countered by the presence of necrotic, infected debris in this longer canal when periapical pathosis is already present. The actual CDJ width or most apical extent of the dentin remains constant with age.[43]

Flaring of the canal should be performed as early in the procedure as possible to provide for a reservoir of irrigation solution and to reduce the stress on metal instruments that occurs when they bind with the canal walls. Thorough and frequent irrigation should be performed to remove the debris

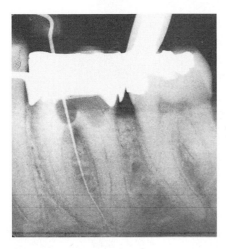

Fig. 24-31 Pain, bleeding, or disorientation of the probing instrument may indicate a perforation and should be immediately investigated radiographically. Repair is possible when the opening is pinpointed and the periodontal tissues are still normal.

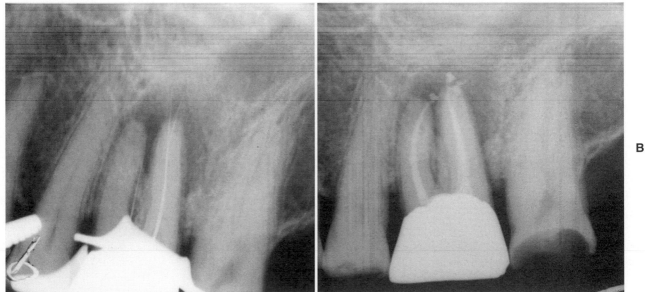

Fig. 24-32 **A**, Perforation occurred during access of these calcified canals. **B**, Endodontic treatment was immediately completed after the perforation repair.

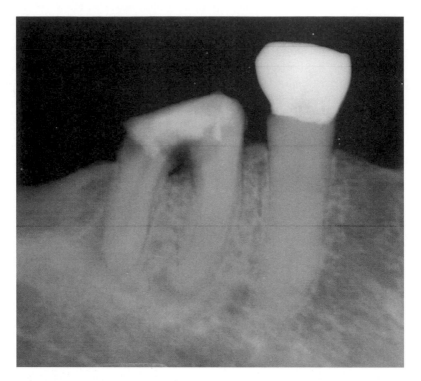

Fig. 24-33 Supraerupted mandibular first molar that was perforated during access.

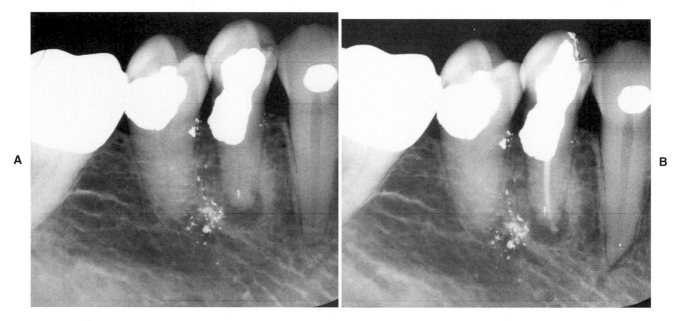

Fig. 24-34 **A**, Midtreatment referral of a mandibular first premolar only after perforation and repair with amalgam.
B, Canal was still detectable with enhanced vision technique and treatment completed.

that could block access. Files with a triangular or square cross section may penetrate into the walls with greater force than the fracture resistance of small files (when used with a reaming action) and result in instrument fatigue and fracture. The benefits of instruments with no rake angle and a crown down technique should be considered.

Because this CDJ is the narrowest constriction of the canal, it is the ideal place to terminate the canal preparation. This point may vary from 0.5 to 2.5 mm from the radiographic apex and be difficult to determine clinically. Calcified canals reduce the clinician's tactile sense in identifying the constriction clinically, and reduced periapical sensitivity

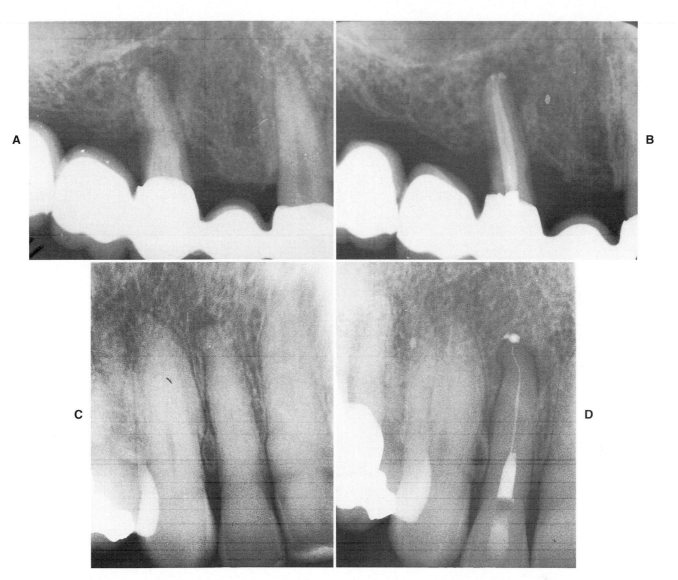

Fig. 24-35 **A,** Strategic middle abutment for a long fixed bridge presents a challenge to the most skilled clinician to perform predictable root canal treatment (**B**). Poor crown-to-root ratio makes root end surgery a poor option. Root canal treatment should have been considered before using this lone-standing premolar as an abutment. **C,** Calcified canals can usually be detected and treated when a nonvital pulp and chronic apical periodontitis is present, even when it is not apparent on the radiograph. Asymptomatic, calcified canals on teeth with vital pulps are much more difficult to find and negotiate. **D,** This access attempt was terminated at midroot, but the presence of a small canal was demonstrated with sealer when the access was filled.

in older patients reduces the patient's response that would indicate penetration of the foramen. Increased incidence of hypercementosis, in which the constriction is even farther from the apex, makes penetration into the cemental canal almost impossible. Achieving and maintaining apical patency is more difficult. Apical root resorption associated with periapical pathosis further changes the shape, size, and position of the constriction. The use of electronic, apex-finding devices is sometimes limited in heavily restored teeth when contact with metal can bleed off the current.

The frequency and intensity of discomfort after instrumentation has not been shown to be related to the amount of preparation, the type of interappointment medication or temporary filling, the pulp or periapical status, the tooth number or age, or whether the root canal filling is completed at the same appointment.[46] The more constricted dentin and cementum junction (DCJ) permits a much smaller pulp wound and resists penetration, even with the initial small files. Patency is difficult to establish and maintain. Dentin debris creates a matrix early in the preparations[53] and further

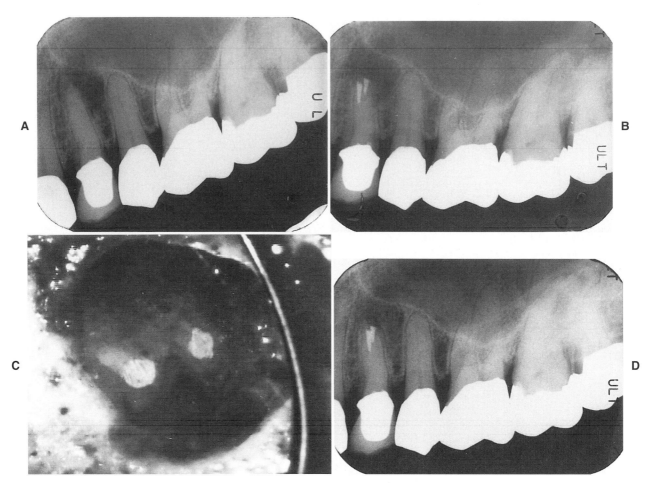

Fig. 24-36 **A**, Completely calcified canals, thin roots, and porcelain fused-to-metal restoration makes risk of perforation high. **B**, Surgical access and root end fillings (**C**) resulted in healing and an intact restoration (**D**).

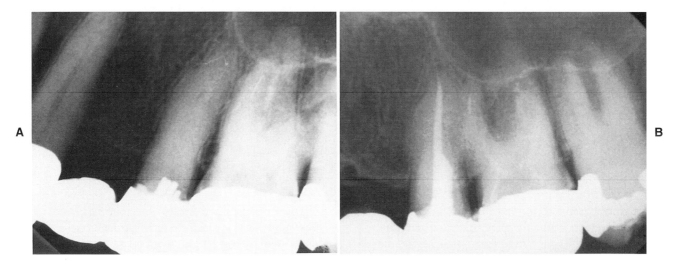

Fig. 24-37 **A**, Multiple pins were used to restore this middle abutment on a fixed bridge. **B**, Extreme care and exceptional skill are required to maintain proper alignment to find and treat the canal with a deep access opening.

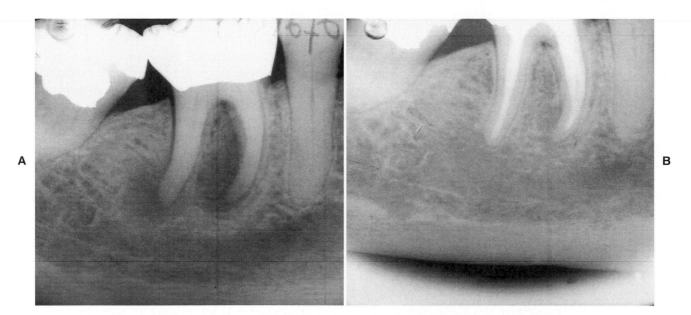

Fig. 24-38 **A**, Long-standing periapical radiolucency with a draining sinus tract indicated the need for endodontic treatment on this crowned mandibular first molar of an 82-year-old patient. **B**, One-year recall examination shows remineralization.

reduces the risk of overinstrumentation or the forcing of debris into the periapical tissues,[32] which could cause an acute apical periodontitis or abscess. Further access to periapical tissues through the canal is likewise limited.

Obturation

For the older patient the prudent clinician selects gutta percha–filling techniques that do not require unusually large midroot tapers and do not generate pressure in this area, which could result in root fracture. (See Chapter 9 for the most appropriate technique to use to seal the canal.)

The coronal seal plays an important role in maintaining the apically sealed environment, and it has significant impact on long-term success.[45] Even a root filled tooth should not have its canals exposed to the oral environment. Permanent restorative procedures should be scheduled as soon as possible, and intermediate restorative materials should be selected and properly placed to maintain a seal until that time. When mechanical retention is not ensured with the preparation, glass ionomer cements are of value for this purpose.

Success and Failure

Repair of periapical tissues after endodontic treatment in older patients is determined by most of the same local and systemic factors that govern the process in all patients. With vital pulps, periapical tissues are normal and can be maintained with an aseptic technique, confining preparation and filling procedures to the canal space. Infected, nonvital pulps

with periapical pathologic abnormalities must have this process altered in favor of the host tissue, and repair is determined by the ability of this tissue to respond. Factors that influence repair have their greatest effect on the prognosis of endodontic therapy when periapical abnormalities are present. With aging, arteriosclerotic changes of blood vessels increase and the viscosity of connective tissue is altered, making repair more difficult. The rate of bone formation and normal resorption decreases with age, and the aging of bone results in greater porosity and decreased mineralization of the formed bone. A 6-month recall period to evaluate repair radiographically may not be adequate; it may take as long as 2 years to produce the healing that would occur at 6 months in an adolescent (Fig. 24-38).

Studies that suggest a difference in success between age groups must note the smaller numbers (usually in this older treatment group) and the local factors that make treatment difficult. Overlooked canals are a more common cause of failure in older patients (Fig. 24-39), which explains the increased clinical indications for retrograde fillings when surgical treatment is attempted.[1] As an isolated symptom, heat sensitivity may indicate a missed canal. (For further information on assessing failures and possible retreatment, see Chapter 25.)

ENDODONTIC SURGERY

Generally considerations and indications for endodontic surgery are not affected by age. The need for establishment of drainage and relief of pain are not common indications for surgery. Anatomic complications of the root canal system, such as small (Fig. 24-40) or completely calcified canals, nonnegotiable root curvatures, extensive apical root resorption, or pulp stones, occur with greater frequency in older patients. Perforation during access, losing length during instrumentation, ledging, and instrument separation are iat-

rogenic treatment complications associated with treatment of calcified canals.

Medical considerations may require consultation but do not contraindicate surgical treatment when extraction is the alternative (Fig. 24-41). In most instances surgical treatment may be performed less traumatically than an extraction, which may also result in the need for surgical access to complete root removal. A thorough medical history and evaluation should reveal the need for any special considerations, such as prophylactic antibiotic premedication, sedation, hospitalization, or more detailed evaluation.

Local considerations in treatment of older patients include an increase in the incidence of fenestrated or dehisced roots and exostoses (Fig. 24-42). The thickness of overlying soft and bony tissue is usually reduced, and apically positioned muscle attachments extend the depth of the vestibule. Smaller amounts of anesthetic and vasoconstrictor are needed for profound anesthesia. Tissue is less resilient, and resistance to reflection appears to be diminished. The oral cavity is usually more accessible with the teeth closed together because the lips can more easily be stretched. The apex can actually be more surgically accessible in older patients. Ability to gain such access varies with the skill of the surgeon; however, some areas are unreachable by even the most experienced clinicians.

The position of anatomic features, such as the sinus, floor of the nose, and neurovascular bundles, remains the same, but their relationship to surrounding structures may change when teeth have been lost. The need may arise to combine endodontic and periodontic flap procedures, and every

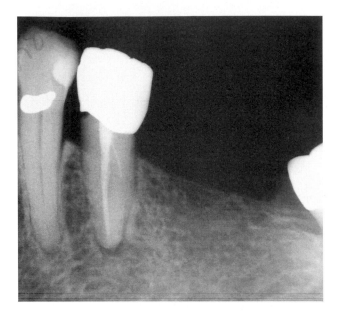

Fig. 24-39 Overlooked canals are a more common cause of failure in older patients than in younger patients, which explains the increased clinical indications for retrograde fillings when surgical treatment is performed.

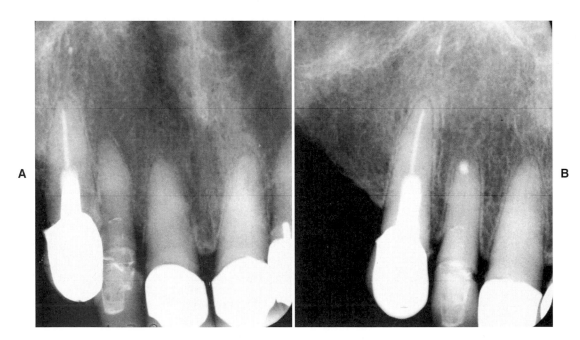

A

B

Fig. 24-40 **A**, Even though a small canal is detectable on the radiograph, it appears that an earlier unsuccessful attempt has been made to find it. **B**, It was decided that the risk of damage to a satisfactory restoration justified surgical treatment for this patient.

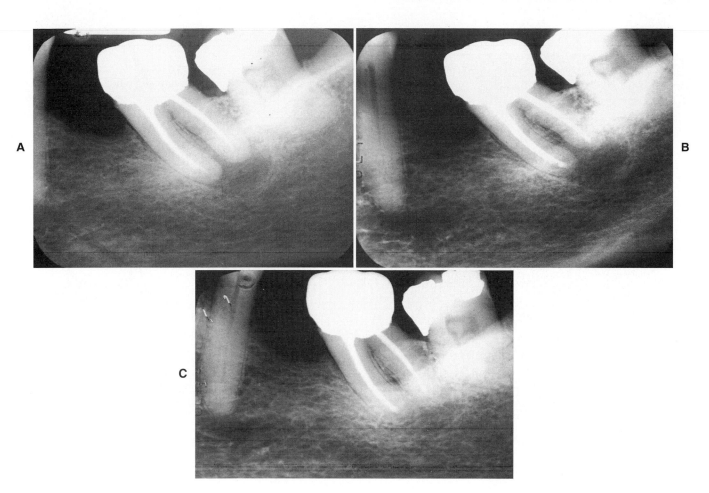

Fig. 24-41 **A**, Unsuccessful and symptomatic treatment on a mandibular second molar of a 78-year-old patient was surgically treated (**B**) with less trauma than the extraction alternative. **C**, Complete healing at 1 year, apparently unaffected by age.

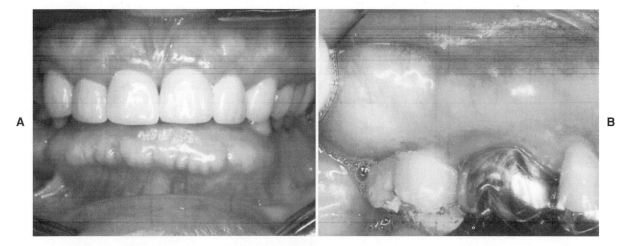

Fig. 24-42 Exostoses, as illustrated in this mandibular anterior (**A**) and maxillary molar (**B**) covered with thin tissue that can easily be torn during flap reflection, as well as the more obvious heavy bone and its effect on surgical access.

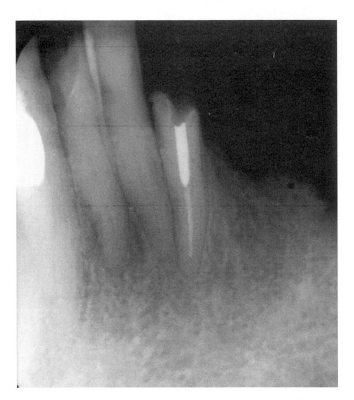

Fig. 24-43 This fracture of a cast post presents a very difficult challenge to remove.

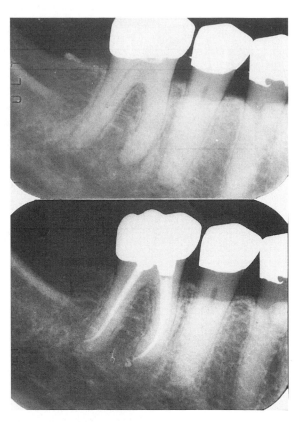

Fig. 24-44 *Top,* Intact margins permitted the continued use of this crown and the access was restored with an amalgam-bond core (*bottom*).

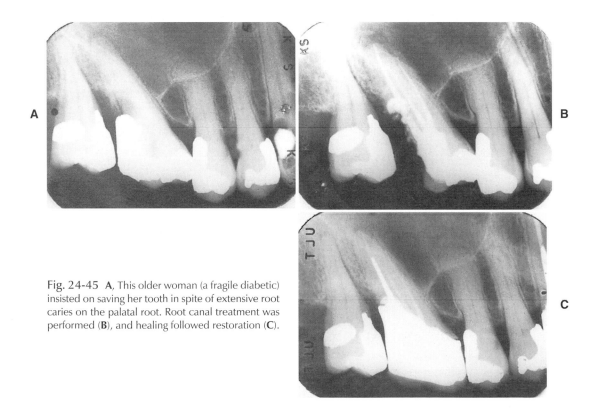

Fig. 24-45 **A**, This older woman (a fragile diabetic) insisted on saving her tooth in spite of extensive root caries on the palatal root. Root canal treatment was performed (**B**), and healing followed restoration (**C**).

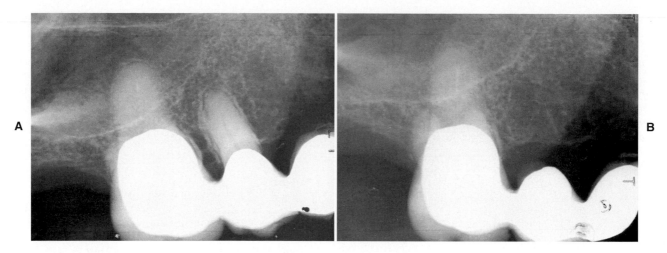

Fig. 24-46 **A,** Unrestorable caries contraindicated endodontic therapy on this second premolar abutment. **B,** Root was surgically extracted from beneath the bridge, which was still functional at this 3-year recall period.

effort should be made to complete these procedures in one sitting.

When apicoectomy is to be performed, the surgeon must consider whether the root that will be left is long enough and thick enough for the tooth to continue to remain functional and stable. This factor is especially important when the tooth will be used as an abutment. (Detailed surgical procedures are presented in Chapter 19.)

Ecchymosis is a more common postoperative finding in older patients and may appear to be extreme. The patient should be reassured that this condition is normal and that normal color may take as long as 2 weeks to return. The blue discoloration will change to brown and yellow before it disappears. Immediate application of an ice pack after surgery reduces bleeding and initiates coagulation to reduce the extent of ecchymosis. Later, application of heat helps to dissipate the discoloration.

RESTORATION

Root canal treatment saves roots, and restorative procedures save crowns. Combined, these procedures are returning more teeth to form and function than was thought possible just a few decades ago. Special consideration must be given to post design, especially when small posts are used in abutment teeth; root fracture is common in older adults when much taper is used. Post failure or fracture occurs when small-diameter parallel posts are used (Fig. 24-43). Posts are not usually needed when root canal treatment is performed through an existing crown that will continue to be used (Fig. 24-44). (General considerations and procedures for post-endodontic restoration are detailed in Chapter 22.)

The value of the tooth, its restorability, its periodontal health, and the patient's wishes should be part of the evaluation preceding endodontic therapy. The restorability of older

teeth can be affected when root decay has limited access to sound margins or reduced the integrity of remaining tooth structure (Fig. 24-45). There can also be insufficient vertical and horizontal space when opposing or adjacent teeth are missing. Patient desires to save appliances can sometimes be fulfilled with creative attempts that may outlive them (Fig. 24-46).

In conclusion, it can be seen that geriatric endodontics will gain a more significant role in complete dental care as our aging population recognizes that a complete dentition, and not complete dentures, is a part of their destiny.

References

1. Allen RK, Newton CW, Brown CE Jr: A statistical analysis of surgical and nonsurgical endodontic retreatment cases, *J Endod* 15:261, 1989.
2. American Association of Retired Persons: *A profile of older Americans*, Washington, DC, 1995, The Association.
3. Barbakow FH, Cleaton-Jones P, Friedman D: An evaluation of 566 cases of root canal therapy in general dental practice: postoperative observations, *J Endod* 6:485, 1980.
4. Baum BJ: Evaluation of stimulated parotid saliva flow rate in different age groups, *J Dent Res* 60:1292, 1981.
5. Berkey DB et al: The old-old dental patient, *J Am Dent Assoc* 127:321, 1996.
6. Bernick S: Effect of aging on the nerve supply to human teeth, *J Dent Res* 46:694, 1967.
7. Bernick S, Nedelman C: Effect of aging on the human pulp, *J Endod* 3:88, 1975.
8. Bhaskar SN: *Orban's oral histology and embryology,* ed 11, St Louis, 1990, Mosby.
9. Browne RM, Tobias RS: Microbial microleakage and pulpal inflammation: a review, *Endodont Dent Traumatol* 2:177, 1986.

10. Campbell PR: *Bureau of the Census, population projections for states, by age, race, and Hispanic origin: 1993 to 2020,* Washington, DC, 1994, US Government Printing Office.

11. Delzangles B: Scanning electron microscopic study of apical and intracanal resorption, *J Endod* 14:281, 1989.

12. Dolan TA, Berkey DB, Mulligan R, Saunders ML: Geriatric dental education and training in the United States: 1995 white paper findings, *Gerodontology* 13:94, 1996.

13. Douglas CW, Furino A: Balancing dental service requirements and supplies: epidemiologic and demographic evidence, *J Am Dent Assoc* 121(5):587, 1990.

14. Douglas CW, Gammon MD, Orr RB: Oral health status in the U.S.: prevalence of inflammatory periodontal disease, *J Dent Educ* 49:365, 1985.

15. Ettinger R, Beck T, Glenn R: Eliminating office architectural barriers to dental care of the elderly and handicapped, *J Am Dent Assoc* 98(3):398, 1979.

16. Fedele DJ, Sheets CG: Issues in the treatment of root caries in older adults, *J Esthet Dent* 10:243, 1998.

17. Frank ME, Hettinger TP, Mott AK: The sense of taste: neurobiology, aging, and medication effects, *Crit Rev Oral Biol Med* 3(4):371, 1992.

18. Joshipura KJ, Willett WC, Douglass CW: The impact of edentulousness on food and nutrient intake, *J Am Dent Assoc* 127:459, 1996.

19. Kier DM et al: Thermally induced pulpalgia in endodontically treated teeth, *J Endod* 17:38, 1991.

20. Klein A: Systematic investigations of the thickness of the periodontal ligament, *Ztschr Stomatol* 26:417, 1928.

21. Kuttler Y: Microscopic investigation of root apexes, *J Am Dent Assoc* 50:544, 1955.

22. Lowman JV, Burke RS, Pelleu GB: Patent accessory canals: incidence in molar furcation region, *Oral Surg* 36:580, 1973.

23. MacNeil RC: The geriatric patient: a periodontal perspective, *J Indian Dent Assoc* 70:24, 1991.

24. Manski RJ, Goldfarb MM: Dental utilization for older Americans aged 55-75, *Gerodontology* 13:49, 1996.

25. Meskin LH: Economic impact of dental service utilization by older patients, *J Am Dent Assoc* 120:665, 1990.

26. Miller CS: Documenting medication use in adult dental patients: 1987-1991, *J Am Dent Assoc* 123:41, 1992.

27. Miller WA, Massler M: Permeability and staining of active and arrested lesions in dentine, *Br Dent J* 112:187, 1962.

28. Moeller TM: Sensory changes in the elderly, *Dent Clin North Am* 33:29, 1989.

29. National Institute on Aging: *Personnel for health needs of the elderly through year 2020: report to Congress,* Washington, DC, 1987, US Government Printing Office.

30. Palmer C: New federal law will ban discrimination, *ADA News* 21(11):1, 1990.

31. Pantera EA, Anderson RW, Pantera CT: Use of dental instruments for bridging during electric pulp testing, *J Endod* 18:37, 1992.

32. Patterson SM et al: The effect of an apical dentin plug in root canal preparation, *J Endod* 14:1, 1988.

33. Philippas GG, Applebaum E: Age changes in the permanent upper canine teeth, *J Dent Res* 47:411, 1968.

34. Polson AM: Periodontal destruction associated with vertical root fracture, *J Periodontol* 48:27, 1977.

35. Replogle K et al: Cardiovascular effects of intraosseous injections of 2 percent lidocaine with 1:100,000 epinephrine and 3 percent mepivacaine, *J Am Dent Assoc* 130:649, 1999.

36. Rossman I: *Clinical geriatrics,* ed 3, Philadelphia, 1986, JB Lippincott.

37. Rubach WC, Mitchell DF: Periodontal disease, accessory canals and pulp pathosis, *J Periodontol* 36:34, 1965.

38. Selvig KF: The fine structure of human cementum, *Acta Odontol Scand* 23:423, 1965.

39. Smith GN, Walton RE: Periodontal ligament injections: distribution of injected solutions, *Oral Surg* 55:232, 1983.

40. Sreebny LM, Schwartz SS: A reference guide to drugs and dry mouth, *Gerodontology* 14:33 1997.

41. Stanley HR, Ranney RR: Age changes in the human dental pulp. I. The quantity of collagen, *Oral Surg* 15:1396, 1962.

42. Stanley HR et al: The detection and prevalence of reactive and physiologic sclerotic dentin, reparative dentin and dead tracts beneath various types of dental lesions according to tooth surface and age, *J Oral Pathol* 12:257, 1983.

43. Stein TJ, Corcoran JF: Anatomy of the root apex and its histologic changes with age, *Oral Surg Oral Pathol Oral Med* 69:238, 1990.

44. Strindberg L: The dependence of the result of pulp therapy on certain factors: an analytic study based on radiographic and clinical follow-up examinations, *Acta Odontol Scand* 14(suppl 21): 1956.

45. Swanson K, Madison S: An evaluation of coronal microleakage in endodontically treated teeth. I. Time periods, *J Endod* 13:56, 1987.

46. Swartz DB, Skidmore AK, Griffin JA: Twenty years of endodontic success and failure, *J Endod* 9:198, 1983.

47. Tenovuo J: Oral defense factors in the elderly, *Endod Dent Traumatol* 8:93, 1992.

48. US Department of Health and Human Services: *Personnel for health needs of the elderly through year 2020: September 1987 report to Congress,* Bethesda, MD, 1987, US Public Health Service.

49. US Department of Health and Human Services: *Use of dental services and dental health, United States: 1986,* Washington, DC, 1988, US Government Printing Office.

50. Wallace MC, Retief DH, Bradley EL: Prevalence of root caries in a population of older adults, *Geriodontics* 4:84, 1988.

51. Walton RE: Endodontic considerations in the geriatric patient, *Dent Clin North Am* 41:795, 1997.

52. Woodly L, Woodworth J, Dobbs JL: A preliminary evaluation of the effect of electric pulp testers on dogs with artificial pacemakers, *J Am Dent Assoc* 89:1099, 1974.

53. Yee RDS et al: The effect of canal preparation on the formation and leakage characteristics of the apical dentin plug, *J Endod* 10:308, 1984.

54. Yokota ET, Miles DA, Newton CW, Brown CE: Interpretation of periapical lesions using Radiovisiography, *J Endod* 20:490, 1994.

55. Zander H, Hurzeler B: Continuous cementum apposition, *J Dent Res* 37:1035, 1958.

Chapter 25

Nonsurgical Endodontic Retreatment*

Clifford J. Ruddle

Chapter Outline

In recent years the number of people seeking endodontic treatment has dramatically increased because of the public's choice of root canal treatment over tooth extraction. General dentists and endodontists are better trained because of advances in technology. Graduate students are also better trained. The growing use of endodontics can be described as the "good-news, bad-news dilemma." The good news is that hundreds of millions of teeth are salvaged through combinations of endodontics, periodontics, and restorative dentistry.

The bad news is that tens of millions of teeth are endodontically failing for a variety of reasons.

Many failures can be attributed to an abundance of misinformation and misconceptions about endodontics. Additional failures occur because clinicians tend to resist change; these practitioners hesitate to embrace relevant, new-and-emerging technologies, instruments, and materials. Unfortunately, the accelerating rate of change in the field of endodontics has left many dentists in the gap between current training and new possibilities.

This chapter is intended to close the endodontic gap by focusing on the concepts, strategies, and techniques that will produce superior results in nonsurgical retreatment. During the last decade significant procedural refinements have increased the ability of endodontics to fulfill the public's higher expectations for predictable results. When the best of what endodontics has to offer is intelligently integrated, it can clinically drive new practice-building techniques and improve success.

RATIONALE FOR RETREATMENT

There are a great number of articles reporting the success rates of endodontic treatment, ranging between 53% and 94%.[89] However, even if 90% of all endodontic treatment is successful over time, the reciprocal failure rate is still 10%. In the United States alone, where the number of teeth treated per year now exceeds 50 million,[22] a 10% failure rate would represent 5 million treatment failures per year. Extrapolating these numbers over the past 3 to 4 decades reveals that the number of failing endodontically treated teeth is massive and could approach tens of millions!

Root canal system anatomy plays a significant role in endodontic success and failure. These systems contain branches that communicate with the periodontal attachment apparatus furcally, laterally, and often terminate apically into multiple portals of exit (Fig. 25-1).[29] Improvement in the diagnosis and treatment of lesions of endodontic origin occurs with the recognition of the interrelationships that exist between pulpal disease flow and the egress of irritants along these anatomic pathways.[76] It is fundamental to associate radiographic lesions of endodontic origin as arising secondary to pulpal breakdown and as forming adjacent to the portals of exit (Fig. 25-2).

Endodontic failures can be attributable to inadequacies in cleaning, shaping and obturation, iatrogenic events, or reinfection of the root canal system when the coronal seal is lost after completion of root canal treatment.[5,85,93] Regardless of the initial cause, the sum of all causes is leakage.[69,78,100] When appropriate, nonsurgical endodontic retreatment efforts are directed toward eliminating microleakage. The

rationale for nonsurgical retreatment is to remove the root canal space as a source of irritation to the attachment apparatus (Fig. 25-3).

Criteria for Success

The healing capacity of endodontic lesions is dependent on many variables, including diagnosis, complete access, identification of all orifices and canal systems, and use of concepts and techniques directed toward three-dimensional (3-D) cleaning, shaping, and obturation.[68,82] The standard for success could be defined by the four following criteria:

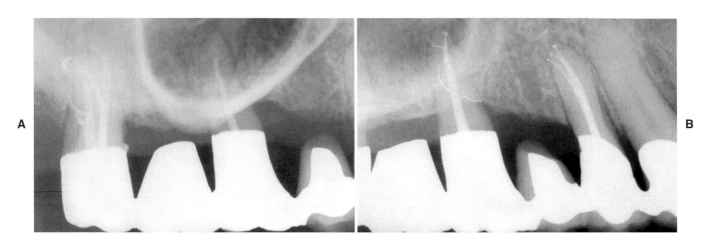

Fig. 25-1 **A**, Preoperative film shows multidisciplinary treatment. The maxillary left first molar's remaining palatal root is endodontically failing. **B**, 3-D endodontic retreatment is the foundation of periodontic prosthetics.

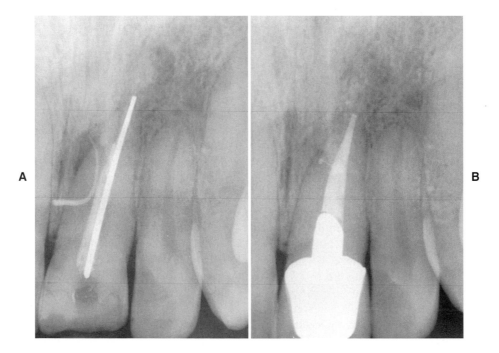

Fig. 25-2 **A**, Preoperative film of an endodontically failing maxillary central incisor. A gutta-percha point traces a fistulous tract to a large lateral root lesion. **B**, 5-year recall film demonstrates osseous repair after 3-D endodontics.

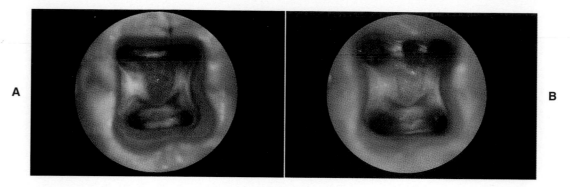

Plate 25-1 A, A view into an access cavity suggests that there are four orifices or systems in this mandibular first molar. **B,** Photograph demonstrating a third mesial orifice and the importance of exploring the isthmus connecting the mesiobuccal and mesiolingual systems.

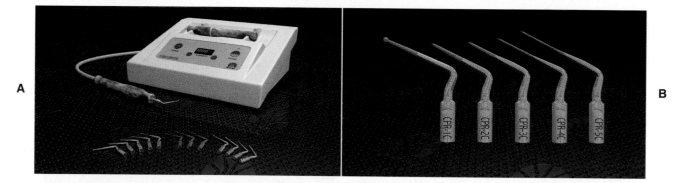

Plate 25-2 A, The P-5 piezoelectric ultrasonic system (Dentsply, Tulsa, Okla.) with an endodontic and periodontic autoclavable handpiece. This unit powers a variety of innovative ultrasonic instruments. **B,** The CPR 1-5 zirconium nitride-coated ultrasonic instruments are uniquely designed to improve vision, access, and control when performing clinical procedures.

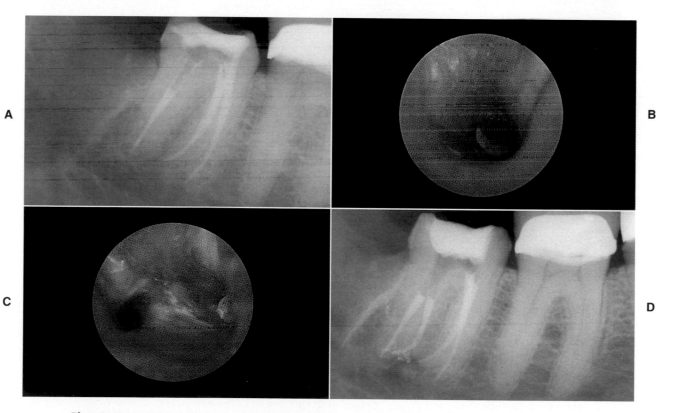

Plate 25-3 A, Radiograph shows a mandibular right second molar with three canals treated endodontically. The obturation material is not centered within the distal root. **B,** A view into the centered distal orifice reveals obturation material positioned subcrestally in a fin off this canal. **C,** Photograph shows improved straight-line access to the DL orifice and gutta-percha deep within the previously treated DB system. **D,** Posttreatment radiograph demonstrates the packed DL root canal system.

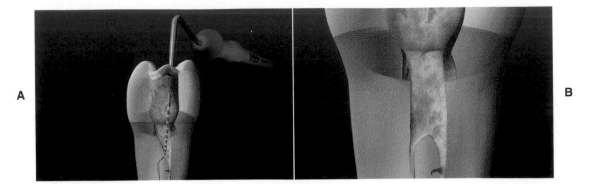

Plate 25-4 A, Distal view of a mandibular molar animation. The microopener's offset handle affords unobstructed vision and is used to initiate treatment in areas where access is difficult and restricted. **B,** Animation showing that the microopener has carved away the triangle of dentin and has created straight-line
access to the second distal system.

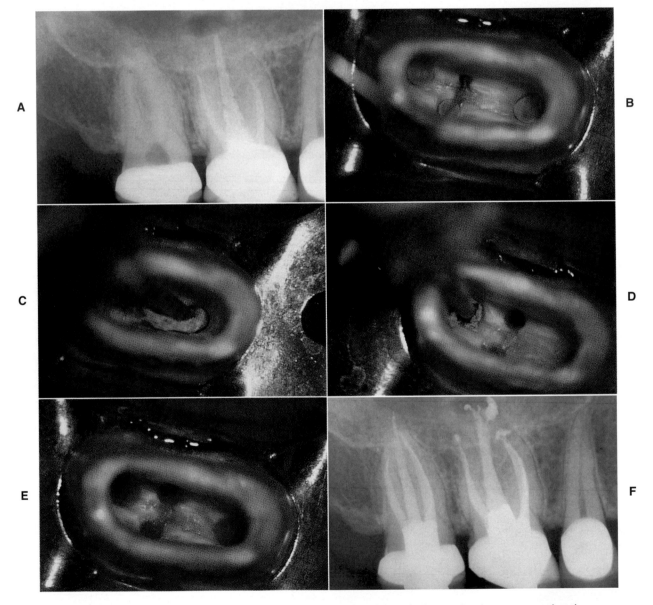

Plate 25-5 A, Radiograph of an endodontically failing maxillary right first molar demonstrates that the
previously treated canals are underfilled and underextended. **B,** Photograph at 15 × demonstrates crown
removal, straight-line access, and the identification of an MB^{II} system. **C,** Photograph at 15 × demonstrates
the removal of gutta-percha from the palatal canal with a .06 tapered, NiTi rotary profile. **D,** Photograph at
15 × demonstrates the removal of gutta-percha from the MB canal with a smaller-sized, .06-tapered, NiTi rotary profile. **E,** Photograph at 15 × shows the pulpal floor and orifices after canal preparation procedures.
F, The postoperative radiograph demonstrates the value of nonsurgical retreatment in its potential to address root canal systems.

1. The patient should be asymptomatic and able to function equally well on both sides.
2. The periodontium should be healthy, including a normal attachment apparatus.
3. Radiographs should demonstrate healing or progressive bone fill over time.
4. The principles of restorative excellence should be satisfied.

Nonsurgical Versus Surgical Retreatment

Endodontic failures must be carefully evaluated so that a decision can be made among nonsurgical retreatment (NSRCT), surgical retreatment (SRCT), or extraction.[3,46,88] *NSRCT is an endodontic procedure used to remove materials from the root canal space and, if present, address deficiencies or repair defects that are pathologic or iatrogenic in origin. These disassembly-and-corrective procedures then allow the clinician to 3-D clean, shape, and pack the root canal system.* Historically, regretfully, and still too often, endodontic surgery is selected as the primary approach to resolve failures (Fig. 25-4). Even with the vast improvements achieved in surgical endodontics in recent years, these techniques are restricted in their ability to eliminate pulp, bacteria, and related irritants from the root canal system.[14,38,75]

Many significant advantages result when failing endodontic cases are nonsurgically reentered. Endodontic failures can be evaluated for coronal leakage, fractures, and missed canals. Importantly, these root canal systems can be cleaned, shaped, and packed in 3-D.[52,74] In fact, many pathologic-and-iatrogenic events can be repaired nonsurgically (Fig. 25-5).[73,78] Infrequently, but on occasion, surgery may still be necessary; however, the clinician will have greater confidence in the surgical outcome if the root canal space has been addressed in

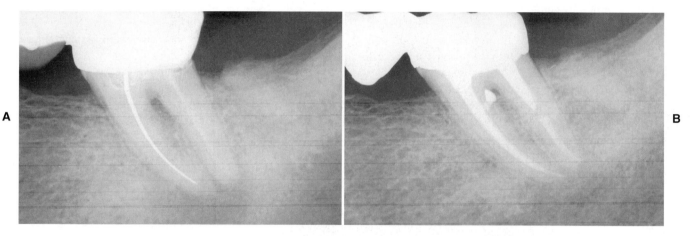

Fig. 25-3 **A**, Radiograph of a mandibular left second molar reveals a poor-fitting bridge, canals holding a silver point and paste, and furcal and apical pathology. **B**, 10-year recall radiograph shows the importance of 3-D endodontics and restorative excellence.

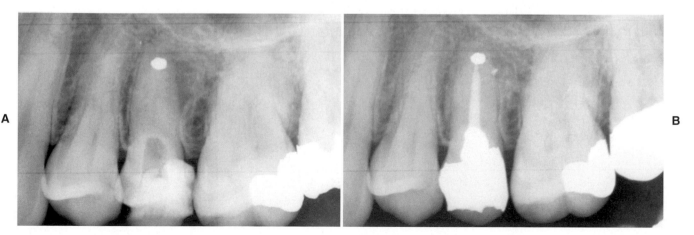

Fig. 25-4 **A**, Preoperative film reveals a failing maxillary bicuspid with a laterally positioned lesion of endodontic origin. Note the "calcified" canal and history of surgery. **B**, 1-year recall film demonstrates healing and the importance of nonsurgical retreatment.

3-D (Fig. 25-6). Consultation with the patient should be directed toward communicating the critical importance of disassembly, the cost of this approach compared with potentially less-effective treatment choices, and the fact that this modality of treatment generally improves long-term results.

Factors Influencing Retreatment Decisions

Currently long-term endodontic success can approach 100%.[77] This phenomenal improvement is related to a multitude of factors. Clinicians now have a better understanding of biologic principles and a greater knowledge, appreciation, and respect for root canal system anatomy and the role it plays in success and failure. Improved training, breakthrough techniques, new technologies, and attention to restorative excellence enable clinicians to obtain superior results. The following factors influence whether a tooth should be retreated or extracted.

1. When should retreatment be considered? Certain teeth may exhibit inadequate endodontic treatment based on present-day criteria; however, they may fulfill the definition of success. These teeth may be "watched" rather than retreated, unless the tooth is to receive a new restoration or lies within the field of anticipated comprehensive dentistry. If, however, the patient is symptomatic, has periodontal disease that appears secondary to an endodontic cause, or exhibits a radiographic lesion of endodontic origin, then a decision needs to be made between retreatment and extraction.[26,81,95] Before initiating retreatment procedures, the prognosis for the retreatment and associated restorative dentistry should be at least equal to that of the alternative treatment plan.

2. What does the patient want? It is profoundly important to understand patients' wants, needs, and overall expectations related to their oral health. The clinician needs to spend sufficient time with patients before treatment to establish rapport and trust, to fully explain the treatment options, and to discuss possible outcomes.[104] Second opinions should be invited and costs of treatment fully disclosed. Equipped with this knowledge, patients can choose the treatment options that best fulfill their wishes. Patient relations are enhanced with this approach because there are "no surprises." On occasion, patients may *want* to proceed with the prescribed treatment, but may be physically or psychologically unable to tolerate the time or uncertainty of some retreatment efforts. These patients may be candidates for retreatment using sedation procedures or, in certain instances, extraction may be the treatment of choice.

3. Is it a strategic tooth? Clinicians need to look carefully at a tooth that is failing endodontically and decide with the patient and the other members of the dental team if the tooth is essential. It is necessary to explore other treatment possibilities that may be, for whatever reason, better or more predictable for this particular patient.[87] Consultation with the appropriate specialists enhances the appreciation for the time, energy, effort, cost, and prognosis associated with the treatment alternatives. It is wise to have this information available before making specific recommendations to the patient.

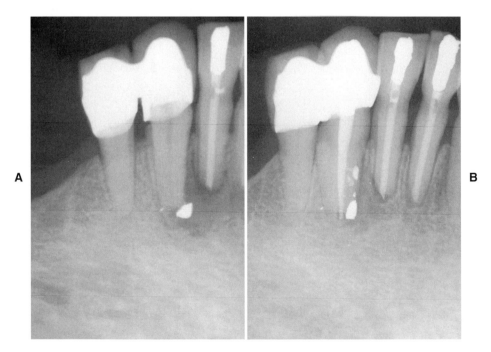

Fig. 25-5 **A,** Radiograph reveals a failing mandibular right canine with a floating retrograde amalgam and large asymmetric lesion. **B,** 2-year recall radiograph demonstrates healing and the significance of nonsurgically treating root canal systems.

4. Restorative evaluation. Fundamental to endodontic treatment is the ability to produce an esthetic, well-designed, and clinically functional restoration.[18,41,105] Often, broken-down teeth should be evaluated for crown-lengthening procedures so that the restorative dentist can achieve the ferrule effect and establish a healthy biologic width.[49,61,83] Indeed, certain teeth fracture after restoration of the endodontically treated tooth because clinicians rely too much on the post and core to retain the coronal restoration, rather than having restorative margins gripping a 2 to 3 mm collar of circumferential tooth structure.[11,57,67] Crown lengthening improves all phases of ensuing interdisciplinary treat-ment. Endodontically, crown lengthening addresses isolation issues, creates pulp chambers that retain solvents, irrigants, and later, if required, interappointment temporaries. This periodontal procedure assists in placing well-defined margins, improves accuracy in impressions, enhances laboratory procedures, allows for accurately fitting restorations, and promotes the health of the attachment apparatus.[42] Clinicians must recognize that crown-lengthening procedures dramatically improve prognosis, and they should integrate this service, when necessary, into restorative excellence procedures.

5. Periodontal evaluation. Practitioners need to know a great deal about the supporting tissues (i.e., their health

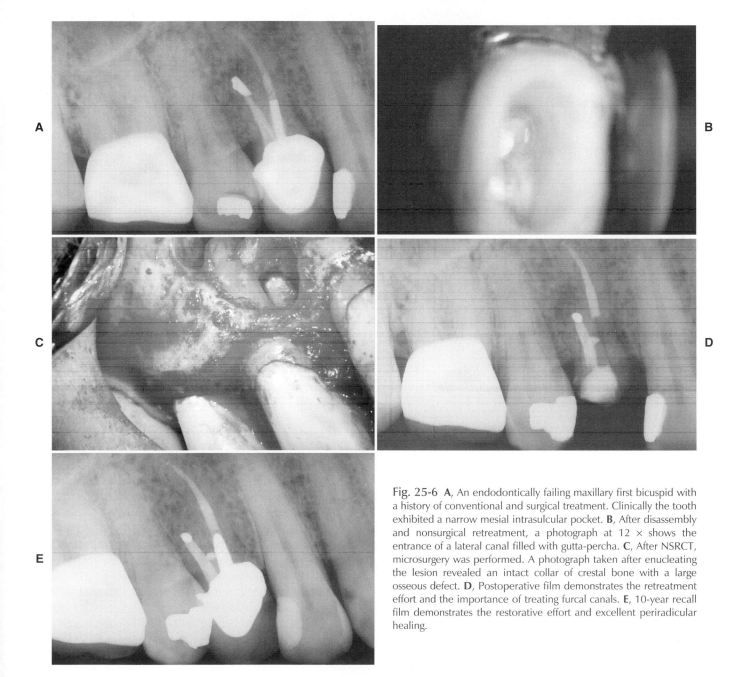

Fig. 25-6 **A**, An endodontically failing maxillary first bicuspid with a history of conventional and surgical treatment. Clinically the tooth exhibited a narrow mesial intrasulcular pocket. **B**, After disassembly and nonsurgical retreatment, a photograph at 12 × shows the entrance of a lateral canal filled with gutta-percha. **C**, After NSRCT, microsurgery was performed. A photograph taken after enucleating the lesion revealed an intact collar of crestal bone with a large osseous defect. **D**, Postoperative film demonstrates the retreatment effort and the importance of treating furcal canals. **E**, 10-year recall film demonstrates the restorative effort and excellent periradicular healing.

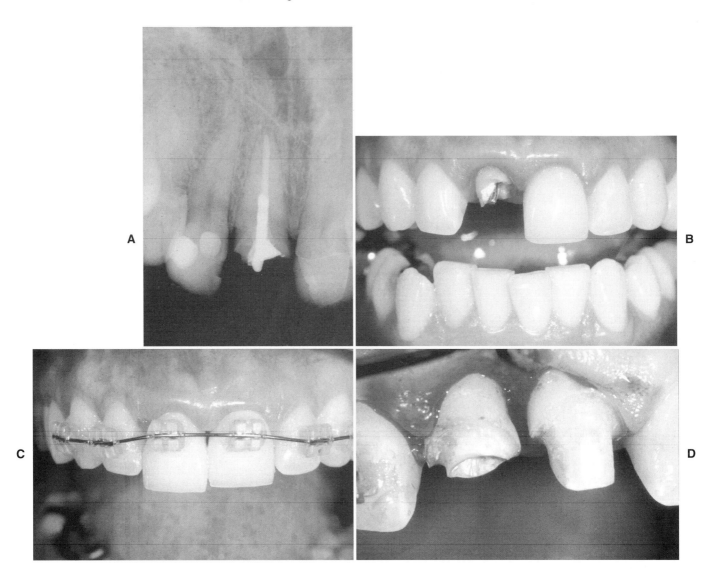

Fig. 25-7 **A**, Pretreatment radiograph of a maxillary central incisor reveals a history of endodontics, a broken post, and no clinical crown. **B**, Pretreatment photograph shows the coronal fracture and esthetic issues. **C**, Photograph demonstrates the provisionalized crown and the initiation of orthodontic forced eruption procedures. **D**, Photograph reveals that the provisionals have been removed to facilitate periodontal microsurgery crown-lengthening procedures.

Continued

or potential for health). Endodontically failing teeth that are being evaluated for retreatment need to be examined for pocket depth, mobility, crown-to-root ratios, hard- and soft-tissue defects, and any other anomalies that could preclude a healthy attachment apparatus. Periodontal treatment can provide numerous treatment modalities that, in concert with other disciplines, can afford excellent longitudinal success.[43,62,79]

6. Other interdisciplinary evaluations. Most endodontically failing teeth can be successfully retreated with the skill, experience, and technologies that are present today. However, clinicians should not just focus on a specific tooth, rather they should appreciate how this tooth fits into a treatment plan that promotes oral health.

The strategic nature of any tooth must be evaluated from a variety of dental disciplines, and the clinician must carefully analyze restorability, the periodontal condition, occlusion, the potential for orthodontic extrusion or uprighting, and the ability to perform successful endodontic retreatment (Fig. 25-7).[44,80,86] The value of any tooth is only as good as the sum of its disciplinary parts and, as such, each discipline must be viewed separately, then collectively, before instituting any treatment. Certainly it is valuable and, at times, critical to obtain additional opinions from other members of the dental team to better appreciate the complex issues that must be understood before commencing with any treatment.

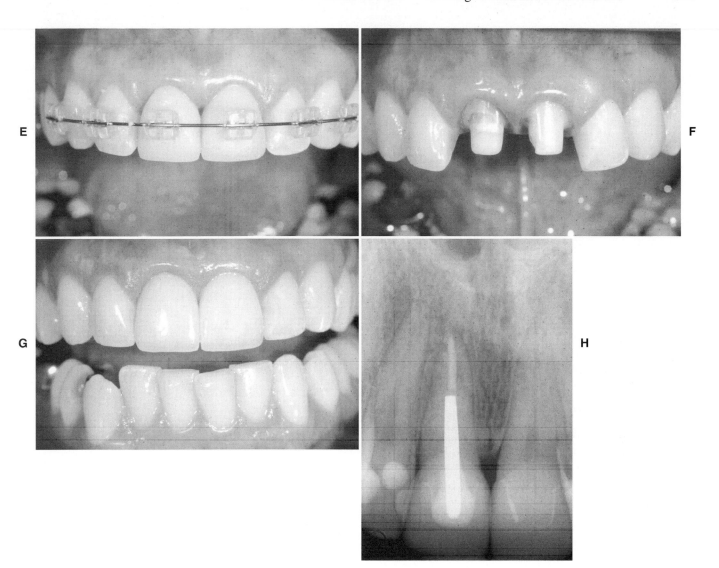

Fig. 25-7, cont'd **E,** Photograph taken one month postsurgery shows orthodontics completed, excellent periodontal healing, and new provisionals. **F,** The maxillary right central incisor received a zirconium oxide post and core, and a photograph shows the completed preparations. **G,** Both teeth were restored with Empress crowns and a posttreatment photograph shows the attention to esthetic excellence. **H,** 1-year recall radiograph shows excellent healing. (Courtesy Dr. Robert R. Winter.)

7. Chair time and cost. The chair time and cost associated with any procedure must be carefully analyzed and understood by the clinician and completely communicated to the patient. With experience, clinicians will begin to appreciate the time required to predictably and safely disassemble an endodontic failure and therefore determine the cost to the patient. Philosophically, the combined fees of endodontic retreatment and restorative procedures should at least equal the alternative fee (i.e., NSRCT + restorative ≥ alternative). Frequently, more time is expended and a lower fee quoted for the combination of endodontic retreatment and restorative procedures as compared with the time and cost of an alternative comprehensive treatment plan. Conscientious clinicians need to quote an adequate "disassembly fee" to compensate themselves for the chair time often required to perform these endodontic retreatment procedures.[70] Regretfully, too many teeth are extracted because of existing insurance compensation tables that favor and promote alternative treatments.

8. Referral. Clinicians should look at all the previously discussed issues and remember that the Hippocratic oath states, "Do no harm while doing good." When evaluating teeth for endodontic retreatment, a series of challenges must be addressed to produce predictably successful outcomes. Ethical questions arise as to who is best qualified to address these challenges and produce the desired result. Colleagues should ask the question,

"Would it be better to refer the patient to a specialist who has more experience, better training, and the technology necessary to achieve more predictable success?" Certainly, clinicians should treat patients as they would like to be treated themselves. Therefore, it is important to remember that, at times, referral is the most ethical and prudent course of action.

CORONAL DISASSEMBLY

Clinicians typically access the pulp chamber through the existing restoration if it is judged to be functionally designed, well fitting, and esthetically pleasing. Endodontically, the decision to remove any restoration is based primarily on whether additional access is required to facilitate disassembly and retreatment.[74,78] If the restorative is deemed inadequate or additional access is required, the restoration should be sacrificed. However, on specific occasions it is desirable to preserve and remove the existing restorative dentistry.[15] A variety of new technologies allow clinicians to eliminate coronal restorations more predictably.

Factors Influencing Restorative Removal

The removal of a restoration is dramatically enhanced when there is knowledge, respect, and appreciation for the concepts, materials, and techniques used in restorative and reconstructive dentistry. The safe dislodgment of a restoration is dependent on five factors that must be considered:

1. Preparation type. Preparations vary in retention, depending on the total surface area of the tooth covered and the height, diameter, and degree of taper of the axial walls.
2. Restoration design and strength. The design and ultimate strength of a restorative is dependent on its physical properties, thickness of material, and the quality and techniques of the laboratory technician.
3. Restorative material. The composition of a restoration ranges from different metals to tooth-colored restoratives, such as porcelain. How these materials react to the stresses and strains required during removal must be appreciated.
4. Cementing agent. The retention of cements ranges from weak to strong, generally progressing from zinc oxide–eugenol to polycarboxylate to silicon phosphate to zinc phosphate to glass ionomers to resin-modified glass ionomers to bonded resins.[1] Clearly, the new generation of bonding materials, in conjunction with well-designed and retentive preparations, have made restorative removal more difficult and, at times, unwise.
5. Removal devices. The safe and successful dislodgment of prosthetic dentistry requires knowledge in the selection and use of a variety of devices. Clinicians need to identify and become familiar with each device, its safe application, effectiveness, limitations, and costs.[74]

A clinician must obtain a good history, confer with the original treating dentist (if appropriate), consult with the patient, and clearly define the risk versus benefit when entertaining the intact removal of an existing restoration.

Coronal Disassembly Devices

Although there are many tools available for coronal disassembly, the following represent the preferred instruments for the removal of restorations. The tools used for disassembly have been arbitrarily divided into three categories. They can be used alone; however, they may also be used in combination to attain removal success synergistically.[63]

Grasping Instruments   In general, this class of hand instruments works by applying inward pressure on two opposing handles. Increasing the handle pressure proportionally increases the instrument's ability to grip a restoration. The actual grasping instrument selected should protect the restoration and provide a strong purchase while reducing dangerous slippage. These grasping devices are best used in removing provisionalized dentistry and include the Trident Crown Placer/Remover (CK Dental Specialties, Orange, CA), K.Y. Pliers (G.C. America, Alsip, IL), and the Wynman Crown Gripper (Miltex Instrument Co., Lake Success, N.Y.). An example of one of these grasping instruments is shown in Fig. 25-8.

Percussive Instruments   This method of prosthetic disassembly involves using a selected and controlled percussive removal force. This family of instruments delivers an impact either directly to a restorative or indirectly to another securely engaged prosthetic removal device. Although these devices are valuable removal instruments, caution must be exercised when considering the disassembly of tooth-colored restoratives. Examples of percussive devices include Ultrasonic Energy (Dentsply Tulsa Dental, Tulsa, Okla.), the Peerless Crown-A-Matic (Henry Schein, Port Washington, N.Y.), and the Coronaflex (KaVo America, Lake Zurich, Ill.), all of which are used to remove provisionalized and potentially definitively cemented dentistry. An example of one of these percussive instruments is shown in Fig. 25-9.

Active Instruments   The instruments in this category actively engage a restorative, enabling a specific dislodgment force to potentially lift off the prosthesis. These devices require a small occlusal window to be cut through the restorative to facilitate the mechanical action of the instrument. In this method of removal, the slight disadvantage of making and repairing the occlusal hole is significantly offset by the advantage of saving the patient's existing restorative dentistry. Active devices among the most effective for removing permanently placed restorations intact are the Metalift (Classic Practice Resources, Baton Rouge, LA), the Kline Crown Remover (Brassler, Savanna, GA), and the Higa Bridge Remover (Higa Manufacturing, West Van-

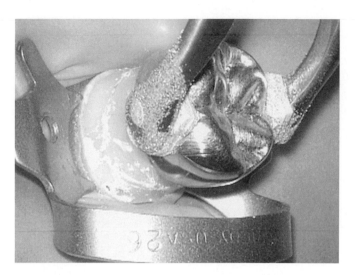

Fig. 25-8 Photograph demonstrates removal of a crown using the K.Y. Pliers. Note the grasping pads have been dipped in emery powder to reduce slippage.

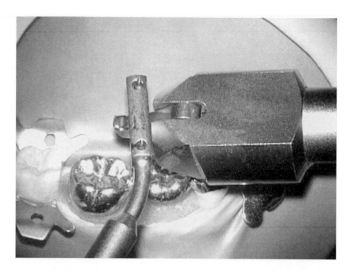

Fig. 25-9 Photograph demonstrates bridge removal using the Coronaflex. The air-driven hammer generates the removal force against various prosthetic attachment devices.

couver, BC, Canada). An example of one of these active instruments is shown in Fig. 25-10.

MISSED CANALS

The cause of endodontic failure is multifaceted, but a statistically significant percentage of failures are related to missed root canal systems. Missed canals hold tissue and, at times, bacteria and related irritants that inevitably contribute to clinical symptoms and lesions of endodontic origin (Fig. 25-11).[8,21,28] Historically and still too often, surgical treatment has been directed toward "corking" the end of the canal with the hopes that the retrograde material will incarcerate biologic irritants within the root canal system over the life of the patient (see Figs. 25-4 through 25-6).[14,38,74] Although this clinical scenario occurs anecdotally, it is not nearly as predictable as nonsurgical retreatment. Endodontic prognosis is maximized in teeth with root canal systems that are cleaned, shaped, and packed in *all* their dimensions.[68,78]

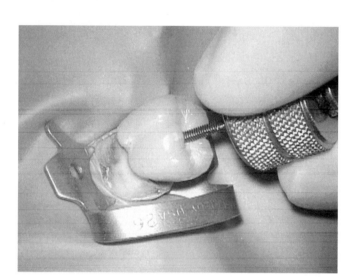

Fig. 25-10 Photograph demonstrates the removal of a PFM crown using the Metalift. This system works because a force is applied between the crown and the tooth.

Canal Anatomy

Several tooth groups have roots that notoriously hold additional systems[13,51]:

- Maxillary central incisors, on occasion, may contain one or more extra canal.[36,71]
- Maxillary first bicuspids are, at times, three rooted and have mesiobuccal (MB), distobuccal (DB), and palatal root canal systems.[35]
- Maxillary second bicuspids contain broad roots buccal to lingual; although the orifices are commonly ribbon shaped, clinicians need to expect deep canal divisions or multiple apical portals of exit.[96]

- Maxillary first molars have an MB root that usually contains two root canal systems that oftentimes anatomically communicate via an isthmus.[91,99] This system can be identified and treated in over 75% of the cases without a microscope and in approximately 90% of the cases with a microscope.[72,91]
- Maxillary second molars should be suspected of having a second canal in the MB root until proven otherwise.[91]
- Mandibular incisors have broad roots facial to lingual and have a second, more lingual canal approximately 45% of the time.[53] Access cavities should be carried more lingual

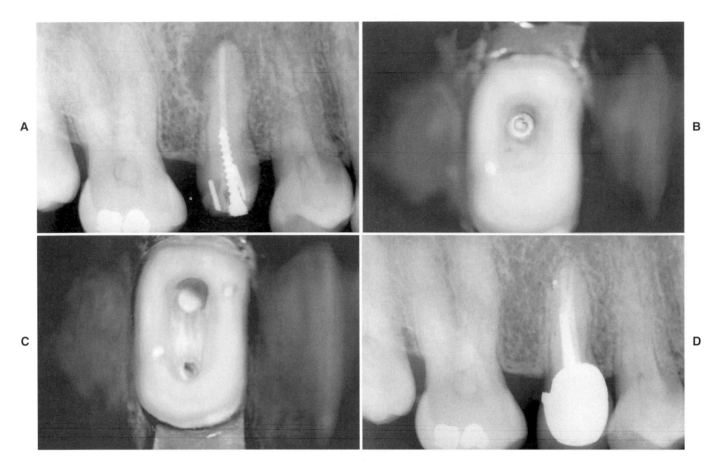

Fig. 25-11 **A**, Radiograph of a maxillary right second bicuspid reveals pins, a post, incomplete endodontics, and an asymmetric lesion. **B**, Photograph at 12 × shows the post is out of the buccal canal, thread marks in the gutta-percha from the screw post, and evidence of a missed lingual system. **C**, Photograph at 12 × demonstrates complete access and identification of the lingual orifice and system. **D**, 1-year recall radiograph shows excellent osseous repair, the importance of 3-D endodontics, and a well-designed-and-sealed restorative.

at the expense of the cingulum to address this potential system.

- Mandibular premolars have roots that frequently hold complex root canal systems. The anatomic variations include displaced orifices, deep divisions, loops and branches, and multiple portals of exit apically.[96]
- Mandibular first and second molars routinely have significant variations within what has become known as "normal anatomy."[13,29] Clinicians need to check the mesial root for a third system that may be displaced or located within the groove between the MB and mesiolingual (ML) orifices.[73] The broad distal root commonly contains an extra canal that may be separate along its length or become contiguous after cleaning-and-shaping procedures. However, even when DB and distolingual (DL) systems become common, deep branching with multiple apical portals of exit are normal.
- C-shaped molars pose challenges in endodontic treatment, and clinicians need to be familiar with this aberrant canal form. Clinicians must also be well aware of radio-

graphic features and the incidence of C-shaped molars within various population groups.[56]

(For a more complete discussion of canal anatomy, see Chapter 7.)

Armamentarium and Techniques

When one is searching for missed canals, the following concepts, armamentarium, and techniques are the most helpful:

- Anatomic familiarity is essential before preparing the access cavity or reentering a tooth that has been previously treated endodontically.[13]
- Radiographic analysis is critical when evaluating an endodontic failure.[37,65] Well-angulated periapical films should be taken with the cone directed straight on, mesioblique, and distoblique. This technique oftentimes reveals and clarifies the 3-D morphology of the tooth. In cases where complete endodontic treatment has been performed, obturation materials are seen radiographically as "centered" within the root, regardless of the selected

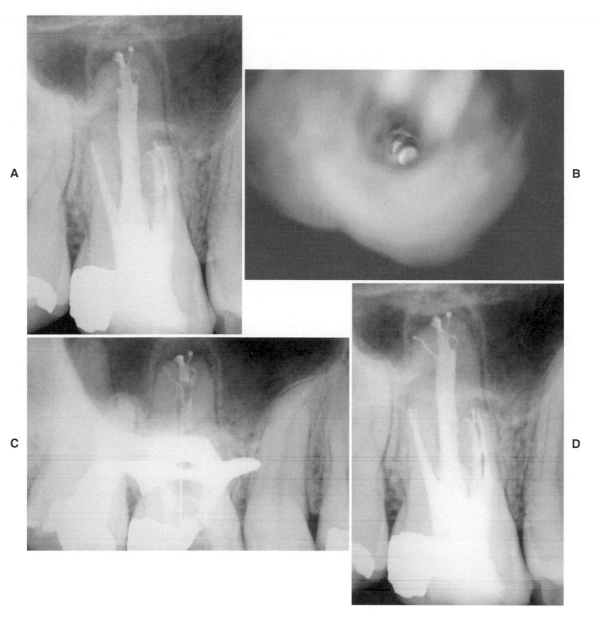

Fig. 25-12 **A**, Radiograph of a maxillary right first molar with a failing palatal root. **B**, A deep look into the apical one third of the palatal canal reveals debris in the entrance to a lateral canal. **C**, Working film demonstrates a no. 10 file moving through this ramification to its terminus. **D**, Posttreatment radiograph depicting the retreatment effort.

angle of the radiograph. Conversely, if the obturation materials appear positioned asymmetrically within the long axis of the root, a missed canal should be suspected (see Fig. 25-11).[37]

- Computerized digital radiography (CDR) (Schick Technologies, Long Island City, NY) affords a variety of software features, significantly enhancing radiographic diagnostics in identifying hidden, calcified, or untreated canals.
- Vision is enhanced with magnification glasses, headlamps, and transilluminating devices. The dental operating microscope (Global Surgical Corp., St. Louis, MO)

affords extraordinary light and magnification, and it gives the clinician unsurpassed vision, control, and confidence in identifying or chasing extra canals (Fig. 25-12).[15,73] Surgical length burs enhance direct vision by moving the head of the handpiece further away from the occlusal table and improving the line of sight along the shaft of the bur.

- Access cavities should be prepared and expanded so that their smallest dimensions are dictated by the separation of the orifices on the pulpal floor and their widest dimensions are at the occlusal table. The isthmus areas or developmental grooves or both are firmly probed with an explorer in an effort to find a "catch" (Fig. 25-13).

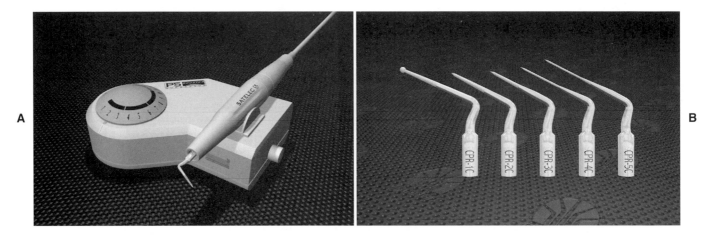

Fig. 25-13 **A**, A view into an access cavity suggests that there are four orifices or systems in this mandibular first molar. **B**, Photograph demonstrating a third mesial orifice and the importance of exploring the isthmus connecting the mesiobuccal and mesiolingual systems.

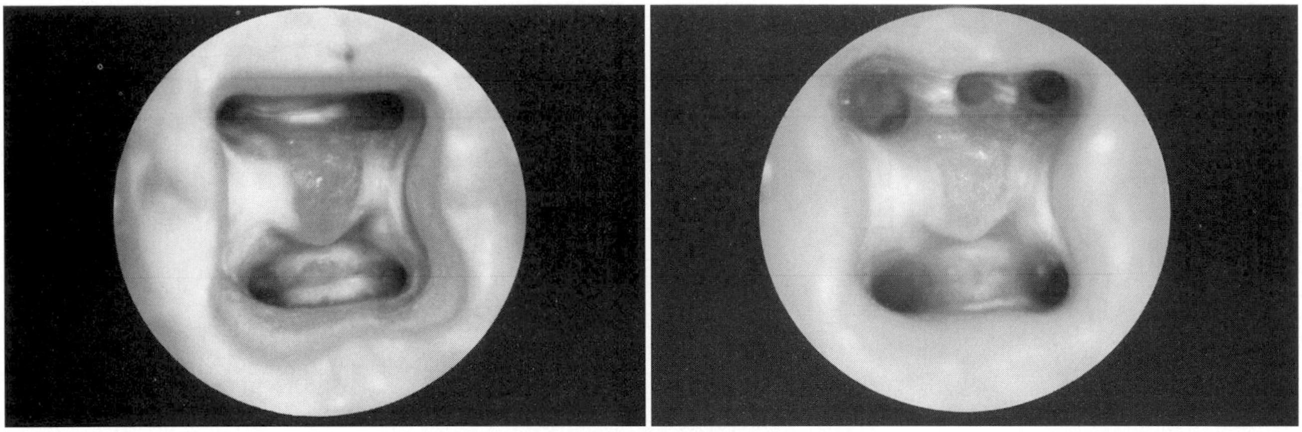

Fig. 25-14 **A**, The P-5 piezoelectric ultrasonic system (Dentsply Tulsa Dental, Tulsa, Okla.) with an endodontic autoclavable handpiece. This unit powers a variety of innovative ultrasonic instruments. **B**, The CPR 1-5 zirconium nitride–coated ultrasonic instruments are uniquely designed to improve vision, access, and control when performing clinical procedures.

- Piezoelectric ultrasonics (Dentsply, Tulsa, Okla.), in conjunction with the innovative new CPR ultrasonic instruments (Dentsply Tulsa Dental, Tulsa, Okla.), provides a breakthrough for exploring and identifying missed canals (Fig. 25-14). Ultrasonic systems eliminate the bulky head of the conventional handpiece, which notoriously obstructs vision. The working ends of these ultrasonic instruments are 10 times smaller than the smallest round burs, and their abrasive coatings allow them to sand away dentin when exploring for missed canals (Fig. 25-15).
- Micro-Openers (Dentsply Maillefer, Tulsa, Okla.) are flexible, stainless steel (SS), ISO-sized hand instruments that feature ergonomically designed offset handles. Micro-Openers have limited-length cutting blades that, in conjunction with their 0.04 and 0.06 tapers, enhance tensile strength, making it easier to locate, penetrate, and

perform initial canal enlargement procedures. These instruments provide unobstructed vision when operating in difficult teeth with limited access (Fig. 25-16).
- Various dyes, like methylene blue, can be irrigated into the pulp chambers of teeth to aid in diagnosis. The chamber is subsequently rinsed thoroughly with water, dried, and visualized to see where the dye has been absorbed. Frequently the dye will be absorbed into orifices, fins, and isthmus areas (and it will "roadmap" the anatomy). This technique can aid in the identification and treatment of missed canals and enhance diagnostics, including the visualization of fractures.
- Sodium hypochlorite (NaOCl) can aid in the diagnosis of missed or hidden canals by means of the "champagne test."[15,73] After cleaning-and-shaping procedures, the access cavity is flooded with NaOCl and the solution is

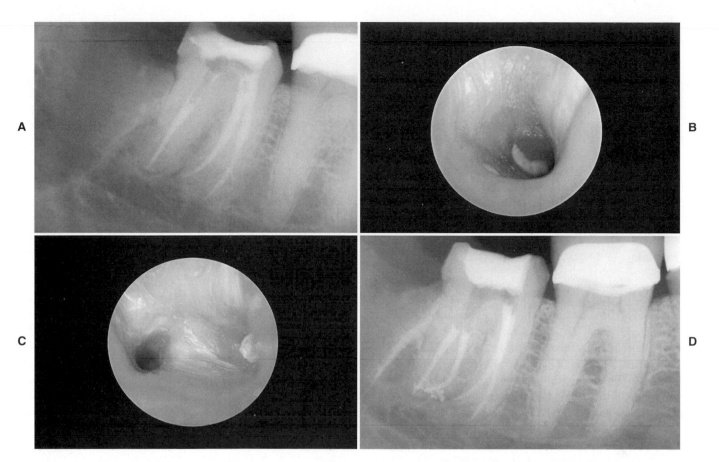

Fig. 25-15 **A**, Radiograph shows a mandibular right second molar with three canals treated endodontically. The obturation material is not centered within the distal root. **B**, A view into the centered distal orifice reveals obturation material positioned subcrestally in a fin off this canal. **C**, Photograph shows improved straight-line access to the DL orifice and gutta-percha deep within the previously treated DB system. **D**, Posttreatment radiograph demonstrates the packed DL root canal system.

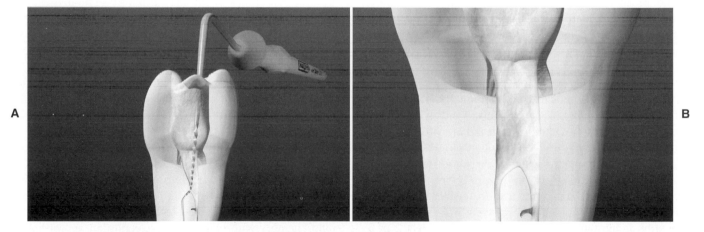

Fig. 25-16 **A**, Distal view of a mandibular molar animation. The microopener's offset handle affords unobstructed vision and is used to initiate treatment in areas where access is difficult and restricted. **B**, Animation showing that the microopener has carved away the triangle of dentin and has created straight-line access to the second distal system.

observed to see if bubbles are emanating toward the occlusal table. A positive, "bubble" reaction signifies that sodium hypochlorite is either reacting with residual tissue within a canal in treatment, reacting with a missed canal, or reacting with a residual chelator that is still present within the canal preparation.

If discovered, missed canals can usually be 3-D cleaned, shaped, and packed. However, if a missed canal is suspected but cannot be readily identified, then an endodontic referral may be prudent to avoid further complications. Caution should be exercised when contemplating surgery because of the aforementioned concerns; however, at times it may be necessary in an effort to salvage the tooth.

REMOVAL OF OBTURATION MATERIALS

Gutta-Percha Removal

The relative difficulty in removing gutta-percha varies according to the canal's length, cross-sectional dimensions, and curvature. Regardless of technique, gutta-percha is best removed from a root canal in a progressive manner to prevent inadvertent displacement of irritants periapically. Dividing the root into thirds, gutta-percha is initially removed from the canal in the coronal one third, then the middle one third, and finally eliminated from the apical one third. In canals that are relatively large and straight, single cones can, at times, be removed with one instrument in one motion. For other canals, there are a number of possible gutta-percha removal schemes. The techniques include rotary files, ultrasonic instruments, heat, hand files with heat or chemicals, and paper points with chemicals.[103] Of these options, the best technique for a specific case is selected after reviewing preoperative radiographs and clinically assessing the diameter of the orifices (after reentering the pulp chamber). Certainly, a combination of methods is generally required; this provides safe, efficient, and potentially complete elimination of gutta-percha and sealer from the internal anatomy of the root canal system.

Rotary Removal   Nickel and titanium (NiTi) 0.04 and 0.06 tapered rotary files (Dentsply Tulsa Dental, Tulsa, OK) are the most effective and efficient group of instruments for removing gutta-percha from a previously treated root canal (Fig. 25-17). Rotary instruments should be used with caution in underprepared canals and are generally not selected for removing gutta-percha in canals that do not accept them passively. When attempting gutta-percha removal, it is useful to mentally divide the root into thirds and then select 2 or 3 appropriately sized rotary instruments that will fit passively within these progressively smaller regions. To soften and engage gutta-percha mechanically, rotary instruments must turn at speeds ranging between 1200 and 1500 RPM. Ultimately, the rotational speed selected is based on the friction required to mechanically soften and effectively auger gutta-percha coronally. Rapidly eliminating gutta-percha benefits

the early acceptance of solvents into the canal or canals and facilitates subsequent cleaning and shaping procedures.

Ultrasonic Removal   The piezoelectric ultrasonic system represents a useful technology to rapidly eliminate gutta-percha. The energized instruments produce heat that thermosoftens gutta-percha. Specially designed ultrasonic instruments are carried into canals that have sufficient shape to receive them and will float gutta-percha coronally into the pulp chamber where it can be subsequently removed.

Heat Removal   Traditionally, a power source in conjunction with specific heat carrier instruments, such as 5004 Touch-N-Heat (Kerr Corp., Glendora, CA) or System B (Analytic Endodontics, Orange, CA) has been used to thermosoften and remove "bites" of gutta-percha from root canal systems.[77] The cross-sectional diameter of the heat carrier limits its ability to plunge into underprepared systems and around pathways of curvature; however, in larger canals, this method works quite well. The technique is to activate the instrument so that it is red-hot; then plunge it into the coronalmost aspect of the gutta-percha. The heat carrier is then deactivated and, as it cools, will freeze a bite of gutta-percha on its working end. Instrument withdrawal generally results in the removal of an attached "bite" of gutta-percha. This process is repeated as long as it continues to be productive.

Heat and Instrument Removal   Another way to remove gutta-percha employs heat and Hedström files (Fig. 25-18). In this method of removal, a hot instrument is plunged into the gutta-percha and immediately withdrawn to heat-soften the material. A size 35, 40, or 45 Hedström file is then selected and quickly, but gently, screwed into the thermosoftened mass.[78] When the gutta-percha cools, it will freeze on the flutes of the file. In poorly obturated canals, removing the file can, at times, eliminate the engaged gutta-percha in one motion. This technique is especially good in those cases where gutta-percha extends beyond the foramen.

After removing as much of the gutta-percha as possible, the clinician must recognize that residual gutta-percha and sealer are entrapped within the canal system. *Chemical* removal techniques are then used to address this issue.

File and Chemical Removal   The file and chemical removal option is best used to remove gutta-percha from *small* and *curved canals*. Chloroform is the reagent of choice and plays an important role in chemically softening gutta-percha.[7,34,92] This sequential technique involves filling the pulp chamber with chloroform, selecting an appropriately sized K-type file, and then gently "picking" into the chemically softened gutta-percha. Initially, a size 10 or 15 SS file is used to "pick" into the gutta-percha occupying the coronal one third of the canal. Frequent irrigation with chloroform (in combination with a "picking" action) creates a pilot hole and sufficient space for the serial use of larger files to remove gutta-percha in this portion of the canal. This method is con-

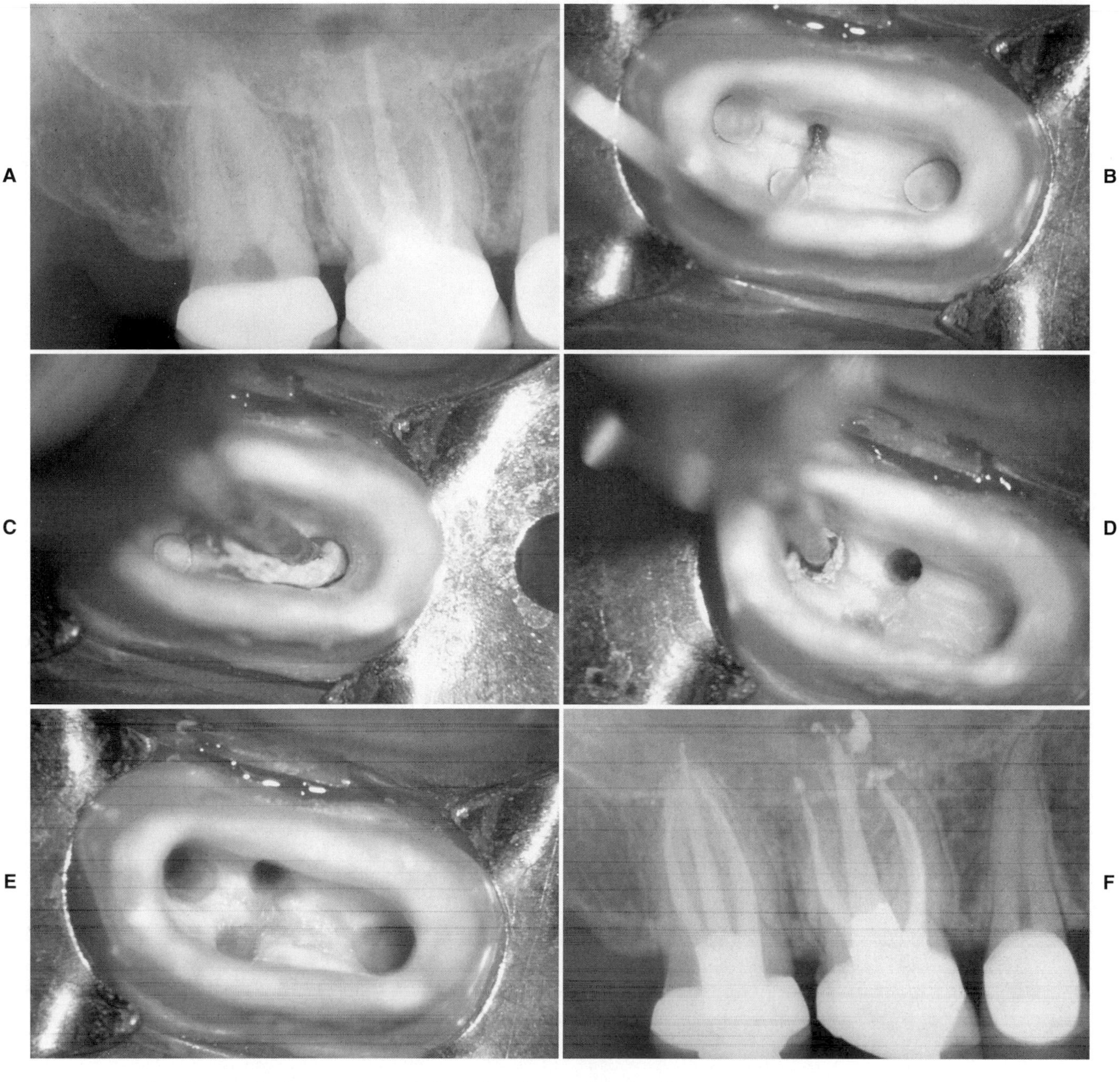

Fig. 25-17 **A**, Radiograph of an endodontically failing maxillary right first molar demonstrates that the previously treated canals are underfilled and underextended. **B**, Photograph at 15 × demonstrates crown removal, straight-line access, and the identification of an MB^{II} system. **C**, Photograph at 15 × demonstrates the removal of gutta-percha from the palatal canal with a .06 tapered, NiTi rotary profile. **D**, Photograph at 15 × demonstrates the removal of gutta-percha from the MB canal with a smaller-sized, 0.06-tapered, NiTi rotary profile. **E**, Photograph at 15 × shows the pulpal floor and orifices after canal preparation procedures. **F**, The postoperative radiograph demonstrates the value of nonsurgical retreatment in its potential to address root canal systems.

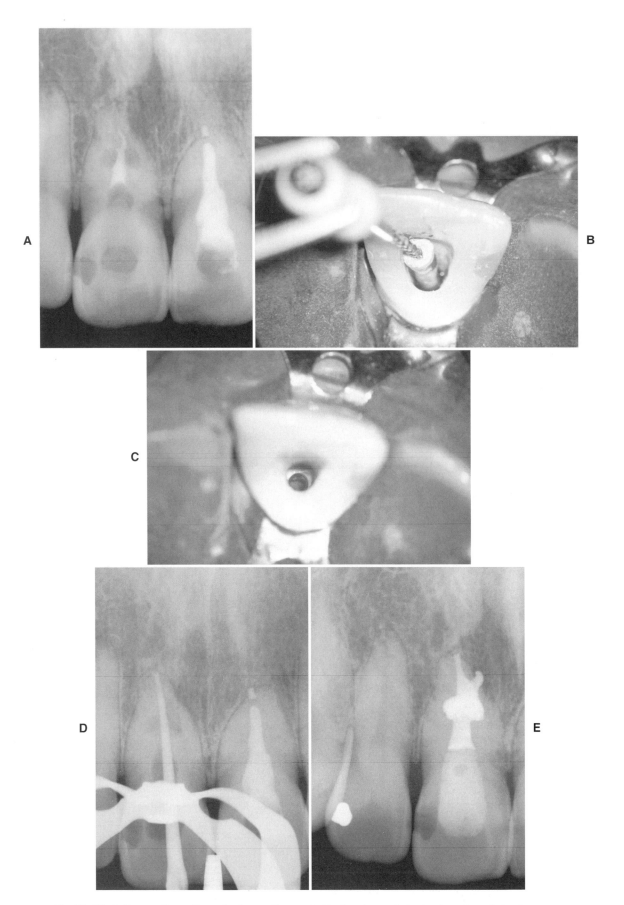

Fig. 25-18 **A**, Preoperative radiograph of a maxillary central incisor demonstrates inadequate endodontics, resorption, and apical one-third pathology. **B**, Photograph at 8 × shows a 45 Hedström mechanically removing the heat-softened single cone of gutta-percha. **C**, Photograph at 8 × shows a portion of the recleaned-and-shaped canal and the position of the resorptive defect. **D**, A cone-fit film suggests the need to laterally inject warm gutta-percha with the Obtura II to enhance hydraulics before initiating the pack. **E**, Postoperative radiograph shows the nonsurgical retreatment result and 3-D obturation.

tinued until gutta-percha is no longer evident on the cutting flutes when the files are withdrawn from the solvent-filled canal. Only after gutta-percha has been removed from the coronal one third of the canal should the clinician repeat the technique in the middle one third and finally in the apical one third. This progressive removal technique helps prevent the needless extrusion of chemically softened gutta-percha periapically. Once the *"file and chemical"* gutta-percha removal technique has been completed, clinicians need to appreciate that they still need to address the residual sealer and gutta-percha that remains in the irregularities of the root canal system.

Paper Point and Chemical Removal   Gutta-percha and most sealers are miscible in chloroform and, once in solution, can be absorbed and removed with appropriately sized, paper points. Drying solvent-filled canals with paper points is known as *"wicking"* and is always the final step of gutta-percha removal.[102] The wicking action is essential in removing residual gutta-percha and sealer out of fins, cul-de-sacs, and aberrations of the root canal systems. In this technique, the canal is first flushed with chloroform and the solution is then absorbed and removed with appropriately sized paper points. Paper points *"wick"* by pulling dissolved materials from peripheral to central, and their use in this manner liberates the residual gutta-percha and sealer from the root canal system. This process is repeated as long as it continues to be visibly productive.

Even when the points come out of the canal clean, white, and dry, the clinician should assume residual gutta-percha and sealer are still present. At this point the chamber is again flooded with chloroform, but the chloroform is now introduced with more of a *"flushing action."* The irrigating cannula is placed below the orifice, and the solvent is passively and repeatedly irrigated then aspirated. This alternating method of irrigating then aspirating creates a vigorous back-and-forth turbulence that powerfully promotes the elimina-

tion of the root canal–filling materials. After chloroform wicking procedures, the canal is liberally flushed with 70% isopropyl alcohol and wicked to further encourage the elimination of chemically softened gutta-percha residues. Removal of all residual material in this manner will enhance the efficacy of sodium hypochlorite when it is used during subsequent cleaning-and-shaping procedures.

Silver Point Removal

The relative ease of removing failing silver points is based on the fact that chronic leakage greatly reduces the seal and, hence, lateral retention. Before a given silver-point retrieval technique is selected, it is useful to recall the canal preparation prescribed for this method of obturation. Typically, the apical 2 to 3 mm of the canal was prepared relatively parallel and then flared coronal to this apical zone. When clinicians evaluate silver point failures, they should recognize that the silver point is parallel over length, hope for a coronally shaped canal, and take advantage of this space discrepancy when approaching retreatment.[98]

Many techniques have been developed for removing silver points, primarily because of their varying lengths, diameters, and the positions they occupy within the root canal space.[24,25,73] Certain removal techniques evolved to address silver points that bind in unshaped canals over distance. Other techniques arose to remove silver points with large cross-sectional diameters (i.e., those approaching the size of smaller posts). Finally, other techniques are necessary to remove the split cone or intentionally sectioned silver points lying deep within the root canal space.

Access   Typically, the coronal heads of silver points are within pulp chambers and are entombed in cements, composites, or amalgam cores (Fig. 25-19). Access preparations must be thoughtfully planned and carefully performed so as to minimize the risk of inadvertently foreshortening the silver points. Initial access is accomplished with high-speed, surgical-length cutting tools. Subsequently, ultrasonic instruments may be carefully used within the pulp chamber to brush cut away restorative materials and progressively expose the silver point.

Pliers Removal   After completing access and fully exposing the part of the silver point confined to the pulp chamber, a suitable grasping instrument, such as Stieglitz Pliers (Henry Schein, Port Washington, NY) is selected. To identify the best removal strategy, the clinician should obtain a strong purchase on the silver point and gently pull to confirm its relative tightness. Many colleagues make the mistake of overmanipulating the head of the silver point, which needlessly foreshortens it. This makes subsequent retrieval efforts difficult, if not impossible. When grasping a silver point, rather than trying to pull it straight out of the canal, the pliers is *rotated* using *fulcrum mechanics* and levered against the restoration or tooth structure to enhance removal efforts (Fig. 25-20).[73]

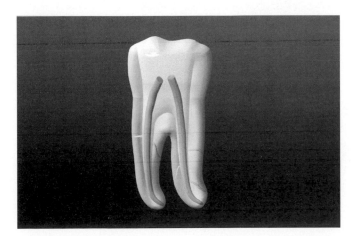

Fig. 25-19 Mandibular-molar animation reminding the clinician to exercise caution not to inadvertently shorten the silver points upon reentering the pulp chamber.

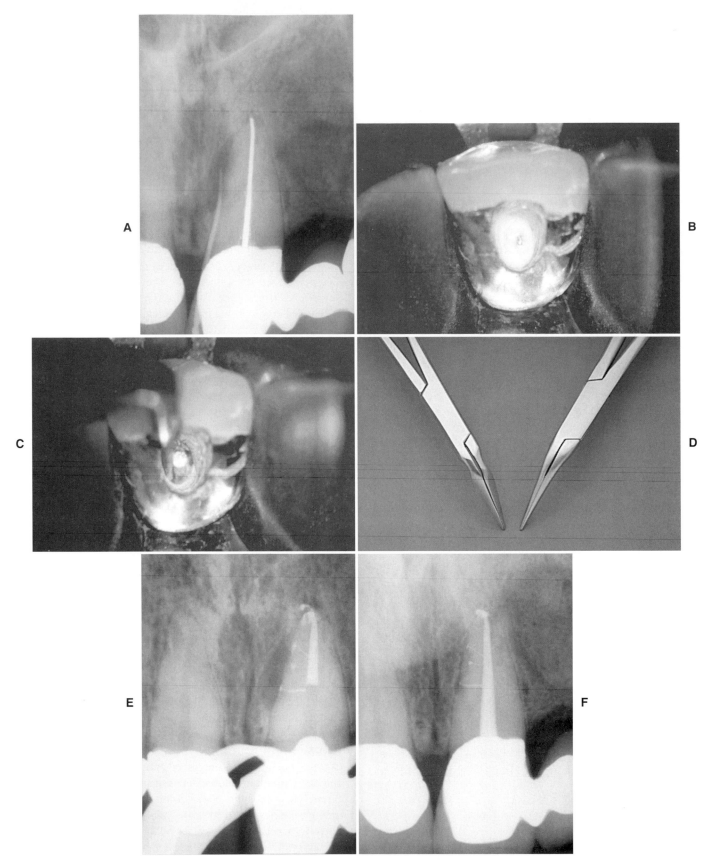

Fig. 25-20 **A**, Preoperative radiograph depicting an endodontically failing maxillary central incisor bridge abutment, a gutta-percha point tracing a fistulous tract to a large lateral root lesion, and a canal underfilled and slightly overextended. **B**, Magnification at 15 × reveals lingual access and restorative build-up around the most coronal aspect of the exposed silver point. **C**, Magnification at 15 × demonstrates a CPR-3 ultrasonic instrument removing material lateral to the silver point. **D**, The left image shows a Stieglitz Pliers used for grasping intracanal obstructions. The right image shows a "modified" Stieglitz Pliers with a working end that has been machined down to enhance access. **E**, Working radiograph during the down pack reveals apical-and-lateral corkage. Note the thermosoftened and compacted gutta-percha is apical to the most coronally positioned lateral canal. **F**, 5-year review demonstrates that 3-D endodontic treatment promotes healing.

Indirect Ultrasonics   When a segment of a silver point is encountered below the orifice and space is restricted, the CPR-3, 4, and 5 ultrasonic instruments may be used. These ultrasonic instruments have parallel walls and provide progressively longer lengths and smaller diameters. The appropriate instrument is selected based on its anticipated depth of use and the available canal diameter. The ultrasonic instruments are used to trephine circumferentially around the obstruction, break up cement, and safely expose as much of the silver point as possible. Caution should be exercised so that ultrasonic instruments are not used *directly* on silver points because elemental silver is soft and rapidly erodes during mechanical manipulation. Once the surrounding material is removed, ultrasonic energy may then be transmitted directly on a grasping pliers to synergistically enhance the retrieval efforts. This form of *indirect* ultrasonics advantageously transfers energy along the silver point, breaks up material deep within the canal, and enhances removal efforts.

Files, Solvents, and Chelators   If grasping techniques or indirect ultrasonics are unsuccessful, then the clinician should immediately abort this approach and appreciate that silver points are perfectly round and root canal systems are typically irregular in their cross-sectional shapes. This discrepancy between the round silver wire and an irregularly shaped canal provides the clinician with an opportunity to use solvents and a size 10 or 15 SS file. In a solvent-filled chamber, files are used laterally to the silver point to break up cements and to undermine and loosen the silver point for removal. In underprepared canals, chelators are, at times, better than solvents by allowing the instrument to "slip and slide" and work laterally to the silver point. If space exists or can be created between the silver point and the canal wall, a 35, 40, or 45 Hedström file can be inserted into this space. The "Hedström displacement technique" powerfully promotes the removal process because the instrument's positive rake angle bites, engages, and establishes a strong purchase on any metallurgically soft silver point (Fig. 25-21).

Microtube Removal Options
   The microtube tap-and-thread option.   The Post Removal System (PRS) (Analytic Endodontics, Orange, Calif.) contains certain smaller microtubular taps that allow the clinician to mechanically tap, thread, and engage the most coronal aspect of any obstruction with a diameter of 0.6 mm or greater (Fig. 25-22). These microtubular taps contain a reverse thread and engage an obstruction by turning in a counterclockwise (CCW) motion. Because intracanal space is often restrictive, this system is generally used to engage obstructions that extend into the pulp chamber. The PRS is discussed in greater detail later in this chapter.
   The microtube mechanics option.   Traditionally, a technique was employed to remove broken instruments using a microtube (Ranfac, Avon, MA) and an appropriately sized Hedström file. In this removal method, a microtube was selected that could be placed over the exposed, coronal-most

aspect of the obstruction. A Hedström file was then passed down the length of the tube until it engaged itself tightly between the obstruction and the internal lumen of the microtube (Fig. 25-23). When properly performed this method of removal was quite successful.

Carrier-Based Gutta-Percha Removal

The techniques for removing carrier-based gutta-percha are the same as has been previously described for gutta-percha and silver point removal. Carrier-based obturators were originally metal and filelike, yet over the past several years they have been manufactured from easier-to-remove plastic materials. Metal carriers, although no longer distributed, are occasionally encountered clinically and are more difficult to remove than silver points because their cutting flutes, at times, engage lateral dentin (Fig. 25-24).[9]

   After careful access and complete circumferential exposure of the carrier, a suitable grasping pliers is selected and a purchase is obtained on the carrier. The relative tightness of the carrier within the canal can then be tested using the pliers. Recognizing that the carrier is frozen in a sea of hardened gutta-percha enhances successful removal in these cases. With this in mind, the following techniques are used to remove carriers:
- The carrier is grasped with the pliers and extrication is attempted using *fulcrum mechanics,* rather than a straight pull out of the tooth.
- If enough canal shape exists, a CPR-3, 4, or 5 ultrasonic instrument can be used alongside the carrier to produce heat and thermosoften the gutta-percha. The activated ultrasonic instrument is gently moved apically, and the carrier is oftentimes displaced and floated out coronally.
- Indirect ultrasonics can be performed by grasping the exposed carrier with a pliers and then placing an ultrasonic instrument against the pliers.
- Rotary instrumentation can be used to auger a plastic carrier effectively and efficiently from a canal. This should only be attempted if there is sufficient space to passively accommodate the rotary instrument without engaging lateral dentin.

   The Instrument Retrieval System (IRS) (Dentsply Tulsa Dental, Tulsa, Okla.) may be considered, in certain cases, to remove a carrier. This method of removal is especially appropriate if the core of the carrier is metal and has cutting flutes that are engaging lateral dentin. For further discussion on this device, see "Broken Instrument Removal" later in this chapter.

   Solvents will chemically soften the gutta-percha and allow small files to work deeper, progressively undermining and loosening a carrier for removal.

   If any of these efforts are successful, the carrier will move and be extricated from the canal. The canal can then be retreated as if it were a gutta-percha case using any of the gutta-percha removal strategies followed by chemical and paper point wicking procedures.

Text continued on p. 897

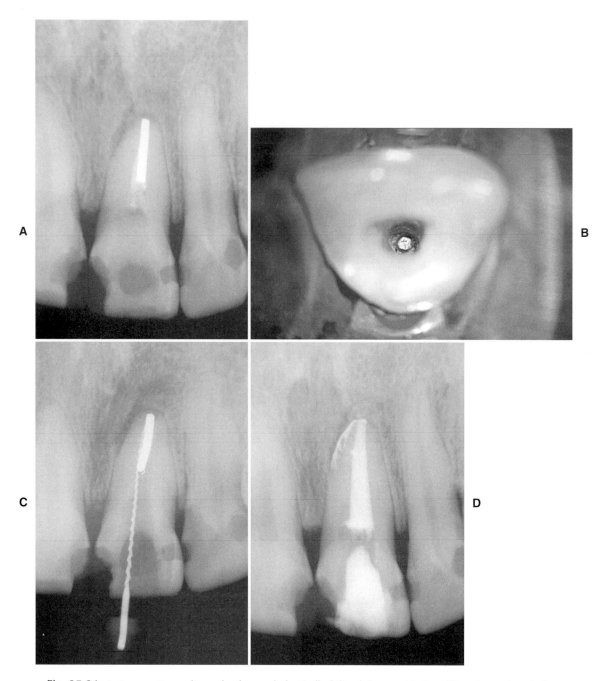

Fig. 25-21 **A**, Preoperative radiograph of an endodontically failing left central incisor. Note the sectioned silver point and asymmetric lesion apically. **B**, Photograph shows the deeply positioned and exposed silver point. **C**, Working film shows a 35 Hedström bypassing the silver point and to length. **D**, Postoperative film demonstrates obturation control, apical corkage, and filling of many lateral canals. (Courtesy Dr. Michael J. Scianamblo.)

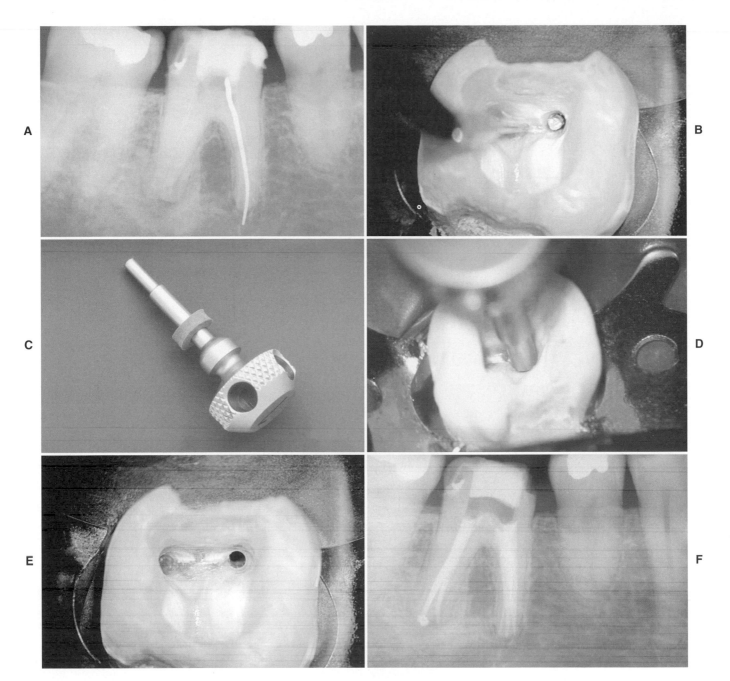

Fig. 25-22 A, Radiograph of a mandibular right first molar reveals a silver point in the mesial root that is coronally foreshortened and apically overextended. **B**, Photograph at 15 × shows a CPR-3 ultrasonic instrument brush cutting away pulpal roof and improving access to the silver point. **C**, A microtubular tap from the Post Removal System kit. The tap may be used to engage an obstruction, and the rubber cushion protects the tooth during the extracting forces. **D**, The microtubular tap engages the silver point by turning the instrument CCW. Care is exercised not to over-thread and shear off the point within the tap. **E**, Photograph at 15 × shows the elimination of the silver point. **F**, Postoperative radiograph shows the nonsurgical retreatment, a packed third mesial system, and corkage of five apical portals of exit.

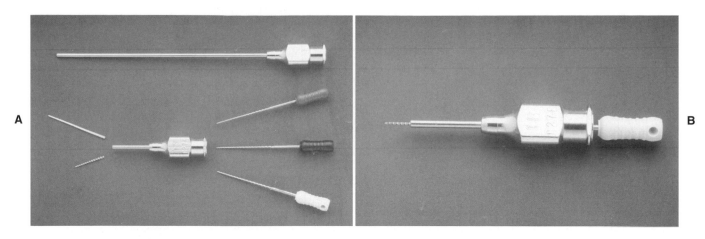

Fig. 25-23 **A**, Photograph showing a full-length spinal tap needle (STN). The STN is shortened and placed over a coronally exposed object. Hedström files are passed through the proximal end of the STN to engage an obstruction. **B**, Photograph demonstrating the assembled STN. A 45 Hedström is engaging a broken-file segment.

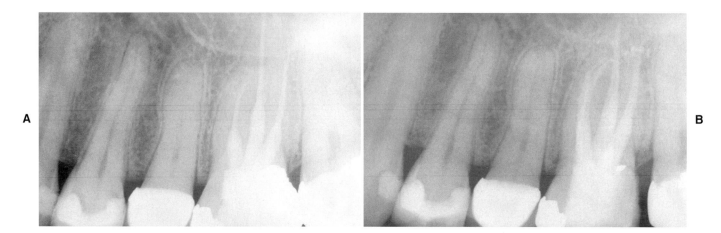

Fig. 25-24 **A**, Radiograph of a maxillary right first molar demonstrates "coke bottle" preparations and carrier-based obturation of three canals. **B**, Postoperative radiograph reveals the retreatment efforts, including the identification and treatment of a second MB root canal system.

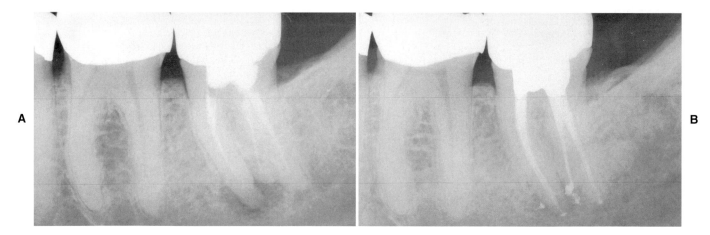

Fig. 25-25 **A**, Preoperative radiograph of an endodontically failing, paste-filled mandibular left second molar. Note the extra DL root. **B**, 5-year recall film shows the treatment of multiple apical portals of exit and excellent osseous healing.

Paste Removal

A great variety of paste types exist; they differ only in chemical formulation. Originally, the intention for paste use was for those patients who could not afford conventional endodontics, and this modality of treatment was considered a benevolent alternative to extraction. Regretfully, countless cases were unsuccessful and too often the "magic" paste was used with hopes of overcoming deficiencies in the removal of irritants during canal preparation (Fig. 25-25).

When evaluating a paste case for retreatment, it is useful to clinically understand that pastes can generally be divided into soft, penetrable, and removable versus hard, impenetrable, and, at times, unremovable.[20,52] Typically, the paste used in the United States remains soft within the canal and is readily removed. Notoriously, the whitish-colored paste oftentimes used in Russia and the reddish-brown resin paste commonly used in Eastern Europe and the Pacific Rim pose formidable challenges in removal because they set-up brick

hard. However, it is important to understand that, because of the method of placement, the coronal portion of the paste in the canal is most dense (the material is progressively less dense moving apically) (Fig. 25-26). In addition, retreatment of paste-filled cases is often wrought with surprises because clinicians frequently encounter calcifications, resorptions, and flare-ups that should be anticipated and communicated (Fig. 25-27).

Ultrasonic Energy   Ultrasonic instruments, in conjunction with the microscope, afford excellent control in removing paste from the straightaway portions of a canal.[32,45,101] Specifically, the CPR-3, 4, and 5 zirconium nitride–coated, ultrasonic instruments may be used below the orifice to remove brick-hard, resin-type paste. To remove paste apical to a canal curvature, a precurved file is attached to a specially designed adapter (Satelec, Inc., Cherry Hill, N.J.) that mounts on and is activated by the ultrasonic handpiece (Fig. 25-28).

Heat   Certain resin pastes soften with heat. Heat carriers can be selected if this modality of removal is chosen.

Rotary Instruments   SS 0.02 tapered hand files may be used to negotiate through paste fillers. These files can potentially create a pilot hole for safe-ended, NiTi rotary instruments to follow and effectively auger the toxic material coronally. Dangerous, but at times helpful, is the use of end-cutting, NiTi rotary instruments (Analytic Endodontics, Orange, CA) to penetrate paste.

Solvents and Hand Files   Reagents like Endosolv "R" and Endosolv "E" (Endoco, Memphis, TN) can be helpful in chemically softening hard paste.[20] The "R" designates the solution of choice for the removal of resin-based pastes, and the "E" is the solution for the elimination of eugenate-based

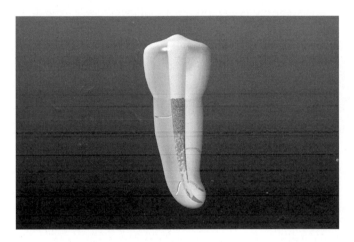

Fig. 25-26 A graphic animation demonstrates that paste fillers generally decrease in density over length.

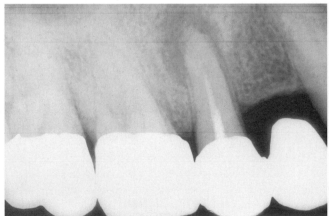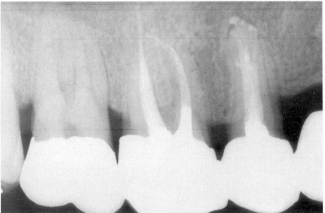

Fig. 25-27 **A**, Radiograph demonstrating splint dentistry, incomplete endodontics associated with the maxillary second premolar, and an asymmetric lesion apically. **B**, 10-year recall film demonstrates that complete endodontic treatment promotes healing and long-term success.

pastes (Fig. 25-29). These reagents can be placed interappointment against a paste-type material via paper points or cotton pellets to promote shrinkage and facilitate subsequent removal.

Micro-Debriders   After removing the paste filler and cleaning and shaping the canal, it is axiomatic that residual paste will still be noted within the irregularities of the root canal preparation. Micro-Debriders (Dentsply Maillefer, Tulsa, OK) are specially designed instruments to precisely remove residual paste materials from a root canal system. Because of their ergonomically designed offset handles, these SS instruments enhance vision; they have D_0 diameters of 0.20 and 0.30 mm, and are available in 0.02 tapers with 16 mm of efficient Hedström-type cutting blades (Fig. 25-30).

Solvents and Paper Points   After paste removal, paper point wicking in the presence of specific paste solvents is

important to further remove and liberate material from the irregularities of the root canal system.

POST REMOVAL

It is common for clinicians to encounter endodontically treated teeth that contain posts.[90] Frequently, when endodontic treatment is failing, the need arises to remove a post to facilitate successful nonsurgical retreatment. In other instances, the endodontic treatment is successful, but the restoration needs require the removal of an existing post to improve the design, mechanics, or esthetics of a new restoration significantly. Over time, many techniques have been advocated for removal of posts and other intracanal obstructions, such as large silver points.[4,52,55]

Factors Influencing Post Removal

The most critical factors required in successful post removal are operator judgment, training, and experience, as well as using the best technologies and techniques.[73] Clinicians must also have knowledge and respect for the anatomy of teeth and be familiar with the range of variation typical within each tooth type. It is important to know each root's morphology, including external concavities, root wall thickness, and the length, shape, and curvature of the canal.[25] This information is best appreciated by obtaining three well-angulated, preoperative radiographs. Films also assist the clinician in visualizing the length, diameter, and direction of the post, and help in determining if it extends coronally into the pulp chamber.

Other factors influencing post removal is the post type and cementing agent.[106] Posts can be catalogued into parallel versus tapered, actively engaged versus nonactively retained, and metallic versus new, nonmetallic compositions (Fig. 25-31). Posts retained with the classic cements (e.g., zinc phosphate) can generally be removed; however, posts bonded into

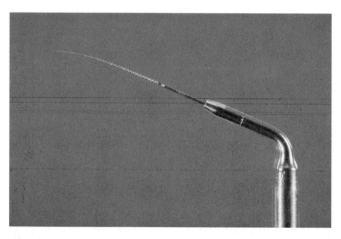

Fig. 25-28 Photograph shows that when the handle of an endodontic file is removed, its shaft can be quickly secured into the ultrasonically activated adapter.

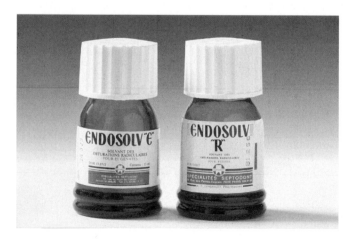

Fig. 25-29 Endosolv "E" is a solvent for eugenate-based pastes, whereas Endosolv "R" is the solvent for resin-based pastes.

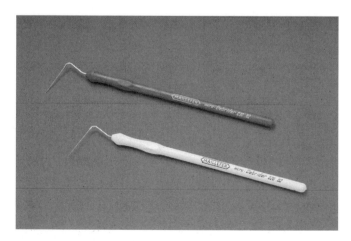

Fig. 25-30 Micro-Debriders have offset handles to enhance vision; 16 mm of efficient Hedström-type cutting blades and are used to remove residual obturation materials from the irregularities of canal systems.

the root canal space with materials like composite resins or glass ionomers are substantially more difficult to remove. In addition, other important factors that impact post removal are the available interocclusal space, existing restorations, and whether the position of the coronal-most aspect of the post is supracrestal or subcrestal. In general, post removal becomes increasingly more challenging moving from anterior to posterior teeth.

Techniques for Post Removal

Successful post removal requires eliminating all circumferential restorative materials from the pulp chamber. Once straight-line access into the pulp chamber is established, the restoratives circumferential to the post are removed. High-speed, surgical-length burs are selected to section and eliminate cores because their added lengths improve vision during reentry into the pulp chamber. These cutting tools remove the greatest bulk of restorative materials that commonly entomb various post head configurations (Fig. 25-32).

Piezoelectric ultrasonic systems, in conjunction with specific instruments, afford the clinician certain advantages in endodontic disassembly and retreatment (see Fig. 25-14). The CPR-2 ultrasonic instrument is used on *full intensity* within the pulp chamber to eliminate the remaining core materials circumferential to the post. The smaller, parallel-sided CPR-3, 4, and 5 ultrasonic instruments are more delicate and should be used on *low intensity*. These instruments are designed to work in small, restricted, and confined spaces (e.g., between a post and an axial wall; below the orifice, between the post and the dentinal wall in irregularly shaped canals).[74]

If space is severely restricted within the field of operation, the CPR-6, 7, or 8 titanium ultrasonic instruments can be selected and used on *low intensity* (Fig. 25-33). These instruments provide the clinician thinner diameters and longer lengths as compared with any other ultrasonic instrument line. The CPRs may be used to safely "brush" and "sculpt" away materials (e.g., cements, composites, amalgams) that, upon elimination, undermine the stability of the post. It should be emphasized that all nonsurgical ultrasonic work is performed dry to optimize vision. When ultrasonic work is performed in a wet field, the debris that is generated quickly accumulates and becomes a slurry of "mud." The assistant advantageously uses the Stropko three-way adapter (Obtura-Spartan Corp., Fenton, MO) with the White Mac tip (Ultradent, Salt Lake City, UT) to direct and control a continuous stream of air into the field (Fig. 25-34). This clinical action blows out debris and, importantly, provides the clinician with constant vision.[73]

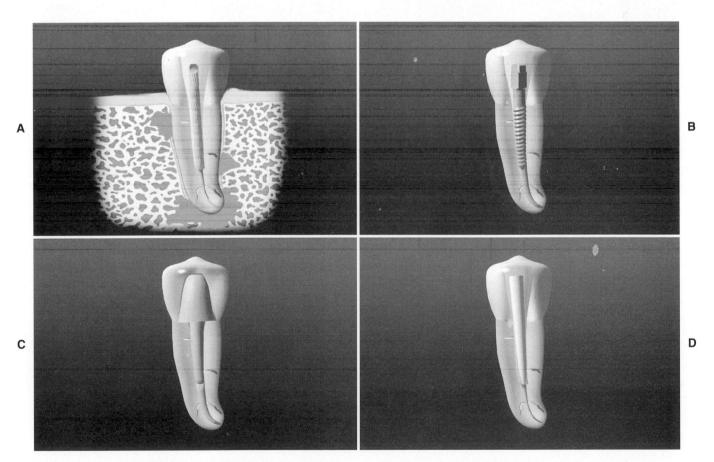

Fig. 25-31 **A**, Parallel post. **B**, Tapered screw post. **C**, Cast-gold post and core. **D**, Composite post.

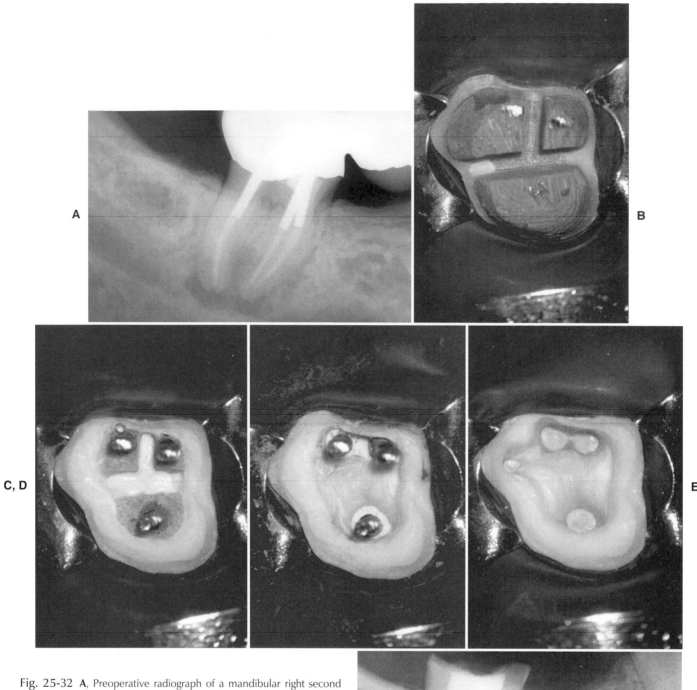

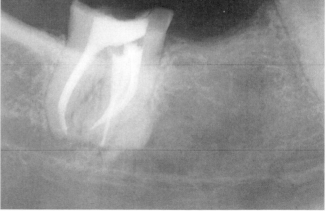

Fig. 25-32 **A,** Preoperative radiograph of a mandibular right second molar bridge abutment demonstrates three posts, previous endodontics, and apical pathology. **B,** After coronal disassembly, the isolated tooth reveals the core sectioned into thirds, the heads of three posts, and a marked mesiolingual protuberance. **C,** Progressively deeper sectioning with rotary cutting tools reduces the build-up. Ultrasonics may then be used to eliminate all restorative materials. **D,** The pulpal floor is exposed and the posts are free above the orifices. **E,** The pulpal floor is shown after 3-D cleaning, shaping, and obturation procedures. Note the displaced most lingual orifice. **F,** A mesially angulated postoperative radiograph confirms the disassembly efforts and demonstrates the pack and displaced lingual system.

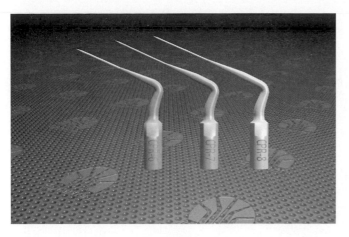

Fig. 25-33 The CPR-6, 7, and 8 are titanium ultrasonic instruments primarily used with a microscope. Their longer lengths and smaller profiles facilitate "microsonic" techniques.

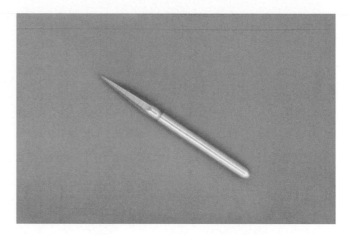

Fig. 25-35 Regular-tip Roto-Pro bur.

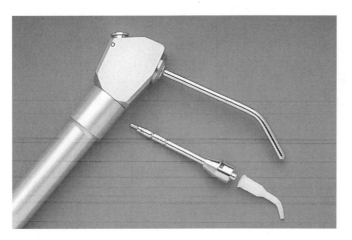

Fig. 25-34 The Stropko 3-way adapter with White Mac tip can be placed on a triplex syringe to deliver controlled-and-directed airflow.

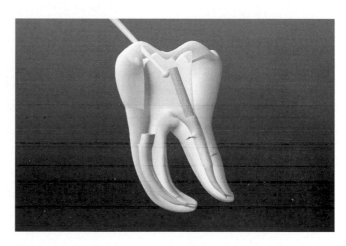

Fig. 25-36 The CPR-1 has a working-end ball that, when ultrasonically energized, can be used to powerfully vibrate against all aspects of the exposed post.

Once the post has been fully exposed, rotosonics is an easy and economic method to potentially loosen and remove it. The regular-tip Roto-Pro bur (Ellman International, Hewlett, NY) is a high-speed, friction-grip, six-sided instrument (Fig. 25-35). When rotated, its edges produce six vibrations per revolution to potentially loosen and remove a post. The bur is kept in intimate contact with the obstruction and is generally carried CCW around the post.[52] Clinically, this action is continued for 2 to 3 minutes in an attempt to first loosen, then remove, the post.

If rotosonic efforts are unsuccessful, the clinician should select a specific ultrasonic instrument, such as the CPR-1, because its superb energy transfer will dislodge most posts. The CPR-1 has a ball at its working end, which is kept in intimate contact with the post to maximize energy transfer (Fig. 25-36). This instrument is used at *full intensity* and is moved

around the post circumferentially and up and down along its exposed length. Experience suggests that after removing all circumferential restorative materials, the majority of posts can be safely and successfully removed in approximately 10 minutes or less using the CPR-1. However, certain posts resist removal even after ultrasonic efforts using the *"10-Minute Rule."* As such, clinicians need a fallback position to liberate these posts from the canal.

The PRS Option   The PRS kit affords simplicity in use and provides extraordinary opportunity in predictably removing different kinds of post systems and other intracanal obstructions (Fig. 25-37, *A*).[73,74] The preparatory procedures for the PRS require straight-line access and complete circumferential visualization of the post within the pulp chamber from the occlusal table to the orifice level.

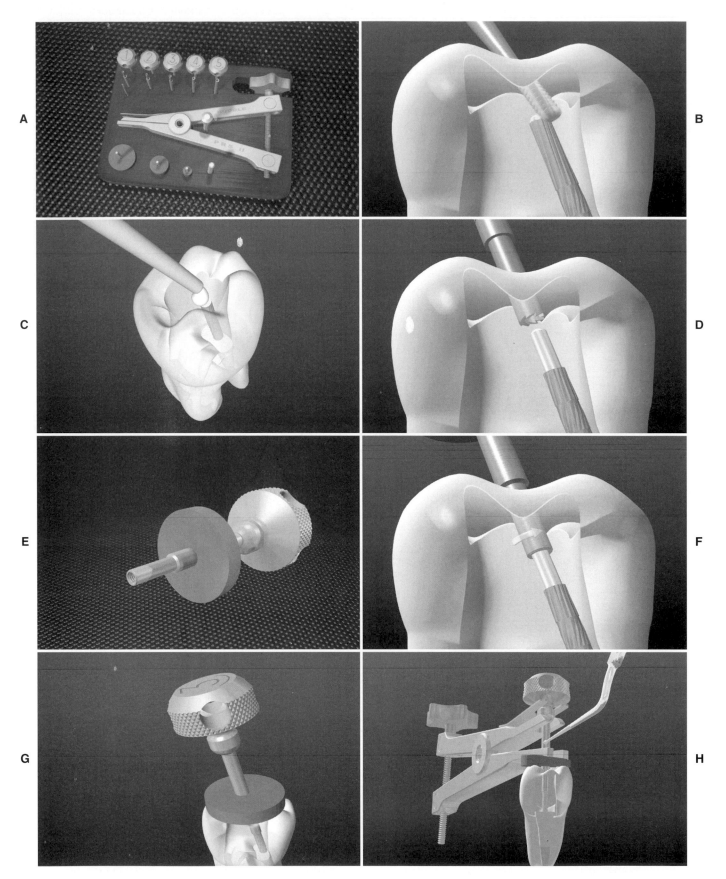

Fig. 25-37 **A**, The PRS kit is comprised of 5 variously sized trephines and corresponding taps, a transmetal bur, rubber bumpers, a torque bar, and the extracting pliers. This system is designed to safely remove virtually any post. **B**, Graphic depicting a transmetal bur efficiently doming the post head. **C**, Graphic shows the placement of a drop of lubricant, such as RC Prep, on the post head. **D**, Graphic depicts that a trephine has precisely machined-down the coronal 2 to 3 mm of the post. **E**, A PRS microtubular tap with an inserted protective bumper. **F**, Graphic demonstrating the tubular tap turning CCW to form threads and engage the post. **G**, Graphic showing a post-engaged tap and a rubber bumper protecting the occlusal surface of the tooth. **H**, Graphic demonstrates the mounted and activated extracting pliers with the energized CPR-1 ultrasonic instrument vibrating on the tap.

Once access has been achieved, the transmetal bur is used to round off and taper the coronal-most aspect of the post (Fig. 25-37, *B*). "Doming" the head of the post in this manner will guide the subsequent instruments over the post. A drop or two of a chelator is then placed on the head of the post to act as a lubricant to facilitate the subsequent machining process (Fig. 25-37, *C*). To ensure circumferential milling, the largest trephine that will just engage the post is selected. The trephine is used with a "peck" drilling motion to maintain RPMs and to keep the head of the post cooler so that it does not work-harden. The trephine is carried down over the head of the post ideally 2 to 3 mm and machines a precisely round, cross-sectional diameter (Fig. 25-37, *D*).

The trephine used for machining the post dictates the subsequent selection of a correspondingly sized tubular tap. Before the tap is placed, a rubber bumper is inserted on the tap to protect and cushion the tooth and restorative during subsequent removal efforts (Fig. 25-37, *E*). The tubular tap is then firmly pushed against the milled down post head and is screwed onto the post in a CCW direction (Fig. 25-37, *F*). Firm apical pressure and small quarter turn, CCW motions will draw down the tubular tap, resulting in its forming threads and securely engaging the post. The tap should be screwed over the post as little as 1 to 3 mm. Caution should be exercised so that the tap is not drawn down too far, because its maximum internal depth is 4 mm. If the tap bottoms out against the post head, it can predispose to stripping the threads, breaking the wall of the tap, or shearing off the obstruction inside the lumen of the tap. When the tubular tap has snugly engaged the post, the protective rubber bumper is pushed down onto the biting surface of the tooth (Fig. 25-37, *G*).

The post removal pliers is then selected and its extracting jaws are mounted onto the tubular tap. The instrument is held firmly with one hand, while the fingers of the other hand begin opening the jaws by turning the screw knob *clockwise* (CW). As the jaws slowly begin to open, increasing pressure will be noted on the screw knob. The clinician should verify that the compressing rubber cushion is properly protecting the tooth. If turning the screw knob becomes increasingly difficult, the clinician should either hesitate a few seconds before continuing or vibrate the CPR-1 ultrasonic instrument on the tubular tap as close to the post as possible (Fig. 25-37, *H*). This combination encourages the screw knob to turn further and is a potent adjunct to successful post removal. Ultimately, the PRS provides clinicians an important post removal method that is employed when ultrasonic techniques are unsuccessful (Fig. 25-38).

Clinicians also encounter actively engaged, threaded posts that require removal. The PRS is specifically designed to address this scenario because each tubular tap turns in a CCW rotation.[74] The post head is milled down as previously described, and a tubular tap is threaded until tight. In instances where threaded posts are encountered, the use of the extracting pliers is contraindicated. Typically, the clinician backs the post out of the canal using a CCW rotation

with finger pressure. If the post is strongly anchored, the CPR-1 ultrasonic instrument is vibrated on the tap and, if necessary, the torque bar is inserted into the handle port to increase leverage (Fig. 25-39).

BROKEN INSTRUMENT REMOVAL

During root canal preparation procedures, the potential for instrument breakage is always present. Many clinicians associate *"broken instruments"* with separated files, but the term could also apply to a silver point, a lentulo, a Gates-Glidden (GG) bur or any manufactured obstruction inadvertently left behind in the canal.[17,23] Historically, the consequences of leaving or bypassing broken instruments have been discussed in the literature, and a variety of approaches for removing these obstructions have been presented.[31,54,59] Because of technologic advancements in vision, ultrasonic instrumentation, and microtube delivery methods, separated instruments can usually be removed. The dental operating microscope affords remarkable vision into most aspects of the root canal system and fulfills the age-old adage, "If you can see it, you can probably do it" (Fig. 25-40). In combination, microscopes and ultrasonics have driven *"microsonic"* techniques that have dramatically improved the potential for and predictability of removing broken instruments safely (Fig. 25-41).[73]

Factors Influencing Broken Instrument Removal

Before discussing the techniques used for broken instrument removal, several factors need to be appreciated. The ability to nonsurgically access and remove a broken instrument will be influenced by the cross-sectional diameter, length, and curvature of the canal (and further guided and limited by the root morphology, including the thickness of dentin and the depth of external concavities). A general rule is if one third of the overall length of an obstruction can be exposed, it can usually be removed. Instruments that lie in the straightaway portions of the canal can usually be removed. When a separated instrument lies partially around the canal curvature, and if access can be established to its most coronal extent, then removal may still be possible. If the *entire* segment of the broken instrument is apical to the curvature of the canal and safe access cannot be accomplished, then removal is usually not possible; in the presence of signs or symptoms, surgery will, at times, be required.

The *type of material* comprising an obstruction is another important factor to be considered. SS files tend to be easier to remove because they do not further fracture during the removal process. Broken NiTi instruments may explode and break again (deeper within the canal) because of heat buildup caused by ultrasonic devices. Additionally it is also useful to know if the *separated file's cutting action* was CW versus CCW before attempting to retrieve a broken instrument.

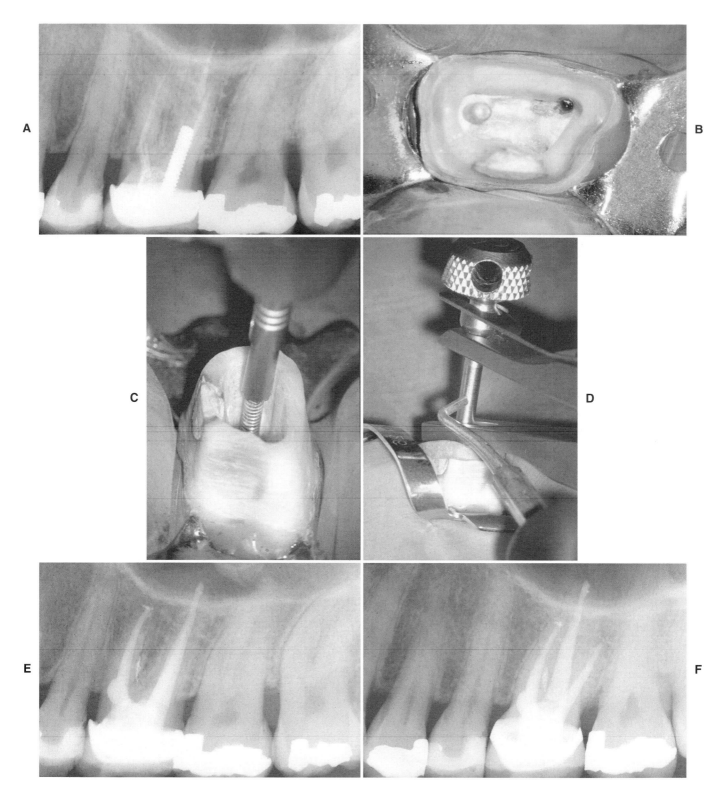

Fig. 25-38 **A**, Radiograph shows incomplete endodontics and resultant failure. Note the poor-fitting crown, internal resorption, furcal involvement, and the large post. **B**, Straight-line access demonstrates the fully exposed post, bleeding from the MB¹ orifice, and evidence of an MBᴵᴵ orifice or system. **C**, A selected trephine precisely machines the coronal 2 to 3 mm of the post. **D**, Photo depicts the mounted extracting pliers, a first generation CPR-1 ultrasonic instrument vibrating on the engaged tap, and the protective-and-compressed, rubber cushion. **E**, An off-angled radiograph reveals a well-packed resorptive defect, a furcal canal, and the PFM crown provisionalized. **F**, 4-year recall shows the new crown and endodontic healing.

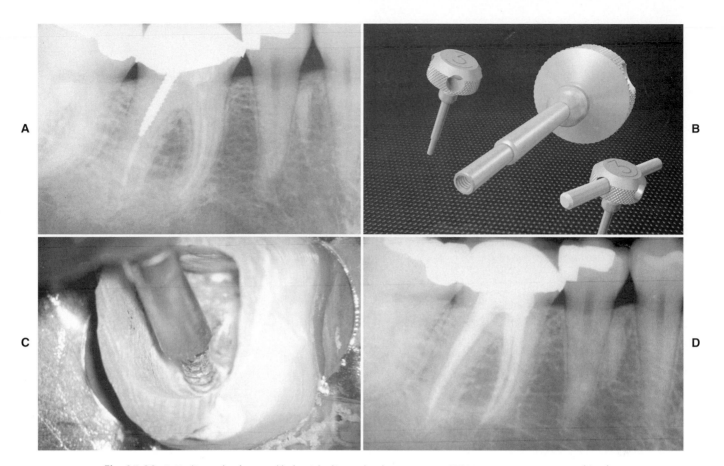

Fig. 25-39 **A**, Radiograph of a mandibular right first molar demonstrates a PFM crown, a screw post, and inadequate endodontic treatment. **B**, Close-up photo of a PRS tap shows the handle design, internal thread pattern, and a torque bar inserted through the handle port to facilitate leverage. **C**, Clinical photo shows the tap is being drawn down to tightly engage and back the post out of the canal. **D**, Postoperative radiograph shows the recemented crown and the retreatment efforts.

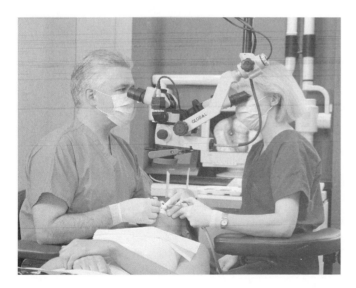

Fig. 25-40 All phases of endodontic treatment are significantly improved when the dental team uses the microscope.

Techniques for Broken Instrument Removal

Before beginning retrieval efforts, specific attention is directed toward preoperative radiographs and working films that reveal the thickness of the dentinal walls and, if present, the depth of an external concavity. Coronal access is the first step in the removal of broken instruments. High-speed, friction-grip, surgical-length burs are selected to create straight-line access to all canal orifices with special attention on the orifice and system containing the obstruction. Radicular access is the second step required in the successful removal of a broken instrument (Fig. 25-42).[15] If radicular access is limited, hand files are used serially (small to large, coronal to the obstruction), to create sufficient space to safely introduce GG drills (Dentsply Maillefer, Tulsa OK). These GGs are then used like "brushes" to create additional space and maximize visibility coronal to the obstruction. Increasingly larger GGs are stepped out of the canal to create a smooth, flowing funnel that is largest at the orifice and narrowest at the obstruction.

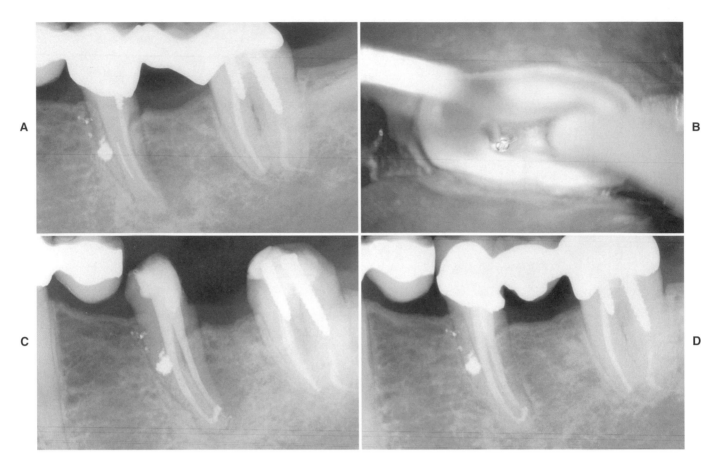

Fig. 25-41 **A**, Preoperative radiograph shows a strategic and endodontically failing mesial root of a mandibular left first molar. Note a short screw post, a separated instrument, and amalgam debris from the hemisection procedures. **B**, Photograph shows the splint removed, the post out, and an ultrasonic instrument trephining around the broken file. **C**, Posttreatment radiograph reveals 3-D retreatment. Note the third mesial system between the MB and ML canals. **D**, An 8-year recall film demonstrates a new bridge and excellent periradicular healing.

Fig. 25-42 Graphic demonstrates coronal and radicular straight-line access to the most coronal aspect of the broken instrument.

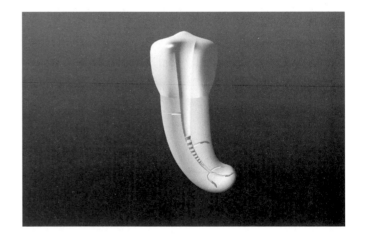

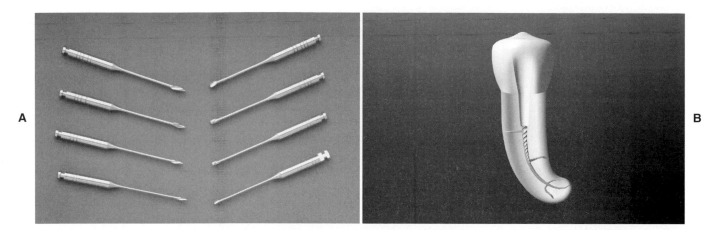

Fig. 25-43 **A**, Photograph showing selected GG drills and their subsequent modification. **B**, Graphic illustrates that after the use of a modified GG, a staging platform has been created at the most coronal aspect of the broken file.

If greater access is required lateral to the most coronal aspect of the obstruction, then the bud-shaped tip of a GG can be *"modified"* and used to create a circumferential "staging platform." The staging platform is made by selecting a GG with a maximum cross-sectional diameter that is slightly larger than the visualized instrument. The bud of the GG is altered by cutting it perpendicular to its long axis at its maximum cross-sectional diameter (Fig. 25-43, *A*). The "modified" GG is rotated at 300 RPM, gently carried into the canal, and directed apically until it "lightly" contacts the most coronal aspect of the obstruction. This clinical action creates a small staging platform that facilitates the introduction of the zirconium nitride–coated CPR-3, 4, 5 or, if restricted by space, the longer and thinner titanium CPR-6, 7, and 8 ultrasonic instruments (Fig. 25-43, *B*).

Before performing any radicular removal techniques, it is wise to place cotton pellets over any other exposed orifices, if present, to prevent the nuisance reentry of the fragment into another canal system. An ultrasonic instrument is selected based on the depth of the broken file and space availability. It is activated at the *lowest* power setting and used *dry* so that the clinician has constant vision between the energized tip and the broken instrument. To maintain vision, the dental assistant uses the Stropko three-way adapter with the appropriate luer-lock tip to direct a continuous stream of air and blow out dentinal dust (see Fig. 25-34). The selected CPR instrument is moved lightly in a CCW direction around the obstruction, except when removing reverse-screw files. This ultrasonic action sands away dentin and trephines around the coronal few millimeters of the obstruction (Fig. 25-44, *A* and *B*). Typically, during ultrasonic use, the obstruction begins to loosen, unwind, and spin. Gently wedging the energized tip between the tapered file and the canal wall oftentimes causes the broken instrument to abruptly "jump-out" of the canal. In the instance where a broken instrument lies deep and access is restricted by root bulk and form, the clinician should select the appropriately sized titanium CPR ultrasonic tip. These instruments' longer lengths and smaller profiles allow clinicians to safely trephine deeper (Fig. 25-44, *C*).

On occasion the clinician may create excellent coronal and radicular access, identify and expose the separated instrument, perform ultrasonic trephining procedures, and still be unable to loosen and "jettison" the instrument out of the canal (Fig. 25-44, *D*). In many instances a microtube device can be selected to engage and potentially remove the obstruction mechanically.

The IRS Option   The IRS provides a breakthrough in the retrieval of broken instruments lodged deep within the root canal space.[19] The IRS is composed of variously sized microtubes and insert wedges that are scaled to fit and work deep within the root canal space (Fig. 25-45). The microtube has a small handle to enhance vision, and its distal end is constructed with a 45-degree, beveled end, and cutout window. Before the IRS can be used, straight-line, coronal and radicular access is required to expose and subsequently visualize the most coronal end of the broken instrument. After establishing access, the clinician uses ultrasonic instrumentation (as previously described) to circumferentially expose 2 to 3 mm of the separated file or, if possible, about one third of its overall length. A microtube is then selected that can passively slide into the canal and drop over the exposed, broken instrument. The microtube is inserted into the canal and, in instances of canal curvature, the long part of its beveled end is oriented to the outer wall of the canal to "scoop-up" the head of the broken instrument and guide it into its lumen (Fig. 25-46, *A* and *B*).

The insert wedge is then placed through the open end of the microtube and passed down its internal lumen until it contacts the broken obstruction (Fig. 25-46, *C*). The broken instrument is engaged and secured by turning the insert wedge's handle screw in a CW rotation. Progressive rotation tightens, wedges, and often displaces the head of the broken file through the microtube's cutout window (Fig. 25-46, *D*).

Text continued on p. 910

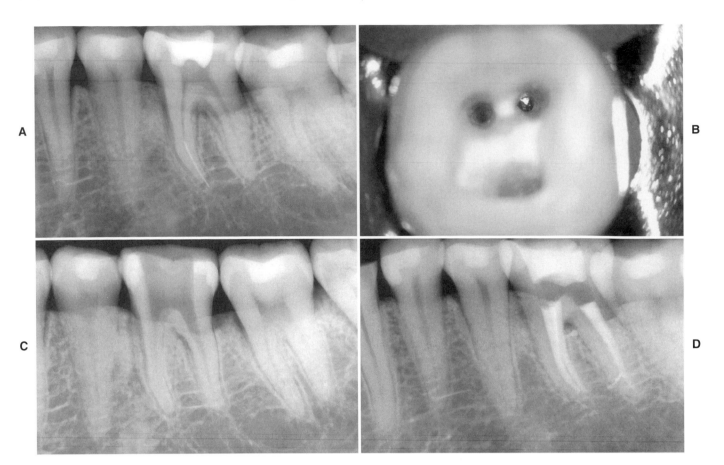

Fig. 25-47 **A**, Preoperative film of a mandibular left first molar with a broken instrument in the apical one third of the mesial root. **B**, Photograph at 12 × shows straight-line access. The head of the broken NiTi file is predictably on the outer wall. **C**, Radiograph confirms the broken file has been removed. **D**, Posttreatment film demonstrates the pack. Note the furcal canal and that the distal system bifurcates apically.

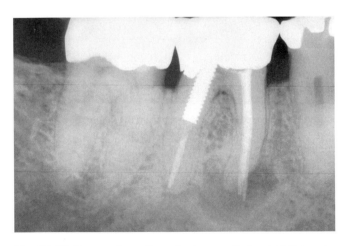

Fig. 25-48 Preoperative radiograph of a mandibular right first molar demonstrates a variety of restorative and endodontic breakdowns.

The obstruction is retrieved by either lifting the microtube and insert wedge assembly or by rotating the IRS in the appropriate direction based on the thread design of the broken instrument (Fig. 25-46, *E* and *F*). A clinical case using the IRS option is shown in Fig. 25-47.

BLOCKS, LEDGES, AND APICAL TRANSPORTATIONS

Failure to respect and appreciate the biologic-and-mechanical objectives of cleaning and shaping increases frustration and predisposes to needless complications, such as blocks, ledges, apical transportations, and, potentially, perforations (Fig. 25-48). These iatrogenic events can be attributable to inappropriate cleaning and shaping concepts. (See Chapter 8 for the concepts, strategies, and techniques used to prevent iatrogenic mishaps.)

On occasion, blocks, ledges and apical transportations *occur* and are clinically encountered. Perhaps the most powerful unsaid method to negotiate a blocked canal, bypass the

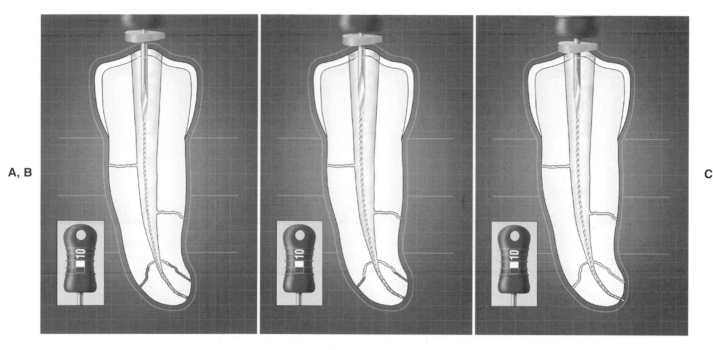

A, B

C

Fig. 25-49 **A**, Graphic demonstrates that a preenlarged canal holds a greater volume of irrigant, improves dexterity, and facilitates the placement of a precurved no. 10 file. **B**, Graphic depicts the working end of the no. 10 file engaging debris and approaching the terminus. **C**, This graphic demonstrates apical patency that is verified by sliding a no. 10 file "to" and gently "through" the foramen.

ledge, or manage a transportation is the attitude "I will," which requires determination, perseverance, and patience.

Techniques for Managing Blocks

When encountering a blocked canal, the tooth is first flooded with sodium hypochlorite. Well-angulated radiographs are observed, and the root curvature and apical pathology, if present, are noted. The clinician should appreciate that disease flow in a root canal system occurs in a coronal-to-apical direction, and the connection should be made that lesions of endodontic origin form adjacent to the portals of exit. As such, and if applicable, files are directed toward apical lesions.

Generally when managing blocked or ledged canals, the shortest file that can reach working length is selected. Shorter instruments provide more stiffness and move the clinician's fingers closer to the tip of the instrument, resulting in greater tactile control. Appreciate that canals are frequently more curved than the roots that hold them. As such, a no. 10 file is precurved to simulate the expected curvature of the canal and a unidirectional rubber stop is oriented to match the file curvature. An attempt is then made to gently slide the file to length. If this is unsuccessful the clinician should preenlarge the canal, irrigate, and slightly overcurve the file to facilitate moving it to length (Fig. 25-49, *A*). If an obstruction is encountered, the precurved file is used in an apically directed picking action. While picking, the clinician

should continuously reorient the unidirectional stop, which will automatically redirect the apical aspect of the precurved file in the hopes of negotiating the rest of the canal.

Clinicians should use very *short amplitude, light, pecking strokes* to negotiate the canal terminus. Short pecking strokes ensure safety, carry irrigant deeper, and increase the possibility of canal negotiation (Fig. 25-49, *B*). The handle of a file with a tip that is engaged should *never* be excessively rotated, because the tortional loads over length will predispose the instrument to break. If the apical extent of the file "sticks" or engages, then the handle motion is a minimal back and forth wiggle. If a no. 10 file begins to move apically, it may be useful to move to a smaller instrument with a D_0 diameter of 0.08 or 0.06 mm. The clinician should obtain a working film or frequently remove the file to see if its curve is following the expected root canal morphology. Depending on the severity of the blockage, these efforts often allow the clinician to reach the foramen passively and establish patency.

If no progress is made after diligent efforts over a timeframe of approximately 3 minutes, then the sodium hypochlorite is removed from the root canal system and replaced with a viscous chelator. The same techniques as described previously are then used, recognizing that it takes a few minutes to work the chelator deep into the canal and benefit from its desirable attributes. If the no. 10 file sticks and engages into the debris, then a smaller instrument, such as an 0.08 file is, at times, useful.

has been either reduced or eliminated. A clinical case depicting ledge management is illustrated in Fig. 25-53.

Ultimately the clinician must make a decision (based on preoperative radiographs, root bulk, and experience) whether to continue shaping procedures in hopes of eliminating the ledge or abort if continued efforts will weaken or perforate the root. Not all ledges can or should be removed. Clinicians must weigh risk versus benefit and make every effort to maximize remaining dentin. (The four *Mechanical Objectives* of cleaning and shaping, described in Chapter 8, should guide each clinician's actions.)

In the instance when the ledge cannot be removed, fitting the master gutta-percha cone can be challenging. In these cases, the master cone is trimmed so that its terminal diameter equals the D_0 diameter of the file that was snug at length. The cone is then precured to simulate the curvature of the

canal, and the radicular portion is placed in a dappen dish of 70% isopropyl alcohol. When the master cone is removed after a few seconds, its rigidity will be increased significantly. An orientational notch is then placed on the butt end of the master cone so that the clinician can identify working length and the direction of the cone's curvature. This technique greatly facilitates the placement of the master cone during the packing procedure.

Techniques for Managing Apical Transportations

Moving the position of the canal's physiologic terminus to a new iatrogenic location on the external root surface equates to a transportation of the foramen. Foraminal rips, zips, or tears are caused by carrying progressively larger and stiffer

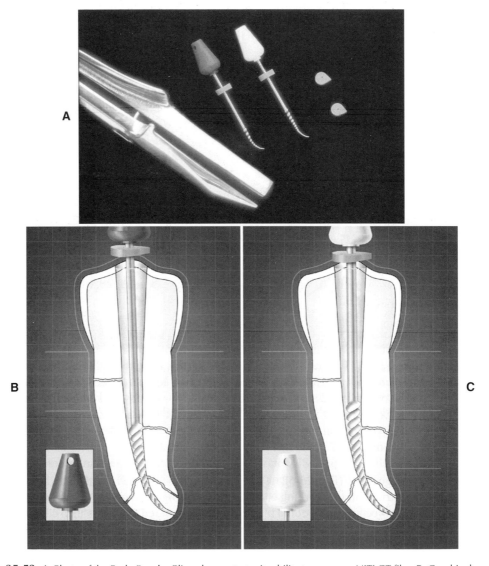

Fig. 25-52 **A**, Photo of the Endo Bender Pliers demonstrates its ability to precure NiTi GT files. **B**, Graphic demonstrates a precured 0.10 tapered GT file is apical to the ledge. **C**, Graphic demonstrates a precured 0.08 tapered GT file has eliminated the ledge and is at length.

files to length.[12,76] If a transportation has occurred, then the canal exhibits reversed apical architecture and fails to provide resistance form for gutta-percha. This contributes to poorly packed cases that are vertically overextended but internally underfilled.[74,77] In general, apical transportations can be categorized into three types, each requiring a specific treatment.

Type I   A Type I transportation represents a minor movement of the physiologic foramen to a new iatrogenic location (Fig. 25-54, *A*). In these instances the clinician must weigh risk versus benefit when trying to create positive apical canal architecture (Fig. 25-54, *B*). Generating shape coronal to the foramen requires the additional removal of dentin and could predispose to root weakening or a lateral strip perforation. If sufficient residual dentin can be maintained and shape created above the foramen, then some of these iatrogenic cases can be 3-D cleaned, shaped, and packed (Fig. 25-54, *C*). Regretfully, many canals with foramens that have been trans-

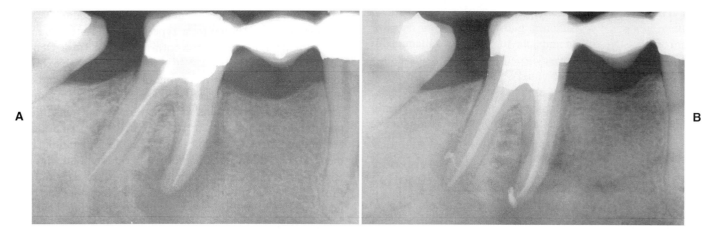

Fig. 25-53 **A**, Preoperative radiograph shows an endodontically failing posterior bridge abutment. Note the amalgam in the pulp chamber and that the mesial root appears to have been ledged. **B**, Posttreatment film demonstrates ledge management with the obturation materials following the root curvature.

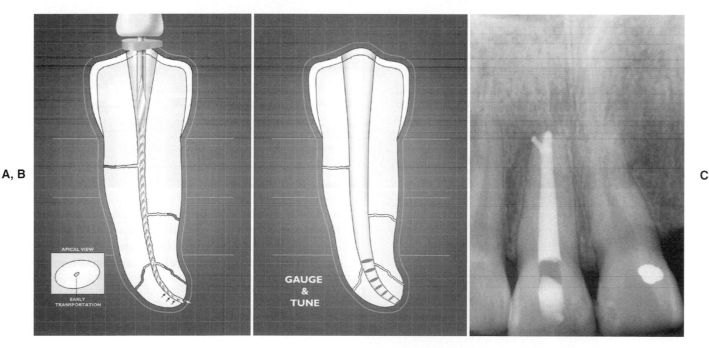

Fig. 25-54 **A**, Graphic demonstrating a Type I transportation. Note there has been a minor movement of the foramen. **B**, Management of a Type I transportation is directed toward creating shape above the foramen. **C**, Posttreatment film demonstrates treatment of a Type I transportation. Shaped canals provide resistance form to hold gutta-percha.

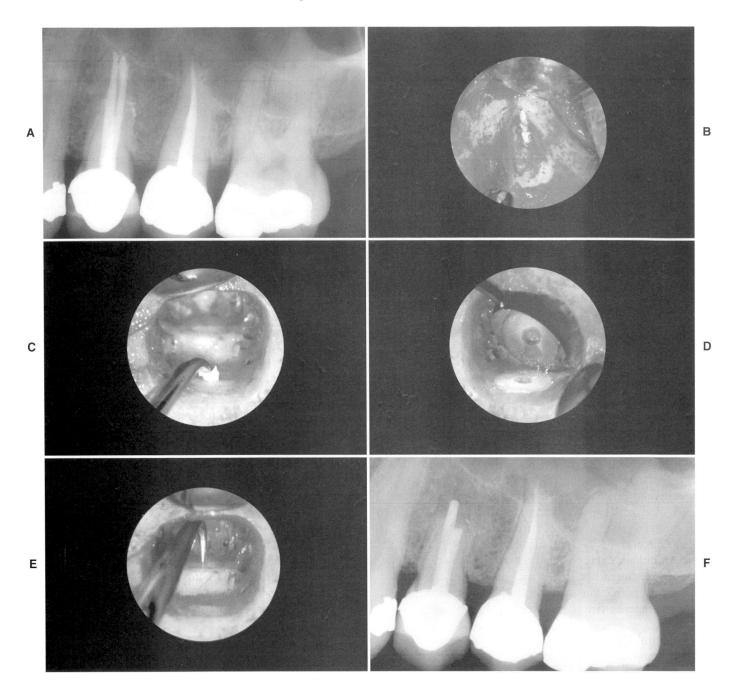

Fig. 25-59 **A,** Preoperative film of a maxillary left first bicuspid. Note the packed buccal canal does not conform to the mechanical objectives of cleaning and shaping. **B,** After flap elevation, a surgical photograph at 12 × shows gutta-percha exiting through a significantly ripped, torn, and relocated foramen. **C,** Surgical photograph at 12 × shows the osteotomy, apicoectomies, and ultrasonic root end preparation of the buccal canal. **D,** Surgical photograph at 12 × through a sapphire-plus micromirror depicts the finished buccal root end preparation. **E,** Surgical photograph at 12 × shows ultrasonic root end preparation of the lingual canal. **F,** 4-year recall film demonstrates the apically corked canals and excellent osseous repair.

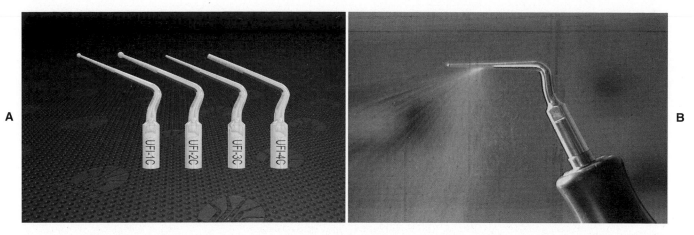

Fig. 25-60 **A**, Photograph shows the four Ultrasonic Finishing Instruments. Their geometries, coatings, and port technologies facilitate many procedures. **B**, Close-up photo of the UFI no. 1 demonstrates a fine, controlled mist exiting from its water port.

calcium sulfate, freeze-dried bone, and MTA.[6,19,84] Other hemostatics exist that are not generally selected because of factors such as cost, ease of handling and placement, or their byproducts. Ironically, some of the best hemostatics, such as ferric sulfate, leave a coagulum behind that may promote bacterial growth, compromise the seal at the tooth and restorative interface, and jeopardize the prognosis.[48]

Barrier Materials   The two main challenges a clinician faces when attempting to repair a perforation are hemostasis and the controlled placement of a restorative material. Barriers help produce a "dry field" and also provide an internal matrix or "back stop" to condense restorative materials against.[73] In general, barriers can be divided into resorbable and nonresorbable; however, it is critical to note that the restorative material used oftentimes dictates the barrier that is selected.

Resorbable barriers.   Internal bleeding into the tooth must be managed; this is accomplished by passing a "resorbable" barrier nonsurgically through the access cavity and internally through the perforation defect into, ideally, a three-walled osseous defect. Resorbable barrier materials are intended to be placed in the bone, not left within tooth structure. The barrier should conform to the anatomy of the furcation or root surface involved. Although a variety of resorbable barriers exist, collagen and calcium sulfate materials are best employed because of ease of handling, research, and observed clinical results.

- Collagen materials, such as Collacote (Sulger Dental, Carlsbad, CA), exhibit excellent working properties that provide complete hemostasis.[39] Collacote is biocompatible, supportive of new tissue growth, resorbable in 10 to 14 days, and left *in situ*.[10,19,33] Based on the size of the defect and the available access, pieces of Collacote are cut to appropriate sizes and carried into the access cavity. The material is incrementally placed through the tooth and into the osseous defect until a solid barrier corresponding to the cavosurface of the root is established. Hemostasis is typically achieved in 2 to 5 minutes. Collagen barriers have been widely used in conjunction with amalgam, Super EBA, and other nonbonded restoratives.[64] Collacote is contraindicated as a barrier if adhesion dentistry is contemplated because it absorbs moisture and will contaminate the restorative.

- Calcium sulfate, such as Capset (Lifecore Biomedical, Chaska, MN), can be used as both a barrier and hemostatic material in perforation management.[2,64,84] Calcium sulfate creates a tamponade effect, mechanically plugging the vascular channels once it sets. Capset is remarkably biocompatible, does not promote inflammation, and is bioresorbable in 2 to 4 weeks. This material is syringed through the tooth and into the osseous defect using a microtube delivery system. During the placement of calcium sulfate, it will fill the osseous defect and a portion of the space within the root defect. Calcium sulfate rapidly sets brick hard and is easily sanded flush to the external root surface with selected Ultrasonic Finishing Instruments (UFI) (Dentsply Tulsa Dental, Tulsa, Okla.). UFIs are coated for sanding, scaled to work deep within the root canal space, and their port technologies dispense irrigant precisely into the field of action (Fig. 25-60). Calcium sulfate is the barrier of choice when using the principles of wet bonding.[1,30,64] Importantly, the perforation defect can be rinsed of contaminants and prepared for adhesion dentistry.

Nonresorbable barriers.   MTA exhibits excellent tissue biocompatibility and can be used both as a nonresorbable barrier and restorative material (see Fig. 25-56).[40] It has many clinical applications and represents an extraordinary breakthrough for managing radicular repairs.[6,47] MTA is the barrier of choice when there is potential moisture contamination or when there are restrictions in technical access and visibility. Furthermore, MTA can be used as the sole

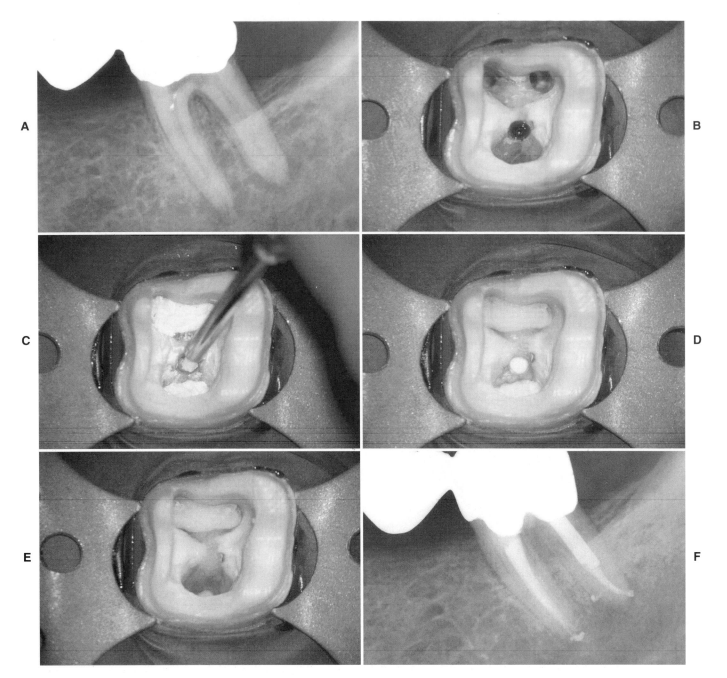

Fig. 25-61 **A**, Preoperative radiograph of an endodontically involved mandibular left second molar bridge abutment. Note the previous access and possible floor perforation. **B**, Photograph demonstrates the identified orifices and a frank furcal-floor perforation. **C**, Photograph demonstrates pieces of Collacote overlying the orifices and calcium sulfate being introduced into the perforation via an STN. **D**, Photograph demonstrates furcal management and the absorbable barrier finished flush to the external cavosurface. **E**, Photograph shows the perforation repair using a dual-cured, composite restorative. **F**, 5-year recall film shows a new bridge and osseous repair furcally and apically.

restorative material radically, or it can be used as a barrier against which to pack another material. (See "Techniques for Managing Apical Transportations" earlier in the chapter.)

Restoratives   Central to success when repairing a perforation is to select a restorative material that is easy to use, nonresorbable, biocompatible, esthetically pleasing, and that provides a complete seal. The materials commonly employed to repair perforations include the time-honored (but decreasing in popularity) amalgam, Super EBA resin cement (Bosworth Co., Skokie, IL), composite bonded restoratives (Den-Mat Corp., Santa Maria, CA), calcium phosphate cement, and MTA.[16,58,60] The choice of the restorative repair material is based on the technical access to the defect, the ability to control moisture, and the esthetic considerations.

Techniques for Repairing Perforations

The specific barrier and restorative selected to repair a perforation site should be based on sound research, judgment, experience, training, esthetics, ease of handling, and the advantages or disadvantages of a particular material in a specific clinical setting. This section describes the armamentarium, materials, and techniques required to repair perforations.

Management of Coronal One-Third and Furcal Perforations   The major difference between coronal one-third and furcal-floor perforations is the shape of the resultant root defect. Mechanical perforations that occur in the furcal floor are generally round, whereas those occurring in the lateral aspects of roots are ovoid by nature of occurrence. When managing these perforations, the clinician must first isolate the perforation site. Generally, if the perforation is mechanical and has just occurred, it is probably clean. In this situation and if hemostasis is present, the defect can be immediately repaired. However, if the perforation is chronic and exhibits microleakage, it needs to be cleaned and prepared before receiving the restorative material. Ultrasonic finishing instruments are ideal for preparing perforation sites because of their geometries, coatings, and port technologies.

Once the defect has been properly prepared, an appropriate barrier material and restorative are then selected based on the following esthetic considerations:
- In a coronal one-third perforation where esthetics is a concern, a calcium sulfate barrier in conjunction with adhesion dentistry is generally used.[30]
- Historically amalgam and, more recently, Super EBA have been used to repair coronal one-third perforations when esthetics was not an issue. Presently, MTA is rapidly becoming the barrier and restorative of choice for repairing nonesthetic coronal one-third defects because of its many desirable attributes.

After perforation repair, the case can be 3-D cleaned, shaped, and packed if this has not already been accomplished (Fig. 25-61).

Management of Perforations in the Middle One Third   Iatrogenic perforations in the middle one third of roots are generally caused by endodontic files, GG drills, or large, misdirected posts. By nature of occurrence, these defects are ovoid in shape and typically represent relatively large surface areas to seal. In multirooted teeth, perforations into the furcation area are termed *furcal strips*.

Middle one-third perforations have the same technical considerations as coronal one-third perforations, *except* that the clinician is now dealing with defects located deeper and further away from the access cavity. The factors that must be addressed to successfully treat these more apically positioned perforations are hemostasis, access, use of microinstrumentation techniques, and selection of best materials in a challenging environment. When managing deeper defects that are positioned on the lateral walls of canals, vision is enhanced when direct access exists or can be safely created. In some instances direct access may not be possible without irreversibly compromising the structural integrity of the tooth and will likewise require indirect repair techniques. Generally perforations that occur secondary to overzealous canal instrumentation are sterile and do not require modification using microinstrumentation procedures. However, failing endodontic cases are associated with microleakage and may require UFI instrumentation to clean and refine the defect in preparation for repair.

In middle one-third perforations with a small defect, if the bleeding can be arrested and the canal dried, the perforation can then be sealed and repaired during 3-D obturation. However, if the defect is large and there is nuisance moisture or if the canal cannot be definitively dried, the perforation must first be repaired before 3-D obturation. It is wise to prepare the canal as optimally as possible before initiating the perforation repair procedures. As has been stated earlier, a prepared canal will facilitate access to the defect and minimize postrepair instrumentation. To prevent obstructing the root canal space during the repair procedures, any readily retrievable material is placed in the canal and apical to the defect before the perforation is repaired.

Because of the difficult technical access, limited visibility, and uncertainty of a moisture-free environment in these cases, MTA is the restorative-and-barrier material of choice. MTA is mixed and carried into the field and managed in accordance with the technique discussed earlier in this chapter. Upon reappointment, MTA will invariably be hard and the clinician can proceed with the required treatment (Fig. 25-62).

Management of Perforations in the Apical One Third   Perforations occurring in the apical one third of roots primarily result from breakdowns that occur during cleaning-and-shaping procedures. Blocks and ledges invite deep perforations and result from inadequate irrigation, inappropriate instrumentation, and failure to maintain patency. Roots perforated in their apical one third can pose surprises and frustration during nonsurgical retreatment. It is

Text continued on p. 926

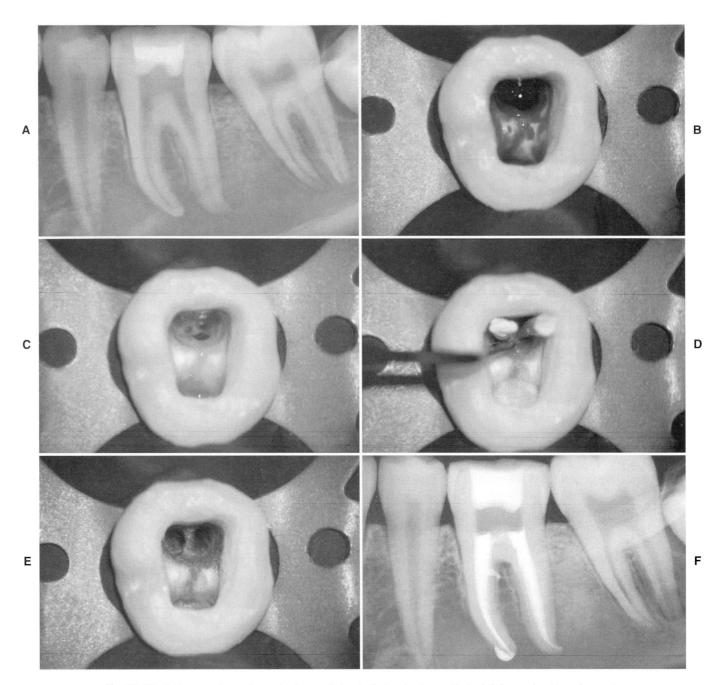

Fig. 25-62 **A**, Preoperative radiograph of an endodontically involved mandibular left first molar. Note the previously overenlarged mesial root. **B**, Photograph taken upon reentry shows significant bleeding emanating from the mesial root. **C**, Photograph demonstrates hemostasis and identifies the position of the strip perforation. **D**, Photograph reveals gutta-percha cones in the MB and ML systems to prevent their blockage. MTA is being vibrated into the perforation defect. **E**, Photograph at a subsequent visit shows the gutta-percha cones removed, the perforation repaired, and the canals ready to pack. **F**, Postoperative film shows the provisionalized tooth, four systems packed, and the apical one-third anatomy.

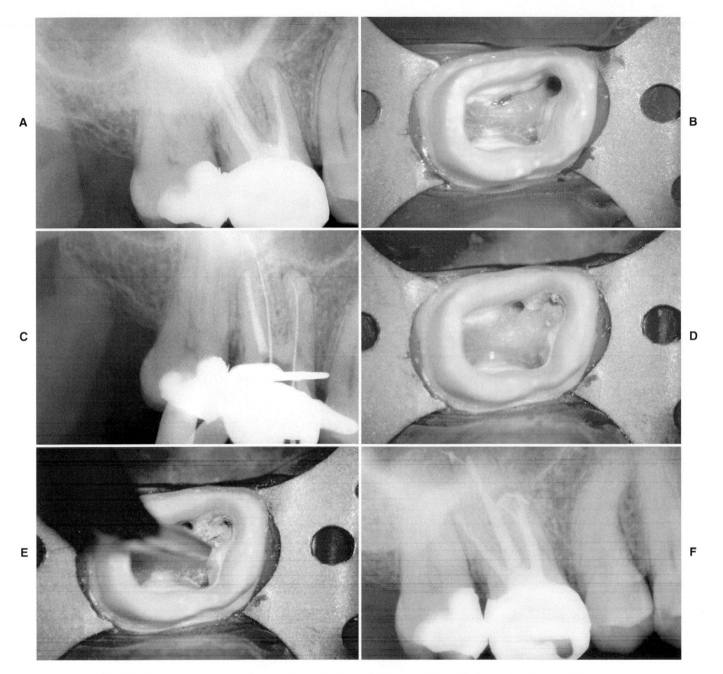

Fig. 25-63 **A,** Preoperative radiograph of an endodontically failing maxillary right first molar. Note the MB root is perforated in its apical one third. **B,** Photograph demonstrates crown removal, the MB^I orifice, and bleeding emanating from the MB^{II} system. **C,** Photograph demonstrates a no. 10 file at the terminus of the MB^{II} system. **D,** Photograph illustrates the prepared MB^{II} system, a holding file within the MB^I canal (intentionally sectioned below the occlusal surface), and MTA used to repair the perforation defect. **E,** At a subsequent visit the MTA was brick hard, and a photograph shows the removal of the holding file from the MB^I system. **F,** Posttreatment radiograph demonstrates the treated MB^I and MB^{II} systems, the perforation repair, and the block-and-ledge management of the DB and palatal systems.

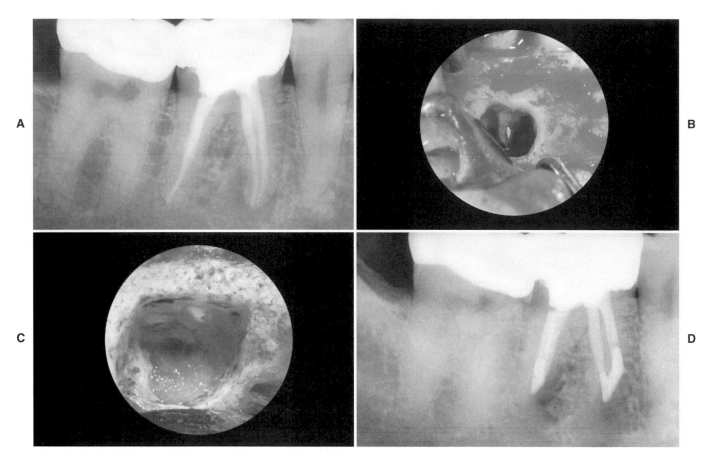

Fig. 25-64 **A**, Preoperative radiograph of an endodontically failing mandibular right first molar. This specific radiographic angle does not reveal the cause of failure. **B**, Photograph reveals gutta-percha perforating the buccal aspect of the mesial root. **C**, Photograph reveals the apicoectomy and retrograde procedures. Note the management of the isthmus between the MB and ML foramina. **D**, Posttreatment radiograph demonstrates the surgical efforts.

quite common that a root perforated in its apical one third holds a canal that is both blocked and ledged. Recognizing the cause of this type of perforation has led to surgical correction using apicoectomy and retrograde-type procedures. However, it is generally best for clinicians to first attempt nonsurgical retreatment to enhance the existing endodontic treatment and, if present, to identify and treat missed canals.

The clinician should attempt to negotiate the physiologic terminus with the concepts, instruments, and techniques previously discussed (see "Techniques for Managing Blocks" and "Techniques for Managing Ledges" in this chapter). On occasion, the apical extent of the file will stick, the handle flutter will be noticed, and the instrument will begin to track along the true canal pathway. The file is gently worked to negotiate the physiologic pathway, establish patency, and pave the way for the next successively larger instrument. The next sequentially larger, precurved file is then inserted and carried apical to the perforation but not necessarily to length. This "holding file" maintains the pathway of the true canal and prevents it from being blocked during subsequent repair.

ProRoot is the material of choice for repairing deep perforations, especially when a dry environment and technical access are not possible. ProRoot is placed as has been previously described. To prevent the holding file from being frozen in a sea of MTA as it hardens, the instrument is grasped with a Stieglitz Pliers and moved up and down in short, 1- to 2-mm amplitude strokes. The loosened holding file is then sectioned so that its most coronal aspect is below the occlusal table. A radiograph should be taken to confirm the position of the MTA and the quality of the repair. A wet-cotton pellet is placed within the pulp chamber against the MTA, the tooth is provisionalized, and the patient dismissed. Upon reentry, the holding file is removed; if the MTA is brick hard, then the clinician should voluminously irrigate and gently finalize the preparation, fit a gutta-percha master cone, and 3-D obturate. It is wise to provisionalize these cases and follow-up periodically before placing a definitive restoration. The clinical steps for managing apical one-third perforations are illustrated in Fig. 25-63. It is also important to acknowledge that not all perforations can be corrected nonsurgically, even when the best technologies are being used in the hands of the most skilled practitioners. Certain cases will still require surgical treatment or extraction (Fig. 25-64).

CONCLUSION

Training, practice, and technology allow clinicians to greatly expand their abilities in nonsurgical endodontic retreatment. As this chapter has shown, a great variety of techniques exist to address endodontically failing teeth. However, not all failures are amenable to successful nonsurgical retreatment. Clinicians need to weigh risk versus benefit and recognize that, at times, surgery or extraction might be in the patient's best interest. When retreatment procedures are appropriate, disassembled teeth create an opening for predictable and corrective repairs. Critical to long-term endodontic success is the placement of a well-designed restoration that prevents microleakage, provides a ferrule effect, promotes periodontal health and harmonious occlusion, and is esthetically pleasing. Interdisciplinary excellence is the foundation for professional fulfillment, patient satisfaction, and long-term success. As the health of the attachment apparatus around endodontically treated teeth becomes fully appreciated, the naturally retained root will be recognized as the ultimate dental implant. Properly performed, endodontic treatment is the cornerstone of restorative and reconstructive dentistry.

References

1. Albers H: *Tooth-colored restoratives,* ed 8, Santa Rosa, Calif., 1996, Alto Books.
2. Alhadainy HA, Abdalla AI: Artificial floor technique used for the repair of furcation perforations: a microleakage study, *J Endod* 24(1):33, 1998.
3. Allen RK, Newton CW, Brown CE: A statistical analysis of surgical and nonsurgical endodontic retreatment cases, *J Endod* 15:6, 1989.
4. Altshul JH, Marshall G, Morgan LA, Baumgartner JC: Comparison of dentinal crack incidence and of post removal time resulting from post removal by ultrasonic or mechanical force, *J Endod* 23(11):683, 1997.
5. Alves J, Walton R, Drake D: Coronal leakage: endotoxin penetration from mixed bacterial communities through obturated, post-prepared root canals, *J Endod* 24(9):587, 1998.
6. Arens DE, Torabinejad M: Repair of furcal perforations with mineral trioxide aggregate, *Oral Surg Oral Med Oral Pathol Oral Radiol Endod* 82:84, 1996.
7. Barbosa SV, Burkard DH, Spangberg LS: Cytotoxic effects of gutta-percha solvents, *J Endod* 20:1, 1994.
8. Barkhordar RA, Stewart GG: The potential of periodontal pocket formation associated with untreated accessory root canals, *Oral Surg Oral Med Oral Pathol* 70:6, 1990.
9. Bertrand MF, Pellegrino JC, Rocca JP, Klinghofer A, Bolla M: Removal of Thermafil root canal filling material, *J Endod* 23:1, 1997.
10. Blumenthal N: The use of collagen membranes for guided tissue regeneration, *Compend Contin Educ Dent* (supp 13), March, 1992.
11. Bragger U, Lauchenauer D, Lang NP: Surgical lengthening of the clinical crown, *J Clin Periodontol* 19:58, 1992.
12. Briseno BM, Sonnabend E: The influence of different root canal instruments on root canal preparation: an *in vitro* study, *Int Endod J* 23:15, 1991.
13. Burns RC, Herbranson EJ: Tooth morphology and cavity preparations. In Cohen S, Burns RC, editors: *Pathways of pulp,* ed 7, St Louis, 1998, Mosby.
14. Carr GB: Surgical endodontics. In Cohen S, Burns RC, editors: *Pathways of pulp,* ed 6, St Louis, 1994, Mosby.
15. Carr GB: Retreatment. In Cohen S, Burns RC, editors: *Pathways of pulp,* ed 7, St Louis, 1998, Mosby.
16. Chau JY, Hutter JW, Mork TO, Nicoll BK: An *in vitro* study of furcation perforation repair using calcium phosphate cement, *J Endod* 23:9, 1997.
17. Chenail BL, Teplitsky PE: Orthograde ultrasonic retrieval of root canal obstructions, *J Endod* 13:186, 1987.
18. Chiche G, Kokich V, Caudill R: Diagnosis and treatment planning of esthetic problems. In Pinault A, Chiche G, editors: *Esthetics in fixed prosthodontics,* Chicago, 1994, Quintessence Publishing Co.
19. Chung KM et al: Clinical evaluation of a biodegradable collagen membrane in guided tissue regeneration, *J Periodontol* 61:732, 1990.
20. Cohen AG: The efficiency of solvents used in the retreatment of paste-filled root canals, master's thesis, Boston 1986, Boston University.
21. DeDeus QD: Frequency, location, and direction of the accessory canals, *J Endod* 1:361, 1975.
22. Endodontic trends reflect changes in care provided, *Dental Products Report* 30(12):94, 1996.
23. Fors UG, Berg JO: Endodontic treatment of root canals obstructed by foreign objects, *Int Endod J* 19:2, 1986.
24. Glick DH, Frank AL: Removal of silver points and fractured posts by ultrasonics, *J Prosthet Dent* 55:212, 1986.
25. Goon WWY: Managing the obstructed root canal space: rationale and techniques, *J Calif Dent Assoc* 19:5, 1991.
26. Haitt WH: Pulpal periodontal disease, *J Periodontol* 48:598, 1977.
27. Hammerstrom LE, Blomloef LB, Feiglin B, Lindskog SF: Effect of calcium hydroxide treatment on periodontal repair and root resorption, *Endod Dent Traumatol* 2:184, 1986.
28. Hess JC, Culieras MJ, Lamiable N: A scanning electron microscope investigation of principal and accessory foramina on the root surfaces of human teeth: thoughts about endodontic pathology and therapeutics, *J Endod* 9:7, 1983.
29. Hess W, Zürcher E: *The anatomy of the root canals of the teeth of the permanent and deciduous dentitions,* New York, 1925, William Wood & Co.
30. Himel VT, Alhadainy HA: Effect of dentin preparation and acid etching on the sealing ability of glass ionomer and composite resin when used to repair furcation perforations over plaster of Paris barriers, *J Endod* 21(3):142, 1995.
31. Hulsmann M: Removal of fractured instruments using a combined automated/ultrasonic technique, *J Endod* 20:3, 1994.
32. Jeng HW, El Deeb ME: Removal of hard paste fillings from the root canal by ultrasonic instrumentation, *J Endod* 13:6, 1987.
33. Johns L, Merritt K, Agarwal S, Ceravolo F: Immunogenicity of bovine collagen membrane used in guided tissue regeneration, *J Dent Res* 71:298, 1992 (abstract).
34. Kaplowitz GJ: Evaluation of gutta-percha solvents, *J Endod* 16:11, 1990.

35. Kartal N, Ozcelik O, Cimilli H: Root canal morphology of maxillary premolars, *J Endod* 24(6):417, 1998.

36. Kasahara E et al: Root canal system of the maxillary central incisor, *J Endod* 16:4, 1990.

37. Kersten HW, Wesselink PR, Thoden van Velzen SK: The diagnostic reliability of the buccal radiograph after root canal filling, *Int Endod J* 20:20, 1987.

38. Kim S: Principles of endodontic microsurgery, *Dent Clin North Am* 41(3):481, 1997.

39. Kim S, Rethnam S: Hemostasis in endodontic microsurgery, *Dent Clin North Am* 41(3):499, 1997.

40. Koh ET, McDonald F, Pitt-Ford TR, Torabinejad M: Cellular response to mineral trioxide aggregate, *J Endod* 24(8):543, 1998.

41. Kois J, Spear FM: Periodontal prosthesis: creating successful restorations, *J Am Dent Assoc* 10:123, 1992.

42. Kois JC: Altering gingival levels: the restorative connection. Part I: biological variables, *J Esthet Dent* 6(1):3, 1994.

43. Kois JC: The restorative-periodontal interface: biological parameters, *Periodontol 2000* 11:29, 1996.

44. Kokich VG et al: Guidelines for managing the orthodontic-restorative patient, *Semin Orthod* 3(1):3, 1997.

45. Krell KV, Neo J: The use of ultrasonic endodontic instrumentation in the retreatment of paste-filled endodontic teeth, *Oral Surg* 60:100, 1985.

46. Kvist T, Reit C: Results of endodontic retreatment: a randomized clinical study comparing surgical and nonsurgical procedures, *J Endod* 25(12):814, 1999.

47. Lee SJ, Monsef M, Torabinejad M: The sealing ability of a mineral trioxide aggregate for repair of lateral root perforations, *J Endod* 19:11, 1993.

48. Lemon RR, Steele PJ, Jeansonne BG: Ferric sulfate hemostasis: effect on osseous wound healing. Part I: left *in situ* for maximum exposure, *J Endod* 19:170, 1993.

49. Lenchner NH: Restoring endodontically treated teeth: ferrule effect and biologic width, *Pract Periodontics Aesth Dent* 1:19, 1989.

50. Machtou P: *Endodontie - guide clinique,* ed CDP, Paris, 1993, CDP.

51. Machtou P: Que faire face aux canaux inaccessibles: faut-il passer a tant prix, *Rev Odontoestomatol,* 13:4, 1984.

52. Machtou P, Sarfati P, Cohen AG: Post removal prior to retreatment, *J Endod* 15:11, 1989.

53. Madeira MC, Heten S: Incidence of bifurcations in mandibular incisors, *Oral Surg* 36:4, 1973.

54. Masserann J: The extraction of instruments broken in the radicular canal: a new technique, *Acta Odontol Stomatol* 47:265, 1959.

55. Masserann J: The extraction of posts broken deeply in the roots, *Acta Odontol Stomatol* 75:329, 1966.

56. Melton DC, Krall KV, Fuller MW: Anatomical and histological features of C-shaped canals in mandibular second molars, *J Endod* 17:8, 1991.

57. Milot P, Stein RS: Root fracture in endodontically treated teeth related to post selection and crown design, *J Prosthet Dent* 68:428, 1992.

58. Moloney LG, Feik SA, Ellender G: Sealing ability of three materials used to repair lateral root perforations, *J Endod* 19:2, 1993.

59. Nagai O, Tani N, Kayaba Y, Kodama S, Osada T: Ultrasonic removal of broken instruments in root canals, *Int Endod J* 19:298, 1986.

60. Nakata TT, Bae KS, Baumgartner JC: Perforation repair comparing mineral trioxide aggregate and amalgam using an anaerobic bacterial leakage model, *J Endod* 24(3):184, 1998.

61. Nevins M, Mellonig JT, editors: *Periodontal therapy, clinical approaches and evidence of success*, Chicago, 1998, Quintessence Publishing Co.

62. Nevins M, Skurow HM: The intracrevicular restorative margin, the biologic width, and the maintenance of the gingival margin, *Int J Periodontics Restorative Dent* 4(3):31, 1984.

63. Parreira FR, O'Connor RP, Hutter JW: Cast prosthesis removal using ultrasonics and a thermoplastic resin adhesive, *J Endod* 20:3, 1994.

64. Pecora G, Baek S, Rethnam S, Kim S: Barrier membrane techniques in endodontic microsurgery, *Dental Clinics of North America* 41(3):585, 1997.

65. Pineda F, Kuttler U: Mesiodistal and buccolingual roentgenographic investigations of 7275 root canals, *Oral Surg* 33:101, 1972.

66. Pitt-Ford TR, Torabinejad M, Hong CU, Kariyawasam SP: Use of mineral trioxide aggregate for repair of furcal perforations, *Oral Surg* 79:756, 1995.

67. Ross SE, Garguilo A: The surgical management of the restorative alveolar interface, *Int J Periodontics Restorative Dent* 2(3):8, 1982.

68. Ruddle CJ: Three-dimensional obturation: the rationale and application of warm gutta-percha with vertical condensation. In Cohen S, Burns RC, editors: *Pathways of pulp*, ed 6, St Louis, 1994, Mosby.

69. Ruddle CJ: Endodontic failures: the rationale and application of surgical retreatment, *Revue Odontostomatol (Paris)* 17(6):511, 1988.

70. Ruddle CJ: How to profit from endo: finding the fair fee for endodontics, *Dent Econ* 88(11):30, 1998.

71. Ruddle CJ, Mangani F: Endodontic treatment of a "very particular" maxillary central incisor, *J Endod* 20:11, 1994.

72. Ruddle CJ: Microdentistry: identification & treatment of MB[II] systems, *J Calif Dent Assoc* 25:4, 1997.

73. Ruddle CJ: Microendodontic nonsurgical retreatment, *Dental Clinics of North America* 41(3):429, 1997.

74. Ruddle CJ: Nonsurgical endodontic retreatment, *J Calif Dent Assoc* 25:11, 1997.

75. Ruddle CJ: Surgical endodontic retreatment, *J Calif Dent Assoc* 19(5):61, 1991.

76. Schilder H: Canal débridement and disinfection. In Cohen S, Burns RC, editors: *Pathways of pulp*, ed 1, St Louis, 1976, Mosby.

77. Schilder H: Filling the root canals in three dimensions, *Dent Clin North Am* 723, 1967.

78. Scianamblo MJ: Endodontic failures: the retreatment of previously endodontically treated teeth, *Revue Odontostomatol (Paris)* 17(5):409, 1988.

79. Shanelec DA, Tibbetts LS: A perspective on the future of periodontal microsurgery, *Periodontol 2000* 11:58, 1996.

80. Sheets CG: The periodontal-restorative interface: enhancement through magnification, *Pract Periodontics Aesthet Dent* 11(8):925, 1999.

81. Simon JHS, Glick DH, Frank AL: The relationship of endodontic-periodontic lesions, *J Periodontol* 43:202, 1972.

82. Smith CS, Setchel DJ, Harty FJ: Factors influencing the success of conventional root canal therapy—a five year retrospective study, *Int Endod J* 26:321, 1993.

83. Sorensen JA, Engelman MJ: Ferrule design and fracture resistance of endodontically treated teeth, *J Prosthet Dent* 63:529, 1990.

84. Sottosanti J: Calcium sulfate: a biodegradable and biocompatible barrier for guided tissue regeneration, *Compend Contin Educ Dent* 13(3):226, 1992.

85. Southard DW: Immediate core buildup of endodontically treated teeth: the rest of the seal, *Pract Periodontics Aesthet Dent* 11(4):519, 1999.

86. Spear FM: Occlusal considerations for complex restorative therapy. In McNeill C, editor: *Science and practice of occlusion,* Chicago, 1997, Quintessence Publishing Co.

87. Spear FM: When to restore, when to remove: the single debilitated tooth, *Compendium* 20(4):316, 1999.

88. Stabholz A, Friedman S: Endodontic retreatment—case selection and technique. Part 2: treatment planning for retreatment, *J Endod* 14:12, 1988.

89. Stabholz A, Friedman S, Tamse A: Endodontic failures and retreatment. In Cohen S, Burns RC, editors: *Pathways of pulp,* ed 6, St Louis, 1994, Mosby.

90. Stamos DE, Gutmann JL: Survey of endodontic retreatment methods used to remove intraradicular posts, *J Endod* 19:7, 1993.

91. Stropko JJ: Canal morphology of maxillary molars: clinical observations of canal configurations, *J Endod* 25(6):446, 1999.

92. Tamse A, Unger U, Metzger Z, Rosenberg M: Gutta-percha solvents—a comparative study, *J Endod* 12:8, 1986.

93. Torabinejad M, Ung B, Kettering JD: *In vitro* bacterial penetration of coronally unsealed endodontically treated teeth, *J Endod* 16:566, 1990.

94. Torabinejad M, Watson TF, Pitt-Ford TR: The sealing ability of a mineral trioxide aggregate as a retrograde root filling material, *J Endod* 19:591, 1993.

95. van Nieuwenhuysen JP, Aoular M, D'Hoore W: Retreatment or radiographic monitoring in endodontics, *Int Endod J* 27:75, 1994.

96. Vertucci FJ: Root canal morphology of mandibular premolars, *J Am Dent Assoc* 97:47, 1978.

97. Vertucci F, Seelig A, Gillis R: Root canal morphology of human maxillary second premolar, *Oral Surg* 38:456, 1974.

98. Weine FS, Rice RT: Handling previously treated silver point cases: removal, retreatment, and tooth retention, *Compend Contin Educ Dent* 7:9, 1986.

99. Weller RN, Niemczyk SP, Kim S: Incidence and position of the canal isthmus. I. Mesiobuccal root of the maxillary first molar, *J Endod* 21:380, 1995.

100. West JD: The relation between the three-dimensional endodontic seal and endodontic failure, master's thesis, Boston, 1975, Boston University.

101. Wilcox LR: Endodontic retreatment: ultrasonics and chloroform as the final step in reinstrumentation, *J Endod* 15(3):125, 1989.

102. Wilcox LR: Endodontic retreatment with halothane versus chloroform solvent, *J Endod* 21(6):305, 1995.

103. Wilcox LR, Krell KV, Madison S, Rittman B: Endodontic retreatment: evaluation of gutta-percha and sealer removal and canal reinstrumentation, *J Endod* 13:9, 1987.

104. Winter R: Visualizing natural teeth, *J Esthet Dent* 5:3, 1993.

105. Wright WE: Prosthetic management of the periodontally compromised dentition, *J Calif Dent Assoc* 17:9, 1989.

106. Yoshida T, Gomyo S, Itoh T, Shibata T, Sekine I: An experimental study of the removal of cemented dowel-retained cast cores by ultrasonic vibration, *J Endod* 23:4, 1997.

Chapter **26**

Digital Technologies in Endodontic Practice

Martin D. Levin

Chapter Outline

To communicate with patients, assess patient status, evaluate treatment options, and determine treatment outcomes, clinicians depend on images, words, and numerical data. This chapter helps the clinician design office systems that use the latest computer, digital-radiographic, photographic, charting, and management tools to gather and document this vital information.

STRATEGIC PLANNING FOR TECHNOLOGY ACQUISITION

Information technology (IT) systems are changing every day and at an ever-increasing rate. Deciding what equipment to purchase for clinical, front desk, and administrative needs can be daunting. Clinicians should begin by establishing clear goals for the systems they want to implement. Generally, such technology planning can be divided into three areas: (1) strategic, (2) operational, and (3) measurement.

Strategic Plan

The strategic plan should be based on a list of goals for the seamless integration of all the clinical, front desk, and administrative functions in the office. Clinicians should focus on what is necessary to provide the best service to patients and establish clear priorities. The more sophisticated the system, the more customization can take place to provide exactly what patients and clinicians most value (Box 26-1).

The goal may be to create a paperless office, assemble a local area network (LAN) in one office location, or create a wide area network (WAN) connecting several office locations. A priority may be to enhance communication with colleagues or access Internet resources. The strategic plan is the place to list these objectives and set up a schedule for achieving them over a 2-year period or more.

A comprehensive strategic technology plan should address all the information generated and processed in the practice and how it will be handled. The clinician must be prepared to manage information from patients and referring clinicians and to document and communicate all pretreatment, treatment, and posttreatment materials via local storage, mail, fax, e-mail, and the Internet. An ideal system to

Box 26-1   THE VIRTUAL OFFICE: READY NOW

The new paradigm for exceptional patient care calls for sophisticated communication and customization that can be accomplished most efficiently in the integrated digital office. The following steps outline the process, or "patient loop," from introduction of endodontic treatment to the last follow-up visit.

1. The process begins when patients need an endodontic procedure. The endodontic office should make these options available:
   a. Website for patient education and referral materials
   b. "Referral kit" for referring doctors with brochure, map to the office, customized referral forms, and business reply envelopes
   c. Informational meetings with referring clinicians to enhance communications and set expectations
2. When patients call for appointments, the office should be ready to do the following:
   a. Preregister patients using the front desk software
   b. Set up an appointment
   c. Refer patients to the office website where they can fill out the secure patient demographic and medical history data forms
   d. Mail, fax, or e-mail a "welcome kit" with welcome letter, brochure, procedure explanation, map, clinician biography, and fee policy
3. When patients arrive for their initial visits, they can also fill out the personal information sheets on a reception room computer terminal connected to the network, or they can watch educational material while waiting. Any film-based radiographs can be scanned into the patient database. Patient status can be indicated in the endodontic time and patient-tracking module, so every member of the dental team knows the status of all patients from their first visit until they are discharged.
4. When patients are seated in the operatory, an assistant can take a digital radiograph and capture a VL image of any teeth or area in question using an intraoral camera. The assistant then can enter the patient's chief complaint and medical history into the digital chart on the chair side computer workstation. The clinician performs pulp tests and records the endodontic findings in the charting module. Then treatment can commence, with each step of the procedure recorded by voice command or mouse or keyboard input. If desired, patients can be reappointed while still in the operatory, and their insurance information can be sent to the office financial coordinator or directly to their insurance company.
5. Patients are discharged at the front desk departure station with all pertinent information already entered into the computer. This is an opportunity for patients to receive customized information about their treatment, next appointment, follow-up care, and any medications prescribed or dispensed.
6. Patient treatment reports and other correspondence can be created by the front desk staff, reviewed by the clinician at a computer terminal, forwarded to the print queue, and sent by mail, fax, or e-mail. Of course, follow-up notification materials can then be scheduled.
7. When patients return for follow-up visits, digital radiographs can be exposed and comparisons of immediate postoperative and check-up films can be made to assess healing. Reports can then be generated.

accomplish all this has clinical, front desk, and administrative components. Each, in turn, has its own shopping list of equipment.

Clinical Systems   Clinical chair side workstations (Fig. 26-1) contain clinical and other patient information. They can be used to record charting data; store and display digital radiographs, photographic images from microscopes, and intraoral cameras; provide reference information on pharmacology; and even keep patient education-and-entertainment modules for patients to view. A cart-based or built-in system should include a fast multimedia central processing unit (CPU) with plenty of random access memory (RAM). It should have a digital versatile disk (DVD), a large-screen monitor, a keyboard, a pointing device (i.e., touch pad, mouse, digitizing tablet, light pen), speakers, and an uninterruptible power supply (UPS). Additional input devices, such as voice control and visible light (VL) imaging from the microscope and intraoral camera, can be added to the system. Stand-alone systems should have a photo quality printer. Networked systems do not need a printer in the oper-

atory, because a front desk workstation connected to the server can control the printing.

Front Desk Systems   The computer setup at the front desk (Fig. 26-2) is used primarily to process patient accounting and insurance, manage scheduling, and generate patient treatment reports. A well-equipped front desk workstation includes a computer with large-screen monitor, ergonomic keyboard, flatbed scanner with a transparency adapter and optional dedicated film scanner, laser printer, color printer, label printer, and a modem for faxing, and an Internet connection. Additional considerations are setting up the LAN and WAN infrastructure, backup, archiving strategies, and ergonomics (Box 26-2).

Administrative Systems   Basic management functions are handled with an administrative computer (Fig. 26-3). These systems run an array of software programs, such as trend analysis, word processing, marketing, accounting, payroll, and time clock; they also maintain the employee handbook, job descriptions, and OSHA documentation. Adminis-

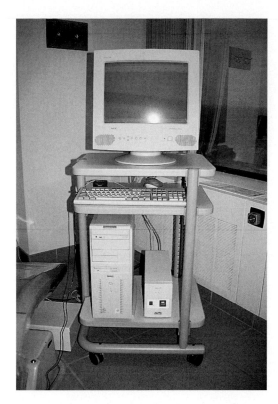

Fig. 26-1 The clinical chair side workstation is the information center for today's dental office.

trative workstations should include adequate RAM, a large-screen, high-quality monitor, ergonomic keyboard, a UPS, and a high capacity black and white laser printer to generate all forms, business cards, and general correspondence. In addition, a sheet-fed scanner should be included. Equipped with a backup tape drive, DVD recordable, or both, this administrative system can also act as the server and workstation in a peer-to-peer network. By connecting the computer to the Internet, the clinician will be able to perform reference searches, order supplies, and get on-line system support. Smaller offices can combine the administrative and front desk computer systems into one workstation.

Operational Plan

The operational strategy covers the planning and day-to-day practices that ensure a smooth-running IT system. Training and cross training of staff are essential elements of a complete plan. To begin with, at least one staff member needs to be knowledgeable in basic computer operations, with special emphasis in word processing. Training courses are available nationwide to teach these basic skills. Books and video self-study materials can augment the classroom training. Of course, purchase of most clinical and front desk software systems should include ample opportunity for training. Once initial training has been accomplished, a second training session, preferably on site, is advisable. Clinicians should try to

schedule this second visit several months after the initial installation. This second visit will allow the clinician and staff to fine-tune the program by customizing certain preferences; it will also ensure that they are taking full advantage of all of the program's features. To get the most out of software, clinicians and staff should periodically reread the training manual that came with the program to discover features and shortcuts that may have been overlooked.

Management of database security is another important aspect of a good operational plan. As with any system open to numerous users, password protection should be established to control access to each level of information. For example, control over deletion of files should be protected to allow only senior staff, the clinician, or both to make changes.

Purchase and continuation of hardware and software maintenance contracts are another area where diligence is important. The clinician should create a procedure for monitoring the status of the maintenance plans for key elements of the IT system, especially digital radiography and front desk software.

Establishing insurance coverage for computer hardware, software, and data also requires special attention. General office insurance policies are limited in computer coverage; therefore clinicians should discuss policies with a knowledgeable insurance agent. To record purchases for insurance purposes, staff should keep a file of purchase documents and digital photographs of the equipment.

Marketing a practice is another place where an IT system can prove invaluable. It is important to upgrade referral and educational materials on an ongoing basis. Clinicians should periodically ask patients and referring clinicians for feedback on the effectiveness of communication materials and act on their suggestions. A proactive approach to these operational issues is the hallmark of an efficient and well-managed office.

Measuring Success

Once various technological systems have been implemented, clinicians should learn how to measure their progress toward achieving goals. For example, if premedication instructions are included in a "welcome kit" sent to new patients or on an Internet "welcome" page, staff should see an improved compliance with those instructions. Enhanced communication with patients and other clinicians should lead to improved satisfaction and increased loyalty.

CLINICAL SYSTEMS

The core function of an endodontic office is to provide the best clinical care for patients, yet most offices today do not have a computer in the operatory! The chair side clinical system is the natural place to begin the most important gathering of data.

In endodontics, clinical systems represent a very broad category that can be divided into two groups: (1) input

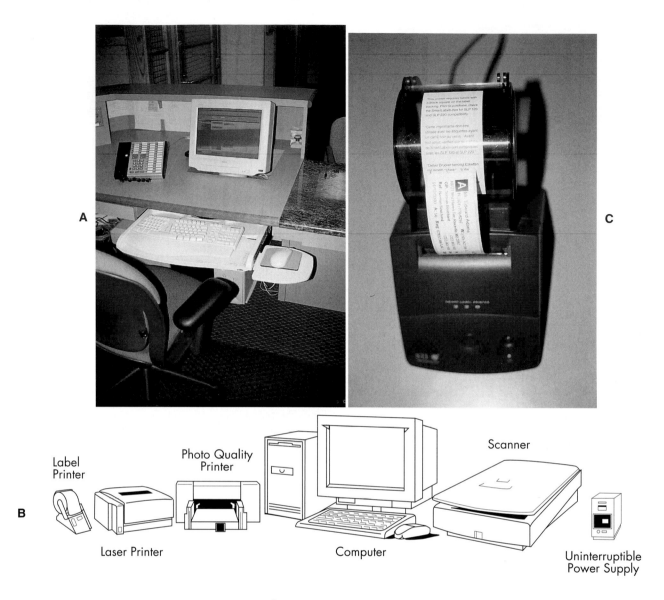

Front Desk Computer System

Fig. 26-2 A and **B**, Typical front desk systems. **C**, A dedicated label printer is useful for mailing labels and maintaining paper charts.

devices and (2) charting software. Input devices can be classified further into radiographic and photographic imaging equipment.

Microscopic Imaging

Medical-grade single-frame digital cameras[28] are available from several manufacturers. Attached to dental microscopes, the cameras (Fig. 26-4) produce high quality VL images. These high-tech cameras provide single frame capture and motion digital video from the operating microscope directly to the computer via the Universal Serial Bus (USB),[38] the FireWire (IEEE 1394, see Box 26-4) port, or a memory card. They also let the clinician preview an image on the camera's

integral display. The cameras attach to the microscope via a beam splitter and camera adapter. Although 35-mm, film-based cameras (Fig. 26-5) will continue to be popular for the highest resolution VL images, digital cameras afford an instant picture with image resolution that can approach that of conventional photography.

Solid-state analog video cameras[29] also can be purchased with an adapter for microscopic videography (Fig. 26-6). These cameras produce analog output (either a *composite* signal or an *S-Video* signal). Composite signals (Box 26-3) in the 280 lines-of-resolution range, usually are less expensive than S-Video models, but they produce images of inadequate resolution. Cameras capable of S-Video output can produce images in the range of 480 lines and are preferred

Box 26-2   HEALTH AND SAFETY FACTORS FOR EMPLOYEES

In the past, concern for worker safety involved primarily avoiding accidental injuries or deaths resulting from hazards in the factory or other industrial environments. With the office as the most common work setting, attention is turning toward subtler but still serious health problems associated with office work—especially cumulative trauma disorders (CTDs) and vision disorders.[36] These disorders are occurring with increasing frequency.

CTDs of the muscles, tendons, or nerves can be caused, by repetitive movements of the body. As the frequency and duration of a repetitive task increases, so does the likelihood of CTD development. Although most CTDs can occur in any part of the body, they most often refer to disorders of the hands, wrists, arms, or shoulders. Carpal tunnel syndrome is one example of a CTD. Typical symptoms of CTDs include pain, swelling, tingling, numbness, or heat around the affected area while both working and resting. These disorders differ from simple fatigue, which disappears after rest. With a CTD, a person may continue to experience symptoms after days or even weeks of inactivity.

Ergonomists often note that computers themselves are not really to blame; repetitive, unvarying work is the cause of most CTD. Individual physiology plays a big part in whether a person develops a CTD. However, experts recognize the importance of workstation design and layout in the prevention of CTDs. For example, work surface height and work process issues (e.g., a company's break policies) affect the incidence of CTDs. For a worker involved in repetitive motion, frequent breaks, even short ones of 30 seconds every 10 minutes, help reduce the probability of developing a CTD. Task variety is also important. Therefore clinicians should design their office duties to allow clerical workers to alternate among different types of work (some of it computer based and some of it non-computer work) or to alternate computing tasks that require different motions and muscle groups.

Front Desk and Administrative Computer Workstations: General Specifications

Work-surface. A desktop height of 28.3 inches (with a keyboard tray below the work surface that places hands and wrists in a wrist neutral position) is a good compromise height for front desk and administrative workstations. Placing a bull nose edge on countertops will help to avoid sharp corners. In addition, the monitor should be placed far enough away from the user to reduce ELF exposure.

Keying. Elbows should position at 90 degrees and arms and hands parallel to the floor to reduce the incidence of CDTs. Using a Microsoft "Natural Keyboard,"[20] wrist rests, locating mouse, and writing platforms within the primary reach zone may also contribute to a more comfortable work environment. Work surface space must allow for efficient organization of documents, papers, and other materials. Try to place peripheral equipment in easy-to-reach locations.

Seating. Seat height should be adjustable to allow for positioning in the range of 16 to 20.5 inches above the floor. Seat depth should be between 15 and 17 inches and have a "waterfall" contour just behind the user's knee and underside of the thigh to avoid excessive pressure in this area. Seat width minimum should be 18.2 inches. Seat pan angle (when user has feet flat on floor) should ensure an angle between the upper and lower leg of between 60 and 100 degrees. Seat pan and pan angle should range from 90 to 105 degrees. A seat back rest and lumbar support should also be provided.

Acoustics and Lighting. Ambient or background noise (i.e., white noise) is desirable at a level that does not interfere with task performance (between 40 and 55 dba).

Lighting sources should be designed and located to minimize glare and provide luminance in the range of 200 to 500 lux on the work area. Task or local lighting may be needed for reading documents. A combination of indirect overhead, natural, and task lighting is preferable. For close-up work, light should be directed sideways onto documents to avoid producing glare on the monitor, which helps prevent eye fatigue and headaches. According to the American Optometric Association, eyestrain is the leading complaint among computer users.[3] It is recommended that users take frequent breaks, have their vision checked, and design the workspace to reduce visual stress.

Setting the monitor's refresh rate to reduce flicker is another way to reduce eyestrain. A higher refresh rate will improve eye comfort. Also, replacing plastic prism coverings with grids that break up the light pattern can reduce fluorescent glare. Choose office color schemes that are neutral and pleasing to the eye.

Ventilation. Proper ventilation requires about two air exchanges per hour—temperature and humidity should be kept constant, with temperature range adjustable from 68° F to 75° F.

for microscopic imaging. They can be connected to video capture cards for incorporation into imaging databases or connected to a video splitter to provide several S-Video outputs. One output can be connected to a computer, a second to an analog monitor, and a third to a videocassette recorder. Even more sophisticated cameras with three charged-coupled devices (CCDs) and *component* outputs are available for the highest-level resolution, but they are not necessary for routine clinical documentation.

Intraoral Cameras

Dental cameras that can photograph a single tooth, a group of teeth, or a patient's full face are now available in analog format, with either a composite or an S-Video output (Fig. 26-7). These cameras are very useful in recording the condition of soft and hard tissues for documentation and patient education. The cameras are available with barrier sheaths to ensure against cross contamination.

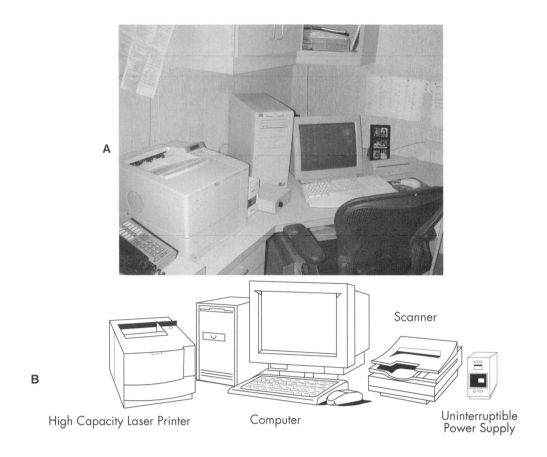

Scanner

High Capacity Laser Printer   Computer   Uninterruptible Power Supply

Administrative Computer System

Fig. 26-3 **A** and **B**, An administrative computer that can be used as an adjunct to the front desk unit.

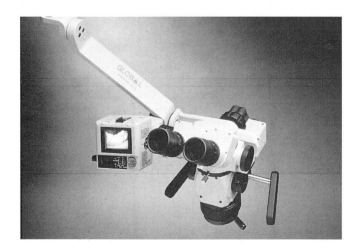

Fig. 26-4 A microscope with a digital camera produces high quality VL images for capture to the clinical chair side workstation. (Courtesy Global Surgical, Inc., St. Louis, Mo.)

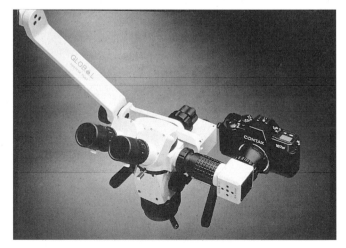

Fig. 26-5 A film-based 35-mm camera attached to a microscope. (Courtesy Global Surgical, Inc., St. Louis, Mo.)

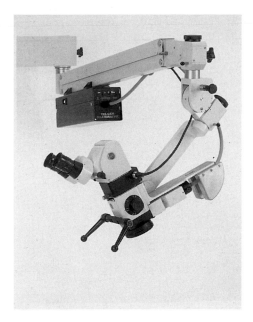

Fig. 26-6 This microscope incorporates a miniature solid-state camera (S-Video format, 480 lines) into the beam splitter. (Courtesy JEDMED Instrument Co., St. Louis, Missouri.)

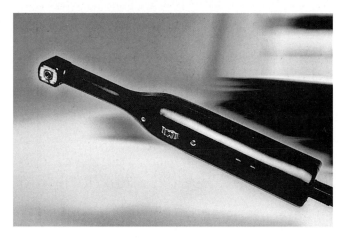

Fig. 26-7 Intraoral cameras, available in composite or S-Video formats, can be wired directly to a capture board in the clinical chair side workstation. (Courtesy Schick Technologies, Inc., Long Island City, New York.)

Box 26-3   A SHORT PRIMER ON VIDEO SIGNALS

It is important to understand the basics of video signal technology to assemble the photographic components of the digital office.

Video cameras generate red, green, and blue (RGB) signals to create video images. If the RGB signals were sent as three separate signals, it would require huge storage and bandwidth capacities. Instead, it is possible to take advantage of the human visual system to reduce storage requirements. This is done by transforming the RGB signals into new video signals that can be band limited with minimal loss of perceived picture quality. In Europe the dominant television standards are PAL and SECAM. The United States has three common NTSC (National Television Standards Committee) signal formats in general use:

Composite video signals (single 75 ohm cable terminated at each end with RCA connectors) mix the red, blue, and green signals together. This architecture is present in almost all contemporary home video equipment; when modulated with audio onto an RF carrier, is used by over-the-air broadcast stations or on coax by cable TV systems. These systems present the lowest quality signals.

S-Video, short for Super-Video (appears as a single cable but internally has two 75 ohm coax or twisted pair cables terminated at each end with a four-pin, DIN connector), is a technology for transmitting video signals over a cable by dividing the video information into two separate signals: one for color (i.e., chrominance) and the other for brightness (i.e., luminance). Professionals refer to this as Y/C video rather than S-Video, because it is more descriptive of the signal format. These systems produce midrange-quality signals.

Component video (analog component video uses three 75 ohm coax cables, terminated at each end with RCA connectors, usually color coded and bundled together) reduces artifacts and color errors by minimizing the number of video signal format conversions between the source and the display device, and it transmits its video signal by dividing the Y, R-Y, and B-Y signals separately. These component video systems produce the highest-quality signals.

In professional and industrial video equipment, impedance-matched, 75 ohm BNC connectors are used for all of these signal formats. Also, each of these analog signal formats can be stored, processed, and transported in the digital domain in professional applications. Digital home satellite systems receive MPEG compressed digital component signals, but they provide only composite and S-Video output. The DVD format, also based on MPEG technology, is available with analog component video for highest possible picture quality.

Computer monitors, on the other hand, are designed for RGB signals. Most digital video devices, such as digital cameras and game machines, produce video in RGB format. The images look best, therefore, when shown on a computer monitor. When seen on a television, however, they look better in S-Video format than in composite format. To use S-Video, the sending and receiving devices and the interconnect cable must be S-Video compatible.

When coupled with professional-grade analog components, this technology can provide high-quality images. Clinicians can integrate the cameras into an office system with analog networks that attach to television monitors, VCR tape decks, and dye-sublimation printers; however, storage of the videotapes and paper prints of screen captures can be cumbersome. A computer-based, direct-capture system is much more efficient and is recommended. When VL images from the intraoral cameras are transmitted directly to a clinical chairside workstation, they can be stored along with radiographic images in the patient database for easy retrieval. This type of camera can be a valuable adjunct to the microscope camera because of its lower cost. Although a microscope can be somewhat difficult for staff to position and use with mirrors, these small and easily positioned intraoral cameras are easy to position.

Fiber-Optic Imaging

Recent introduction of *fiber-optic endoscopes* specifically for use in the oral cavity takes endodontic imaging into the root canal.[5,6] The OraScope[13] (Sitca, Inc., Ann Arbor, MI) consists of a 0.7-mm and 1.8-mm diameter lighted, fiber-optic probe. The 0.7-mm probe can be inserted into the root canal for internal viewing. This scope sends images to a solid-state video camera, a medical-grade video monitor, and digital-image capture device. Other documentation options are a digital video recording system and a standard 35-mm photo camera that can be attached to the proximal end of the scope for very high-resolution images.

Each probe consists of a flexible fiber-optic bundle with fibers that emit light generated by the metal halide light source and others that transmit the image. The digital signal-processing unit filters the image to produce an enhanced, consistent image. Storage and retrieval of images can be accomplished with connection to the clinical chair side workstation. Infection control is provided by placing disposable, optical-grade, plastic sheaths over the distal end of the probe.

Digital Photography

Many practitioners routinely take images of their patients for identification purposes with consumer-grade digital cameras[27] (Fig. 26-8). In addition, intraoral and perioral imaging are valuable documentation tools if the patient presents with skin lesions or swelling. Instant digital photography is relatively inexpensive and can record these images with a high degree of accuracy. Image quality of digital, still cameras is superior to intraoral cameras because of its higher resolution, accurate color values, and no ghosting or distortion. The minimum resolution for acceptable images is 1600×1200 pixels. Although the resolution of digital images is currently inferior to film-based images, digital images do provide important benefits. Advantages include no film to purchase or process, absolute archiveability, instantaneous evaluation of the image, and the ability to catalogue and search the image database. In addition, the clinician can print multiple, high-quality copies in only a few minutes.

Clinicians should choose a camera with "point-and-shoot" controls. They should also select a megapixel camera with flash, macro capabilities (adjustable from about 2 inches to infinity), and a convenient pathway for inputting the image data into the clinical chair side workstation. The industry standard methods of image transfer are direct wiring via the USB port, and use of a small memory card. Most digital radiography and front desk management programs that accept images will store and display these VL files directly in the patient database.

Radiographic Imaging

The three methods of producing digital images are (1) CCD/CMOS sensors,[15] (2) phosphorus plates,[39] and (3) scanning of conventional film. All three systems are available in periapical and panoramic sizes. This digital-radiography equipment uses conventional generation devices to produce x-ray energy. Direct digital radiography and phosphorus plates have many advantages over silver halide film, such as speed, reduced radiation, environmental waste reduction, elimination of darkroom costs, e-mail image transfer,[21] and enhanced practice image.

CMOS-APS sensors technology is literally a camera on a chip (Fig. 26-9). It has a full-digital interface, so no analog signals are generated by the chip. Although CCD systems require many supporting components, such as timing generators and signal-processing chips, CMOS-APS sensors integrate all of these functions onto a single chip. Therefore, any personal computer (PC) with a USB port can accept this sensor without installing a separate processing board. With this being said, Dentsply/Gendex has recently introduced its GX-S USB digital imaging system with a USB interface. Both the Schick and Dentsply/Gendex sensors, when placed in the patient's mouth, detect the onset of x-ray irradiation,

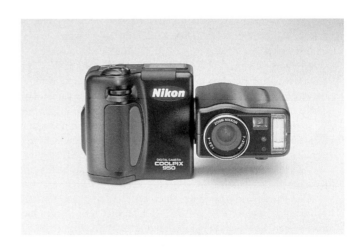

Fig. 26-8 Consumer-grade digital still camera. (Courtesy Nikon, Inc., Melville, N.Y.)

integrate the radiographic image, and initiate the readout of the pixel data.

Storage phosphor plate technology allows these systems to produce radiographic images using a flexible, wireless plate. With the DenOptix system (Dentsply International, Gendex Division, Des Plaines, Ill.) (Fig. 26-10), plates are loaded into a sheath, exposed, mounted in a carousel, and then placed in the scanner. As many as eight images are ready for viewing in about 90 seconds. The plates are available in periapical, panoramic, and cephalometric sizes, and they support a wide range of exposure settings.

For the truly paperless office, a film scanner (Box 26-4) is necessary because it allows input of historic, film-based radiographic images. Two categories of silver halide film scanners exist. The ScanRite (Smith Companies Dental Products, Freemont, Calif.) dedicated film scanner (Fig. 26-11, *A*) provides a single image in about 10 seconds. This high-resolution image can be enhanced and imported into any TWAIN-compliant software (i.e., standard software protocol and applications programming interface that regulates communications between software applications and imaging devices) via the small computer system interface (SCSI) or USB port on the CPU. The TigerView (rdental.com, Los Gatos, Calif.) flatbed scanner (Fig. 26-11, *B*) can accept film sizes ranging from periapical to panoramic to cephalometric, and it uses special software to align and enhance the images.

Flatbed scanners use transparency adapters for film-based images. They also can be used to scan paper documents and append them to the patient's digital chart.

The value of instant digital imaging in the modern dental office, especially for endodontic and implant procedures, is well known. "Several phosphorus and CCD/CMOS digital systems have good to very good image quality, plus ease of use and image enhancement capabilities that make them competitive with conventional film in overall usefulness."[9] However, according to the Clinical Research Associates (CRA), the image quality of digital radiographs still does not measure up to the sharpness and detail of silver halide film.[10] Conventional film provides a finer grade of detail through continuous shades of black-and-white images, rather than discrete shades of gray used by digital systems. Advances are being made though (e.g., digital subtraction radiography,[26] improved resolution), and digital image quality may equal or surpass that of film in the future. As Dunn and Kantor[11] stated in their review of the subject, "digital imaging has many potential benefits yet to be fully explored or demonstrated."

Resolution   One of the most critical and misunderstood issues concerning digital representation of image data is resolution. Although computer screen selection, ambient lighting, and image compression all affect resolution, the most compelling issue is the *image quality of dental structures as viewed by the clinician*. According to a study by CRA[9] on dental-imaging quality, some currently available systems were ranked using a scale of 1 to 10. Film ranked highest at 8.7. The second highest ranking was a film scanner that achieved an image quality score of 7.0 (but is dependent on the quality of the original film-based image). The digital

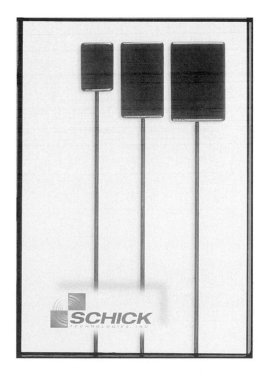

Fig. 26-9 CMOS-APS sensors technology is literally a camera on a chip that connect to the PC via the USB port, thereby eliminating a processing board. (Courtesy Schick Technologies, Inc., Long Island City, N.Y.)

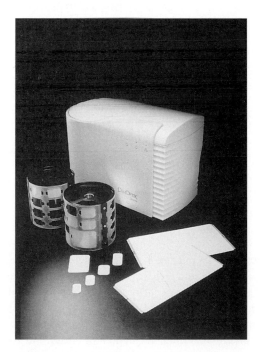

Fig. 26-10 The DenOptix system of storage phosphor plate technology. (Courtesy Dentsply International, Gendex Division, Des Plaines, Ill.)

Box 26-4   DENTAL FILM SCANNING

A scanner can be used as a complement or an alternative to a sensor- or phosphor-based, digital radiography system. Scanned film images can either be saved in digital-radiography system software, patient management software, or imaging software (e.g., Windows 98 operating software).

Complimentary System
To compliment a sensor- or phosphor-based digital radiography system, it is important that both the scanner and the system software be TWAIN compliant. Being TWAIN compliant allows images to be scanned directly into the digital patient file or exam. Some system software will even automatically name the file to simplify the process to a two-click procedure.

Alternative System
Scanners are used as an alternative to sensor- or phosphor-based digital radiography system because the investment cost is less and, in some cases, the image quality is better. If the office is networked or wired for monitors in the operatories, the image can be scanned at any location and shown on any computer linked to the network.

Two major classes of scanners are of interest to the dental practitioner: (1) the relatively inexpensive *flatbed scanner* configuration and (2) the more expensive *dedicated film scanner*.

Flatbed scanners. Certain models of flatbed scanners offer a *transparency adapter* to allow the scanning of radiographic film. Flatbed scanners are typically best used for documents, photographs, panoramic films, and cephalometric films. Flatbed scanners are usually slow to preview, slow to scan, and their image quality and resolution are inferior to film scanners.

Film scanners. Film scanners are typically best used for 35-mm slides, 35-mm film, and periapical/bitewing radiographs. ScanRite Systems makes a fast, high-quality film scanner specifically for periapical and bitewing films, mounted 35-mm color slides, and 35-mm color film.

The primary considerations when choosing a scanner for dental film include resolution, levels of gray scanned, speed, software, and convenience. Scanner resolution is typically quantified using dots per inch (dpi). Quantification of sensor-based digital radiography is typically specified in line pairs per millimeter (506 dpi is equal to 10 line pairs per millimeter). Higher resolutions result in better clarity when images are enlarged. *Optical resolution* describes the capability of the hardware. *Interpolated resolution* is the ability of the scanner software to place additional dots among the data scanned. This process can artificially improve the image quality. Additionally, image quality can be adversely affected by "noise" during image processing of either a scanned or direct digital image.

The levels of gray or number of colors scanned is important because each scanned dot is assigned a "color." The more grays or colors scanned will improve the image quality. Fewer grays or colors result in "blotchy" images. This can be demonstrated by adjusting the computer monitor settings to a low color palette or depth while viewing a digital image.

The scanning speed is dependent on many factors. Better scanners have built-in buffer memory so the data does not have to be sent in multiple "bursts" to the computer. Better scanners will scan in one pass without stopping and also have a Small System Computer Interface (SSCI)[33] or FireWire (a data transfer protocol and interconnection system, standardized by the Institute of Electrical and Electronic Engineers as IEEE 1394)[1] connection to maximize the speed of the data transfer from the scanner to the computer. Scanning speed also depends on the resolution selected, the physical size of the original, whether color or grayscale, the speed of the microprocessor, and the amount of RAM in the computer.

The better scanners will save the user time by automatically optimizing the brightness, contrast, and color for each scanned image. Most scanner software includes the ability to preview an image before saving it to disk. An important feature is that the preview image is large and clear. Low-cost scanners will typically have a small preview image shown at a very low resolution. This small preview image makes it difficult to accurately make image enhancements. Most scanners will allow changing of the brightness, contrast, and exposure before saving to disk. Better scanners will include the capability to change the color, select film calibrations, sharpen the image, rotate the image, scale the output, match the output (i.e., gamma level) to other software applications, invert colors or grayscale levels, and save settings for various types of originals.

---

radiography systems ranked slightly lower for image quality in dental applications, with a high score of 6.5 (Table 26-1).

The quality of many film-based images, on the other hand, is compromised by operational problems, such as chemical and film freshness, developing inconsistencies, light leaks, and shipment handling. Detection of gross and moderate caries can be performed with both conventional film and digital-imaging systems with a great degree of surety. For incipient caries detection, film sharpness and detail can still be

helpful adjuncts to digital systems. Unfortunately, the presence of caries is always more extensive than depicted by either digital or film systems. Incipient caries and some periapical lesions continue to present a challenge for both film- and digital-based systems.

In the detection of periapical bone lesions created in cortical-and-trabecular bone, no difference was detected by Paurazas et al[30] between E-speed film (Kodak, Rochester, N.Y.), CCD, and CMOS sensors. Furthermore, "cortical

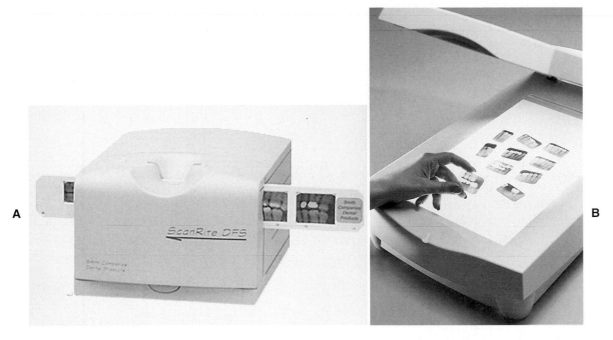

Fig. 26-11 The two categories of silver halide film scanners. **A**, The ScanRite Dental Film Scanner. **B**, The TigerView flatbed scanner. (*A*, Courtesy ScanRite Systems, Fremont, Calif.; *B*, Courtesy rdental.com, Los Gatos, Calif.)

bone lesions were detected with significantly higher accuracy once the junction of the cortical plate was involved or perforated."[30]

Radiation   Digital imaging generally requires less radiation than film-based systems. According to the CRA Newsletter, CCD/CMOS sensors can reduce exposure by up to 82%. Phosphorous plates reduce radiation by up to 22%, compared with conventional film.[9] Foroughi et al noted reduced radiation averaging 55% when compared with Kodak D speed film and an average of 45% reduction when compared with E speed film.[14] However, recently introduced Kodak F Speed film requires less radiation than E speed along with improved image quality; this will continue to make film-based products competitive. Film scanning provides no reduction in radiation because a conventional film image must first be produced.

Time to Image and Time to Retake   Conventional film and phosphorous plates take at least a minute to process after the film is transported to the developing site and unwrapped, whereas CCD/CID/CMOS sensors are virtually instant, with "paint times" usually completed in just a few seconds. If the image is unsatisfactory or a second view is required, this image can be generated using the direct digital sensor by simply repositioning the tube head and/or sensor and exposing another image. Phosphor plates and films require considerably more time to produce the first image; time to retake is thereby increased, with less assurance that the second image

will be at the desired angle. This improved workflow pattern using CCD/CMOS sensors will enhance efficiency and reduce patient waiting time for images and, if necessary, retakes. Dedicated film scanners generally take 10 seconds to process a developed film.

Optimization   All digital radiographic systems allow for image optimization (Fig. 26-12). Optimizing digital radiographs and VL images is relatively easy using currently available software. Most feature the ability to change contrast and brightness to view images that are underexposed or overexposed, create an inverse image, equalize density, magnify, and allow for image rotation and mirror imaging. Image annotation is another advantage of digital radiography. Some programs allow creation of "markers" or notes that will place descriptive annotation with numbered pointers to call attention to specific details in the image. Algorithms that can sharpen and enhance caries are also present in a number of systems, holding promise for even more future improvements. Another enhancement, pseudo coloring, ascribes false colors based on brightness of pixels and can help with patient visualization of images.

Measurement   Three types of measurement available with digital images are (1) linear measurement, which allows the practitioner to measure the distance between two points in millimeters; (2) angle measurement, which measures the angle between two lines; and (3) area measurement, which measures the area of the image or a segment of the image.

Table 26-1   How Do Current Digital Systems Compare with Each Other?

Brand (Listed by type & overall ranking within method)	A-Image Quality	B-Software Ease of Use	C-Correct Orientation as Image First Appears on Screen	D-Ease of Sensor Transfer Between Ops	E-Ease of Sensor Size Change	F-Delay Between Exposure & Image	G-Number of Sensor Sites	H-Panoramic Capability	I-Active Area Size (#2 sensor or only sensor)	J-Sensor Comfort	K-Has 3 Most Used Features •	L-Warranty	Overall ranking*
Conventional film	8.7	N/A	No	N/A	E	P	5 intraoral 3 extraoral	Yes	1271 mm²	F	N/A	N/A	G-E
Scanners													
TigerView	7.0	E	No	N/A	E	P	Same as film	Yes	1271 mm²	F	Yes	30 day return	G
ScanRite DFS	6.5	G	No	N/A	E	P	Same as film	Yes	1080 mm²	F	No	1 year parts & labor	F-G
Phosphorus													
Denoptix	6.5	E	No	E	E	F	9 sizes	Yes	1240 mm²	G	Yes	2 year parts & labor	G-E
Digora	3.0	E	No	E	E	F-G	2 sizes	No	1131 mm²	F	Yes	1 year parts & labor	F-E
CCD/CMOS													
CDR	6.2	G-E	Yes	G-E	G	E	3 sizes	Yes	875 mm²	G	Yes	1 year parts & labor	G-E
Dexis	5.3	E	Yes	G-E	N/A	E	1 size	Yes	800 mm²	E	Yes	1 year parts & labor	G-E
GX-S	4.0	E	No	G-E	N/A	E	1 size	Yes	600 mm²	E	Yes	2 year	G
QuickRay DSX 730	5.3	E	Yes	G-E	N/A	E	1 size	No	693 mm²	G	Yes	1 year parts & labor	G
RVGui	4.0	G-E	No	G	F-G	E	2 sizes	Yes	927 mm²	F	Yes	2 year sensor	G
Sens-A-Ray 2000	5.2	G-E	Yes	F	F	E	2 sizes	No	621 mm²	G	Yes	2 year parts & labor	G

• 3 most used features indicated by survey of owners:

(1) Magnification

(2) Contrast

(3) Measurement

*Overall ranking determined by averaging scores across columns, A, B, C, D, E, F, G, H, I, J, & K

Image Quality graded on 1-10 scale, 10 = Best

E, Excellent = 4; G, good = 3; F, fair = 2; P, poor = 1; Yes = 4, No = 1

Number of sensor sizes graded as follows: 1 = Fair, 2-3 = Good, 4 or more = Excellent

(Modified from CRA Newsletter, September 1999, Page 4.)

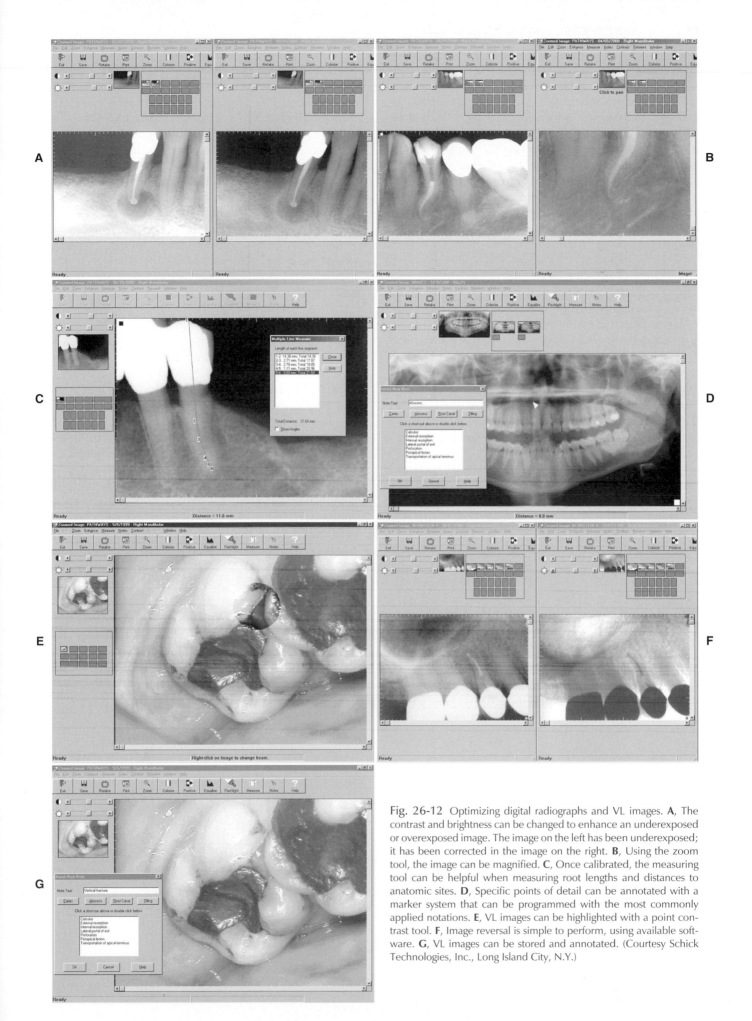

Fig. 26-12 Optimizing digital radiographs and VL images. **A**, The contrast and brightness can be changed to enhance an underexposed or overexposed image. The image on the left has been underexposed; it has been corrected in the image on the right. **B**, Using the zoom tool, the image can be magnified. **C**, Once calibrated, the measuring tool can be helpful when measuring root lengths and distances to anatomic sites. **D**, Specific points of detail can be annotated with a marker system that can be programmed with the most commonly applied notations. **E**, VL images can be highlighted with a point contrast tool. **F**, Image reversal is simple to perform, using available software. **G**, VL images can be stored and annotated. (Courtesy Schick Technologies, Inc., Long Island City, N.Y.)

Because magnification and distortion error play a significant role in all radiographic measurement accuracy, both film and digital systems are subject to error. A recent study by Eikenberg and Vandre demonstrated that "measurement error was significantly less for the digital images than the film-based images"[12] when comparing file length images of human skulls taken with a custom jig. However, the authors point out that in clinical situations these measurement differences may not be clinically significant. Sophisticated calibration algorithms are under development, so accurate measurement of parallel images should be more feasible in the future.[7]

Security   Although film-based images can easily be produced in duplicate, each subsequent rendition of the image will be reduced in quality. Digital images, on the other hand, can be reproduced in unlimited quantity because the images are stored and produced without loss of any detail. Furthermore, digital images can be stored on *and* off-site and on many types of media, thereby helping to mitigate loss from theft, fire, or other causes.

Paradoxically, the ease of reproduction and storage of digital images allows for the alteration of radiographs without a trace.[39] The ease of producing an altered image is controversial, but improved safeguards are under development.[32] Archiving radiographic images in the form of CD, DVD, and other writable formats is one of the current solutions to this issue. These optical media can be stored off site by a third-party archivist for extra protection. When sent through the Internet, this data is also vulnerable. The two technologies available today to encrypt this data, either Secure Socket Layer (SSL)[38] or digital certificates, can provide at least 128-bit encryption and virtually eliminate the chance of alteration or fraud. SSL connections to Internet servers can be recognized by the prefix "https://" in the address line.

Markers   Occasionally, radiographs and VL images warrant a tag so that the operator can return to them later to assemble teaching or patient education materials. Most software today allows markers to be placed so that a computer search can call up the images efficiently. These customized tags can be useful in organizing cases that require special follow-up to evaluate postoperative healing. In addition, readily available software enables the clinician to create notes and diagrammatic annotation of important features of an image (Fig. 26-13).

Computer Interface   Although each of the intraoral direct digital-radiography systems requires connection to the computer, at this time only the CDR Schick Technologies, Inc. ((Long Island City, N.Y.) system connects directly to the USB port of the clinical chair side workstation, thereby eliminating the processing board and simplifying installation and maintenance. Laptop configurations (Fig. 26-14) add flexibility if the practitioner wants to move the equipment between different operatories and office locations or use it for off-site procedures at hospitals and nursing homes. They also benefit from the elimination of special cards for sensor connection. Although the screens on most laptops allow somewhat limited viewing angles, they can be connected to large, high-resolution, cathode ray tube (CRT) monitors. System backup strategies are particularly impor-

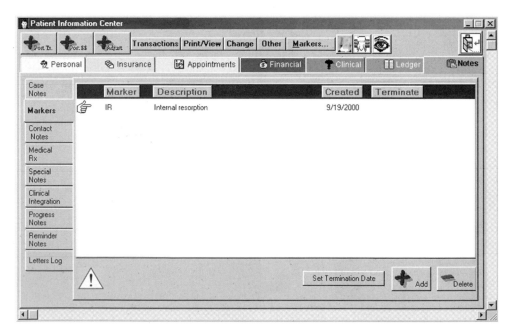

Fig. 26-13 Searchable "markers" or notes. (Courtesy Discus Dental Software, Culver City, Calif.)

tant for laptops because of the increased risk of theft or being dropped.

Charting

Good record keeping in a dental practice is critical. Electronic charting does everything paper systems do and much more. Presently, there are numerous systems available for endodontists, including (1) The Digital Office for Endodontists (PERF, San Diego, Calif.), (2) EndoVision 2000 (Discus Dental Software, Culver City, Calif.), and EndoChart (PBS Endo, ProBusiness Systems, Cedar Park, Tex). A discussion of the charting module of EndoVision 2000 (endorsed by the American Association of Endodontists [AAE]) will reveal how software can automate record keeping.

Basically, electronic charting serves two purposes: (1) it accurately records diagnostics and treatment data for individual patients, and (2) it indicates trends by analyzing and reporting from the patient's records based on user-defined queries.

An electronic charting system includes the following:

- Integration with the general practice management software
- Extensive trend analysis and reporting
- Voice integration (i.e., the ability of the computer to understand natural speech and record findings)
- Comprehensive, easy-to-use interface (includes user programmable "required fields" so that certain information, such as a diagnosis, must be inserted in the patient record before the software will allow the user to save and exit)
- Macro automation (i.e., ability of the program to automate common functions by playing back a series of recorded actions)
- Scanner integration, allowing the user to scan in supporting documents, radiographs, and other paper records

Tabbed pages prompt the user through a logical diagnostic and treatment sequence that include eight steps:

1. General demographic and health information (patient demographics and medical history)
2. Chief complaint and history of present illness
   a. Chief complaint (notes field to record, in the patient's words, what inspired the trip to the office)
   b. History of present illness (notes field to record the history of the current illness in the patient's words)
3. Examination—clinical (describes findings by tooth numbers with user-defined criteria)
4. Examination—radiographic (includes radiographic analysis [essential because analyzing the radiographic findings will be important when measuring treatment outcomes])
5. Etiology—user-defined list of causative factors
6. Diagnosis and treatment plan
7. Treatment notes—based on user-defined criteria and including information about
   a. File-lengths
   b. Type of injection and type and amount of anesthesia medication
   c. Tooth number
   d. Rubber dam clamp
   e. Number and names of canals
   f. Trial length and actual length
   g. Reference point
   h. Instrumentation technique, irrigants
   i. Final instrument each visit
   j. Post space
   k. Obturation material and technique, including cement
   l. Prescribed medications (may include over-the-counter drugs)
   m. Temporization method and materials
8. Postoperative and recall notes and data to send postoperative reports and contact log (notes and data entered to compare results with previous findings)

Integration of Third-Party Products

Digital radiography and VL imaging products are very important to the modern endodontic practice, especially if the goal is to create a paperless environment. Several software packages specific to dentistry are available that can acquire, store, annotate, manipulate, and output images of many types. Comprehensive packages, such as ViperSoft (Integra Medical, Camarillo, Calif.) and TigerView (rdental. com, Los Gatos, Calif.) work with analog and digital still and video cameras, scanners, and digital-radiography programs. Once the image is acquired, these sophisticated software programs allow the clinician to label and annotate the images and even simulate the repair and restoration of teeth (i.e., cosmetic imaging). As operatory-based computers become the norm, dental imaging systems are becoming mainstream.

Imaging software can be an invaluable aid in cataloging images for easy retrieval, case presentation to other dentists and patients, and analysis and magnification of images for improved diagnosis. Sophisticated practice management

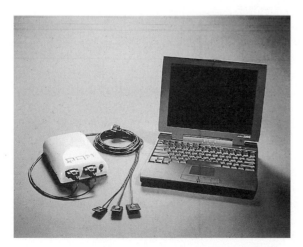

Fig. 26-14 Laptop computers add flexibility to the digital-radiography system, especially if the clinician works at several office sites or remote locations. (Courtesy DMD Systems, Westlake Village, Calif.)

software integrates intimately with these systems, extending the functionality of the office software and creating a complete patient record.

FRONT DESK SYSTEMS

Practice management software for an endodontist has some of the same features as software for the generalist. In addition, there are several key requirements for a specialty market, especially endodontics. Considerations of hardware and networking, as well as product features (e.g., scheduling, referral tracking, preregistration, advanced reporting and analysis) have poor analogues in general practice management software and necessitate the selection of a product written specifically for the endodontic specialist. Another important factor in the selection of software is the recent consolidation trends in the dental software industry.[17] Careful investigation of software companies should include a look at the parent companies to predict which ones will survive in the future.

Great software, like a great building, is constructed on a solid foundation. Although there are many techniques to build software, some are superior. The 1990s saw the delivery of incredible power to the desktop. We now have client/server models that eclipse all others. Put simply, it features a powerful database engine run on a central computer (i.e., a dedicated file server) that controls access to data requested by client workstations. The standard in databases for this model is Structured Query Language (SQL),[16] delivering data more rapidly than any other database system; it does so with far greater efficiency, safety, and simplicity.

Client/server systems result in less network traffic and greater performance because, unlike other systems that move data back and forth between the network server and client workstations, virtually all data manipulation in a SQL system is done at the server. This also decreases the chance that data will become corrupt, because data never leaves the server and the SQL engine actively controls access to the data. In previous models, each client workstation read data from the server, manipulated it, then wrote it back. Because no client was aware of the activity of any other client and the network operated more or less like an independent system, two or more workstations writing data to the server at the same moment was commonplace. In addition, older models look at data one row at a time. However, SQL engines grab chunks of data in response to queries issued by the client and send these *result sets* in their entirety to the client. The resulting performance increases in terms of speed are significant, especially to remote offices.

One would imagine, then, that all of today's systems would use the client/server model. Virtually the opposite is true. Almost none of the systems used by medium and large businesses, hospitals, universities, government and military agencies, and few of the small-business systems used by dentists, physicians, lawyers, accountants, and other profes- sionals employ this advanced, standard technology. In contrast, EndoVision 2000 is a true 32-bit client/server product with an SQL database.

Computer Industry Standards

Open Database Connectivity (ODBC)   One of the classic problems in the computer industry is that each vendor stores and manipulates its data differently. The result is that you can only read your data using tools created by the same company. To "fix" this problem, Microsoft introduced Open Database Connectivity (ODBC). With ODBC in place, software programs connecting to databases first connect to ODBC (another software product called a *driver*) and ODBC connects to the database. This makes ODBC (and other derivative standards like JDBC and OLE DB[22]) a translator (of sorts) between software programs and databases. The "magic" of ODBC is that developers of software can plug into different databases without changing their program codes. In addition, ODBC-compliant databases are accessible from many programs.

How does this help clinicians? Because of ODBC, clinicians can read and analyze the database from spreadsheet programs, report writers, graphics programs, and other database programs. In today's open-standards world, *it is unwise to purchase any product that is not ODBC compliant.* Unfortunately, most databases and programs in dentistry are not fully compliant at this time.

Digital Imaging and Communications in Medicine (DICOM)   Although the aforementioned standards are important from a global IT standpoint, dental-imaging programs need specific standards so that they can interact with programs in the clinician's Enterprise Information System (EIS) and with systems outside each dental office. The first such standard, Digital Imaging and Communications in Medicine (DICOM), established in 1985 by the American College of Radiology (ACR) and the National Electrical Manufacturers Association[31](NEMA), addressed the issue of vendor-independent data formats and data transfers for digital medical images.[2] This industry standard for transferal of radiographic images and other medical information among computers enables digital communication between systems from various manufacturers (e.g., Dexis, Gendex, and Schick) and across different platforms (e.g., Macintosh, Windows). The DICOM standard provides for several hundred attribute fields in the record header, which contains information about the image (e.g., pixel density, dimensions, number of bits per pixel) and relevant patient data and medical history. Although earlier versions did not specify the exact order and definition of the header fields, each vendor is now required to publish a DICOM conformance statement, which gives the location of pertinent data. The DICOM standard will also support a form of SSL (see section on "Security" earlier in this chapter) for the transmission of digital images. The big hurdle is to support a common language that permits medical and dental consultations between two or more locations with different imaging software. Another benefit of DICOM conformance is the freedom to change vendors and maintain database continuity.

Although most of the software vendors are striving to achieve full DICOM compliance, some vendors have at least achieved partial compliance. In the future, advances will continue to be made in medical and dental imaging and charting, yielding obvious benefits in system communication. Based on the DICOM international standard, the ADA Standards Committee on Dental Informatics has recently identified four basic goals for electronic standards in dentistry: (1) interoperability, (2) electronic health record design, (3) clinical workstation architecture, and (4) electronic dissemination of dental information.[2] DICOM is an example of an interoperability standard.

Systematized Nomenclature of Dentistry (SNODENT)

SNODENT is an ADA-sponsored,[35] comprehensive set of standardized terms for defining dental disease in an electronic environment. SNODENT is part of a larger code set called Systematized Nomenclature of Medicine (SNOMED),[19] that was developed by the College of American Pathologists. The codes will allow dentists to document a wide range of conditions and risk factors using standard terms to aid communication among dental and medical practitioners. In addition, SNODENT will allow dentists and researchers to better assess the long-term benefits of certain treatment modalities by standardizing the measurement of outcomes and the documentation of evidence-based care.[25]

Graphics and Imaging

For most dental practitioners this is a confusing area. Windows has many graphics standards, and it has been difficult to sort out which ones to use; however, this is beginning to change. Although some dental imaging software stores graphics data in nonstandard ways, most products are beginning to support computer industry norms. It is less important that clinicians understand the peculiarities of the different graphics storage categories than which ones to look for in a program. The importance of standards is simply that if the graphics are stored in a standard manner, clinicians will be able to manipulate the image and drop it directly into the dental software.

Following are the most common image formats:
- Bitmap (BMP). This is the Microsoft standard for Windows. It is used and understood by almost all imaging software and is the format of most pictures delivered with a Windows computer. Its strengths are universal distribution and very high quality. Its chief weakness is that the files it creates are not compressed, and they will cause the hard drive to get filled-up quickly.
- Joint Photographic Experts Group (JPEG or JPG). This is probably the most popular standard for personal com-

puters (PCs) and the Internet. It has good quality and supports compressed formats (allowing for smaller files).
- Tagged Image File Format (TIFF or TIF). This is also a very popular standard. The images are usually very high quality and typically support minimal compression.
- Graphic Interchange Format (GIF). This is a very compressed format that is most popular on the Internet and on-line services but not helpful in storing digital images.

Single Locations—Local-Area Networking

LANs enable the sharing of data and network-attached devices to improve workflow efficiency. The simplest form of LAN is the peer-to-peer model. Connected by a hub and simple wiring, two or more computers can network to share resources and data (Fig. 26-15). The drawbacks of this type of system are the limited number of workstations that can be adequately supported and the necessity to restart the entire system if a program fault occurs. A much more robust solution requires a dedicated server connected with cabling to each workstation via a central hub (Fig. 26-16). The utility of a network cannot be underestimated. For example, a central repository of digital radiographs will allow clinical chairside workstations in each operatory to call up all patient images so that a patient does not have to be in the same operatory for each subsequent visit. A server-based LAN has several additional advantages. In addition to greater reliability and faster overall speed, server-based LANs allow individual stations to be rebooted without restarting the entire system, secludes the server in a safe location, and supports a large number of workstations at one or multiple sites.

Multiple Locations—Wide-Area Networking

The efficiency of the client/server model also allows practices with multiple facilities to set up high-speed communications between those locations, keeping the database on a single server. Client/server-based systems allow the practice to provide a virtual separation of the data into two or more locations. Typically, this is accomplished by leasing a full T1 phone line from a local telephone company. T1 moves data between the server and the remote clients at speeds up to 1.5 megabits per second. Competing technologies, especially Digital Subscriber Line (DSL), are becoming more prominent. DSL currently has the advantage of delivering performance equal to T1 at an increasingly lower cost. In the near future, DSL promises to deliver performance equal to that achieved on a local-area network. DSL signals travel over existing copper phone cable, obviating the need for communications companies to lay new cable. This means that the entire country—and most of the world—is already wired. Unfortunately, the disadvantage of using copper cable is that copper pushed at high speeds builds up a great deal of resistance. In fact, after three miles, the quality of DSL degrades to the point of not being useful. Therefore only customers within 3 miles of the local telephone company switch are

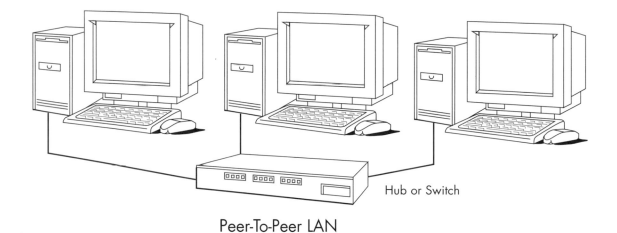

Peer-To-Peer LAN

Fig. 26-15 A peer-to-peer LAN supports only a limited number of work stations and must be entirely restarted if a program fault occurs.

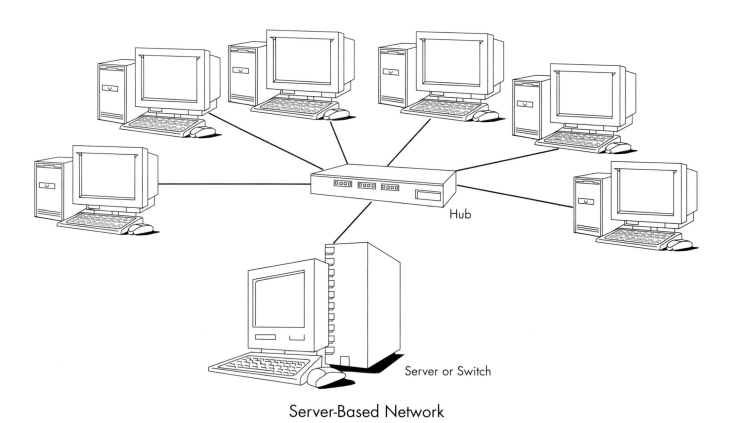

Server-Based Network

Fig. 26-16 A server-based LAN can support a large number of work stations; individual stations can be rebooted without restarting the entire system.

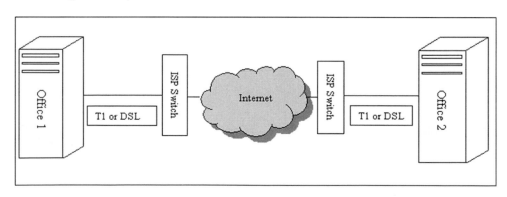

Fig. 26-17 VPNs use wide-bandwidth technology to connect two or more office locations.

able to use DSL. However, the bright side of the picture is that the research to overcome this barrier is so intense that communications companies see this as their "holy grail."

Virtual Private Networks

For very long distances, neither T1 nor DSL alone is practical or affordable. Rather, a Virtual Private Network (VPN)[18] (Fig. 26-17), used in conjunction with T1 or DSL and the internet, is the solution. VPNs use encryption technology to connect two or more office locations. "Firewalls" need to be installed at each location to guard against unwanted "hacking." Unfortunately, DSL service is limited to offices located within a set distance from the local telephone switching center (see previous section on DSL).

VPNs use the Internet as their long-distance backbone. Essentially the process looks like this:
- Each office gets a short-range T1 or DSL line to an Internet Service Provider (ISP).
- The ISP passes the signal through the Internet to another ISP switch that is connected (via T1 or DSL) to the second office. VPNs are private because the signal that passes through the Internet is encrypted to prevent others from intercepting and reading the traffic.

As VPNs become more commonplace, you will hear more about Transmission Control Protocol/Internet Protocol (TCP/IP)[34] (often simply referred to as *IP*). IP is the language of the Internet and is used in networks of almost any size. Each computer on the Internet has a unique IP address. When using the Internet browser, an operator types in a web address, and the browser translates that into that site's IP address. A WAN, whether using a VPN or not, uses IP to connect all the computers in the network. Because each computer server has a unique address known by the workstations, traffic can flow freely between them. Although other communications protocols exist (e.g., Netbeui, IPX/SPX), IP is the clear standard, especially in the client/server world.

Routers are another piece of the multioffice connection puzzle. They do for WANs what modems do for dial-up services (i.e., they convert computer signals into telephone signals and vice-versa). Routers connect networks together. In the multiple-office model discussed earlier, routers sit in each office, connected to the server with a network cable and to the outside world with a link to the T1 or DSL cable.

Citrix and Windows Terminal Server

Just a few years ago all networking was wide area, combining mainframe-like servers at one location with remote dumb terminals at other locations. The difference between these systems and the current technology is that the old networks are just receiving-and-transmitting stations and are capable of only displaying text. But the advantage of these systems is that they are highly efficient. Because there is only one central computer, no data moves through the network; only

screens and key clicks move between server and terminal. These systems require only low-speed, inexpensive data lines. In fact, most Internet servers run on a UNIX platform.

By comparison, Windows-based networks are highly inefficient. *Because everything in Windows is an image, all workstations are computers; real data are moving across the network, and higher performance communications lines are required to carry the signals.* A company called Citrix has provided the closest approximation (in the Windows world) of the mainframe model of computing. Citrix software (known by names such as WinFrame, MetaFrame, and Windows Terminal Services) keeps all data and programs on a single server. In other words, the client workstations, PCs in most cases, are *not* running any software; they are simply sending and receiving Windows screens and transmitting keyboard and mouse activity. Because a great deal less data is moving around the network, Citrix systems can perform well with much lower-speed communications lines.

No matter which WAN model clinicians choose, the client/server, SQL-based system is preferred, because very little real data travel on the network. This is vastly different from other software systems, which transmit data to the workstation for change and then transmit the data back for storage. In these nonclient/server systems, the server is simply a passive storage system. Client/server systems feature a dynamic, active server that controls access. This can be likened to a busy intersection. In a client/server system, traffic lights and police officers (i.e., the SQL database engine) control access. In a nonclient/server system no such controls exist, so each car (i.e., workstation) entering the intersection makes its own decisions as to when to stop and when to go; this makes collisions and accidents (i.e., corrupted data) more common.

Fat- and Thin-Client Computing and the Internet

Software written for PCs and Windows often is referred to as a fat-client model. This unattractive label signifies that software written for the PC must be installed and run separately from each client computer; only the database is centralized. Each fat-client model has to be a powerful PC with the software individually installed. Because data need to travel to and from the client, the bandwidth of the communications channel needs to be significant. *Bandwidth* is a term used to specify the speed of a communications channel. For example, T1 is considered *wide* bandwidth because it can transmit at 1.5 megabits per second. A 56 k modem connection is *narrow* bandwidth because it can only transmit at speeds up to 56 kilobits per second. Specialists in communications often refer to bandwidth as "the size of the pipe."

The other disadvantage of the fat-client model is that it is very expensive for businesses to maintain. For example, imagine for a moment a large law office with 200 desktop computers all running the same software. If the company

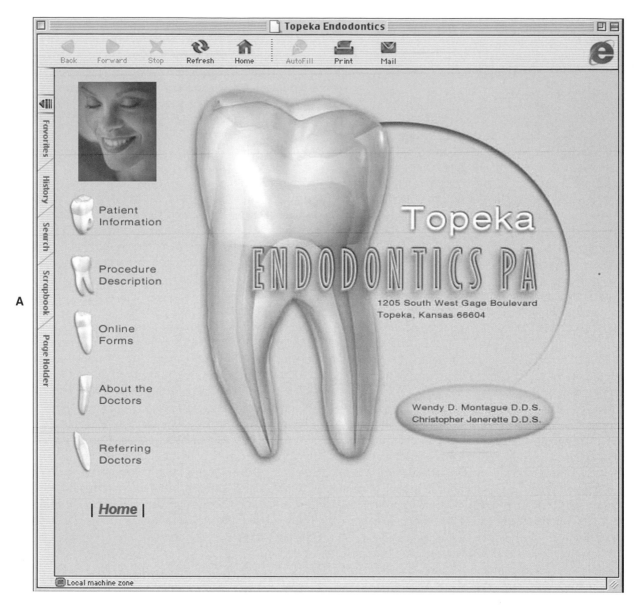

Fig. 26-18 The Internet has proven to be the most important communication tool of the new century. **A,** The main index page of "Topeka Endodontics, P.A.," a fictitious endodontic office, demonstrates the esthetic possibilities of a professionally designed site.   *Continued*

making the law office's software released an update, the practice would have to install the update separately on each workstation. In addition, each of those 200 workstations would have to be powerful PCs that would carry their own maintenance headaches.

The thin-client model is simpler. It is, incidentally, not a new model. UNIX and many mainframe networks have always been *thin*. In fact, the fat-client model is a side effect of the PC age. The Internet, the ultimate thin-client network, has become so pervasive that thin-client computing has again become the preferred model. Within the next few years, developers of software for dental practitioners will probably reengineer their software and hardware to run on the Internet as a thin-client solution, with imaging, charting, and patient demographic data stored and archived remotely.

The Internet, however, represents a great deal more to clinicians than just a different place to run office software. Functionality never available before will become commonplace in a world where everyone is connected on one vast network. The remarkable innovations, to name just a few are:

1. Multiprovider networks. Clinicians will be part of multiprovider networks that can send patient records and images between colleagues in a secure area on the Internet.
2. On-line scheduling. Patients will have limited use of a clinician's schedule on-line.

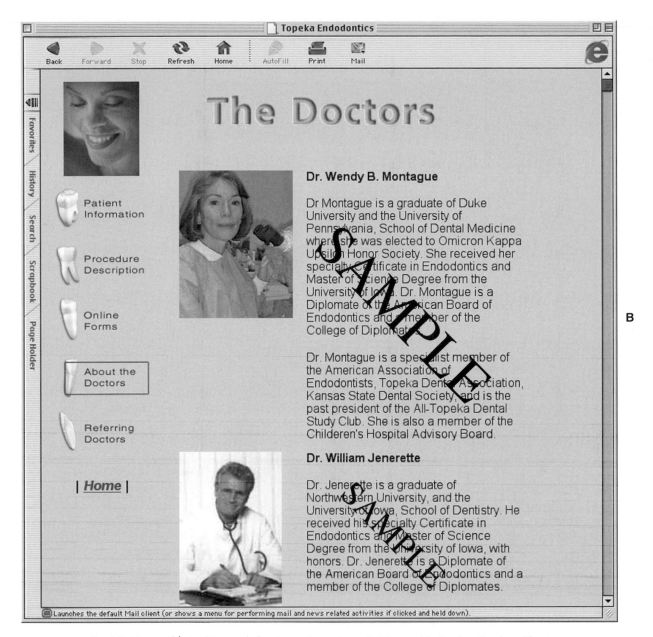

Fig. 26-18, cont'd **B**, This page helps viewers learn about clinicians and their educational qualifications.

Continued

3. On-line payments. Patients will be able to pay their bills on-line.
4. On-line insurance. Eligibility, claims transmission, and automatic electronic explanation of benefits (EOBs) will be available to patients on-line.
5. Data analysis. Clinicians may participate with other clinicians in providing anonymous data-to-data banks that will analyze the information and report back statistics regarding their practices.
6. Data backup. Because data will be housed at a central server, often outside the facility, backup will be done for the clinician.
7. On-line ordering. Clinicians will order all their supplies via the World Wide Web.
8. Automated preregistration over the Internet. Several vendors provide on-line patient registration and health history forms that can securely transfer information over the Internet directly into an endodontic software database.

Internet Websites

The World Wide Web has already proven itself as a cost-effective communication and marketing tool in dentistry (Fig. 26-18). For current and prospective patients, an Internet site can provide a wealth of information and can greatly speed communications. When designing a site, it is a good

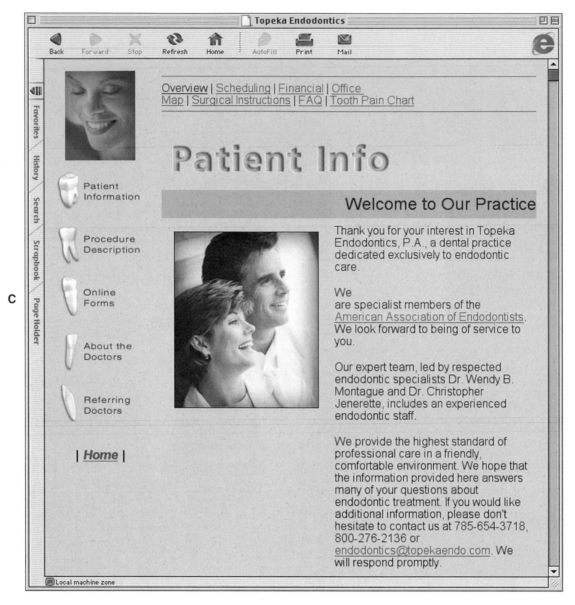

Fig. 26-18, cont'd **C**, The "Patient Info" page introduces the practice and lists contact information.

Continued

idea to include information that will convey what is unique about the practice. Also, if clinicians are trying to attract new patients who "surf the web," they should list themselves with as many web search engines as possible.

A clinician's web page can contain searchable educational material for study clubs and referring clinicians. Websites can be transformed into a communication center, a scientific reference library, and clinical and business information resource. This can provide fast and convenient access to resources like MEDLINE, on-line continuing education (CE) courses, product catalogs, and practice management information.

Several vendors currently provide services for site construction and hosting that include creative patient education modules, maps with customized directions, clinician biographies, and animated procedure descriptions. In addition, some sites include referral forms that automate attachment of digital radiographs and interactive study clubs with on-line chat and bulletin boards. Clinicians can customize referral forms to provide data fields that *require* inclusion of certain information for submission to their e-mail addresses. This will help eliminate incomplete referral information being transmitted from referring sources.

Important Software Features

Financial Security   Although fraud in dental offices is not often discussed, even conservative statistics indicate that

Text continued on p. 957

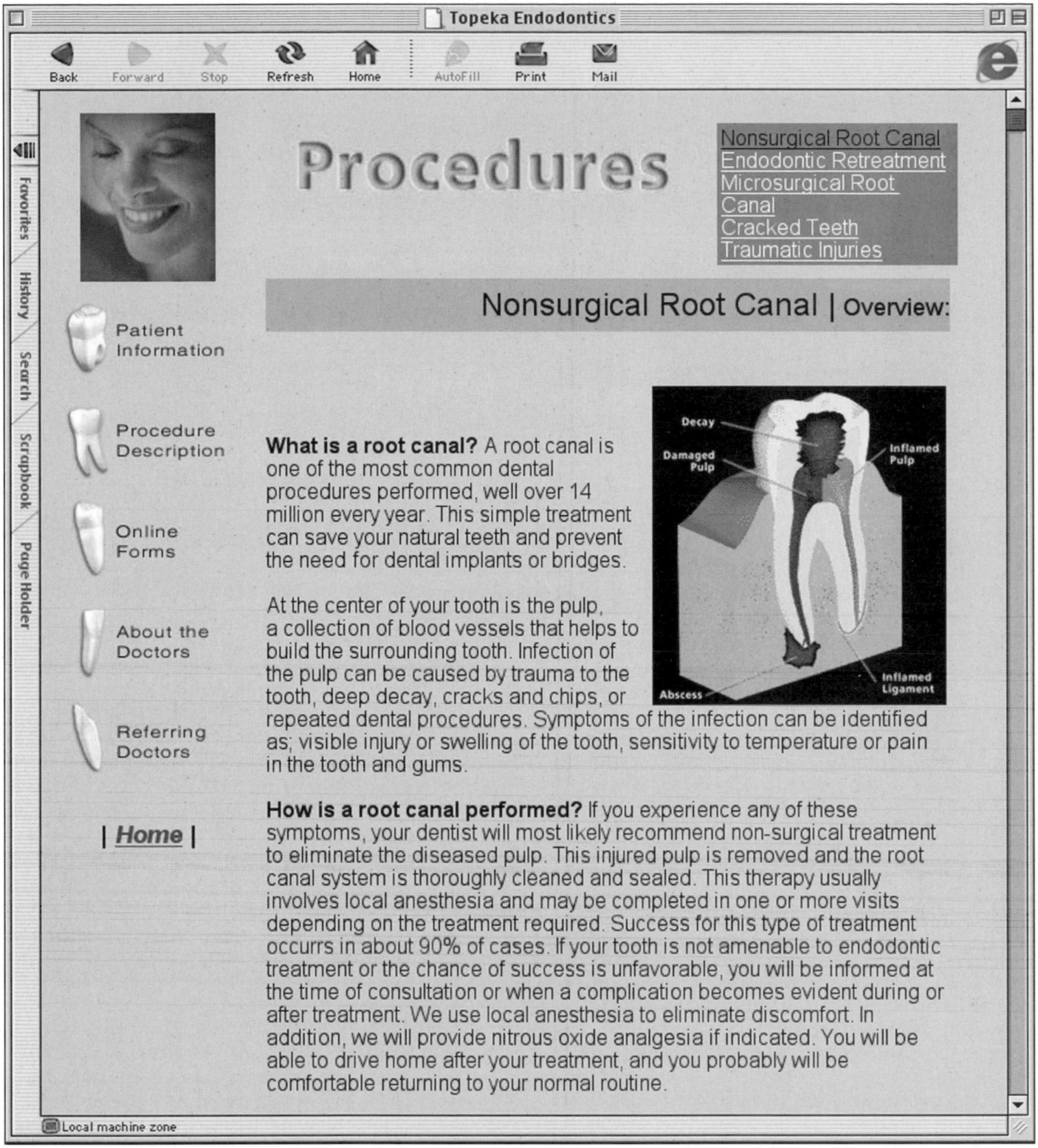

Topeka Endodontics
Back
Forward
Stop
Refresh
Home
AutoFill
Print
Mail
Favorites
History
Search
Scrapbook
Page Holder
Procedures
Nonsurgical Root Canal
Endodontic Retreatment
Microsurgical Root Canal
Cracked Teeth
Traumatic Injuries
Nonsurgical Root Canal | Overview:
Patient Information
Procedure Description
Online Forms
About the Doctors
Referring Doctors
| Home |
Decay
Damaged Pulp
Inflamed Pulp
Abscess
Inflamed Ligament
What is a root canal? A root canal is one of the most common dental procedures performed, well over 14 million every year. This simple treatment can save your natural teeth and prevent the need for dental implants or bridges.
At the center of your tooth is the pulp, a collection of blood vessels that helps to build the surrounding tooth. Infection of the pulp can be caused by trauma to the tooth, deep decay, cracks and chips, or repeated dental procedures. Symptoms of the infection can be identified as; visible injury or swelling of the tooth, sensitivity to temperature or pain in the tooth and gums.
How is a root canal performed? If you experience any of these symptoms, your dentist will most likely recommend non-surgical treatment to eliminate the diseased pulp. This injured pulp is removed and the root canal system is thoroughly cleaned and sealed. This therapy usually involves local anesthesia and may be completed in one or more visits depending on the treatment required. Success for this type of treatment occurrs in about 90% of cases. If your tooth is not amenable to endodontic treatment or the chance of success is unfavorable, you will be informed at the time of consultation or when a complication becomes evident during or after treatment. We use local anesthesia to eliminate discomfort. In addition, we will provide nitrous oxide analgesia if indicated. You will be able to drive home after your treatment, and you probably will be comfortable returning to your normal routine.
Local machine zone

D

Fig. 26-18, cont'd **D**, Patients can view animated illustrations and video sequences to help understand procedures. Here, the nonsurgical phase of therapy is explained. *Continued*

Fig. 26-18, cont'd **E**, Patient demographics, medical history, and financial information can be encrypted and fed directly into an endodontic software database.   *Continued*

Fig. 26-18, cont'd F, The "Referral Form" enhances communication with other practitioners. It can even be configured to include the seamless transmission of digital radiographs via the Internet. (Courtesy PBHS, Inc., Pomona, N.Y.)

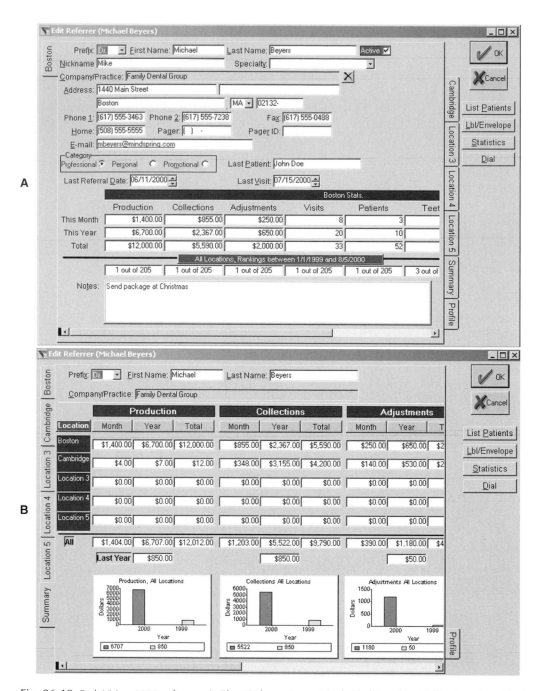

Fig. 26-19 EndoVision 2000 software. **A**, The "Referrer Screen" is divided into five "Office Location Tabs," a "Summary Tab," which consolidates statistics from all locations, and a "Profile Tab," which sets defaults for preregistration. In this figure the Boston "Location Tab" is displayed, showing the referring clinician's statistics. Rankings on this screen compare the referrer to all others from January 1 of the previous year to the present. **B**, The "Summary Tab" page consolidates statistics from all five of the referrer's locations and graphs each of the statistical categories. (Courtesy Discus Dental Software, Culver City, Calif.)

it is a significant problem. There is no absolute solution, and vigilance is the key. But most experts agree that clinicians should do three things:

1. Become educated. Clinicians should find out how people embezzle from a dental office. Sometimes this means taking a course or two, hiring a fraud expert to review the office systems, or both.
2. Pay attention to the business. Too many dental professionals abdicate the function of their front office to trusted "office managers." This dynamic, in which the owner of the business ignores the business, is ill conceived and invites fraud.
3. Select software with a security log. Use an office computer system that carefully tracks all deletions, edits, and other potentially suspicious behavior automatically and prevents anyone except the administrator (i.e., the clinician) from viewing the security log. In addition, each user is logged on and off the system so that the software knows when a particular person was on the system; what station the person was using; and which transactions they created, edited, or removed.

Referral Tracking   Sophisticated referral tracking and trend analysis is critical to the success of a specialized practice. It also is what is lacking in software created for the general dentist. Software designed using SQL tracks financial and other statistics associated with referrers in the practice at the moment transactions are posted (Fig. 26-19). Therefore the statistics are always current and accurate.

Key features of referral tracking include:

1. Real-time statistics. The software should give the clinician up-to-the-second statistics (without having to run reports) in the key areas of:
   a. Production
   b. Collections
   c. Adjustments
   d. New patients
   e. Patient visits
   f. Teeth treated
   g. Production-collections ratio, the collections percentage
2. Real-time ranking of all referrers relative to all others in any of the previously mentioned categories.
3. Sophisticated, flexible reports based on production, collections, procedures, etc. that can be filtered and sorted on almost any imaginable permutation.
4. Generation of correspondence, labels, and envelopes to one referrer or a selection of referrers, based on queries.
5. Availability of referrer data from the patient screen, the schedule, and other key areas so that the practitioner can make rapid decisions and see the juxtaposition of referrer and other system information.
6. Charts and graphs on referrer and patient activity associated with referrers.
7. Tracking of multiple-referrer categories:
   a. Referral source
   b. General dentist
   c. Cotherapists
8. Collection of the previously mentioned data by multiple facilities of the referrer. In other words, if the referral source has multiple facilities, the clinician should be able to track statistics for each of those facilities and summarize a consolidated set of numbers for all facilities.
9. Collection of the previously mentioned data by practice. If several referral sources are employed by the same practice, this feature lets the clinician discern statistical data by practice.

Preregistration   Using a specialized system, EndoVision 2000's preregistration (i.e., the process of recording information for patients referred but not yet seen by a clinician) can be accomplished at almost any level of detail (Fig. 26-20, A-C). This sophisticated system replaces the venerated call slip most dental offices use. It goes much further than the call slip, because it is tightly woven into the fabric of the rest of the program.

The major features associated with preregistration are:

1. The ability to record all pertinent data about a referred patient, including insurance, referral source, and medical conditions before an appointment is made. There are ample notes fields to record comments from both the patient and other clinicians. A direct link to e-mail and home and work phone icons facilitates quick communication. A "welcome letter" and information about the patient's first appointment can be produced automatically and sent out with a brochure (see Fig. 26-20, A).
2. An integrated link to the schedule, allowing the clinician to easily drag and drop the preregistration record into the appointment book, complete with all of the relevant information from preregistration.
3. Automatic correspondence to the patient after creation of the preregistration record.
4. An integrated link to the registration module so that the system automatically creates both the patient record and the insurance records without reentering the data. Sophisticated algorithms continually update insurance data based on previous cases submitted. When the system automatically registers the patient later, this information will create the patient's insurance record (see Fig. 26-20, B).
5. Printing of preregistration data as a call slip.

COMPUTER WORKSTATIONS

There are two kinds of computer workstations: (1) the clinical chair side workstation and (2) the front desk and administrative workstation. The clinical chair side workstation is located in the operatory to store and display clinical information, whereas the front desk and administrative unit is located at the front desk, in the management office, and in the clinician's office, if applicable. Unlike the administrative

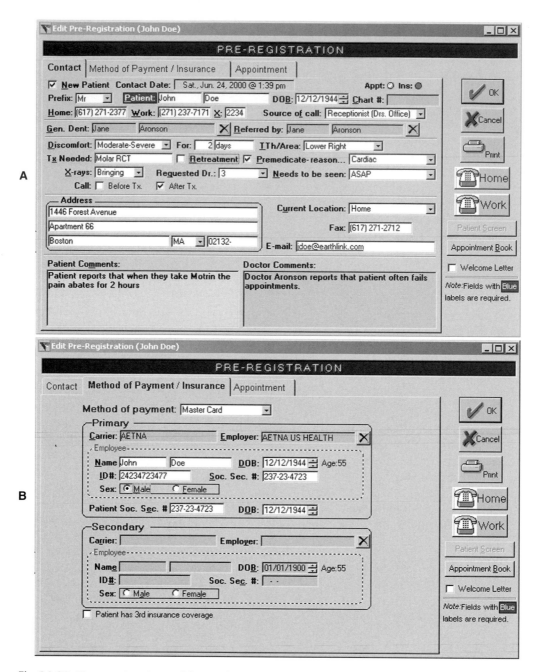

Fig. 26-20 The preregistration module in EndoVision 2000. **A,** The "Contact Tab" records all pertinent data about the patient. **B,** The "Method of Payment/Insurance Tab" allows the clinician to prerecord the patient's insurance information.   *Continued*

stations, the clinical chair side workstation has no printer and uses a touch pad or digitizing tablet, mouse, or light pen, and a keyboard protected by barrier techniques. A single clinical chairside workstation may support two monitors using a Matrox G450 dual-monitor display board: one for the assistant and one for the clinician. In addition, it may display the schedule, charting, and digital radiography at the same time.

CPU

The CPU should use one of the fastest processors available, have enough RAM to allow several programs to run simultaneously, and include at least two peripheral component interconnect (PCI) slots and one drive bay for additional peripheral components. As a general rule, a faster processor will add to a machine's useful life, and upgrading the system's RAM to at least one level more than required to run the com-

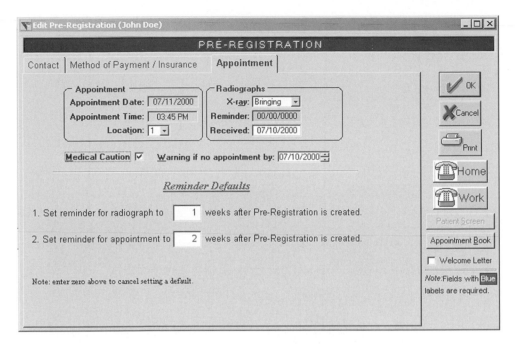

Fig. 26-20, cont'd **C**, The "Appointment Tab" records data on the patient's appointment and permits the clinician to set up automatic warnings. (Courtesy Discus Dental Software, Culver City, Calif.)

puter's Operating System (OS) (e.g., Windows 2000, Windows XP) is advisable. Increasing RAM to at least 128 MB (megabyte) will improve speed for today's graphic intensive software. Fortunately, RAM is now relatively inexpensive and will be worth the additional investment.

The hard drive is where the computer stores software programs, the OS, and patient education materials. As hard drive capacity continues to increase and price per MB declines, choosing a large hard drive of at least 30-GB (gigabyte) is adequate for most purposes.

Monitor

The monitor's size and image quality are critical to image resolution. Clinicians should invest in the best-quality unit they can afford. In all likelihood, the monitor will have longevity well past any single CPU. Minimum recommended specifications are *dot pitch* (the distance between dots on the screen) of 0.25 mm or less and screen resolution of at least 1024 × 768 pixels. However, monitor specifications can be confusing. For example, horizontal pitch measurements are not the same as conventional *stripe pitch* or dot pitch. Horizontal stripe or dot pitch measures a shorter distance from one blue stripe to another or one blue dot to another than conventional diagonal measurements. Therefore a conventional dot pitch of 0.26 mm is the equivalent of a 0.22 mm horizontal dot pitch.

Clinicians should try to choose a true, flat-screen model that will reduce distortion and provide the best nonglare surface for viewing images. Because the monitor position is typically 48 inches or more from the operator, the largest-size monitor that will fit in the operatory is advisable. A 19-inch or larger monitor is recommended. Integral speakers also are helpful when space for separate speakers is at a premium. These speakers will allow for showing patient education materials and entertainment programs.

Because monitor "footprint" is a critical issue for most dental offices, clinicians should consider a CRT monitor that has a reduced depth "space saver" design or a Liquid Crystal Display (LCD) flat panel. The LCDs are more expensive and do not allow as wide a viewing angle as CRT monitors, but the reduced size and heat produced by these displays are big advantages. Because the most precise images on flat panels are found in digital rather than analog units, a monitor that allows for analog and digital inputs will provide the most flexibility. The digital input will require a special digital video card in the CPU to operate. All types of monitors dim with age, but the longevity of the backlighting on the flat-panel units is particularly limited and is a maintenance issue that needs to be evaluated.

Accessories

When choosing pointing devices and keyboards, location and ease of use should be considered along with infection control. In the operatory, clinicians should choose touch pads that allow barrier protection and can be attached with Velcro to the work surface to conserve space. Wireless keyboards are another useful adjunct for clinicians and their assistants to interface with their computers. Most wireless units are

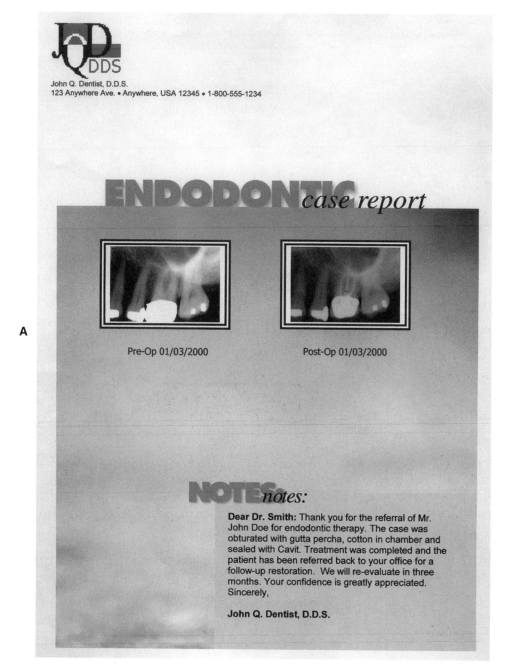

Fig. 26-21 **A**, The printer used for this patient treatment report was the ALPS MD5000, with 2400 dpi resolution and archival "Micro Dry" ink technology.   *Continued*

infrared (IR), so the accessory must be able to "see" the receiver. Remote IR-signal distribution systems can be placed to relay the signal to its intended receiver.

Printers

The right printers are crucial to the usefulness of the entire computer system. The front desk computer should have a monochrome laser for printing reports, insurance materials, and general word processing tasks. Clinicians will also need a photo quality ink jet printer for letter-size patient treatment reports (Fig. 26-21) and a label printer for chart labels. Connecting several printers to one CPU can be accomplished via USB or networked connections for shared printers.

Power and Cabling

Each workstation in the office should be plugged into an uninterruptible power supply (UPS), also known as a "battery backup" power protection system.[23] UPS units (Fig. 26-

John Q. Dentist, D.D.S.
123 Anywhere Ave.
Anywhere, USA 12345
1-800-555-1234

ENDODONTIC CASE REPORT

Dear Dr. Smith:

Re: John Doe, Tooth #3

Thank you for referring Mr. Doe for endodontic treatment. Endodontic re-evaluation was completed on June 15, 2001. Mr. Doe reports no symptoms and endodontic healing is within normal limits. We plan to re-evaluate Mr. Smith in one year.

Thank you for your confidence in our office.

Sincerely,

John Q. Dentist, D.D.S.

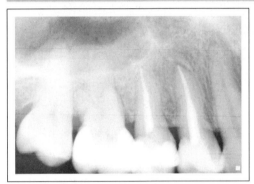

Pre-Op February 12, 2001

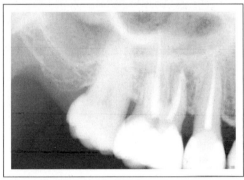

Post-Op March 15, 2001

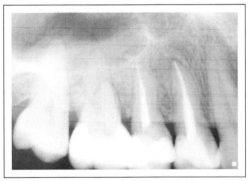

Re-Eval May 12, 2001

Fig. 26-21, cont'd **B**, An Epson 980 ink jet printer with 2880 × 720 dpi resolution and "Micro Piezo" ink technology printed this report. (*A*, Courtesy Alps Electric (USA), Inc., San Jose, Calif.; *B*, Courtesy Schick Technologies, Inc., Long Island City, N.Y.)

22) protect the CPU and peripheral equipment from voltage sags, interruptions, and surges by using advanced technology to smooth out the power. Clinicians should make sure that computers and monitors are plugged into sockets that are surge and battery backup protected. Laser printers should not be plugged into these devices because they draw too much current. Any system that receives telephone service also should be protected from "back door" lightning strikes by passing the line through a surge protector.

Clinicians should place power and *Ethernet* (i.e., a LAN technology that transmits information between computers at speeds of up to 100 Mbps [mega bits per second]) wall jacks near the clinical chair side workstation. In addition, they should specify a double-duplex power outlet at each location,

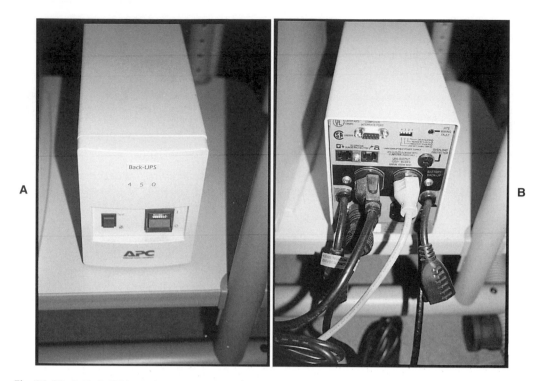

Fig. 26-22 **A**, Each CPU, monitor, power source for cameras, and appropriate peripherals should be protected by a UPS. **B**, Plugging critical equipment into battery outlets will enhance system reliability and help avoid corruption of data or files caused by power irregularities.

along with a combination wall plate containing two Ethernet and one telephone outlet. Internal wiring for the Ethernet should be run with copper unshielded twisted-pair (UTP) Cat 5E wire that is terminated in RJ45 outlets. The Cat 5E and Cat 6 will support data rates of up to 1 Gbps.

Cart or Built-In

Another major consideration is whether to use a cart-based clinical chair side workstation or a built-in configuration. The cart-based system allows flexibility in positioning, especially for offices with both left- and right-handed operators. Remote placement of monitors with ceiling or wall mounts also is helpful, especially in areas where space is at a premium. Provisions for Ethernet and power to the cart need to be located so that the system can be positioned without risk of injury from a fall. If the clinician chooses a built-in system, the cabinet housing the CPU must be ventilated to allow air circulation and easy access to the DVD drive and other peripherals.

Consulting and Support

It is best to hire local consultants to plan any network system. These vendors are usually certified by Microsoft, Novel, or both to provide support in the event of system failures. Because technology changes constantly, clinicians will need someone who can update their system's hardware and soft-

ware, upload "patches" and "firmware," and generally be available for help with equipment purchase decisions. These vendors usually work on an hourly basis and may offer blocks of time per month or per quarter at discounted rates and guaranteed response times.

Backup Strategies

Because "data is only as good as the last backup," it is imperative that a consistent backup protocol be followed because *all hard drives fail eventually*. The best way to back up data is to configure an automatic backup as part of the computer's scheduled routine. Along with automated defrag and scandisk routines, a nightly backup is essential. Most offices use tape backup, but on-line Internet backup[8] and disaster recovery programs are becoming more reliable and simpler to use.

Pharmacology Reference Software

Many programs are available to serve as clinical pharmacology references. Clinical Pharmacology (Gold Standard Multimedia, Inc., Tampa, Fla.) features extensive indexing, cross-referencing, and linking of drugs for optimal quick search functions. For example, the clinician simply types in the name of a drug and the program calls up every reference to the drug in the compendium. Users can search alphabetical listings, a main index of drug classifications, product identification (by description of the drug), adverse reactions, drug interactions, and more. This product contains clinically oriented monographs on all U.S. drugs and allows for quick, accurate identification of drug interactions and contraindications. Available with quarterly updates, it can be kept current with a continuing subscription. Online reference to this program may be found at www.gsm.com. Another online reference is the Physicians Desk Reference (Medical Economics Co., Inc., Montvale, N.J) at www.pdr.net.

Patient Education Software

Patient education is an important part of modern dental treatment. It is clear from research performed by Chandler and Silversin[33] for the AAE that there is a positive statistical correlation between patient education and their endodontic treatment experience. To this end, several vendors have created informational software programs for the web and local computer use. These programs can be observed by the patient on the Internet, at a computer station in the reception room, or at the clinical chair side workstation.

Internet Access

Accessing the Internet from the dental office is another important benefit of an up-to-date computer system. Clinicians are able to connect to continuing education courses, e-mail colleagues, purchase dental supplies, and download the latest software. Patients will also benefit by being able to contact the clinician when a question arises, even from overseas when time zones preclude other forms of communication.

CONCLUSION

Computers and associated software are proving to be invaluable aids to practice operations. Most clinicians would not consider practice without some of these sophisticated systems. However, technology is not a substitute for treatment excellence, and clinicians must continue to strive to provide quality treatment *and* experiences for patients regardless of the equipment they use.

References

1. 1394 Trade Association. ta.org (website), accessed Jan 1, 2000.
2. ADA moves forward on electronic standards, *ADA News*, Aug 23, 1999.
3. American Optometric Association, aoanet.org (website), accessed Jan 1, 2000.
4. American Power Conversion Corp., apc.com (website), accessed Jan 1, 2000.
5. Bachall J, Barss J: Orascopy: a vision for the new millennium, part 1, *Dent Today* 18(5):66, 1999.
6. Bachall J, Barss J: Orascopy: a vision for the new millennium, part 2, *Dent Today* 18(9):82, 1999.
7. Burger CL, Mork TO, Hutter JW, Nicoll B: Direct digital radiography versus conventional radiography for estimation of canal length in curved canals, *J Endod* 25:260, 1999.
8. Chandler L, Silversin J: What do patients think of you? Building relationships, Chicago, American Association of Endodontists (videotape).
9. Clinical Research Associates, cranews.com (website), accessed Jan 1, 2000.
10. Digital radiographs, state-of-art, *CRA Newsletter* 23(9):1, 1999.
11. Dunn SM, Kantor ML: Digital radiology facts and fictions, *J Am Dent Assoc* 124:39, 1993.
12. Eikenberg S, Vandre R: Comparison of digital dental x-ray systems with self-developing film and manual processing for endodontic file length comparison, *J Endod* 26:65 1999.
13. Sitca, Inc., sitca.com (website), accessed Jan 1, 2000.
14. Foroughi K et al: Comparison of radiation exposure rates necessary to produce computerized images and conventional radiographs, *J Endod* 25:305 1999 (abstract).
15. Fossum, Eric: CMOS evolution: the digital camera-on-a-chip gets active, *Advanced Imaging* 12:13,1997.
16. Fronckowiak JW: *OLE and ADO*, Indianapolis, IN, 1991, Sams Publishing.
17. Levato C: Advancing the state of the art, *Dental Practice and Finance* 7(8), 1999.
18. Loshin P: *TCP/IP*, ed 2, San Diego, CA, 1997, AP Professional.
19. McKee L: SNODENT to provide inclusive means of transmitting dental information, *ADA News* 30(9):1, 1999.
20. Microsoft, microsoft.com (website), accessed Jan 1, 2000
21. Mistak EJ et al: Interpretation of periapical lesions comparing conventional, direct, and telephonically transmitted radiographic images, *J Endod* 11:262, 1998.
22. National Electric Manufacturers Association, nema.org/standards (website), accessed Jan 1, 2000.
23. Nemzow M: *Fast Ethernet, implementation and migration solutions*, New York, 1997, McGraw-Hill.
24. IBM, networking.ibm.com (website), White paper: *thin server feature*, accessed Jan 1, 2000.
25. IBM, networking.ibm.com, (website), White paper: *virtual private network overview*, accessed Jan 1, 2000.
26. Nummikoski PV et al: Digital subtraction radiography in artificial recurrent caries detection, *Dentomaxillofac Radiol* 21:59, 1992.
27. Olympus, olympusamerica.com (website), accessed Jan 1, 2000.
28. Olympus, olympusamerica.com (website), accessed Jan 1, 2000.
29. Panasonic, panasonic.com/medical_industrial/index.html (website), accessed Jan 1, 2000.
30. Paurazas SB et al: Comparison of diagnostic accuracy of digital imaging and E-speed film in the detection of periapical bone lesions, *J Endod* 25:285 1999 (abstract).
31. The Radiological Society of North America, Inc., rsna.com (website), *DICOM: the value and importance of an imaging standard*, accessed Jan 1, 2000.
32. Schick D: Letter to the editor: alteration of computer dental radiography images, *J Endod* 25:475 1999.
33. SCSI Trade Association, scsita.org (website), accessed Jan 1, 2000.
34. Sinclair JT, Merkow M: *Thin clients*, New York, 2000, Academic Press.

35. College or American Pathologists, snowmed.org (website), accessed Jan 1, 2000.

36. Technology and Health: Compaq to put warnings on keyboards about risk of repetitive-stress injuries, *The Wall Street Journal*, section B, p. 6, February 1995.

37. The TWAIN working group, twain.org (website), accessed Jan 1, 2000.

38. USB Implementers Forum, Inc., usb.org (website), accessed Jan 1, 2000.

39. Vandre RH, Webber RL: Future trends in dental radiology, *Oral Surg Oral Med Oral Pathol* 80:471, 1995.

40. VeriSign, Inc. Enterprise & Internet Security Solutions, www.verisign.com (website), accessed Jan 1, 2000.

41. Visser H, Kruger W: Can dentists recognize manipulated digital radiographs? *Dentomaxillofac Radiol* 26(1):67, 1997.

42. Worden DJ: *Sybase developers handbook*, San Diego, 1999, AP Professional.

Conclusion: Tomorrow

Stephen Cohen

As eloquently outlined in Dr. Gutmann's "Introduction" to this eighth edition of *Pathways of the Pulp,* the specialty of endodontics stands strong today, fully expressive of its rich-and-layered past and poised to define clinical excellence in the future. The dynamic admixture of basic science and technologic innovation that has characterized the field, will continue to drive developments and advances in the future.

This continuum of exploration and discovery is most evident in the fact that the innovations and technical advances considered the most significant and exciting for endodontics today are, in some cases, simply the elaborations and refinements of ideas proposed, researched, and published by dental scientists generations ago.

Predictable, pain-free root canal therapy is the application of Alfred Einhorn's discovery of acetylsalicylic acid (i.e., aspirin) and Novocaine (i.e., Procaine). Advances in post-endodontic-treatment pain prevention are becoming the next extension of Einhorn's work: painless endodontic therapy from the beginning to the end.

The dramatic reduction in ionizing radiation achieved by digital radiography is the refinement of the *x-ray films* brought to dentistry by Otto Walkhoff and C. Edmund Kells. Based on current trends, it appears likely that within the next few years, digital radiography will completely replace conventional, film-based radiography in most dental offices.

One-visit endodontic treatment, increasingly supported by evidence-based findings of its efficacy and benefit, is the reappearance of a radical concept first proposed and practiced in the nineteenth century. Currently, there is a general consensus that one-visit endodontic treatment for vital teeth is the preferred treatment plan whenever possible. The next frontier is one-visit endodontic treatment for asymptomatic, nonvital teeth. It is clear that international research about single-visit treatment for nonvital teeth will remain robust; based on well-designed studies that have been published in refereed dental journals, it appears increasingly likely that reproducible studies will eventually validate this paradigm shift in endodontic therapy.

Even gutta-percha, the icon of endodontic materials, will likely be replaced in the next few years with a biocompatible, leak-resistant (i.e., bonded) material. Currently, research is focused on the development of a delivery system that will allow clinicians to pack a more refined particle size of non-staining MTA into the apical third of most canals, thus achieving a tighter, hard seal with superior biocompatibility.

Ongoing testing to find a more sophisticated, easily applied method of determining the presence of early pulp inflammation will lead to the development of a harmless chemical that can be applied to the exudate of dentinal tubules from freshly cut dentin. Like a litmus test, a color change of the chemical will indicate pulp inflammation, enabling the restorative dentist to know whether or not endodontic therapy should be performed before the placement of a final restoration.

Although endodontics as a profession will continue to be defined by its inherent passion for excellence and for its steadfast support of the highest quality research to drive its revolution in methods and materials, it is now essential that this be seen in the context of the most significant and pervasive advance of all—the communications revolution.

Computer technology, especially the Internet and the World Wide Web, means that every new discovery, further development, and clinical innovation will be universally available immediately. This new knowledge, available to us as it is found, will inspire us as clinicians and healers. This new information will be accessible as never before to our patients, and it will motivate them to ask for the best treatment that can be provided. This is our new millennium challenge as a profession and our new covenant as doctors.

CHALLENGE

A Self-Assessment Exam

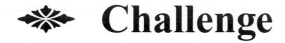

Challenge

Richard E. Walton, William T. Johnson, Lisa R. Wilcox

CHAPTER 1: DIAGNOSTIC PROCEDURES

1. Anesthetic testing is most effective in localizing pain to which of the following?
   a. Specific tooth
   b. Mandible or maxilla
   c. Across the midline of the face
   d. Posterior tooth

2. Areas of rarefaction are evident on radiographic examination in which of the following?
   a. When the tooth is responsive to cold
   b. When the tooth is responsive to percussion
   c. When a tooth fracture has been identified
   d. When the cortical layer of bone has been eroded

3. Irreversible pulpitis is often defined by which of the following?
   a. Moderate response to percussion
   b. Painful, lingering response to cold
   c. Short, painful response to cold
   d. Short, painful response to heat

4. The majority of patients with symptoms of severe odontogenic pain have a diagnosis of which of the following?
   a. Periodontal abscess
   b. Irreversible pulpitis
   c. Acute apical periodontitis
   d. Acute apical abscess

5. Medical history of coronary heart disease is significant for which of the following reasons?
   a. It contraindicates endodontic treatment.
   b. Many heart medications impact dental treatment.
   c. It indicates the need for premedication with antibiotics.
   d. It contraindicates local anesthetic with epinephrine.

6. The best approach for diagnosis of odontogenic pain is which of the following?
   a. Radiographic examination
   b. Percussion
   c. Visual examination
   d. A step-by-step, sequenced examination and testing approach

7. Of the following, which is the most likely to have referred pain?
   a. Irreversible pulpitis
   b. Reversible pulpitis
   c. Acute apical periodontitis
   d. Phoenix abscess

8. A sinus tract that drains out on the face (through skin) is mostly likely from which of the following?
   a. Nonodontogenic pathosis
   b. A periodontal abscess
   c. Periradicular (i.e., endodontic) pathosis
   d. Pericoronitis of a mandibular, third molar

9. Which of the following statements regarding a test cavity is accurate?
   a. It is the first test in diagnostic sequence.
   b. It often results in a dull-pain response.
   c. It is used when all other test findings are equivocal.
   d. It should be performed with local anesthetic.

10. Percussion of a tooth is a test for which of the following?
    a. Pulpal inflammation
    b. Pulpal necrosis
    c. Acute periradicular inflammation
    d. Chronic periradicular inflammation

11. Pulp stones are consistent indicators of which of the following?
    a. Periodontal inflammation impacting the pulp
    b. Pulpal inflammation
    c. Older patient
    d. Pulp that has been injured in the past but has recovered
    e. None of the above

12. Radiographically, which of the following statements regarding acute apical abscess is most accurate?
    a. It is generally of larger size than other lesions.
    b. It has more diffuse margins than other lesions.
    c. It often contains radiopacities (i.e., calcification).
    d. It may not be evident.

13. In which of the following may a false-negative response to the pulp tester occur?
    a. Primarily in anterior teeth
    b. In a patient with a history of trauma
    c. Most often in teenagers
    d. In the presence of periodontal disease

14. The lateral periodontal abscess is best differentiated from the acute apical abscess by which of the following?
    a. Pulp testing
    b. Radiographic appearance
    c. Location of swelling
    d. Probing patterns

15. The acute apical abscess is best differentiated from the acute apical periodontitis by which of the following?
    a. Pulp testing
    b. Radiographic appearance
    c. Presence of swelling
    d. Degree of mobility

16. Chronic apical periodontitis is best differentiated from acute apical periodontitis by which of the following?
    a. Pulp testing and radiographic appearance
    b. Pulp testing and nature of symptoms
    c. Radiographic appearance and nature of symptoms
    d. Pulp testing, radiographic appearance, and nature of symptoms

17. The abrupt change (*arrow*) in radiographic appearance in the following illustration probably indicates which of the following?

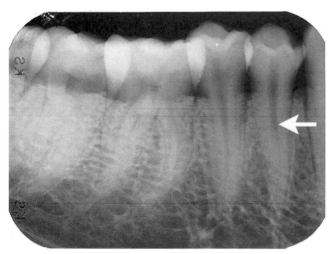

    a. Calcific metamorphosis
    b. A dense accumulation of diffuse calcification
    c. An increased density of overlying bone
    d. A bifurcation into two canals

18. The patient in the following illustration reports severe, throbbing pain in the mandibular right molar region. The pain is exaggerated by cold. Which tooth and which tissue is *likely* the source of pain?

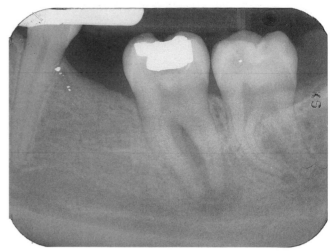

    a. First molar and pulp
    b. First molar and periapex
    c. Second molar and pulp
    d. Second molar and periapex

19. Of the following cold-testing agents, which is the least effective in producing a response?
    a. Bathing a tooth in ice water
    b. Dicholorodifluoromethane (DDM)
    c. CO_2 snow (i.e., dry ice)
    d. Ethyl chloride

20. Which of the following statements regarding internal resorption is accurate?
    a. The condition is usually accompanied by symptoms.
    b. It is continuous.
    c. It is self-limiting.
    d. It is usually visible in its early stages.
    e. It is treated only if time shows it to be progressive.

CHAPTER 2: OROFACIAL DENTAL PAIN EMERGENCIES: ENDODONTIC DIAGNOSES AND MANAGEMENT

1. Which of the following statements regarding the degree of pulp pathosis is accurate?
    a. It can be determined by the level of pain a patient experiences.
    b. It can be related to the level of response of the electrical pulp tester.
    c. It can be correlated best when a diagnosis of irreversible pulpitis is established.
    d. It does not correlate well with the level of pain a patient perceives.

2. A key measure as to the degree (i.e., intensity) of pain is to determine which of the following?
   a. Painful stimulus with cold
   b. Painful stimulus with heat
   c. Painful stimulus on biting
   d. Increasing pain
   e. Pain affecting patient's lifestyle

3. In describing the sensory innervation of the dental pulp, which of the following statements is accurate?
   a. A-delta fibers are high-threshold, myelinated fibers that transmit sharp, momentary pain.
   b. C fibers are low-threshold, unmyelinated fibers that produce pain in response to inflammatory mediators.
   c. The domination of C-fiber stimulation produces pain that is not well localized.
   d. The sharp, well-localized pain to cold testing is conducted by both A-delta and C-fiber stimulation.

4. Which of the following induces hyperalgesia in local-nerve fibers?
   a. Prostaglandin and serotonin
   b. Lysosomal enzymes
   c. Calcitonin gene-related peptide
   d. Substance P

5. Each of the following statements is correct regarding trigeminal neuralgia, *except for* one. Which is the *exception*?
   a. The onset occurs in midlife and is unilateral in location.
   b. The pain occurs unilaterally but often involves more than one division of the trigeminal nerve.
   c. The pain is characteristically sharp, lasts for several hours, and is induced by a trigger point.
   d. The pain mimics pain of pulpal origin in that thermal sensitivity and tingling is often encountered just before an attack.

6. A patient complains of dull and constant pain that lasts 3 days on the left side of the face. The patient notes the pain increases on positional changes, such as bending over and when jogging. The most likely diagnosis is which of the following?
   a. Myocardial infarction
   b. Maxillary sinusitis
   c. Atypical facial pain
   d. Irreversible pulpitis

7. Which of the following most likely indicates pain that is not of pulpal origin?
   a. Unilateral pain that radiates over the face to the ear
   b. Pain that has paresthesia as a component
   c. Pain that is described as throbbing and intermittent
   d. Pain that is increased during mastication

8. A complete medical history is essential when treating an emergency dental patient for which of the following reasons?
   a. To identify patients with conditions that would contraindicate root canal treatment
   b. To determine conditions that might require modifications in the approach to treatment
   c. To protect the health care team from potential blood-borne pathogens and other infectious diseases the patient may have
   d. For medical and legal protection and to determine if the medical status will affect the prognosis for root canal treatment

9. When a patient complains of severe pain that cannot be localized:
   a. The pain is most likely periradicular in origin and likely to persist even when the necrotic pulp is removed.
   b. Treatment procedures should be delayed and the condition managed with analgesic medications.
   c. The cause is most likely nonodontogenic in origin.
   d. Selective administration of local anesthesia can lead to a definitive diagnosis.
   e. The pulp of more than one tooth will be involved and the pathosis produce a synergistic-hyperalgesia response within the central nervous system (CNS).

10. A patient's chief complaint is severe pain from the mandibular, right first molar (tooth no. 30) when eating ice cream and drinking iced tea. Clinical examination reveals MOD amalgam restorations in all posterior teeth. The margins appear intact and no cracks or caries is detected. Pulp testing indicates all teeth in the quadrant are responsive to electrical-pulp testing. Application of cold fails to reproduce the symptoms. Which of the following actions should be taken?
   a. The patient should be dismissed and asked to return when the symptoms increase and the pain to cold becomes prolonged.
   b. Initiate root canal treatment by performing a pulpotomy or pulpectomy on tooth no. 30.
   c. Place a rubber dam on individual teeth and apply ice water.
   d. Remove the restoration in tooth no. 30, place a sedative restoration, and prescribe a nonsteroidal, anti-inflammatory agent.

11. A patient complains of pain to biting pressure and sensitivity to cold in the maxillary, left, posterior quadrant that subsides within seconds of removal of the stimulus. Clinical examination reveals teeth nos. 2 and 3 exhibit occlusal amalgams. Which of the following test or actions is most appropriate based on the chief complaint?
    a. Periapical radiographs of the posterior teeth
    b. Examination with transillumination
    c. Electrical pulp testing
    d. Percussion and palpation testing

12. A practitioner refers a patient for root canal treatment. The clinician should obtain a new preoperative radiograph during which of the following situations?
    a. When the film from the referring dentist is more than 1 month old
    b. In cases when an emergency treatment procedure was performed
    c. When the film from the referring dentist reveals a radiolucent area that has a "hanging drop" appearance
    d. Immediately before examining the patient

13. Which of the following is true regarding the periodontal ligament injection when treating a tooth with a pulpal diagnosis of reversible pulpitis?
    a. There will be a decrease in pulpal blood flow when anesthetic agents with a vasoconstrictor are used.
    b. Damage to the supporting structures can cause continued symptoms.
    c. The periodontal-ligament injection is contraindicated when block or infiltration injections are not effective.
    d. The periodontal ligament injection can be used as primary anesthesia in teeth that exhibit single roots, regardless of the number of canals.

14. A patient describes pain on chewing and sensitivity to cold that goes away immediately with removal of the stimulus. The mandibular, left, second molar (tooth no. 18) exhibits a mesial, occlusal crack. The tooth is caries free, and no restorations are present. Periodontal probing depths are 3 mm or less. Which of the following statements is correct?
    a. The pulpal diagnosis is normal pulp, and the tooth should be prepared and restored with a MO-bonded amalgam.
    b. The pulpal diagnosis is reversible pulpitis, and the tooth should be restored with a crown.
    c. The pulpal diagnosis is irreversible pulpitis, and root canal treatment should be performed, a bonded amalgam placed, and a crown fabricated.
    d. A radiograph will likely reveal a radiolucent area associated with the mesial root.
    e. The prognosis for the tooth is unfavorable.

15. Treatment of severe, throbbing pain associated with the maxillary, left, first molar (tooth no. 14) is best managed by which of the following?
    a. Pulpotomy
    b. Partial pulpectomy
    c. Pulpectomy
    d. Analgesic agents
    e. Analgesic and antibiotic agents

16. Which of the following statements regarding leaving a tooth open for drainage in cases of an acute, apical abscess is accurate?
    a. It is the recommended method of managing the emergency patient.
    b. It may adversely affect the outcome of treatment.
    c. It is appropriate, providing the patient is also placed on an antibiotic.
    d. It should be considered in addition to soft tissue incision and drainage.

17. With acute, apical abscess, antibiotic administration is indicated in which of the following?
    a. Primarily only when there is diffuse swelling
    b. When there is swelling to any degree (i.e., localized or diffuse)
    c. 2 to 3 days before beginning treatment of the tooth
    d. Only if there is purulence draining from an incision

18. A 21-year-old model requires emergency treatment of a soft, fluctuant swelling over the facial alveolar process of the maxillary, left, lateral incisor (tooth no. 10). The swelling is visible because of a high-lip line. Which of the following statements is correct regarding performing incision and drainage?
    a. The incision should be placed vertically and go directly to bone.
    b. The incision should be horizontal in the attached gingiva at the base of the swelling.
    c. If drainage occurs with the initial incision, blunt dissection is not necessary.
    d. The placement of a drain is necessary for 24 to 48 hours.

19. Which of the following statements regarding incision and drainage of an indurated swelling is accurate?
    a. They should be delayed until it becomes fluctuant.
    b. They can reduce pain caused by tissue distention.
    c. They provide a purulent exudate for culture and sensitivity testing.
    d. They are not indicated, because antibiotic treatment will result in resolution of the lesion.

20. Flare-ups during root canal treatment are more commonly associated with which of the following?
    a. Teeth with vital-pulp tissue when compared to teeth with pulp necrosis
    b. Teeth with apical radiolucent areas when compared to teeth with normal periapical tissues
    c. With single-visit endodontic procedures
    d. Symptomatic teeth exhibiting pulp necrosis
    e. Multirooted teeth

21. Of the following reasons, when is apical trephination through the faciobuccal, cortical plate advocated?
    a. To release exudate
    b. As a routine procedure for relief of pain when the offending tooth has been obturated
    c. For treatment of severe, recalcitrant pain
    d. Between multiple-visit endodontic procedures to prevent the occurrence of a flare-up

22. A 22-year-old, white man requires root canal treatment for pain and swelling in the mandibular, anterior area (see illustration). He notes that his dentist has been treating teeth nos. 25 and 26 for several months and that swelling has occurred after each visit for cleaning and shaping. Clinical examination reveals swelling located on the alveolar process in the area of the incisor teeth. Teeth nos. 25 and 26 are tender to palpation and percussion. The clinician should perform which of the following?

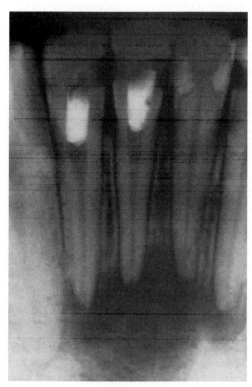

a. Diagnostic tests on the other incisor
b. Open teeth nos. 25 and 26, débride these teeth, and place calcium hydroxide as an antimicrobial intracanal medicament
c. Open teeth nos. 25 and 26, débride these teeth, and perform incision and drainage
d. Open teeth nos. 25 and 26, débride these teeth, and leave the teeth open for drainage
e. Perform incision and drainage and prescribe an antibiotic for supportive care

23. A cusp fractures in a noncarious, nonrestored premolar so that dentin is exposed. When this exposed dentin is contacted by cold fluids, the patient experiences brief, sharp pain. Which of the following pulp status is likely?
    a. Normal and uninflamed
    b. Reversibly inflamed
    c. Irreversibly inflamed
    d. Innervated only by A-delta fibers

24. Corticosteroids have their major pharmacologic effect as which of the following?
    a. Antimicrobial agent
    b. Analgesic
    c. Antiinflammatory agent
    d. Agent to reduce swelling
    e. Agent to prevent spread of infection

CHAPTER 3: NONODONTOGENIC OROFACIAL PAIN AND ENDODONTICS: PAIN DISORDERS INVOLVING THE JAWS THAT SIMULATE ODONTALGIA

1. Peripheral pain impulses in the dental pulp are transmitted centrally via which of the following pathways?
    a. Peripheral nerve, trigeminal nucleus, trigeminal ganglion, thalamus, cortex
    b. Peripheral nerve, trigeminal ganglion, mesencephalic nucleus, thalamus, cortex
    c. Peripheral nerve, trigeminal ganglion, trigeminal nucleus, mesencephalic nucleus, cortex
    d. Peripheral nerve, trigeminal ganglion, trigeminal nucleus, thalamus, cortex

2. Each of the following statements regarding trigeminal neuralgia is correct, *except for one*. Which is the *exception*?
    a. The empiric evidence suggests vascular compression of the trigeminal ganglion as a cause of trigeminal neuralgia.
    b. The pain involves all three divisions of the trigeminal nerve equally.
    c. There is an electrical quality of the pain.
    d. The pain is severe, often shooting into the bone and teeth.
    e. The standard medical therapy is carbamazepine (i.e., Tegretol).

3. Which of the following statements regarding cluster headaches is correct?
   a. Vessels that encircle nociceptive fibers compress the fibers during vasoconstriction, causing pain.
   b. The pain is usually unilateral and involves the maxilla, sinus, and retro-orbital area.
   c. Cluster headaches frequently involve females between 40 and 60 years of age.
   d. The pain, which is severe and lasts for 30 to 45 minutes, can occur at anytime.

4. Each of the following has been shown to benefit patients with cluster headaches, *except for one*. Which is the *exception*?
   a. Nifedipine
   b. Prednisone in combination with lithium
   c. Hyperbaric oxygen
   d. Alcohol
   e. Sumatriptin

5. A 57-year-old man complains of pain in the mandibular, left, posterior quadrant. The patient relates sporadic, spontaneous pain during his waking hours for the past 1 to 2 weeks. Upon examination no dental cause can be identified. Which of the following would be the most likely cause of the pain?
   a. Cluster headache
   b. Myalgia
   c. Cardiogenic jaw pain
   d. Temporal arteritis
   e. Otitis media

6. Each of the following statements regarding maxillary sinusitis is correct, *except for one*. Which is the *exception*?
   a. Pain is often referred to all teeth in the maxillary, posterior quadrant with percussion sensitivity being a common finding.
   b. The maxillary sinusitis may be initiated by a tooth with a necrotic pulp located in the maxillary, posterior area.
   c. Treatment of the sinusitis requires referral to an otolaryngologist and antibiotic therapy.
   d. The Waters view radiograph may be of diagnostic value in demonstrating fluid.
   e. An allergen-induced inflammation of the sinus is an immediate-type hypersensitivity reaction mediated by IgE.

7. Which of the following statements regarding sialolithiasis is correct?
   a. The sialolith develops in patients that often exhibit increased levels of serum calcium.
   b. Pain may mimic pulpal pain in the maxillary, posterior teeth because sialolithiasis is most frequently noted in parotid duct.

c. An occlusal radiograph provides more diagnostic information than a panoramic film.
d. Sialolithiasis has been associated with kidney stones and gallbladder stones, so patient's exhibiting this disorder should be referred to a physician for evaluation.

8. Which of the following statements regarding myofascial pain is correct?
   a. Trigger points found in the superficial aspect of the masseter may refer pain the maxillary teeth and mandibular teeth.
   b. Trigger points have been noted only in the masseter muscles and temporalis muscles.
   c. Initial treatment consists of finding occlusal discrepancies and performing an equilibration.
   d. Meniscus displacement and intraarticular adhesions are the cause, and corrective surgery provides long-term success.

9. Each of the following statements regarding malignant lesions of the head and neck is correct, *except for one*. Which is the *exception*?
   a. Although paresthesia is an ominous symptom, motor deficits are rare.
   b. Metastatic lesions may develop from the lung, breast, and colon.
   c. Radiolucent areas detected on radiographs are frequently poorly marginated.
   d. Multiple myeloma may produce pain in the affected bone.

10. Which of the following statements regarding atypical orofacial pain is false?
    a. The pain is often chronic, difficult to localize, and there is no identifiable cause.
    b. The pain has no specific symptoms that lead to a diagnosis.
    c. Patient's with atypical orofacial pain may give a history of having endodontic treatment that did not alleviate the pain.
    d. Patient's with atypical orofacial pain complain of pain in other areas of the body.
    e. Neuralgia-inducing cavitational osteonecrosis (NICO) is distinct from atypical orofacial–pain disorders.

11. Which of the following statements accurately describe phantom tooth pain?
    a. It occurs in 10% of the patients having endodontic treatment.
    b. It may be a form of deafferentation pain.
    c. It has been shown to have a psychopathologic component.
    d. It has been associated with tooth extraction but does not occur with extirpation of the pulp.

CHAPTER 4: CASE SELECTION AND TREATMENT PLANNING

1. Which of the following statements regarding the use of electronic-apex locators is accurate?
   a. The patient is physically impaired.
   b. Anatomic structures overlay the root apex.
   c. A pregnant patient wishes to avoid exposure to x-rays.
   d. All of the above statements are accurate.

2. Antibiotic prophylaxis is suggested for patients with a history of which of the following?
   a. Coronary bypass surgery
   b. Atrial fibrillation
   c. Artificial heart valve replacement
   d. Myocardial infarction
   e. Rheumatic fever

3. Elective endodontic treatment is contraindicated in which of the following?
   a. Patient is a borderline diabetic.
   b. Patient has had a heart attack within the last 6 months.
   c. Patient has had numerous opportunistic infections secondary to HIV infection.
   d. Patient has an implanted pacemaker.

4. Which of the following accurately describes external resorptions?
   a. They are untreatable.
   b. They can only be distinguished surgically from internal resorptions.
   c. They appear to be superimposed over the root canal.
   d. They always require root canal treatment.

5. Referral of difficult cases is indicated in which of the following?
   a. The general dentist does not have the indicated equipment.
   b. The general dentist does not have the indicated training and experience.
   c. The general dentist is not sure what procedures are indicated.
   d. All of the above

6. Which of the following statements regarding one-appointment root canal treatment is accurate?
   a. It is best performed in association with trephination or root end surgery.
   b. It may predispose the patient to postoperative flare-ups.
   c. It is equally successful as multiple-appointment root canal treatment.
   d. All of the above statements are accurate.

7. Single visit is equivalent in outcome to multiple visits (to complete RCT) with what situation?
   a. Vital pulp with acute pain
   b. Necrotic pulp with acute pain
   c. Necrotic pulp without pain
   d. Necrotic pulp with a draining sinus tract

8. Root end surgery is indicated for endodontic failure in which of the following?
   a. The dentist suspects a missed canal.
   b. There has been coronal leakage.
   c. A cast post and core and a well-fitting crown are present.
   d. All of the above

9. Prognosis for root canal treatment is worse when the patient is experiencing which of the following?
   a. Pain as a symptom
   b. Interappointment flare-up
   c. Class III mobility and loss of bone support (i.e., probing defects)
   d. Small, periradicular, radiolucent lesion

10. When is endodontic treatment is contraindicated?
    a. The patient has no motivation to maintain the tooth.
    b. The canal appears to be calcified.
    c. A large periapical lesion is present.
    d. The tooth needs periodontal crown lengthening before restoration.

11. With pregnancy, the safest period to provide dental care is during which month?
    a. First
    b. Second and third
    c. Fourth to the sixth
    d. Seventh and eighth
    e. There is no period that is most safe.

12. A preoperative finding that predisposes to a decreased prognosis (i.e., lower-success rate) is which of the following?
    a. The tooth is in hyperocclusion.
    b. The pulp is vital.
    c. The pulp is necrotic with no periradicular lesion.
    d. The pulp is necrotic with a periradicular lesion present.
    e. Treatment is in an elderly patient.

CHAPTER 5: PREPARATION FOR TREATMENT

1. Which of the following statements describes human immunodeficiency virus (HIV)?
   a. HIV is more easily transmissible than Hepatitis B.
   b. HIV is more fragile than the Hepatitis B virus.
   c. HIV is a good model for infection control practices.

2. Which of the following statements regarding Occupational Safety and Health Administration (OSHA) standards is accurate?
   a. The standards are established to protect the dentist.
   b. They mandate that employees be offered the HIV vaccine.
   c. They include engineering and work practice controls.
   d. They do not impose financial penalties.

3. Which of the following statements regarding informed consent information for endodontic therapy is accurate?
   a. It must be freely given.
   b. It includes prognosis for the recommended treatment and also the alternatives.
   c. It includes the opportunity to ask questions.
   d. All the above statements are accurate.

4. Which of the following statements regarding radiation exposure from a single, full-mouth survey is accurate?
   a. It is half that of a single chest film.
   b. It is comparable to a barium study of the intestines.
   c. It would be sufficient to cause skin cancer if all exposures were at one site.

5. While exposing films, dental personnel should do which of the following?
   a. Stand back at least 6 feet in an area that is 90 to 135 degrees from the beam
   b. Stand behind a plaster, cinderblock, or 1-inch drywall barrier
   c. Wear a lead apron

6. The recommended antibiotics for a patient with a total joint replacement who is allergic to penicillin or cephalosporin is which of the following?
   a. Amoxicillin
   b. Erythromycin
   c. Clindamycin
   d. Tetracycline

7. The most effective method for controlling pain that often occurs after cleaning and shaping is to administer which of the following?
   a. Analgesic shortly before the procedure
   b. Equal amounts of the analgesic before and during the procedure
   c. Analgesic at the conclusion of the procedure
   d. Analgesic with instructions to the patient to take if necessary

8. Which of the following statements regarding the long-cone paralleling technique is accurate?
   a. It minimizes distortion of tooth dimension.
   b. It minimizes superimposition of the infraorbital rim for maxillary molars.

   c. It requires the film be placed directly touching the tooth without bending the film.

9. Radiographic contrast can be directly affected by altering which of the following?
   a. Milliamperage
   b. Exposure time
   c. Kilovoltage
   d. Angulation

10. An advantage of digitized radiography in endodontic treatment is which of the following?
    a. Image quality is better for working length radiographs.
    b. X-ray generating source is not required.
    c. Radiation exposure is reduced.

11. In which of the following situations is a rubber dam not placed?
    a. When the clamp impinges on the gingiva, causing discomfort
    b. When the chamber or canal may be difficult to locate on access
    c. When the tooth is rotated, preventing placement of a clamp on the indicated tooth
    d. None; there are no situations in which a rubber dam is not placed.

12. To enhance crown preparation and retention when an infrabony defect exists, crown lengthening is completed by which of the following?
    a. Electrosurgery
    b. Gingivectomy
    c. Laser surgery
    d. Apically positioned flap, reverse bevel

13. Of the following, which statement accurately describes radiograph units?
    a. It should be optimally capable of using 70 kVp.
    b. It should be pointed (i.e., cone) in shape.
    c. It should be collimated to reduce exposure level, not to exceed 7 cm at the skin surface.
    d. It should have a filtration equivalent of 10 mm of aluminum.

14. With the cone moved to the distal and directed toward the mesial, which of the following accurately describes the mesiobuccal root of the first molar?
    a. It is projected mesially on the film.
    b. It is projected distally on the film.
    c. It does not move.
    d. It is projected lingually on the film.

15. The cone angulation in the following illustration is which of the following?

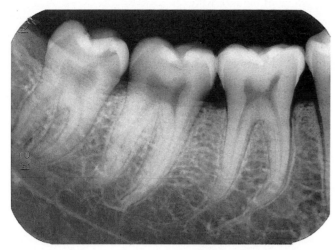

   a. Mesial
   b. Distal
   c. Parallel
   d. Bisecting

16. The radiopaque structure overlying the buccal roots in the following illustration is which of the following?

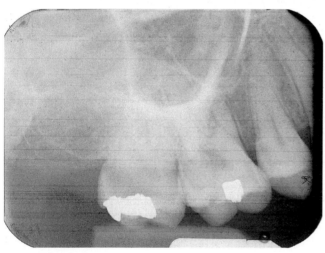

   a. Zygoma
   b. Floor of the maxillary sinus
   c. Coronoid process
   d. Eyeglass frame

17. Which of the following is the best way to "move" the structure in the previous illustration away from the buccal apexes of both molars? Reposition the cone
   a. Inferiorly (i.e., decrease the vertical angle)
   b. Superiorly (i.e., increase the vertical angle)
   c. Mesially (i.e., the beam is directed more distally)
   d. Distally (i.e., the beam is directed more mesially)

18. Why does the tooth in the following illustration appear elongated?

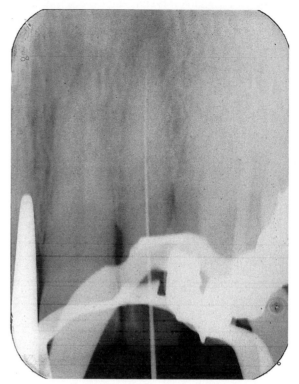

   a. There was excessive, positive-and-vertical angle to the cone.
   b. There was insufficient, positive-and-vertical angle to the cone.
   c. The film was not parallel to the tooth.
   d. The film was bent.

19. The radiopaque structure (*arrow*) in the following illustration is which of the following?

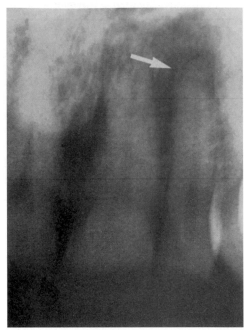

    a. Condensing osteitis
    b. Trabeculation
    c. Lamina dura
    d. Root surface

20. The view in the following radiograph is a mesially angled (beam is directed distally) film. The unobturated root is which of the following?

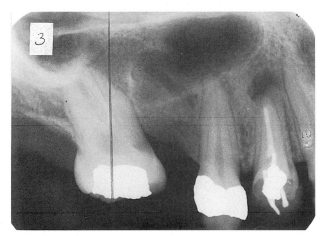

    a. Buccal root
    b. Lingual root

21. Of the following, the best way to identify the source of the radiolucency (*arrow*) in the following illustration is which of the following?

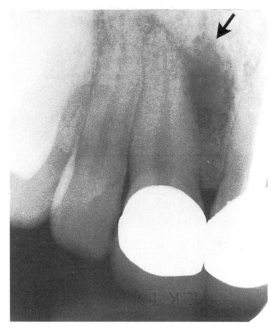

    a. Pulp test
    b. Incisional biopsy
    c. Excisional biopsy
    d. Observation over time to evaluate for changes

CHAPTER 6: ARMAMENTARIUM AND STERILIZATION

1. The patient is exposed to the least amount of radiation when which of the following is used?
    a. Digital imaging
    b. Ektaspeed film
    c. Ultraspeed film

2. Patients with a latex allergy can be treated how?
    a. Safely without a rubber dam
    b. With a rubber dam if there is no direct skin contact
    c. With a nonlatex, rubber dam

3. The temporary restorative material, Cavit, is which of the following?
    a. Type of zinc oxide–eugenol (ZOE) material
    b. Superior to other materials in *in vitro* resistance to bacterial leakage
    c. Prepared by mixing a powder and liquid
    d. More durable than intermediate restorative material (IRM) or composite

4. The best way to clean dental instruments before sterilization is by which of the following?
   a. Ultrasonic cleaning for 5 minutes in a perforated basket
   b. Hand scrubbing, using a brush and heavy rubber gloves
   c. Rinsing under a forceful water spray

5. Steam sterilization is achieved when the load has reached which of the following?
   a. 250° C for 15 minutes
   b. 250° F for 15 minutes
   c. 250° C for 30 minutes
   d. 250° F for 30 minutes

6. An advantage of rapid-steam autoclave over traditional autoclave is which of the following?
   a. Rapid-steam autoclave will not corrode steel instruments.
   b. Rapid-steam autoclave is safe for all types of materials.
   c. Instruments do not have to be air dried at the end of the cycle.
   d. Rapid-steam autoclave has a shorter sterilization cycle than traditional autoclave.

7. Of the following, which statement accurately describes a chemical vapor sterilizer?
   a. It uses a reusable chemical.
   b. It requires adequate ventilation in the area where it is used.
   c. It achieves sterilization when heated to 270° F at 20 psi for 10 minutes.
   d. It does not destroy heat-sensitive materials.

8. An approved method for reducing microorganisms in water output from dental units is which of the following?
   a. Filters at the water source
   b. Flushing the water line before attaching it to the hand piece or syringe
   c. Retrograde (i.e., reverse) flushing of all water lines
   d. Careful sterilization of water lines within hand pieces and syringes between patients
   e. Installation of sterile water delivery systems

9. Gutta-percha is best sterilized by which of the following?
   a. Immersion in full-strength sodium hypochlorite
   b. Immersion in rubbing alcohol
   c. Dry heat
   d. Bead sterilizer

10. The effect of sterilization on endodontic files is which of the following?
    a. Negative and proportional to the number of times sterilized
    b. Neutral; no effect is seen on physical properties
    c. Positive; it restores to the files flexibility lost over time

11. The most reliable agent for destroying microorganisms is which of the following?
    a. Chemical sterilizing agents
    b. Hot water
    c. Ultrasonics
    d. X-ray irradiation
    e. Heat

12. A good, two-stage technique (i.e., two burs in sequence) for access through a porcelain fixed-to-metal crown is which of the following?
    a. Stainless steel (SS), round-diamond, coated fissure
    b. Diamond-coated, round-carbide, end-cutting fissure
    c. SS fissure, carbide, end-cutting fissure
    d. carbide, round-diamond, coated, round fissure
    e. SS, round-carbide, end-cutting fissure

13. An advantage that nickel titanium (NiTi) has over SS for intracanal instruments is which of the following?
    a. Lower cost
    b. More resistance to breakage
    c. Sharper
    d. More uniform in shape
    e. More flexibility

CHAPTER 7: TOOTH MORPHOLOGY AND CAVITY PREPARATION

1. Which of the following statements describes dens-en-dente?
   a. It occurs primarily in maxillary, lateral, incisor teeth.
   b. It requires the use of a long-shank bur for access because the pulp chamber is located in the middle portion of the root.
   c. It results in an untreatable, periodontal pocket.
   d. It produces an evagination of dentin and enamel in mandibular premolars.

2. The incidence of three roots and three canals in maxillary first premolars is which of the following?
   a. Less than 1%
   b. 3%
   c. 6%
   d. 10%

3. Vertucci noted in maxillary second premolars which of the following?
   a. When two canals were present and join at the apex, the lingual canal is the straightest.
   b. The incidence of two canals at the apex was high, approaching 75%.
   c. The incidence of accessory canals found in the furcation was 59%.
   d. Histologically, calcification correlated with the radiographic narrowing of the canal space.

4. In their study of maxillary molars, Kulild and Peters noted which of the following?
   a. Although two canals were often present in the mesiobuccal roots, the canals merged apically.
   b. The use of magnification did not increase the number of canals found clinically in this tooth group.
   c. The orifice to a second canal in the mesiobuccal root was distal to the main orifice in a line connecting the mesiobuccal canal to the palatal canal.
   d. A high incidence of two canals with separate foramina in the mesiobuccal root (71%).

5. When treating a mandibular incisor with two canals evident on the preoperative radiograph, which of the following statements are true?
   a. The internal morphology of the canals will be ribbon shaped.
   b. A facial-access opening might be considered.
   c. The canals often remain separate and distinct throughout the root.
   d. The access opening should be triangular with the apex at the cingulum.

6. Which of the following teeth is most likely to exhibit C-shaped morphology?
   a. Maxillary first premolar
   b. Maxillary first molar
   c. Mandibular first premolar
   d. Mandibular first molar

7. In their study of mandibular molars, Skidmore and Bjorndal noted which of the following?
   a. The access opening should be rectangular.
   b. When there were two canals in the distal root, they remained distinct with separate apical foramina.
   c. The incidence of four canals was over 50%.
   d. The mesiobuccal canal was located under the mesiobuccal cusp tip and exhibited the straightest morphology.

8. The mandibular, second molar should be restored with a crown after endodontic treatment for which of the following reasons?
   a. The pulp chamber is relatively large in comparison to the crown, making the tooth susceptible to fracture.
   b. The tooth is in close to the insertion of the muscles of mastication, and the percentage of preexisting fractures is high.
   c. There is a tendency for the buccal cusps to shear off under occlusal loading.
   d. Providing a post can be placed in the distal root to strengthen the root.

9. Which of the following statements regarding the mandibular, second molar exhibiting a C-shaped morphology is correct?
   a. The root morphology varies with two separate-and-distinct roots being a common finding.
   b. Research indicates that the presence of a C-shaped canal is most common in Caucasians.
   c. The C-shaped molar exhibits a ribbon-shaped orifice with a 180-degree arc beginning in the mesiobuccal area and forming an arch extending lingually to the distobuccal.
   d. The mesiolingual canal is often noted to be separate and distinct, exhibiting a separate foramen.

10. A 30-year-old male patient is being treated for a maxillary central incisor that he traumatized as a teenager. Radiographically, the canal appears calcified and there is evidence of apical pathosis. After attempting access the canal cannot be located despite drilling into the middle third of the root. Which of the following statements regarding further treatment is false?
   a. Radiographs may indicate the orientation of the access opening within the root.
   b. The risk of perforation will be greatest on the lingual surface, should the clinician continue.
   c. The clinician should consider obturating the coronal segment and performing root end surgery.
   d. Because canals become less calcified as they proceed apically, a pathfinder might be used to negotiate the residual canal space.

CHAPTER 8: CLEANING AND SHAPING THE ROOT CANAL SYSTEM

1. Which of the following statements regarding shaping procedures is false?
   a. Shaping is performed after cleaning of the apical one third of the canal to ensure patency.
   b. Shaping facilitates placement of instruments to the working length by increasing the coronal taper.
   c. Shaping permits the a more accurate assessment of the apical, cross-sectional canal diameter.
   d. Shaping is a necessary procedure because calcification occurs from the coronal portion of the canal to the apex.

2. Which of the following statements best describes the Profile Series 29 files?
   a. The Profile Series 29 files conform to the International Standards Organization (ISO) specifications for instrument design.
   b. The instruments exhibit a constant percentage change between successive instruments.
   c. The Profile Series 29 files were designed to facilitate preparation of the coronal portion of the radicular space.
   d. The instruments are most useful in the larger sizes because there is a smaller change in diameter between the files.

3. Each of the following are direct advantages of pre-enlarging the radicular space, *except for one*. Which is the *exception*?
   a. It provides better tactile control of instruments when negotiating a small, curved canal.
   b. It removes the bulk of tissue and contaminants before apical preparation.
   c. It facilitates obturation.
   d. It provides a reservoir for the irrigant.

4. The result of root canal treatment in establishing patency is which of the following?
   a. It revents procedural errors, such as canal blockage and transportation.
   b. It causes irritation of the periodontal attachment apparatus and increased postoperative pain.
   c. It enlarges the apical terminus and increases the potential for extrusion of obturating materials.
   d. It requires insertion of a file 1.0 to 2.0 mm beyond the canal terminus.

5. Which of the following statements regarding gauging and tuning is correct?
   a. Gauging is performed in the coronal portion of the canal to confirm the coronal enlargement is complete.
   b. Tuning identifies the most apical, cross-sectional diameter of the canal.
   c. Gauging and tuning verify the completed shaping of the apical portion of the canal.
   d. Gauging and tuning produces a uniform, cylindric diameter to the canal in the apical 2 to 3 mm that enhances obturation and sealing.

6. Which of the following statements best describes the Quantec files?
   a. The instruments have a constant helical angle and three flutes.
   b. The recommended rotational speed is 1000 to 2000 RPM.
   c. The instruments exhibit a constant rate of taper along their length.
   d. The instruments exhibit varied tapers with a constant D_0 diameter of 0.25 mm.

7. Which of the following statements regarding the use of chelating agents in canal preparation is correct?
   a. Aqueous solutions are preferred to viscous suspensions in canal preparation.
   b. Viscous suspensions are more effective in preventing accumulation of tissue and dentinal debris.
   c. Viscous suspensions contain the highest concentration of ethylenediaminetetracitic acid (EDTA) and are most effective in removing the smear layer.
   d. Aqueous solutions are most efficient as lubricants and, therefore, preferred to viscous suspensions during canal preparation.
   e. EDTA, in concert with sodium hypochlorite, causes a nascent release of oxygen, which kills anaerobic organisms.

8. Which of the following statements regarding an endogram is false?
   a. An endogram would provide information on the extent of internal resorptive lesion.
   b. The visualization of fractures and leaking restorations is attributed to the incorporation of Hypaque in the irrigating solution.
   c. Conventional radiography and digital radiography may both be used in producing an endogram.
   d. The endogram is used to confirm the correct working length.

9. During the early phase of root canal preparation, which of the following is true?
   a. The initial scouter file that moves easily through the canal should be advanced to the estimated working length.
   b. The initial scouter file may not advance to the estimated working length because of the rate of instrument taper.
   c. The initial scouter file should be advanced with a reciprocating action using apical pressure when resistance is encountered.
   d. The initial scouter file is used before the introduction of a viscous chelator in cases exhibiting vital tissue.

10. Which of the following statements is correct regarding coronal canal preparation in endodontic treatment?
    a. Nickel-and-titanium (NiTi) rotary instruments are preferred to Gates-Glidden (GG) drills because they remove dentin uniformly from the canal wall.
    b. NiTi rotary instruments are best used in a step-back fashion.
    c. Both GG drills and NiTi rotary instruments should be used large to small, because this develops a preparation that is centered in the root.
    d. GG drills used in a step-back technique can relocate the canal away from the furcal wall.

11. When using the balanced-force technique for canal preparation, which of the following statements is accurate?
    a. The cutting stroke involves apical pressure and a counterclockwise rotation.
    b. Clockwise rotation balances the tendency of the file to be drawn into the canal during the cutting stroke.
    c. Dentin is engaged with a counterclockwise rotation and cut with a 45- to 90-degree, clockwise rotation.
    d. It requires the use of a crown down technique.

12. Extending a no. 10 file with a 0.02 taper 1.0 mm beyond the apical foramen will result in which of the following?
    a. It opens the apical foramen to a minimum diameter of 0.12 mm.
    b. It increases postoperative discomfort to occlusal forces.
    c. It reduces the percentage of change from a no. 10 file to a no. 15 file by 50%.
    d. It eliminates the natural constriction of the foramen and increases the chance for an overfill.

CHAPTER 9: OBTURATION OF THE CLEANED AND SHAPED ROOT CANAL SYSTEM

1. Of the following, the least important determinant of root canal treatment success is which of the following?
   a. Proper placed restoration after root canal treatment
   b. Healthy periodontium
   c. Three-dimensional (3-D) obturation of the root canal system

2. Paraformaldehyde-containing obturating materials result in which of the following?
   a. Eliminate bacteria that remains in the canals
   b. Mummify tissue remnants in the canals
   c. Reduce posttreatment pain
   d. Are below the standard of care for root canal treatment

3. It is preferable to not extrude sealer beyond the apex for which of the following reasons?
   a. The sealer usually does not resorb.
   b. The sealer often stains or tattoos the tissue.
   c. The sealer is a tissue irritant and may delay healing.
   d. The sealer promotes bacterial growth.

4. Gutta-percha in contact with connective tissue is which of the following?
   a. Relatively inert
   b. Immunogenic
   c. Unstable
   d. Carcinogenic

5. The primary reason to use a sealer and cement is which of the following?
   a. Attainment of an impervious seal
   b. Canal disinfection
   c. Lubrication of the master cone
   d. Adhesion to dentin
   e. All of the above

6. Considering lateral versus vertical condensation, studies have shown which of the following?
   a. Lateral condensation results in a better seal.
   b. Vertical condensation results in a better seal.
   c. Both consistently fill lateral canals.
   d. Sealability with either largely depends on the shape of the prepared canal.

7. A problem with nickel-and-titanium (NiTi) spreaders is which of the following?
   a. Tendency to buckle under compaction pressure
   b. Tendency to break during condensation
   c. Creation of greater wedging forces, leading to root fracture
   d. They do not penetrate as deeply as stainless steel (SS) spreaders under equal force

8. Moderate extrusion of obturating materials beyond the apex is undesirable because of which of the following?
   a. There is more likelihood of postoperative discomfort.
   b. Sealer and gutta-percha cause a severe, inflammatory reaction in periradicular tissue.
   c. The prognosis is poorer.
   d. All of the above

9. In which of the following is one-visit root canal treatment not recommended?
   a. The pulp is necrotic and not symptomatic.
   b. The pulp is necrotic and symptomatic.
   c. The pulp is necrotic and there is a draining sinus tract.
   d. The pulp is vital and symptomatic.

10. When is an application of heater-injected gutta-percha potentially beneficial?
    a. When there is an open apex
    b. When there are aberrations or irregularities of the canal
    c. When the clinician cannot master lateral condensation
    d. When the canals are curved and small after preparation

11. Which of the following statements accurately describe an adequate apical seal?
    a. It can only be achieved with lateral condensation.
    b. It depends on placing the compacting instrument close to the apical terminus.
    c. It can be achieved in small, nontapering canal preparations.

12. Which of the following statements accurately describe the continuous-wave technique?
    a. It uses a heat carrier that can both compact and heat gutta-percha.
    b. It is superior to other warm-compaction techniques.
    c. It has been shown to provide a better prognosis than cold-compaction techniques.
    d. It has been shown to have no adverse effects on the periodontium.

13. An advantage of the continuous-wave technique over warm, vertical compaction is which of the following?
    a. The continuous-wave technique is faster.
    b. The continuous-wave technique adapts better to canal irregularities.
    c. The continuous-wave technique is not technique sensitive.
    d. No special devices are necessary.

14. The most likely cause of a gross overfill is which of the following?
    a. Lack of an apical seat or stop
    b. Use of excessive amounts of sealer
    c. Use of excessive apical pressure on the spreader
    d. Use of a master cone that is too small

15. The obturation of the incisor shown in the following illustration is inadequate because of which of the following?

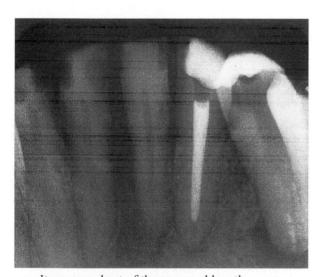

    a. It appears short of the prepared length.
    b. There is variable radiodensity (i.e., incomplete condensation) throughout its length.
    c. There is a space between the temporary restoration and the gutta-percha.
    d. The diagnosis was pulp necrosis and chronic apical periodontitis; the canal should be filled to the apical foramen.

16. The dark tooth in the following illustration has a history of trauma and root canal treatment. It is likely that the discoloration is primarily caused by which of the following?

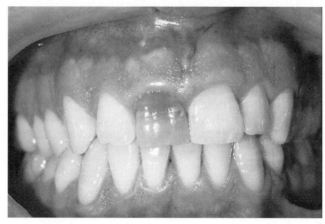

    a. Remnants of necrotic tissue
    b. A leaking restoration
    c. Blood pigments in the dentinal tubules
    d. Obturating materials not removed from the chamber

17. Of the following, what is the most likely cause of failure of root canal treatment on the lateral incisor in the illustration?

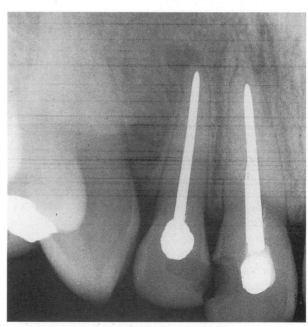

    a. The silver point corrodes.
    b. The canal is filled too close to the apex.
    c. There is coronal leakage.
    d. The silver point does not adapt to the prepared space.

CHAPTER 10: RECORDS AND LEGAL RESPONSIBILITIES

1. Concerning making changes in a patient record, which of the following statements is accurate?
   a. Any changes are forbidden.
   b. Deletions are permitted if erased completely as soon as they occur.
   c. Corrections are permitted, if dated.

2. Standard of care, as defined by the courts, is which of the following?
   a. Requires absolute perfection
   b. Describes what any careful-and-prudent clinician would do under similar circumstances
   c. Does not allow for individual variations of treatment
   d. Is equivalent to customary practice

3. The doctrine of informed consent does not require which of the following?
   a. Patients to be advised of reasonably foreseeable risks of treatment
   b. Patients to be advised of reasonable alternatives
   c. Patients forfeit their right to do as they see fit with their body.
   d. Patients be advised of the consequences of nontreatment.

4. Which of the following statements accurately describe a periodontal examination of a patient referred for endodontic treatment?
   a. It should performed on the entire dentition.
   b. It must be performed at least on the tooth to be treated.
   c. It is necessary only if there is evidence of periodontal disease.
   d. It is necessary only if requested by the referring dentist.

5. A dentist may legally do which of the following?
   a. Refuse to treat a new patient, despite severe pain and infection
   b. Be bound to see a former patient on recall after treatment is completed
   c. Discharge a patient from the practice at any time
   d. Refuse to treat a patient who has an outstanding account balance

6. If a patient with human immunodeficiency virus (HIV) requests that the dentist not inform the staff of the condition, the dentist should do which of the following?
   a. Refuse to treat the patient
   b. Tell the staff in private, and then treat the patient with extra precautions
   c. Not tell the staff but treat the patient with great caution
   d. Not tell the staff and require the patient to assume liability should anyone contract the virus

7. A specialist may be held liable if which of the following occurs?
   a. Informs the patient that the general practitioner performed substandard care
   b. Fails to disclose to the patient or referring dentist evident pathosis on teeth other than those the specialist is treating
   c. Fails to locate a small canal that is not evident radiographically
   d. Mistakenly initiates treatment on the wrong tooth in a difficult diagnostic situation

8. Of the following, which is the best way for clinicians to avoid legal actions by patients?
   a. Tell patients they have no malpractice insurance.
   b. Attend continuing education courses to remain informed of current techniques.
   c. Refer all major patient complaints to peer review.
   d. Demonstrate genuine interest in the welfare of the patient.

9. Computerized treatment records may not be signed electronically.
   a. True
   b. False

10. Suing to collect fees is a proven route to being counter sued for malpractice.
    a. True
    b. False

11. Standard of care for routine endodontics is set by which of the following?
    a. The state's dental licensing agency
    b. Endodontists
    c. The community of general dentists

12. A patient continues to have pain after a dentist uses the technique of Paraformaldehyde paste pulpotomy on a tooth with a necrotic pulp and apical pathosis and then places a crown. In this situation, which of the following statements is true?
    a. The dentist is liable for malpractice because unacceptable treatment procedures were followed.
    b. The dentist is not liable if the patient is now referred to the appropriate specialist who can treat the case.
    c. The dentist is not liable if the dentist performs additional treatment for no fee.

CHAPTER 11: STRUCTURE AND FUNCTIONS OF THE DENTIN AND PULP COMPLEX

1. In the process of tooth development, which of the following statements are true?
   a. The basement membrane separating the inner dental epithelium from the dental mesenchyme is composed of type I and III collagen.
   b. Blood vessels become established in the dental papilla during the cap stage.
   c. Mature ameloblasts appear before odontoblasts mature. However, the formation of enamel takes place following the deposition of dentin.
   d. Type II collagen mRNA increases with odontoblastic differentiation.
   e. Ameloblasts form enamel spindles near the future dentinoenamel junction (DEJ).

2. von Korff fibers are best described as which of the following?
   a. The first-formed collagen fibers formed between pre-odontoblasts.
   b. Unmyelinated sensory fibers in the cell-free zone of Weil
   c. Odontoblastic processes interposed between ameloblasts
   d. Silver-stained ground substance located between odontoblasts

3. Which of the following statements regarding root development is false?
   a. Root development begins after completion of enamel formation.
   b. The inner epithelium, the stellate reticulum, and outer enamel epithelium form Hertwig's epithelial root sheath.
   c. The dental sac disintegrates upon induction of dentin formation and remnants persist as the Epithelial Rests of Malassez.
   d. Accessory canals in the root are formed when there is discontinuity in the root sheath.

4. Which of the following statements regarding dentin is correct?
   a. Mantle dentin is the first formed dentin and has collagen fibers that run perpendicular to the DEJ.
   b. Dentin deposited after eruption is termed secondary dentin.
   c. Dentinal tubules make up 50% of the dentin volume and they exhibit extensive terminal ramifications.
   d. Calcification of dentin results in an organic component composed of noncollagenous matrix components.

5. Which of the following statements regarding the tubular structure of dentin is correct?
   a. Peritubular dentin and intertubular dentin are the same composition, except for the fact peritubular dentin lines the tubule.
   b. Peritubular dentin has a lower-collagen content when compared to intertubular dentin and is more susceptible to removal by acids.
   c. Intertubular dentin is more highly mineralized when compared to peritubular dentin.
   d. Peritubular dentin defines the tubule size and is common to all mammals.

6. Which of the following statements regarding dentin permeability is true?
   a. Remains constant regardless of the depth of a cavity preparation because of a pulpal tissue pressure of 10.3 mm Hg
   b. Increases as the pulp and dentin border is approached (primarily because the tubular surface area increases)
   c. Is lower in radicular dentin because of tubular sclerosis
   d. Increases near the pulp and dentin border as the hydrostatic pressure in the tubules decreases

7. Which of the following statements regarding tight junctions in the odontoblastic layer is true?
   a. They regulate permeability of extracellular substances between the odontoblastic layer and the predentin.
   b. They permit low-resistance pathways for electrical excitation when the odontoblastic process is distorted.
   c. They provide a mechanism for intracellular materials to be exchanged.
   d. They are infrequent but when found are located in the basal portion of the cells.

8. Which of the following statements regarding production of collagen by the odontoblast is correct?
   a. Type I collagen is manufactured in the cellular cytoplasm, packaged by the Golgi complex, and released by reverse pinocytosis.
   b. Tropocollagen is synthesized in the rough endoplasmic reticulum (RER) and packaged in the Golgi complex. Vesicles consisting of collagen fibrils migrate into the odontoblastic process and are released.
   c. The Golgi complex packages collagen precursors (e.g., proline) into vesicles that are released into the predentin. These then precipitate to form tropocollagen and, eventually, collagen fibrils.
   d. Synthesis begins in the RER with procollagen being packaged in the Golgi complex. Vesicles are formed and release tropocollagen in the predentin matrix.

9. Which of the following statements regarding dendritic cells is false?
   a. Dendritic cells are similar to Langerhans' cells and play a significant role in induction of T-cell immunity.
   b. Although not normally present in the healthy pulp, dendritic cells appear during inflammation and, like macrophages, are phagocytic.
   c. Considered accessory cells, the dendritic cell participates in antigen recognition and presentation.
   d. Dendritic cells are primarily found in lymphoid tissues.

10. Which of the following statements regarding the extracellular matrix of the pulp is false?
    a. The extracellular matrix changes with eruption of the tooth as the chrondroitin sulfate concentration decreases and the hyaluronic acid and dermatan sulfate fractions increase.
    b. The proteoglycans regulate the dispersion of interstitial solutes.
    c. The state of polymerization of the ground substance regulates osmotic pressures.
    d. The water content of the extracellular matrix is relatively low, giving the tissue a colloidal consistency and limiting movement of components within the tissue.

11. Teeth with immature root development often are unresponsive to electrical pulp testing because which of the following?
    a. Myelinated fibers are the last structures to appear in the developing pulp.
    b. Predentin and intratubular fibers are not present until root formation is complete.
    c. There is a relative hypoxic condition of the pulp during developmental glycolysis.
    d. Electrical stimulation of autonomic fibers decreases blood flow and depresses A-delta fiber activity.

12. Each of the following statements support the hydrodynamic theory for pain, *except for one*. Which is the *exception*?
    a. Odontoblasts have a low-membrane potential and do not respond to electrical stimulation.
    b. Placement of local anesthetics on dentin does not alter the pain response.
    c. There is a positive correlation between fluid movement in the tubules and the discharge of intradental nerves.
    d. Forty percent of the tubules in the area of pulp horns contain intratubular nerve endings.
    e. The presence of a smear layer decreases dentinal sensitivity.

13. Which of the following statements regarding a patient that has a sharp, short sensation to cold that resolves immediately with removal of the stimulus is correct?
    a. The patient's response indicates inflammation and tissue damage.
    b. A-delta and C fibers are responsible for the painful sensation.
    c. A-delta and A-beta fibers are being stimulated.
    d. C-fibers are responding to the release of inflammatory mediators, such as bradykinin and substance P.

14. Which of the following statements regarding pulpal blood flow is correct?
    a. Blood flow within the pulp is homogenous with arteriovenous anastomoses maintaining an even flow.
    b. Unmyelinated, sympathetic fibers innervating the arterioles and venules produce vasoconstriction.
    c. The pulpal blood flow is the highest of oral tissues because of the relatively high metabolic activity of the pulp.
    d. Accessory and lateral canals provide adequate collateral circulation.

15. Which of the following statements outlines the most significant factor influencing the pulp's response to injury and compromised healing?
    a. Inflammatory cells, such as polymorphonuclear leukocytes and B-lymphocytes, are not found in the normal pulp.
    b. There is a lack of a collateral circulation.
    c. Odontoblasts are end line cells incapable of replication.
    d. The fact that the pulp may not have a lymphatic system.
    e. The environment of the dental pulp is low compliant.

16. Which of the following statements regarding age changes in the pulp are false?
    a. There is a decrease in the cellularity and collagenous fibers, especially in the radicular pulp.
    b. Odontoblasts decrease in size and may disappear completely in some areas, particularly the pulpal floor of multirooted teeth.
    c. There is a reduction in the nerves and vasculature of the pulp.
    d. There is an increase in peritubular dentin.
    e. The pulp demonstrates an increased resistance to the action of proteolytic enzymes.

CHAPTER 12: PATHOBIOLOGY OF THE PERIAPEX

1. Inflammation of the periapical tissue is sustained by which of the following?
   a. Stagnant tissue fluid
   b. Necrotic tissue
   c. Microorganisms
   d. All of the above

2. Acute, apical periodontitis is characterized by which of the following?
   a. A focus of neutrophils within the lesion
   b. A focus of granulomatous tissue in the lesion
   c. A focus of lymphocytes, plasma cells, and macrophages in the lesion

3. A periapical, true cyst communicates with the root canal; however, a periapical-pocket cyst does not.
   a. True
   b. False

4. The most important route of bacteria into the dental pulp is from which of the following?
   a. The general circulation via anachoresis
   b. Exposure to the oral cavity via caries
   c. The gingival sulcus

5. The least important factor influencing the pathogenicity of endodontic flora is which of the following?
   a. Microbial interaction
   b. Endotoxins released after bacterial death
   c. Exotoxins released by living bacteria
   d. Enzymes produced by bacteria

6. Which of the following statements regarding neutrophils is accurate?
   a. They are nonspecific phagocytes.
   b. They have a single pathway for intracellular killing.
   c. They are mobilized primarily to neutralize bacterial endotoxins.
   d. All of the above are accurate.

7. Which of the following statements regarding T-lymphocytes are accurate?
   a. They are thyroid-derived cells.
   b. They concentrate in the cortical area of lymph nodes and also circulate in the blood.
   c. They are responsible for the cell-mediated arm of the immune system.
   d. All of the above statements are accurate.

8. Which of the following statements regarding B-lymphocytes are accurate?
   a. They were originally discovered in an avian gut-associated organ.
   b. They account for the majority of circulating lymphocytes.
   c. They produce antibodies.
   d. All of the above statements are accurate.

9. The function(s) of macrophages include(s) which of the following?
   a. Phagocytosis of microorganisms
   b. Removal of small foreign particles
   c. Antigen processing and presentation
   d. All of the above

10. Which of the following statements regarding osteocytes is accurate?
    a. They originate as monocytes in the blood.
    b. They respond only to mediators released by osteoblasts.
    c. They are mononuclear cells capable of bone demineralization.
    d. They form a ruffled border away from the bone surface.

11. Which of the following statements regarding acute apical periodontitis is accurate?
    a. It is limited to the periodontal ligament (histologically).
    b. It is detectable radiographically.
    c. It may heal if induced by a noninfectious agent.
    d. All of the above statements are accurate.

12. Which of the following statements regarding chronic, apical periodontitis is accurate?
    a. It is a neutrophil-dominated lesion encapsulated in a collagenous connective tissue.
    b. It may contain epithelial arcardes or rings.
    c. It represents a continuous, slow process that is asymptomatic.
    d. It as a predominance of B-cells over T-cells.

13. Which of the following statements regarding cholesterol crystals is accurate?
    a. They may induce granulomatous lesions.
    b. They are potentially associated with nonresolving apical periodontitis.
    c. They are difficult for macrophages and multinucleated giant cells to remove.
    d. All of the above statements are accurate.

14. Which of the following statements regarding periapical actinomycosis is accurate?
    a. It is caused by gram-negative organisms exhibiting branching filaments that end in clubs or hyphae.
    b. It is a fungal disease characterized by filamentous colonies called sulphur granules.
    c. It is most commonly an endodontic infection resulting from dental caries.
    d. All of the above statements are accurate.

15. Extraradicular infections are not found in which of the following?
    a. Solid, apical granulomas
    b. Periapical-pocket cysts with cavities open to the root canal
    c. Periapical actinomycosis
    d. Acute, apical periodontitis

**CHAPTER 13: ENDODONTIC MICROBIOLOGY
AND TREATMENT OF INFECTIONS**

1. Pulpal and periradicular pathosis results primarily from which of the following?
   a. Traumatic injury caused by heat during cavity preparation
   b. Bacterial invasion
   c. Toxicity of dental materials
   d. Immunologic reactions

2. Which of the following statements regarding the organism producing pulpal pathosis is correct?
   a. The organisms are primarily facultative streptococci.
   b. Single isolates (i.e., monoinfection) produce the most severe reactions.
   c. Isolates tend to be polymicrobial and anaerobic.
   d. Organisms infecting the pulp tend to be aerobic, compared to organisms infecting the periapex.

3. Which of the following best describes anachoresis?
   a. The attraction of bloodborne microorganisms to inflamed tissue during a bacteremia
   b. The process of carious invasion, cavitation, and exposure of the pulp from bacteria
   c. Bacteria located in dentinal tubules, and the pulp that are seeded to the systemic circulation, inducing disease in other areas of the body

4. Which of the following statements regarding strict anaerobes is accurate?
   a. They are missing enzymes, catalase, and superoxide dismutase.
   b. They function best at high oxidation–reduction potentials.
   c. They can grow in the presence of oxygen.
   d. All of the above statements are accurate.

5. The most common black-pigmented bacteria cultivated from endodontic infections is which of the following?
   a. Bacteroides melaninogaster
   b. Fusobacterium nucleatum
   c. Prevotella nigrescens
   d. Porphyromonas intermedia

6. Treatment of actinomycosis israelii may include which of the following?
   a. Root canal treatment
   b. Root end surgery
   c. Antibiotics
   d. All of the above

7. Which is true regarding microbial virulence factors?
   a. Fimbriae assist in bacterial aggregation.
   b. Pili break off and form extracellular vesicles filled with enzymes.
   c. Lipopolysaccharides is found in the liposomes of gram-positive bacteria.
   d. All of the above.

8. Which of the following statements regarding polyamines is accurate?
   a. They are produced by bacteria and host cells.
   b. They may be found in infected root canals.
   c. They are more concentrated in teeth with spontaneous pain.
   d. All of the above statements are accurate.

9. Which of the following statements regarding fascial space infections is accurate?
   a. They are associated with radiographically visible periradicular lesions.
   b. They occur in potential spaces between fascia and underlying tissue.
   c. They occur when a tooth apex is located coronal to a muscle attachment.
   d. All of the above statements are accurate.

10. Which of the following statements regarding Ludwig's angina is accurate?
    a. It involves the submental, sublingual, and submental space of the right or left side.
    b. It can progress into the canine and infraorbital space.
    c. It can result in airway obstruction.
    d. All of the above statements are accurate.

11. Antibiotics are recommended for which of the following?
    a. Sinus tracts
    b. Acute, apical periodontitis
    c. After root end surgery
    d. None of the above

12. Incision and drainage is indicated which of the following?
    a. For sinus tracts
    b. When the swelling is diffuse and indurated
    c. For acute, apical periodontitis
    d. All of the above

13. Incision and drainage of cellulitis is effective because of which of the following?
    a. It provides a pathway of drainage to prevent spread of infection.
    b. It relieves increased tissue pressure.
    c. It provides relief of pain.
    d. It increases circulation to the area and improves delivery of antibiotics.
    e. All of the above statements are accurate.

14. Which of the following statements regarding potassium penicillin V is accurate?
    a. It has a broader spectrum than amoxicillin.
    b. It may be dosed at 4-hour intervals for severe infection.
    c. It will select for resistant organisms, especially in the GI tract.
    d. It has up to a 25% allergy rate.

15. Which of the following statements regarding metronidazole is accurate?
    a. It is effective against facultative and anaerobic bacteria.
    b. It cannot be given with penicillin because of disulfuram reaction.
    c. It cannot be taken with lithium or alcohol.
    d. All of the above statements are accurate.

16. Which of the following statements regarding clindamycin is accurate?
    a. It is an alternative to potassium penicillin V in allergic individuals.
    b. It is effective against facultative and anaerobic bacteria.
    c. It is rarely associated with pseudomembranous colitis in doses recommended for endodontic infections.
    d. All of the above statements are accurate.

17. Which of the following statements regarding the American Heart Association (AHA) guidelines for prophylactic antibiotic coverage is accurate?
    a. They are the standard of care for clinicians.
    b. They are based on controlled clinical studies.
    c. They are not a substitute for clinical judgment.

18. The AHA recommends antibiotic prophylaxis for which of the following?
    a. Surgery
    b. Instrumentation beyond the apex
    c. Periodontal-ligament injection
    d. All of the above

19. Which of the following statements regarding he theory of focal infection is accurate?
    a. It was propounded by Dr. William Hunter in 1910.
    b. It was referred to infections found around poorly made restorations.
    c. It was used to explain diseases for which there was no cure.
    d. It results in needless tooth extraction.
    e. All of the above statements are accurate.

20. Which of the following is correct in relation to the periradicular lesion formed in response to dental caries and subsequent pulp necrosis?
    a. Bacteria are commonly found in the granuloma.
    b. T-helper cells predominate over T-suppressor cells.
    c. Formation of the granuloma is mediated through a specific immunologic response.
    d. The release of interleukins can mediate bone resorption.

CHAPTER 14: INSTRUMENTS, MATERIALS, AND DEVICES

1. Which of the following statements regarding pulp stimulation with cold is accurate?
    a. It is best accomplished with carbon dioxide snow (i.e., dry ice).
    b. It is an accurate assessment of pulp vitality.
    c. It directly stimulates the pain fibers in the pulp.
    d. It is best determined with a blast of air.

2. With regard to electrical pulp testing, which of the following is true?
    a. Positive responses can be used for differential diagnosis of pulp pathosis.
    b. The device uses a pulsating, alternating current with a duration of 1 to 15 ms.
    c. The device uses a low current with a high-potential difference in voltage.
    d. Gingival and periodontal tissues are more sensitive to testing than the pulp.

3. Which of the following statements regarding digital radiographs is accurate?
    a. They are produced by a charged coupled device and do not require x-rays.
    b. They have the advantage of being manipulatable, which facilitates interpretation.
    c. They have greater resolution than traditional film.
    d. They are captured by a sensor that has a greater surface area than traditional film.

4. Which of the following statements regarding nickel and titanium (NiTi) instruments is accurate?
    a. They exhibit a high elastic modulus, which provides flexibility.
    b. When stressed, they exhibit transformation from the austenitic crystalline phase to a martensitic structure.
    c. They cannot be strained to the same level as stainless steel (SS) without permanent deformation.
    d. They are easier to prebend before placement in the canal than SS.

5. A barbed broach is most useful for which of the following?
   a. Removal of cotton, paper points, and other objects from the canal
   b. Removal of vital tissue from fine canals
   c. Initial planing of the canal walls
   d. Coronal-orifice enlargement before establishing the correct working length

6. In comparing K-type files with reamers, which of the following statements regarding K-type files is accurate?
   a. They have more flutes per millimeter, which increase flexibility.
   b. They differ, because the file is manufactured by twisting a tapered, square blank.
   c. They are more effective in removing debris.
   d. They are the least flexible when comparing instruments of the same size.

7. Based on instrument design and method of manufacturing, which of the following is most susceptible to fracture?
   a. K-type file fabricated from tapered, square SS blank
   b. K-flex file fabricated from rhomboidal SS blank
   c. Hedström file fabricated from round SS blank
   d. Reamer fabricated from triangular SS blank

8. Which of the following statements regarding Hedström files are accurate?
   a. They are manufactured by machining a round cross-sectional wire.
   b. They are effective when used in a reaming action.
   c. They are safer than K-type files, because external signs of stress are more visible as changes in flute design.
   d. They are aggressive because of a negative-rake angle that is parallel to the shaft.

9. Which of the following statements regarding the Profile rotary instruments is accurate?
   a. They are used at a range of 1500 to 2000 rpm.
   b. They are NiTi instruments manufactured in half sizes.
   c. They exhibit sizes that are ISO and ANSI standardized.
   d. They incorporate radial lands in the flute design.

10. Which of the following statements regarding the best apex locators is accurate?
    a. They require training with the instrument to become proficient.
    b. They are sensitive to canal contents.
    c. They measure the impedance between the file and the mucosa.
    d. On average, they are accurate to within 0.5 mm of the apex.
    e. All of the above statements are accurate.

11. Piezoelectric, ultrasonic devices differ from magnetostrictive devices in which of the following?
    a. The piezoelectric unit transfers more energy to the files.
    b. The piezoelectric unit produces heat that requires a coolant.
    c. The piezoelectric unit uses a RispiSonic, ShaperSonic, and TrioSonic file system.
    d. The piezoelectric unit vibrates at 2 to 3 kHz.

12. Which of the following statements regarding ultrasonic root canal instrumentation is accurate?
    a. It should be performed in a dry environment.
    b. It poses little risk of file breakage.
    c. It is not very useful for dentin removal.
    d. It is most useful in small canals where file contact with the wall is maximized.

13. Which of the following statements regarding sodium hypochlorite used as a root canal irrigating solution is accurate?
    a. It is buffered to a pH of 12 to 13, which increases toxicity.
    b. It exhibits a chelating action on dentin.
    c. It should be used in higher concentrations because of the increased free chlorine available.
    d. It is a good wetting agent that permits the solution to flow into canal irregularities.

14. When ethylenediaminetetraacetic acid (EDTA) is used as an endodontic irrigant, which of the following statements is accurate?
    a. It must be completely removed after use to prevent continued action and destruction of dentin.
    b. It is a rapid-and-efficient method of removing the smear layer.
    c. It acts on organic-and-inorganic components of the smear layer.
    d. It penetrates deep into dentin and enhances root canal preparation.

15. Calcium hydroxide is advocated as an interappointment medication primarily because of which of the following
    a. Its ability to dissolve necrotic tissue
    b. Its antimicrobial activity
    c. Its ability to stimulate hard-tissue formation
    d. Its ability to temporarily seal the canal

16. Which of the following statements is accurate regarding gutta-percha points is accurate?
    a. They contain 40% to 50% pure gutta-percha.
    b. They adhere to dentin when compacted.
    c. They can be heat sterilized.
    d. They are not compressible.

17. An advantage to AH26 as an endodontic sealer is which of the following?
    a. The release of formaldehyde on setting
    b. Low toxicity
    c. Long working time, but quick setting (i.e., 1 to 2 hours) at body temperature
    d. It can be distinguished from gutta-percha radiographically

18. N2, Endomethasone, and Reibler's paste are sealers that do which of the following?
    a. Produce liquefaction necrosis in the periradicular tissues
    b. Induce healing in the apical pulp wound after vital pulp extirpation
    c. Can cause periapical inflammation
    d. Do not produce a seal when used in combination with a core material

19. Which of the following statements is accurate regarding TERM is accurate?
    a. It seals as well as Cavit.
    b. It is the material of choice when strength is a requirement.
    c. It is a zinc oxide–reinforced material that can be light cured.
    d. It has a eugenol component that is antibacterial.

20. The root end is ultrasonically prepared during endodontic surgery for which of the following reasons?
    a. It results in apical cracks at low settings.
    b. It results in larger, but cleaner, cavity walls.
    c. It can make a deeper cavity more safely than a bur.
    d. It does not require as acute an angle of root resection.

CHAPTER 15: PULPAL REACTION TO CARIES AND DENTAL PROCEDURES

1. The most common response in the dentin deep to caries is which of the following?
   a. Increased permeability
   b. Alteration of collagen
   c. Dissolution of peritubular dentin
   d. Dentinal sclerosis

2. Relatively few bacteria are found in a pulp abscess because of which of the following?
   a. Immune response of pulp tissue
   b. High tissue pH in the adjacent inflammation
   c. Mechanical blockage of sclerotic dentin
   d. Antibacterial products of neutrophils

3. A periodontal ligament injection of 2% lidocaine with 1:100,000 epinephrine causes which of the following?
   a. The pulp circulation ceases for about 30 minutes.
   b. The pulp circulation remains the same.
   c. The pulp circulation increases markedly.
   d. The pulp circulation decreases slightly.

4. The highest incidence of pulp necrosis is associated with which of the following?
   a. Class V preparations on root surface
   b. Inlay preparations
   c. Partial veneer restorations
   d. Full-crown preparations

5. A disadvantage of acid etching dentin (regarding effects on the pulp) is which of the following?
   a. Dentinal tubules are opened, thereby increasing permeability.
   b. Acid penetrates to the pulp and kills large numbers of cells.
   c. Acid penetrates to the pulp and damages the vessels.
   d. Acid softens the dentin and increases microleakage at the restoration dentin interface.

6. The response of the pulp to a recently placed amalgam without a cavity lining is usually which of the following?
   a. Slight-to-moderate inflammation
   b. Moderate-to-severe inflammation
   c. Slight but increasingly severe with time
   d. None

7. The smear layer on dentin walls acts to prevent pulpal injury for which of the following?
   a. It reduces diffusion of toxic substance through the tubules.
   b. It resists the effects of acid etching of the dentin.
   c. It eliminates the need for a cavity liner or base.
   d. Its bactericidal activity acts against oral microorganisms.

8. A reaction that tends to protect the pulp from injury from dentinal caries is which of the following?
   a. A predictable stimulation of sensory nerves resulting in pain
   b. A decrease in permeability of dentin
   c. An increase in numbers of odontoblasts under the tubules affected by the caries
   d. A buffering (i.e., neutralization) by ground substance of bacterial toxins
   e. A decrease in pulpal metabolism

9. Hypersensitivity is best relieved or controlled by which of the following?
   a. Opening the tubules to permit release of intrapulpal pressure
   b. Root planing to remove surface layers that are hypersensitive
   c. Applying antiinflammatory agents to exposed dentin
   d. Blocking exposed tubules on the dentin surface

10. Deeper cavity preparations have more potential for pulpal damage because of which of the following?
    1. Tubule diameter and density increases; therefore there is increasing permeability.
    2. There is more vibration to pulp cells.
    3. Odontoblastic processes are more likely to be severed.
       a. 1 only
       b. 3 only
       c. 1 and 3
       d. 2 and 3
       e. 1 and 2

11. Agents that clean, dry, or sterilize the cavity are which of the following?
    a. Best used in deep cavities
    b. Indicated when a patient reports symptoms
    c. Generally very damaging to the pulp
    d. Generally not useful

12. Of the following, which is the best way to prevent pulp damage during cavity preparation?
    a. Retain the smear layer
    b. Use sharp burs with a brush stroke
    c. Use adequate air coolant
    d. Use adequate water coolant

13. Which is the major reason why Class II restorations with composite are damaging to the pulp?
    a. Microleakage occurs at the occlusal surface.
    b. Microleakage occurs at the gingival margin.
    c. Toxic chemicals are released from the composite and diffuse into the pulp.
    d. Polymerization shrinkage distorts cusps and opens gaps.

14. A pulp has been damaged and is inflamed because of deep caries and cavity preparation. What material placed on the floor of the cavity aids the pulp in resolving the inflammation?
    a. Calcium hydroxide
    b. Zinc oxide–eugenol
    c. Steroid formulations
    d. None; there is no material that promotes healing.

15. A cusp fractures and exposes dentin but not the pulp. What is the probable response in the pulp?
    a. Severe damage with irreversible inflammation
    b. Mild-to-moderate inflammation
    c. Pain but no inflammation
    d. No pulp response

16. The following illustration shows a section of pulp and dentin underlying an area of cavity preparation, which was done 1 day previous. The best description of the pulp reaction is which of the following?

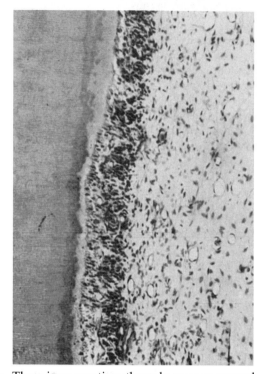

   a. There is no reaction; the pulp appears normal.
   b. The odontoblast layer is disrupted, and there is mild inflammation.
   c. Odontoblasts are aspirated into tubules, and there is mild inflammation.
   d. Odontoblasts are absent, and there is extravasation of erythrocytes.

17. This is an area of pulp close to a carious exposure (see the following illustration). The inflammatory response is primarily which of the following?

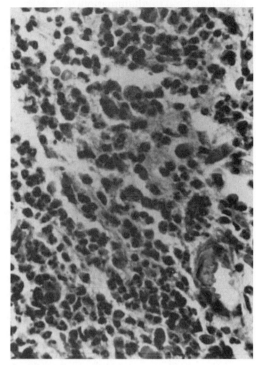

   a. Acute
   b. Chronic
   c. Giant cell
   d. Vascular

18. The early inflammatory cell infiltrate response of the pulp to caries involves primarily which of the following?
   a. Neutrophils
   b. Macrophages
   c. Neutrophils, plasma cells, and lymphocytes
   d. Macrophages and lymphocytes
   e. Lymphocytes, plasma cells, and macrophages

19. Hypersensitivity of the pulp after restoration placement indicates which of the following?
   a. Acute inflammation in the pulp
   b. Chronic inflammation in the pulp
   c. Microleakage at the restoration and tooth interface
   d. Stimulation of sensory nerves by hydrodynamics
   e. Tubules are blocked by restorative material or smear layer or both

CHAPTER 16: TRAUMATIC INJURIES

1. If several teeth are out of alignment after trauma, the most reasonable explanation is which of the following?
   a. Luxation
   b. Subluxation
   c. Alveolar fracture
   d. Root fracture

2. Initial vitality testing of traumatized teeth is most useful to which of the following?
   a. It establishes a baseline for comparison with future testing.
   b. It determines whether root canal treatment is indicated.
   c. It determines if the blood supply to the pulp is compromised.
   d. It predicts the prognosis.

3. A normal periapical radiograph of a traumatized tooth is useful for which of the following?
   a. It visualizes most root fractures.
   b. It visualizes concussion injuries.
   c. It gathers baseline information.
   d. It locates foreign objects.

4. Which of the following statements regarding crown infraction is accurate?
   a. It may indicate luxation injuries.
   b. It is rarely seen on transillumination.
   c. It seldom requires a follow-up examination.
   d. It describes the process of coronal pulp necrosis.

5. Which of the following statements regarding uncomplicated crown fracture is accurate?
   a. It is an indication for a dentin-bonded restoration.
   b. It requires baseline pulp testing.
   c. It involves root canal treatment if the exposed dentin is sensitive to cold stimulus.
   d. It has a questionable long-term prognosis.
   e. It is managed differently in young versus older patients.

6. Which of the following statements regarding complicated crown fractures is accurate?
   a. Exposure to the oral cavity permits rapid bacterial penetration through the pulp.
   b. Inflammation is limited to the coronal 2 mm of the exposed pulp for the first 24 hours.
   c. The tooth is normally managed by root canal treatment and restoration.

7. Which of the following statements regarding replacement resorption is accurate?
   a. It results from direct contact between root, dentin, and bone.
   b. It is managed by surgical exposure and repair with a biocompatible material.
   c. It results when at least 75% of the root surface is damaged.
   d. It can be avoided by timely endodontic intervention.

8. Pulp necrosis is most likely to occur after which of the following?
   a. Midroot fracture
   b. Intrusive luxation
   c. Concussion
   d. Complicated crown fracture

9. Which of the following statements regarding cervical root resorption is accurate?
   a. It is a common, self-limiting result of luxation injury.
   b. It causes significant pulpal symptoms.
   c. It can be arrested by root canal treatment.
   d. It may extend coronally to present as a pink spot on the crown.

10. Which of the following statements regarding internal root resorption is accurate?
    a. It is more common in permanent than deciduous teeth.
    b. It is simple to differentiate from other types of resorption.
    c. It is characterized histologically by inflammatory tissue with multinucleated giant cells.
    d. It is ruled out when there is no response to pulp testing.

11. A luxated tooth should be splinted in which of the following situations?
    a. If the tooth is mobile after splinting
    b. Until the root canal treatment is completed
    c. With the composite as close to the gingiva as possible
    d. All of the above

12. Which medium of storage for an avulsed tooth is best for prolonged extraoral periods?
    a. Hanks balanced salt solution
    b. Milk
    c. Distilled water
    d. Saliva

13. The most important factor for managing avulsions is which of the following?
    a. Extraoral time
    b. Decontamination of the root surface
    c. Prompt initiation of root canal treatment
    d. Proper preparation of the socket

14. Tooth mobility after trauma may be because of which of the following?
    a. Displacement
    b. Alveolar fracture
    c. Root fracture
    d. Crown fracture
    e. All of the above

15. Which of the following is true about thermal and electrical tests after trauma?
    a. Sensitivity tests evaluate the nerve and circulatory condition of the tooth.
    b. False-positive tests are more likely than false-negative tests.
    c. It may take up to 9 months for normal blood flow to return.
    d. None of the above statements are accurate.

16. Which of the following statements regarding internal root resorption is accurate?
    a. It is rare in deciduous teeth.
    b. It is initiated by odontoblasts.
    c. It is seldom confused with external resorption.
    d. It is usually asymptomatic.

17. Which of the following statements regarding avulsed teeth is accurate?
    a. They can be treated endodontically outside the mouth in limited circumstances.
    b. They should be rigidly splinted for 3 to 4 weeks to allow periodontal support to mature.
    c. They generally do not require antibiotic treatment at the time of replantation.
    d. They should have apexification attempted when the apex is not closed.

CHAPTER 17: ENDODONTIC AND PERIODONTIC INTERRELATIONSHIPS

1. According to Gutmann, molar teeth are most likely to have accessory and lateral canals:
   a. Branching from the main canal to form an apical delta
   b. In the apical one third of the root
   c. On the lateral surface of the root
   d. In the furcation

2. Which of the following statements regarding palatogingival grooves is false?
   a. The incidence of palatogingival grooves ranges from 10% to 20% of the population.
   b. The maxillary lateral incisor is affected more that the central incisor.
   c. The grooves extend apically in varying distances, with less than 1% reaching the apex.
   d. Pulp necrosis frequently occurs in teeth with palatogingival grooves because of the lack of cementum covering the dentin.

3. The prognosis for a tooth with a perforation is affected by all of the following factors, *except for one*. Which is the *exception*?
   a. Location of the perforation
   b. The time of repair
   c. The ability to seal the defect
   d. The ability to perform root canal treatment on the remaining canals
   e. The placement of a post to retain the core after perforation repair

4. Which of the following statements best describes retrograde periodontitis?
   a. Inflammation from the periodontal sulcus migrates apically, causing pulp inflammation and eventually pulp necrosis.
   b. Pulp necrosis occurs, and the toxic irritants cause inflammation that migrates to the gingival margin, creating a periodontal pocket.
   c. Irritants gain access to the periodontal tissues at the site of a vertical-root fracture, producing tissue destruction that mimics periodontitis.
   d. Pulp necrosis results in the formation of an apical, radiolucent lesion characterized by the loss of the apical lamina dura.

5. Which of the following statements best describes the effect periodontal disease has on the dental pulp?
   a. There is a direct correlation between the severity of the periodontal disease and the percentage of pulps that become necrotic.
   b. When periodontal disease or the treatment of the disease exposes a lateral or accessory canal, complete pulp necrosis will result.
   c. Although periodontitis can cause pulp inflammation and necrosis, treatment procedures have little effect on the pulp.
   d. Periodontal disease that does not expose the apical foramen is unlikely to produce significant damage to the pulp.

6. Which of the following statements regarding the primary endodontic lesion with secondary periodontic involvement is correct?
   a. Pulp necrosis occurs initially and an apical lesion forms. Apical migration of periodontal disease results in communication between the two lesions.
   b. Treatment consists of performing endodontic treatment, which is followed by a 6-month recall examination. If the periodontal component is still present, periodontal therapy is initiated.
   c. The primary endodontic lesion with secondary periodontic involvement exhibits a poorer prognosis when compared with the primary periodontal lesion with secondary endodontic involvement.
   d. Pulp necrosis occurs and forms a sinus tract through the periodontal ligament that, over time, permits the accumulation of plaque and calculus on the root.

7. Which of the following statements regarding root resection is false?
   a. Success depends primarily on treatment planning and case selection.
   b. Failures occur primarily because of continued periodontal breakdown.
   c. The long-term prognosis for the pulp in teeth with vital-root resection is poor.
   d. Endodontic treatment should precede resection of a root.

8. Which of the following statements regarding guided tissue regeneration (GTR) is false?
   a. GTR is an effective adjunct to treatment of periodontal disease but has limited value in treating endodontic pathosis.
   b. The combined endodontic periodontic lesion has the least favorable prognosis for GTR because of the relationship of the lesion to the gingival margin.
   c. Bioresorbable membranes exhibit results similar to nonresorbable membranes.
   d. Evidence suggest that GTR enhances bone formation by preventing contact of connective tissue with the bone.

9. A 24-year-old female patient has drainage from the gingival sulcus of her maxillary, right, central incisor (tooth no. 8). Three years ago she relates a porcelain fused-to-metal bridge (nos. 6 to 8) was placed because of a congenitally missing, lateral incisor. Clinical examination reveals a 12 mm probing defect on the lingual aspect of tooth no. 8. Additional probing depths are 3 mm or less. Pulp testing reveals that no. 6, no. 8, no. 9, no. 10 are responsive to CO_2 snow. Radiographic examination reveals a diffuse radiolucent area along the mesial lateral root surface extending from the crestal tissue to the apex. Which of the following is the most likely cause of this lesion?
   a. Vertical-root fracture
   b. Palatogingival groove
   c. Pulp necrosis
   d. Periodontitis
   e. Osteogenic sarcoma

10. A 51-year-old woman seeks evaluation of swelling of the buccal tissue opposite her mandibular, right, first molar (tooth no. 30). She relates a history of having a full-gold crown placed 2 months ago. She states that she has had pain for the past week and that the swelling began yesterday. Clinical examination reveals swelling in the buccal furcation area of tooth no. 30. Probing depths are 3 to 4 mm, except for a 6-mm defect in the furcal area of tooth no. 30. Pulp testing with CO_2 snow reveals teeth nos. 28, 29, and 31 respond. Tooth no. 30 is not responsive. Radiographic examination reveals normal apical structures, however, there is a radiolucent area in the furcation of tooth no. 30. This area was not evident on the film taken before placement of the crown. Based on this information what diagnostic classification is most appropriate?
   a. Primary endodontic lesion
   b. Primary periodontic lesion
   c. Primary endodontic lesion with secondary periodontic involvement
   d. Primary periodontic lesion with secondary endodontic involvement
   e. Concomitant endodontic and periodontic lesion

CHAPTER 18: ENDODONTIC PHARMACOLOGY

1. Odontogenic pain is usually caused by which of the following?
   a. Noxious physical stimuli
   b. The release of inflammatory mediators
   c. Stimulation of sympathetic fibers in the pulp
   d. Edema produced in a ridged, noncompliant root canal system

2. Which of the following best describes the neural innervation of the dental pulp?
   a. A-delta fibers transmit pain to the trigeminal nucleus.
   b. C fibers transmit pain to the superior cervical ganglion.
   c. Sympathetic fibers are not blocked with application of local anesthetic agents.
   d. A-delta fibers play the predominant role in encoding inflammatory pain.

3. Nociceptive signals are transmitted primarily to which of the following?
   a. Nucleus caudalis
   b. Limbic system
   c. Reticular system
   d. Superior cervical ganglion

4. Pain that refers from an inflamed maxillary sinus to maxillary molars is likely to the phenomenon of which of the following?
   a. Convergence
   b. Sublimation
   c. Nociception
   d. Information transfer
   e. Projection

5. Which of the following statements is true regarding descending fibers?
   a. They inhibit transmission of nociceptive information.
   b. They are not affected by endogenous opioid peptides.
   c. They transmit information from the cerebral cortex to the thalamus.
   d. They are sympathetic fibers that modulate blood flow in the pulp after sensory stimulation.

6. Hyperalgesia is characterized by the following, *except for one*. Which is the *exception*?
   a. Hyperalgesia is primarily a central mechanism.
   b. Spontaneous pain is present.
   c. The pain threshold is reduced.
   d. Hyperalgesia produces an increased pain perception to a noxious stimuli.

7. Regarding etodolac (i.e., Lodine), which of the following statements is correct?
   a. The drug exhibits minimal gastrointestinal irritation when compared to ibuprofen.
   b. When compared with ibuprofen, etodolac has a more profound analgesic action.
   c. Studies indicate etodolac is unique, because the drug does not have a peripheral analgesic mechanism of action.
   d. This drug can be prescribed for adult patients with aspirin hypersensitivity.

8. Which of the following statements regarding activation of the opiate receptor is accurate?
   a. It blocks nociceptive signals from the trigeminal nucleus to higher brain centers.
   b. It blocks transmission of signals from the thalamus to the cerebral cortex.
   c. It induces the release of endorphins.
   d. It blocks the release of dynorphins.

9. Opioids are frequently used in combination with other drugs because which of the following?
   a. The nonsteroidal, antiinflammatory drugs in combination with the opioid act synergistically on the opiate receptor.
   b. The combination permits a lower dose of the opioid, which can reduce side effects.
   c. Opioids do not act peripherally.
   d. Opioids are not antipyretic.

10. Which of the following is true for the use of codeine as an analgesic agent?
    a. Codeine prescribed in 60-mg doses is more effective than 650 mg of aspirin.
    b. Codeine prescribed in 30-mg doses is more effective than 600 mg of acetaminophen.
    c. Codeine prescribed in 30-mg doses is more effective than a placebo.
    d. Codeine prescribed in 60-mg doses is more effective than a placebo.

11. Management of pain of endodontic origin should focus on which of the following?
    a. Removing the peripheral mechanism of hyperalgesia
    b. Providing an adequate level of nonsteroidal, antiinflammatory analgesic agent
    c. Prescribing an appropriate antibiotic in cases where pain is the result of infection
    d. Using long-acting, local anesthetic agents to break the pain cycle

12. Which of the following best describes a "flexible plan" for prescribing analgesic agents?
    a. A maximal dose of an opioid is administered. If pain persists, the opioid is supplemented with a nonsteroidal, antiinflammatory agent or acetaminophen. Doses are then alternated.
    b. A maximal dose of a nonsteroidal, antiinflammatory agent or acetaminophen is administered. If pain persists, the drug is supplemented with an opioid. Doses are then alternated.
    c. Patients are advised to take the maximal dose of a nonsteroidal, antiinflammatory agent a day before the appointment and then as necessary for postoperative pain.
    d. Patients are advised to take an opioid agent a day before the appointment and then as necessary for postoperative pain.

13. Nonsteroidal, antiinflammatory agents administered in combination with cyclosporine may result in which of the following?
    a. They increase the risk of nephrotoxicity.
    b. They induce bone marrow suppression.
    c. They decrease the activity of the cyclosporine.
    d. They result in increased concentrations of the nonsteroidal agent in the blood plasma.

14. Nonsteroidal, antiinflammatory agents administered in combination with anticoagulants may result in which of the following?
    a. Increase the prothrombin time
    b. Result in a decreased bleeding time
    c. Increase the bioavailability of the anticoagulant
    d. Produce no adverse effect

15. Indomethacin administered in combination with sympathomimetic agents results in which of the following?
    a. Decreased blood pressure
    b. Increased blood pressure
    c. Decreased water retention
    d. Decreased absorption of indomethacin, requiring a higher dose

16. Peripheral afferent nerve fibers in an inflamed pulp may respond to mediators by which of the following?
    a. Reducing the concentration of those mediators
    b. Decreasing responsiveness to nociceptive stimuli
    c. Decreasing the number of anesthetic molecule receptors
    d. Decreasing numbers of ion channels
    e. Sprouting of terminal fibers

17. Two nonsteroidal antiinflammatory drugs (NSAIDs) that have minimal adverse gastrointestinal side effects are which of the following?
    a. Etodolac and ibuprofen
    b. Etodolac and rofecoxib
    c. Ibuprofen and ketoprofen
    d. Ketoprofen and etodolac
    e. Ibuprofen and rofecoxib

18. To minimize posttreatment pain, when are analgesics most effective when administered?
    a. As a pretreatment
    b. Immediately after treatment
    c. When the anesthetic begins to wear off
    d. When the patient first perceives pain
    e. When the pain is the most intense

19. Prophylactic administration of antibiotics to control adverse posttreatment symptoms in prospective, controlled, clinical trials on asymptomatic patients has been shown to be which of the following?
    a. Ineffective
    b. Effective if given in high doses
    c. Effective only if given pretreatment
    d. Effective if given in conjunction with intracanal antibiotics

CHAPTER 19: ENDODONTIC MICROSURGERY

1. A 45-year-old man has a radiolucent area associated with his maxillary, right, central incisor (tooth no. 8) and facial swelling. He relates traumatic injury as a child with root canal treatment during his teenage years. Subsequent to this treatment he fractured tooth no. 8 playing basketball in his early thirties. Root canal retreatment was necessary and the tooth was restored with a cast post, core and crown. Which of the following is the most appropriate treatment sequence?
   a. Incision and drainage followed by nonsurgical retreatment and fabrication of a new restoration
   b. Root end surgery and a postsurgical antibiotic
   c. Management of the infection and performance of root end surgery when the swelling subsides
   d. Incise and drain the swelling, prescribe an antibiotic, and follow the patient on recall examinations
   e. Tooth extraction and implant placement

2. Each of the following statements on the reasons two radiographs are recommended for evaluation of a tooth to be treated surgically is correct, *except for one*. Which is the *exception*?
   a. Two films permit the evaluation and location of normal anatomic structures.
   b. The root length can be assessed.
   c. The size of the lesion can be determined.
   d. Root curvatures can be viewed.
   e. The depth of the overlying bone can be determined.

3. When a vessel is severed, initial hemostasis results from which of the following?
   a. Contraction of the vessel wall
   b. Formation of a platelet plug
   c. The conversion of prothrombin to thrombin
   d. The conversion of fibrinogen to fibrin

4. The anesthetic of choice when performing endodontic root end surgery on a patient with mild cardiovascular disease is which of the following?
   a. 1.5% etidocaine 1:200,000 epinephrine
   b. 0.5% marcaine 1:200,000 epinephrine
   c. 2% lidocaine 1:100,000 epinephrine
   d. 2% lidocaine 1:50,000 epinephrine
   e. 4% prilocaine plain

5. The primary beneficial action of epinephrine when performing root end surgery is which of the following?
   a. It effects the drug on alpha-1 receptors in the alveolar mucosa.
   b. It effects the drug on beta-1 receptors of skeletal muscle.
   c. It decreased systemic uptake of the anesthetic solution.
   d. It prolonged the duration of anesthesia.

6. Which of the following statements regarding flap reflection is correct?
   a. The horizontal incision for the mucogingival flap is made perpendicular to the cortical bone.
   b. The rectangular flap design is most appropriate in the posterior areas.
   c. The mucogingival flap with an anterior-releasing incision is preferred in posterior areas.
   d. The type of vertical-releasing incisions distinguish the mucogingival flap from the Luebke-Oschsenbein flap.
   e. The semilunar flap has the advantage of providing an esthetic result without scar formation.

7. Which of the following hemostatic agents activates the intrinsic coagulation pathway?
   a. Ferric sulfate
   b. Calcium sulfate paste
   c. Microfibrillar collagen
   d. Bone wax
   e. Epinephrine pellets

8. Which of the following is the recommended hemostatic technique to control bleeding during root end surgery?
   a. Local anesthesia with 2% lidocaine 1:50,000 epinephrine, epinephrine saturated pellets, ferric sulfate, calcium sulfate paste
   b. Local anesthesia with 2% lidocaine 1:50,000 epinephrine, ferric sulfate, microfibrillar collagen, bone wax
   c. Local anesthesia with 2% lidocaine 1:100,000 epinephrine, ferric sulfate, microfibrillar collagen, Telfa pad
   d. Local anesthesia with 0.5% marcaine 1:200,000 epinephrine, ferric sulfate, calcium sulfate paste

9. Each of the following statements is correct regarding the use of the H 161 Lindemann bone cutter for root end surgery is correct, *except for one*. Which is the *exception*?
   a. It reduces frictional heat when resecting bone.
   b. It has more flutes that conventional burs, so cutting is faster and more efficient.
   c. When used with the Impact Air 45 hand piece splatter is decreased.
   d. It has fewer flutes and is less likely to clog.

10. Which of the following statements regarding root end resection is correct?
    a. The root should be resected at a 45-degree angle to ensure adequate access and visibility.
    b. The apical 2 mm should be removed to ensure that apical ramifications are not present.
    c. Root end resection should precede apical curettage.
    d. Resection of the root should be as perpendicular to the long access of the root as possible.

11. Which of the following statements regarding the isthmus between canals is correct?
    a. Although often noted between canals, failure to include this area in the preparation does not affect the prognosis of a tooth.
    b. The incomplete isthmus should be prepared with a tracking groove before ultrasonic preparation.
    c. Isthmus incidence is not affected by the amount of the root resection but increases as the bevel approaches 45 degrees.
    d. When using a surgical operating microscope, the absence of an isthmus at $16 \times$ to $25 \times$ is evidence that no connection between canals exist.

12. Which of the following statements regarding ferric sulfate is correct?
    a. Ferric sulfate acts by producing a tamponade effect and is absorbed by the body over 2 to 3 weeks.
    b. Ferric sulfate exhibits an alkaline pH.
    c. Applied to the osseous surface, ferric sulfate causes agglutination of blood proteins.
    d. Ferric sulfate induces osseous tissue formation.

13. Which of the following statements regarding root end preparation is false?
    a. The ideal preparation should extend 3 mm into the root and follow the long axis of the tooth.
    b. The lingual wall of the preparation is the most difficult area to evaluate.
    c. Ultrasonic preparation has the potential to induce micofractures in the dentin.
    d. KiS tips have enhanced cutting efficiency for root end preparations because of a zirconium nitride coating.
    e. Ultrasonic root end preparation may thermoplasticize the remaining gutta-percha.

14. Which of the following statements regarding root end filling materials is false?
    a. Super EBA is preferred as a root end filling material over IRM because it lacks eugenol.
    b. IRM is preferred over amalgam.
    c. Mineral trioxide aggregate (MTA) is not adversely affected by contamination with blood.
    d. Periapical healing with MTA results in cementum formation over the material.
    e. Composite resins appear to be acceptable, providing a dry-operating field can be maintained.

15. Which of the following statements is correct regarding treatment for a 73-year-old woman who develops ecchymosis after root end surgery?
    a. Instruct the patient to place warm compresses over the area three to four times daily.
    b. Place the patient on an antibiotic to prevent infection of the area.
    c. Prescribe an antiinflammatory analgesic to enhance the healing process.
    d. Explain the cause of the problem to the patient and provide reassurance.

CHAPTER 20: MANAGEMENT OF PAIN AND ANXIETY

1. The majority of life-threatening systemic complications arise in which of the following?
    a. During or immediately after injection of local anesthetics
    b. In conjunction with surgical procedures, such as tooth extraction
    c. During the pulp extirpation phase of root canal treatment
    d. As a result of bleeding from patients with known bleeding disorders

2. Which of the following tooth groups is the most difficult to anesthetize?
    a. Mandibular premolars
    b. Maxillary premolars
    c. Maxillary molars
    d. Mandibular molars

3. Which of the following is *not* a factor affecting the onset of local anesthesia?
    a. Diffusion of the local anesthetic through the lipid-rich nerve sheath
    b. The pKa for the anesthetic agent
    c. The pH of the tissue
    d. The protein-binding ability of the local anesthetic

4. A decrease in the tissue pH causes which of the following?
    a. It increases the free base of the local anesthetic agents.
    b. It results in fewer anesthetic molecules entering the nerve sheath.
    c. It changes the pKa value for a given local anesthetic.
    d. It cecreases the protein-binding of the local anesthetic.

5. Failure to obtain adequate anesthesia after an appropriately administered nerve block is most likely the result in which of the following?
   a. pH changes in the pulp tissue caused by inflammations
   b. Morphologic neurodegenerative changes and inflammatory mediators
   c. Insufficient volume of local anesthetic injected
   d. Tolerance to the anesthetic agent

6. When comparing amide and ester local anesthetic agents, which of the following is true?
   a. Esters are more likely to produce systemic toxicity when compared to amides.
   b. Amides are more allergenic when compared to esters.
   c. Amides are more effective than esters.
   d. Esters and amides are equally effective.

7. A patient is anesthetized using a posterior superior alveolar (PSA) nerve block to perform endodontic treatment on the maxillary, first molar. Adequate anesthesia is not obtained. In this situation the clinician should consider which of the following?
   a. Anesthetizing the anterior, superior nerve
   b. Anesthetizing the middle, superior nerve
   c. Performing a palatal infiltration
   d. Repeating the PSA

8. An infiltration injection is given for a maxillary, second premolar. Adequate anesthesia is not obtained. Which injection should be considered?
   a. Anterior superior alveolar (ASA) block
   b. PSA block
   c. Palatal infiltration
   d. Maxillary (division II) block
   e. Greater palatine nerve block

9. Infiltration in the mandible may be an effective technique in treating the which of the following?
   a. Central incisor
   b. Canine
   c. First premolar
   d. Second molar

10. In performing the Akinosi technique, which of the following are accurate?
    a. The needle is inserted at the height of the mucogingival junction of the most posterior, maxillary tooth.
    b. The needle is passed lingual to the mandibular ramous until is bone is contacted.
    c. Injection at the neck of the mandibular condyle is the objective.
    d. All of the above statements are accurate.

11. The Stabident local anesthesia system is used for which one of the following reasons?
    a. As a true intraosseous injection
    b. As a modified periodontal ligament injection
    c. To limit the adverse reactions to vasopressor components of local anesthetic cartridges
    d. As a method to administer intrapulpal injections painlessly

12. Prescriptions for analgesic agents should provide which of the following?
    a. Instructions for administration at regular intervals
    b. Instructions for taking the medication when patients experience pain
    c. Administration instructions for patients in pain the day before initiating root canal treatment to ensure adequate blood levels
    d. Immediate preoperative administration of opiates when pulpal pain is present

13. For emergency treatment of patients with pulp pathosis, oral sedation should be considered during which of the following?
    a. When deep sedation of the fearful patient is desired
    b. When barbiturates with oral sedation should be considered
    c. When oral sedation with midazolam may provide an amnesia effect
    d. When a short-acting agent permits the patient to leave without an escort

14. Which of the following statements regarding the use of nitrous oxide inhalation sedation is accurate?
    a. It produces significant analgesic effect when used in conjunction with local anesthetics.
    b. It is difficult in managing endodontic patients because of the application of the rubber dam.
    c. It should be considered if oral sedation cannot be used.
    d. It should be used only when an auxiliary of the same sex as the patient is present to assist.

15. Which of the following statements regarding supraperiosteal injection (infiltration) is accurate?
    a. It is effective for most maxillary teeth.
    b. It is more effective in the presence of infection.
    c. It is ineffective for both adults and children in anesthetizing mandibular teeth.
    d. It is targeted mesial and distal to the apex of the involved tooth.

16. Which of the following statements regarding regional nerve block is accurate?
    a. It achieves anesthesia by blocking efferent nerve impulses.
    b. It may be more effective because it is deposited in normal, rather than inflamed, tissue.
    c. It is exemplified by the long buccal nerve block.
    d. It requires use of an agent without vasoconstrictors.

17. Which of the following statements regarding the anterior middle superior alveolar (AMSA) nerve block is accurate?
    a. It anesthetizes all branches of the maxillary nerve.
    b. It can be delivered by a computer-controlled system or by traditional needle and syringe.
    c. It anesthetizes buccal and palatal bone, but not soft tissue.
    d. It occasionally anesthetizes the orbicularis oris.

18. If the dentist thinks there may be considerable posttreatment pain, the clinician may do which of the following?
    a. Prescribe antibiotics
    b. Reanesthetize with a long-acting anesthetic
    c. Prescribe antianxiety medications
    d. All of the above

19. Which of the following statements regarding oral sedation is accurate?
    a. It has a quick onset of action.
    b. It has a significant number of adverse reactions.
    c. It has a reasonably short duration.
    d. It is difficult to titrate to ideal levels.

CHAPTER 21: TOOTH-WHITENING MODALITIES FOR PULPLESS AND DISCOLORED TEETH

1. The whitening mechanism for bleaching teeth is thought to be which of the following?
    a. A result of the degradation organic molecules of high molecular weight that reflect a specific wavelength of light
    b. Related to changes in the inorganic hydroxyapitite crystals
    c. Related to the dissolution of the stain
    d. A result of removal of free-metal ions, such as iron and copper

2. Which of the following statements is correct regarding the incidence of cervical resorption after internal bleaching?
    a. Cervical resorption can be as high 25% when Superoxyl and heat are used.
    b. Lesions develop rapidly and can be detected 1 to 2 months after bleaching.
    c. The incidence of cervical resorption increases in patients who are 25 years old and older.
    d. Although cervical resorption is often attributed to bleaching, it is more likely caused by a previous traumatic injury to the involved tooth.

3. Each of the following is an intrinsic form of tooth discoloration, *except for one*. Which is the *exception*?
    a. Endemic fluorosis
    b. Hereditary opalescent dentin
    c. Tetracycline staining
    d. Peridex staining

4. Which of the following statements regarding microabrasion is correct?
    a. The agent used in the technique is 30% hydrogen peroxide, which can be obtained in proprietary products, such as Prema.
    b. The technique is useful in treating white-and-brown-spot surface lesions.
    c. Microabrasion should not be used before placement of bonded restorations.
    d. Requires a local anesthetic and frequently produces postoperative thermal sensitivity.

5. When performing a walking bleach procedure, which of the following statements is accurate?
    a. The dentin should be etched before placement of the bleaching agent to increase permeability of the tubules and enhance the bleaching action.
    b. The sodium perborate paste should be covered by a minimum of 2 mm of Cavit or IRM.
    c. A barrier over the obturating material is not required.
    d. The definitive bonded restoration should be placed at the visit in which the sodium perborate paste is removed.

6. Which of the following statements regarding power bleaching is false?
    a. Power bleaching often uses a liquid rubber dam composed of a light cured resin gel.
    b. Vitamin E can be used to neutralize the oxidizing effects of hydrogen peroxide that comes in contact with soft tissues.
    c. Power bleaching can often be performed by trained dental auxiliary personnel.
    d. After fabrication of custom trays with appropriate reservoirs, patients apply a bleaching gel every 2 hours during their waking hours.

CHAPTER 22: RESTORATION OF THE ENDODONTICALLY TREATED TOOTH

1. Which of the following statements regarding the density of dentinal tubules (per square millimeter) is accurate?
   a. It remains constant as they progress from the periphery to the pulpal dentin junction with a decreasing diameter.
   b. It remains constant as they progress from the periphery to the pulpal dentin junction with an increasing diameter.
   c. It decreases as they progress from the periphery to the pulpal dentin junction, maintaining a constant diameter.
   d. It increases as they progress from the periphery to the pulpal dentin junction with an increase in diameter.
   e. It increases as they progress from the periphery to the pulpal dentin junction, maintaining a constant diameter.

2. Which of the following statements regarding teeth restored with crowns is correct?
   a. When teeth exhibiting no caries, fracture, or other causative factors are restored with crowns, those serving as abutments exhibit a higher rate of necrosis.
   b. The periodontal status of teeth restored with crowns is not a significant factor in the pulpal prognosis.
   c. Should pulp necrosis occur in teeth restored with crowns, the process occurs rapidly, usually within the first 3 years after cementation.
   d. The amount of occlusal reduction is a more significant factor in inducing pulpal pathosis when compared to axial reduction.
   e. Pulpal pathosis becomes significant when the remaining thickness of dentin is less than 1.5 mm.

3. Which of the following would best fit the definition of the "stressed pulp syndrome"?
   a. A tooth recently prepared for a porcelain fused-to-metal crown that (with placement of a provisional crown) exhibits severe pain to thermal stimulation
   b. A tooth that is asymptomatic but has had numerous restorations placed over a period of years because of recurrent caries
   c. A nonrestored tooth that exhibits probing depths of 4 to 5 mm
   d. A tooth that is not responsive to pulp testing with CO_2 and EPT

4. Each of the following is a concern when restoring an endodontically treated molar with minimal remaining tooth structure, *except for one*. Which is the *exception*?
   a. Increased chance for root fracture
   b. Greater potential for recurrent caries
   c. Infringement on the biologic width
   d. The altered light refraction
   e. Changes in collagen cross linking

5. A tooth requires a post, core, and crown for adequate restorative treatment. Which of the following is the most important factor in the restorative equation?
   a. Dowel length
   b. Dowel width
   c. The surface configuration of the dowel
   d. The core material
   e. An adequate ferrule

6. A patient requires a post and core for restoration of a narrow, mandibular, central incisor tooth with 1 mm of structure above the gingival level. Which of the following would be the most appropriate dowel for this situation?
   a. Cast post and core
   b. Carbon fiber post with a composite core
   c. Parallel stainless steel (SS) post with an amalgam core
   d. Threaded dowel with a composite core

7. Which of the following statements regarding the carbon fiber dowels is false?
   a. They are radiolucent.
   b. They have a modulus of elasticity similar to dentin.
   c. They provide esthetic qualities similar to metal dowels.
   d. The carbon fiber dowels are more resistant to fracture.

8. Which of the following statements regarding the zirconia dowel is accurate?
   a. It is easily removed from the canal by ultrasonics and special burs.
   b. It is readily seen on radiographs.
   c. It requires a composite core.
   d. It is similar to dentin in elasticity.

9. The most appropriate time to determine the precise method for restoring the endodontically treated tooth is which of the following?
   a. When the initial diagnosis and treatment plan is established
   b. During the endodontic treatment procedures
   c. After completion of the root canal treatment
   d. After the initial-crown preparation

10. Which of the following statements regarding post space is correct?
    a. The post space for passive dowels must provide intimate contact between the dowel and the dentin wall.
    b. Post space should extend into the root to a depth 3 to 5 mm from the apex.
    c. The post space required for fabrication of a dowel and core using a direct technique requires removal of more tooth structure than the proprietary dowel systems because of the need to remove undercuts.
    d. Direct composite–reinforced systems require the least amount of preparation.

CHAPTER 23: PEDIATRIC ENDODONTICS: ENDODONTIC TREATMENT FOR THE PRIMARY AND YOUNG, PERMANENT DENTITION

1. The basic morphologic difference between primary and permanent teeth is which of the following?
   a. Thickness of dentin between pulp and enamel is greater in primary teeth
   b. Enamel is thicker in primary teeth
   c. The pulp chamber is comparatively smaller in primary teeth
   d. The pulp horns are higher in primary molars

2. Radiographically, which of the following statements regarding primary teeth is accurate?
   a. Pathologic changes in the periradicular tissues are most often apparent at the apexes than the furcation of molars.
   b. The presence of calcified masses within the pulp is indicative of acute pulpal disease.
   c. By the time internal resorption is visible the only treatment is extraction.
   d. Pathologic bone-and-root resorption is always indicative of nonvital pulp.

3. Which of the following diagnostic tests is usually reliable for determining pulpal status of primary teeth?
   a. Thermal pulp tests
   b. Electrical pulp tests
   c. Percussion
   d. None are reliable in children.

4. Which of the following statements regarding indirect pulp therapy is accurate?
   a. It is indicated only in the treatment of teeth with deep carious lesions in which there is no clinical evidence of pulpal degeneration or periapical pathosis.
   b. It removes much of the bacteria present in dentin.
   c. It includes placing calcium hydroxide or zinc oxide–eugenol (ZOE) over the remaining caries and permanently restoring the tooth with amalgam.
   d. It involves all of the above.

5. Direct pulp capping is recommended for primary teeth with which of the following?
   a. Carious exposures
   b. Mechanical exposures
   c. Calcification in the pulp chamber
   d. All of the above

6. Symptoms of pulp abnormalities in primary teeth include which of the following?
   a. Pain to percussion
   b. History of spontaneous pain
   c. Variations in mobility
   d. All of the above

7. A calcium hydroxide pulpotomy performed on a young, permanent tooth is judged to be successful during which of the following?
   a. When the patient is asymptomatic
   b. When the tooth responds to pulp testing
   c. When normal root development continues
   d. All of the above statements are accurate.

8. Formocresol pulpotomy on a primary tooth is indicated during which of the following?
   a. When there is a history of spontaneous toothache
   b. When the inflammation or infection is confined to the coronal pulp
   c. When the pulp does not bleed
   d. When there is only apical pathosis

9. The effect of formocresol on the pulp tissue is controlled by which of the following?
   a. Concentration used
   b. Method of application
   c. Length of time applied
   d. All of the above

10. An increasingly popular technique for pulpotomy in primary teeth is which of the following?
    a. Formocresol
    b. Calcium hydroxide
    c. Electrosurgery
    d. Laser surgery

11. Glutaraldehyde may be preferred to formocresol for primary pulpotomy because of which of the following reasons?
    a. It has less systemic distribution beyond the pulp.
    b. It has a better prognosis.
    c. It is not antigenic.
    d. It is less readily metabolized.

12. Which of the following is an indication for root canal treatment of primary teeth?
    a. Radiographic evidence of internal root resorption
    b. Periapical lesion
    c. Dentigerous cyst
    d. Mechanical or carious perforation of the chamber floor

13. Which of the following statements regarding access opening on primary incisors is accurate?
    a. They are from the facial surface.
    b. They are from the lingual surface.
    c. They are from the incisal edge.
    d. They are different for maxillary teeth and mandibular teeth.

14. Which of the following is true in placing zinc oxide–eugenol in a primary tooth?
    a. Technique is not important.
    b. The overfill has a poorer prognosis than a flush fill.
    c. The paste should be mixed to a thick consistency.
    d. All are true.

CHAPTER 24: GERIATRIC ENDODONTICS

1. As related to dental visits by the older patient, which of the following statements are accurate?
    a. Older patients have fewer visits per year than younger patients.
    b. The number of visits by older patients should decrease in the future.
    c. Most visits are for comprehensive procedures.
    d. Dental visits of older patients are for less-complicated procedures when compared to younger patients.

2. Which of the following statements regarding secondary dentin formation in the radicular pulp in an older patient is accurate?
    a. It is less likely to occur in response to abrasion than in younger patients.
    b. It may result in complete pulp obliteration.
    c. It may compromise the blood supply and cause pulp necrosis.
    d. It does not require an irritant.

3. In the older patient (as compared with a younger patient), regarding pulpal inflammation from caries, which of the following statements is accurate?
    a. It is less likely to be as painful as in a younger patient.
    b. It usually progresses more slowly.
    c. It is less likely to occur.
    d. It is more likely to be acute than chronic.

4. Pulps in older patients tend to be less responsive to thermal stimuli because of which of the following reasons?
    a. Sensory nerves in dentin degenerate with time.
    b. Sensory nerves in pulp lose their myelin sheath as a result of long-term, repeated injuries.
    c. With age, patients become less alert and, therefore, less responsive to external stimuli.
    d. Pulpal calcifications block external stimuli from reaching receptors.
    e. Pulps tend to have less sensory innervation in older teeth.

5. An abrupt midroot radiographic disappearance of a canal usually indicates which of the following?
    a. Bifurcation in the canal
    b. Secondary dentin formation apically
    c. Concentrations of dystrophic calcifications apically
    d. Diminished (often unnegotiable) sized canal

6. In the older patient (as compared with the younger patient) the exit of the canal (i.e., apical foramen) is which of the following?
    a. Closer to the radiographic apex
    b. Closer to the true apex
    c. Easier to detect tactilely
    d. More variable because of cementum formation

7. Which of the following statements regarding single-visit root canal treatment in an older patient is accurate?
    a. It should be avoided because there is more likely to be an increase in postappointment pain.
    b. It should be avoided because it decreases successful prognosis.
    c. It is acceptable if it is more convenient for the patient.
    d. It should be avoided to place an intracanal medicament.

8. Success of root canal treatment in older patients (as compared with younger patients) is which of the following?
    a. Better
    b. Poorer
    c. Equivalent
    d. Unknown (has not been investigated)

9. In the older patient root canal treatment (as compared to extraction) is which of the following?
    a. Usually more emotionally traumatic
    b. Usually more tissue traumatic
    c. Often less expensive in the long run
    d. More likely to result in postappointment complication

10. A postsurgical condition that tends to occur more frequently in older patients is which of the following?
    a. Ecchymosis (i.e., discoloration) of soft tissues
    b. Infection of the surgical site
    c. Loss of sutures because of more friable tissues
    d. Continued hemorrhage of the incision site
    e. Loss of consciousness

11. When should periapical radiographs be prescribed?
    a. Before discussion of the chief complaint
    b. After discussing the chief complaint with the patient
    c. Just before the clinical examination
    d. After completing the clinical examination

12. With aging, which of the following statements are accurate?
    a. Lateral canals enlarge and become more clinically significant.
    b. Gingival recession exposes cementum and dentin, which is less resistant to caries.
    c. The cementodentinal junction locates progressively more coronally.
    d. All of the above occur.

13. In geriatric patients, which of the following statements are accurate?
    a. There is a direct correlation between the nature of response to electrical-pulp testing and the degree of inflammation.
    b. There is a reduced volume and increased neural component of the pulp.
    c. Tooth discoloration usually is not indicative of pulpal death.
    d. Diffuse pain of vague origin is unlikely to be odontogenic.

14. In evaluating success and failure of endodontic treatment in aged patients, a consideration is which of the following?
    a. The bone of the aged patient is more mineralized than that of a younger patient.
    b. Overlooked canals are seldom a problem because they are usually calcified.
    c. There may be failure even though the patient has no symptoms.
    d. Cold sensitivity is the usual symptom that indicates a missed canal.

15. Which of the following statements regarding endodontic surgery in older patients is accurate?
    a. It requires more anesthetic and vasoconstrictor than in younger patients.
    b. It may be somewhat easier because the vestibule is deeper.
    c. It is risky because inadequate blood supply may result in postsurgical osteomyelitis.
    d. It has been demonstrated to be much less successful than in younger patients.

16. The radiolucent structure at the periapex of the premolar in the following illustration is likely which of the following?

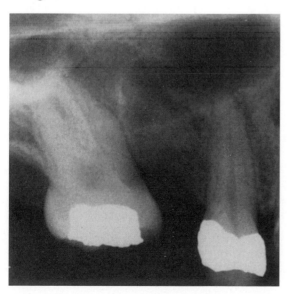

a. A maxillary sinus
b. An endodontic apical pathosis
c. A fibroosseous lesion
d. A bony trabecular pattern

17. The elevated structure facial to the crowned first molar in the following illustration is likely which of the following?

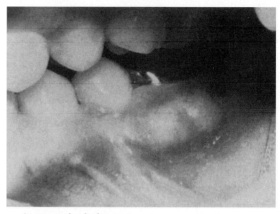

a. Acute apical abscess
b. Periodontal abscess
c. Fibroma
d. Exostoses

CHAPTER 25: NONSURGICAL ENDODONTIC RETREATMENT

1. Canals may be missed during treatment because of which of the following?
   a. Calcification
   b. Anomalous location
   c. Inadequate access
   d. All of the above

2. Radiographically, which of the following statements regarding canals that appear calcified are accurate?
   a. They are seldom able to be instrumented.
   b. They have a different appearance than the surrounding dentin.
   c. They should be opened up with rotary rather than ultrasonic instruments.

3. The *major* reason for failure, requiring retreatment, is which of the following?
   a. Persistent pain
   b. Draining sinus tract
   c. Restorative indications
   d. Microleakage

4. Presence of excess gutta-percha beyond the apex is usually caused by which of the following?
   a. Use of too small a master cone
   b. Excessive heating and compaction during warm, vertical condensation
   c. Destruction of the natural apical constriction

5. Lateral or furcal canals are which of the following?
   a. Commonplace
   b. Not able to be mechanically cleaned
   c. Not routinely obturated
   d. Seldom the sole cause of endodontic failure
   e. All of the above

6. Retreatment has the most favorable prognosis during which of the following?
   a. When the cause of failure is identified and is correctable
   b. When the patient is asymptomatic
   c. When gutta-percha was used instead of paste
   d. When a surgical microscope is used

7. For silver point removal, ultrasonics are used for which of the following reasons?
   a. To break up cement surrounding the point
   b. To reduce the level of dentin on the floor of the chamber to expose the point
   c. To break up the silver point into small pieces, which can then be flushed out
   d. To loosen the silver point by applying the vibrating instrument directly to the silver cone

8. How should rotary instruments be used for the removal of gutta-percha?
   a. To remove all the gutta-percha the length of the canal
   b. At the highest speeds
   c. In reverse of the canal preparation direction
   d. In portions of the canal where the instruments fit passively
   e. In portions of the canal where the instruments fit snugly

9. If a cervical root perforation occurs during the treatment and the canal preparation is incomplete, the generally preferred time for repairing the defect is which of the following?
   a. Immediately, that is, before proceeding with further preparation
   b. After cleaning and shaping is complete but before obturation
   c. Immediately after obturation
   d. After an appropriate recall period, to assess the status of the tissues

10. Removal of objects can be facilitated by:
    a. Straight-line access
    b. A good light source
    c. Magnification
    d. All of the above

11. Carrier-based gutta-percha removal and retreatment is:
    a. Generally easy, because all components are soluble
    b. Very difficult, because the gutta-percha is insoluble
    c. Usually by using a combination of techniques
    d. Impossible

12. Type III transportation is best managed by:
    a. Extraction
    b. Apexification with calcium hydroxide
    c. Forming an artificial barrier with a material, such as MTA
    d. Obturation, as best as possible, then surgery

CHAPTER 26: DIGITAL TECHNOLOGIES IN ENDODONTIC PRACTICE

1. A disadvantage of digital cameras relative to film-based cameras is that the digital cameras:
   a. Are very expensive to purchase
   b. Are more expensive to operate
   c. Have inferior image resolution
   d. Have a greater delay in obtaining images
   e. Are very complicated to operate

2. An advantage of conventional radiographic film relative to digital radiographic imaging is that film:
   a. Generally produces an image of superior quality
   b. Is easier to duplicate (reproduce)
   c. Requires less radiation exposure
   d. Accurately depicts the extent of caries
   e. Produces an image more quickly

3. The Internet is usable in dentistry for all of the following except:
   a. Inter-doctor consultations
   b. Online scheduling of patients
   c. Patient access to his/her dental records
   d. Online ordering of supplies
   e. Transmission of insurance claims

4. The Clinical Chairside Workstation is used for:
   a. Storing and displaying clinical information
   b. Electronically determining shades for porcelain crowns
   c. Selecting and mixing cements
   d. Communicating by voice with the front desk

5. The pre-registration specialized system is designed to:
   a. Obtain early registration for professional meetings
   b. Remind patients of recall appointments
   c. Automatically contact insurance companies to determine coverage limits of a patient
   d. Record pertinent data on a referred patient prior to any appointment
   e. Any of the above are possibilities

TEST YOUR KNOWLEDGE

Questions 1 to 3 relate to the following radiograph.

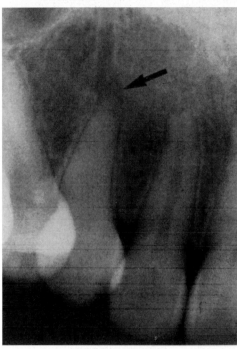

The patient does not have symptoms. All teeth shown in the radiograph respond to pulp testing, except the canine.

1. The radiolucent structure (*arrow*) at the apex of the canine is likely which of the following?
   a. Maxillary fracture
   b. Apical pathosis
   c. Nasopalatine duct
   d. Nutrient canal

2. The radiographic appearance internally indicates which of the following?
   a. Two likely superimposed canals
   b. Dentinogenesis imperfecta
   c. Dense accumulations of linear calcifications
   d. Calcific metamorphosis

3. The recommended treatment and reason for the treatment is which of the following?
   a. Root canal treatment; there is pulp pathosis.
   b. Root end resection and root end filling; there is pathosis, but the pulp space is too small to attempt root canal treatment.
   c. No treatment; there is no pathosis.
   d. Extraction is prescribed.

Questions 4 to 8 relate to the following illustration.

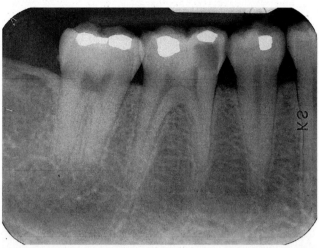

Tooth no. 30 (first molar) causes the patient prolonged pain to cold and episodes of spontaneous pain. The tooth responds to probing with an explorer into the carious lesion. There is no pain to percussion or palpation and no swelling. Periodontal probing is within normal limits.

4. What is the pulpal diagnosis?
   a. Reversible pulpitis
   b. Irreversible pulpitis
   c. Necrosis
   d. Unknown, pending further information

5. What is the periapical diagnosis?
   a. Normal
   b. Acute apical periodontitis
   c. Chronic apical periodontitis
   d. Acute apical abscess

6. What is the likely appearance of the pulp histologically?
   a. Coronal pulp is necrotic; radicular pulp is inflamed.
   b. Coronal pulp is inflamed; radicular pulp is normal.
   c. The entire pulp is inflamed.
   d. The entire pulp is necrotic.

7. What is the likely appearance of the periapex histologically?
   a. Normal structures
   b. Acute inflammation; no bone resorption
   c. Acute inflammation; bone resorption
   d. Chronic inflammation; bone resorption

8. What *minimal* immediate treatment is indicated?
   a. None. Schedule the patient for future evaluation.
   b. Complete canal preparation at this visit.
   c. Remove the caries and place a sedative temporarily.
   d. Perform pulpotomy or partial pulpectomy.

Questions 9 to 13 relate to the following photograph and radiograph.

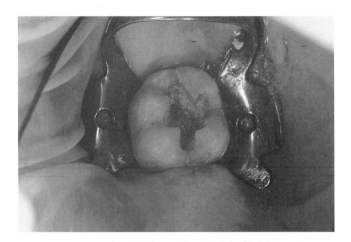

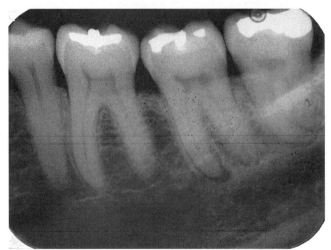

A 50-year-old woman comes to the clinic complaining of sharp sensitivity with chewing on the lower left second molar. She reports a period of cold sensitivity 6 months prior but has not had any cold tenderness for several months. The third and first molars respond to pulp testing; the second molar does not respond. There is no pain to palpation, but the tooth is tender to percussion on the cusps and tender to biting on a bite stick. There is an isolated 6-mm probing defect on distal. (*Photograph:* The shallow occlusal alloy has been removed.)

9. What is the pulpal diagnosis for tooth no. 18?
   a. Normal
   b. Hypersensitive
   c. Irreversible pulpitis
   d. Necrosis

10. What type of bacteria would likely be found in the pulp?
    a. Gram-positive aerobes
    b. Gram-negative anaerobes
    c. Mixed flora
    d. None

11. What is the likely cause of the patient's pain?
    a. Inflamed pulp
    b. Apical abscess
    c. Cracked tooth
    d. Periodontal abscess

12. What additional tests are indicated?
    a. Cold test
    b. Heat test
    c. Test cavity
    d. Transillumination

13. What type of permanent restoration is indicated?
    a. Occlusal amalgam
    b. Occlusal bonded composite
    c. Pin-retained amalgam
    d. Full-cast crown

Questions 14 to 20 relate to the following photograph and radiograph.

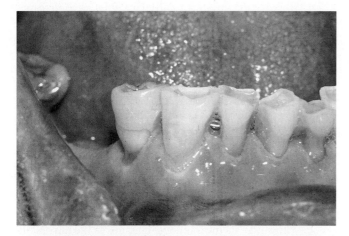

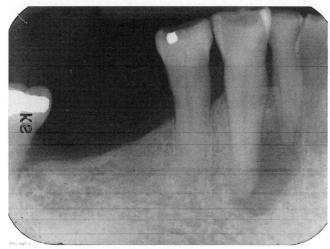

The patient reports "a bad toothache for 2 days. I can't bite on these lower, right, front teeth." There is pain on pressure and palpation in the region of the lateral incisor and canine. The premolar (small amalgam) is asymptomatic. The lateral and premolar respond to pulp testing; the canine does not respond. There is no swelling. There is an aphthous ulcer on the facial attached gingiva of the lateral. All probings are normal. The lateral and canine have moderate mobility.

14. Which tooth and tissue are the probable source of pain?
    a. Lateral incisor and pulp
    b. Canine and pulp
    c. Canine and periapical tissue
    d. Lateral incisor, canine, and periapical tissue

15. What is the likely pulpal and periapical diagnosis for the lateral incisor?
    a. Irreversible; phoenix abscess
    b. Normal; chronic apical periodontitis
    c. Necrosis; phoenix abscess
    d. Reversible; normal

16. What is the likely pulpal and periapical diagnosis for the canine?
    a. Irreversible pulpitis; phoenix abscess
    b. Normal; chronic apical periodontitis
    c. Necrosis; phoenix abscess
    d. Necrosis; suppurative apical periodontitis

17. Which teeth (tooth) require(s) endodontic treatment?
    a. Lateral incisor only
    b. Canine only
    c. Both the lateral incisor and canine
    d. Neither at present

18. Which bacteria have been related to this pathosis?
    a. Gram-negative rods; anaerobic
    b. Gram-positive rods; anaerobic
    c. Gram-negative cocci; aerobic
    d. Gram-positive cocci; aerobic

19. Of the following inflammatory cells, which would likely predominate periapically?
    a. Lymphocytes
    b. Polymorphonuclear neutrophilic leukocytes
    c. Plasma cells
    d. Macrophages

20. Looking at the radiograph and clinical photograph, what is the likely cause of the pulpal and periapical pathosis?
    a. Incisal attrition
    b. Cervical erosion
    c. Caries
    d. Impact trauma

Questions 21 to 25 relate to the following radiograph.

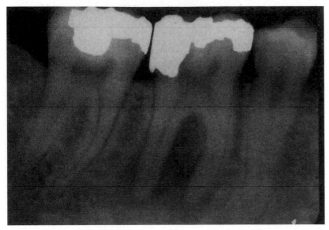

The patient reports severe, continuous pain in the mandibular, right quadrant. She states that the pain began when she was drinking iced tea last evening and the pain has not subsided. She slept poorly last night. Medical history is noncontributory.

Amalgams were placed a few months earlier after removal of deep caries on both molars. She has increased pain on lying down. The pain is not relieved with analgesics. She cannot localize the pain to an individual tooth. Pulp testing shows response on the premolar and second molar. The first molar does not respond. Cold-water application causes intense, diffuse pain in the region. Percussion and palpation are not painful. Probings are normal.

21. Which tooth (teeth) is (are) the most likely cause of her pain?
    a. Premolar
    b. First molar
    c. Second molar
    d. First and second molars

22. What is the pulpal and periapical diagnosis for the first molar?
    a. Necrosis; chronic apical periodontitis
    b. Necrosis; phoenix abscess
    c. Irreversible pulpitis; chronic apical periodontitis
    d. Irreversible pulpitis; acute apical periodontitis

23. What is the pulpal and periapical diagnosis for the second molar?
    a. Irreversible pulpitis; normal
    b. Irreversible pulpitis; acute apical periodontitis
    c. Irreversible pulpitis; acute apical abscess
    d. Normal; normal

24. What should be the minimal emergency treatment on the offending tooth (teeth)?
    a. Remove the amalgam and place a sedative dressing. Prescribe analgesics and antibiotics.
    b. Do a complete canal preparation. Place a cotton pellet of formocresol.
    c. Reduce the occlusion and prescribe antibiotics.
    d. Perform a pulpotomy and place a dry-cotton pellet.

25. Inferior alveolar injection is indicated. If the offending tooth (teeth) is (are) not anesthetized, what is the likely reason?
    a. There is a decreased pH in the region favoring formation of cations.
    b. The anesthetic solution is diluted by the inflammatory fluids.
    c. There may be morphologic changes in the nerves that originate in the inflamed areas; these nerves becomes more excitable.
    d. Because of inflammation, there is increased circulation in the area; this carries away the anesthetic very rapidly.

Questions 26 to 28 relate to the following radiograph.

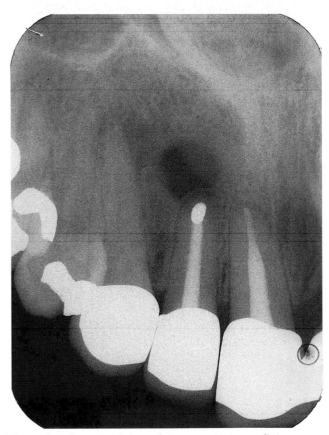

The patient has no adverse signs or symptoms. Surgery was several years ago. There are no probing defects. The canine responds to pulp testing.

26. What diagnosis is likely?
    a. Chronic apical periodontitis
    b. Foreign-body reaction
    c. Apical radicular cyst
    d. Scar tissue

27. What is the likely cause?
    a. Continued irritation from an undébrided, unsealed canal
    b. Adverse reaction to corrosion of the amalgam
    c. Coronal leakage
    d. Perforation of both cortical plates.

28. What should the treatment plan be?
    a. Replace the crown; retreat the canal.
    b. Perform another surgery and place another root end material.
    c. Place the patient on antibiotics to resolve the lesion.
    d. No treatment is needed.

Questions 29 to 35 relate to the following clinical photograph and radiograph.

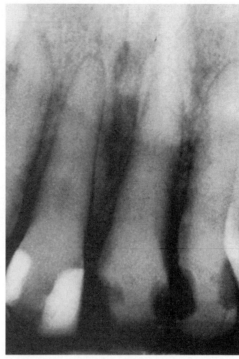

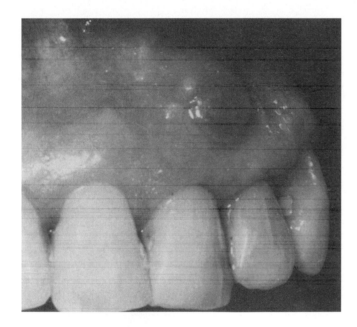

A 58-year-old woman has swelling in the maxillary anterior area that has steadily increased for 2 days. She denies thermal sensitivity and tenderness to biting pressure. The swelling is between teeth nos. 9 (central incisor) and 10 (lateral incisor). There is normal mobility, and probing depths are 4 to 5 mm with the distofacial surface of tooth no. 9 probing 8 mm. There is no tenderness to percussion, but there is tenderness to palpation. Pulp tests reveal that teeth nos. 8, 9, 10, and 11 are responsive to electrical-pulp testing and to thermal stimulation with carbon dioxide snow (i.e., dry ice).

29. Based on this information, the clinical photograph, and the radiograph, what is the pulpal diagnosis for tooth no. 9?
    a. Normal
    b. Reversible pulpitis
    c. Irreversible pulpitis
    d. Necrotic

30. Based on this information, the clinical photograph, and the radiograph, what is the pulpal diagnosis for tooth no. 10?
    a. Normal
    b. Reversible pulpitis
    c. Irreversible pulpitis
    d. Necrotic

31. What is the periradicular diagnosis for tooth no. 9?
    a. Normal
    b. Chronic apical periodontitis
    c. Chronic suppurative, apical periodontitis
    d. Acute apical periodontitis
    e. Acute periodontal abscess

32. Which of the following is the most likely the cause of swelling associated with teeth nos. 9 and 10?
    a. Pulp necrosis
    b. Periodontal disease
    c. A developmental groove defect
    d. Vertical-root fracture
    e. Peripheral giant-cell granuloma

33. Which of the following is most important in determining if this lesion is of periodontal origin or of pulpal origin?
    a. Percussion
    b. A periapical radiograph
    c. Periodontal mobility and mobility assessment
    d. Pulp testing
    e. Periodontal probing

34. Treatment of this case requires which of the following?
    a. Periodontal scaling, root planing of the area, and drainage
    b. Root canal débridement of tooth no. 9, followed by incision and drainage
    c. Analgesic treatment and antibiotic treatment until the involved tooth can be localized
    d. Flap reflection to inspect the root for a vertical root fracture or lateral canal
    e. Surgical excision and biopsy

35. Which of the following statements is *true* regarding the effects of periodontal treatment procedures on the dental pulp?
    a. Scaling and root-planing procedures remove cementum, expose dentinal tubules, which are invaded and result in pulp inflammation.
    b. Citric acid application appears to produce pulpal inflammation when used in conjunction with reattachment procedures.
    c. Hypersensitivity may result from scaling but is a sign of pulpal pathosis or inflammation or both.
    d. Scaling and root-planing procedures may produce deposition of tertiary dentin.

ANSWER KEY

Chapter 1
1. b; 2. d; 3. b; 4. b; 5. b; 6. d; 7. a; 8. c; 9. c; 10. c; 11. e; 12. d; 13. b; 14. a; 15. c; 16. d; 17. d; 18. c; 19. d; 20. b.

Chapter 2
1. d; 2. e; 3. c; 4. a; 5. b; 6. b; 7. b; 8. b; 9. b; 10. c; 11. b; 12. b; 13. a; 14. b; 15. c; 16. b; 17. a; 18. a; 19. b; 20. d; 21. c; 22. a; 23. b; 24. c.

Chapter 3
1. d; 2. b; 3. b; 4. d; 5. c; 6. c; 7. c; 8. a; 9. a; 10. e; 11. b.

Chapter 4
1. d; 2. c; 3. b; 4. c; 5. d; 6. c; 7. d; 8. c; 9. c; 10. a; 11. c; 12. d.

Chapter 5
1. b; 2. c; 3. d; 4. b; 5. a; 6. c; 7. d; 8. a; 9. c; 10. c; 11. c; 12. d; 13. c; 14. a; 15. c; 16. a; 17. a; 18. d; 19. c; 20. b; 21. a.

Chapter 6
1. a; 2. c; 3. b; 4. a; 5. b; 6. d; 7. b; 8. c; 9. a; 10. b; 11. e; 12. b; 13. e.

Chapter 7
1. a; 2. c; 3. a; 4. d; 5. b; 6. c; 7. a; 8. b; 9. d; 10. b.

Chapter 8
1. a; 2. b; 3. c; 4. a; 5. c; 6. d; 7. b; 8. d; 9. b; 10. d; 11. a; 12. a.

Chapter 9
1. c; 2. d; 3. a; 4. c; 5. e; 6. d; 7. a; 8. d; 9. c; 10. b; 11. b; 12. a; 13. a; 14. a; 15. a; 16. d; 17. d.

Chapter 10
1. c; 2. b; 3. c; 4. b; 5. a; 6. a; 7. b; 8. d; 9. b; 10. a; 11. b; 12. a.

Chapter 11
1. c; 2. a; 3. b; 4. a; 5. b; 6. b; 7. a; 8. d; 9. b; 10. d; 11. a; 12. d; 13. c; 14. b; 15. b; 16. a.

Chapter 12
1. c; 2. a; 3. b; 4. b; 5. c; 6. a; 7. c; 8. a; 9. d; 10. a; 11. c; 12. b; 13. b; 14. c; 15. a.

Chapter 13
1. d 2. c 3. a 4. a 5. c 6. d 7. b; 8. d 9. b; 10. c 11. d 12. b; 13. e 14. b; 15. c; 16. c; 17. c; 18. d; 19. e; 20. b.

Chapter 14
1. a; 2. c; 3. a; 4. b; 5. a; 6. a; 7. c; 8. a; 9. c; 10. e; 11. a; 12. c; 13. a; 14. b; 15. b; 16. d; 17. b; 18. c; 19. a; 20. d.

Chapter 15
1. d; 2. d; 3. a; 4. d; 5. a; 6. a; 7. a; 8. b; 9. d; 10. c; 11. d; 12. d; 13. b; 14. d; 15. b; 16. b; 17. a; 18. e; 19. d.

Chapter 16
1. c; 2. a; 3. c; 4. a; 5. b; 6. b; 7. a; 8. b; 9. d; 10. c; 11. a; 12. a; 13. a; 14. e; 15. c; 16. d; 17. b.

Chapter 17
1. b; 2. a; 3. e; 4. b; 5. d; 6. d; 7. b; 8. a; 9. b; 10. a.

Chapter 18

1. a; 2. a; 3. a; 4. a; 5. a; 6. a; 7. a; 8. a; 9. b; 10. d; 11. a; 12. b; 13. a; 14. a; 15. b; 16. e; 17. b; 18. a; 19. a.

Chapter 19

1. c; 2. e; 3. a; 4. d; 5. a; 6. d; 7. c; 8. a; 9. b; 10. d; 11. b; 12. c; 13. b; 14. a; 15. d.

Chapter 20

1. a; 2. d; 3. d; 4. b; 5. c; 6. c; 7. b; 8. a; 9. d; 10. a; 11. a; 12. a; 13. c; 14. d; 15. a; 16. b; 17. c; 18. b; 19. d.

Chapter 21

1. a; 2. a; 3. d; 4. b; 5. b; 6. d.

Chapter 22

1. d; 2. a; 3. b; 4. d; 5. e; 6. a; 7. d; 8. b; 9. d; 10. d.

Chapter 23

1. d; 2. c; 3. d; 4. d; 5. b; 6. d; 7. c; 8. b; 9. a; 10. c; 11. a; 12. b; 13. b; 14. d.

Chapter 24

1. c; 2. d; 3. a; 4. e; 5. a; 6. d; 7. c; 8. c; 9. c; 10. a; 11. d; 12. b; 13. c; 14. c; 15. b; 16. a; 17. d.

Chapter 25

1. d; 2. b; 3. d; 4. c; 5. e; 6. a; 7. a; 8. d; 9. a; 10. d; 11. c; 12. d.

Chapter 26

1. c; 2. a; 3. c; 4. a; 5. d

Test Your Knowledge

1. d; 2. d; 3. c; 4. b; 5. a; 6. b; 7. a; 8. d; 9. d; 10. c; 11. c; 12. d; 13. d; 14. c; 15. d; 16. c; 17. b; 18. a; 19. b; 20. a; 21. c; 22. a; 23. a; 24. d; 25. c. 26. d; 27. d; 28. d; 29. a; 30. a; 31. e; 32. b; 33. d; 34. a; 35. d.

INDEX

❧ Index